UNDERSTANDING PHARMACOLOGY FOR PHARMACY TECHNICIANS

UNDERSTANDING PHARMACOLOGY FOR PHARMACY TECHNICIANS

2nd Edition

Mary Ann Stuhan, PharmD, RPh

Pharmacy Program Director
Cuyahoga Community College
Highland Hills, OH

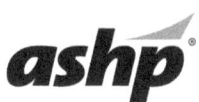

Any correspondence regarding this publication should be sent to the publisher, American Society of Health-System Pharmacists, 4500 East West Highway, suite 900, Bethesda, MD 20814, attention: Special Publishing.

The information presented herein reflects the opinions of the contributors and advisors. It should not be interpreted as an official policy of ASHP or as an endorsement of any product.

Because of ongoing research and improvements in technology, the information and its applications contained in this text are constantly evolving and are subject to the professional judgment and interpretation of the practitioner due to the uniqueness of a clinical situation. The editors and ASHP have made reasonable efforts to ensure the accuracy and appropriateness of the information presented in this document. However, any user of this information is advised that the editors and ASHP are not responsible for the continued currency of the information, for any errors or omissions, and/or for any consequences arising from the use of the information in the document in any and all practice settings. Any reader of this document is cautioned that ASHP makes no representation, guarantee, or warranty, express or implied, as to the accuracy and appropriateness of the information contained in this document and specifically disclaims any liability to any party for the accuracy and/or completeness of the material or for any damages arising out of the use or non-use of any of the information contained in this document.

Vice President, Publishing Office: Daniel J. Cobaugh, PharmD, DABAT, FAACT

Editorial Director, Special Publishing: Ryan E. Owens, PharmD, BCPS

Editorial Coordinator, Special Publishing: Elaine Jimenez

Director, Production and Platform Services, Publishing Operations: Johnna M. Hershey, BA

Cover Design: DeVall Advertising

Cover Art: ASHP

Page Design: David Wade

Print ISBN: 978-1-58528-662-1

PDF ISBN: 978-1-58528-663-8

ePub ISBN: 978-1-58528-664-5

DOI: 10.37573/9781585286638

10 9 8 7 6 5 4 3 2

DEDICATION

To my husband, Rick Stuhan, who has supported all my professional endeavors with love and encouragement.
To my parents, Don and Mary Ann Cipriano, who knew even before I did that I would love being a pharmacist.

ACKNOWLEDGMENTS

I would like to acknowledge the following groups and individuals for their contributions to this book:

- The students, faculty, and administration of Cuyahoga Community College—especially Lorraine Gaston and Gregory Malone—who supported and enhanced this undertaking.

- The staff at ASHP—especially Elaine Jimenez, Johnna Hershey, and Daniel Cobaugh—for their encouragement and assistance throughout the process.

- The late Jack Bruggeman, who, as ASHP Special Publishing Director, conceived of this text and guided publication of the first edition.

- Editorial consultant Toni Fera, PharmD, whose patience and expertise enabled the completion of this book, and Lynn Gohn, who ensured the quality of the final product.

- All of the contributing authors and reviewers, who lent their expertise and experience to the authority of our book and patiently and continually revised their work to include the most current and complete information in an ever-changing field.

Mary Ann Stuhan, PharmD, RPh

TABLE OF CONTENTS

DOI 10.37573/9781585286638.FM

As pharmacists become increasingly engaged in direct patient care, pharmacy technicians are assuming new responsibilities to support that involvement while promoting medication safety. Both traditional (dispensing) and advanced technician roles (including immunization, medication reconciliation, and patient history collection) require a strong foundation knowledge of drug actions, doses, routes of administration, side effects, and interactions.

As our population ages and our healthcare system changes, more demands are being asked of the pharmacy technician. Once limited to "lick-stick-pour" duties, today's pharmacy technicians are becoming part of the modern healthcare team. In most states, pharmacy practice acts limit certain roles and responsibilities to technicians who have demonstrated their knowledge of pharmacy; some even require specific training or examinations for them. To prepare for a future that will demand more from them, pharmacy technicians will need an understanding of the medications they are handling—their actions, doses, routes of administration, and interactions.

Pharmacology is the study that includes the medication knowledge technicians need to function in modern pharmacy. Pharmacists learn pharmacology in the context of patient care from textbooks and articles authored by healthcare professionals with specific expertise in the areas in which they are writing. Since these materials are based on a background in physical and life sciences broader than currently required of technicians, as well as explore clinical decision-making on a level usually reserved for physicians and pharmacists, they are not appropriate for technician students. That should not mean, however, that pharmacy technician education should be limited to paraphrased editions from less authoritative sources. This text has been written by professionals who have specialized in the types of treatment they are covering (in some cases, the same respected authors who have contributed to prominent pharmacy references). The material contained here has been written specifically for pharmacy technicians, with their backgrounds and duties as guides for both breadth and depth, and with full respect for its importance to them, their careers, and the patients they serve.

HOW THIS BOOK IS ORGANIZED

The Introduction communicates the rationale for the study of pharmacology by pharmacy technicians, as explained by an experienced technician. It is followed by a lesson in basic pharmacokinetics, giving a basis for the medication information delivered in subsequent chapters. In this edition, a new chapter on pharmacogenomics discusses the science of precision medicine and relates its concepts to testing and dosing protocols that are becoming increasingly common in everyday pharmacy.

As in the first edition, the medication chapters are organized around body systems and disease states, presented in an order similar to that of pharmacists' textbooks, with sections on the nervous, endocrine, musculoskeletal, cardiovascular and renal, respiratory, gastrointestinal, and hematologic systems, followed by treatments for infectious diseases, cancer, and conditions of the skin, eye, ear, nose, and throat. All chapters have been updated to reflect the most current medications and information at the time of publication.

HOW EACH CHAPTER IS ORGANIZED

Each chapter begins with clearly defined learning objectives and highlights key terms with their definitions. Each chapter also includes:

- An introduction reviewing the body system and conditions covered, giving a context for subsequent material.

- Discussion of medications, divided as appropriate, into subclasses and groups, detailing their mechanisms of action, routes of administration, and side effects.

- Medication tables summarizing important information including generic and brand names, dosage forms and products, as well as doses and indications for quick and efficient reference and study.

DOI 10.37573/9781585286638.FM

- A chapter summary that relates the material to the learning objectives and stresses key points.

- References list resources used in compiling the chapter.

LEARNING FEATURES YOU WILL FIND IN THIS BOOK

A variety of pedagogical, or learning features, are found throughout the book to assist the student. They include:

- *Case studies*: Case studies are based on the issues of patients that pharmacy technicians encounter in various practice settings, and help them relate the abstract knowledge conveyed in each chapter to real people and real-life scenarios. Discussion questions based on these cases are distributed throughout the chapters, giving students examples of how the concepts being developed may apply to their work.

- *Alerts*: Key points relevant to patient or occupational safety are emphasized in marginal notes highlighted "Alert." These include look-alike/sound-alike issues, allergy precautions, and contraindications.

- *Practice points*: Practical advice and real-world applications related to technician work with the medications being discussed are highlighted throughout each chapter, giving immediate emphasis and impact to the material.

- *Pronunciations*: Generic drug names are accompanied by phonetic pronunciations using common spellings and capitals for accented syllables, requiring no knowledge of diacritical markings or symbols.

- *Illustrations*: Anatomy and drug action are illustrated with figures throughout the text, giving visual representation to the concepts presented.

Mary Ann Stuhan
September 2022

CONTRIBUTORS

EDITOR

Mary Ann Stuhan, PharmD, RPh
Pharmacy Program Director
Cuyahoga Community College
Highland Hills, OH

CONTRIBUTORS

James Adams, PharmD, BCCCP
Clinical Pharmacist II
SCL Health
Erie, CO

Kathleen K. Adams, PharmD, BCPS
Assistant Clinical Professor of Pharmacy Practice
Department of Pharmacy Practice
University of Connecticut School of Pharmacy
Storrs, CT

Christopher M. Archangeli, MD
Child and Adult Psychiatrist
Munson Medical Center
Traverse City, MI

Toy S. Biederman, PharmD
Pharmacist, retired
Pharmacy Systems, Inc.
Worthington, OH

Shelby P. Brooks, PharmD, BCPS
Assistant Professor
University of Louisiana Monroe
College of Pharmacy, Shreveport Campus
Clinical Instructor, LSUHSC-Shreveport
Shreveport, LA

Sherrill J. Brown, DVM, PharmD, BCPS
Director, Drug Information Service
Professor, Pharmacy Practice
University of Montana
Skaggs School of Pharmacy
Missoula, MT

Richard Chan, PharmD, BCPS
Assistant Professor, Pharmacy Practice
NEOMED College of Pharmacy
Rootstown, OH

Rachael Craft, PharmD, BCIDP
Clinical Pharmacy Specialist–Infectious Disease/
Internal Medicine
Banner Boswell Medical Center
Sun City, AZ

Julie Cunningham, MPH, RDN, LDN, CDCES, IBCLC
Registered Dietitian Nutritionist
Certified Diabetes Care and Education Specialist
International Board-Certified Lactation Consultant
Hendersonville, NC

Devra Dang, PharmD, CDCES, FNAP
Associate Clinical Professor of Pharmacy Practice
Department of Pharmacy Practice
University of Connecticut School of Pharmacy
Storrs, CT

Sandra B. Earle, PharmD
Associate Professor of Pharmaceutical Science
Associate Dean of Assessment and Student Success
College of Pharmacy
University of Findlay
Findlay, OH

DOI 10.37573/9781585286638.FM

Lori J. Ernsthausen, PharmD, BCPS
Associate Dean of Curricular Affairs
Department Chair of Pharmacy Practice
University of Findlay
Findlay, OH

Jeffery D. Evans, PharmD
Director and Associate Professor
Louisiana Independent Pharmacists Association Endowed
    Professor
School of Clinical Sciences, College of Pharmacy
University of Louisiana Monroe
Monroe, LA

Richard G. Fiscella, PharmD, MPH
Clinical Professor Emeritus
Pharmacy Practice
College of Pharmacy–Chicago
University of Illinois Chicago
Rockford, IL

John Flanigan, PharmD
Pharmacy Supervisor
Director, PGY-1 Residency Program
Intermountain Health–Good Samaritan Medical Center
Lafayette, CO

Patrick J. Gallegos, PharmD, BCPS
Vice Chair, Pharmacy Practice Based Research
Associate Professor of Pharmacy Practice
Associate Professor of Internal Medicine Fellow,
    Master Teachers Guild
Northeast Ohio Medical University
Rootstown, OH
Clinical Pharmacy Specialist of Internal Medicine
Cleveland Clinic Akron General
Akron, OH

Katherine S. Hale, PharmD, BCPS, MFA
Clinical Pharmacist
Kadlec Regional Medical Center
Richland, WA

Bianca Harris, PharmD
Clinical Pharmacist
William S. Middleton Memorial Veterans Hospital
Madison, WI

Catherine W. Hebert, PharmD, BCPS
Clinical Pharmacist, Infectious Diseases
Exempla Good Samaritan Medical Center
Lafayette, CO

Brian A. Hemstreet, PharmD, FCCP, BCPS
Associate Dean for Student Affairs and Professor
University of Colorado Skaggs School of Pharmacy and
Pharmaceutical Sciences
Aurora, CO

Marcia E. Honisko, PharmD, RPh, BCOP
Clinical Oncology Pharmacy Specialist
ProMedica Cancer Institute
Sylvania, OH

Tibb F. Jacobs, PharmD, BCPS
Clinical Professor
University of Louisiana Monroe
Shreveport Campus
Shreveport, LA

Ashley M. Jones, PharmD, BCPS
Emergency Medicine Clinical Pharmacy Specialist
University Hospitals Geauga Medical Center
Chardon, OH

Megan A. Kaun, PharmD, RPh, BCACP
Director of Experiential Education
Senior Lecturer
Department of Pharmacy Practice
University of Toledo
Toledo, OH

Allison R. King, PharmD, FASHP
Investigational Drug Pharmacist
PGY1 Residency Director
Children's Mercy Hospital
Kansas City, MO

Michael E. Klepser, PharmD, FCCP, FIDP
Professor, Pharmacy Practice
Ferris State University
Big Rapids, MI

Stephanie A. Klepser, PharmD
Clinical Pharmacist, Clinical Program Oversight
CVS/Caremark
Kalamazoo, MI

Jayden Lee, PharmD, BCACP
Ambulatory Clinical Pharmacist
Banner Health
Phoenix, AZ

Joseph S. Marchiano, PharmD, BCPS, BCGP
Assistant Professor of Pharmacy Practice
Clinical Lead Pharmacist, Geriatrics
Summa Health
NEOMED
Rootstown, OH

Amanda R. Margolis, PharmD, MS, BCACP
Assistant Professor
Pharmacy Practice and Translational Research Division
University of Wisconsin–Madison School of Pharmacy
Clinical Pharmacy Specialist
William S. Middleton Memorial Veteran's Hospital
Madison, WI

Andrew Meador, BS, CPhT
Clinical Education Specialist–Pharmacy Technician Program
IU Health Methodist Hospital
Indianapolis, IN

Karen A. Newell, MMSc, PA-C, DFAAPA
Emory University School of Medicine
Assistant Professor, retired
Emory University School of Medicine
Physician Assistant Program
Atlanta, GA

Nikola Paulic, PharmD
Clinical Pharmacy Specialist, Medical Oncology
University Hospitals Geauga Medical Center
Chardon, OH

Chris Paxos, PharmD, BCPP, BCPS, BCGP
Professor of Pharmacy Practice
Associate Professor of Psychiatry
NEOMED
Rootstown, OH

Laura A. Perry, PharmD, BCPS
Professor of Pharmacy Practice
University of Findlay
Findlay, OH

Steve W. Plogsted, PharmD, BCNSP, CNSC, FASPEN
Clinical Pharmacist, retired
Nationwide Children's Hospital
Columbus, OH

Benjamin A. Pontefract, PharmD, BCPS
Assistant Professor
Ferris State University College of Pharmacy
Director of Research
Collaboration to Harmonize Antimicrobial Registry
Measures
Grand Rapids, MI

Kendra Keeley Procacci, PharmD, BCPS, AE–C
Professor
Department of Pharmacy Practice
University of Montana–Missoula
Missoula, MT

Prabodh Sadana, PhD
Associate Professor of Pharmacy Practice and
    Pharmaceutical Sciences
College of Pharmacy
NEOMED
Rootstown, OH

Kelly L. Scolaro, PharmD
Pharmacy Manager
Good Samaritan Pharmacy and Health Services
Venice, FL
Clinical Pharmacist
Turning Points
Bradenton, FL

Mate M. Soric, PharmD, BCPS, FCCP
Chair and Professor, Pharmacy Practice
NEOMED
Rootstown, OH

Jamie M. Terrell, PharmD
Clinical Professor
University of Louisiana Monroe
School of Clinical Sciences
Shreveport, LA

Celeste Voight, PharmD, BCPS
Assistant Professor of Pharmacy Practice
University of Findlay
Findlay, OH
Per Diem Pharmacist
Select Medical
Sylvania, OH

Jamie L. Woodyard, PharmD, BCACP
Director of Professional Skills Laboratories
Clinical Assistant Professor of Pharmacy Practice
Purdue University College of Pharmacy
West Lafayette, IN

Bethany Baker, PharmD, MHA
Director
Pharmacy Clinical Services
Children's Mercy Kansas City
Kansas City, MO

Carly Copeman, PharmD, BCPS
Ambulatory Care Pharmacist
Hospice Service
Kaiser Permanente South Sacramento Service Area
Sacramento, CA

S. Dee Melnyk Evans, PharmD, MHS
Independent Consultant
Burlington, NC

Mort Goldman, PharmD, FCCP, BCPS
Independent Consultant
Cleveland, OH

Mitra Habibi, PharmD
Clinical Associate Professor
Neuroscience Clinical Pharmacist
University of Illinois at Chicago
Chicago, IL

Lauren M. Hynicka, PharmD
Associate Professor
University of Maryland
School of Pharmacy
Baltimore, MD

Colleen D. Lauster, PharmD, BCPS, CDCES
Ambulatory Care Clinical Pharmacist
Beaumont Health
Royal Oak, MI

Cindy Magrini, PharmD, AAHIVP
Senior Program Manager
Positive Health Clinic
Allegheny Health Network
Pittsburgh, PA

Kimberly J. Novak, PharmD, BCPS, BCPPS, FPPA
Advanced Patient Care Pharmacist–Pediatric and Adult
    Cystic Fibrosis
Director, PGY2 Pharmacy Residency–Pediatrics Nationwide
    Children's Hospital
Department of Pharmacy
Columbus, OH

Raynold Yin, PharmD, BCACP, APh, CDCES
Clinical Supervisor
Sharp Central Pharmacy Services
Sharp Grossmont Hospital
San Diego, CA

Spencer K. Yingling, PharmD, BCOP
Oncology Pharmacy Specialist
WVU Medicine
Morgantown, WV

DOI 10.37573/9781585286638.FM

Part 1

INTRODUCTION

Chapter 1

Why Technicians Need to Study Pharmacology and Therapeutics

Andrew Meador, BS, CPhT

KEY TERMS AND DEFINITIONS

Medication—a substance that is used to diagnose, cure, mitigate, treat, or prevent a disease state in a human or animal.

Pharmacokinetics—the study of the movement of a drug through body systems, including its absorption, distribution, metabolism, and excretion.

Pharmacology—the study of drugs and medications, including their origins, properties, actions, and effects on the body.

Precipitate—solid particles, usually insoluble, that settle out of a solution.

Therapeutics—a branch of medicine that deals with the application of remedies to disease states.

LEARNING OBJECTIVES

After completing this chapter, you should be able to

1. Define *medication, pharmacology,* and *therapeutics* and explain how they are related to one another.

2. Describe reasons why it is important for pharmacy technicians to study pharmacology and how it provides benefit to pharmacy practices.

DOI 10.37573/9781585286638.001

3. Explain how an understanding of pharmacology enhances a technician's abilities to better help patients and other pharmacy staff.

4. List examples of how a pharmacy technician's professional development and career advancement are related to understanding pharmacology.

5. Explain how pharmacy professional development has changed from the past to today.

All across the country, every day, thousands of prescriptions and medication orders are filled. In a hospital, the medications, or drugs, will be taken to the bedside and administered by a nurse, and in a retail pharmacy patients will collect the medication to take at home as prescribed. Every single dose is prescribed with an intended purpose. Each prescription has been evaluated on many different levels before it ever reaches the patient. Drug researchers are constantly developing new medications with the intent of alleviating a specific disease state. Prescribers are evaluating patients' needs to determine what medications will be necessary. Finally, pharmacists are reviewing the prescriptions and dispensing the medications to the patients to provide them the therapeutic effects they need. Along the way, each of these professionals has an obligation to do their best to provide care to the patient. They are part of a team of professionals united to provide care to a patient. A pharmacy technician is an integral part of that team and provides care to each and every patient with each and every dose.

Being a pharmacy technician means taking on the responsibility to provide the best care to every patient. To accomplish that task, it is important to develop a unique set of skills. These include knowing the different brands and generics, understanding the basics of prescription insurance, and calculating doses based upon what is prescribed. To perform these duties professionally, it is important to have a knowledge of pharmacology. Pharmacology is the study of drugs, and includes where medications originate, how they are developed, and their effects in the body. Having a basic understanding of pharmacology provides the technician with the ability to provide great care to the patients. Without that understanding, a technician is like a carpenter who doesn't know what a hammer is.

In a community pharmacy, during a typical work shift technicians will be responsible for numerous prescriptions or orders. In a retail pharmacy, prescriptions will be sent electronically or handed over in person. Upon receipt, the technician reviews each prescription to ensure it is complete before updating a patient's profile with the medication and directions for use and processing it through any insurance. Then the technician will count the correct amount to dispense, prepare the prescription with the correct package information, and prepare it for review by the pharmacist. The technician will also prepare the prescription for shipping, delivery, or for pick up by the patient. Once the patient comes to pick up the prescription, the technician will verify what the patient is receiving and confirm the patient understands the prescription directions. If a patient needs counseling, it is the responsibility of the technician to have the pharmacist explain particulars of the prescription, its directions, administration technique, and even side effects.

In a hospital setting, the process for handling a medication order starts after it has been verified by the pharmacist. When the medication label is printed the technician will review it and begin preparing the order for the patient. This means selecting the correct medication from stock, performing dose calculations, and, for oral medication, preparing a unit dose at the processing counter. For sterile intravenous solutions, the technician will mix the solution in a clean room, and finally, making sure it is delivered to the correct nursing unit medication room and placed in the proper area for the nurses to retrieve. In almost every pharmacy, the technician plays a vital role in preparing medications. Proper performance of each of the steps to prepare a medication is enhanced by a knowledge of pharmacology.

Why is it so important to have an understanding of pharmacology? The answer seems straightforward, yet many technicians will simply state that it is the responsibility of the pharmacist, not the technician, to know why and how the medications are used. In reality, knowing the basics of pharmacology will allow a pharmacy technician the opportunity to provide a better quality of care to patients, become a vital asset to the pharmacist, and advance his or her career opportunities.

With a basic understanding of pharmacology, a technician gains a plethora of valuable knowledge that can be used to assist patients every day. Application of that knowledge allows the technician to make an impact on a patient's life and provide the best care possible. For example, if Mrs. Smith calls the pharmacy and asks the technician for a refill on her "water pill," a technician with a knowledge of pharmacology will be able to identify the diuretic medication in the patient's profile. This technician knows that diuretics are used to help remove excess water from a patient's body, which will decrease the patient's blood pressure. Mrs. Smith also needs to refill her "sugar pills." The technician will know to check the patient's profile for her diabetes medication. Understanding the different types of medications, their chemical structure, and the intended use of each of the medications allows the technician a level of independence that a pharmacist can count on.

Each medication has its own unique set of storage, handling, and compounding guidelines. These guidelines are related to a medication's classification and other properties. Some medications, for instance, must be protected from light, while others might need to be refrigerated. If a medication is not placed under the proper storage conditions, it could possibly deteriorate or even undergo a chemical change. When compounding sterile products, a technician must be aware that some medications require reconstitution with specific fluids. If the incorrect fluid is used, a precipitate could form, exposing the patient who receives it to dangerous particulate matter. While it might sound trivial, disregarding the proper procedure when storing, handling, or compounding a medication can make a dramatic difference and lead to considerable harm to a patient.

Within pharmacology is a branch called pharmacokinetics. This is the study of the absorption, distribution, metabolism, and excretion of medications within the body. Pharmacokinetics can influence several aspects of a prescription. Medications being administered orally by a tablet or via injection of a solution have different pathways and even different mechanisms for how they work in the body. An experienced and educated technician is able to discern what routes of administration are most effective for each medication. For example, vancomycin is not absorbed via the gastrointestinal tract. Therefore, if a systemic course of vancomycin is needed, it will be administered intravenously (IV),[1] while if it is being used to treat an intestinal infection, it may be given orally. Knowing this can give insight into the disease state that a patient has, and can be applied to better meet the needs of the patient.

With an understanding of pharmacology, technicians are able to help pharmacists more safely and effectively. Pharmacists must be confident in placing their trust in the technicians with whom they work. In today's healthcare environment, pharmacists are taking on increasingly advanced roles. They are responsible for many nontraditional duties that, years ago, were not considered pharmacists' responsibilities. Nowadays, many people count on their local pharmacist to administer flu shots, help with Medicare enrollment, and even counsel on smoking cessation. With the ever-evolving functions that pharmacists are assuming, it is expected that the role of the technician will advance as well. Accountability for safe, legal, and efficient pharmacy operations is shared between the pharmacist

and the technician. As current trends continue, technicians' responsibilities are expected to expand and increase.

With pharmacists spending more and more time meeting the clinical needs of patients, the daily operations of the pharmacy have transitioned to become the obligation of the technician. All across the country pharmacists administer flu vaccines (and many other immunizations), and it is common for the technician to prepare the patient and ask appropriate screening questions. While the technician assists with the vaccination record, a pharmacist will counsel a patient seeking a cold remedy. In a hospital setting this concept is no different. Relying on a technician to complete an order can allow the pharmacist to step away and discuss the needs of the patient with other healthcare providers.

Technicians today are breaking out of their traditional job descriptions into new roles and duties. Such new career opportunities would not be available today if technicians had not pushed for advancement and prepared for new tasks. In a number of states, technicians are already able to administer immunizations, provide final reviews of medication refills, and transcribe new prescriptions called in from a doctor's office.[2] Each of these innovations came from professionals realizing the potential of pharmacy technicians. With the proper training, advanced technician roles in pharmacy operations have become more prevalent. It is important that technicians are good stewards of these positions, which requires application of checks and balances. Technicians can use their knowledge of pharmacology to provide checks for themselves. For example, when immunizing a patient, knowing the length of the needle is important for proper administration. When providing a final check on a refill, knowing the difference between the variations of formulations can ensure the correct product is chosen. When transcribing a medication order, knowing the indication of the drug will provide context for the complete prescription, including dosage form, route of administration, and schedule. A knowledge of pharmacology provides the ability to enhance the care technicians provide with every task.

As technicians assume additional responsibilities, expectations will shift regarding what a technician is required to do and know. This shift in focus is nothing new to pharmacy. In the early twentieth century, for example, Abraham Flexner, a renowned educator at the time, was asked by the American Medical Association to evaluate the state of medical colleges.[3] In his report, he noted that being a pharmacist was not a professional occupation because the pharmacist simply submitted to the wishes of the physician. In response to those remarks, the Association of Colleges of Pharmacy altered educational practices and required a more rigorous curriculum for pharmacy students. This reform led to pharmacists becoming more autonomous and taking additional roles not traditionally considered. As technicians begin to take on new skills and new knowledge, their autonomy will increase just as it did with pharmacists. Technicians will be asked to do more because they know more.

When patients go to a hospital, they expect to receive the best care and believe that the doctors who treat them have studied and understand the basics of medicine. This expectation applies to pharmacy care as well. Patients needing prescriptions believe that taking medications will give them the therapeutic effects that are intended, and they trust the pharmacy staff to apply their skills to be sure this occurs. The only way to fulfill these expectations is to be competent and knowledgeable in pharmacy. Part of being a professional technician is taking on the responsibility of knowing aspects of pharmacy that will make you more effective at your job. The American Association of Pharmacy Technicians Code of Ethics[4] states that it is the first consideration of the technician "to ensure the health and safety of the patient, and to use knowledge and skills to the best of his/her ability in serving others." Taking on this responsibility to the patients requires extensive knowledge and learning.

Technicians' capabilities are elevated by the study of pharmacology. With a basic foundational knowledge of how medications impact the body, a technician can make decisions that positively affect the health of their patients. Technicians should be a valuable resource to any pharmacist with whom they work, and with the proper degree of passion, a technician can continue to expand their profession into new areas. It is a large responsibility to take on, but when lives are at stake it is important to know that the person who is dispensing medications has been educated to meet the obligations of their duties.

REFERENCES

1. Rao S, Kupfer Y, Pagala M, et al. Systemic absorption of oral vancomycin in patients with Clostridium difficile infection. *Scand J Infect Dis*. 2011;43(5):386-388. doi: 10.3109/00365548.2010.544671.

2. Peshek SC. *Professional Skills for the Pharmacy Technician*. Burlington, MA: Jones & Bartlett Learning; 2017:17-19.

3. DiPiro J. The 21st century Abraham Flexner. *Am J Pharm Educ*. 2008;72(4):79. doi: 10.5688/aj720479.

4. American Association of Pharmacy Technicians. Code of Ethics for Pharmacy Technicians. https://www.pharmacytechnician.com/pharmacy-technician-code-of-ethics/. Accessed May 24, 2021.

REVIEW QUESTIONS

1. How does a technician having a basic understanding of pharmacology provide a benefit to the technician, patient, and pharmacist?

2. What direct impact does the pharmacy technician's role have on the care that a patient receives? Is there also an indirect impact?

3. What are some ways that technicians have been able to advance their professional development, and how is that dependent upon understanding pharmacology? How do you see the technician's role advancing in the future?

4. Explain how the Pharmacy Technician Code of Ethics promotes the ideal of learning pharmacological principles.

Chapter 2

Pharmacokinetics

Sandra B. Earle, PharmD

KEY TERMS AND DEFINITIONS

Bioavailability (F)—the fraction of the administered dose that is available to the systemic circulation. Units are expressed as a fraction in decimal form (eg, 4/5 = 0.8) or percentage (eg, 80%).

Clearance (CL)—the volume of serum, plasma, or blood that has all of the drug removed per unit of time by the eliminating organ. Total body clearance is the sum of the clearances of all the eliminating organs. Units are expressed as volume per time (eg, mL/hour).

Dosage regimen—how much drug will be given how often when multiple doses of the drug will be given (eg, 10 mg every day).

Elimination rate constant (k; it may also be signified as ke or kd)—the fraction of drug removed from the blood in a given time. Units are expressed as a fraction per time.

First-pass drugs—drugs that have a large fraction of the active drug metabolized in the liver as it passes through the liver before reaching the systemic circulation.

Half-life ($t\frac{1}{2}$)—the time it takes for one half of the drug to be removed from the body. Units are in time (usually hours).

Prodrug—a drug that has to be converted into an active form by the body, usually by an enzyme in the liver.

Route of administration—the method used to give the drug to the patient during treatment.

Steady state (ss)—the point in therapy when the amount of drug administered exactly replaces the amount of drug removed. Steady state is never technically achieved, but

DOI 10.37573/9781585286638.002

for clinical purposes, five half-lives, which is when 97% of steady state is achieved, is considered to be at steady state. Units are in time.

Systemic—having a distribution or effect throughout the body.

Therapeutic range—a statistical range of desirable drug concentrations, for which the *majority* of patients show an effective therapeutic response with minimal drug-related side effects.

Volume of distribution—describes the volume into which the drug distributes in the body. Units are expressed in volume (mL or L).

LEARNING OBJECTIVES

After completing this chapter, you should be able to

1. Define pharmacokinetics and relate its principles to the work of a pharmacy technician.

2. Relate the route of administration to the actions of a drug and define at least eight routes of administration.

3. Define absorption, distribution, metabolism, and excretion and describe the relevance of each of these.

4. Discuss how pharmacokinetics contributes to choosing dosage regimens.

5. Relate pharmacokinetic principles to the prediction of drug interactions.

When using medication, the first concern is *the effect of that medication on the body.* Pharmacokinetics is the study of the *body's effect on the medication.* As soon as a drug is introduced to the body, it goes on a trip through the body on its way to elimination. Mathematical models can be used to predict this "trip" and, therefore, determine how much drug will be in the body at any time. When certain concentrations cause predictable outcomes or effects ("pharmacodynamics"), the models can be used to set target levels (concentrations) to produce the desired effects of drugs in patients. These principles are applied to improve patient outcomes.

Using pharmacokinetics, the pharmacist can properly evaluate measured drug concentrations and design good dosage regimens for patients. These dosage regimens

are intended to increase efficacy while avoiding toxicity in patients treated with medications. In addition, pharmacokinetic principles help to predict and avoid drug-drug and drug-disease interactions.

ROUTES OF ADMINISTRATION

There are several methods of giving drugs to patients, commonly called routes of administration. While some routes are created for convenience, others may be needed due to a patient's or drug's limitations or characteristics. The routes of administration are reviewed in the following section.

Oral Route

The oral (PO) route of administration is the most commonly prescribed route, as well as the route most associated with taking medications. Oral medications are beneficial for individuals taking medications on a daily basis, and medication for oral use can easily be carried along for dosing throughout the day. However, not all drugs can be given orally because of the rigorous journey from administration to site of action.

After being swallowed, a drug in a capsule, tablet, or liquid travels down the esophagus and into the stomach. Once it enters the stomach it comes in contact with various digestive enzymes and stomach fluids that are acidic in nature. The acidic environment, enzymes, and physical mixing require that the medication be formulated to withstand the conditions or it could be rendered ineffective. Most absorption of drugs occurs in the small intestine. The finger-like villi found there increase the surface area, improving the chances for drugs and nutrients to be absorbed. When the drug is absorbed it enters the gut wall, which contains drug-metabolizing enzymes and efflux pumps. If the drug makes it through the gut wall without being metabolized, it will travel via the bloodstream to the liver before finally making it to the systemic circulation. By going through the gut wall and liver before reaching the systemic circulation, some drugs are significantly metabolized before reaching the site of action. This is called the first-pass effect. Not all drugs can be given orally because they all cannot "survive" this rigorous journey.

Some drugs given orally are formulated to release their contents slowly. This may be done for many reasons. In these cases, the drug may have "sustained release" or "controlled release" in the name of the preparation. Some preparations may also have a coating ("enteric coating"), which will protect the drug from being destroyed in the journey to the absorption site. These types of medications should never be crushed or chewed or split unless the product is specifically formulated and labeled to allow this. Otherwise, the patient could be at risk for toxicity from the entire dose being available at once or lack of efficacy if the drug is destroyed.

Sublingual and Buccal

These medications are formulated to be given through the mucosa in the mouth. Sublingual (SL) administration designates administration under the tongue, and in buccal administration, the drug is placed between the gums and the cheek. This type of formulation is not chewed or swallowed but placed in the mouth to dissolve. These routes of administration provide quicker absorption and, for some drugs, greater bioavailability, because the drug is absorbed directly into the bloodstream without going to the gut and liver first, thereby avoiding the first-pass elimination. After the medication is dissolved and absorbed, it is immediately available in the bloodstream, which may lead to a quicker onset of action than would occur with an oral dose. An example of an SL product is the Nitrostat® tablet. These are administered if a patient is experiencing chest pain due to angina. The formulation allows for an abrupt onset of action that will quickly diminish the chest pain.

Inhalation

Inhalation (INH) affords local delivery of the drug directly to the lungs or nasal passages. Following INH, an aerosolized or powdered drug can be available quickly and completely to the lungs, the nasal passages, and/or the blood vessels in these areas. This is beneficial for patients with respiratory illnesses, who can have the drug delivered to the site of action without exposing the whole body to its effects. Many drugs for the treatment of asthma or chronic obstructive pulmonary disease (COPD) come in a form to be inhaled to deliver the drug to the site of action without exposing the whole body to the drug. The INH route may also be used for the systemic delivery of drugs that cannot be given orally. Examples of this are the nasal spray of calcitonin used to deliver a bone hormone for the treatment of osteoporosis and immediate-release insulin given by oral inhalation for the treatment of type one diabetes mellitus.

Rectal

The rectal (PR) route of administration is not one most patients prefer, but it does have a place in therapy. Suppositories are solid medication dosage forms that are given rectally and may be advantageous for patients who are vomiting or for patients who are not conscious and do not have intravenous (IV) access, as well as if needed for local action. Enemas are liquid dosage forms delivered rectally; most are intended to act locally. Most medications in suppositories will not go through the liver and therefore will not have the first-pass effect.

Vaginal

While the vaginal (PV) route of administration is also not highly used, it is beneficial for local treatment of vaginal conditions. Formulations that may be used include vaginal suppositories, creams, and even some tablets. Patients who benefit from PV administration include those being treated for vaginal infections, menopause, and infertility.

Topical

Topical application includes preparations intended for use directly on the skin (dermal), into the eye (ophthalmic), into the ear (otic), and into the nose (nasal). This route is quite common and there are a variety of products available for topical administration, with subtle differences. Preparations made for direct application to the skin include creams, ointments, lotions, gels, shampoos, and solutions. Both creams and ointments have oil bases, but ointments have higher oil content than creams and provide a protective layer on top of the skin. Lotions and gels have a water base and are more easily spread on top of the skin. Solutions contain the highest liquid content and are most readily absorbed through the skin. Shampoos are soap solutions intended for use on the head and body. Both ophthalmic and otic preparations come in solutions and suspensions. A suspension is different than a solution because a suspension suspends small particles of an insoluble drug in a liquid that is usually water based. It is a good way to administer a drug that is insoluble in water. A solution, in contrast, has a soluble drug dispersed in a solvent, which is also usually water based. It is important to realize that there is a difference between them because the use of some preparations may not be appropriate for a given medical condition. For example, solutions may contain alcohol, whereas suspensions do not, and, therefore, otic drops formulated into a solution should not be used in a patient with a ruptured eardrum due to the risk of worsening the injury because of the alcohol. Ophthalmic preparations are specially formulated for comfort and safety of sensitive eye tissues and must be sterile to prevent infection.

Topical nasal preparations are commonly drops or gels that are applied directly into the nose. The nasal route is beneficial for patients suffering from allergies as the drug is delivered directly to the site of the symptoms.

Intravenous/Intramuscular/ Subcutaneous Injections

Injection routes of administration deliver the medication directly into the vein (IV), muscle (IM), or subcutaneous (SUBQ) tissue of the patient. Injection methods require delivery by a needle. Because the drugs bypass the gastro-intestinal (GI) tract, lack of absorption and destruction in the journey to the systemic circulation is not an issue for IV medications, and is less problematic for IM formulations than for those administered PO.

Transdermal

The application of patches is considered transdermal drug delivery. After a patch is applied to unbroken skin, the drug travels across the layers of skin and is absorbed by the body. This route is beneficial because of the ease of administration of the drug. Also, while most oral medications require everyday dosing, patches allow for multiple-day and longer dosing. For a patient who is unable to take pain medications

due to effects on the GI system, the transdermal application allows the administration of an effective analgesic without many of the adverse effects associated with the oral form. Transdermal dosage forms are described in more detail in Chapter 32.

ADME (ABSORPTION, DISTRIBUTION, METABOLISM, EXCRETION): A TRIP THROUGH THE BODY

Absorption

If a drug is given by any route other than intravenously, it must first be absorbed. For the drug, the trip from the site of administration to the systemic circulation can be difficult. Medications taken orally must pass through and withstand the conditions of the stomach and then travel to the small intestine for absorption. There are enzymes found in the wall of the small intestine that can metabolize (break down or change) the drug. Also, in the wall of the small intestine, there are pumps that can transport the drug back into the GI tract. After absorption, the drug must travel to the liver, where it again may be metabolized. With routes of administration other than IV, it is possible that not all of the drug given will be available to the body. The percent of medication available to the body from a given dose is known as the drug's bioavailability. This is a property specific to each drug and depends on many factors, including dosage form and route of administration. If the drug is able to bypass the absorption step, as with those given intravenously, drug absorption is not an issue and the bioavailability of the drug is 100%. Some drugs are so highly affected before reaching the systemic circulation that it is not useful to give them by the oral route. In most cases, however, a larger dose can be given when administered orally to overcome any decrease in bioavailability related to poor absorption or the first-pass effect (described in the section on Metabolism that follows). Drug-drug and drug-food interactions can occur at many points in the absorption process (details are described later on in the section on Drug and Disease Interactions).

Distribution

Distribution describes the process by which the drug is spread throughout the body and to what extent it is concentrated in various tissues. This property is also unique to each drug, as some drugs distribute widely throughout the body and have large distributions and others do not travel much beyond the bloodstream and therefore have small distributions. Common sites of distribution are the blood, muscles, fat tissue, bones, and organs. These may become important when treating certain conditions that require the drug to penetrate tissues to be effective. Besides this, the volume of distribution of a drug also helps pharmacists determine the rate at which the drug is removed from the body. Drugs having a larger volume of distribution will take longer to be eliminated from the body, whereas drugs with smaller volumes of distribution will take less time to be removed.

Metabolism

As soon as drugs enter the body, elimination begins. Some drugs need to be changed into a new compound to enhance their elimination. Metabolism is the process by which the drug is broken down or changed by various enzyme systems. The compounds formed as a result of the interaction between the drug and enzymes are known as metabolites. Metabolites may be *active* (with a therapeutic effect) or *inactive* (with little or no therapeutic effect) when compared to their precursors (the original drug compounds) and *some* may even be responsible for toxic side effects. Some drugs are inactive until they are activated by being metabolized. These are called prodrugs. Recall that drugs taken orally are absorbed and transported to the liver before reaching the rest of the body. This is an important safeguard built into our bodies, to ensure than anything eaten must go through the liver for possible metabolism before being utilized by the body. This, however, may result in significant metabolism of drugs before reaching the site of action. This is called the first-pass effect because drugs taken orally must "first pass" through the liver before reaching the systemic circulation. If a drug intended for systemic effect is highly eliminated by the first pass, (ie, nitroglycerin, lidocaine), it may be ineffective when given orally and, therefore, should be given via a "non-first-pass route" such as SL or IV.

Several liver enzymes are responsible for the metabolism of drugs. They are categorized into two groups: phase I and phase II enzyme systems. The most common phase I drug-metabolizing enzymes are known collectively as the cytochrome P450 enzymes, sometimes abbreviated CYP P450 (pronounced "sip P four-fifty"). The CYP P450 family of enzymes includes a large number of individual enzymes. Other enzyme systems that can metabolize drugs include phase II enzymes, which act by conjugating (chemically combining) drugs with glucuronic acid or glutathione, or modifying the drug by the transfer of methyl, acetyl, or sulfa groups from donor compounds. Most enzymes can be upregulated and downregulated by inducing or inhibiting the enzymes. There are drugs and diseases that can induce and inhibit

enzymes. This is a major source of drug and disease interactions (as described later in the section on Drug and Disease Interactions).

There are also some enzymes that are genetically controlled and could exist in greater or lesser amounts in individual patients. For example, if a patient has a large amount of enzymes available to metabolize a drug, he or she will be a fast metabolizer and will have a more rapid clearance of the drug. In this case, the patient may suffer from a lack of efficacy because of this genetically determined increase in the enzyme. This patient would possibly need a higher dose of the drug compared to patients without this genetic trait. On the other hand, slow metabolizers would have genetically less enzyme available and would need lower doses of drugs metabolized by that enzyme. Pharmacogenomics is a relatively new and exciting field of study that examines how to accurately predict and react to such potential over- or under-dosing of drugs based upon the genetic make-up of the patient. Tests are available to predict the genetic types for some critical metabolizing enzymes. This information can be utilized to determine if some drugs can or should be used, and to help tailor the proper dosages of drugs to ensure that they are safe and effective. Chapter 3 examines this field in detail.

Excretion

Excretion is the process by which the drug and its metabolites are eliminated from the body. The main routes of excretion are through the urine and feces. Drugs may also exit the body through exhalation and sweating but to a much lesser extent. How readily drugs and metabolites are excreted in the urine or feces is dependent on their physiochemical properties and the function of the excreting organ. A drug excreted primarily by the kidneys will likely require dose adjustment for a patient with kidney failure. If the dose is not adjusted, the concentration of the drug may increase to a range that is toxic to the patient. Similarly, if two drugs are cleared by the same mechanism, one drug may be preferentially eliminated over another, resulting in hindering the elimination of the other drug. This may result in an increased concentration of the drug that had its elimination reduced. There are even drug interactions that can occur in the kidneys (as described in the section on Drug and Disease Interactions).

PHARMACOKINETIC MODELING

Mathematical models can be used to predict concentrations of drug in the body and when they will occur. If there is a known effect that is targeted and related to drug concentration, dosage regimens can be designed to deliver a given concentration-time profile. Most drugs are eliminated in a *log linear* fashion. This may sound complicated, but it simply means that, instead of a drug being removed by a certain number of milligrams or grams each minute or hour, a given fraction or percentage of the drug is removed each hour. For example, 50% of the drug may be removed per hour. In this case, after 1 hour 50% would be left, after 2 hours 25% would be left, after 3 hours 12.5% would remain, etc. The amount of time it takes for half of the drug to be removed is called the half-life. The half-life is a measure of how long the drug hangs around in the body and is, therefore, an important element in determining how often a drug should be given. The shorter the half-life, the more often the drug must be given and vice versa. Half-life also determines how long it takes for the drug to reach a steady state. Steady state is a state of equilibrium that occurs when the drug administered replaces the drug removed. It takes four or five half-lives to reach a "clinical" steady state.

The line formed by a plot of drug concentrations after administration versus time will be curved, if the drug follows what is termed a linear, "one-compartment" model (see Figure 2-1). If the same drug concentrations versus time are plotted on a log linear plot or the log normal (ln) concentration versus time is plotted, the resulting line will be straight.

To determine the half-life and elimination rate constant (*k*), the slope of the elimination line must be determined. The elimination rate constant (*k*) is a measure of the

fraction of the drug that is removed per unit of time. The units for half-life are in terms of time (hours, minutes, etc.). The units for the elimination rate constant will be the inverse of half-life, per unit of time (per hour, etc.). This is because it is signifying the fraction of removal in that time. The elimination rate constant (*k*) is the slope of the straight line formed in the log linear plot in Figure 2-1. Therefore, a simple "rise over run" method can be used to determine the elimination rate constant (*k*):

$$k = \frac{rise}{run} = \frac{\ln C_2 - \ln C_1}{t_2 - t_1} \qquad \text{Eq. 1}$$

The elimination rate constant (*k*) is closely related to the half-life.

$$t\tfrac{1}{2} = \frac{0.693}{k} \qquad \text{Eq. 2}$$

These equations are complex but pharmacy technicians are not usually expected to do such calculations. The important point to take from them is that removal of a drug from the body is often described using numbers (the elimination rate constant and, more commonly, the half-life) that give us an idea of how long it takes to remove the drug and how long it takes to reach a steady state. This will influence how frequently a drug must be dosed.

DOSAGE REGIMEN DESIGN

A dosage regimen is how much drug will be given in a period of time when multiple doses of the drug will be given (eg, 10 mg every day). It is usually designed to ensure that the drug concentrations resulting from the dosage regimen will be within the therapeutic range. The therapeutic range is a range of concentrations that describes the best chance for the patient to achieve therapeutic efficacy and avoid toxicity. The dosage regimen is made up of two parts, the dose rate (how much drug is given per unit of time) and the dosing interval (how often the drug is given).

Determination of the Dosing Rate

The dosing rate can be defined as the amount of drug given per unit of time. For example, if a drug's dosage regimen is 10 mg once daily, the dose rate would be 10 mg per day. However, if the drug were given 10 mg twice daily, the dose rate would be 20 mg per day. Pharmacists are able to determine an ideal dose rate for a given patient if some parameters

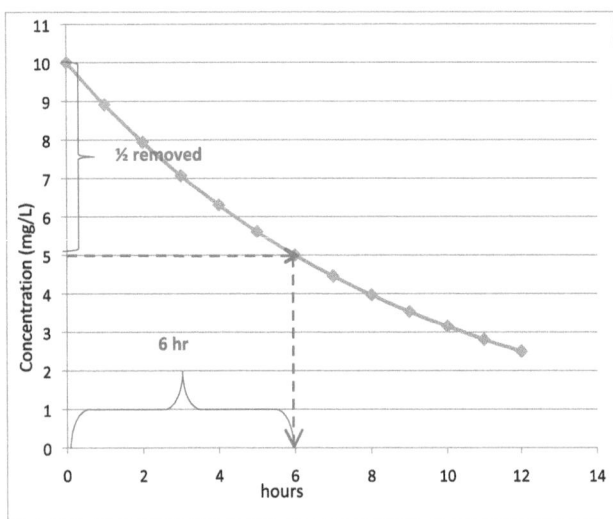

FIGURE 2-1. Concentrations after a dose given where it takes 6 hours for half of the drug to be removed; therefore, the half-life of this drug is 6 hours.

are known. The ideal dosing rate will be targeting a chosen average concentration at steady state (Css,avg). This is as it states, the average concentration measured over the dosing interval once at steady state. This concentration will likely be toward the middle of the therapeutic range.

$$C_{ss,\,avg} = \frac{F \times DR}{CL} \qquad \text{Eq. 3}$$

The average concentration over a dosing interval at steady state ($C_{ss,avg}$) is determined by the clearance (CL), bioavailability (F), and dose rate (DR) of the drug given. While bioavailability is important in most routes of administration, it is not necessary to consider it when determining a dosing rate for a drug given intravenously. (Recall that the bioavailability of these drugs is 100%.)

Once the drug is at steady state and assuming that the F and CL remain constant, the average concentration at steady state will be proportional to the amount of drug given per unit of time (dose rate). Therefore, if the concentration is too low, the dose rate can be increased proportionally to raise the concentration to the target range. If the concentration is too high, the dose rate should be proportionally lowered to ensure that the patient doesn't suffer from toxicity. This is only true for drugs that exhibit linear clearance. This is when a given fraction of the drug is removed per unit of time.

There are some drugs that are eliminated in a nonlinear fashion. In this case, an amount of drug is removed per unit of time, not a fraction of the drug per unit of time. Drugs that are eliminated this way will have a clearance that is concentration dependent. The $C_{ss,avg}$ will not be proportional to the dose rate in this case. Phenytoin (Dilantin®), a drug used for seizures, is cleared this way. If the dose rate of phenytoin is doubled, the resulting concentration would be much more than double. This is a concern as it could result in toxicity.

Determination of the Dose Interval

The dose interval is how often the drug is given (ie, daily, twice a day, etc.). The longer the dosing interval, the more variation there will be in the concentrations over the dosing interval. For most drugs, the goal is to minimize the difference between the maximum concentration (C_{max}) achieved, usually at or near the beginning of the dosing interval, and the minimum concentration (C_{min}) achieved at the end of the dosing interval. The longer the dosing interval, the larger the difference between C_{max} and C_{min}. Figure 2-2 demonstrates the difference when giving 150 mg every 12 hours (blue line) compared to giving 75 mg every 6 hours (red line). The amounts given per time are the same (12.5 mg/hr), so the patient will get the same amount of drug per time (same dose rate) but the C_{max} and C_{min} will differ.

As a rule of thumb, dosing every one or two half-lives works well for most drugs. Since it takes one half-life to eliminate half the drug, this means that there will be half (one half-life) or a quarter (two half-lives) of the drug at the end of the dosing interval when compared to the beginning of the dosing interval. Therefore, drugs with longer half-lives can be given less often. This is usually desirable to improve patient adherence to the dosage regimen.

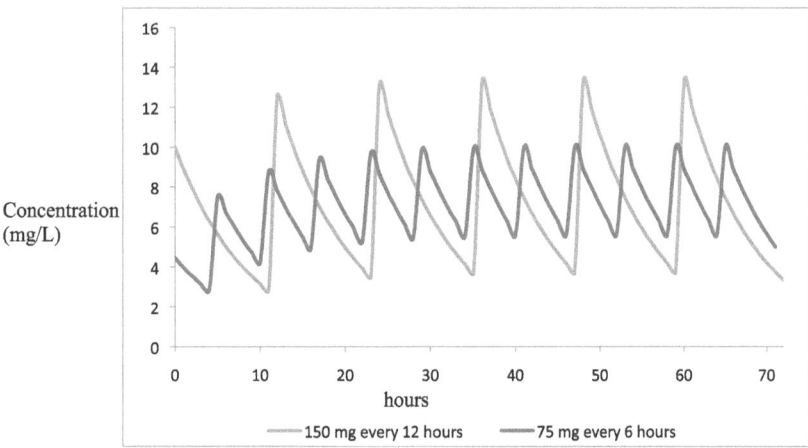

FIGURE 2-2. Concentration time curves when giving the same dose rate but differing dose intervals. Half-life is 6 hours.

MONITORING

One of the benefits of applying pharmacokinetics to patient drug regimens is the ability of the pharmacist to monitor drug concentrations that correlate with drug effects, both therapeutic and toxic. These concentrations can be measured through blood draws. Of course, determining whether a patient has either subtherapeutic or toxic drug effects is not determined by a drug concentration level alone. Drug concentration should always be viewed in the context of the patient's signs and symptoms. If the concentrations are too high, indicating possible toxicity, is the patient exhibiting signs and symptoms of toxicity? If the concentrations are too low, is the patient showing signs of lack of efficacy? Once this has been established, calculations can be utilized to estimate concentrations at any time after a drug is given. For most drugs a log linear relationship allows any concentration to be determined when one concentration and the half-life (or the elimination rate constant, k) are known.

$$C_t = C_0 e^{-\frac{0.693}{t^{1/2}} \times t} \ or \ C_t = C_0 e^{-k \times t} \qquad \text{Eq. 4}$$

where C_t = concentration that occurs t amount of time after C_0

C_0 = concentration that occurs "t" amount of time before C_t

$t^{1/2}$ = half-life

k = elimination rate constant

t = amount of time between C_t and C_0

e^{-kt} = fraction of drug remaining at time t

Note: equation 4 is a rearrangement of equation 1.

$$k = \frac{rise}{run} = \frac{\ln C_2 - \ln C_1}{t_2 - t_1}$$
$$k(\Delta t) = \ln C_2 - \ln C_1$$
$$\ln C_2 = \ln C_1 - k(\Delta t)$$
anti-log each side
$$C_2 = C_1 \cdot e^{-k \Delta t}$$

These equations look challenging, but they are very useful. For example, if it is known that a drug has a therapeutic range from 5 mg/L to 20 mg/L, a dosage regimen can be designed to keep the concentrations within that range. If the $t^{1/2}$ of the drug is known to be 6 hours and a concentration is measured 8 hours after the drug is given and is found to be 7.94 mg/L, it can be determined when the concentration will fall below 5 mg/L and the next dose must be administered.

$$C_t = c_0 e^{-\frac{0.693}{t^{1/2}} t}$$
$$5\frac{mg}{L} = \frac{7.94 mg}{L} e^{-\frac{0.693}{6hr} t}$$

When solved for t: $t = 4$ hr.

Thus, the concentration will fall to 5 mg/L in 4 hours, which will be 12 hours after the drug is given. This drug should be dosed every 12 hours to stay within the therapeutic range (Figure 2-3).

Utilizing pharmacokinetic modeling in choosing the proper dosing regimen for a patient can result in better

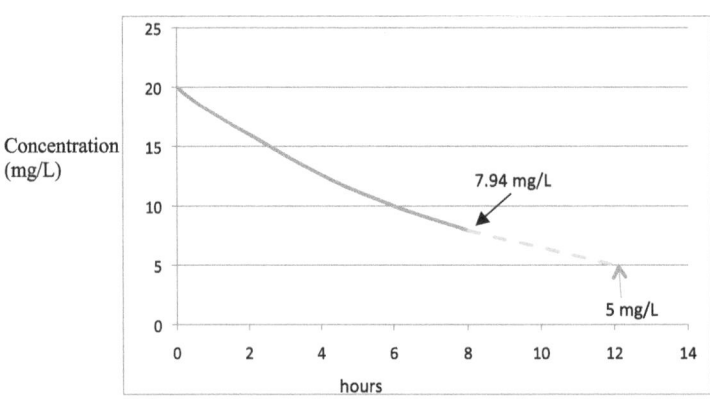

FIGURE 2-3. Concentration-time curve demonstrating the determination of when the next dose should be given.

TABLE 2-1. Representative Drugs with Narrow Therapeutic Range

Central Nervous System	Cardiovascular
Acetaminophen	Digoxin
Amitriptyline	Disopyramide
Carbamazepine	Flecainide
Desipramine	Lidocaine
Ethosuximide	Procainamide
Imipramine	Quinidine
Lithium	
Nortriptyline	
Phenobarbital	
Phenytoin	
Primidone	
Valproic acid/divalproex	
Antibiotics	Immunologic/ Immunosuppressive
Amikacin	Cyclosporine
Chloramphenicol	Methotrexate
Gentamicin	Sirolimus
Tobramycin	Tacrolimus

patient care because there is more confidence in predicting a regimen that will be effective while avoiding toxicity. This is based on the Css,avg, Css,max, and Css,min all being within the therapeutic range. Drugs with relatively small ("narrow") therapeutic ranges are the ones that most commonly require drug level monitoring and specialized dosing because the differences between the Cmax that is needed to avoid toxicity and the Cmin that is needed to ensure efficacy is small. These are also the drugs that are highly vulnerable to drug, food, and disease interactions. A representative list of these drugs can be found in Table 2-1.

DRUG AND DISEASE INTERACTIONS

Drug Interactions in Absorption

Absorption can be increased or decreased depending on disease states, the drugs, or the foods that are administered at the same time. This can pose a problem for individuals who have multiple disease states requiring the use of multiple medications. Absorption drug interactions may result in either more or less drug being absorbed and, therefore, leave some therapies possibly toxic and some possibly ineffective. It is important to understand that drug, food, and disease interactions do not just happen when an interfering drug or food is

added but the reverse effect will often happen when the drug or food is stopped.

One such interaction occurs when drugs given orally bind with other compounds, decreasing their ability to be absorbed. An example of this is ciprofloxacin (Cipro®), an antibiotic. When calcium is given with oral ciprofloxacin, it will decrease the amount of ciprofloxacin available for absorption. This could result in suboptimal concentrations of this antibiotic, possibly resulting in therapeutic failure. If you add the auxiliary label that says do not take with antacids, this is likely the reason why.

When grapefruit or grapefruit juice comes into contact with the intestinal tract, it can decrease the effectiveness of some of the enzymes in the intestinal wall. By decreasing the enzyme activity, drugs that are subject to this enzyme can have an increase in the amount of drug that is bioavailable or the amount that makes it to the systemic circulation. This increase in bioavailability will increase the concentration of drug in the body, possibly putting the patient at risk for toxicity. An example of this drug-food interaction happens with grapefruit juice and a group of cholesterol-lowering medications called statins, as well as with cyclosporine, an immunosuppressant used to block the rejection of transplanted organs.

These are only a few examples of many types of interactions that can occur in the process of absorption. There are many others. These are most significant for drugs with small therapeutic ranges (Table 2-1).

Drug Interactions in Metabolism

Metabolism may also be the source of drug-disease, drug-drug, and drug-food interactions. Recall from earlier discussion, the importance of the CYP P450 system of enzymes. Many, but not all, drugs require metabolism by these enzymes to become active or inactive. There are many drugs that can induce or inhibit CYP P450 enzymes. If an enzyme inhibitor of the CYP P450 3A4 enzyme, such as fluconazole (Diflucan®), is added to the regimen of a patient who is already taking a drug like phenytoin (Dilantin®) that is metabolized by this system, the phenytoin will not be metabolized as quickly and will increase the concentration of the phenytoin, putting the patient at risk for toxicity. Conversely, if erythromycin, a CYP P450 3A4 inducer is added to the regimen of a patient on phenytoin, the clearance of phenytoin will increase, causing a decrease in the concentration of phenytoin. This could result in therapeutic failure.

Enzymes that metabolize drugs can be induced or inhibited by other drugs and diseases. Recall that genetic predispositions for being fast and slow metabolizers will also enter into the determination of the dosing regimen for metabolized drugs. A more detailed discussion can be found in chapter 3.

Drug Interactions in Excretion

When a patient who has kidney disease is taking a drug for which the body relies on the kidneys for elimination, it would be expected that the clearance would decrease. This would result in an increase in the amount of drug in the body, possibly putting the patient at risk for toxicity unless the dose rate is decreased.

There are drug interactions that can occur as well. Some drugs are eliminated by utilizing transport systems or "carriers" that move them from the blood into the nephron and out of the body in the urine. Drugs may compete with each other for the carrier taking them from the blood into the nephron. If two drugs are competing for the same carrier, one may be preferentially carried into the nephron and one left behind. The one left behind will not be cleared, thereby decreasing drug clearance and increasing concentrations and half-life. This drug interaction is utilized for a beneficial therapeutic effect when probenecid is added to the regimen of a patient who is already on penicillin. The probenecid will be preferentially carried into the nephron leaving the penicillin behind, purposefully increasing the concentrations and duration ($t\frac{1}{2}$) of the antibiotic penicillin. There are other similar drug interactions that are not always considered to be beneficial.

There are also drug interactions associated with changes in the pH of the urine that could increase or decrease the clearance of a drug eliminated in the urine. If a patient with renal impairment is taking a drug that is cleared by the kidneys, the patient is at risk for toxicity. Adding or stopping a drug that affects the carrier of another drug for secretion into the nephron could alter the clearance of drugs susceptible to these interactions.

Knowing about all these interactions will be helpful to ensure that patients are properly warned or advised by the pharmacist. However, it is ultimately the pharmacist's role to evaluate the situation and confer with the prescriber for suggested changes in the dosing regimen or warn the patient about potential problems.

SUMMARY

Pharmacokinetics provides an important set of tools for pharmacists to ensure that their patients have optimal dosage regimens. Utilization of these concepts can help pharmacists predict and avoid the possible dangerous effects of drug-drug,

drug-food, and drug-disease interactions and, therefore, avoid possible problems of inefficacy or toxicity. It is important to recognize that utilizing drug concentrations and pharmacokinetics is only a tool. This information must be coupled with clinical information and evidence in order to get a true picture of the patient. Understanding and using these principles will result in better outcomes in patients.

REVIEW QUESTIONS

1. You see that one of your patients is buying some St. John's Wort OTC (over-the-counter) for depression. You want to be sure that there are no drug interactions. You recall the pharmacist saying that this drug can be an enzyme inhibitor. What should you do?

2. A patient is well controlled on a drug that is totally cleared by the kidneys, and then the patient becomes renally impaired. Is the patient at risk? What will this mean for the patient's drug regimen?

3. A patient is on a drug that has a half-life of 8 hours. How long will it take for the patient to reach steady state?

4. The concentration after an IV dose is given is 80 mg/L. Twenty-four hours later the concentration of this drug is measured to be 10 mg/L. What is the half-life of this drug? If the therapeutic range of this drug is 20–80 mg/L, how often should the drug be given?

5. A patient on an antihypertensive medication has had a change in her insurance coverage, which means the patient must change brands of her blood pressure medication. The patient would be happy with this because it is much cheaper for her. However, it is known that this brand of the drug has a lower bioavailability. How would this likely affect the clearance, volume, half-life, and concentrations of this drug in your patient? What dosage regimen changes should be recommended?

6. A patient is taking 200 mg twice daily of a drug called "Nemo" for cholesterol lowering. The average target concentration is 10 mg/L. The patient's cholesterol has not improved, and the average concentration is measured to be 5 mg/L. What dosage regimen changes should be recommended? (Assume the patient is at steady state and that F and CL are stable. "Nemo" is a linearly cleared drug.)

7. How could pharmacokinetic principles be used to help determine how often a drug is given to a patient?

8. How might pharmacokinetic principles be used to anticipate drug interactions?

Chapter 3

Pharmacogenomics

Prabodh Sadana, PhD

KEY TERMS AND DEFINITIONS

Allele—a particular type of DNA sequence at a specific location in the genome. Such a sequence can be a wild-type or variant sequence.

DNA or deoxyribonucleic acid—the double-stranded molecule found in the nucleus of cells that carries the genetic blueprint of an organism.

Gene transcription—the biological process of making an RNA copy from the DNA sequence of the gene. The RNA produced is called the messenger RNA (mRNA) which provides information for making the protein coded by the gene.

Gene—a basic unit of heredity made of DNA and found on chromosomes in the nucleus.

Genotype—broadly, refers to the entire genetic makeup of an individual. More specifically, it refers to the pair of alleles found at a particular genomic location.

Heterozygous genotype—the presence of two different alleles at a particular genomic location.

Homozygous genotype—the presence of identical alleles (either wild-type or variant) at a particular genomic location.

Metabolizing enzymes—proteins that facilitate, enhance, or accelerate chemical reactions in the body. These enzymes convert the drug molecules to either inactive or active products in the body.

Pharmacogenomics—the study of how the entire genome affects the response to a drug therapy.

Phenotype—the physical or functional manifestation of the genotype in an organism.

DOI 10.37573/9781585286638.003

Polymorphism—a gene variant that occurs at a frequency greater than 1% in a population.

RNA or ribonucleic Acid—a single-stranded molecule with multiple functions, including allowing genes that make up the DNA to be expressed in the form of proteins.

Single nucleotide polymorphism or SNP—a sequence variation at a single position in a DNA sequence.

Variant—a specific region of the genetic material that differs from the most common DNA sequence and that may or may not lead to altered function.

Wild-type—phenotype or allele that is in the form most commonly found in the population, and that is assumed to result in the "typical" function for an organism.

LEARNING OBJECTIVES

After completing this chapter, you should be able to

1. Define pharmacogenomics and key terms related to this subject.

2. Outline basic forms of genetic variability that affect medication action.

3. Identify common gene variants in drug-metabolizing enzymes and drug transporters.

4. Describe how genetic variability influences enzyme activities and metabolizer status in individual patients.

5. Discuss how prodrugs are affected differently than standard bioactive drugs by the influence of genetic variants in metabolizing enzymes.

6. Describe the pharmacogenetic interaction between at least three different medication-gene pairs and the appropriate dose or therapy adjustments needed in such interactions.

Efficacy and safety are the defining characteristics of any drug approved for human administration. While the drug development process entails the evaluation of drug candidates in a sizable patient population, there can still be patient-specific or subpopulation-specific pharmacological effects that may be observed only after the drug has been deployed in clinical practice. A complex interplay of factors influences the therapeutic window within which the drug

produces its intended pharmacological effect. However, a one-size-fits-all drug therapy frequently fails. Drug therapy is often modified based on several patient-specific factors (Table 3-1). Each person's genetic makeup is a unique biological blueprint, and it can profoundly influence not only susceptibility to specific diseases, but also response to drug therapies. The modification of drug therapies after inefficacy or adverse events are evident has always been possible. However, this trial-and-error approach can come at the expense of delay in appropriate treatment and, at times, serious health consequences. Pharmacogenomics provides preemptive ways to avoid these scenarios and increases the likelihood of successful drug therapy for a given condition and its treatment.

Pharmacogenomics and the related term "pharmacogenetics" refer to the study of how genes in an individual or in a population affect the response to drug therapy. Another term that has commonly been used is "precision medicine" which refers to the use of a systematic approach to disease treatment and prevention that takes into account a patient's genes, environment, and lifestyle. Pharmacogenomics is a component of the broader precision medicine approach. Several factors have helped to increase the attention on pharmacogenomics as a tool to improve the clinical outcomes of drug therapy. Despite an increase in targeted drug therapies, the health and economic burden of ineffective drug treatments remain high. In addition, drug therapies are often associated with frequent and predictable adverse effects that are responsible for significant mortality, especially in the hospital setting. The cost of prescription drugs has increased rapidly over the past few decades which has justifiably increased patient expectations of safe, proven, and effective drug treatments. The advent of large-scale gene-sequencing technologies and data analysis tools have also fueled the rise of pharmacogenomics in mainstream medicine. This chapter provides a basic explanation of the

TABLE 3-1. Common Factors Influencing Modification or Tailoring of Drug Therapy

Factors
Age/weight
Presence of other diseases or conditions
Hepatic or renal function
Other co-administered drugs
Disease severity or progression
Cost of therapy

science of pharmacogenomics and its application in clinical practice, using discrete examples.

THE FUNDAMENTALS OF GENETICS

DNA is organized into chromosomes and packaged into the nucleus of cells, encoding the genetic information that serves as the "blueprint" of life. Adult human cells have 23 pairs of chromosomes, including a pair of sex chromosomes. One chromosome in each pair is inherited from the father and one from the mother. Fertilization of the egg with the sperm followed by the pairing of the chromosomes from the mother and father results in the regeneration of the two sets of chromosomes. DNA is made of four nucleotide bases—two purine bases (adenine [A] and guanine [G]) and two pyrimidine bases (cytosine [C] and thymine [T]). In the RNA molecule, a nucleotide called uracil (U) replaces T. The nucleotide bases in DNA are attached to a sugar (deoxyribose)-phosphate backbone. Two such strands of polymeric chains coil together to form the classical double helical form of DNA. In the DNA double helix, the nucleotide bases on the two strands are joined to each other following the base-pairing rules (A pairs with T, and G pairs with C; A pairs with U in RNA). The organization of nucleotides in a specific sequence forms the genetic message that form genes, which encode proteins responsible for carrying out all the bodily functions—from structural proteins of the body to enzymes, transporters, receptors, etc. The basic structure of DNA is illustrated in Figure 3-1.

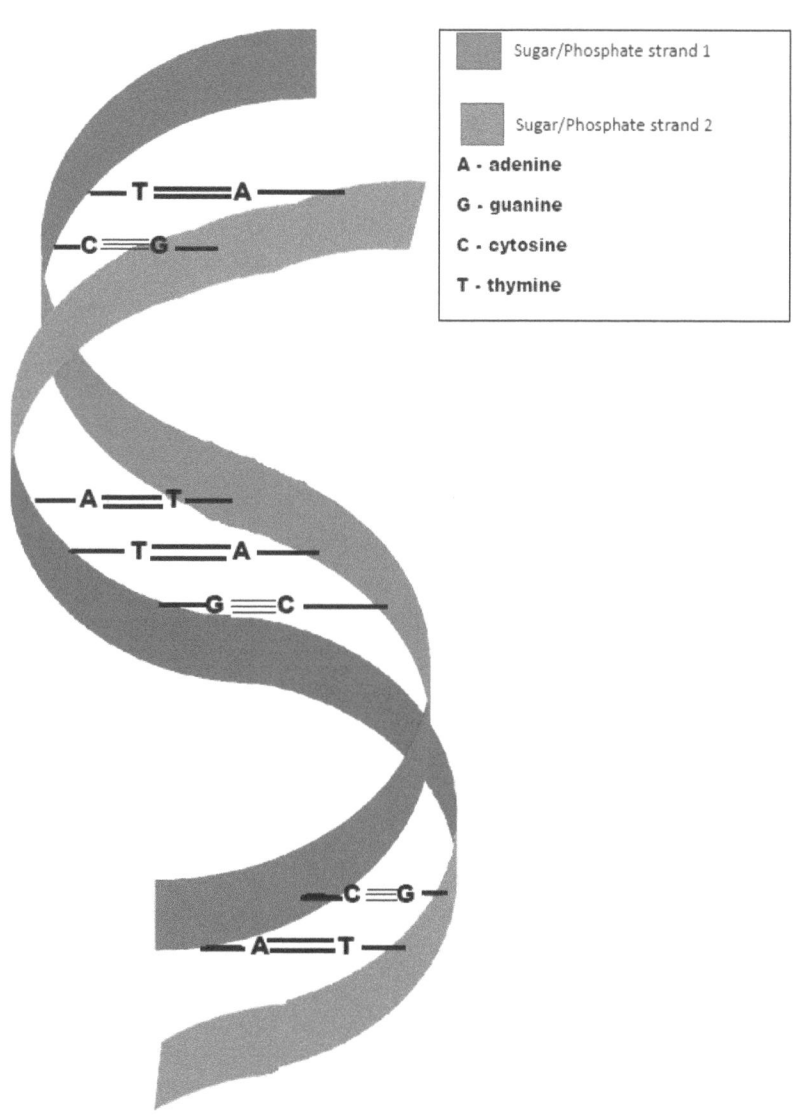

Sugar/Phosphate strand 1

Sugar/Phosphate strand 2

A - adenine

G - guanine

C - cytosine

T - thymine

FIGURE 3-1. Representation of deoxyribonucleic acid (DNA).

Genes are the parts of the human genome that carry the information that affects an individual's characteristics and/or phenotype. Humans have two copies of each gene, one inherited from each parent. Overall, the human genome is believed to code for approximately 20,000 to 25,000 proteins, a number far lower than was once believed. Using the genetic information carried in the DNA to form proteins entails the molecular processes of transcription and translation.

During transcription, the genetic information in the DNA is copied to generate a single-stranded messenger RNA (mRNA) molecule by the enzyme RNA polymerase. This mRNA molecule generated in the nucleus then leaves the nucleus to enter the cytoplasm, where it is used in the process of protein synthesis or translation. The genetic information in the mRNA molecule forms a script that is read three letters (A, T, G, or C) at a time (known as codons) in a process involving organelles called ribosomes and another specialized RNA molecule called the transfer RNA or tRNA. Each of the 64 codons (the number of possible combinations of four bases in a three-letter format) codes for a specific amino acid. The mRNA sequence information is "read" in a specific order of three-letter codons known as the open reading frame, defined by a start codon (typically *AUG*, which codes for the amino acid methionine) and that ends with a stop codon (*UGA*, *UAA*, or *UAG*). The tRNA transfers the appropriate amino acid coded by a specific codon to the ribosome for assembly and thereby the mRNA sequence is translated into the polypeptide sequence of amino acids to form proteins. There is redundancy in the genetic code, with multiple possible codons for a specific amino acid. For example, the amino acid arginine (Arg) is coded by codons *CGU, CGC, CGA, CGG, AGA*, and *AGG*. Overall, this process of transcription and translation is called the "central dogma of molecular biology," which is simply defined as *DNA makes RNA, and RNA makes protein*.

Genetic Variations

There is a vast similarity in the DNA sequence among the 6 billion bases that make up the human genome. In fact, 99.5% of the DNA sequence is believed to be identical across the human race. At the scale of billions of bases, the 0.5% difference still accounts for millions of bases and is sufficient for meaningful differences in the genetic predisposition to diseases and variable drug response. Differences occur at the rate of one change in every 1,000 bases. Various types of genetic variations have been identified (Figure 3-2). Among the most important types of sequence variations or mutations are the single nucleotide polymorphisms

Genetic variation

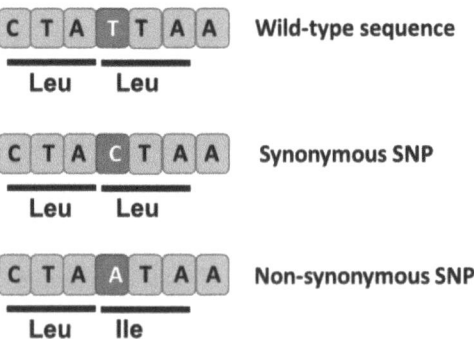

FIGURE 3-2. Types of genetic variations illustrated using an example wild-type sequence. SNP = single nucleotide polymorphisms; Leu = leucine; Ile = isoleucine.

or SNPs (pronounced as "snips"). SNPs refer to variations in a sequence at a single position in a DNA sequence. For example, rather than a stretch of sequence such as *AATGCTAG*, an individual may have *AAAGCTAG*. The *T* in the third position, in this case, is changed to an *A*. A population frequency of >1% is used as a threshold to define variations at a single nucleotide position as a polymorphism. When population frequency is <1%, the variations are classified as mutations. Approximately 12 million SNPs have been identified to date. Importantly, a vast number of these SNPs are "silent"—that is, they do not alter or affect the function or expression of genes. However, in certain cases, these SNPs can have a profound effect on the expression or activity of the specific protein coded by the gene harboring the SNP.

The SNPs are of different types, broadly classified as:

1. Synonymous—these SNPs do not result in a change in the encoded amino acid. For example, an *A→G* substitution in *AGA* to *AGG* still results in the Arg amino acid in the polypeptide chain.

2. Nonsynonymous: These SNPs alter the amino acid encoded by the codon. For example, a *C→A* substitution in *CCG* to *CAG* results in a change in the amino acid encoded from proline to glutamine. This type of SNP is also sometimes called a missense substitution. Another type of nonsynonymous SNP is a nonsense substitution wherein a single nucleotide change in the DNA sequence results in the generation of a stop codon, which causes the termination of the transcription process.

SNPs can also be in noncoding parts of the DNA, such as in the promoter regions of the genes. The promoter region of a gene is the DNA sequence that flanks the gene and to which critical proteins called transcription factors and RNA polymerase bind, ultimately resulting in the expression of the gene. So, while variants in these regions do not alter the sequence of the encoded protein, they have the potential to affect the expression levels of the proteins by affecting the normal transcriptional rate of a gene. It is important to note that based on the presence or absence of variant(s) at a particular site, a gene can be present in one of the two or more alternate forms. Each of these forms of a gene is called an allele. An allele can be a wild-type allele, which refers to the most common version of the gene sequence in a population, or it can be a variant allele. A copy of a gene inherited from a parent can be in wild-type or variant form. Each pair of alleles represents the genotype of a specific gene. Genotypes are described as homozygous if there are two identical alleles at a particular genetic location and as heterozygous if the two alleles differ. The genotype that an individual has for a specific gene (wild type/wild type; wild type/variant; variant/variant) eventually determines the phenotype that the patient exhibits for that gene function.

Because of the existence of millions of SNPs, a naming system is in place to ensure that individual SNPs are accurately referred to in the scientific literature and clinical practice. A few different nomenclature conventions have been used for designating SNPs. The two most common ones are—a star-allele-based convention and a RefSNP-based naming convention (Table 3-2).

While SNPs are the most common types of genetic variations, another type of genetic variation are the copy number variations (CNVs). The CNVs in genes result in an individual carrying multiple copies of a gene on a chromosome. A significant example of CNV is observed in the *CYP2D6* gene, with multiple functional copies of the *CYP2D6* gene reported in certain individuals. The typical annotation of gene duplication or multiplication is, for example, *1xN or *2xN where xN is the number of copies. These multiple copies can be of a normal function allele, an increased function allele, or a decreased function allele.

Effects of Genetic Variations

As mentioned earlier, the genotype for a specific gene influences the observed phenotype. Broadly, the variants produce either a loss-of-function or a gain-of-function effect on the gene activity. The loss-of-function effect is more common. An individual may have inherited one or both copies of a gene in its variant form. Based on the possible combinations of inheritance patterns for the wild-type and variant allele, significant differences in gene function can be observed. In the case of a loss-of-function variant the following phenotypical effects would be observed for the corresponding genotypes:

Wild type/Wild type (homozygous for wild type): normal function

Wild type/Variant (heterozygous): reduction in function

Variant/Variant (homozygous for variant): significant reduction in function

Thus, while normal gene function is expected when both the inherited alleles are wild-type, a significant reduction in function is seen when both the inherited alleles are loss-of-function variants. Analogously, carrying both alleles which are gain-of-function variants is expected to produce a significant increase in gene function compared to the homozygous wild-type inheritance. It is also important to acknowledge the relative prevalence of a gene variant in a given population or allele frequency. There can be significant differences in the prevalence of a variant based on a specific genetic ancestry. So, while some variants may be more common in the Caucasian population, they may be missing or less prevalent in populations of African or Asian ancestry and vice versa. Population-wide genetic screening

TABLE 3-2. Commonly Used Nomenclature System for Single Nucleotide Polymorphisms (SNPs)

System	Description	Example
Star-allele based	Uses the standard gene symbol followed by a star symbol and an arbitrary number. The wild-type allele is generally designated as *1. Variants are assigned other designations (*2, *3, *4, . . ., etc.).	*CYP2C9*2* is a SNP in the *CYP2C9* gene that results in an arginine to cysteine substitution at the 144th position of the CYP2C9 protein
RefSNP based	Uses accession numbers in a specific database of SNPs called the dbSNP. The dbSNP accession numbers are written as the prefix "rs" followed by a number.	rs1799853 refers to the CYP2C9*2 SNP

has yielded important observational data on the prevalence patterns of specific gene variants, and in some cases, have shaped population-specific medication therapy guidelines and recommendations. However, ethnicity only predicts the likelihood of carrying specific genetic variants. Individual patient sequencing is still necessary to confirm the presence or absence of the variants of interest.

The effect of having a genetic variant is also largely dependent on the gene that carries that variant and the natural function of the gene. While the variants can occur in any gene, for the purpose of pharmacogenomics, the following discussion will only consider the genes that have a role in regulating a medication's drug-body interactions. Broadly, the drug-body interactions can be grouped according to either the pharmacokinetic or the pharmacodynamic properties of the medication. Recall from Chapter 2 that pharmacokinetics describes the effect that the body has on a medication. For the medication to produce its effects on the human body it must navigate through several membrane barriers (absorption or A), effectively use the circulatory system to travel through the body (distribution or D), and survive enzymatic transformation (metabolism or M), and the processes that are designed to remove it from the body (elimination or E). These ADME characteristics of a given medication comprise its pharmacokinetic profile and determine the levels of the active medication found at the target action site.

Once the medication is at the active site (for example, the heart cells or myocytes for an anti-arrhythmic medication), the medication has a chance to exert its therapeutic effect. These effects that the medication produces on the body are classified as its pharmacodynamic effects. The pharmacodynamics of a medication characterize the biochemical and physiological effects it exerts via its ability to bind and modify the function of various target proteins in the body, including receptors, enzymes, ion channels, or transporters. In the context of pharmacogenomics, the vast majority of currently known and clinically important variants are found in the genes encoding for proteins that determine the pharmacokinetics of medications.

To understand the implications of gene variants for pharmacogenomics, it is important to review which genes and their corresponding proteins govern the concentrations of drug molecules in the body. The concentration of the drug in the body determines not only the therapeutic efficacy of the drug but also the adverse effect potential of the treatment. Therefore, any increase or decrease in the levels of the drug in the body beyond the therapeutic range has the potential to compromise the efficacy or exacerbate the adverse effects of the medication. A major role in regulating

these levels is ascribed to the metabolizing enzymes, which are proteins that promote or accelerate chemical reactions in the body. Human beings have hundreds of drug-metabolizing enzymes. The chemical reactions catalyzed by the drug-metabolizing enzymes can be classified into either phase I metabolism or phase II metabolism.

Phase I Metabolism

The phase I reaction is an enzymatic reaction that often occurs in the liver wherein polar modifications are introduced to the molecules of the drug by the processes of oxidation, reduction, or hydrolysis. Phase I reactions facilitate the conversion of lipophilic (dissolving in lipids or fats) drug molecules to hydrophilic (dissolving in water). This group of reactions is catalyzed predominantly by the cytochrome P450 superfamily of mixed-function oxidases (CYPs).

The sequencing of the human genome has identified 57 *CYP* genes. Together, they account for the metabolism of >75% of prescription pharmaceuticals. The majority of *CYP* genes are polymorphic (exist in variant forms) and these polymorphisms are found at significant levels in the population. These polymorphisms result in either a decrease or increase in enzymatic activity leading to an increase or decrease in the levels of the drugs that are metabolized by these enzymes. Among the numerous CYP enzymes, the most important polymorphisms are seen in CYP2C9, CYP2C19, and CYP2D6. Collectively, the genes that code for these enzymes are responsible for the way biotransformation of 60% to 70% of all medications occurs. The following discussion will cover the relevant genetic variants found in each of these phase I metabolizing enzymes (Figure 3-3).

CYP2C9

This is one of the most abundant enzymes in the human liver and is responsible for the metabolism of 15% to 20% of prescribed and over-the-counter drugs (Table 3-3). The most clinically important variants of *CYP2C9* are *2 and *3, both of which have a significantly lower frequency in the African and Asian populations than the Caucasian population.

- *CYP2C9*2*: A variant seen in 10% to 20% for Caucasian populations and considerably less in African (0 to 6%) and Asian (1% to 3%) populations. This variant results in a 50% reduction in enzymatic activity compared to *1 (wild type).

- *CYP2C9*3*: This variant is seen at a frequency of 4% to 10% in Caucasians, 1% in Africans, and 3% in Asians. This variant results in an 80% reduction in enzymatic activity compared to *1.

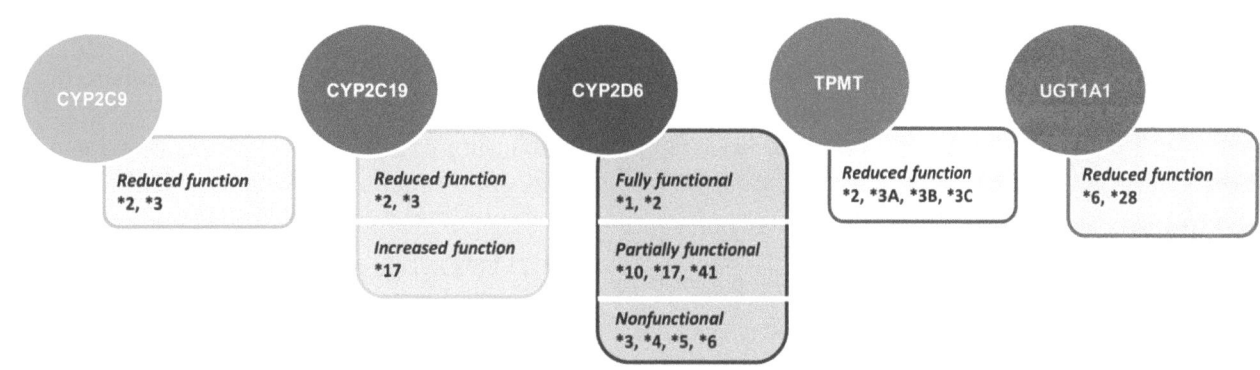

FIGURE 3-3. Important gene variants found in drug-metabolizing enzymes.

TABLE 3-3. Common Drug-Metabolizing Enzymes and the Medications They Metabolize

CYP2C9	CYP2C19	CYP2D6	TPMT	UGT1A1
Tolbutamide	Omeprazole	Haloperidol	6-Mercaptopurine	Irinotecan
Glipizide	Phenytoin	Clozapine	Azathioprine	Raloxifene
Phenytoin	Proguanil	Risperidone		Etoposide
Warfarin	Diazepam	Flecainide		
Losartan	Citalopram	Perphenazine		
Torsemide	Imipramine	Imipramine,		
Ibuprofen	Amitriptyline	Clomipramine		
Diclofenac	Clomipramine	Nortriptyline		
Piroxicam	Clopidogrel	Amitriptyline		
Tenoxicam		Metoprolol		
Mefenamic acid		Propranolol		
		Bupranolol		
		Carvedilol		
		Codeine		
		Tramadol		
		Tamoxifen		

CYP2C19

This enzyme is another major polymorphic CYP450 enzyme. There are three clinically important variants in the *CY2C19* gene: two loss-of-function variants (*2 and *3) and one gain-of-function variant (*17).

- *CYP2C19*2*: The allele frequencies of the *2 variant are 12% in Caucasians, 15% in Africans, and 29% to 35% in Asians.

- *CYP2C19*3*: This variant is most common in Asians (2% to 9%), with <1% allelic frequency in Caucasians and Africans.

- *CYP2C19*17*: This variant results in increased transcription and expression of *CYP2C19*. It has a frequency of 21% in Caucasians, 16% in Africans, and 3% in Asians.

CYP2D6

This major member of the P450 family has been shown to be involved in the metabolism of 25% of prescribed drugs. Several variants of CYP2D6 have been identified, including some that exist in multiple copies ranging from 2 to 13.

- Fully functional CYP2D6 variants: *1 and *2

- Partially functional CYP2D6 variants: *10, *17, and *41

- Nonfunctional CYP2D6 variants: *3, *4, *5, and *6

Among the nonfunctional CYP2D6 variants, the most common expression is seen for *4 in the Caucasian population (~20%); *3 is more common in the Caucasian population than others, although found at low frequencies (~1%); *5 is more common in African and Asian populations (5% to 7%) than Caucasian populations (<1%); and *6 is more common in African (3%) than other populations.

Phase II Metabolism

Among the phase II metabolizing enzymes, important pharmacogenetic associations have been shown for thiopurine S-methyltransferase (TPMT) and uridine diphosphate (UDP) glucuronosyltransferases 1A1 (UGT1A1).

TMPT

This enzyme causes S-methylation of thiopurine drugs (6-mercaptopurine [6-MP] and azathioprine), a modification that leads to their inactivation. Because 6-MP and azathioprine are narrow therapeutic index drugs used in the treatment of cancers and autoimmune and inflammatory disorders, the variants in the TPMT gene can have a profound impact on their pharmacological effects. The most clinically relevant TPMT variants are *2, *3A, *3B, and *3C.

- TPMT*2: This is a rare variant that results in a 100-fold reduction in TPMT activity.

- TPMT*3A: This is a combination of two SNPs and results in a significant decrease in TMPT activity. This is the most common variant in the Caucasian population.

- TPMT*3B: This is a rare variant commonly inherited together with a SNP in exon 10 (*3C) leading to the generation of the *3A variant.

- TPMT*3C: This variant is most common in populations of African or East Asian ancestry.

UGT1A1

UGT enzymes attach a glucuronic acid moiety to the drugs and endogenous substances (like bilirubin) that enhances their solubility in water, thereby allowing them to be excreted in bile or urine. The variants of UGT1A1 known to be clinically relevant include *28 and *6.

- UGT1A1*28: This variant has significant expression in Caucasians, with approximately 10% being homozygous and about 40% heterozygous. Also, it is present at 42% to 56% population frequency in African and 9% to 16% in Asian populations.

- UGT1A1*6: This variant is common in populations with East Asian ancestry (~20%).

This background in drug-metabolizing enzymes is useful to understand the functional consequences of the presence of genetic variants in these enzymes. Individuals can be classified into the following standard phenotypes of metabolizer status for each metabolizing enzyme gene.

- Ultra-rapid metabolizer (UM): markedly increased metabolic activity.

- Normal metabolizer (NM): previously referred to as extensive metabolic (EM) activity.

- Intermediate metabolizer (IM): patients with reduced metabolic activity.

- Poor metabolizer (PM): markedly lower metabolic activity.

Importantly, the metabolizer phenotypes are determined by genotype for a particular enzyme that an individual may have. As mentioned earlier, this is dependent on the different combinations of allele pairs (wild type and variant) that an individual has for a specific gene. An increase in metabolic activity or UM phenotype is usually a result of gain-of-function variants. In contrast, the decrease in metabolic activity of an enzyme or PM is usually a result of loss-of-function variants. The amplitude of gain or loss of function is dependent on whether an individual is homozygous or heterozygous for the gain- or loss-of-function variants. Individuals homozygous for gain-of-function variants are usually UM and those homozygous for loss-of-function are usually PM. The exact genotype-phenotype relationship may vary for different genes (Table 3-4).

An important concept to understand regarding drug metabolism is the effect it has on the biological activity of

TABLE 3-4. The Assignment of Metabolizer Phenotype for the CYP Enzymes Based on Genotype

Gene	Phenotype	Genotype
CYP2C9	NM	*1/*1
	IM	*1/*2, *1/*3, *2/*2
	PM	*2/*3, *3/*3
CYP2C19	UM	*1/*17, *17/*17
	NM	*1/*1
	IM	*1/*2, *1/*3, *2/*17
	PM	*2/*2, *2/*3, *3/*3
CYP2D6[a]	UM	*1/*1xN, *1/*2xN, *2/*2xN
	NM	*1/*1, *1/*2, *1/*9, *1/*41, *2/*2
	IM	*4/*10, *4/*41, *5/*9
	PM	*3/*4, *4/*4, *5/*5, *5/*6

CYP, cytochrome P450; NM, normal metabolizer; IM, intermediate metabolizers; PM, poor metabolizers; UM, ultra-rapid metabolizers.
[a] xN denotes the number of copies of the CYP2D6 gene.

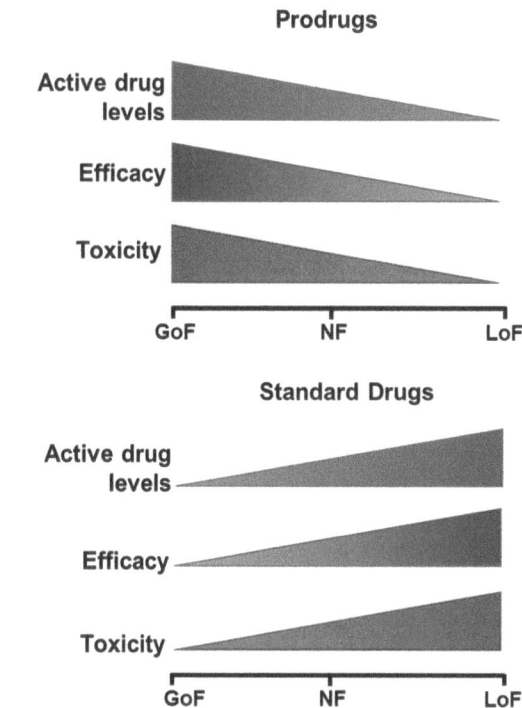

FIGURE 3-4. The effect of functional status of metabolizing enzymes on the drug levels, efficacy, and toxicity of prodrugs and active drugs. GoF, gain of function; NF, normal function; LoF, loss of function.

the drug molecules. Typically, the drugs are bioactive molecules capable of producing the desired therapeutic effect in their native unmodified forms. The modifications of the chemical structure of the parent drug molecule in the process of metabolism often result in a reduction in the activity of the drug. However, this is not always true. For certain drugs, the process of undergoing metabolism in the body results in the activation of the drug molecule. These drugs are called prodrugs—they are administered in their inactive precursor forms and get converted to active moieties by virtue of the chemical modification that occurs in the body. Therefore, the effect of pharmacogenetic variants in the drug-metabolizing enzyme is dependent on the type of drug molecule being examined (Figure 3-4).

For a standard drug (eg, warfarin) with a bioactive parent moiety, a loss-of-function variant results in decreased conversion to the inactive form and an increase in the levels of the active drug molecule that can exceed the intended therapeutic range. This situation can result in increased toxicity of the drug directly related to increased levels of the drug in the circulation. On the other hand, a gain-of-function variant for an enzyme metabolizing the bioactive parent moiety will result in increased metabolism of the drug to inactive forms and as a result, there is a risk of loss of therapeutic efficacy.

For a prodrug (eg, clopidogrel), wherein the drug metabolite is the active form, a loss-of-function variant results in decreased conversion to the active form and as a result, a loss of efficacy. On the other hand, a gain-of-function variant for an enzyme metabolizing the prodrug will result in increased metabolism of the drug to active forms and as a result, an increased risk of causing a toxic drug response.

Both scenarios are observed in clinical practice. Therefore, a knowledge of the basic pharmacological characteristics of the drug is critical to understanding the potential pharmacogenetic interactions.

It is important to consider the information about genetic variants in drug-metabolizing enzymes in the context of the specific role that the enzyme plays in the metabolism of a given drug. Often, drug molecules may have multiple metabolic pathways, each contributing to the breakdown of a specific fraction of the drug. If the variant is found in an enzyme that does not contribute significantly to the breakdown of the drug, then having genetic variants in that enzyme will not have a measurable clinical impact on the pharmacological effect of the drug. A variation of this rule is when the minor metabolic pathway may be more important for the pharmacological effect of the drug. For example, the antiplatelet drug clopidogrel is broken down by enzymes called esterases (accounting for 85% of clopidogrel metabolism) and by CYP2C19 (accounting for 15% of clopidogrel metabolism). In this case, although CYP2C19 is responsible for a much smaller fraction of clopidogrel metabolism, this metabolic pathway converts the prodrug clopidogrel to its active moiety responsible for antiplatelet action; esterases convert clopidogrel to inactive metabolites. Therefore, in this case, loss-of-function variants in CYP2C19 are clinically important although the contribution of CYP2C19 to the metabolic fate of clopidogrel is relatively minor.

While metabolizing enzymes are a major focus of pharmacogenetic interactions, variants in other types of proteins such as transporters and the proteins of the immune system are also clinically relevant.

Transporters are proteins that allow the uptake of drugs and other molecules into cells. Genetic variants that affect the functional activity of transporters can prevent a drug from accumulating in the target tissue and lead to greater off-target adverse effects of drugs. Among transporters, organic anion transporting polypeptide 1B1 (OATP1B1), the protein product of a gene called *SLCO1B1*, is especially important in the context of pharmacogenetics. OATP1B1 is found in the liver cells and is responsible for the transport of widely used drugs such as statins, angiotensin-converting enzyme (ACE) inhibitors, and angiotensin II (AT II) receptor blockers into the liver cells (Figure 3-5). The two known variants of

SLCO1B1 that are associated with reduced OATP1B1 transport function are *5 and *15.

The immune response to drug therapy can have significant implications. Drug-induced hypersensitivity reactions or drug allergies account for 10% of all adverse drug reactions. For a given drug, these reactions would occur only in a small fraction of patients. Predicting which patients would show a hypersensitivity reaction is not easy but certain genetic markers can be useful in this determination. The human leukocyte antigen B (HLA-B) protein is a component of the immune system that has been implicated in drug-induced hypersensitivity. Normally, HLA-B is expressed on the surface of cells and presents cellular peptides to T cells, a major type of immune cell. Certain *HLA-B* alleles are associated with susceptibility to severe skin reactions (Stevens-Johnson syndrome [SJS] or toxic epidermal necrolysis [TEN]) to drugs such as abacavir or carbamazepine. These include variants *57:01 and *15:02. The *15:02 variant is reported at a higher allelic frequency in those with Han Chinese ancestry.

EXAMPLES OF PHARMACOGENOMICS IN ACTION

The application of complex genetic information to guide therapeutic decisions in clinical practice remains a challenge. A consortium of pharmacogenetic experts called the Clinical Pharmacogenetics Implementation Consortium (CPIC), founded in 2009, has led the efforts to formulate guidelines and recommendations for the use of genetic information in

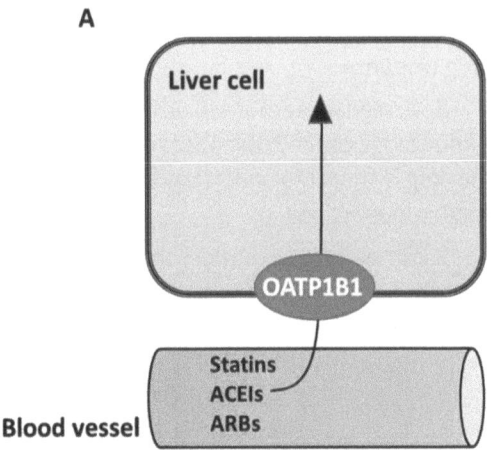
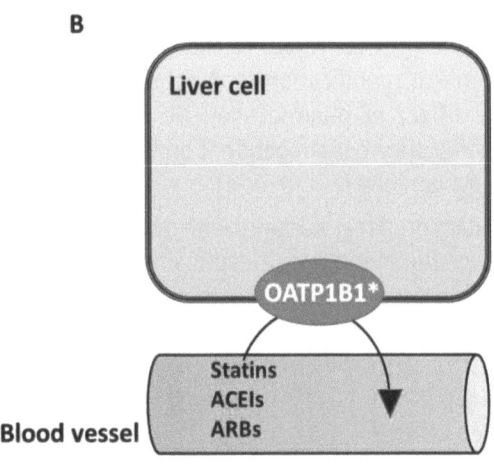

FIGURE 3-5. Organic anion transporting polypeptide 1B1 (OATP1B1) transporter-mediated uptake of medications in the liver. *A*, Normal or wild-type OATP1B1 allows medications such as statins, angiotensin-converting enzyme inhibitors, and angiotensin receptor blockers to be taken up into the liver cells. *B*, OATP1B1 with certain sequence variations (designated OATP1B1*) is unable to allow the entry of medications into the liver cells. The blood levels of the medications increase, resulting in an increased likelihood of adverse effects.

clinical practice guidelines for drug therapy. So far, guidelines for 37 drug/drug class-gene pairs have been published. On the regulatory side, the Food and Drug Administration (FDA) also includes pharmacogenomic information in the various sections of the drug label. Currently, 457 FDA-approved therapeutic products contain pharmacogenomic information in different sections of the drug label, although not all of them are associated with a specific action required based on genetic information. While pharmacogenetic interaction evidence exists for several drug-gene pairs, the actual number of such pairs where that information is "actionable" and requires therapy modifications is much smaller. Even in this group of actionable pharmacogenetic associations, fewer drug-gene pairs require or mandate pharmacogenetic testing; the majority provide recommendations with the assumption that the sequence of the specific interacting gene is already known for a patient, which is very often not the case. These recommendations are based on the strength of the pharmacogenetic evidence reported in the literature. Naturally, pharmacogenomics application is still in its early stages. However, with an increased focus on gene sequencing from healthcare systems and the end consumers, an enhanced utilization of pharmacogenetic evidence in therapeutic decisions is expected to occur.

The power of pharmacogenomics to affect medication therapy is best illustrated by reviewing the drug-gene pair associations. The scope of this chapter does not allow a description of all known drug-gene pharmacogenetic associations. However, the following examples will serve to provide a good overview of some well-established drug-gene pharmacogenetic pairs (Table 3-5).

Clopidogrel-*CYP2C19*

Clopidogrel is a widely prescribed antiplatelet drug that functions as an irreversible inhibitor of a receptor found on the surface of platelets. Clopidogrel binding to this receptor prevents adenosine diphosphate (ADP) from binding to it and activating the platelets. The key feature of clopidogrel pharmacology is that it is administered as an inactive prodrug that must be metabolized to its active form by the action of the enzyme CYP2C19. This process is affected by genetic polymorphisms in *CYP2C19*, as indicated in an earlier section. Variants that decrease the CYP2C19 activity decrease the formation of the active metabolite of clopidogrel and thereby decrease its antiplatelet effect. Increased variability in clopidogrel response is observed in such individuals and therapy modifications may be required.

Carriers of *CYP2C19* loss-of-function alleles are at risk of more cardiovascular events (myocardial infarction [MI],

stroke, stent thrombosis, etc.) due to inadequate antiplatelet effect with clopidogrel usage. Based on their genotypes, they can be classified as EM (*1/*1), UM (*1/*17, *17/*17), IM (*1/*2, *1/*3, *2/*17), and/or PM (*2/*2, *3/*3, *2/*3). Current guidelines suggest using standard clopidogrel dosing in UM and EM but considering an alternative antiplatelet agent such as ticagrelor or prasugrel for IM and PM patients. These recommendations are most beneficial and applicable for patients with acute coronary syndrome (ACS) and those undergoing percutaneous coronary intervention (PCI). Patients with stable ischemic heart disease are less likely to derive benefit from these recommendations.

Codeine-*CYP2D6*

Codeine is an analgesic that belongs to the opioid class of drugs. It is indicated for mild to moderately severe pain and also finds use as an antitussive medication. Codeine is a prodrug that is metabolized by CYP2D6 leading to its bio-activation to morphine in the liver. The analgesic effect of codeine is almost entirely dependent on the generation of morphine in this reaction. As indicated earlier, CYP2D6 is a polymorphic phase I enzyme, with known fully functional (*1 and *2), partially functional (*10, *17, and *41), and non-functional (*3, *4, *5, and *6) variants. Based on the inherited alleles, the possible phenotypes of CYP2D6 activity include UM, EM, IM, and PM.

CYP2D6 UM carriers possess multiple functional copies of the *CYP2D6* gene, with reports of 2 to 13 copies present in some individuals. In patients with PM CYP2D6 phenotype, codeine is not activated to morphine. Such patients would experience inadequate pain relief from codeine and fewer uncomfortable gastrointestinal side effects although the sedation, nausea, and dry mouth are reported to be comparable between PM and EM patients. On the opposite end of the activity spectrum, the UM phenotype will result in an increased generation of morphine, making patients more susceptible to codeine's analgesic effect as well as its serious adverse effects of drowsiness and respiratory depression, even at standard doses. The CPIC guidelines suggest avoiding codeine in both CYP2D6 UM and PM patients. The FDA label for codeine, while describing the pharmacogenetic influence on codeine pharmacology, does not recommend a specific course of action.

Simvastatin-*SLCO1B1*

Statins are prescribed to reduce serum cholesterol, specifically the low-density lipoprotein cholesterol (LDL-C). Due to their LDL-C-lowering property, statins have a significant effect of decreasing cardiovascular disease risk. The mechanism of action of statins involves inhibition of HMG-CoA

TABLE 3-5. Classical Pharmacogenetic Interaction Examples

Drug	Gene	Gene Variants	Pharmacogenetic Mechanism	Effect on Pharmacology	Recommendations
Clopidogrel	CYP2C19	*2 (loss-of-function) *3 (loss-of-function) *17 (gain-of-function)	Clopidogrel is a prodrug that is converted to its active form by CYP2C19	Carriers of CYP2C19 loss-of-function variants are susceptible to increased cardiovascular events due to inadequate antiplatelet effect of clopidogrel	Using alternate antiplatelet agents (like ticagrelor or prasugrel) in CYP2C19 IM and PM carriers; standard clopidogrel dosing suggested in CYP2C19 EM and UM patients
Codeine	CYP2D6	*1 and *2 (fully functional) *10, *17, and *41 (partially functional), *3, *4, *5, and *6 (nonfunctional). Multiple copies of functional genes (hyper-functional)	Codeine is a prodrug that is bioactivated to morphine by CYP2D6	CYP2D6 PM would have inadequate pain relief from codeine due to a decrease in its conversion to morphine; CYP2D6 UM are more susceptible to morphine's analgesic effect and serious adverse effects of drowsiness and respiratory depression	Avoid codeine in both CYP2D6 UM and PM
Simvastatin	SLCO1B1	*5 and *15 (loss-of-function)	OATP1B1 (the protein product of SLOC1B1) is responsible for the transport of statin drugs into liver cells where statins produce their pharmacological effect	Loss of function of SLCO1B1 causes an increase in plasma levels of simvastatin; carriers of SLCO1B1 loss-of-function variants are more likely to experience the muscle toxicity of simvastatin	Using low-dose simvastatin or alternate statin agent (rosuvastatin or pravastatin) in SLCO1B1 loss-of-function carriers
Abacavir	HLA-B	*57:01	HLA-B proteins are responsible for the presentation of endogenous proteins and certain drug molecules on the surface of cells for recognition by the immune system	HLA-B*5701 is able to bind to abacavir and presents it on the cell surface; using abacavir in HLA*57:01 carriers results in an immune-mediated hypersensitivity reaction particularly in the form of Stevens-Johnson syndrome	HLA-B*57:01 screening in all patients starting abacavir for the first time before the initiation of therapy is recommended; in patients lacking the HLA-B*57:01, abacavir can be used at standard doses; in patients carrying HLA-B*57:01, abacavir is not recommended
Warfarin	CYP2C9	*2 (loss-of-function) *3 (loss-of-function)	Warfarin is metabolized by CYP2C9 to inactive metabolites	Loss of function of CYP2C9 causes an increase in sensitivity to warfarin as its metabolism to inactive metabolites is decreased	Patients with CYP2C9 *2 and *3 or VKORC1 1639G>A SNP require less warfarin dose to achieve target INR. Patients with both CYP2C9 *2 and *3 and VKORC1 1639G>A SNP have the lowest warfarin dose requirements; using validated algorithms for warfarin dosing in the non-African carriers of VKORC1 −1639G>A and CYP2C9*2 and *3 variants is recommended
	VKORC1	−1639G>A (decrease in expression)	VKORC1 is the molecular target of the anticoagulant action of warfarin and is inhibited by warfarin	Patients carrying the VKORC1 1639G>A SNP have a greater sensitivity to warfarin and thereby lower dose requirement	

CYP = cytochrome P450; EM = extensive metabolizer; HLA = human leukocyte antigen; INR = international normalized ratio; OATP1B1 = organic anion transporting polypeptides 1B1; PM = poor metabolizers; SLCO1B1 = solute carrier organic anion transporter family member 1B1; SNP = single nucleotide polymorphism; UM = ultra-rapid metabolizers; VKORC1 = vitamin K epoxide reductase 1.

reductase in the liver. HMG-CoA is the rate-limiting enzyme that catalyzes an early step in the synthesis of cholesterol. In response to the reduced free cholesterol content within the liver cells, the expression of the LDL receptor gene is increased. An increase in the number of LDL receptors on the surface of liver cells causes increased removal of LDL from the blood, thereby lowering LDL-C levels. While statins enjoy widespread usage, statin-associated muscle symptoms (SAMS) can limit their use, at least in certain groups of patients. The incidence of SAMS is reported to range between 7% and 29%. These muscle toxicities often lead to noncompliance with statin therapy, resulting in an increased risk of cardiovascular disease and mortality.

The LDL-C-lowering pharmacological effect of statins requires their uptake and concentration in the liver cells. The OATP1B1 transporter facilitates the liver uptake of statins in addition to several other medications (Figure 3.5). The OAT1B1 protein is encoded by the *SLCO1B1* gene. The *SCLO1B1*5* variant is associated with a decrease in the transport function of OATP1B1 attributed to a decrease in the expression of the transporter on the surface of liver cells. The heterozygous and homozygous carriers of the **5* variant have higher plasma concentrations of statins. This increased systemic exposure of statins is associated with an increase in the risk of development of myopathy. Among the statin drug class, this pharmacogenetic interaction is primarily ascribed to simvastatin. The risk of myopathy is higher with the 80 mg dose of simvastatin than for those on lower doses. Using a low dose of simvastatin or considering an alternative statin (such as pravastatin or rosuvastatin) is recommended by the CPIC guidelines in patients with intermediate or low function of OAT1B1. The availability of low-cost alternate statins as well as generally low incidence of adverse effects with statins has made the use of pharmacogenetic testing before statin initiation unnecessary. However, pharmacogenetic testing can help identify underlying reasons for the observation of muscle toxicity with simvastatin use and can help to guide statin switching in such patients.

Abacavir-*HLA-B*

Abacavir is a medication used in the treatment of acquired immunodeficiency syndrome (AIDS) caused by the human immunodeficiency virus (HIV). The use of abacavir is associated with skin hypersensitivity reactions, particularly SJS. A genetic mechanism for these reactions has been elucidated with the identification of the *HLA-B* gene variants. HLA-B belongs to the major histocompatibility complex (MHC) family of proteins that are expressed on the surface of almost all cells and participate in antigen presentation to the immune system. The protein breakdown products are attached to the MHC molecules for presentation on the cell surface. Physiologically, the presentation of "self" proteins or the body's own proteins does not activate the immune system, whereas infection by pathogens results in the presentation of "non-self" proteins and elicitation of an immune response. Certain drug molecules also get processed in a manner similar to proteins and are presented on cell surfaces complexed with MHC molecules.

In the case of abacavir, such complexation with HLA protein occurs in patients with certain variants of *HLA-B*. In particular, the *HLA-B*57:01* allele binds abacavir and presents the drug along with other peptide fragments on the surface of cells. This presentation results in the recognition of peptide fragments on the cell surface as non-self and causes the development of a hypersensitivity reaction due to immune system activation. This pharmacogenetic mechanism does not affect drug pharmacokinetics or pharmacodynamics; rather it affects only the risk of hypersensitivity reactions. The presence of even just one *HLA-B*57:01* allele is associated with an increased risk of hypersensitivity reactions and there are no intermediate phenotypes. The evidence supporting the role of *HLA-B*57:01* in abacavir-induced hypersensitivity reaction is quite strong; CPIC recommendations call for *HLA-B*57:01* screening in all patients starting abacavir for the first time before the initiation of therapy. In patients lacking the *HLA-B*57:01*, abacavir can be used at standard doses. In patients carrying *HLA-B*57:01*, abacavir is not recommended.

Another HLA-B variant with known pharmacogenetic interaction is *HLA-B*15:02* which is implicated in carbamazepine-associated SJS and TEN.

Warfarin-*CYP2C9-VKORC1*

Warfarin is an oral anticoagulant that has been in clinical usage for more than six decades and is frequently called by its former brand name Coumadin. The initiation of warfarin therapy for its anticoagulation effect is characterized by frequent dose adjustments needed to achieve target international normalized ratio (INR) values in each patient. If the dose of warfarin is too high, it increases the risk of bleeding, whereas if the dose is too low, there is an increased risk of thromboembolism. The dose of warfarin required to achieve the therapeutic INR can be highly variable between patients; up to 10- to 20-fold differences (0.5 to 7 mg) in the warfarin dose required have been observed. Genetic factors have been shown to account for a significant portion of warfarin's dose variability.

Variants in three genes have been shown to influence warfarin response: *CYP2C9*, vitamin K epoxide reductase 1 (*VKORC1*), and *CYP4F2*. The role of these genes in warfarin

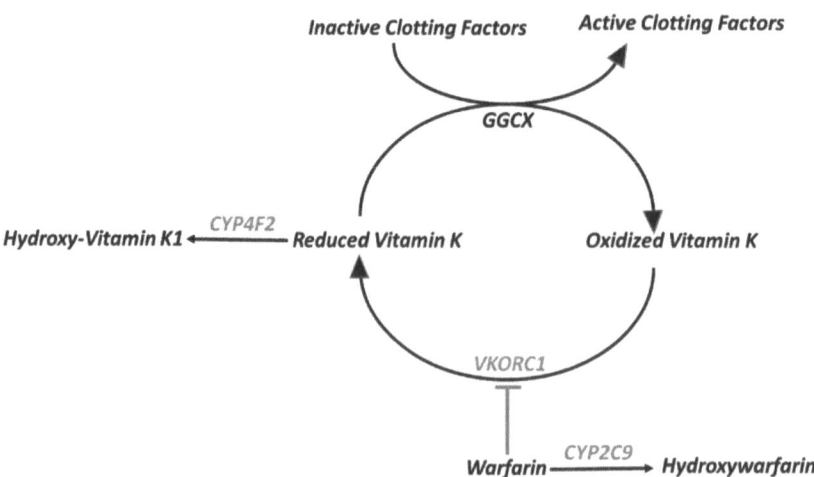

FIGURE 3-6. The mechanism of action of warfarin. *CYP* = cytochrome P450; *GGCX* = gamma-glutamyl carboxylase; *VKORC1* = vitamin K epoxide reductase 1.

response is evident in examining warfarin's mechanism of action (Figure 3-6). The *S* enantiomer of warfarin (the active stereoisomer) is metabolized by the enzyme CYP2C9 to inactive metabolites. Warfarin's molecular target protein is VKORC1, a protein that warfarin inhibits. VKORC1 is responsible for converting vitamin K (in its epoxide form) to reduced vitamin K, which functions as a cofactor in the activation of clotting factors. The reduced vitamin K is converted back to epoxide vitamin K by the action of the enzyme gamma-glutamyl carboxylase (GGCX). These conversion reactions between epoxide and reduced vitamin K catalyzed by VKORC1 and GGCX are termed the vitamin K cycle. The enzyme CYP4F2 removes reduced vitamin K from the vitamin K cycle by converting it to hydroxy-vitamin K1. Overall, warfarin inhibition of VKORC1 prevents the generation of reduced vitamin K, which leads to the inhibition of clotting factor activation. CYP2C9 prevents warfarin activity by converting it to inactive metabolites. The action of CYP4F2 is consistent with the warfarin effect as it limits the amount of reduced vitamin K available for clotting factor activation.

The *CYP2C9* genetic variants have been indicated earlier. Especially important are the loss-of-function alleles—*2 and *3. Patients with these alleles have a higher sensitivity to warfarin due to decreased metabolism of warfarin to inactive metabolites. Such patients need lower doses of warfarin to achieve the therapeutic INR. With regard to *VKORC1*, the most common variant is seen in the promoter region of the gene. The SNP at the −1639 position causes a decrease in the transcription of the *VKORC1* gene and hence, a decrease in the expression of the VKORC1 protein. Since the target protein of the warfarin effect is reduced, patients carrying the *VKORC1 1639G>A* SNP have a greater sensitivity to warfarin and thereby lower dose requirement. The allelic frequency of

CYP2C9 and *VKORC1* across different races shows important differences: *CYP2C9 *2* and *3 are seen at higher levels in the white population (13% and 7%, respectively) as compared to Asian (0 and 4%) and Black populations (3% and 2%); *VKORC1−1639G>A* is seen at a frequency of 40% in Whites, 91% in Asians, and 11% in Black populations. In patients with African ancestry, *CYP2C9*5, *6, *8*, and *11 are important in the determination of warfarin dose. A SNP in the *CYP4F2* gene (*rs2108622*; designated as *3) has been shown to be associated with a higher warfarin dose requirement.

The recommendations from CPIC guidelines include using published and validated algorithms for warfarin dosing in the non-African carriers of *VKORC1 −1639G>A* and *CYP2C9*2* and *3 variants. The carriers of either *VKORC1 −1639G>A* or *CYP2C9*2* and *3 have lower dose requirements, whereas those with the loss-of-function *CYP2C9* variants as well as *VKORC1−1639G>A* have the lowest warfarin dose requirements. In contrast, wild-type *CYP2C9* and *VKORC1* carriers require higher warfarin doses. The incorporation of *CYP4F2* genetic information has also been shown to improve the accuracy of warfarin dose prediction. The warfarindosing.org website contains the two major dosing algorithms developed for the determination of warfarin dose: the Gage algorithm and the International Warfarin Pharmacogenetics Consortium (IWPC) algorithm. These algorithms integrate genetic as well as nongenetic factors in the determination of warfarin dose. Warfarin dose determination shows that the pharmacogenetic factors, although important, are not always sufficient to explain the variability in drug response. Nongenetic factors such as the patient's age, race, weight, height, and clinical factors such as the history of smoking, presence of liver disease, and use of other co-administered drugs (statins, amiodarone, antifungals, antibiotics, etc.) can have a significant effect on the warfarin dose required in each patient. This integrated approach that factors pharmacogenomic evidence into therapeutic decision making along with patient and clinical characteristics represents the spirit of precision medicine.

The pharmacogenetics of warfarin is unique in two different ways. First, it is one of the few examples showing how pharmacogenetic variants in pharmacodynamic proteins can influence drug response. The majority of the well-studied pharmacogenetic interactions are based on variants in pharmacokinetic proteins such as metabolizing enzymes and transporters. *VKORC1* variants show that there likely are several more clinically meaningful variants in the pharmacodynamic proteins that have not been discovered yet. Second, the pharmacogenetics of warfarin illustrates the polygenic nature of warfarin response—ie, genetic variants in multiple genes influence response to warfarin. Frequently, how individual genes, in isolation, influence drug response has been the focus of attention. However, the drug response in the body is a composite of multiple proteins made by multiple genes, some affecting the active levels of the drugs and others affecting the pharmacological effect produced. These proteins/genes can be of the same functional class (e.g., metabolizing enzymes) or divergent protein classes (metabolizing enzymes vs. receptors). In a specific patient, the observed genetic influence on drug response is a net effect of all genes with which that drug interacts in the body to produce its pharmacological activity.

As illustrated by the above examples, pharmacogenomics-guided drug therapy has the potential to improve clinical outcomes of both efficacy and adverse effects. However, the application of this guidance is often dependent on the availability of a patient's genetic sequence information. The genetic sequencing tests are available in different formats: single-gene tests, gene panels, and whole-genome sequencing. The cost of getting the genetic sequencing and the turnaround time for getting the genetic information to the prescribers often impede the full adoption of pharmacogenetic guidance. However, if this information were already available, then many of the pharmacogenomic recommendations could be readily applied in the selection of the right drug at the right dose. Such preemptive genetic testing would enable the application of pharmacogenomic-guided drug therapies over the lifetime of a patient. Unlike other diagnostic tests (blood sugar, lipid panels, etc.), genetic tests for each specific gene need to be performed only once and can provide immense value throughout a patient's lifespan. The proliferation of such tests and services will expand the patient population who have their genetic information available to use in therapeutic decision making.

SUMMARY

Efforts to lay the foundation for the application of pharmacogenomics in clinical practice have long been underway. The field of pharmacogenomics finally has enough momentum to gain mainstream prominence in medicine. The tailwinds helping the field are the converging forces of big data/data science, artificial intelligence, advances in sequencing technology, and an increase in consumer expectations of healthcare. All of these are, of course, propelled by an accumulating body of scientific evidence supporting drug-gene interactions, as well as the formation of a consortium of experts systematically evaluating this vast body of evidence and proposing appropriate recommendations and guidelines. At its very core, pharmacogenomics is a tool to maximize the benefit of drug therapy and minimize the associated risk. While there are still significant implementation barriers to overcome the promise of pharmacogenomics to unlock the full potential of targeted drug treatments is getting closer to fulfillment.

ADDITIONAL RESOURCES

1. Pharmacogenomics knowledgebase or PharmGKB: This is a pharmacogenomics database that curates scientific and clinical evidence supporting drug-gene pharmacogenetic associations along with links to clinical guidelines, drug labels, individual drug and gene information, and visualization of drug pathways and mechanisms of pharmacogenetic interactions. Website: https://www.pharmgkb.org/ (accessed August 5, 2022).

2. CPIC or Clinical Pharmacogenetics Implementation Consortium: This is an international consortium of volunteers and experts who participate in the creation, curation, and dissemination of peer-reviewed, evidence-based detailed drug/gene clinical practice guidelines. These guidelines enable the translation of genetic laboratory test results into actionable prescribing decisions for affected drugs. Website: https://cpicpgx.org/ (accessed August 5, 2022).

3. Food and Drug Administration (FDA): Maintains two different tables for pharmacogenomics information: a) Table of pharmacogenomic biomarkers in drug labeling (https://www.fda.gov/drugs/science-and-research -drugs/table-pharmacogenomic-biomarkers-drug -labeling); b) Table of pharmacogenetic associations (https://www.fda.gov/medical-devices/precision -medicine/table-pharmacogenetic-associations) (accessed August 5, 2022).

Part 2

THE NERVOUS SYSTEM

Chapter 4

The Autonomic Nervous System

Mary Ann Stuhan, PharmD, RPh

KEY TERMS AND DEFINITIONS

Adrenal medulla—the endocrine gland situated on top of each kidney, which produces and releases epinephrine (also known as adrenaline) to stimulate functions of the sympathetic autonomic nervous system (SANS).

Adrenergic—related to the actions of epinephrine (adrenaline); sometimes used to designate actions and responses to the sympathetic autonomic nervous system.

Afferent neuron—a neuron carrying nerve impulses to the central nervous system (brain and spinal cord) from the periphery (other parts of the body).

Autonomic nervous system—the system of nerves that controls automatic bodily actions, such as the functions of glandular tissues, the heart and smooth muscle, and involuntary movements and body functions (including secretions, pulse, and blood pressure).

Axon—an elongated protrusion of the neuron that conducts impulses away from the cell.

Catecholamines—characterization of substances, such as epinephrine and norepinephrine, that exert their effect in the sympathetic autonomic nervous system and agents that are chemically similar to these substances.

DOI 10.37573/9781585286638.004

Cholinergic—related to the actions of the neurotransmitter acetylcholine. Cholinergic effects include slowed heart rate, increased secretion, and increased activity of the gastrointestinal tract.

Effector organ—cells or tissues that perform their functions in response to a stimulus (such as a nerve impulse); sometimes called *target* organs. Those receiving stimulation from the nervous system are designated by the term neuroeffector.

Efferent neuron—a neuron carrying nerve impulses toward an effector organ.

Endocrine secretion—the release of substances (hormones) synthesized by glands directly into the bloodstream to circulate throughout the body. (Contrasts with paracrine secretion, in which substances are released to act locally on nearby tissues.)

Endogenous—refers to an agent synthesized or produced within the organism.

Exocrine secretion—the release of glandular products to ducts or tracts that lead directly to the outside of the body. Examples are sweat and tears.

Exogenous—refers to an agent introduced to an organism from an outside source, even if the same as substances also produced or synthesized endogenously.

Ganglion—a mass of neuron bodies (nerves). Plural = ganglia.

Homeostasis—physiologic equilibrium required for life processes and maintained by several systems and biologic mechanisms.

Innervation—the function of supplying an organ or tissue with nerves. ("Innervate" means to supply an organ or tissue with nerves.)

Neuron—a nerve cell.

Neurotransmitters—chemical compounds produced by the body ("endogenous") that relay, amplify, and/or modulate signal transmission between two neurons or between neurons and other cells.

Parasympathetic—pertaining to autonomic functions mainly governing body systems at rest, including glandular secretions, tone and contractility of smooth muscle, and slowing the heart rate.

Secretion—the process of production and release of chemical compounds from a tissue (gland). The secreted product has a function, as opposed to an excreted waste.

Sympathetic—pertaining to autonomic functions related to stress situations, often called the *fight or flight response*. This includes suppressing glandular secretions, reducing tone and contractility of smooth muscle, and increasing the heart rate.

Synapse—the space between the axon terminal of a neuron and the dendrite body of another neuron where a functional connection between them occurs.

Tachycardia—rapid heart rate that exceeds 100 beats per minute in adults.

Tone—the state of tension of tissues or organs in the body.

LEARNING OBJECTIVES

After completing this chapter, you should be able to

1. Define the autonomic nervous system (ANS) and its divisions, the parasympathetic and sympathetic autonomic nervous systems (PANS and SANS, respectively).

2. Outline the anatomy, physiology, and functions of the ANS, PANS, and SANS.

3. Describe the targets/sites of action of endogenous neurotransmitters and of exogenous drugs that act on the ANS,

4. Review the classification and mechanisms of action of drugs acting on the ANS.

5. List therapeutic applications of the primary drug classes acting on the ANS.

6. State the brand and generic names of representative therapeutic agents acting on the ANS, together with their routes of administration, side effects, and potential drug interactions.

The nervous system is the most complex system in the human body. It has two main anatomical and functional divisions: the central nervous system (CNS), discussed in Chapter 5, and the peripheral nervous system (PNS). The PNS is divided into two subsystems: the somatic and autonomic nervous systems. The somatic nervous system involves voluntary movement such as walking or talking. It is discussed in more detail in Chapter 12. The autonomic

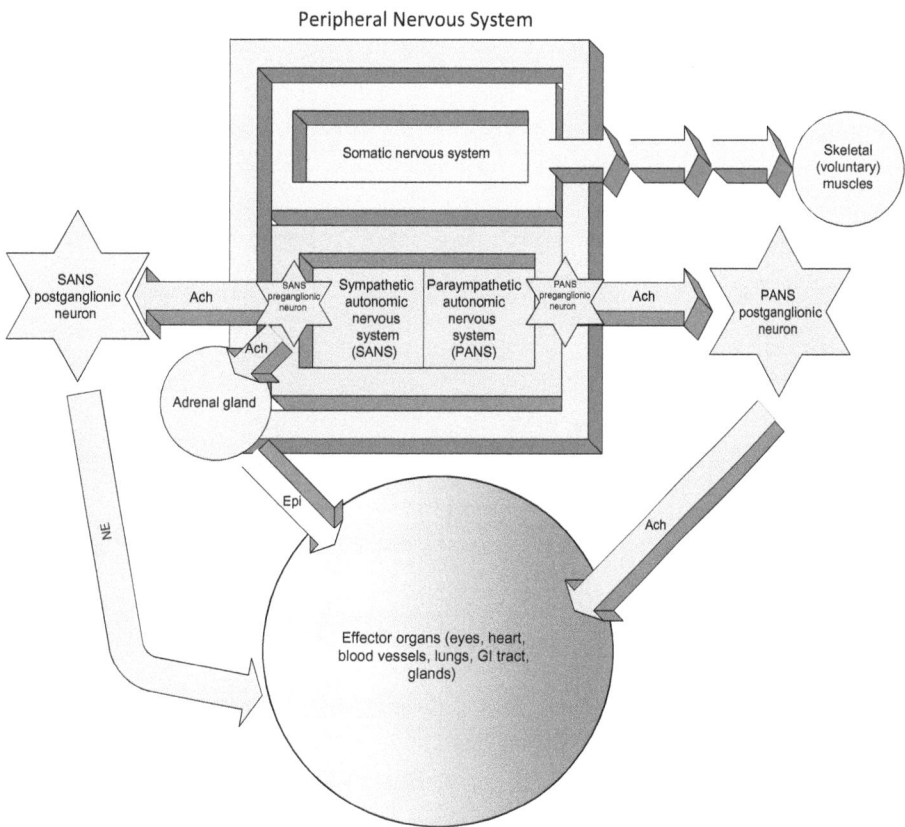

FIGURE 4-1. The peripheral nervous system.
Ach = acetylcholine; NE = norepinephrine; Epi = epinephrine.

nervous system (ANS) is the major involuntary, unconscious, automatic portion of the PNS. For example, the ANS keeps the heart beating. The heart doesn't need to be "told" by the conscious mind to continue beating, it just does so. Other examples of the ANS at work include regulation of blood pressure, saliva secretion, sweating, gastrointestinal motility, and bronchial air exchange. The ANS relies on neurotransmitters acting on certain receptors to cause its effects on body systems.[1] See Figure 4-1 for a graphical representation of the relationships between the divisions of the nervous system. Knowledge of the anatomy and physiology, neurotransmitter synthesis and release, signal termination, receptor characteristics, and functional integration of the ANS is important to an understanding of how many drugs act on many systems and organs of the body.

ANATOMY AND PHYSIOLOGY

The ANS has two functional divisions: the sympathetic autonomic nervous system (SANS) and the parasympathetic autonomic nervous system (PANS). These two divisions have opposite effects and serve to keep the body in a balanced state called homeostasis. The PANS is involved in conserving body processes such as digestion and resting (causing decreased heart rate and increased secretions). The SANS contributes to the provision of energy and stamina in emergency situations such as fighting or escape from danger (sometimes called the *fight or flight reactions*). For example, both the SANS and PANS stimulate muscles in the eye to change pupil size. The SANS increases pupil size (mydriasis), resulting in better far-range vision for emergency situations or night/low light conditions. The PANS decreases pupil size (miosis), which produces better shortrange vision for reading or viewing fine details.[1]

All body systems are affected by ANS neurons, but not all organs have both PANS and SANS innervation. Innervation is described as the distribution of nerve fibers to a specific body system or organ. The overall response of an organ to ANS stimulation will equal the sum of influences from both PANS and SANS fibers. This means that if more SANS nerves are activated in a specific organ, then the SANS actions will predominate there. Sensory nerves (afferent neurons) communicate the happenings in the

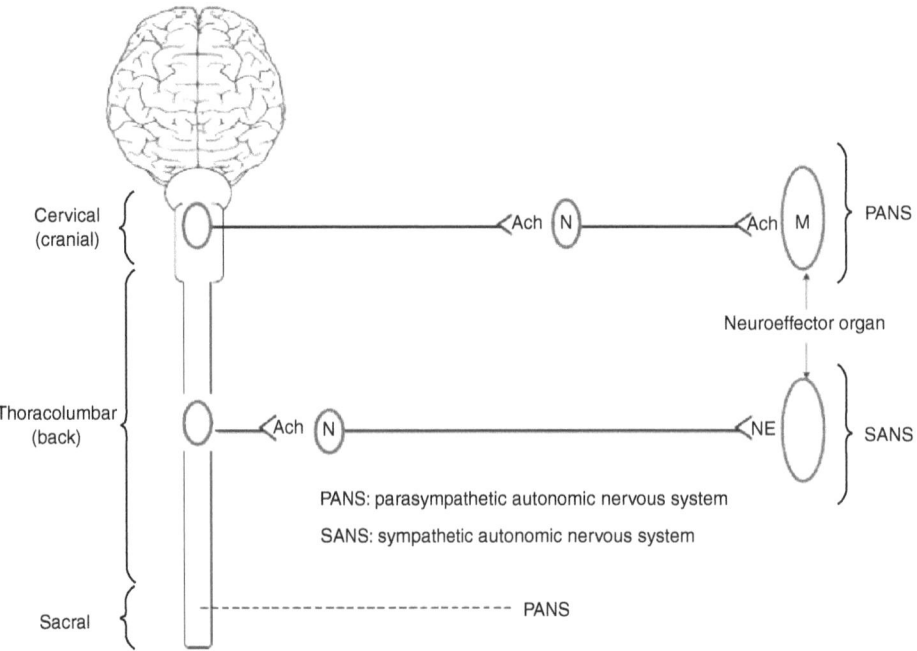

FIGURE 4-2. Anatomical representation of the ANS, its divisions, and nerve fibers. Ach = acetylcholine; NE = norepinephrine; Epi = EPI = epinephrine.

periphery (outside the CNS) back to the brain through the spinal cord. This communication allows the appropriate ANS actions to occur in a given situation. These responses are also integrated with the somatic nervous system so appropriate voluntary movements can occur. Figure 4-2 is an anatomical representation of the ANS. The variety of effects of the ANS on effector organs in the human body is summarized in Table 4-1.

Nerve Fibers

A nerve cell is called a neuron. It has the ability to carry impulses and is much like an electrical wire in which a signal can be transmitted. Innervation in the ANS is composed of two neurons: a *preganglionic* efferent neuron, with a body in the CNS and an axon extending to a ganglion; and a *postganglionic* neuron, with a cell body in a ganglion (mass of several neuron bodies) and the axon extending to an effector organ. Neurons communicate with one another across a connection called a synapse. A ganglion contains several synapses, and all ganglia are located between the spinal cord and the effector organ. Figure 4-3 shows the parts of the nerve cell and its connections. Axons and synapses are discussed in more detail in Chapter 5. The adrenal gland is innervated only by sympathetic neurons. The adrenal medulla acts as a sympathetic ganglion, but its primary

function is the release of epinephrine into the systemic circulation (endocrine secretion).

Neurotransmitters

Neurotransmitters are chemical compounds synthesized and stored in neurons, which allow nerve cells to communicate with each other. A neurotransmitter can produce either an

TABLE 4-1. Autonomic Nervous System Effects[1]

Organ	PANS Effect	SANS Effect
Blood vessels	Dilation	Constriction
Eye	Miosis (pupil constriction)	Mydriasis (pupil dilation)
Endocrine glands	Increased secretion	Decreased secretion
Exocrine glands	Increased secretion	(Minor effects)
Gastrointestinal tract	Increased motility	Decreased motility
Heart	Decreased heart rate	Increased heart rate and force of contraction
Lungs (bronchi)	Constriction	Dilation
Urinary bladder (sphincter)	Relaxation	Contraction

PANS = parasympathetic autonomic nervous system; SANS = sympathetic autonomic nervous system.

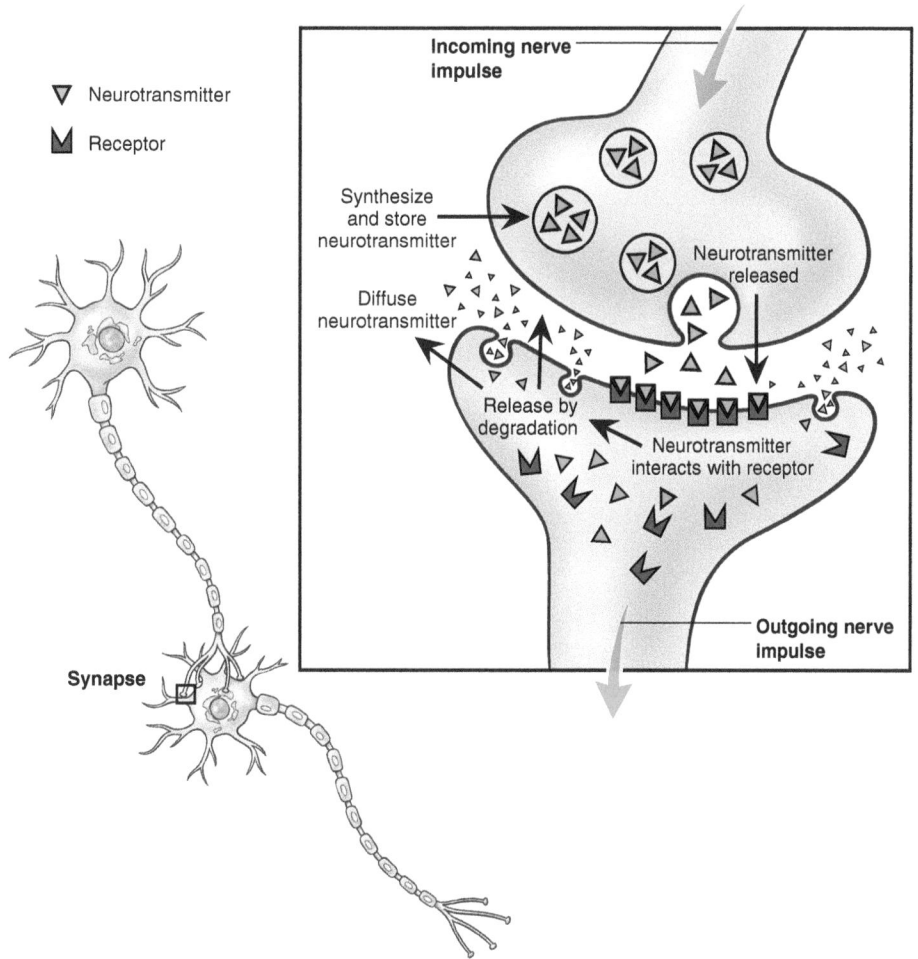

FIGURE 4-3. The parts of the nerve cell and its connections. Neurotransmitters at synapse.

TABLE 4-2. Neurotransmitters in the Autonomic Nervous System[1]

Neuron	Neurotransmitter	Neuron	Neurotransmitter
PANS presynaptic	Acetylcholine (Ach)	PANS postsynaptic	Ach
SANS presynaptic	Ach	SANS postsynaptic	Norepinephrine (NE)

PANS = parasympathetic autonomic nervous system; SANS = sympathetic autonomic nervous system.

excitatory or an inhibitory response. An excitatory response causes action at the effector site; an inhibitory response stops or slows an action. Additional information about neurotransmitters and receptors can be found in Chapter 5.

In the ANS, there are three main neurotransmitters involved in conduction and signaling: acetylcholine (Ach), epinephrine (Epi), and norepinephrine (NE).[1] Ach is released by all presynaptic (preganglionic) nerve terminals in both the PANS and SANS and activates the adrenal medulla. The major difference between the PANS and SANS, besides anatomy, is the neurotransmitter released by postganglionic neurons. PANS postganglionic neurons release Ach to activate effector organs or tissues. The PANS is designated as a cholinergic system because this neurotransmitter is the final messenger acting on organs and tissues. The SANS postganglionic neurons release NE to activate organs and tissues. Table 4-2 lists the ANS neurons and their corresponding neurotransmitters. Epi is also a messenger for the activation of organs and tissues innervated by the SANS. NE and Epi are sometimes known as *noradrenaline* and *adrenaline*, respectively. This is the reason for the designation of the SANS as the adrenergic system.

Receptors

The interaction between a neurotransmitter and its receptor is specific and depends on the chemical structure of both. Neurotransmission, however, is not continuous. There are two ways the action of a neurotransmitter is stopped. The first is through "reuptake"—transport of the neurotransmitter back into the neuron by special pumps on the presynaptic neuron. The other mechanism by which neurotransmission is ended is through degradation or breakdown of the neurotransmitter by enzymes. Cholinergic neurons have a mechanism of degradation in which the enzyme acetylcholinesterase (AchE) hydrolyzes Ach to form acetic acid and choline. Both of these inactive metabolites can be recycled by the cell to produce new Ach or to maintain other processes. AchE is present near the receptor and prevents overactivation of the PANS.

Adrenergic neurons terminate the action of NE by utilizing both mechanisms. NE reuptake is accomplished by a specific NE transporter (NET) present in the neuronal membrane. NE that undergoes reuptake can be recycled for future use or metabolized by enzymatic degradation. One mechanism of NE degradation utilizes the enzyme monoamine oxidase (MAO), which is present inside the nerve cell. Another degradative enzyme is catechol-*O*-methyltransferase (COMT). The overall processes of reuptake and degradation contribute to a decrease in adrenergic activity in the SANS.[2]

Ach binds to two types of receptors: nicotinic and muscarinic (or cholinergic) receptors. These designations were made based on the chemicals (nicotine and muscarine) that were first used to demonstrate the presence of these receptors and to study them. Nicotinic receptors are present on all the preganglionic neurons in both the PANS and SANS, while muscarinic receptors are present on organs only for the PANS. There are several different subtypes of muscarinic receptors, each with its own location and function.

Receptors for NE and Epi are present in effector organs and tissues innervated by the SANS, and they are designated adrenergic receptors. There are three main classes of adrenergic receptors: α_1 (alpha one), β_1 (beta one), and β_2 (beta two), which are located in different organs and tissues and can produce different actions. Another type of adrenergic receptors is the α_2 (alpha two) type; these receptors are located in the presynaptic membrane terminals, and they control or inhibit NE release.

PHARMACOLOGICAL INTERVENTION AT THE AUTONOMIC NERVOUS SYSTEM

The use of medications to activate or inhibit any specific division of the ANS is designated as pharmacological intervention. The ANS acts as a regulator of body functions, and a balance of the activities of the PANS and SANS is required to maintain homeostasis. Pathological disorders can arise from excessive activation or inhibition of either the PANS or SANS and pharmacological interventions can increase or decrease activity by different mechanisms of action. A variety of ANS chemicals and functions can be targets for pharmacological intervention.

PANS Activation

As discussed earlier, Ach is the primary mediator of PANS activity. There are two mechanisms by which the actions of Ach can be mimicked by medications (increasing PANS activity). One mechanism is that the medication can *look like* (chemically resemble) Ach and bind its receptor. Another mechanism of increasing PANS activity is by blocking the degradation of Ach, allowing more of it to be present for a longer time (so increasing its action). In both cases direct- or indirect-acting drugs are designated cholinergic agents (also known as cholinomimetic or parasympathomimetic agents).

Direct-Acting Cholinergic (Parasympathomimetic) Agents

Ach is the simplest choline derivative, so the easiest way to increase PANS activity would be to administer Ach. However, when administered by conventional routes such as orally or intravenously, Ach is very unstable and not bioavailable. As such, more stable esters can be administered to mimic the effects of Ach and to activate the PANS.

PRACTICE POINT

The cholines that are active in the body are known as esters, a term used to describe a particular type of chemical molecule.

Bethanechol is a choline ester drug. It binds selectively to the muscarinic cholinergic receptor (found only in the PANS) without affecting nicotinic receptors (present in both SANS and PANS), making it selective for the PANS. Its effects on body organs can be predicted from the PANS Effect column in Table 4-1. Bethanechol is administered orally and is used to treat urinary retention (by its action on bladder muscle tone). It is administered three to four times per day and is contraindicated in patients with asthma, epilepsy, or a bladder or gastrointestinal blockage. Common adverse effects are also predictable from its cholinergic activity and include miosis, increased tear production (exocrine gland secretion), and diarrhea (increased GI motility).

Another choline ester is carbachol (Miostat), which is used as an intraocular instillation in cataract surgery. Carbachol activates the pupillary sphincter and the ciliary muscles (which cause pupil contraction) to obtain miosis during surgery and decrease intraocular pressure afterward. Because they decrease intraocular pressure, carbachol and other choline esters were once a mainstay of glaucoma treatment (see Chapter 34), but they are used infrequently at this time because more specific therapies with fewer toxicities are available.[3] When administered in the eye, there are limited adverse effects since the action is local and only a small amount of the medication is absorbed into the body. However, when choline esters are administered orally, adverse effects include increased sweating, diarrhea, and runny nose.

Indirect-Acting Cholinergic (Parasympathomimetic) Agents

This group includes agents that act by binding and inhibiting the enzyme AchE, which degrades Ach, thereby indirectly increasing the concentration of Ach in the synapses. As a result, they activate both nicotinic (found in PANS and SANS) and muscarinic (PANS-only) receptors. They can be subdivided into three categories: very long acting (organophosphates), intermediate acting (carbamates or alkaloids), and short acting (edrophonium). Very-long-acting agents include malathion (Ovide) and echothiophate. Malathion is a pesticide and has no clinical use as a cholinergic agent (although it is available as a scalp lotion for the treatment of head lice). Echothiophate, which reduces intraocular pressure, is used as a last-line option in the treatment of glaucoma.

Intermediate-acting agents include physostigmine, neostigmine, and pyridostigmine. Physostigmine was once used as an eye drop for glaucoma, but now is only indicated for use as an antidote administered intravenously for anticholinergic toxicity. It has a fairly short half-life of 1–2 hours, so repeated doses (every 30–60 minutes) may be necessary if anticholinergic symptoms return. Physostigmine is preferred over neostigmine and pyridostigmine for anticholinergic toxicity due to its high lipid (fat) solubility, which allows the medication to cross the blood–brain-barrier (BBB). Adverse effects from physostigmine are similar to those of the previous agents that act on the PANS. Neostigmine is used in the reversal of neuromuscular blockade used in surgery.

ALERT!

Patients who intentionally or accidentally ingest overdoses of medications with potent anticholinergic properties may receive physostigmine in the emergency room. Administration is by intravenous push, but the administration rate should not exceed 1 mg/min to avoid potential cholinergic toxicity if too much is administered too quickly. Whenever it is used, atropine (an anticholinergic agent) should be readily available to reverse any excess effects caused by physostigmine administration.[4]

Myasthenia gravis is an autoimmune disorder in which antibodies reduce available Ach receptors, inhibiting the actions of Ach and resulting in muscle weakness because of decreased Ach stimulation. While immunotherapy is the primary treatment, pyridostigmine is used to treat myasthenia gravis symptoms, overcoming, to a certain extent, the decreased stimulation by increasing the amount of Ach available. This medication is very similar to physostigmine in its actions and adverse effects, except that pyridostigmine has a longer half-life (8 hours).[5]

Other AchE inhibitors include donepezil (Aricept), rivastigmine (Exelon), and galantamine (Razadyne ER), which are used to prevent the progression of Alzheimer disease. They are orally bioavailable and are highly lipid soluble, resulting in enhanced penetration through the BBB. These medications are discussed in more depth in Chapter 6.

Edrophonium is the shortest-acting (15 minutes) AchE inhibitor and is not orally bioavailable. It has little clinical application other than for the diagnosis of myasthenia gravis. (Its short action makes it useless in treating myasthenia gravis; the longer-acting agents mentioned above are used instead.) Drugs with cholinergic activity (both direct and indirect) are used in a variety of ways. Medication Table 4-1 lists some representative agents from this class (Medication Tables are located at the end of the chapter).

Adverse or Toxic Reactions

Adverse reactions associated with the administration of cholinergic agents are essentially extensions of their pharmacologic effects. The adverse or toxic effects are described by the acronym BAD SLUDGE. They are summarized in Table 4-3. Large doses can result in neuromuscular paralysis and CNS effects and can ultimately lead to death.

Contraindications for cholinergic agents include asthma, gastrointestinal or urinary obstruction, cardiac disease, or peptic ulcer disease. These conditions may be either caused or exacerbated by increasing cholinergic activity.

PANS Inhibition

PANS inhibition refers to the blockade of cholinergic (acetylcholine-mediated) conduction, and the agents that do this are termed *anticholinergic*. They prevent the activity of Ach primarily at the postganglionic nerve endings. Some of the agents block cholinergic signaling by interfering with the synthesis and release of Ach. Botulinum toxins are proteins produced by the bacteria *Clostridium botulinum* that are extremely neurotoxic (poisonous at the nerve level). This bacterium is responsible for causing botulism, which some patients may get from eating improperly stored food. Botulinum toxins inhibit the release of Ach from vesicles; the lack of Ach causes paralysis in skeletal muscle. While botulinum toxins are not classified as anticholinergic medications, they do have various clinical uses, such as for blepharospasm (eyelid muscle spasm), cervical dystonia (muscle tone impairment), and for cosmetic procedures ("Botox").

TABLE 4-3. Cholinergic Adverse Effects

	Symptom	Parasympathetic Autonomic Nervous System (PANS) Effect
B	Bradycardia	Decreased heart rate
A	Anxiety	(non-PANS effect related to central nervous system arousal with excess acetylcholine [Ach])
D	Delirium/confusion	(non-PANS effect related to central nervous system arousal with excess Ach)
S	Salivation (drooling)	Increased exocrine secretion
L	Lacrimation (tears)	Increased exocrine secretion
U	Urination	Relaxation of bladder sphincter
D	Defecation	Increased gastrointestinal (GI) motility, anal sphincter relaxation
G	Gastrointestinal distress	Increased GI motility
E	Emesis (vomiting)	Increased GI motility

In contrast to botulinum toxins, anticholinergic agents currently used systemically cause blockade or antagonism of Ach at its receptors, resulting in decreased stimulation of the PANS. Most anticholinergic medications are competitive inhibitors (antagonists) at the muscarinic (PANS) receptor, meaning they interact with receptors normally stimulated by Ach, preventing that stimulation. Anticholinergic agents can be divided into two groups: antimuscarinic and antinicotinic. Antinicotinic medications have little therapeutic use, except as neuromuscular blockers. Medications such as pancuronium, vecuronium, and atracurium bind to cholinergic receptors and are used to produce skeletal muscle blockade resulting in paralysis pre- and perioperatively to assist in anesthesia. These actions are detailed in Chapter 12.

Antimuscarinic Agents

Because cholinergic innervation and muscarinic receptors are so widespread throughout the body, drugs that block activity at these sites (antimuscarinics/anticholinergics) are used in the treatment of a variety of conditions. Some clinical applications of antimuscarinic drugs are shown in Medication Table 4-2. Medication Table 4-3 lists a representative group of anticholinergic agents and their clinical applications.

Atropine is the prototype antimuscarinic agent. It is a natural alkaloid extracted from the plant *Atropa belladonna*. Atropine is relatively fat soluble and readily crosses cell membranes, including the BBB, resulting in central nervous system activity in addition to its PANS actions. The drug is well absorbed when taken orally. It is eliminated by liver metabolism and renal excretion and the half-life is approximately 2 hours. The duration of action of oral doses is 4–8 hours, longer in the eye, where the effects can last for 72 hours or more. As an eye drop, atropine is used to dilate the pupil (by interfering with the miosis caused by PANS stimulation) and paralyze the accommodating effects of the eye to aid in performing eye examinations. Other anticholinergic eye drops for eye examinations are covered in Chapter 34.

Parenteral atropine has long been used to reduce airway secretions during surgery. Atropine is also administered in patients who are in cardiac arrest and have severe bradycardia, although the most recent guidelines state that atropine

is no longer a first-line option. Scopolamine (Transderm Scop) is an alkaloid substance derived from the same plant as atropine. It represents the standard therapy for prevention of motion sickness in the form of a transdermal patch. This patch is applied behind the ear every 3 days and is usually the treatment of choice for prolonged sea voyages.

Benztropine (Cogentin) and trihexyphenidyl are antimuscarinic agents that are active in the CNS. They are representative of anticholinergic agents used to treat symptoms of Parkinson disease (PD) and similar symptoms caused by some CNS drugs. They work by combating the overactivity of cholinergic neurons that results from the low activity of CNS dopamine in patients with PD. Anticholinergics can result in decreasing the movement symptoms associated with PD. (See Chapter 6 for more on the use of these agents in PD treatment.)

Ipratropium (Atrovent) is an agent used to reduce bronchoconstriction in asthma and chronic obstructive pulmonary disease (COPD). It is administered directly to the respiratory tract either through a metered dose inhaler or by a nebulizer. Because inhaled ipratropium is poorly absorbed from the lungs, most of its action is confined to the bronchi, which prevents antimuscarinic side effects in other parts of the body. It is less likely to cause cardiac arrhythmias in patients sensitive to adrenergic drugs. The use of anticholinergics in respiratory disease is discussed at length in Chapter 19.

Methscopolamine (Pamine) and similar agents were once commonly used in the treatment of gastrointestinal disorders due to their ability to block Ach-stimulated gastric secretion. Since they are not as effective as newer medications such as histamine$_2$ receptors or proton pump blockers (discussed in Chapter 21), they are no longer indicated for these conditions.

Methscopolamine, oxybutynin (Ditropan), tolterodine (Detrol), darifenacin, solifenacin (Vesicare), and trospium are agents that can be used to reduce urgency in mild cystitis (inflammation of the urinary bladder), to reduce bladder spasms following urologic surgery, or to treat an overactive bladder. Newer agents in this class, such as tolterodine, darifenacin, solifenacin, and trospium are more specific for muscarinic receptors in the bladder, resulting in fewer systemic and CNS adverse effects. Drugs with anticholinergic activity that are useful in treating bladder conditions are listed in Medication Table 4-4.

Adverse/Toxic Reactions

The adverse reactions that can result from anticholinergic agents are extensions of their pharmacological effects. These can include xerostomia (dry mouth due to a lack of saliva), blurred vision, photophobia (excessive sensitivity to light producing eye pain or discomfort during light exposure), confusion, reflex tachycardia, decreased sweating, urinary retention, and constipation. Fever is caused by decreased sweating, which can result in hyperpyrexia (severely increased body temperature) that is potentially lethal in infants. A popular list of anticholinergic reactions is included in Table 4-4. Many drugs used primarily for actions other than those in the autonomic nervous system also have some anticholinergic activity that can cause unwanted side effects. This is particularly true of older antihistamines.[6]

Contraindications for the antimuscarinic drugs include narrow angle glaucoma (because these drugs can increase intraocular pressure), benign prostatic hyperplasia (potential worsening of urinary retention), and intestinal or mechanical

obstruction of the GI or urinary tract. They are used with caution in patients who have cardiovascular disease due to the increased risk of tachycardia and in patients who have irritable bowel syndrome.

SANS Activation

The important endogenous messengers in the SANS include NE and Epi. NE is the primary neurotransmitter released at nerve terminals of the SANS. Epi is released from the adrenal medulla into the bloodstream to act at adrenergic receptors throughout the body. NE, Epi, dopamine (DA), and some adrenergic drugs such as isoproterenol, belong to the chemical class of catecholamines.

Drugs that activate the SANS are designated adrenergic drugs or sympathomimetics. These drugs are classified according to their mechanism of action, as either direct-acting or indirect-acting adrenergic medications. Direct-acting adrenergic agents bind to and have activity on the adrenergic receptors of the SANS. Indirect-acting adrenergic agents are drugs that cause the release of NE or block the termination of NE signaling. They are subdivided as releasers, reuptake inhibitors, and enzyme inhibitors. Mixed-acting agents act by both mechanisms to directly activate adrenergic receptors and to increase NE concentrations at synapses.

TABLE 4-4. Toxic Anticholinergic Reactions[7]

	Symptom	Parasympathetic Autonomous Nervous System (PANS) Effect Antagonized
"Hot as Hades"	Increased body temperature/decreased sweating	Exocrine gland secretion
"Dry as a bone"	Dry mouth and dry mucous membranes	Exocrine gland secretion
"Red as a beet"	Tachycardia with skin flushing	Heart rate lowering
"Blind as a bat"	Blurred vision	Ocular muscle tone
"Mad as a hatter"	Agitation, confusion, hallucinations	(Non-PANS effect related to actions of acetylcholine in central nervous system)

Endogenous NE and Epi are rapidly metabolized by MAO and COMT. As a result, NE and Epi are inactive when orally administered. Synthetic catecholamines and synthetic non-catecholamine sympathomimetics are resistant to MAO and COMT, and some have activity when administered orally.

Adrenergic receptors are distributed differentially on various effector organs and tissues and have been classified in two types: α (alpha) and β (beta) (see Medication Table 4-5). Additionally, there are two subtypes of each, known as α_1, α_2, β_1, and β_2. When discussing the pharmacologic effects of adrenergic drugs, it is important to note the proportion of activity at α or β receptors and the subclasses of receptors involved. For example, Epi is active at both α and β receptors, while NE is active primarily at α receptors but also at β_1 receptors in the heart. Several newer drugs are very selective, acting primarily on α or β subclasses of receptors. The more selective an agent's activity is, the narrower its spectrum of actions and side effects will be. Table 4-5 summarizes the actions of the SANS on the human body. An agent such as Epi, which is active on all four subclasses of receptors, can be expected to stimulate SANS receptors throughout the body when administered systemically. In contrast, a drug such as dobutamine, which is only active at β_1 receptors, specifically increases the heart rate and force of contraction of the heart. This mechanism explains its use as an emergency drug to treat cardiac arrest.

Adrenergic or sympathomimetic medications are available to treat pathologies in which any type of SANS stimulation is required. Examples of drugs with clinical applications are detailed in Medication Table 4-5.

CASE?

What type of autonomic action does albuterol have that makes it effective for wheezing?

General Agonists

Epinephrine (Epi) is the endogenous agent released from the adrenal medulla (and also known as adrenaline) in emergency situations. Epi can act at all four subclasses of adrenergic receptors. Epi is clinically indicated in cases of anaphylactic shock (a widespread and very serious allergic reaction) by intramuscular (IM) or intravenous (IV) administration. It is also administered IV to produce vasoconstriction (narrowing of the blood vessels), increase blood pressure and the force of contraction of the heart, and induce bronchodilation. Other clinical applications of Epi include asthmatic crises and in combination with local anesthetics to prolong their duration of action. Epi is quickly metabolized in the tissues by both monoamine oxidase and catechol-*O*-methyltransferase, so it has a short duration of action. It does not reach the CNS and its potential toxicity is an extension of its pharmacological activities, causing adverse effects such as cardiac arrhythmia, excessive vasoconstriction, hypertension, and pulmonary edema.

TABLE 4-5. Adrenergic Receptors, Distribution in the Body, and Effects of Their Activation

Receptor Type	Effector Tissue/Organ	Action
General	All SANS-innervated Tissues	All in List
α_1	Vascular smooth muscle	Vasoconstriction
	Pupillary dilator muscle	Mydriasis
	Pilomotor smooth muscle	Erects hair
α_2	Adrenergic nerve terminals	Inhibits NE release
β_1	Heart	Rate and force of contraction
	Kidney	Renin release
β_2	Bronchi	Bronchodilation
	Uterus	Relaxation
	Vascular smooth muscle	Vasodilation
	Liver	Glycogenolysis (increases blood sugar by releasing it from storage)

Selective Agonists

Phenylephrine (Neo Synephrine), oxymetazoline, naphazoline, and similar agents are primarily α_1 agonists that produce vasoconstriction and are used clinically to reduce nasal congestion or to treat conjunctivitis. These agents are primarily used locally as eye or nasal drops or nasal sprays. Side effects are extensions of their pharmacological effects if the drugs reach the systemic circulation. The vasoconstriction produced by these agents can lead to increases in blood pressure, but since they normally act locally at the site where they are administered, this is rarely an issue.

Clonidine (Catapres) and guanfacine are typical α_2 agonists. They are used to lower blood pressure and can act in the CNS. Clonidine is available in tablet form and as a patch, which is applied once weekly. If stopped abruptly clonidine can cause reflex hypertension, which may be quite severe. More information about its use as an antihypertensive is available in Chapter 15. The CNS actions of these agents are useful in treating attention deficit hyperactivity disorder (ADHD—see Chapter 7).

Isoproterenol (Isuprel) is a nonselective β agonist with activity at both β_1 and β_2 receptor types. It is poorly absorbed when administered orally and is usually administered intravenously to treat heart block and cardiac arrest. It was previously used to treat asthma, but its activity at β_1 receptors produced many unwanted side effects, so that it has been supplanted by specific β_2 agonists. Dobutamine is a more specific β_1 agonist with important activities on the heart. This agent is used clinically to treat cardiac decompensation and heart failure, as well as some types of shock. It increases cardiac output and blood flow to tissues. Dopamine is also useful in cardiac patients but doesn't have the selectivity that dobutamine does for the heart.

Salmeterol (Serevent), albuterol (Ventolin, Proventil), levalbuterol (Xopenex), and other specific β_2 agonists (considered in detail in Chapter 19) have primary actions on the bronchi, with few effects on the heart, making them the drugs of choice to treat asthma. These agents are absorbed orally, but they are used in the form of inhalers or nebulizers to reduce systemic adverse effects, including tachycardia and CNS stimulation.

Indirect Releasers

Amphetamines (Adderall), methylphenidate (Ritalin or Concerta), dexmethylphenidate (Focalin), and lisdexamfetamine (Vyvanse) are agents that can cross the BBB and, while they have little or no effect on the SANS, they induce the release of the neurotransmitters NE and DA in the brain. These agents have a spectrum of stimulant effects, beginning with increasing alertness and reducing fatigue. Higher doses can produce anorexia, euphoria, and insomnia. They are used clinically to treat ADHD in both children and adults. Toxicity and adverse effects are extensions of their pharmacological effects and include nervousness, insomnia, decreased appetite, and, rarely, paranoia and convulsions.

Ephedrine and pseudoephedrine (Sudafed) are mixed-acting agents that can act directly on adrenergic receptors and may also induce NE release. Pseudoephedrine is less able to penetrate the BBB and therefore has fewer CNS effects. Pseudoephedrine, which alleviates nasal congestion, is used clinically to treat common colds and allergies and is available over the counter. Ephedrine is administered intravenously in emergency situations, and is also available in combination with guaifenesin, in an oral tablet for asthma relief. The adverse effects of pseudoephedrine include increased blood pressure, tachycardia, and excitability. Misuse or overdoses of these agents produce CNS stimulation, insomnia, anxiety, and psychotic episodes.

PRACTICE POINT:

Ephedrine or pseudoephedrine can be used as a precursor in the illicit manufacture of methamphetamine. Federal law limits quantities sold and requires that even nonprescription dosage forms of these drugs be kept "behind the counter." Some state laws are even more restrictive.

Indirect Reuptake Inhibitors

Cocaine is a natural agent with a mechanism of action combining the inhibition of reuptake transporters of NE in the body and DA in the CNS. Cocaine crosses the BBB and increases the concentration and signaling of NE and DA in the synapses there but can also cause increased blood pressure and tachycardia by peripheral effects on the ANS, as well as produce local anesthesia. One clinical application for cocaine is as an anesthetic in facial surgery. In addition, antidepressants are inhibitors of the NE reuptake transporter and act by increasing both concentration and signaling of NE as well as those of other neurotransmitters in the brain. See Chapter 7 for more information on antidepressants.

Enzyme Inhibitors

Monoamine oxidase (MAO) and catechol-*O*-methyl transferase (COMT) inhibitors such as selegiline and entacapone prevent the enzyme-mediated degradation of NE, dopamine, and chemically similar neurotransmitters. These agents are used to treat Parkinson disease and for their antidepressant actions, and their side effects are mostly a result of stimulation of the SANS by the excess (undegraded) NE. See Chapters 6 and 7 for more information on COMT and MAO inhibitors.

SANS Inhibition

Adrenergic antagonists (*blocking agents*) are drugs that decrease or prevent the stimulation of SANS receptors. Some adrenergic antagonists can cause blockade at all types of adrenergic receptors, while others are specific and act at one type or subtype. α- and β-blocking drugs are considered separately because they exhibit markedly different pharmacological effects. Representative adrenergic antagonists are listed in Medication Table 4-6.

Alpha-Adrenergic Blocking Agents

Nonspecific α Blockers

Agents of this type have affinity for both α_1- and α_2-adrenergic receptors. They attach to the receptors without stimulating them and competitively block the physiological effects of both NE and Epi at these sites. The most important effect of nonselective alpha blockers on the cardiovascular system is reduced blood pressure. They do not produce direct cardiac effects but may produce a reflex tachycardia.

Phentolamine is a nonselective, competitive, and reversible blocking agent that binds to both α_1- and α_2-adrenergic receptors, preventing the binding of NE and Epi at those spots. Phentolamine (OraVerse) has a duration action of about 2–4 hours when taken orally and 20–40 minutes when administered parenterally. Phentolamine is used to treat hypertension associated with pheochromocytoma (a tumor of the adrenal medulla that secretes excessive Epi and NE), and to prevent the effects of norepinephrine extravasation, as well as to reverse the effects of some oral anesthesia. Another medication used in the treatment of hypertension due to pheochromocytoma is phenoxybenzamine. Phenoxybenzamine has a longer duration of action than phentolamine since the binding of phenoxybenzamine to α receptors is irreversible.

α_1-Selective Blockers

Prazosin (Minipress), terazosin, and doxazosin (Cardura) are very selective, reversible α_1 blockers that have little or no effect on the other SANS receptors. Their duration of action is about 8–10 hours. They have clinical applications in the management of hypertension and prevention of urinary retention in men with benign prostatic hyperplasia. These medications cause much less tachycardia than nonselective α blockers but do cause orthostatic hypotension. For more information on the use of these drugs for hypertension see Chapter 15, and for benign prostatic hyperplasia see Chapter 11.

α₂ Blockers

Yohimbine has affinity for α_2-adrenergic receptors, where it acts as a competitive antagonist; however, it also has affinity for serotonin and DA receptors. This drug had been used clinically to treat male impotence and sexual dysfunction caused by antidepressants, but it has been replaced by newer, non-SANS agents with fewer and less intense side effects. Yohimbine has significant side effects, such as anxiety, hypertension, tachycardia, insomnia, hallucinations, and skin flushing. It has a narrow therapeutic index; overdoses can be harmful and dangerous. While it no longer has FDA-approved indications, it is a component of some OTC herbal supplements containing yohimbe derivatives.

Beta-Adrenergic Blocking Agents

These drugs, commonly called *beta blockers*, competitively block β receptors in the SANS. As mentioned above, β-receptor activation results in vasodilation, bronchodilation, and tachycardia; therefore, β blockers antagonize these effects, producing lower heart rates and bronchoconstriction. The primary applications of these agents are the treatment of cardiovascular pathologies such as hypertension, angina pectoris, arrhythmia prophylaxis after myocardial infarction, and congestive heart failure. Pheochromocytoma is sometimes treated with combined α and β blockers, especially if the tumor is producing large amounts of both Epi and NE. Some of these agents are used in the form of eye drops to treat glaucoma.[7] The toxicities of these agents are extensions of the β blockade and can include bradycardia, atrioventricular blockade, and arrhythmia. Some of these agents, such as propranolol, metoprolol, pindolol, timolol, and labetalol can cross the BBB and result in sedation, fatigue, and sleep alterations. Patients with asthma or other reactive airway diseases may have worsening of their condition unless a selective β_1 blocker is used, but β blocker use is generally cautioned in these patients.

Nonspecific Blockers

These agents have effects on the heart and cardiovascular system (β_1 receptors) and on the bronchi (β_2 receptors). More information on these medications can be found in the chapters covering the conditions they are used to treat. Carteolol, levobunolol, and metipranolol are nonselective β blockers administered as eye drops in the treatment of glaucoma, and they work by decreasing aqueous humor production.[3] Nadolol (Corgard), propranolol (Inderal), and timolol are all used to treat hypertension or other cardiovascular conditions. Carvedilol (Coreg) and labetalol are antagonists at both β receptors and at α_1 receptors and are also used to treat high blood pressure.

β₁-Selective Blockers

These agents have more antagonist effects on the actions of the SANS in the heart and blood vessels, and little action in the lungs. This specificity results in fewer side effects and a lower risk of exacerbating asthma symptoms. Medications in the class include atenolol (Tenormin), metoprolol (Lopressor), and others. These agents are all used to treat high blood pressure and prevent heart failure; more information on them can be found in Chapters 15 and 16.

SUMMARY

The autonomic nervous system (ANS) is the part of the nervous system that is responsible for the coordination and regulation of body functions. The ANS has two functional divisions, the parasympathetic autonomic nervous system (PANS) and the sympathetic autonomic nervous system (SANS), which have opposing functions but work in a coordinated manner to maintain homeostasis. The ANS functions by rapid transmission of nerve impulses through innervations that terminate at organs or tissues releasing a neurotransmitter. The effector cells respond to the release of neurotransmitters, which activate specific receptors. Pathological disorders or diseases can arise from excessive activation or inhibition of either division of the ANS. Medications used to treat these disorders act at the level of the neurotransmitters and receptors, working to balance the functions of the ANS.

ACKNOWLEDGMENTS

The author wishes to acknowledge and thank Raymond A. Lorenz, PharmD, BCPP, Alejandro Pino-Figueroa, PhD, Mark Böhlke, PhD, Timothy J. Maher, PhD, Karen A. Newell, MMSc, PA-C, and Elizabeth P. Rothschild, MMSc, PA-C, contributors to this chapter in the first edition of this book.

REFERENCES

1. Westfall TC, Macarthur H, Westfall DP. Neurotransmission: The autonomic and somatic motor nervous systems. In: Brunton LL, Hilal-Dandan R, Knollmann BC., eds. *Goodman & Gilman's The Pharmacological Basis of Therapeutics.* 13th ed. New York, NY: McGraw-Hill; 2017.

2. Westfall TC, Macarthur H, Westfall DP. Adrenergic agonists and antagonists. In: Brunton LL, Hilal-Dandan R, Knollmann BC., eds. *Goodman & Gilman's The Pharmacological Basis of Therapeutics.* 13th ed. New York, NY: McGraw-Hill; 2017.

3. Fiscella, RG, Lesar, TS, Owaidhah OA, Edward, DP. Glaucoma. In: DiPiro JT, Yee GC, Posey L, et al., eds. *Pharmacotherapy: A Pathophysiologic Approach.* 11th edition. New York, NY: McGraw-Hill; 2020.

4. Hayes BD, Chyka PA. Clinical toxicology. In: DiPiro JT, Yee GC, Posey L, et al., eds. *Pharmacotherapy: A Pathophysiologic Approach.* 11th ed. New York, NY: McGraw-Hill; 2020.

5. Amato AA. Myasthenia gravis and other diseases of the neuromuscular junction. In: Jameson J, Fauci AS, Kasper DL, et al., eds. *Harrison's Principles of Internal Medicine.* 20th ed. New York, NY: McGraw-Hill; 2018.

6. Skidgel RA. Histamine, bradykinin, and their antagonists. In: Brunton LL, Hilal-Dandan R, Knollmann BC., eds. *Goodman & Gilman's The Pharmacological Basis of Therapeutics.* 13th ed. New York, NY: McGraw-Hill; 2017.

7. Feinberg M. The problems of anticholinergic adverse effects in older patients. *Drugs Aging.* 1993;3(4):335-348. doi: 10.2165/00002512-199303040-00004.

REVIEW QUESTIONS

1. Indicate and explain the physiological difference between the PANS and SANS divisions of the ANS.

2. What are the neurotransmitters at the ANS? What are their anatomical locations?

3. What is the primary general mechanism of action of ANS drugs?

4. Explain the terms *indirect agonist* and *indirect antagonist*.

5. Explain the term *beta blocker* and the mechanism of action of drugs in this category.

MEDICATION TABLES

MEDICATION TABLE 4-1. Representative Cholinergic Agents[a]

Generic Name	Brand Name	Mechanism of Action	Route of Administration/ Dosage Form	Usual Dose[b]	Indication(s)	Notes
Bethanechol (be THAN e kole)	Generics only	Direct: binds and activates muscarinic receptors	Oral: tablet	10–50 mg 3–4 times/day	Urinary retention, neurogenic bladder	Should be administered 1 hr before meals or 2 hr after meals
Carbachol (KAR ba kole)	Miostat	Direct: binds and activates muscarinic receptors	Intraocular: solution	0.5 mL instilled into anterior chamber before or after securing sutures	Cataract surgery: causes miosis during surgery; reduces postsurgical intraocular pressure	Sterile technique must be used
Pilocarpine (pye loe KAR peen)	Isopto Carpine	Direct: binds and activates muscarinic receptors	Sterile ophthalmic solution	1 drop up to 4 times daily (or 1–2 drops to cause miosis)	Elevated intraocular pressure; glaucoma	May cause decreased visual acuity, especially at night
	Salagen		Oral tablet	5–10 mg 3–4 times daily	Xerostomia (dry mouth)	Avoid administration with high-fat meal
Malathion (mal a THYE on)	Ovide	Indirect: prevents degradation of Ach by AchE	Topical: lotion	Sprinkled on hair/scalp	Treatment of head lice and their ova	Use is contraindicated in neonates and infants
Edrophonium (ed roe FOE nee um)	Generics only	Indirect: Prevents destruction of Ach by AchE, resulting in increased cholinergic responses such as miosis	IV, IM, or SUBQ: injection solution	IV: 2 mg test dose administered over 15–30 sec; 8 mg given 45 sec later if no response is seen	Diagnosis of myasthenia gravis; differentiation of cholinergic crises from myasthenia crises; reversal of nondepolarizing neuromuscular blockers	Overdosage can cause cholinergic crisis, which may be fatal
Neostigmine (nee oh STIG meen)	Bloxiverz, Generic available	Indirect: prevents degradation of Ach by AchE	IV Injection: solution	0.03–0.07 mg/kg (up to 5 mg maximum dose)	Reversal of the effects of nondepolarizing neuromuscular-blocking agents; treatment of myasthenia gravis; prevention and treatment of postoperative bladder distention and urinary retention	Should be injected slowly over a period of at least 1 min

Continued next page

MEDICATION TABLE 4-1. Representative Cholinergic Agents[a] *(Continued)*

Generic Name	Brand Name	Mechanism of Action	Route of Administration/ Dosage Form	Usual Dose[b]	Indication(s)	Notes
Physostigmine (fye zoe STIG meen)	Generic available	Indirect: prevents degradation of Ach by AchE	IM, IV: injection solution	0.5–2 mg to start; repeat q 10–30 min until response occurs or adverse effect occurs; repeat 1–4 mg q 30–40 min as life-threatening symptoms recur	Reverse toxic, life-threatening delirium caused by atropine, dimenhydrinate, *Atropa belladonna*, or jimson weed	To be administered slowly at a rate not exceeding 1 mg/min (0.5 mg/min in children) to prevent respiratory distress and seizures; never to be infused continuously
Pyridostigmine (peer id oh STIG meen)	Mestinon	Indirect: prevents degradation of Ach by AchE	Oral: syrup, tablet, extended-release tablet	Oral: 600 mg/day divided into 5–6 doses; sustained release 180–540 mg once or twice daily	Myasthenia gravis	Do not crush sustained-release tablet
	Regonol		IV injection: solution	0.1–0.25 mg/kg/dose	Reversal of nondepolarizing neuromuscular blocking agents	Administered as slow IV push

Ach = acetylcholine; AchE = acetylcholinesterase; IM = intramuscular; IV = intravenous; SUBQ = subcutaneous.
[a]Pronunciations have been adapted with permission from USP Dictionary of USAN and International Drug Names (USP Dictionary) © 2022.
[b]Dosages from AHFS DI® [database]. Bethesda, MD: American Society of Health-System Pharmacists; 2021.

MEDICATION TABLE 4-2. Clinical Applications of Antimuscarinic Drugs[a]

Organ System	Drugs (pronunciation)	Application
Central nervous system	Benztropine (BENZ troe peen), trihexyphenidyl (trye hex ee FEN i dil)	Treat manifestations of Parkinson disease (Chapter 6)
	Scopolamine (skoe POL a meen)	Prevent motion sickness (Chapter 21)
Eye	Atropine (A troe peen), homatropine (hoe MAT roe peen), cyclopentolate (sye kloe PEN toe late), tropicamide (troe PIK a mide)	Mydriasis and cycloplegia for eye examination (Chapter 34)
Bronchi	Ipratropium (i pra TROE pee um)	Bronchodilation in chronic obstructive pulmonary disease (Chapter 19)
Gastrointestinal tract	Glycopyrrolate (glye koe PYE roe late), methscopolamine (meth skoe POL a meen)	Reduce gastric secretion and transient hypermotility (Chapter 21)
Genitourinary tract	Oxybutynin (ox i BYOO ti nin), tolterodine (tole TER a deen), darifenacin (dar ee FEN a sin), solifenacin (sol i FEN a cin), trospium (TROSE pee um)	Treat transient cystitis, postoperative bladder spasms, or overactive bladder (Chapter 4)

[a]Pronunciations have been adapted with permission from USP Dictionary of USAN and International Drug Names (USP Dictionary) © 2022.

MEDICATION TABLE 4-3. Representative Antimuscarinic Drugs[a]

Generic Name	Brand Name	Route of Administration/ Dosage Form	Usual Dose[b]	Indication(s)	Notes	More Information in Chapter
Atropine (A troe peen)	AtroPen, generics	IM/IV: injection	IM, IV, SUBQ: 0.4–0.6 mg 30–60 min preop and repeat q 4–6 hr	Inhibition of salivation and secretions during surgery	Patient must be monitored for tachycardia and hypotension	
			0.5–1 mg q 3–5 min (maximum dose 3 mg)	Sinus bradycardia	Ineffective in heart transplant patients due to lack of vagal (PANS) innervation	16
	Isopto Atropine, generics	Ophthalmic: ointment/solution	1 or 2 drops in the eye(s) or a small amount in the conjunctival sac	Mydriasis (especially for eye exam)		34
Benztropine (BENZ troe peen)	Cogentin	Oral: tablet IM/IV: injection	1–2 mg/day IM/IV/oral (range 0.5–6 mg/day)	Parkinson disease and Parkinson-like side effects of other drugs	May impair body temperature regulation	6
Dicyclomine (dye SYE kloe meen)	Bentyl	Oral: capsule, syrup, tablet IM: solution	80 mg/day in 4 divided doses (20 mg/dose)	Treatment of functional bowel/irritable bowel syndrome	Not to be administered IV	
Glycopyrrolate (glye koe PYE roe late)	Cuvposa, Robinul, Robinul Forte	IM/IV: solution Oral: solution, tablet	Preoperative: 4 mcg/kg 30–60 min before procedure (IM); intraoperative: 0.1 mg repeated as needed at 2–3 min intervals (IV) (Pediatric: 3–16 0.02 mg/kg 3 times per day)	Inhibit salivation and excessive secretions of the respiratory tract preoperatively; control of upper airway secretions	Oral solution to be administered on an empty stomach, 1 hr before or 2 hr after meals	

Continued next page

MEDICATION TABLE 4-3. Representative Antimuscarinic Drugs[a] *(Continued)*

Generic Name	Brand Name	Route of Administration/ Dosage Form	Usual Dose[b]	Indication(s)	Notes	More Information in Chapter
Hyoscyamine (hye oh SYE a meen)	Levsin, Levbid, many other brands and generics	Oral: elixir, solution, tablet (SL, chewable, extended release, orally disintegrating, sustained release, variable release) Injection: solution	Oral or SL: 0.125–0.25 mg q 4 hr or as needed; oral, timed release: 0.375–0.75 mg q 12 hr; IM, IV, SUBQ: 0.25–0.5 mg given 5–10 min prior to procedure	Oral: peptic ulcers, irritable bowel, neurogenic bladder/ bowel; injection: preoperative to reduce secretions and block cardiac vagal inhibitory reflexes; to improve radiologic visibility of the kidneys	Maximum: 1.5 mg/24 hr	
Ipratropium (i pra TROE pee um)	Atrovent	Inhalation: nebulizer solution, dry powder inhaler	2 inhalations 4 times a day up to 12 in 24 hr OR Nebulizer 0.5 mg every 6 to 8 hours as needed	Chronic obstructive pulmonary disease		19
Methscopolamine (meth skoe POL a meen)	Pamine	Oral: tablet	2.5 mg 30 min before meals or food and 2.5–5 mg at bedtime; may increase dose to 5 mg twice daily	Peptic ulcer	To be administered 30 min before meals or food	
Scopolamine (skoe POL a meen)	Transderm Scōp	Transdermal: patch	Apply 1 patch to hairless area behind ear the night before surgery or 1 hr prior to cesarean section	Prevention of nausea/ vomiting associated with motion sickness and recovery from anesthesia and surgery	Once topical patch is applied, it is not to be removed for 3 full days	21

IM = intramuscular; IV = intravenous; SUBQ = subcutaneous; SL = sublingual.
[a]Pronunciations have been adapted with permission from USP Dictionary of USAN and International Drug Names (USP Dictionary) © 2022.
[b]Dosages from AHFS DI® [database]. Bethesda, MD: American Society of Health-System Pharmacists; 2021.

MEDICATION TABLE 4-4. Antimuscarinics for Bladder Spasm and Overactivity[a]

Generic Name	Brand Name	Mechanism of Action	Dosage Form(s)/Route of Administration	Usual Dose[b]	Notes/Uses
Darifenacin (dar ee FEN a sin)	Generics	Antimuscarinic: blockade of muscarinic receptors limits bladder contractions, reducing the symptoms of bladder irritability/overactivity (urge incontinence, urgency and frequency)	Oral: tablet, extended release	7.5–15 mg once daily	Used in the management of symptoms of bladder overactivity; tablet should be taken with liquid and swallowed whole
Fesoterodine (fes oh TER oh deen)	Toviaz	Converted in the body to a competitive Ach antagonist at muscarinic receptors	Oral: tablet, extended release	4 mg once daily; may be increased to 8 mg once daily	Treatment of patients with an overactive bladder with symptoms of urinary frequency, urgency, or urge incontinence; do not crush
Flavoxate (fla VOX ate)	Generic available	Synthetic antispasmodic with a direct relaxant effect on smooth muscles, providing symptomatic relief for a variety of smooth muscle spasms, especially urinary tract	Oral: tablet	100–200 mg 3–4 times/day	Should be taken with water on an empty stomach; may cause CNS depression
Oxybutynin (ox i BYOO ti nin)	Ditropan XL, Gelnique, Oxytrol	Inhibits action of Ach on bladder muscle and acts as a direct antispasmodic; increases bladder capacity, decreases uninhibited contractions, and delays desire to void—therefore, decreases urgency and frequency	Topical: 10% gel (Gelnique); transdermal: 3.9 mg/24 hr patch (Oxytrol); oral: tablet; extended-release tablet (Ditropan XL)	5 mg 2–3 times/day up to maximum of 5 mg 4 times/day; topical: 100 mg application once daily; transdermal: one patch twice weekly	Antispasmodic for neurogenic bladder (urgency, frequency, leakage, urge incontinence, dysuria); do not apply topical application to the same site on consecutive days
Solifenacin (sol i FEN a cin)	VESIcare	Inhibits muscarinic receptors resulting in decreased urinary bladder contraction, increased residual urine volume, and decreased detrusor muscle pressure	Oral: tablet	5 mg once daily; may increase to 10 mg once daily	Treatment of overactive bladder with symptoms of urinary frequency, urgency, or urge incontinence
Tolterodine (tole TER a deen)	Detrol, Detrol LA	Competitive antagonist of muscarinic receptors	Oral: tablet, extended-release capsule	2 mg twice daily (immediate release); 4 mg once a day (extended release)	Treatment of patients with overactive bladder with symptoms of urinary frequency, urgency, or urge incontinence; do not crush
Trospium (TROSE pee um)	Generics	Antagonizes the effects of Ach on muscarinic receptors in cholinergically innervated organs; reduces the smooth muscle tone of the bladder	Oral: tablet, extended-release capsule	20 mg twice daily	Treatment of overactive bladder with symptoms of urgency, incontinence, and urinary frequency; administer 1 hr prior to meals or on an empty stomach

Ach = acetylcholine; CNS = central nervous system.

[a]Pronunciations have been adapted with permission from USP Dictionary of USAN and International Drug Names (USP Dictionary) © 2022.

[b]Dosages from AHFS DI® [database]. Bethesda, MD: American Society of Health-System Pharmacists; 2021.

MEDICATION TABLE 4-5. Subgroups of Adrenergic or Sympathomimetic Drugs, Representative Agents[a]

Group	Subgroup	Molecular Target	Example	Therapeutic Use
Direct acting	General	α and β receptors	Epinephrine (ep i NEF rin)	Anaphylaxis
	α agonists	α receptors		Relief of nasal and ophthalmic congestion
	• α₁ selective	• α₁ receptor	Phenylephrine (fen il EF rin)	
	• α₂ selective	• α₂ receptor	Clonidine (KLOE ni deen)	Blood pressure, CNS conditions (ADHD)
	β agonists	β receptors		
	• β₁ selective	• β₁ receptor	Dobutamine (doe BYOO ta meen)	Heart failure
	• β₂ selective	• β₂ receptor	Albuterol (al BYOO ter ole)	Asthma
	• Nonselective	• β₁ and β₂ receptors	Isoproterenol (eye so proe TER e nole)	Bradycardia, heart block
Indirect acting	Releasers	Vesicles—cell membrane	Methylphenidate (meth il FEN i date)	Stimulant (alertness, ADHD)
	Reuptake inhibitors	NE transporter	Cocaine (koe KANE)	Facial surgery
	Enzyme inhibitors	Monoamine oxidase (MAO), catechol-O-methyl transferase (COMT)	Selegiline (se LE ji leen) Entacapone (en TA ka pone)	Parkinson disease
Mixed	Releasers with agonist activity	Receptors, vesicles	Pseudoephedrine (soo doe e FED rin)	Nasal congestion

ADHD = attention deficit hyperactive disorder; CNS = central nervous system.
[a]Pronunciations have been adapted with permission from USP Dictionary of USAN and International Drug Names (USP Dictionary) © 2022.

MEDICATION TABLE 4-6. Representative Adrenergic Blocking Agents (Antagonists)[a]

Antagonist Type	Receptors Blocked	Representative Agent	Brand	Therapeutic Use(s)	More Information in Chapter
Nonspecific α blocker	α_1 and α_2	Phentolamine (fen TOLE a meen)	OraVerse	Pheochromocytoma, α stimulant extravasation	
α_1 selective blocker	α_1	Doxazosin (dox AY zoe sin)	Cardura	Hypertension, benign prostatic hyperplasia–related urinary retention	10, 14
Mixed adrenergic blocker	β_1 and α_1	Labetalol (la BET a lole)		Hypertension	14
Nonspecific β blocker	β_1 and α_2	Propranolol (proe PRAN oh lole)	Inderal	Hypertension	14
β_1 blocker	β_1	Metoprolol (me TOE proe lole)	Lopressor, Toprol	Hypertension, heart failure	14, 15

[a]Pronunciations have been adapted with permission from USP Dictionary of USAN and International Drug Names (USP Dictionary) © 2022.

Chapter 5

Central Nervous System

Ashley M. Jones, PharmD, BCPS |
Chris Paxos, PharmD, BCPP, BCPS, BCGP

KEY TERMS AND DEFINITIONS

Action potential—a series of electrical and chemical impulses that travel along the neuron and activate other neurons.

Addiction—a behavioral pattern characterized as lack of control over and compulsive use of drugs despite negative consequences from use.

Analgesia—relieving or reducing pain.

Anesthesia—a condition during which a patient forms no new memories, is unconscious, cannot move, and does not respond to pain.

Blood–brain barrier—specialized cells in the blood vessels of the meninges, which keep foreign materials (e.g., microorganisms, medications) from entering the brain.

Brain—organ at the center of the central nervous system.

Central nervous system—composed of the brain and spinal cord; relays and interprets motor and sensory information, as well as higher-order functions such as memory and reasoning.

General anesthetics—medications, administered by inhalation or intravenously, that produce anesthesia.

Local anesthetics—medications applied or administered to a specific part of the body to block the nerves in that part of the body.

DOI 10.37573/9781585286638.005

Meninges—outer layers of the brain that protect it; located below the skull.

Neuron—nerve cell; functional unit of the brain.

Physical dependence—a condition characterized by the occurrence of withdrawal symptoms on abrupt reduction or discontinuation of a drug.

Spinal cord—enclosed within the vertebral column; transmits nerve impulses from the brain to the rest of the body.

Tolerance—the need for larger doses of medication to achieve the same effect that occurred when first starting the drug.

LEARNING OBJECTIVES

After completing this chapter, you should be able to

1. Describe brain and spinal cord anatomy and physiology.

2. Describe common neurotransmitters and their actions in the central nervous system.

3. Identify local and general anesthetics and how each affects the central nervous system.

4. Define analgesia.

5. List opioid medications and differentiate them by drug class and route of administration.

6. Discuss the pharmacological effects and adverse effects of opioid medications.

The nervous system is the communication system through which electrical and chemical signals responsible for the conscious and unconscious functions of the human body are transmitted. The central nervous system (CNS) is composed of the brain and the spinal cord. The brain is the information-processing center for the body and resides within the skull. Different areas within the brain are responsible for a plethora of human function, ranging from language processing, memory, and personality, to movement, speech, and fine motor skills. The brain sends signals to the rest of the body to initiate movement and direction whether these are unconscious or conscious movements. The brain also processes the changing environment around the individual through interpretation of electrical signals from the rest of the body. It communicates signals to and from other parts

of the organism via the nerves. The spinal cord is located in the spinal column, or backbone, and these nerves branch out to the rest of the body. The spinal cord helps to move signals back to the brain and to carry out actions dictated by the brain. A person's emotional state is also determined by the brain and is mediated through a complex balance of neurotransmitters.

The CNS is an elaborate network of communicating cells and chemicals that serve as specific drug targets. Many different medications have their actions in the CNS, and these include anesthetics, analgesics, and other medications such as antidepressants or treatments for Alzheimer disease. This chapter introduces the basic structure and functions of the CNS and examines common medications that are used to modify certain processes in the CNS that lead to anesthesia, pain relief, and addiction.

ANATOMY AND PHYSIOLOGY OF THE CENTRAL NERVOUS SYSTEM

Within the skull, the brain is covered by three protective outer layers called meninges (see Figure 5-1). The meninges are located directly below the skull and protect the brain from injury, form a protective coating around it, and provide blood flow. The meninges also distribute cerebrospinal fluid (CSF) over the outer surface of the brain. The brain and spinal cord are floating in CSF, which is composed of glucose, protein, and water and is a clear color. The CSF is isolated from other areas outside of the body and is therefore considered sterile. It provides nutrients to the brain. The blood vessels that feed the brain and help produce CSF contain a row of specialized cells called the blood–brain barrier (BBB), which keeps foreign organisms and chemicals from entering the brain, while allowing nutrients and oxygen to enter the brain. Medications that have actions in the CNS generally need to "cross" the BBB to reach their desired target and exert their action. The need to penetrate the BBB dictates the way medications intended to act on the CNS are formulated. The BBB can be affected by certain inflammatory disease states that dysregulate the passage of certain substances to the brain. Sometimes, organisms can invade the meninges and make it through the BBB, leading to inflammation of the meninges called meningitis.

The brain is composed of many different structures. It is divided into two halves—"hemispheres"—connected by the corpus callosum, which enables the halves of the brain to communicate. The largest and most complex part of the brain is the cerebrum (or cerebral cortex) (see Figure 5-2).

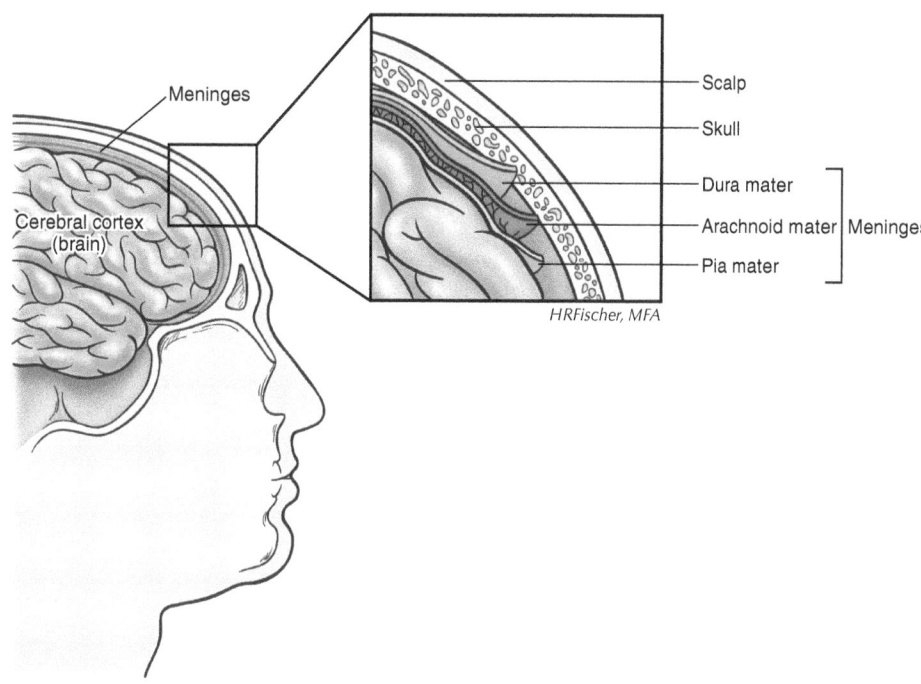

HRFischer, MFA

FIGURE 5-1. Meninges—the different layers of meninges from skull down to brain.

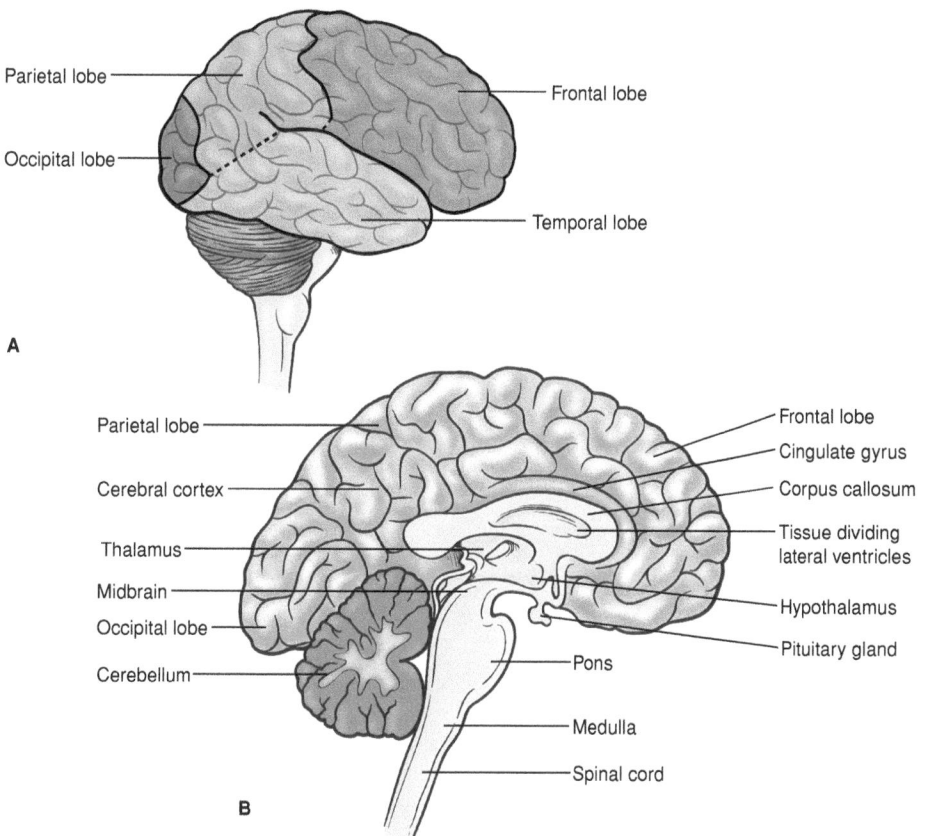

FIGURE 5-2. General brain structures. A. Different lobes of the cerebrum; B. cross-section of the brain with various structures identified.

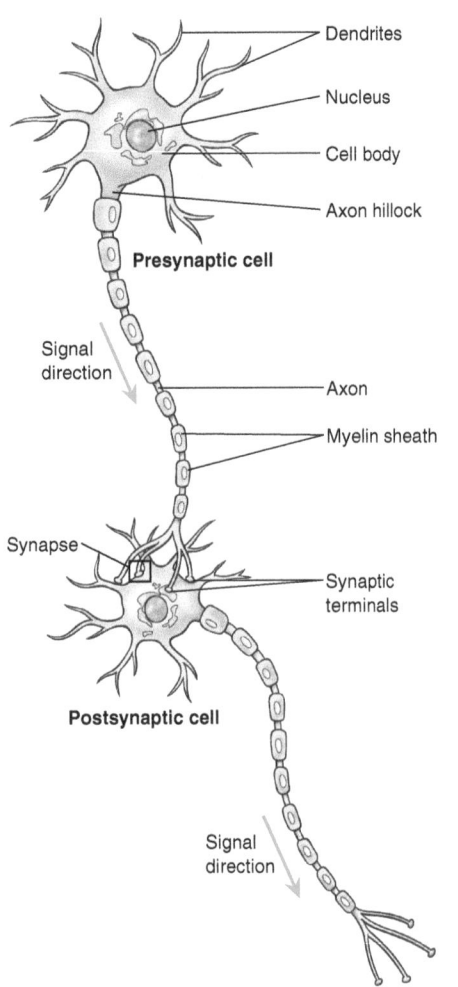

FIGURE 5-3. Synapse—a synapse between two nerve cells with dendrite and cell body.

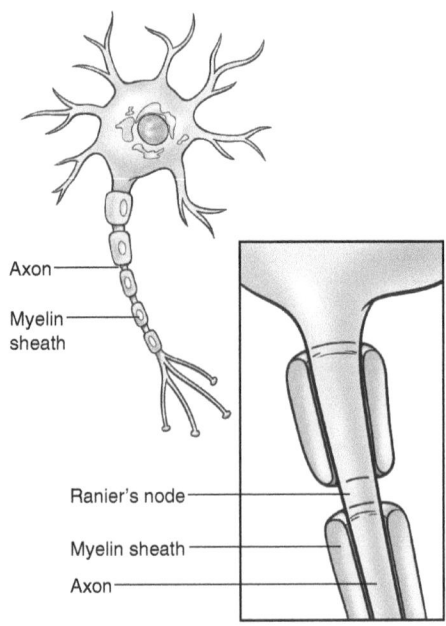

FIGURE 5-4. Axon with myelin sheath.

This is where the majority of reasoning, movement, and sensory information are processed. The cerebrum is divided into four different areas: frontal lobe, parietal lobe, temporal lobe, and occipital lobe. Each of these has unique functions. The frontal lobe deals primarily with reasoning, determining consequences to actions, attention, and other higher mental functions and is commonly characterized as the part of the brain responsible for personality. The parietal lobe is primarily concerned with motor and sensory activity. The temporal lobe helps with memories, hearing, speech, and language. The occipital lobe deals with vision. Other areas of the brain identified in the figure include the cerebellum, which is used for balance and motor movement; the brainstem, which is used for many of the automatic functions of the body such as breathing; the hypothalamus and pituitary gland, which

secrete hormones; and the limbic system, which is responsible for emotions. The brain is a complex organ, and many areas and structures of the brain have overlapping functions. Just because a certain area of the brain is identified as related to a particular function does not mean that the function happens only in that part. All of the different brain regions and sections work together to help us navigate the world around us.

The functional unit of the brain is the neuron or nerve cell (see Figure 5-3). Neurons consist of different parts, each of which has its own function. The cell body of a neuron is called the soma. This is where proteins and neurotransmitters (described in Chapter 4) are made and where the nucleus resides. Branching directly off the soma are structures called dendrites. Dendrites receive information from other cells as transmitted by action potentials and the release of neurotransmitters. Axons are the part of the nerve that stretch away from the body of the nerve cell to carry signals to the next nerve (a little like the wires on a telephone pole). Axons are sometimes coated in a myelin sheath, or a layer of fat and protein (Figure 5-4). The myelin sheath protects the axon and increases the conduction of nerve impulses. The point at which the axon ends is a space called the synapse, or synaptic junction. At the other end of the synapse is the dendrite of another neuron. The synapse is where neurotransmitters are released for the action potential to send information to other neurons. There are also other cells present in the brain called glial cells, which provide a support function to the neurons.[1]

An action potential is a series of electrical and chemical impulses that travel along the neuron and activate other neurons. The action potential is an essential part of neuronal function as without action potentials one part of the brain would not be able to communicate with another part of the brain. The same is true for sensory neurons in the rest of the body; without action potentials, a person would not know that his or her hand was being burned.

The major function of the spinal cord is to send information to, and receive information from, the brain. The basic structure of the spinal cord can be seen in Figure 5-5. It is composed of meninges, CSF, neurons, and support cells just like the brain. Unlike the brain, however, the spinal cord has very long axons, which are the nerves in the peripheral nervous system (see Chapter 4) that enable the brain to receive sensory information such as pain and touch and send motor signals like "move your arm here." As seen in **Figure 5-5**, the spinal cord is composed of gray matter and white matter. Each of these has a specific function: the white matter is where the motor and sensory neurons are located, and the

gray matter is where the nerve cell bodies for the spinal cord are located.

The spinal cord is involved in all voluntary movement and some involuntary movements. The motor nerves projecting to the rest of the body from the spinal cord innervate muscles and end in the neuromuscular junction, a type of synapse that activates muscle instead of other neurons. If the neuromuscular junction is blocked by a medication, such as succinylcholine, this inhibits muscle functioning and causes paralysis.

The spinal cord is also involved in receiving sensory information from the body. There are two types of sensory pathways: the dorsal column-medial lemniscus pathway (or the posterior column-medial lemniscus pathway) and the anterolateral system. The dorsal column-medial lemniscus pathway deals with sensory information in the form of touch, proprioception, and vibration. Proprioception is the awareness of the relative position of neighboring parts of the body. The anterolateral system senses pain and temperature. The spinal cord's role in pain perception allows it to serve as a target for anesthesia and delivery of pain medications.[2]

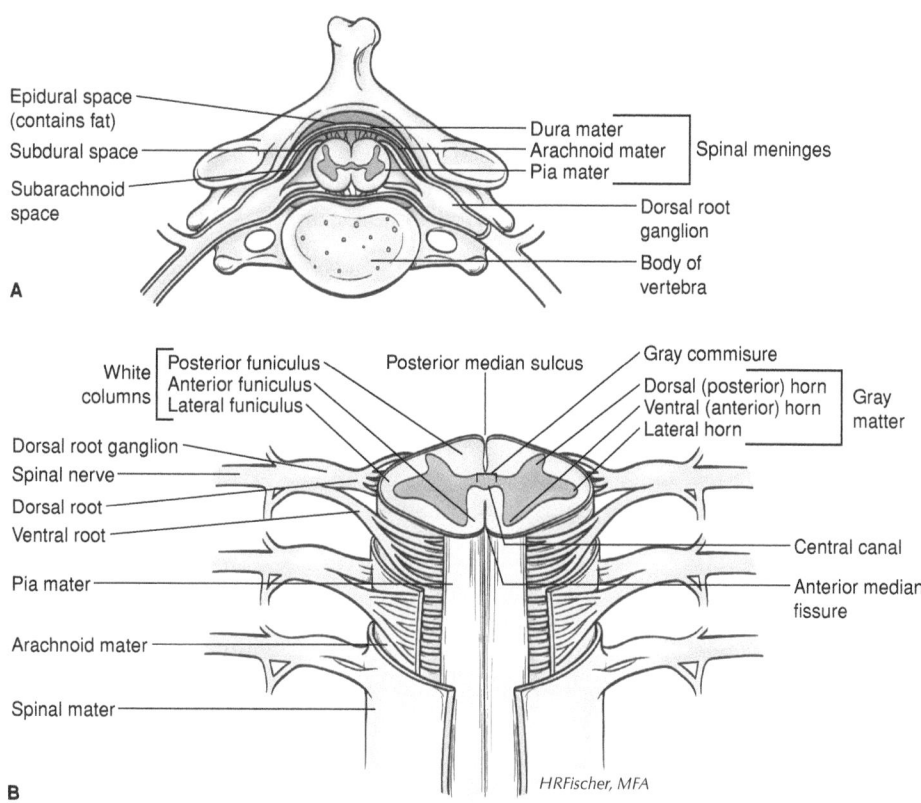

FIGURE 5-5. Spinal cord—general spinal cord structures.

NEUROTRANSMITTERS

Neurotransmitters are chemicals produced by neurons in order for them to communicate effectively.[1] They are stored in vesicles, or pouches, within neurons. Neurotransmitters are released into the synapse in response to an action potential. The neuron releasing the neurotransmitter is called the presynaptic neuron, whereas the neuron receiving the neurotransmitter is called the postsynaptic neuron. Neurotransmitters attach to receptors located on neurons. When a neurotransmitter is released from the presynaptic neuron then binds to receptors on the postsynaptic neuron this generates an action potential on the postsynaptic neuron.

Medications can enhance or diminish the actions of neurotransmitters. This is often accomplished by stimulating or blocking the receptors on the neurons with which the neurotransmitters interact. In general, medications that stimulate—or activate—receptors are called agonists. Agonists duplicate or enhance the actions of neurotransmitters. Medications that block—or inhibit—receptors are called antagonists. Medications that are receptor antagonists reduce the actions of neurotransmitters. Medications are often specific for certain neurotransmitters or receptors, allowing them to precisely affect only one neurotransmitter system.

Gamma-aminobutyric acid (GABA), an amino acid neurotransmitter, is the major inhibitory neurotransmitter of the CNS. This means that GABA generally decreases or slows actions across the CNS because of its restraining role in almost every neuronal circuit in the brain. There are two types of GABA receptors: $GABA_A$ and $GABA_B$. Most medications that affect the GABA system interact with the $GABA_A$ receptor. These medications enhance the inhibitory effects of GABA; therefore, they often produce sleep-promoting, anti-anxiety, and antiseizure effects. Examples of medications that promote the effects of GABA are benzodiazepines and barbiturates. Alcohol also promotes the inhibitory effects of GABA. Another neurotransmitter, glycine, is similar to GABA in its functioning, except it is found only in the spinal cord.

Glutamate, another amino acid neurotransmitter, is the major excitatory neurotransmitter of the CNS. As such, when glutamate is activated, it generally increases activity across the CNS because of its stimulating role in almost every neuronal circuit in the brain. A common receptor that is stimulated by glutamate is the N-methyl-D-aspartate (NMDA) receptor, which is implicated in regulating learning and memory. Several classes of medications influence glutamate neurotransmission in the CNS. Several antiepileptic medications discussed in Chapter 6 reduce the excitatory actions of glutamate to produce their antiseizure effects.

Memantine, a medication that blocks glutamate from binding to its NMDA receptor, is used to treat Alzheimer disease (see Chapter 6). The illicit substance phencyclidine (PCP) also blocks the NMDA receptor.

Acetylcholine is found in varying concentrations throughout the CNS. Acetylcholine activates muscarinic and nicotinic receptors (see Chapter 4), which deal with memory, reward, and learning. Although this neurotransmitter plays a significant role in the autonomic nervous system (in places like the heart, lungs, eyes, sweat glands, and gastrointestinal tract), acetylcholine is also found in the neuromuscular junction, where the neuron acts on the muscle to tell the muscle to contract. Acetylcholine is broken down in the synapse by the enzyme acetylcholinesterase. Several medications either promote or inhibit the effects of acetylcholine. Medications such as donepezil and rivastigmine, known as cholinesterase inhibitors, prevent the breakdown of acetylcholine. Because they increase the availability of acetylcholine for learning and memory, they are useful for the treatment of Alzheimer disease.

Dopamine is a catecholamine neurotransmitter that is found throughout the brain and deals with attention, reward response, movement, and hormone regulation. Dopamine exerts its actions through dopamine receptors, which include D_1, D_2, D_3, D_4, and D_5 receptors. Parkinson disease (Chapter 6) involves a relative lack of dopamine in areas of the brain that regulate movement; therefore, medications that stimulate dopamine receptors, such as levodopa and ropinirole, treat Parkinson disease. Conversely, schizophrenia (Chapter 7) involves high levels of dopamine activity in certain areas of the brain. Antipsychotic medications antagonize D_2 receptors and alleviate some of the symptoms of schizophrenia.

Norepinephrine (also called noradrenaline) and epinephrine (also called adrenaline) are catecholamine neurotransmitters. They activate many different types of receptors in the CNS and peripheral nervous system, including α_1, α_2, β_1, and β_2 receptors. In the CNS, these neurotransmitters have specific actions related to attention and alertness. Medications such as methylphenidate and atomoxetine that increase norepinephrine activity promote attention and alertness when used for attention-deficit/hyperactivity disorder.

Serotonin (5-hydroxytryptamine or 5-HT) is a neurotransmitter characterized as a "monoamine." Although it is distributed throughout the CNS, it is concentrated in the frontal cortex, spinal cord, and limbic system. Serotonin regulates a number of activities in the CNS, including sleep, mood, anger, and appetite. It acts on serotonin receptors, of which there are more than a dozen different subtypes. Serotonin also plays a significant role in the gastrointestinal system. Serotonin and its actions are affected by many medications, including antidepressants (e.g., fluoxetine), antiemetics (e.g., ondansetron), antimigraine agents (e.g., sumatriptan), and illicit substances (e.g., lysergic acid diethylamide, or LSD), which are studied in Chapters 6 and 7.

Histamine is a chemical that has actions within the brain, especially at the hypothalamus, and throughout the body, playing key roles in the sleep/wake cycle and in digestion. Histamine acts on four different receptors: H_1, H_2, H_3, and H_4. The H_1 receptor subtype is found primarily in the CNS. Medications that antagonize H_1 receptors are also called antihistamines (e.g., diphenhydramine). These medications are used for allergic rhinitis, motion sickness, and even for insomnia. Gastric acid secretion is regulated, in part, by the H_2 receptor. Medications such as famotidine and cimetidine, commonly used for gastroesophageal reflux disease (GERD), are H_2 receptor antagonists. They decrease stomach acid secretion and improve GERD symptoms. Finally, pitolisant, an H_3 receptor antagonist, has been found to be helpful for the treatment of narcolepsy, a condition characterized by inordinate daytime sleepiness.

There are other neurotransmitters that play roles in the CNS, but they are not regularly affected by medications and, therefore, are not discussed here.

CASE STUDY

Mr. Jones is a patient in the intensive care unit (ICU). He was admitted for a case of severe pneumonia. He is currently being sedated (a deep sleep, but not full anesthesia) because he is on a mechanical ventilator to aid in the treatment of his pneumonia. Patients who are on mechanical ventilation need to be sedated to prevent normal breathing from interfering with the ventilator. Breathing is a process that happens involuntarily in patients with intact neurological function and the only way to prevent the brain from automatically breathing is through a medically induced deep sleep.

CASE?

What purpose might sedation have for a patient on a mechanical ventilator?

ANESTHETICS

Anesthetics are divided into two types: general and local. General anesthetics are used in surgery and produce general anesthesia, a reversible state in which the patient is unresponsive, does not respond to pain, and does not remember the time during which they were under general anesthesia. Inhaled and intravenous (IV) anesthetics are types of general anesthetics. Each has distinct properties (see Medication Table 5-1; Medication Tables are located at the end of the chapter).

Inhaled anesthetics are used in general anesthesia and are easily administered in the form of a gas, with the patient breathing in air to which the medication (anesthetic) has been added. The medical gas is mixed with a constant flow of oxygen and nitrous oxide, which is then inhaled through either a mask or a ventilator attached to the anesthesia machine. The machine enables the anesthesiologist to monitor the patient's level of anesthesia and regulate the flow of medical gas through the ventilator. The inhaled anesthetics generally produce anesthesia very quickly. The original medication from this class is halothane. Halothane is a volatile general anesthetic that has been used in surgeries for many years. It can cause serious adverse effects, including heart and liver problems, and is no longer commercially available in the United States. Halothane has been replaced by newer, safer, and easier-to-use inhaled anesthetics like isoflurane (Forane), sevoflurane (Ultane), and desflurane (Suprane).

PRACTICE POINT

When stored in the pharmacy, inhaled anesthetics are typically shelved in an area designated for medications utilized in operating rooms.

Intravenous anesthetics belong to various drug classes. Methohexital (Brevital) is a barbiturate, which works by increasing GABA transmission throughout the brain, enhancing its inhibitory action. Methohexital has a very rapid onset of action and a half-life of 2 to 3 hours, making it desirable for outpatient surgical procedures.

The most common side effects from IV barbiturates include injection site reactions, low blood pressure, and headache. Serious adverse effects include respiratory and cardiovascular depression.[2]

Propofol (Diprivan), a nonbarbiturate sedative, is the most commonly administered IV anesthetic. It is used widely for many surgeries, colonoscopies, other nonsurgical procedures, and intubated, mechanically ventilated patients. Propofol is advantageous for procedures where rapid onset of medication effects and quick return of baseline mental status is desired. It works similarly to barbiturates through potentiation of GABA but may have other mechanisms of action as well. Propofol can cause serious blood pressure reduction, and its use is avoided for patients who have preexisting hypotension. Propofol is a fat emulsion with a milky appearance and is available in many different-sized containers. While propofol preparations do contain an antimicrobial agent, they should be used immediately when opened and infusion completed within the time specified (usually 12 hours) to limit infection risk.[2]

PRACTICE POINT

Propofol should be accounted for when calculating total parenteral nutrition (TPN) since it provides 1.1 kcal/mL of lipid nutrition. In addition, triglycerides should be monitored while a patient is receiving a prolonged infusion of propofol.

ALERT!

Patients who are allergic to soy or egg products should not receive propofol.

Many hospitals restrict and monitor access to propofol since it has been misused in the past. This may lead to difficulties in keeping adequate supplies of the medication stocked in a restricted area (e.g., automated dispensing cabinet) in all locations of a hospital, as it is difficult to predict the amount of medication that each patient may require to maintain sedation. The onset of action of propofol is fast (less than 1 minute) with an induction dose of 1.5 to 2.5 mg/kg, and the clinical effects can last up to 2 hours from a bolus dose. The quick onset of propofol given as a bolus allows it to be used as an induction agent for sedation in rapid-sequence intubations. Many sites have rapid-sequence intubation kits that stock the 200 mg/20 mL vial for this reason. Propofol can also be used as a maintenance infusion at much lower doses (100 to 300 mcg/kg/min), but there is considerable inter- and intrapatient variability. For example, propofol is titrated to a desired level of sedation, and each patient may

require a different dose of propofol to reach that desired level for reasons discussed below.[2]

CASE?

Mr. Jones is receiving propofol (Diprivan) for sedation. On the last delivery this morning at 0600, the pharmacy technician left an entire carton of the 50-mL bottles there, which should have lasted until tomorrow. It is 1800 and the nurse is calling for an additional supply. Why might Mr. Jones be in need of more propofol?

ALERT!

LOOK-ALIKE/SOUND-ALIKE—Diprivan (propofol) and Diflucan (fluconazole) have been the subject of confusion.

Varying doses of propofol may be needed to keep a patient sedated, as the medication can accumulate in fat tissue and then "redistribute." Redistribution occurs when a highly fat-soluble medication is deposited in fat tissue after prolonged exposure and, once administration of the medication stops, diffuses away from the fat tissue and reenters the circulation. At this point, the medication is continuing to perform its actions until it is removed from the body. Additionally, effects of other sedatives that the patient is receiving, such as opioid agonists, may necessitate alterations in the infusion rate. After prolonged infusion, propofol may accumulate in the fat tissue of a patient with obesity and prolong recovery time due to redistribution of the medication.

Adverse effects from propofol include hypotension, bradycardia, respiratory depression, injection site pain, involuntary muscle movements, hypertriglyceridemia, and pancreatitis. Rarely, patients who are receiving propofol for more than 48 hours and have additional risk factors may develop propofol-related infusion syndrome. This potentially fatal syndrome is characterized by many different symptoms, including, but not limited to, metabolic acidosis, bradycardia or tachycardia, renal failure, and hyperkalemia. If a patient develops persistent hypotension with propofol infusions, the medication may be changed to an alternative agent such as fentanyl. If the patient needs additional blood pressure support and requires the use of propofol, catecholamine infusions (e.g., norepinephrine) can be used. For transient decreases in blood pressure due to an initial bolus of propofol, patients may receive a bolus of an IV crystalloid fluid (e.g., normal saline, lactated Ringer's) and potentially an IV push of a vasopressor, commonly phenylephrine.[2]

ALERT!

Propofol is not compatible with many other IV infusions and should not be administered in the same IV line as other medications or blood products.

PRACTICE POINT

Propofol may be administered with lidocaine, a local anesthetic, to prevent injection site pain.

Another IV anesthetic is ketamine (Ketalar), which is classified as a dissociative anesthetic. The mechanism of action of this medication is similar to PCP, working as an NMDA receptor antagonist. However, this may not be the only mechanism through which anesthesia is achieved. The onset of action of ketamine is similar to other anesthetics but it has a slightly longer duration of action. The initial dose of ketamine is 0.5 to 2 mg/kg with an infusion dose of 0.25 to 0.35 mg/kg, followed by continuous infusion up to 1 mg/kg/hour. Unlike other anesthetics, ketamine has some analgesic properties. Ketamine is also given by other routes of administration, including the subcutaneous and intramuscular (IM) routes and intranasally as esketamine. Ketamine is utilized for other disease states such as acute agitation, procedural sedation, and refractory status epilepticus, whereas esketamine is used to treat major depressive disorder.[2]

ALERT!

Ketamine is a CIII controlled substance and has been used illicitly. Hence, it may be stored in a special location in the hospital pharmacy. Adverse effects from ketamine include hallucinations, vivid dreams, hypertension, tachycardia, increased muscle movements, and respiratory depression.

Etomidate is an IV anesthetic that is commonly used for patients at an increased risk for hemodynamic instability during anesthesia, as it does not reduce blood pressure and increases cardiac output. Etomidate has a rapid onset of action and a half-life of about 3 hours, making it a good option for starting anesthesia at a dose of 0.2 to 0.6 mg/kg. Etomidate is commonly the anesthetic of choice in patients who have hypo- or hypertension, risk for increased intracranial pressures, and who are in need of sedation for rapid-sequence intubation. While etomidate does not affect the cardiovascular or respiratory systems, postoperative nausea and vomiting is significantly increased. Another adverse effect is the suppression of stress hormone release, leading to decreased cortisol concentrations in the blood and increased mortality.[2]

CASE?

Mr. Jones is admitted to the ICU for new-onset heart failure. He requires the placement of a Swan-Ganz catheter (pulmonary artery catheter) which is used to closely monitor heart function in patients with heart failure. When the Swan-Ganz catheter is being placed into a large vein, patients can experience significant pain at the site. Which local anesthetic should be used and how should it be administered?

Local anesthetics are applied to a specific part of the body to block the nerves in that part of the body. They block all nerves, motor and sensory, in the localized area. These actions are reversible once the anesthetic is removed or metabolized, and the anesthetizing effects diminish over time. Local anesthesia is preferred when it is not necessary for the patient to lose consciousness during a procedure.[3]

Examples of local anesthetics include lidocaine, bupivacaine, mepivacaine, and tetracaine (Medication Table 5-2). They work by blocking the conduction of action potentials along the nerve and can be used in a variety of contexts, including surgery, dental work, and childbirth. The first medication discovered to have local anesthetic properties was cocaine which, due to the potential for misuse, is not commonly used for this purpose except in emergent situations to provide local vasoconstriction and anesthesia in epistaxis (nosebleed). Adverse effects of this drug class include local site reactions such as pain, redness, and tingling. Those administering local anesthetics must be mindful of the area that they are injecting into, as the volume of the medication itself may cause pain and pressure. Systemic adverse effects such as cardiac conduction abnormalities, bradycardia, seizures, and hypotension are rare, unless a large amount of medication is absorbed systemically. Many times, a local vasoconstrictor like epinephrine is administered along with the local anesthetic to prolong the action of the local anesthetic and prevent large amounts of systemic absorption. Metabolism of local anesthetics occurs in the region in which they are administered and are usually broken down by plasma esterases.[3]

ALERT!

Many injectable local anesthetics are available in multiple strengths and as preparations with varying concentrations of epinephrine already added. Pharmacy technicians must be sure not only to choose the correct agent, but also the correct strength, as well as noting whether or not an epinephrine-containing preparation has been ordered (and, if so, in what strength). Local anesthetics used for spinal administration (e.g., epidural) must always be preservative-free and labeled MPF (methylparaben preservative-free).

For topical anesthesia, direct application of the local anesthetic on the desired place of action is often sufficient and desirable. This application would only affect the area to which it is applied and does not extend to the lower structures of the skin. If the local anesthetic is applied to mucus membranes such as the nose or mouth, then systemic absorption is possible, and the effects may be severe. Such absorption and accompanying adverse effects are not likely if the local anesthetic is used in appropriate amounts. Other areas for local anesthesia include entire nerve roots (nerve block) and specific spinal nerve block. These are useful for local surgical procedures. In such cases, the local anesthetics are administered to the desired site by injection. Topical anesthetics can be compounded together in standard products such as LET gel (lidocaine, epinephrine, and tetracaine) and EMLA cream (lidocaine and prilocaine eutectic mixture). Lidocaine 4% IV solution may also be utilized as a topical anesthetic for bronchoscopies and is administered to patients via nebulizer to decrease the pain associated with this procedure.[3]

Epidural anesthesia is the administration of a local anesthetic by injection into the epidural space in the spinal cord to block the spinal nerve roots, thus causing decreased sensation. This is performed in many surgeries but is used most commonly in childbirth. One advantage to using epidural anesthesia is the ability to place a catheter into the epidural space to administer a continuous dose of local anesthetic. This eliminates the need for repeated injections into the epidural space. In patients who have pain, opioids can be administered with the local anesthetic into the epidural space to give even longer lasting pain relief. Even in patients who are postoperative, the combination of an opioid and local anesthetic administered in the epidural space may be enough to provide adequate pain relief.[3]

CASE STUDY

Mrs. Smith presents to the emergency department following a motor vehicle accident. After conducting a physical assessment, the prescriber writes a prescription for an opioid analgesic for the patient's severe, acute pain.

CASE?

What opioid analgesic options are available for the treatment of acute pain? What are the differences in drug class and mechanism of action between different opioid analgesics?

ANALGESICS

Analgesia is also known as pain relief, and medications used for this purpose are called analgesics. Analgesics are effective for both acute and chronic pain. Pain can come from a variety of sources, such as an injury, cancer, or even nerve pain from diabetes mellitus. A commonly accepted precept is that pain should be treated using the simplest dosage regimens and the most effective treatments for the patient's pain. Pain can be rated subjectively by the patient on a 0 to 10 scale, with 0 being no pain and 10 being the worst pain imaginable. The PQRSTU assessment is another tool available to characterize a patient's pain. It includes P (palliative—what makes the pain better or worse), Q (quality—describe the pain), R (radiation—where is the pain and does it radiate), S (severity—rate pain severity), T (temporal—when did the pain start and how long has it been ongoing), and U (you—how are other aspects of health, such as sleep, mood, and general well-being). Some objective measurements like grimacing, increased heart rate and blood pressure, and favoring a limb can be used, but they are likely absent in a patient with chronic pain.

Several routes of administration are available for analgesics, including oral, IV, IM, rectal, transdermal, buccal, and intranasal. Route of administration is determined by various patient characteristics, but the oral route is preferred for most. Some notable exceptions include patients who cannot take oral medication or when immediate relief of pain is needed.[4]

Analgesics include acetaminophen, nonsteroidal anti-inflammatory drugs (NSAIDs), and opioids. Acetaminophen and NSAIDs are covered in more depth in Chapter 13, so the focus of this section will be opioid analgesics.

Opioid analgesics can be grouped by their chemical structures into several different classes: phenanthrenes, phenylpiperidines, diphenylheptanes, and benzomorphans. Opioids may also be grouped by their mechanisms of action: opioid agonists, opioid antagonists, mixed opioid agonists-antagonists, and opioid partial agonists. Opioid analgesics interact with opioid receptors, which include mu (μ), kappa (κ), and delta (δ) receptors.[4] Opioid agonists work by stimulating opioid receptors in the brain and spinal cord, modulating (usually reducing) the impulses from the pain receptors in the body and providing pain relief. Opioid partial agonists also stimulate opioid receptors and provide pain relief. To their advantage, the partial agonists have a lower risk of respiratory depression than the full agonists. Mixed opioid agonists-antagonists are rarely used in practice today. Opioid antagonists block opioid receptors; therefore, they do not provide pain relief. They reverse the effects of opioid agonists and partial agonists. Naloxone and other opioid antagonists are described in more detail below.

Opioid analgesics can differ from one another in several important ways. Opioids differ by potency. Some are highly potent and useful for severe pain, whereas others are less potent and better for moderate pain. Opioids also differ by mechanism of action. In addition to interacting with opioid receptors, several of these medications have additional actions. For example, tramadol inhibits the reuptake of serotonin and norepinephrine, and methadone antagonizes NMDA receptors. Opioids differ in their pharmacokinetic profiles, including the duration of analgesia that a dose of each medication provides. A comparison of opioid analgesics can be found in Medication Table 5-3.

Clinicians are often tasked with converting one opioid analgesic to a different opioid analgesic. Equianalgesic dosing charts are available to assist with these dosing conversions. These dosing charts often use morphine as the reference standard. Equianalgesic dosing assists the clinician with calculating the equivalent dose between formulations (e.g., IV morphine to oral morphine) or when converting to a different opioid (e.g., morphine to hydromorphone). After the new dose is calculated, some sources recommend reducing the calculated dose by 25% or more to avoid adverse effects such as excessive sedation. This comparison calculation is reflected in Medication Table 5.3 in the column labeled "Equianalgesic Dose."

ALERT!

LOOK-ALIKE/SOUND-ALIKE—Tramadol (an analgesic) and Trazodone (an antidepressant) have been confused.

ALERT!

Careless drug abbreviations can cause errors. Morphine sulfate should never be abbreviated as MS or MSO4. This can be confused with other medications, such as magnesium sulfate (MgSO4).

PRACTICE POINT

Opioid analgesics are listed by the Drug Enforcement Administration (DEA) as controlled substances. Controlled substances can produce physical and psychological dependence. Therefore, they may be stored in a locked cabinet or other special location within the pharmacy. The DEA has different categories, or schedules, of controlled substances (Table 5-1). A special form, DEA 222, is used to order CII controlled substances, which can only be acquired by DEA registrants.

CASE?

Mrs. Smith arrives at the outpatient pharmacy with two opioid prescriptions. The prescriber has written prescriptions for oxycodone immediate-release 5 mg by mouth every 6 hours as needed and oxycodone extended-release 10 mg by mouth every 12 hours. Why might a prescriber order two different dosage forms and strengths of the same opioid medication?

The most frequently employed dosing strategy for opioid agonists in the treatment of acute pain is around-the-clock dosing. This method has been shown to be very effective if the medication is titrated appropriately, by starting with the initial dose of the opioid agonist and then increasing or decreasing based on pain control and adverse effects. If the opioid agonist is given only on an as-needed basis, patients may not get adequate pain control due to the varying blood concentrations of the opioid agonist. For chronic pain, the most useful strategy is a basal-bolus-type dosing strategy. This means that there is a long-acting (8 to 12 hours) opioid agonist used for around-the-clock pain control in addition to an as-needed medication for breakthrough pain. Usually, these two medications are the same opioid agonist. For example, a patient may use extended-release morphine sulfate every 12 hours for basal pain control and then use immediate-release morphine for breakthrough pain as needed every 3 to 4 hours. If a consistent pattern of increased use of the as-needed medication is noted, then this amount of medication can be added to the basal (long-acting) pain control, with a goal to eliminate the necessity for as-needed use of opioid agonists. One important note about opioid analgesics is that opioid agonists have no maximum effective dose; their dose is limited only by adverse

TABLE 5-1. Drug Enforcement Administration Controlled Substance Schedules

Schedule	Definition	Example Medications	Special Order Form Required
CI	No current medical use; high abuse potential; no data for safety under medical supervision	3,4-methylenedioxymethamphetamine (MDMA, or "ecstasy") Heroin Lysergic acid diethylamide Phencyclidine	Yes, for research purposes only
CII	Medical use; high abuse potential; abuse of the drug or other substance may lead to severe psychological or physical dependence	Amphetamines Fentanyl Hydromorphone Meperidine Methadone Methylphenidate Morphine Oxycodone Oxymorphone	Yes
CIII	Medical use; abuse potential is less than schedules I and II; abuse of the drug or other substance may lead to moderate or low physical dependence or high psychological dependence	Buprenorphine Esketamine Ketamine Perampanel Sodium oxybate Testosterone	No

Continued next page

TABLE 5-1. Drug Enforcement Administration Controlled Substance Schedules *(Continued)*

Schedule	Definition	Example Medications	Special Order Form Required
CIV	Medical use; abuse potential is low relative to schedule III; abuse of the drug or other substance may lead to limited physical or psychological dependence	Armodafinil Benzodiazepines (alprazolam, clonazepam, diazepam) Modafinil Nonbenzodiazepine sedative/hypnotics (eszopiclone, zaleplon, zolpidem) Phenobarbital Tramadol	No
CV	Medical use; abuse potential is low relative to schedule IV; abuse of the drug or other substance may lead to limited physical or psychological dependence	Cough syrups containing a small amount of codeine Diphenoxylate with atropine Lacosamide Pregabalin	No

effects. Conversely, tramadol, tapentadol, and opioid partial agonists have maximum doses.

The regular use of opioid analgesics can result in tolerance and physical dependence. Tolerance is defined as needing larger doses of medication to achieve the same effect that occurred when first starting the medication. Physical dependence is defined as the occurrence of withdrawal symptoms upon abrupt reduction of dose or discontinuation of the drug. Opioid withdrawal symptoms (e.g., muscle aches, diarrhea, anxiety) may also result from the administration of an opioid antagonist medication, as discussed later on. Both of these phenomena, tolerance and

physical dependence, are expected with long-term, daily use of opioids and are different from addiction. Addiction is a behavioral pattern characterized as a lack of control over—and compulsive use of—drugs despite negative consequences from use.[5] While tolerance and physical dependence may be present in patients with opioid addiction, the rate of addiction among those who are prescribed opioids for pain relief is small. Many factors influence a patient's risk for addiction, including genetics, social factors, and psychological factors. (Addiction is more thoroughly addressed in Chapter 7.) Pseudoaddiction is a phenomenon that occurs when a patient's pain is undertreated. Patients appear to have symptoms of addiction, but these symptoms resolve once the patient's pain is adequately managed.

Opioid analgesics can cause a number of adverse effects. Opioids cause sedation or drowsiness. Tolerance develops to the sedating effects of opioids, and sedation should dissipate with time. Constipation is a common adverse effect that may not resolve with time. Many options are available to treat opioid-induced constipation, including stimulant laxatives. The release of histamine may contribute to the development of rash and pruritis (itching), and this must be distinguished from an allergic reaction. Management of other adverse effects may be achieved by using the lowest possible dose for the shortest amount of time. Other CNS depressants, such as benzodiazepines or alcohol, should not be used along with opioids as the concurrent use increases the risk of respiratory depression. Major adverse effects of opioid medications are listed in Table 5-2.

Patient-controlled analgesia (PCA) is a commonly utilized pain management strategy for patients within a hospital setting and is also prescribed for outpatients suffering from chronic pain. It is initiated in patients requiring high doses of pain medication who need continuous and breakthrough coverage for pain. In institutional settings, it is often prepared in the form of an IV bag or epidural infusion or provided as a commercially manufactured container compatible with the technology in use, and administered with an automated pump programmed to provide a continuous infusion of pain medication and bolus doses. In outpatient settings, the pumps are frequently much smaller, to be worn or implanted, and epidural administration is more common.

The automated pump technology includes a button that the patient uses to self-administer a premeasured dose of opioid analgesia for breakthrough pain, using preset parameters for dose and frequency. Only a prespecified amount of medication is administered with each button press, and the patient is only able to use the button a certain number of times per hour. The period between allowable doses is commonly referred to as a "lock out period." A PCA pump also includes a continuous infusion of a basal dose of analgesic. This method of administration results in better pain control and the patient feeling empowered. Knowing the number of patient-administered doses (or bolus doses) given helps clinicians determine the adjustments that need to be made to the basal infusion rate, and the amount and frequency of bolus doses. Very close monitoring of certain parameters such as respiratory and heart rate, blood pressure, pulse oximetry, and alertness is needed to ensure the safety of this approach. PCA is generally avoided for patients who are unconscious or unable to provide themselves bolus dosing, as this could lead to inappropriate dosing by family members and others based on their perception of the patient's pain.[4]

TABLE 5-2. Adverse Effects of Opioid Agonists

Body System	Adverse Effects
Central nervous system	Euphoria, drowsiness, withdrawal (upon abrupt discontinuation)
Circulatory system	Orthostatic hypotension
Digestive system	Nausea, vomiting, constipation
Genitourinary system	Urinary retention, sexual dysfunction
Integumentary system	Rash, pruritus (itching)
Respiratory system	Decreased respiratory rate

CASE?

Along with the oxycodone prescriptions, the prescriber also orders intranasal naloxone for Mrs. Smith. The pharmacist trains Mrs. Smith and her spouse on the proper use of intranasal naloxone. What type of medication is naloxone? What is the purpose behind providing naloxone to patients taking opioid analgesics?

Opioid antagonists, such as naloxone and naltrexone, block the effects of opioid analgesics. If a patient taking opioid analgesics has developed physical dependence, the administration of an opioid antagonist will precipitate opioid withdrawal symptoms. Therefore, opioid antagonists are administered only in specific circumstances. Naltrexone is a long-acting opioid antagonist used to treat patients with either opioid or alcohol addiction. Naloxone, an opioid antagonist with a more immediate onset and shorter duration of action, is used to reverse life-threatening situations of intentional or unintentional opioid overdose.

When administered promptly, naloxone can prevent opioid overdose–related deaths. It does not reverse overdoses caused by other substances (e.g., benzodiazepines, cocaine). Symptoms of opioid intoxication include slow or shallow breathing, drowsiness or coma, blue lips or fingertips, and slow heart rate. Naloxone reverses opioid-induced respiratory depression. It can be administered by IV, IM, or subcutaneous injection or by intranasal administration. Depending on route of administration, naloxone may start to work in as little as 2 to 5 minutes. Because naloxone is short acting (i.e., duration of approximately 30 to 120 minutes), several doses may be required to reverse the effects of longer-acting opioid analgesics.[6] While individual state laws differ, most have expanded naloxone access in the community setting (e.g., dispensing naloxone without a prescription under a physician collaborative practice agreement). The intranasal formulation is often distributed in the community setting due to ease of administration. Because it is a "bystander-administered" medication, all individuals with access to it (e.g., patient, family members, caregivers) require overdose prevention education, instructions on how to administer the specific naloxone product dispensed, and instructions for responding to an overdose situation.

Responding to an opioid overdose begins with attempting to wake the individual by calling his or her name and by firmly rubbing in the middle of the individual's chest (i.e., sternal rub). Emergency services (i.e., 911) should be contacted. It is important to ensure nothing is in the individual's mouth or throat that can affect breathing. After these steps, naloxone can be administered, and rescue breathing provided if the individual is not breathing. Naloxone doses are repeated as indicated. If the individual begins breathing, the individual should be placed on his or her side in the recovery position to prevent aspiration. Someone should stay with the individual until emergency medical services arrive.[7]

SUMMARY

The CNS is a complex organization of neurons and neurotransmitters that serve as useful medication targets. There are many different neurotransmitters that act on various systems in the brain and spinal cord. Neurotransmitters serve as unique medication targets that can assist with anesthesia and analgesia. Anesthetics are useful for surgery, pain control, and minor procedures. General anesthetics can be administered IV or inhaled, each having different utility in various areas of medicine. Among the most common of these is propofol, which has many characteristics that make it unique. Local and topical anesthetics are utilized for targeted application during simple surgical procedures. Opioid analgesics are among the medications most commonly prescribed for pain and share many similar properties. Opioids can be given by multiple routes of administration. Patients requiring continuous infusions of opioid pain medications and in need of additional doses for breakthrough pain may qualify for patient-controlled analgesia.

REFERENCES

1. Free RB, Clark J, Amara S, Sibley DR. Neurotransmission in the central nervous system. In: Brunton LL, Hilal-Dandan R, Knollmann BC, eds. *Goodman & Gilman's: The Pharmacological Basis of Therapeutics*. 13th ed. New York, NY: McGraw-Hill; 2018:243-266.

2. Patel HH, Pearn ML, Patel PM, Roth DM. General anesthetics and therapeutic gases. In: Brunton LL, Hilal-Dandan R, Knollmann BC, eds. *Goodman & Gilman's: The Pharmacological Basis of Therapeutics*. 13th ed. New York, NY: McGraw-Hill; 2018:387-404.

3. Catterall WA, Mackie K. Local anesthetics. In: Brunton LL, Hilal-Dandan R, Knollmann BC, eds. *Goodman & Gilman's: The Pharmacological Basis of Therapeutics*. 13th ed. New York, NY: McGraw-Hill; 2018:405-420.

4. Schumacher MA, Basbaum AI, Naidu RK. Opioid agonists and antagonists. In: Katzung BG, Vanderah TW, eds. *Basic and Clinical Pharmacology*. 15th ed. New York, NY: McGraw-Hill; 2021:573-595.

5. American Psychiatric Association. *Diagnostic and Statistical Manual of Mental Disorders*. 5th ed. Arlington, VA: American Psychiatric Association; 2013.

6. Lexicomp Online. Lexi-Drugs Online. Hudson, Ohio: Wolters Kluwer; 2021.

7. Substance Abuse and Mental Health Services Administration. SAMHSA Opioid Overdose Prevention Toolkit. https://store.samhsa.gov/sites/default/files/d7/priv/sma18-4742.pdf. Accessed October 24, 2021.

REVIEW QUESTIONS

1. Explain the function of meninges and how the blood–brain barrier is important to medication therapy.

2. Describe the roles of common neurotransmitters, such as dopamine, serotonin, and GABA, and list medications that affect each neurotransmitter.

3. What is anesthesia and why is it important?

4. How do addiction, pseudoaddiction, physical dependence, and tolerance differ?

5. Which adverse effects are common among opioid agonist medications?

FURTHER READING

Becker DE, Reed KL. Local anesthetics: Review of pharmacologic considerations. *Anesth Prog*. 2012;59(2):90-102.

Vearrier D, Grundmann O. Clinical pharmacology, toxicity, and abuse potential of opioids. *J Clin Pharmacol*. 2021;61 (2 Suppl):S70-S88.

MEDICATION TABLES

MEDICATION TABLE 5-1. Intravenous Anesthetics[6]

Generic Name (pronunciation)	Brand Name	Available Preparations (mg)	Induction Dose (IV) (mg/kg)	Induction Dose Duration (minutes)	Uses	Notes
Methohexital (meth oh HEKS i tal)	Brevital	500, 2,500 preservative-free injectable solution	1.0–1.5	4–7	Anesthesia, procedural sedation	Immediate onset of action Used for intracarotid testing (Wada test)
Etomidate (e TOM i date)	Amidate		0.2–0.6	0.5–1	General anesthesia, procedural sedation, rapid-sequence intubation	Used in Cushing syndrome
Propofol (PROE po fole)	Diprivan, Fresenius Propoven, Propofol-Lipuro	100 mg/10mL 200 mg/20 mL 1,000 mg/100 mL, 500 mg/50 mL (Preservative free available)	1.5–2.5	4–8	General anesthesia, sedation for mechanically ventilated ICU patients, sedation and regional anesthesia	Avoid in patients with egg and soy allergy Contains 1.1 kcal/mL
Ketamine (KEET a meen)	Ketalar	10, 50, 100 injectable solution Prefilled IV syringe: 50 mg/5 mL	0.5–2	1–3	Procedural sedation, rapid-sequence intubation, analgesia/sedation/agitation, depression, status epilepticus, chronic pain	Can be administered by intravenous, intramuscular, subcutaneous, intranasal, or intraosseous means

MEDICATION TABLE 5-2. Local Anesthetics[a,6]

Generic Name (pronunciation)	Brand Name	Available Preparations	Onset of Action (minutes)	Duration of Anesthesia (hours)	Uses	Notes
Bupivacaine (byoo PIV a kane)	Marcaine, Sensorcaine	Injectable formulations (available with and without preservatives): 0.25%, 0.5%, 0.75% (without epinephrine) 0.25%, 0.5%, 0.75% (with epinephrine 1:200,000) preservatives—MPF)	5	2–8	Surgery, dental procedures, obstetrics (includes nerve block and epidural)	Available in preservative-free dextrose injection for spinal anesthesia
Bupivacaine (Liposomal) (byoo PIV a kane lye po SO mal)	Exparel	Suspension, injection: 1.3%	Rapid	Up to 72	Local postsurgical analgesia	Single-dose infiltration or nerve block
Lidocaine (LYE doe kane)	Xylocaine, LidaMantle, Lidoderm, others	Injection: 0.5%, 1%, 1.5%, 2%, 4% (with and without epinephrine; with and without preservatives—MPF) Topical: solution, ointment, cream, lotion, gel, patch in various strengths	<2	0.5–1	Injection: nerve block, IV administration Topical: skin, anorectal area, oral area, many others; sterile preparations for ophthalmic use, nebulized inhalation for bronchoscopy	Also used to treat life-threatening cardiac arrhythmias
Mepivacaine (me PIV a kane)	Carbocaine, Polocaine	Injection only: 1%, 1.5%, 2%, 3% with and without preservatives—MPF	3–20	2–2.5	Peripheral nerve block, obstetrics (includes epidural), infiltration, dental procedures, pain management	
Ropivacaine (roe PIV a kane)	Naropin	2 mg/mL (10 mL, 20 mL, 100 mL, 200 mL) 5 mg/mL (20 mL, 30 mL, 100 mL, 200 mL) 7.5 mg/20 mL, 10 mg/mL (10 mL, 20 mL)	3–15	3–15	Surgical anesthesia, epidural for labor pain, postoperative pain management	Reduced toxicity compared to bupivacaine
Tetracaine (TET ra kane)	Altacaine, others	Injection: 0.5%, 1%, 2%, 20 mg for reconstitution Ophthalmic, mouth/throat solution, ointment	<30	10–20 minutes	Injection: spinal anesthesia Topical products: local anesthesia, pain relief	Not used with epinephrine

MPF = methylparaben free

[a]Pronunciations have been adapted with permission from USP Dictionary of USAN and International Drug Names (USP Dictionary) © 2022.

MEDICATION TABLE 5-3. Opioid Analgesics[6]

Generic Name (pronunciation)	Brand Name	Route	Duration of Analgesia (hours)	Equianalgesic Dose (mg)	Notes
Drug Class: Phenanthrenes **Mechanism of Action: Opioid Agonists**					
Codeine (KOE deen)	Various	Oral	3–4	200	Often combined with acetaminophen (Tylenol with codeine #3)
Hydrocodone (hye droe KOE done)	Zohydro ER	Oral	4–6	30	Often combined with acetaminophen (Lorcet, Norco, Vicodin)
Hydromorphone (hye droe MOR fone)	Dilaudid	Oral IV Rectal	3–4	7.5 (oral) 1.5 (IV)	More potent than morphine; IM administration is not recommended
Morphine (MOR feen)	MS Contin, Roxanol, others	Oral IV Rectal Intrathecal	4–5	30 (oral) 10 (IV)	The standard opioid to which other opioids are generally compared
Oxycodone (oks i KOE done)	Oxycontin, others	Oral	3–4	20	Often combined with acetaminophen (Percocet)
Oxymorphone (oks i MOR fone)		Oral	3–4	10	More potent than morphine
Drug Class: Phenanthrenes **Mechanism of Action: Partial Opioid Agonists**					
Buprenorphine (byoo pre NOR feen)	Buprenex, Butrans, Belbuca Sublocade, Subutex	Oral IV IM, sublingual Topical	4–8	0.3 (IV)	Topical formulation (patch) applied once every 7 days; other formulations (Subutex, Sublocade) used to manage opioid addiction
Drug Class: Phenanthrenes **Mechanism of Action: Opioid Agonists-Antagonists**					
Butorphanol (byoo TOR fa nole)		IV IM Intranasal	3–4	2 (IV)	Rarely used; only opioid available as an intranasal formulation
Nalbuphine (NAL byoo feen)		IV IM	3–6	10 (IV)	Rarely used
Drug Class: Phenylpiperidines **Mechanism of Action: Opioid Agonists**					
Fentanyl (FEN ta nil)	Actiq, Duragesic, Subsys, others	Oral IV IM Topical	1–1.5	0.125 (IV)	Topical formulation (patch) not for acute pain; other similar drugs include sufentanil and remifentanil
Meperidine (me PER i deen)	Demerol	Oral IV IM	2–4	300 (oral) 100 (IV)	Less commonly used for analgesia than other drugs; may cause seizures, especially in patients with poor kidney function

Continued next page

MEDICATION TABLE 5-3. Opioid Analgesics[6] *(Continued)*

Generic Name (pronunciation)	Brand Name	Route	Duration of Analgesia (hours)	Equianalgesic Dose (mg)	Notes
Drug Class: Diphenylheptanes **Mechanism of Action: Opioid Agonists**					
Methadone (METH a done)	Dolophine, Methadose	Oral IV IM	8–12	Variable	Used for analgesia; also used to manage opioid addiction; high doses may require heart rhythm monitoring
Drug Class: Miscellaneous **Mechanism of Action: Opioid Agonists**					
Tramadol (TRA ma dole)	Ultram	Oral	4–6	120	Inhibits reuptake of norepinephrine and serotonin; increases risk of seizures
Tapentadol (ta PEN ta dol)	Nucynta	Oral	4–6	100	Inhibits reuptake of norepinephrine; increases risk of seizures

IM = intramuscular; IV = intravenous.

MEDICATION TABLE 5-4. Representative Emergency Opioid Antagonists[6]

Generic Name (pronunciation)	Brand Name	Route	Dose (mg)	Instructions for Use
Naloxone (nal OKS one)	Narcan, others	IM IV Subcutaneous	0.4–2, up to 10	Remove cap from vial and uncover needle; insert needle into vial and pull back on plunger; administer 0.4–2 mg by injection; administer additional doses every 2–3 minutes if needed; evaluate for other causes of respiratory depression if no response following administration of 10 mg total
Naloxone (nal OKS one)	Narcan	Intranasal	2, 4	Tilt the individual's head back and support the neck with one hand; using other hand, insert the nozzle into either nostril; press the plunger firmly to administer a single spray into one nostril; administer additional doses every 2–3 minutes if needed, alternating nostrils, using a new device each time
Naloxone (nal OKS one)	Kloxxado	Intranasal	8	Tilt the individual's head back and support the neck with one hand; using the other hand, insert the nozzle into either nostril; press the plunger firmly to administer a single spray into one nostril; administer additional doses every 2–3 minutes if needed, alternating nostrils, using a new device each time
Naloxone (nal OKS one)	Zimhi	IM Subcutaneous	5	Preferably administered by individuals 12 years and older; administer into anterolateral thigh by IM or subcutaneous injection; may be injected through clothing if needed; administer additional doses every 2–3 minutes if needed using a new device each time

IM = intramuscular; IV = intravenous.

Chapter 6
Neurologic Disorders

Toy S. Biederman, PharmD

KEY TERMS AND DEFINITIONS

Anticonvulsant—a drug that helps to reduce the tendency of the brain to have a seizure. Although their primary use is for epilepsy, anticonvulsants are also used to treat psychiatric disorders, pain syndromes, and migraines.

Aura—a sensory experience that precedes a neurologic event, such as a migraine or seizure. During an aura, the patient may see, smell, or hear something unusual, or have a strange feeling, such as déjà vu (the feeling that one has been in a new place previously). In the case of seizures, the aura is actually a simple partial seizure.

Seizure—a neurological event caused by abnormal electrical activity in the brain. Seizures come in many types. Some cause a patient to fall and thrash about on the floor, and others cause a loss of awareness without falling.

Spasm—a strong, unexpected, often painful muscle contraction.

Tremor—an involuntary, fast musculoskeletal movement. Tremors can be due to neurological conditions, such as Parkinson's disease and multiple sclerosis, excessive intake of stimulants, such as caffeine, or may be a harmless genetic condition, such as essential tremor. Tremors may affect the hands, chin, and other parts of the body.

DOI 10.37573/9781585286638.006

LEARNING OBJECTIVES

After completing this chapter, you should be able to

1. Describe how lesions in the brain and peripheral nervous system are related to neurological diseases.

2. List the causes, symptoms, and expected course of the following illnesses:
    *   Headache—migraine, cluster, and tension.
    *   Stroke.
    *   Parkinson's disease.
    *   Dementia.
    *   Epilepsy.
    *   Multiple sclerosis.
    *   Neuropathic pain.
    *   Sleep disorders.

3. Describe the psychosocial consequences for patients and families of patients with neurologic disorders.

4. State the generic and brand names of representative medications used to treat neurologic disorders, along with dosage forms and available doses.

5. List the mechanism of action, common adverse effects, and special precautions of medications used to treat neurologic disorders.

Neurologic disorders tend to be chronic illnesses, many of which are progressive in the decline of function. They include conditions ranging from those as common as migraine headaches to rare genetic diseases. Some diseases affect memory and reasoning, such as Alzheimer's disease. Others, such as multiple sclerosis and amyotrophic lateral sclerosis, cause deterioration in the body while the mind is mostly intact. And many, such as epilepsy, are subject to social stigma, due to the sudden and often frightening onset of seizures or the muscle rigidity and hallucinations associated with Parkinson's disease. Many of these conditions cause stress not only for the patient but also for caregivers and loved ones. Occasionally, medications can cause neurologic deficits.

In the past 30 years, there has been an enormous increase in the availability of medications to treat many of these diseases but none to cure them. Many of the medications in use are prescribed to delay disease progression; others are indicated to help manage the symptoms. People with neurologic diseases may have life spans close to normal but with 20 years or more of progressing disability. Patients and their families need health workers who understand the difficulties posed by their conditions.

What causes neurologic disorders? As the name implies, there are problems within the nervous system—the brain, spinal cord, and peripheral nerves that communicate with every part of the body. When this system is working well, we can multiply, remember old songs, walk a balance beam, hit a target with an arrow, and carry on a normal conversation. Our chewing and swallowing are coordinated so that we don't choke. Our bowels and bladders do their jobs without stubbornly balking at their tasks. Our fingers can feel hot and cold objects, and we can feel a pebble in our shoe. We can pick up a quarter from the floor without falling over. We readily fall asleep when we are tired at night and wake up rested in the morning. Any of these systems can be thrown off by disease. Sometimes the disease attacks the nerves themselves. Sometimes there is a particular area of the brain that is affected. Often particular neurotransmitters—chemicals that carry messages from one nerve to another—are out of balance.

Many of the medications used to treat neurologic disorders are specific to a certain disease. Others are prescribed for several different conditions. Some medications used to treat epilepsy are also used to treat pain conditions, migraine headaches, and mood disorders. Some medications used to treat depression are also used to treat pain and migraine. There are many overlapping characteristics of neurologic diseases and psychiatric diseases (Chapter 7). Neurologic disorders are more likely to be detected by a physical examination and diagnostic procedures, such as MRI (magnetic resonance imaging) scans and EEGs (electroencephalograms). Psychiatric diseases are more likely to be diagnosed by the patients' descriptions of their emotions, thoughts, and behavior. There is often overlap—patients with neurologic disorders frequently experience depression, for example.

HEADACHE

Headache disorders are one of the most common neurologic conditions we encounter. Many conditions can cause headaches, and we must not treat this condition lightly. In addition, the overuse of over-the-counter (OTC) headache medications can lead to a condition of chronic daily headache, which is difficult to manage. Patients who describe frequent headaches, headaches that accompany certain activities (for example, coughing or sex), or a new headache that is the worst they have ever had, should see a doctor for evaluation. See Medication Table 6-1 for a list of medications commonly prescribed for the treatment of headache. (Medication Tables are located at the end of the chapter.)

CASE STUDY

R. B. is a 32-year-old woman who goes to her doctor because of a 6-month history of throbbing headaches on the right side of her head. She has been having these headaches once or twice a week. Before the headache starts, she sees beams of light that come together to form a figure that looks like the letter c, which floats around changing position and color. When she has the headaches, she also feels sick to her stomach and cannot stand to be around any light or noise. She has to go into a dark room and sleep. The headache is not relieved by two tablets of either aspirin 325 mg or ibuprofen 200 mg and generally lasts all day unless she is able to lie in a dark room and sleep. The headaches usually interfere with her ability to continue work. R. B. does not know what triggers her headaches but says she gets more headaches the week before her period. She says that both her mother and grandmother had "sick headaches."

CASE?

What kind of headache does R. B. most likely have?

For occasional tension headaches, OTC acetaminophen, ibuprofen, or naproxen is usually sufficient. (These medications are covered in detail in other chapters; please consult the index.) The patient can also be questioned about caffeine use. Sudden withdrawal from a daily high intake of caffeine can cause severe headaches, which can be treated by reintroducing a source of caffeine and gradually decreasing the amount ingested over several days.

Migraine headaches are a particularly distressing and incapacitating type of headache that is very common and may even occur in children. Migraines are characterized by throbbing on one side of the head. Patients are sensitive to light, sound, or both. Migraines are also known as "sick headaches" because they are frequently accompanied by nausea. In some patients the headache is preceded by a visual aura. Migraines are often relieved by sleep.

Many migraine sufferers are able to detect headache triggers by charting their headaches on a calendar. They can monitor how often the headaches occur, their intensity,

and if a food or beverage appeared to cause the headache. Women often find that their headaches are more likely to occur at a certain time during their menstrual cycle. As with patients with tension headaches, patients with frequent migraine headaches should be encouraged to see a doctor to help better manage the problem. Infrequent migraines often will respond to OTC pain medications and rest, but more frequent migraines are better treated with medicines that prevent or reduce the frequency of the headaches, as well as medications that are used to stop the headache once it has started.

Cluster headaches are less common than migraine but also very debilitating when they occur. Unlike migraines, which are more common in women, cluster headaches are much more likely to occur in men. The headache is a short but intensely painful sensation. Cluster headache sufferers often describe the pain as feeling as if they had a knife stabbing one eyeball. In addition to intense pain on one side of the head, they often have a reddened, teary eye and runny nose. Cluster headache sufferers are not usually sensitive to light or sound. The headache is not relieved by sleep—in fact, the headache sometimes starts while the patient is asleep. Sometimes the patient will pace around or go outside if the weather is cold in an attempt to get some relief. This kind of headache usually only lasts a few minutes, but the patient experiences clusters of these short headaches—several in a day or over a few weeks—and then they will disappear for an extended period.

CASE?

What medication might R. B.'s doctor prescribe?

Because cluster headaches are very short in duration, oral medications are not useful since they take too long to work. For quick relief, injectable sumatriptan is used. Inhaled oxygen will abort an attack for some people. The strategy is also to prevent the attacks by using medications prophylactically, although not all of the medications used prophylactically for migraines are effective for cluster headaches. Drugs used for cluster headache prophylaxis include verapamil and certain anticonvulsants.

The approach to managing migraine headaches is both to try to prevent them (prophylactic therapy) and to treat the headache when it occurs. Treating the headache at the first sign of onset is usually more effective at getting rid of it than waiting to try to treat a full-blown migraine. Prophylactic medications include several classes of drugs originally intended for other problems (and covered in other chapters of this text). Beta-blockers (eg, metoprolol, propranolol) were originally used to treat high blood pressure. Antidepressants (amitriptyline and venlafaxine) and antiepileptic drugs (valproate and topiramate) can be used to prevent migraines. Usually, drugs used for prevention must be taken by the patient for several weeks to get the best effects. Patients need to be patient and keep a headache diary to monitor benefits. The reduction in headache frequency may take several weeks to occur.

Medications used to stop an attack that has already developed include drugs derived from ergot and the triptan (selective serotonin agonist) class. Both of these classes of drugs act by increasing serotonin activity to constrict blood vessels in the cranium and possibly reduce inflammation that is contributing to the headache.

Ergot-derived drugs include dihydroergotamine, which is available as an injection and as a nasal spray, and ergotamine tablets. Ergot is a fungus that grows on grain. In the Middle Ages, people who consumed this fungus experienced toxic symptoms, such as hallucinations, muscle spasms, and gangrene due to blood vessel constriction. In small doses, drugs derived from ergot cause constriction of blood vessels affected by the migraine reaction. These medications must not be used in women who are pregnant, because they can cause contractions of the uterus, resulting in miscarriage. In addition, they can cause nausea, vomiting, and numbness and tingling in the fingers, toes, and face. They should not be used at the same time or within a day of other ergots or triptans. Patients with heart and blood vessel disease should not use these medications. These medications are only used at the time of the attack and are limited in how often they may be repeated.

The triptan class (selective serotonin agonists) is the most popular drug class used to stop migraine attacks when ibuprofen or other OTC products are not sufficient. There are many drugs in this category: almotriptan, eletriptan, frovatriptan, naratriptan, rizatriptan, sumatriptan, and zolmitriptan. They all act in the same way but differ in how quickly they work, how long their effects last, dosage forms, and some drug interactions. Dosage forms in this class include tablets, orally dissolving tablets, and nasal sprays. Sumatriptan is the only drug in this class available for administration by subcutaneous (SUBQ) injection. These drugs are used at the first sign of migraine. Side effects can include dizziness, chest tightness, nausea, numbness, and sweating.[1]

Lasmiditan (Reyvow) is an oral serotonin receptor agonist that targets a different receptor than the triptans do.[2] It is indicated for the treatment of acute migraine. Lasmiditan may cause intense drowsiness, and patients must not drive or operate machinery for several hours after taking this medication.

Because of the risk of serotonin syndrome, serotonin receptor agonists must be used with caution in patients who are taking other medications with activity affecting serotonin, such as selective serotonin reuptake inhibitors (SSRIs) and some antidepressants. Serotonin syndrome can cause abnormal muscle contractions, incoordination, and cardiovascular problems that can be life threatening.

ALERT!

Patients with ischemic heart disease (angina, coronary heart disease, and others) should not use medications from the triptan class.

A newer class of drugs specifically targets the activity of the trigeminal nerve, which has been implicated in migraine pain. Drugs in this class are called calcitonin gene-related peptide (CGRP) antagonists ("blockers").[2] Unlike ergot derivatives and triptans, drugs that target CGRP activity do not directly cause constriction of blood vessels. Some of these agents are monoclonal antibodies—proteins biologically engineered to bind CGRP or its receptors—and are used for migraine prevention. Most of the monoclonal antibody CGRP antagonists—erenumab, fremanezumab, and galcanezumab—are injected subcutaneously monthly. Fremanezumab may also be administered quarterly (every 3 months). Another CGRP blocking monoclonal antibody, eptinezumab, is administered by intravenous infusion every 3 months. Galcanezumab is also approved for the treatment of episodic cluster headaches. All may cause hypersensitivity reactions, usually mild, and injection site reactions. Erenumab may also cause constipation. Three other CGRP receptor antagonists are approved for use in the treatment of migraine. These agents—atogepant, ubrogepant and rimegepant (also called gepants)—differ from the monoclonal antibodies mentioned earlier, and are smaller molecules that block the ability of CGRP to bind to its receptors. The gepants are administered orally.[2] Atogepant (Qulipta) is a once-daily oral dose for migraine prevention. Ubrogepant (Ubrelvy) is taken as a single oral dose when a migraine begins; the dose may be repeated two hours later if needed. Rimegepant (Nurtec) is an orally disintegrating tablet usually taken every other day to prevent migraine, but has been used to treat attacks in patients for whom triptans are ineffective or contraindicated.[3] The gepants have a low incidence of side effects, but some patients experience nausea and fatigue or drowsiness.

STROKE

CASE STUDY

L. D. is a 72-year-old woman with high blood pressure and diabetes. While dining out with her husband, she suddenly became confused and began slurring her words. Her husband also noticed that her face was droopy on the left side. The restaurant manager called the emergency squad. The paramedics examined her and said that she appeared to be having a stroke. They transported L. D. along with her husband to the hospital in their town that has a stroke treatment center. L. D.'s blood pressure was 180/122 mm Hg on arrival, and her glucose level was 153 mg/dL. The CT scan was normal.

CASE?

Why was it important for L. D. to be rushed to the hospital rather than waiting awhile to see if her symptoms went away?

Stroke is a condition caused by either bleeding or a clot in the brain. A stroke due to bleeding in the brain is called a hemorrhagic stroke. A stroke due to a blood clot, which cuts off the blood supply to a section of the brain, is called a thrombotic stroke. In adults, thrombotic strokes are much more common than hemorrhagic strokes. Both kinds can cause severe debility or death. If a thrombotic stroke is detected early enough, medication may be able to dissolve the clot and resume the blood flow in the brain before permanent damage occurs. It is very important to recognize the symptoms of stroke and get help immediately. Symptoms of a stroke are a sudden severe headache, sudden weakness, or inability to talk or walk. Symptoms are usually on one side of the body. When a stroke is suspected, it is important to call for emergency help to get the patient to a hospital that is equipped to evaluate and treat stroke patients quickly. If the patient meets the qualifications for receiving medication (alteplase, described below) to break up the clot (for a thrombotic stroke that has occurred less than 3 hours ago, in a patient who has not had recent surgery or bleeding problems), the medication can often return the patient to his or her original level of functioning. Risks of stroke include uncontrolled high blood pressure, age, atrial fibrillation (a heart rhythm problem), and diabetes. In addition to treating the stroke, it is also important to treat blood pressure or heart rhythm problems. Patients are also routinely started on antiplatelet or anticoagulant therapy to reduce the risk of another clot forming. Antiplatelet agents used include aspirin, clopidogrel, and dipyridamole. (These agents are discussed in detail in Chapter 16.) The anticoagulant, apixaban, is another option. (See Chapter 26.) In addition, stroke patients are usually started on a statin drug (see Chapter 16), which has been shown to reduce the occurrence of future strokes.

CASE?

Since there was no sign of bleeding, the physician said that L. D. was having a thrombotic stroke. Which treatment could be prescribed to break up the clot? What did the emergency room team need to know about L. D. first?

Alteplase, also called tPA or tissue plasminogen activator, breaks up the clot (details in Chapter 16) that has caused a thrombotic stroke. Alteplase is administered by intravenous (IV) infusion as soon as the patient has been deemed to qualify for its use. Since alteplase can dissolve any clots in the body, a patient who has had recent surgery or bleeding problems usually cannot take this drug. Also, excessively high blood pressure must be brought to a safer level before alteplase is given.

PARKINSON'S DISEASE

Parkinson's disease (PD) is a condition that affects about 1 million people in the United States. This disease is not common in younger patients, but the incidence increases with age. PD is named for an English physician, James Parkinson, who described people he met in the street who had similar characteristics. His description is still considered

W. S. is a 62-year-old man who comes to his doctor's office complaining that he feels achy and tired all the time, and his right hand shakes. He says that he often drops tools or dishes. On examination, W. S. appears in good health, with no previous problems since he broke his arm 2 years ago. His posture is stooped, and he walks with a shuffling gait. Neurological examination shows balance problems and rigidity in his right hand. W. S. also says he has developed constipation even though his diet hasn't changed, and his wife says he thrashes around in his sleep. W. S. works as a construction foreman and likes to do woodworking in his spare time. He says he is thinking of retiring early because he feels like he is slowing down too much.

CASE?

What symptoms of PD does W. S. exhibit?

accurate today. The most common traits associated with PD are bradykinesia (general slowness of movement), muscular rigidity, balance problems, and tremor. The tremor is described as "pill rolling," meaning the fingers (usually the forefinger and middle finger) rub against the thumb at a specific frequency. This tremor usually appears only on one side of the body in the early stages of the disease. Sometimes it is not present at all, but everyone with PD will have problems with slowness and rigidity.

CASE?

What effects might PD have on W. S.'s activities of daily living?

Patients with PD are at a high risk for falls due to the rigidity and balance problems. Medications that can cause orthostatic hypotension (decreased blood pressure when getting out of bed or up from a chair), including some medications used to treat PD, can greatly increase this risk.

The movement problems due to PD are caused by the loss of dopamine activity in the area of the brain called the substantia nigra. By the time symptoms such as tremor and rigidity are detected, the brain has lost more than 80% of its dopamine activity. Some patients report earlier problems, such as loss of the sense of smell, depression, and rapid eye movement sleep behavior disorder in the years preceding the diagnosis of PD. Movement problems are not the only symptoms of PD. Most patients also have problems with oily skin, constipation, and drooling. Some will develop hallucinations (which can also be caused by PD medications), muscle spasms, and dementia.

In treating PD, the challenge is to give adequate amounts of medication so that the patient is able to move for as long as possible during the day without causing side effects due to those medications, such as hallucinations, dyskinesias (excessive abnormal movements), and dystonic reactions (muscle spasms). As the disease progresses, this balance becomes more difficult. In talking with a patient with PD, you may notice that the patient gives you very little nonverbal expressions of understanding. The face often appears mask-like, and the voice may be low in volume and range of expression. Answers may come slowly. These are also common PD traits and, unfortunately, they contribute to patient isolation. The patient's handwriting often becomes very small (micrographia); the patient's posture is usually stooped, and he or she often walks with a slow, shuffling gait. Because PD medications can also cause abnormal movements, the patient may appear to sway or writhe at certain times—usually when the drug is in its peak phase. As the disease progresses, the patient will usually need a cane, walker, or wheelchair.

CASE?

Which drugs might W. S. be taking for PD?

Medications used to treat PD are aimed at increasing the dopamine activity in the brain. These medications fall into several categories. (See Medication Table 6-2.) Anticholinergic drugs are sometimes used. The neurotransmitter, acetylcholine, is in a balance with dopamine, as if they were on the opposing seats of a seesaw. When the level of dopamine is low, acetylcholine is overly active. Using an anticholinergic drug returns this balance closer to normal by reducing the activity of acetylcholine. Anticholinergic drugs are mostly used to reduce tremor activity. They can also be useful in reducing drooling. However, because most PD patients are elderly, anticholinergics must be used very cautiously because they can increase the risk of delirium and falls. Anticholinergic drugs used to treat PD include benztropine (Cogentin), biperiden (Akineton), and trihexyphenidyl (Artane).

Monoamine oxidase inhibitors are another class of medications that have the effect of increasing levels (and, thus, activity) of dopamine in the brain by inhibiting one of the enzymes, monoamine oxidase, that breaks down dopamine. They may be used alone in early stages of PD or in combination with other drugs as the disease progresses. These drugs are similar to amphetamines as they can interfere with sleep. For this reason, they must be dosed early in the day. Drugs in this category include selegiline (Eldepryl and Zelapar), rasagiline (Azilect), and safinamide (Xadago).

Amantadine, a drug that was originally used to prevent influenza A, was found to also have activity in PD patients. It has some anticholinergic activity, so it must be used with caution in elderly patients. In addition, since amantadine is partly removed from the body by the kidneys, patients with decreased kidney function will need lower daily doses. Amantadine is no longer marketed under the Symmetrel brand, but some doctors and patients may still use that name. There are two once-daily (extended-release) amantadine products, Gocovri and Osmolex ER, which are approved for use in Parkinson's disease and also for drug-induced extrapyramidal reactions.

Levodopa is a drug that actually increases the amount of dopamine in the brain. Dopamine itself cannot be used for PD because it cannot enter the brain from the systemic circulation. Levodopa is an alteration of the dopamine molecule that can cross the blood–brain barrier into the brain, where it is converted to dopamine. Carbidopa, which accompanies levodopa in the brand-name products Sinemet, Parcopa, Rytary, and the enteric pump product, Duopa, prevents the conversion of levodopa to dopamine until the drug gets into the brain. Levodopa is one of the most important drugs used in managing PD, but it is not without its drawbacks. It has a fairly short duration of action, so it must be dosed several times daily. There are long-acting carbidopa/levodopa preparations, which can be taken twice a day, but the onset of action for long-acting carbidopa/levodopa is delayed, so the patient may need to take an immediate-release tablet early in the morning in order to be able to get moving sooner. In addition, as PD progresses many patients will take both the long-acting drug (two or three times a day) and also several doses of the immediate-release drug during the day.

PRACTICE POINT

Levodopa comes in a variety of dosage forms and strengths, with and without carbidopa, and some are extended-release preparations. Entacapone is also included in some products. The pharmacy technician must exercise care to choose the product that precisely matches the one that has been prescribed. Combination and extended-release brands are not interchangeable.

Dopamine agonists are medications that mimic the effects of dopamine on the dopamine receptors in the brain. Since they act in a similar manner to dopamine, they can postpone the need for carbidopa/levodopa. They are often an early choice for younger patients with PD. Dopamine agonists include bromocriptine (Parlodel), pramipexole (Mirapex), ropinirole, and the transdermal patch, rotigotine (Neupro). In addition, the injectable dopamine agonist apomorphine (Apokyn) is used to provide relief from "off episodes," in which patients become frozen and unable to move. All drugs that increase dopamine activity, including both dopamine agonists and levodopa, have the potential to cause hallucinations, dyskinesias (abnormal movements), and unusual obsessive behavior. Some patients taking these medicines have developed a new compulsion to gamble or obsession with sex. These effects do not happen in most patients with PD using these medicines, but patients should be counseled to report any unusual thoughts or behavior to the doctor. In addition, these medicines have a side effect known as "sleep attacks." There are reports of patients suddenly, without preliminary drowsiness, falling asleep. Patients should be warned of this possibility, especially if they are still operating automobiles or machinery.

COMT inhibitors (catechol-*O*-methyl transferase) are also used to extend the activity of dopamine by reducing another enzyme responsible for its break down. Available COMT inhibitors include entacapone, opicapone, and tolcapone. Because tolcapone has been reported to cause liver damage and must be monitored with regular liver enzyme tests, and opicapone has no generic equivalent, entacapone is much more commonly used. These drugs have no direct activity on PD and must always be given along with carbidopa/levodopa. There is a combination product, Stalevo, that combines carbidopa, levodopa, and entacapone into one product for ease of use. COMT inhibitors have the potential to cause diarrhea.

As PD progresses, patients may develop "off spells," when they become unable to move. Off spells may occur at random or predictable times during the day. Some PD medications are used only for patients who experience off spells. Daily oral istradefylline (Nourianz), an adenosine receptor antagonist, may be added to a patient's carbidopa/levodopa regimen when off spells become a regular problem. It is not known specifically how this product helps to prevent off spells. Tobacco use may reduce this drug's effectiveness, so a higher dose may be needed if a patient smokes a pack or more of cigarettes daily. For acute treatment, apomorphine (Apokyn) is an injectable product used for off spells. Because of several problematic side effects, it is not often used. Apomorphine causes severe nausea, and the patient needs to take trimethobenzamide (Tigan) for 3 days before beginning apomorphine therapy to prevent nausea. Most drugs used to treat nausea, such as promethazine and metoclopramide, act against dopamine and make PD symptoms worse, so they should not be used in patients with PD. In addition, the type 3 serotonin (5-HT$_3$) receptor antagonists, such as ondansetron (Zofran), are contraindicated with apomorphine. (These agents are addressed specifically in Chapter 21.) Levodopa inhalation powder (Inbrija) is another product for off spells that is effective within about 10 minutes of use and lasts up to one hour. Patients should inhale the powder slowly through their mouths to avoid gagging and coughing. Istradefylline (Nourianz) is also used for off spells.

Patients with PD will often need other medications to help manage constipation, skin problems, depression, sleep disturbances, and pain. Sometimes an antipsychotic medication is needed to help manage hallucinations or delusions that may occur in PD or with PD medications. Most antipsychotics are not good choices due to their activity against dopamine. Most practitioners prefer to use low doses of quetiapine or sometimes clozapine in patients with PD. Pimavanserin (Nuplazid) is an atypical antipsychotic that is approved only for treatment of hallucinations and delusions associated with PD.

DEMENTIA

CASE STUDY

Matilda is a 93-year-old widow who just moved to an assisted-living facility. Matilda is a retired real estate agent. She has three grown sons, eight grandchildren, and two great-grandchildren. Matilda's sons decided that their mother needed more supervision than they were able to give her and persuaded her to move to the assisted-living home. Matilda had been found wandering in the neighborhood in her housecoat and slippers, and she could not find her way home. She also had her telephone and electricity shut off due to not paying the bills. Matilda's checkbook was a mess, with some legible writing mixed with unreadable scribbles. Matilda sometimes calls her sons by her husband's or brothers' names. She usually does not recognize her grandchildren but is happy to see them when they visit.

CASE?

From what type of dementia is Matilda likely suffering?

Dementia is a condition in which a person declines in cognitive, or mental, level of functioning. Some of the characteristics of dementia are impairment of memory, especially of recent events; loss of the ability to do everyday cognitive tasks, such as following a grocery list, paying bills, or managing a checkbook; loss of the ability to follow directions; and decline in the ability to name common objects, such as books, paper clips, and shoelaces. The patient with dementia may become confused or lost in a formerly familiar setting. There are several types of dementia, the most common one being Alzheimer's disease, which is a progressive dementia that ends with the patient being bedfast and unable to walk, talk, or recognize family. Death follows when the patient loses the will to eat or develops an infection such as pneumonia or a urinary tract infection. The duration of the disease varies but averages about 10 years from onset to death. Other types of dementia include vascular dementia, in which the mental decline is due to strokes or other blood vessel disease in the brain; Lewy body dementia, which may exist alone or as part of PD and often includes visual hallucinations (animals, strange people in the house, children playing) and may lead to the patient becoming suspicious of caregivers; and frontotemporal dementia, which involves dramatic changes in personality and the ability to make judgments.

CASE?

Matilda's doctor conducted the Mini Mental Status Exam, on which Matilda scored 19 out of a possible 30, indicating that she has significant dementia. Matilda had problems remembering lists, doing subtraction, repeating a phrase, and drawing a geometric figure. What medication(s) might Matilda be taking? What benefits would be expected from them?

Dementia is assessed by tests such as the Mini Mental Status Exam, in which the examiner asks the patient to repeat phrases, name objects, follow commands, and do simple tasks. The score given is an assessment of the severity of the disease. Because of the expected decline, it is better for a patient to be assessed early in the disease so the patient can make decisions about supportive care, living situation, driving, and other important issues.

Dementia cannot be cured. Medication may help to slow the decline and treat behavioral issues. Currently, nearly one-half of elderly people over the age of 85 years have symptoms of cognitive impairment. Studies are ongoing to see if the incidence of dementia can be lowered with interventions made earlier in life. There are suggestions that good nutrition, regular exercise, lifelong learning, and avoiding or managing diabetes, hypertension, and depression may reduce the likelihood of dementia if these changes are made by middle age.

Medications specifically indicated to treat dementia include cholinesterase inhibitors and memantine. (See Medication Table 6-3.) Most of these agents have a formal Food and Drug Administration (FDA) approval only for Alzheimer's disease, but are usually also useful for Lewy body and vascular dementias. Frontotemporal dementia usually does not respond to medications used for Alzheimer's disease. In addition, other medications, such as antidepressants, mood stabilizers, sedative-hypnotics, and antipsychotics are used for depression, sleep, and behavioral problems. Usually initial doses used are lower than would be used in a younger person. In addition, the use of antipsychotics is controversial—they help with behavioral problems, such as aggression and hallucinations, but they have been shown to increase the risk of stroke and other events in patients with dementia. In addition, most antipsychotics should be avoided in patients with Lewy body dementia, since they can exacerbate PD symptoms that often accompany that condition.

The effects of plaques and nerve tangles in the brain that are characteristic of Alzheimer's disease reduce the activity of acetylcholine, causing many symptoms. The cholinesterase inhibitors work by reducing the metabolism of acetylcholine in the brain, thus increasing its activity. Cholinesterase inhibitors have been shown to slow the decline in mental function by at least several months. The drugs, which include donepezil (Aricept), rivastigmine (Exelon), and galantamine (Razadyne), should be started at a lower dose and titrated up to the desired dose in order to improve patient tolerance. Common side effects are stomach upset, decreased appetite, and weight loss. These drugs may increase the risk of gastrointestinal (GI) bleeding in patients with ulcers and must be used with care in patients with heart rhythm problems.

PRACTICE POINT

Rivastigmine is available as both an oral capsule and a transdermal (patch) system. Namzaric is an oral extended-release combination product containing 10 mg donepezil and varying amounts of memantine. Take care to notice the amount of each ingredient in orders and prescriptions.

CASE?

What side effects might Matilda experience from her treatment?

Memantine (Namenda) is another drug that may be helpful in patients with dementia. Memantine works by decreasing the activity of *N*-methyl-D-aspartate (NMDA) receptors in the brain. These receptors are acted on by glutamate, and the result is believed to worsen some of the symptoms of Alzheimer's disease. Since memantine is mostly eliminated by the kidneys, the dose should be reduced in patients with renal impairment. Memantine has a titration schedule for achieving the desired dosage and is usually well tolerated, but dizziness, headache, constipation, and confusion have been reported in a small percentage of patients.

Herbals and Supplements

Vitamin E and the herb *Gingko biloba* have been studied to see if they would benefit patients with Alzheimer's disease. Vitamin E was hypothesized to work as an antioxidant to reduce the advancement of the disease. *Gingko biloba*, a plant used for centuries in traditional Chinese medicine, was thought to be beneficial by acting to enhance neurotransmitter activity, improve blood circulation in the brain, or other unknown actions. Studies have not shown a clear benefit for either, but some doctors will recommend high doses of vitamin E. A patient with early cognitive impairment may be interested in trying *Gingko biloba* even though effectiveness has not been established. Although not standard medications, both vitamin E and *Gingko biloba* still have the potential for side effects and drug interactions.

EPILEPSY

CASE STUDY

M. J. is a 72-year-old woman who had seizure onset following a stroke 3 years ago. She had been seizure-free for 17 months, but for the last 3 weeks she has been having one to two brief (lasting about 1 minute) complex partial seizures per week. On questioning, she also complains of worsening heartburn problems for the past 6 weeks, which causes her to wake up at night. She feels tired because of the interruption of her sleep.

CASE?

M. J. has been taking the following medications: gabapentin 400 mg TID, Lipitor 10 mg daily (for 3 years), Plavix 75 mg daily, Hyzaar 50/12.5 daily, and omeprazole 40 mg daily. Which of M. J.'s medication was prescribed to treat her seizures?

Epilepsy is a condition that is really a collection of disorders. Due to excessive electrical activity in the brain, a person will partially or completely lose consciousness. The person will have either localized movements, such as an arm shaking, or generalized movements, such as arms and legs jerking wildly. Seizures usually last only a few minutes, and the patient regains consciousness but often feels tired or confused for several hours. If a seizure lasts more than a few (eg, 5) minutes, it can become life threatening and needs to be treated as an emergency.

Epilepsy is diagnosed by taking a history from the patient, doing a neurologic examination, and checking an MRI scan and an EEG. The EEG is the most beneficial tool for detecting abnormal brain waves. Often, a neurologist can detect abnormal brain waves when a patient is not having a seizure, but sometimes the brain looks normal at that time.

There are many medications available to reduce the number of seizures a patient has. The goal is to have no seizures and no side effects. Many patients can be treated successfully with the first drug that is tried. Unfortunately, some patients have epilepsy that is more difficult to treat and will have to try several different medications or use two or three medications together. Many epilepsy medications, especially the older ones, are prone to causing drug interactions with other medications. The physician and pharmacist must always check for these interactions. Some medications will decrease the blood levels of the antiepileptic drug, and that could cause the patient to have a seizure.

Some situations that can increase the possibility of having a seizure are missing doses of medicine, not getting enough sleep, stress or infections, and, for women, different phases of the menstrual cycle. Patients with epilepsy, especially when seizures are not well controlled, often have problems with their memory. It is helpful to use a seizure calendar and medication compliance aids, such as pill boxes, to monitor the effectiveness of the medication and improve adherence to therapy. In addition, patients may contact the Epilepsy Foundation for assistance in meeting the challenges of this condition.

Treatment of epilepsy relies on medication. (See Medication Table 6-4.) There has been a dramatic increase in the number of drugs available to treat epilepsy in the past 20 years, but the older drugs are also commonly used. Certain drugs are more effective for particular types of epilepsy. For example, ethosuximide, valproate, and a few others are effective in treating absence seizures, but some other medications, such as carbamazepine and phenytoin, are not—indeed, these drugs can increase the frequency of seizures in these patients.

For about half of patients with epilepsy, the first drug their doctor tries will be effective in controlling their seizures. If the patient tolerates the drug well, treatment can continue with that medication. For many other patients, their epilepsy is more difficult to control and will require trials of different medications and sometimes combinations of medications. Patients with difficult to control seizures often benefit from a referral to a neurologist who specializes in epilepsy.

Many antiepileptic drugs have the potential for drug interactions. These drugs can interact with other antiepileptics and also other medications the patient may take, such as antidepressants and warfarin. The effects of these interactions must be recognized, especially when adding or withdrawing a drug from the patient's therapy. In addition, some antiepileptics have a narrow range of blood levels between which they are effective but not toxic. Some doctors test the blood of their patients to follow the levels, and others just rely on the patient's response and monitor for side effects. Patients with particular needs in epilepsy management are women who may become pregnant. Some antiepileptic drugs may reduce the effectiveness of hormone contraceptives or have the potential to cause birth defects. The choice of drugs used to treat epilepsy will depend on issues such as these in addition to patient tolerance and effectiveness of a drug in treating the patient's seizures.

The following sections discuss medications used to treat epilepsy, some particular features of the medicine, and possible side effects. Some important drug interactions are listed, but a more complete reference should be consulted for a thorough discussion of possible interactions. In general, antiepileptic drugs should be started at low doses and gradually increased to the desired dose to reduce the chance of undesirable effects. Likewise, when taking a patient off an antiepileptic drug, the dose should be lowered gradually—usually over several weeks—to reduce the risk of seizures. In addition, when drugs that have interactions are used together, attention must be paid to the effect that removal of one drug may have on the levels of the continued drug. In addition to all benzodiazepines and barbiturates, some other antiepileptic drugs (eg, pregabalin, lacosamide) are controlled substances.

Benzodiazepines

In status epilepticus (a seizure that lasts for a prolonged period, which, if not treated immediately, can cause brain damage or death), the seizures must be brought under control as quickly as possible. For that reason, IV medications are used. Only a few antiepileptic drugs are available and approved to be used intravenously for status epilepticus.

A benzodiazepine, such as lorazepam, diazepam, or midazolam, is used initially, because these drugs work quickly (within a few minutes) by increasing the seizure-suppressing activity of gamma-aminobutyric acid (GABA) in the brain. In addition, the patient is started on another antiepileptic drug—usually phenytoin, fosphenytoin, or a barbiturate—which takes longer to administer and to start working. Clonazepam, a long-acting benzodiazepine, is also used sometimes to prevent seizures. Clonazepam is also frequently used for certain sleep disorders. Clobazam (Onfi) is a benzodiazepine approved for a rare epilepsy condition that begins in children (Lennox-Gastaut syndrome). Midazolam (Nayzilam) and diazepam (Valtoco) nasal sprays can be used for breakthrough seizures and seizure clusters, as can diazepam rectal gel (Diastat).

Sudden withdrawal of a benzodiazepine that a patient has been using for a long time—whether it is being used for epilepsy, sleep, or anxiety—can sometimes precipitate seizures. Withdrawal should be done gradually, reducing the dose over several weeks. All benzodiazepines can depress respirations at high levels, or when used with other central nervous system (CNS) depressants, including alcohol.

ALERT!

LOOK-ALIKE/SOUND-ALIKE—Clonazepam and its brand name, Klonopin, can be confused with clonidine, an autonomic nervous system drug used for cardiovascular disorders.

Barbiturates

The main barbiturate used to treat epilepsy is phenobarbital, which is a depressant of the central nervous system. It works by regulating the flow of sodium ions into nerve cells, which slows the conduction of the seizure signals and also enhances GABA, an inhibitory neurotransmitter. It is used for partial seizures and generalized seizures but not for absence seizures. Phenobarbital commonly causes drowsiness. At high doses or in combination with other CNS depressants, such as alcohol, phenobarbital can cause respiratory depression. Phenobarbital has many drug interactions. Primidone (Mysoline) has action resembling that of barbiturates and is, in fact, partially metabolized to a barbiturate.

Phenytoin and Fosphenytoin

Phenytoin is a drug that has been available for many decades. It, too, works by regulating sodium ion flow through openings called gates or channels in nerve cells. It is tricky to dose since the metabolism of this drug may differ greatly from one patient to another. Also, there are many drug interactions with phenytoin, including with other antiepileptic drugs. For this reason, there is no typical dose of this medication. Some patients may take as little as 200 mg daily; others may take 500 mg daily. Many patients tolerate this medication well as long the levels are not too high. At higher blood (serum) phenytoin levels, the patient may have problems walking. The eyes may appear to bounce around (nystagmus). Another unusual effect of this medication is that it may cause increased growth in gum tissue—sometimes to the point of causing the patient to need surgery to free the teeth. Some patients who take phenytoin for a long time may have a coarsening of their facial features. Phenytoin comes in several dosage forms, including capsules, chewable tablets, oral suspension, and IV solution. Phenytoin IV admixtures should only be mixed with normal saline. Adding the drug to dextrose solutions will cause prompt precipitation.

ALERT!

LOOK-ALIKE/SOUND-ALIKE—Cerebyx, the brand name for fosphenytoin, has been confused with Celebrex and Celexa. Fosphenytoin has been misspelled with an initial "ph." This can cause confusion for hospital staff looking for the drug in dispensing machines.

PRACTICE POINT

Many precautions must be taken with IV phenytoin. It is not stable in dextrose solutions and must only be mixed in normal saline solution (and even then carefully examined for precipitation).

IV phenytoin must be administered slowly to avoid problems with the heart and blood pressure. IV phenytoin also can cause serious tissue damage if the drug is accidentally administered out of the vein. For these reasons, fosphenytoin was developed as a *prodrug*. Fosphenytoin is better tolerated on administration and breaks down in the body to phenytoin.

ALERT!

The dosage schedule for phenytoin varies greatly with the dosage form and must be adjusted when a patient's therapy is changed from one dosage form or route of administration to another.

Carbamazepine and Oxcarbazepine

Carbamazepine and oxcarbazepine are related drugs that are used for partial seizures. They are also sodium channel regulators. Oxcarbazepine was developed to take advantage of the benefits of carbamazepine but to reduce the side effects and drug interactions. Carbamazepine may also be used for certain neuropathic pain conditions and to stabilize patients with bipolar disorder. Patients beginning carbamazepine must have their blood and liver function checked during the early weeks of therapy. In addition, early side effects include nausea, dizziness, drowsiness, double vision, and problems walking. An occasional unusual side effect of these medications is hyponatremia, or low sodium levels in the blood. Carbamazepine has many drug interactions, mostly due to its activity as an inducer of enzymes in the liver. Use of carbamazepine can cause levels of certain other medications to decrease, requiring a dose adjustment. In fact, carbamazepine induces its own metabolism. Carbamazepine is contraindicated with nefazodone due to reducing nefazodone levels dramatically. Other important interactions are with warfarin, levothyroxine, methadone, phenytoin, and oral contraceptives.

Ethosuximide

Ethosuximide is an antiepileptic drug that is only used for patients with absence seizures. Its mechanism of action is not clear but may involve regulating ion flow in nerve cells. Absence seizures, also called petit mal seizures, usually occur in children. Characteristically, the child stares or blinks for several moments, and sometimes many times daily. Ethosuximide will not help other types of epilepsy. The most common side effects are nausea and vomiting early in therapy.

Note: Because generalized tonic-clonic seizures are also called grand mal (big sickness) seizures, the lay public often calls less dramatic partial seizures *petit mal (little sickness)* seizures. This is a misuse of the term. The term *petit mal* only refers to absence seizures.

Valproic Acid, Valproate Sodium, Divalproex

Valproate sodium and divalproex are variations of the same original drug product, valproic acid. Valproic acid is the most versatile of all the antiepileptic drugs, which is believed to work by enhancing the activity of GABA in the brain. GABA is the main neurotransmitter that inhibits nerve activity, and increasing GABA activity will prevent or reduce seizure activity. Valproic acid can be used for absence, partial, and generalized tonic-clonic seizures. In addition, valproic acid can help to prevent migraine headaches, reduce neuropathic pain, and manage bipolar disorder. Valproic acid has many possible side effects, including nausea and vomiting, weight gain, hair loss, and tremor, and many potential drug interactions. There are many dosage forms, including tablets, capsules, oral solution, and IV preparations. Valproic acid (Depakene) is dosed three times a day and often causes nausea and other GI side effects. Valproate sodium (Depakote) is a twice-daily, long-acting preparation, but divalproex (Depakote ER) is a once-daily dosage formulation.

ALERT!

Technicians must be careful to distinguish the type of valproic acid product ordered to be sure the patient receives the correct one.

CASE?

What might be causing M. J.'s sudden increase in seizure frequency?

Gabapentin and Pregabalin

Gabapentin (Neurontin) is a usually well-tolerated antiepileptic drug that has few drug interactions. In spite of its name, gabapentin does not increase GABA activity in the brain. It acts by an unknown mechanism. It is also useful in treating neuropathic pain, which is actually its main use. Common side effects include fatigue, dizziness, weight gain, and edema. Pregabalin (Lyrica) is a medication that is similar in activity to gabapentin, and it also can be used for neuropathic pain.

PRACTICE POINT

Taking antacids within 2 hours of a dose of gabapentin can reduce the amount absorbed by the body significantly and patients may suffer from seizures. Patients using antacids, especially OTC products that may not be on the medical or pharmacy profile because they were not prescribed by a physician, should be counseled by the pharmacist about timing them so that the gabapentin is taken at least 2 hours after the antacid.

Lamotrigine

Lamotrigine (Lamictil) works by regulating sodium channels, and it is usually well tolerated and has fewer drug interactions than phenobarbital, phenytoin, carbamazepine, and valproic acid. However, a very important interaction can occur when it is used along with valproic acid. Lamotrigine sometimes causes a serious rash that is potentially life threatening (as well as less serious rashes). To avoid the risk of rash, the starting dose must be very low and gradually increased to the desired dose. Valproic acid reduces the elimination of lamotrigine from the body. For this reason, patients who are taking valproic acid must start lamotrigine at even lower doses and titrate the dosage more slowly. When doses are started low, the side effects of headache, drowsiness, and double vision are less likely to occur or more easily tolerated.

ALERT!

LOOK-ALIKE/SOUND-ALIKE—Lamotrigine and its brand name, Lamictal, have been confused with the antiviral drug lamivudine and with the antifungal drug, Lamisil.

Topiramate and Zonisamide

Topiramate (Topamax) and zonisamide (Zonegran) are medications that work differently than most of the other drugs for epilepsy. Topiramate and zonisamide work by regulating the activity of calcium entering the nerve cells, and they are similar in how they work and in their side effects. They are also potentially useful in a variety of seizure conditions. Zonisamide may cause a reaction in patients who are allergic to sulfa drugs. Other common side effects include dizziness, nausea, and headache. Many patients lose weight when taking these two drugs. They can also occasionally cause kidney stones, so patients should be advised to drink plenty of water while on these medications. Some patients complain of mental slowing and problems finding words. Topiramate and zonisamide may reduce sweating. Since sweating is the way humans cool their bodies, drugs that suppress sweating can cause the body temperature to rise during hot weather or exercise, risking heat stroke. Patients should be advised not to get overheated from exercise or heat exposure.

ALERT!

LOOK-ALIKE/SOUND-ALIKE—Topamax, the brand name for topiramate, is similar to Toprol XL, a medication used for cardiovascular disease.

Tiagabine

Tiagabine (Gabitril) is usually considered a second-line option when other medications have been ineffective in treating a patient's seizures. The way tiagabine works is different from other drugs for epilepsy. It increases the activity of GABA by inhibiting its reuptake into storage sites in nerve cells. Side effects include dizziness, weakness, nervousness, diarrhea, tremor, and depression.

ALERT!

LOOK-ALIKE/SOUND-ALIKE—Tiagabine has been confused with the muscle relaxant drug tizanidine.

Levetiracetam

Levetiracetam (Keppra) is a popular drug in the treatment of epilepsy due to usually good tolerance, effectiveness, and few drug interactions. Levetiracetam works differently than all of the other antiepileptic drugs, but its exact mechanism is not known. It is usually well tolerated and has few drug interactions because it is mostly removed from

the body by the kidneys, rather than primarily through the liver. Common side effects include fatigue, drowsiness, problems with coordination, and occasionally behavior problems. Because of the usually mild side effect profile, the dosage can be titrated to desired levels quicker than with some other medications.

Felbamate

Felbamate (Felbatol) is an antiepileptic drug that may be tried when several others have either not been effective or are not tolerated. Its mechanism of action is unknown. Felbamate is an effective drug but has the rare side effect of causing serious blood and liver problems, which may be fatal. Other more common side effects are nausea and weight loss.[2]

Lacosamide

Lacosamide (Vimpat) is a newer antiepileptic drug whose exact mechanism is uncertain. One facet is believed to be regulation of sodium entrance into nerve cells, which is one factor that controls the transmission of signals through the nerves, but there may also be other areas of activity. Lacosamide is available as a tablet, oral liquid, and IV injection. The dose of lacosamide must be reduced in patients who have severe impairment of their kidney activity. Side effects of lacosamide include nausea, headache, drowsiness, dizziness, double vision, and balance problems; rarely it can cause heart conduction problems and hypersensitivity reactions.

Vigabatrin

Vigabitrin (Sabril, Vigadrone) is approved for use alone for infantile spasms, and as adjunctive therapy for patients with refractory complex partial seizures. Its mechanism is unknown, but it is believed to increase GABA levels in the brain. Patients must have their vision monitored periodically while on this medication, due to reports of effects on the visual field.

Perampanel

Perampanel (Fycompa) is an antiepileptic drug with a novel mechanism of action—it reduces the activity of glutamate, a CNS-stimulating neurotransmitter, on one type of receptor in the brain. It is approved for partial seizures and primary generalized tonic-clonic seizures. Possible side effects include behavior and psychiatric reactions, drowsiness, and falls. This medication also has the potential for several drug interactions.

Cenobamate

Cenobamate (Xcopri) is a new antiepileptic drug that inhibits flow through sodium channels and also enhances GABA activity. It is approved as an add-on treatment for partial seizures. Both initiation and discontinuation must involve careful dose titration. Because of interactions with other medications, doses of other antiepileptic drugs may need to be increased or decreased when cenobamate is added.

Stiripentol and Cannabidiol

The mechanisms of action for stiripentol (Diacomit) and cannabidiol (Epidiolex) are not known. Stiripentol is approved to treat Dravet syndrome. Cannabidiol is approved for both Dravet syndrome and Lennox-Gastaut syndrome. Both are epilepsy syndromes that begin in childhood.

ALERT!

Some antiepileptic drugs are controlled substances under federal law. These include phenobarbital, pregabalin, the benzodiazepines, lacosamide, cenobamate, and cannabidiol. Gabapentin is also a controlled substance in many states and carries special reporting requirements in others.

Nonpharmacologic Therapy

In addition to medications, there are other approaches to controlling seizures. One is the vagal nerve stimulator, an implantable device that sends electrical impulses to the vagal nerve. This device is controlled with a magnetic wand so that the strength and frequency of the impulses can be adjusted. Another approach for some patients is brain surgery to remove the site in the brain where their seizures start. Surgery can be very effective in improving control of seizures, often leading to a seizure-free life. With both the vagal nerve stimulator and epilepsy surgery, the patient must still take antiepileptic drugs, although sometimes the number of medications can be reduced. For some children with difficult-to-control seizures doctors will prescribe a ketogenic diet, which is a diet very high in fat and protein and extremely low in carbohydrates. This diet has been shown to reduce seizures in many children whose seizures have not responded well to drugs. The ketogenic diet is not a "natural" diet. The child cannot have common foods such as milk, bread, and fruit because of the carbohydrate content. The diet is usually started in the hospital in order to closely monitor the child, including blood tests that are frequently done. It is a difficult diet to follow and some children do not tolerate it, but it is a useful tool for many.

MULTIPLE SCLEROSIS

CASE STUDY

Paula is a 43-year-old woman who has had a diagnosis of multiple sclerosis (MS) for 13 years. Initially she noticed numbness and weakness in her right hand that lasted a week or so and then went away on its own. Eight months later she had an episode of optic neuritis, in which she developed blurring in her right eye that progressed to loss of sight within a few hours. After treatment, her vision came back over the following 2 weeks. An MRI showed abnormal areas in the brain that were suspicious for MS. Since then, she has had a flare-up of neurologic symptoms about once a year. Sometimes it is profound tiredness and weakness that makes her unable to do her job as a hotel manager, and on other occasions she has had numbness and tingling in her feet and lower legs. She has problems with constipation, depression, and occasional muscle spasms. When the numbness is severe, she must use a cane to get around.

MS is a disease that affects nerves, causing a dramatic slowing in the conduction of electrical impulses. It is caused by an inflammatory process that attacks myelin, a protective insulator of the axon of nerve cells. When the myelin is damaged or destroyed, the areas innervated by those nerves lose their function (Figure 6-1). The symptoms of MS vary, depending on which area of the brain is having its myelin attacked. These attacks come and go, with disability followed by recovery, or they continue to progress. Eventually many patients become unable to walk without assistance. Muscle weakness, muscle spasms, problems with constipation, bladder incontinence, and vision problems are common developments.

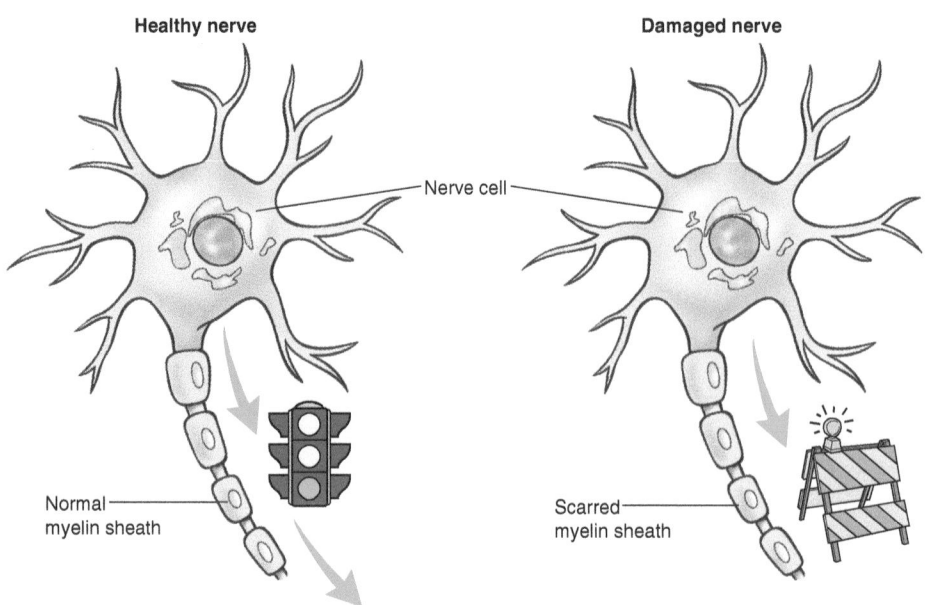

Healthy nerve

Damaged nerve

Nerve cell

Normal myelin sheath

Scarred myelin sheath

FIGURE 6-1. Myelin sheath.

CASE?

Can Paula's physician prescribe a medication or therapy to cure her MS?

The treatment of MS includes treatment of acute exacerbations, the use of disease-modifying therapy to reduce exacerbations, and the use of other medications for symptomatic problems such as pain, spasticity, fatigue, constipation, and urinary problems.

The medications used to treat MS are meant to reduce the number of relapses the patient experiences. These medications are known as immunomodulators. Other medications are used for treatment of the symptoms associated with MS, such as fatigue, depression, constipation, or muscle spasms. None of these medications will cure the disease. (See Medication Table 6-5.)

CASE?

Sometimes Paula's symptoms become especially severe. Should her regular medication doses be increased at these times or might something else be added?

For acute exacerbations, high doses of corticosteroids are used, usually intravenously. Methylprednisolone is given

IV for 3 to 10 days, and symptoms usually improve after 5 days or so. The main key to management of MS is disease-modifying therapy. Several medications are used for this purpose. The specific mechanisms of action are not known for all of these products but, as a group, they interfere, in different ways, with the immune system's attack on myelin. The choice of therapy depends on the characteristics of the patient's disease, such as relapsing or progressive, and how the patient responds and tolerates a medication. A challenge to compliance is that these medications often cause considerable side effects and are inconvenient and expensive. They are intended to reduce the rate of relapses, but the patient may not realize that benefit for a year or more. Interferons (beta$_{1b}$ and beta$_{1a}$) are one class in this category. Their exact mechanism of action is not known, but they are believed to reduce the immune response that attacks myelin. Interferons are administered either intramuscularly (IM) or subcutaneously. When administered according to direction, which varies by product, they can reduce the rate of MS relapses. However, these medications often cause side effects that discourage compliance, including flu-like symptoms, injection site irritation, and depression. Brand names of interferon drugs include Rebif, Plegridy, Extavia, and Betaseron.

Glatiramer acetate (Copaxone, Glatopa) is an alternative to interferons in many patients and may be better tolerated. Its mechanism is not fully understood, but it may act as a substitute for receptors that are attacked by the immune response in MS. Glatiramer is administered as a daily or three times weekly SUBQ injection, and it must be stored in the refrigerator. Glatiramer is very expensive but is gaining more attention as a useful agent for many MS patients. Some patients (about 10%) may develop flushing and tightness in the chest and difficulty breathing the first time they use this medication, but this reaction usually goes away in about 20 minutes.

Natalizumab (Tysabri), ocrelizumab (Ocrevus), and alemtuzumab (Lemtrada) are monoclonal antibodies that work by preventing white blood cells from attacking myelin in the brain. They are alternatives for patients who continue to have relapses while on other medications. All three are administered as IV infusions, but they have different schedules. These products are usually well tolerated, but patients must be monitored during and after infusions for reactions. Common side effects include headache, fatigue, and nausea. These products, because of their action in reducing the immune response, may increase the patient's susceptibility to certain infections.

Mitoxantrone (Novantrone) is a chemotherapy drug that is also used for progressing forms of MS and for difficult cases of MS that have not responded well to other medications. It inhibits white blood cell activity in attacking nerve cells. Because of the possible reduced heart function that can be caused by this medication, there is a maximum total lifetime dosage that should not be exceeded. Other side effects include nausea, vomiting, hair loss, and menstrual problems.[3] Cladribine (Mavenclad) is another drug that resembles a chemotherapy medication. It has approval for certain MS patients who meet its criteria. This medication is taken orally, and only a few days over the course of two years, but has limitations due to several precautions, including the possibility of causing malignancies.

PRACTICE POINT

Mitoxantrone must be prepared with the same precautions as other chemotherapy drugs and is administered every 3 months by IV infusion.

Medications used to manage fatigue, urinary problems, constipation, muscle spasms, depression, and other symptoms of MS are also used to manage these symptoms due to other causes, which are discussed in the appropriate chapters of this text. Dalfampridine (Ampyra) is a medication approved specifically to improve the walking ability of people with MS. It works by blocking potassium channels, which increase nerve signal conduction through axons. Dalfampridine is an oral medication. It is contraindicated in patients who have had seizures and in those who have decreased kidney function.

In addition to medications, patients with MS need to avoid becoming excessively fatigued or overheated. In spite of the difficulties associated with the disease, patients will usually have a normal life expectancy. The degree of disability varies dramatically from one patient to another.

NEUROPATHIC PAIN

Neuropathic pain is a particular pain condition caused by sensitivity, excessive activity, or damage in nerves. Characteristics of neuropathic pain are numbness, burning, tingling, shooting, and electric shock-like pain. Neuropathic pain can occur due to neuropathies caused by diabetes, nerve pain due to MS, pain in a nerve root due to shingles, and pressure on the spinal cord, such as spinal stenosis. Neuropathic pain can be treated with medications that work on the neurotransmitters that transmit pain signals. Medications that we have already discussed include tricyclic antidepressants (used at low doses); many of the anticonvulsants, such as gabapentin, pregabalin, and carbamazepine; and specific analgesics, such as tramadol and methadone.

SLEEP DISORDERS

CASE STUDY

Q. Z. is a 23-year-old college student who comes to the pharmacy looking for something to help him sleep. He says it takes an hour for him to fall asleep at night, and sometimes he wakes up in the middle of the night and can't get back to sleep. Q. Z. is healthy, but says he is worn out trying to keep up with his classes and working part-time. He drinks two or three cups of coffee in the morning and has a couple of Red Bulls in the afternoon to keep going. On days that he isn't working in the evening, he stays up late playing video games or goes out drinking with his friends. On those nights he might not go to bed until 3:00 or 4:00 a.m. instead of his usual midnight bedtime. Some days he has an 8:00 a.m. class but other days he has later classes and he can sleep in until 10:00 a.m. He wants to know what he can take to help him fall asleep when he wants to every night.

When we think of sleep disorders, we usually think of problems falling asleep. That is the most common problem for Americans, but there are many other conditions that cause problems with the sleep cycle. To begin we should discuss normal sleep. Our bodies react to decreasing amounts of light to increase the production of melatonin in the brain. Melatonin causes us to feel drowsy and fall asleep. In addition there is a circadian rhythm that determines periods of time during the day that we sleep or are alert. When we fall asleep, we initially enter a light sleep, then proceed through deeper phases to deep sleep (phases 3 and 4). Then we enter

a lighter sleep in which we do most of our dreaming, the rapid eye movement phase (REM sleep), and then the cycle begins again. We go through this cycle several times every night, with the amount of time in the deep and REM phases changing as the night progresses.

CASE?

What are some of the factors that might be contributing to Q. Z.'s sleep problems?

People with sleep disorders may have problems falling asleep, problems staying asleep, and problems waking up too early and being unable to go back to sleep. Sleep problems may be transient or temporary—resulting from some change or stress in the patient's life—or chronic and continuing for a long period of time. Some patients also have unusual behaviors during sleep in which they may walk, cook, eat, or do other activities that are better left to the waking hours. During REM sleep behavior disorder, a patient will thrash around as he acts out his dreams (normally we do not move during dreaming.)

Nonpharmacologic Therapies

There are many nonpharmacologic interventions that can improve the ability to fall asleep and stay asleep. In general, these methods are known as *good sleep hygiene*. Some of these strategies include maintaining constant times for going to bed and rising, avoiding drinking caffeine or alcohol in the evening, using the bedroom only for sleep and intimacy (ban the TV, computer, etc.), eliminating sources of light in the bedroom, avoiding long naps during the day, and exercising daily but not within 2 hours of bedtime. In addition, counseling, such as cognitive behavioral therapy (CBT), in which the patient brings to light worries that interfere with sleep and develops techniques to deal with them, is helpful for many people. Comfortable bedding and cool room temperature also enhance sleep. In older people, who do not sleep as deeply as the young, increasing the skin temperature very slightly—using a warm bath or electric blanket or mattress pad—may improve sleep structure.

For insomnia, which is the inability to fall asleep or stay asleep, there are several OTC medications that are effective short term. These are in two categories: antihistamines and melatonin. The first-generation antihistamines cause drowsiness as an expected side effect and are also marketed for

CASE?

When Q. Z. tells the pharmacist about his problem, will she tell him he needs to see a doctor if he wants things to improve or are there any OTC remedies she can recommend?

insomnia. These products include doxylamine and diphenhydramine. Diphenhydramine is the "PM" of medications such as Tylenol PM and Advil PM. Side effects include dry mouth, constipation, and possible hangover feeling the next morning. In older people these drugs should be avoided as they can also cause urinary retention and confusion, which older people are more sensitive to.

Melatonin is a synthetic form of the natural product produced in our brains that makes us sleepy. When taken about an hour before the usual bedtime, melatonin can help a patient become drowsy and fall asleep. Patients, especially elderly ones, should try a low dose initially (i.e., cutting the tablet in half). Melatonin may also be helpful in people who expect to experience jet lag while traveling or after returning home. One prescription sleep aid, ramelteon (Rozerem) acts on melatonin receptors in the brain to produce sleep.

CASE?

If OTC remedies do not help Q. Z., what might his doctor prescribe to help him sleep? Is there any reason for him not to take them every night for the rest of his life?

Most of the prescription medications stimulate GABA receptors to cause drowsiness. These include the benzodiazepines—flurazepam and temazepam, quazepam, and triazolam. Benzodiazepines can be habit forming, and they also can cause drowsiness during the next day. For this reason, they are less safe to use in older patients. These medications have fallen from favor in recent years due to the availability of nonbenzodiazepines that also stimulate GABA receptors, such as zolpidem, zaleplon, and eszopiclone. These medications are shorter acting than benzodiazepines and can be used to help a patient fall asleep initially, or for a patient who has problems getting back to sleep during the night. Side effects include headache, dry mouth, strange behavior during sleep, and weight gain (zolpidem).

PRACTICE POINT

Of the prescription sleep medications, all of the ones that are benzodiazepines (or act on benzodiazepine receptors) are controlled substances under federal law. These include estazolam, eszopiclone (Lunesta), zaleplon (Sonata), zolpidem (Ambien), quazepam (Doral), temazepam (Restoril), and flurazepam. Drugs specifically approved for insomnia that are not controlled substances include doxepin (Silenor) and the antidepressants suvorexant (Belsomra) and lemborexant (Dayvigo), both of which block orexin, an alertness chemical in the brain, and ramelteon (Rozerem), which acts on melatonin receptors. Antidepressants that are often used off-label for sleep, such as trazodone, amitriptyline, doxepin, and mirtazapine, are not controlled substances either. Many antihistamines used for insomnia, such as diphenhydramine and doxylamine, are available in OTC products.

Other prescription medications used to help with sleep are usually in the category of sedating antidepressants. These include trazodone, mirtazapine, doxepin, and amitriptyline. These medications are discussed thoroughly in Chapter 7. (See Medication Table 6-6.)

Restless legs syndrome (RLS) is a condition in which a patient feels the need to move his or her legs after going to bed, to relieve crawling or tingling feelings in the legs. (One patient said it felt like he needed to ride a bicycle in bed.) This condition is sometimes associated with iron deficiency anemia or pregnancy, but more often the problem is unexplainable. When iron levels are low, an iron supplement will often improve the symptoms. Otherwise, some nonpharmaceutical approaches are to take a walk or exercise early in the evening and take a warm bath before bed. Medications that are used to treat PD, such as ropinirole and pramipexole, taken at bedtime are the choice agents. As carbidopa/levodopa may cause rebound restlessness later in the night, other alternatives are benzodiazepines, gabapentin, and opioids.

Obstructive sleep apnea is another condition that interferes with a person's ability to get a good night's sleep and can have serious health consequences. It is caused when tissue in the throat relaxes during sleep, closing the airway. The sleeper often snores, stops breathing for several seconds, and then resumes breathing with a snort. This pattern prevents the patient from getting into the restful phases of deep sleep, and the patient often is tired the next day. Sleep apnea contributes to poor control of diabetes and high blood pressure, and the tiredness during the day can lead to accidents. It is diagnosed when a sleep study shows that the patient has periods during sleep in which he or she does not breathe for extended lengths of time. Sleep apnea is managed with machines that force air into the lungs during sleep, and, alternatively, it may be managed with oral appliances that are made by dentists. For patients who have excessive drowsiness during the day, medications such as methylphenidate, modafinil (Provigil), armodafinil (Nuvigil), and solriamfetol (Sunosi) may be used.

There are many other rare sleep disorders, such as narcolepsy and non-24-hour sleep-wake disorder. There are some medications that are specifically directed at these conditions, and are only available through specialty pharmacies. Two such medications are sodium oxybate (Xyrem) for narcolepsy and tasimelteon (Hetlioz) for non-24-hour sleep-wake disorder. Patients must be enrolled in the Risk Evaluation and Mitigation Strategies (REMS) program by their physicians, and the medications are shipped to them at home.

SUMMARY

The central nervous system is complex and is connected to every part of the body in some way. This means there are many different kinds of malfunctions that can occur and many different conditions that can result. Some of these can be completely relieved, while others can be treated to lessen their impact on the patient's daily life. Often, multiple therapies, including medications and other treatments, must be tried and/or continued before the patient's condition improves.

REFERENCES

1. Biederman T. Antimigraine drugs; Neurodegenerative drugs. In: Smith K, Riche D, Henyan N, eds. *Clinical Drug Data*. 11th ed. New York, NY: McGraw-Hill; 2010.

2. Tallian KB, Heinrich NT. Headache disorders. In: DiPiro JT, Yee GC, Posey L, et al. eds. *Pharmacotherapy: A Pathophysiologic Approach*. 12th ed. New York, NY: McGraw Hill; 2021.

3. Lexi-Drugs [Database]. Lexicomp. Hudson, OH. http://online.lexi.com.

CHAPTER RESOURCES

AHFS Drug Information. AHFS Clinical Drug Information. Bethesda, MD: American Society of Health-System Pharmacists.

Bainbridge JL, Miravalle A, Wong P, Makelky MJ. Multiple sclerosis. In: DiPiro JT, Yee GC, Posey L, et al. eds. *Pharmacotherapy: A Pathophysiologic Approach*. 11th ed. New York, NY: McGraw-Hill; 2020.

Nguyen VV, Dergalust S, Chang E. Epilepsy. In: DiPiro JT, Yee GC, Posey L, et al. eds. *Pharmacotherapy: A Pathophysiologic Approach*. 11th ed. New York, NY: McGraw-Hill, 2020.

REVIEW QUESTIONS

1. Describe some differences between disorders described as *neurologic* and those considered *psychiatric*.

2. What are some of the distinguishing characteristics of migraine headaches?

3. List some of the signs of stroke and describe what measures should be taken if stroke is suspected.

4. What causes the symptoms of Parkinson's disease, and what is the common goal of most of the medications used to treat it, regardless of their mechanism of action?

5. What types of medication therapy are used in the treatment of multiple sclerosis?

MEDICATION TABLES WITH REPRESENTATIVE AGENTS FOR EACH DISORDER

MEDICATION TABLE 6-1. Headache[3]

CLASS Generic Name	Brand Name	Route	Forms	Dose	Notes
Ergotamine (er GOT a meen)	Ergomar	Sublingual	Tablet	2 mg at the first sign of attack; may be followed in 30 min	Total daily dose should not exceed 3 tablets; weekly dose up to 10 mg
Almotriptan (al moh TRIP tan)	Axert	Oral	Tablet	6.25–12.5 mg; may be repeated	No more than 4 treatments/month
Eletriptan (el e TRIP tan)	Relpax	Oral	Tablet	40 mg/dose; up to 80 mg/day	No more than 3 treatments/month
Frovatriptan (froe va TRIP tan)	Frova	Oral	Tablet	2.5–7.5 mg/24 hr	No more than 4 treatments/month
Naratriptan (NAR a trip tan)	Amerge	Oral	Tablet	Up to 5 mg/24 hr	No more than 4 treatments/month
Rizatriptan (rye za TRIP tan)	Maxalt	Oral	Tablet	Up to 30 mg/24 hr	No more than 4 treatments/month
	Maxalt-MLT	Oral	Dispersible tablet	Up to 30 mg/24 hr	Disintegrates on tongue
Sumatriptan (soo ma TRIP tan)	Imitrex	Oral	Tablet	25–100 mg/dose up to 200 mg/day	
Zolmitriptan (zohl mi TRIP tan)	Zomig	Nasal, oral	Solution, tablet	2.5–5 mg/dose up to 10 mg/day	No more than 3 treatments/month
	Zomig ZMT	Oral	Dispersible tablet		Disintegrates on tongue
Ergotamine and caffeine (er GOT a meen) (KAF een)	Cafergot	Oral	Tablet	2 tablets/dose up to 6 tablets/attack	Not to exceed 10 tablets/week
	Migergot	Rectal	Suppository	Insert 1 for attack; may repeat	Not to exceed 5 suppositories/week
Acetaminophen, isometheptene, and dichloralphenazone (a seet a MIN oh fen) (eye soe me THEP teen) (dye klor al PHEN a zone)	Various generics	Oral	Capsule	2 capsules to start; then 1 every hr up to 5 in 12 hr	Up to 8 capsules/day
Sumatriptan and naproxen (soo ma TRIP tan) (na PROX en)	Treximet	Oral	Tablet	1 tablet; may repeat × 1	Maximum dose = 2 tablets/24 hr
Ubrogepant (ue BROE je pant)	Ubrelvy	Oral	Tablet	50, 100 mg tablet, may repeat × 1 in 2 hours	Max dose = 200 mg/24 hours
Erezumab-aooe (e REN ue mab)	Aimovig	SUBQ	Solution	70–140 mg monthly	For prevention
Fremanezumab-vfrm (free ma NEZ ue mab)	Ajovy	SUBQ	Solution	225 mg monthly or 675 mg every 3 months	For prevention
Galcanezumab-gnlm (GAL ka NEZ ue mab)	Emgality	SUBQ	Solution	120 mg monthly for migraine; 100 mg monthly for cluster episodes	For prevention of migraine, needs a loading dose; For treatment of cluster, needs a loading dose

SUBQ = subcutaneous.

MEDICATION TABLE 6-2. Parkinson's Disease[3]

CLASS Generic Name	Brand Name	Route	Forms	Dose	Notes
Adamantine					
Amantadine (a MAN ta deen)	Gocovri Osmolex ER	Oral	100 mg capsule, tablet; 50 mg/5 mL oral syrup Gocovri extended-release capsules 68.5 mg and 137 mg Osmolex ER 129 mg, 193 mg, 258 mg tablets	100 mg PO twice daily up to 400 mg/day in divided doses Gocovri: Start with 137 mg at bedtime; titrate to 274 mg Osmolex ER: Start with 129 mg daily, titrate to maximum of 322 mg daily in the morning	May cause anticholinergic symptoms, blurred vision, and increased compulsive behavior; dose for renal insufficiency
Anticholinergics					
Benztropine mesylate (BENZ troe peen)	Generics	IM/IV/oral	1 mg/mL injection solution; 0.5 mg, 1 mg, 2 mg tablet	1–2 mg/day IM/IV/oral (range 0.5–6 mg/day)	May impair heat regulation
Trihexyphenidyl hydrochloride (trye hex ee FEN i dil)	Generics	Oral	2 mg, 5 mg tablet; 2 mg/5 mL elixir	5–15 mg orally daily (divided 3–4 times daily)	Common adverse effects include nausea, xerostomia, dizziness, blurred vision, and nervousness
COMT Inhibitors					
Entacapone (en TA ka pone)	Comtan	Oral	200 mg tablet	200 mg orally (adjunct to levodopa/carbidopa dose)	Max 1,600 mg/day Stalevo contains levodopa, carbidopa, and entacapone
Opicapone (oh PIK a pone)	Ongentys	Oral	25 mg, 50 mg capsule	50 mg once daily at bedtime	
Tolcapone (TOLE ka pone)	Tasmar	Oral	100 mg tablet	100 mg orally 3 times daily (adjunct to levodopa/carbidopa therapy)	Warning: risk of potentially fatal liver failure associated with administration of tolcapone
Dopamine Precursors					
Carbidopa/levodopa (kar bi DOE pa) (lee voe DOE pa)	Sinemet 10–100, Sinemet 25–100, Sinemet 25–250, Sinemet CR Rytary Duopa pump	Oral	Sinemet: 10–100 mg, 25–100 mg, 25–250 mg (tablet and orally disintegrating tablet); 25–100 mg, 50–200 mg and others (extended-release tablet)	Multiple dosing schedules based on pathogenesis of parkinsonism; common: 1 tablet orally 3 or 4 times daily (may be increased)	May cause loss of appetite, nausea, or vomiting; all drugs that enhance dopamine activity may produce hallucinations, especially at drug peaks
Levodopa	Inbrija	Inhaler	42 mg capsules	2 capsules (84 mg) inhaled via mouth up to 5 times/day	Rescue for "off spells"

Continued next page

MEDICATION TABLE 6-2. Parkinson's Disease[3] *(Continued)*

CLASS Generic Name	Brand Name	Route	Forms	Dose	Notes
Dopamine Agonists					
Bromocriptine mesylate (broe moe KRIP teen)	Parlodel	Oral	5 mg capsule, 2.5 mg tablet	2.5–40 mg/day orally, up to 100 mg daily	To be administered with meals; also used for endocrine disorders
Apomorphine hydrochloride (a poe MOR feen)	Apokyn	SUBQ	10 mg/mL solution	0.2–0.6 mL (2–6 mg) SUBQ as needed for "off spells"; maximum 0.6 mL (6 mg)	Should not be administered without use of concomitant antiemetic
Pramipexole dihydrochloride (pra mi PEX ole)	Mirapex, Mirapex ER	Oral	0.125 mg, 0.25 mg, 0.5 mg, 0.75 mg, 1 mg, 1.5 mg tablet; 3 mg, 4.5 mg extended-release tablet	0.5–1.5 mg orally 3 times/day (upward titration)	Abrupt withdrawal, dose reduction, or changes in treatment may result in confusion
Ropinirole hydrochloride (roe PIN i role)	Generics	Oral	0.25 mg, 0.5 mg, 1 mg, 2 mg, 3 mg, 4 mg, 5 mg tablets; 2 mg, 4 mg, 6 mg, 8 mg, 12 mg extended-release tablets	0.25 mg orally 3 times daily	Risk of cardiovascular disease and potential for cardiovascular events
Rotigotine (roe TIG oh teen)	Neupro	Transdermal patch	1 mg, 2 mg, 3 mg, 4 mg, 6 mg, 8 mg	1 patch per day	Also used for restless leg syndrome
MAO Inhibitor					
Rasagiline (ra SA ji leen)	Azilect	Oral	0.5 mg, 1 mg tablet	1 mg orally once daily	Multiple significant drug-drug interactions
Safinamide (sa FIN i mide)	Xadago	Oral	50 mg, 100 mg	50–100 mg daily	Multiple significant drug-drug interactions
Selegeline (suh LEJ uh leen)	Zelapar Emsam	Oral Oral disintegrating tablet Transdermal	5 mg 1.25mg 6 mg, 9 mg, 12 mg	5 mg twice daily 1.25 mg to 2.5mg daily Daily	Multiple significant drug-drug interactions Emsam's approved indication is depression

COMT = catechol-*O*-methyltransferase; IM = intramuscular; IV = intravenous; MAO = monoamine oxidase; PO = by mouth; SUBQ = subcutaneous.

MEDICATION TABLE 6-3. Dementia[3]

CLASS Generic Name	Brand Name	Route	Forms	Dose	Notes
Cholinesterase Inhibitors					
Donepezil hydrochloride (doe NEP e zil)	Aricept, Aricept ODT	Oral (tablet and orally disintegrating tablet)	5 mg, 10 mg, 23 mg tablet (23 mg not available as ODT)	5–10 mg once daily at bedtime	May cause diarrhea, anorexia, nausea, vomiting, muscle cramps, insomnia, or fatigue
Galantamine (ga LAN ta meen)	Razadyne, Razadyne ER	Oral	4 mg/mL oral solution; 4 mg, 8 mg, 12 mg tablet (Razadyne); 8 mg, 16 mg, 24 mg (Razadyne ER)	Start tablets and oral solution at 4 mg orally twice daily for a minimum of 4 weeks, then titrate	Patient should maintain adequate hydration
Rivastigmine (ri va STIG meen)	Generics	Oral	1.5 mg, 3 mg, 4.5 mg, 6 mg capsule; 2 mg/mL oral solution	1.5 mg orally twice daily	Max dose 6 mg twice daily
	Exelon	Transdermal	4.6 mg/24 hr, 9.5 mg/24 hr	One patch topically once daily	Patch should not be directly exposed to external heat sources
NMDA Antagonist					
Memantine (MEM an teen)	Namenda	Oral	2 mg/mL oral solution; 5 mg, 10 mg tablet	20 mg/day target dose	Attention should be given to proper dose escalation
	Namenda XR	Oral	ER capsules	7–28 mg daily	May be sprinkled on applesauce
Memantine + Donepezil	Namzaric	Oral	ER capsule: 7 mg/10 mg, 14 mg/10 mg, 21 mg/10 mg, 28 mg/10 mg	One tablet daily	See package insert for titration or conversion schedule

ER = extended release; NMDA = N-methyl-D-aspartate; ODT = orally disintegrating tablet.

MEDICATION TABLE 6-4. Seizures/Epilepsy[3]

CLASS Generic Name	Brand Name	Route	Forms	Dose	DEA Schedule/ Regulatory Status	Notes
Barbiturates						
Phenobarbital (fee noe BAR bi tal)	Generics	Oral, IV, IM	Oral elixir, tablet, solution; injection	30–120 mg/day in 2–3 divided doses	Schedule IV controlled substance (CIV)	No more than 400 mg should be given during a 24-hr period
Primidone (PRI mi done)	Mysoline	Oral	50 mg, 250 mg tablet	250 mg 3 times/day	Rx only	Common gastrointestinal adverse effects include nausea and vomiting
Benzodiazepines						
Clonazepam (kloe NA ze pam)	Klonopin, Klonopin Wafers	Oral	0.5 mg, 1 mg, 2 mg tablet (Klonopin); 0.125 mg, 0.25 mg, 0.5 mg, 1 mg, 2 mg (disintegrating tablet)	0.5–1 mg orally 3 times/day	CIV	Max total daily dose 20 mg divided into 3 doses
Diazepam (dye AZ e pam)	Diastat, Diastat Pediatric, Diazepam Intensol, Valium Valtoco nasal spray	Oral, IM, IV, rectal	Generic: 5 mg/mL injection solution; 5 mg/5 mL oral solution; 2 mg, 5 mg, 10 mg tablet (Valium); 5 mg/mL oral solution (Diazepam Intensol)	5–10 mg IV every 10–15 min up to a maximum dose of 30 mg	CIV	Status epilepticus, seizure clusters
Lorazepam (lor A ze pam)	Ativan, Lorazepam Intensol	IM, IV, oral	2 mg/mL, 4 mg/mL injection solution (Ativan); 0.5 mg, 1 mg, 2 mg tablet (Ativan); 2 mg/mL oral solution (Lorazepam Intensol); generic: 2 mg/mL, 4 mg/mL injection solution; 2 mg/mL oral solution: 0.5 mg, 1 mg, 2 mg tablets	4 mg IV given slowly at 2 mg/min; may repeat dose in 10–15 min if needed for status epilepticus or seizure cluster	CIV	Status epilepticus, seizure clusters
Midazolam (mi DAZE oh lam)	Generics, Nayzilam	IV, IM, Preservative-free injection, Oral syrup, nasal spray	Injection 2 mg/mL and 5 mg/mL; Oral syrup 2 mg/mL; Nayzilam spray 5 mg/0.1 mL	Injection: Dose varies by age and weight One spray into nostril; may repeat in 10 min	CIV	For sedation, status epilepticus, seizure clusters; IV form comes in 2 concentrations
Clobazam (KLOE ba zam)	Onfi, Sympazan	Oral tablets, oral suspension	Tablets 10 mg, 20 mg Oral suspension 2.5 mg/mL	Dose by weight, 5–40 mg/day; titrate	CIV	Suspension: shake well

Continued next page

MEDICATION TABLE 6-4. Seizures/Epilepsy[3] (Continued)

CLASS Generic Name	Brand Name	Route	Forms	Dose	DEA Schedule/ Regulatory Status	Notes
Hydantoins						
Fosphenytoin sodium (fos FEN i toyn)	Cerebyx	IV, IM	50 mg PE/mL (PE = phenytoin equivalents), 75 mg/mL	10–20 mg PE/kg IV or IM; maximum IV rate of 150 mg PE/min	Rx only	For short-term administration when oral phenytoin is not feasible
Phenytoin (FEN i toyn)	Dilantin, Dilantin Infatabs, Dilantin-125	Oral, IV	Oral capsule, suspension, chewable tablet (Dilantin Infatab); injection	100–300 mg oral or IV every 6–8 hr	Rx only	Dose should be adjusted every 7–10 days as necessary
Succinimides						
Ethosuximide (eth oh SUX i mide)	Zarontin	Oral	Zarontin: 250 mg liquid-filled capsule; 250 mg/5 mL oral syrup (both forms available generic)	500 mg/day orally adjusted by 250 mg increments every 4–7 days	Rx only	Dosages exceeding 1.5 g daily should be administered only under the strictest supervision of a physician
Miscellaneous Anticonvulsants						
Cannabidiol (kan na bi DYE ol)	Epidiolex	Oral	Oral solution 100 mg/ml	2.5–10 mg/kg twice a day; titrate dose	Schedule V controlled substance (CV)	For Lennox-Gastaut or Dravet syndrome
Carbamazepine (kar ba MAZ e peen)	Carbatrol, Epitol, Equetor, Tegretol, Tegretol-XR	Oral	Oral tablets, suspension, capsule, chewable, extended-release	400–1,200 mg/day in divided doses; children are dosed by weight; titrate dose	Rx	Indicated for the management of epilepsy, neuralgia, and bipolar disorder
Cenobamate (sen o BAM ate)	Xcopri	Oral	Oral tablets 12.5 mg, 25 mg, 50 mg, 100 mg, 150 mg, 200 mg	Titrate dose from 12.5 mg daily to target over several weeks; maximum dose is 400 mg/day	CV	Slow discontinuation recommended over several weeks
Gabapentin (GA ba PEN tin)	Neurontin, Gralise (extended release)	Oral	100 mg, 300 mg, 400 mg capsule; 250 mg/5 mL oral solution; 300 mg, 600 mg, 800 mg oral tablet	300 mg orally 3 times/day; Gralise: once daily, for neuropathic pain	Rx only Gabapentin is a controlled substance in many states, but not federally	Drug may cause peripheral edema, myalgia, ataxia, nystagmus, tremor, or fatigue

Continued next page

MEDICATION TABLE 6-4. Seizures/Epilepsy[3] *(Continued)*

CLASS Generic Name	Brand Name	Route	Forms	Dose	DEA Schedule/ Regulatory Status	Notes
Lacosamide (la KOE sa mide)	Vimpat	IV, oral	10 mg/mL IV solution; 10 mg/mL oral solution; 50 mg, 100 mg, 150 mg, 200 mg tablets	50 mg orally twice daily; increase weekly by 100 mg/day in 2 divided doses up to 200–400 mg/day	CV	Discontinuation may cause seizures (this is true of all antiepileptics as quick discontinuation can cause exacerbation of seizures)
Lamotrigine (la MOE tri jeen)	Lamictal, Lamictal CD, Lamictal ODT, Lamictal XR	Oral	Lamictal CD: 2 mg, 5 mg, 25 mg oral chewable tablet; Lamictal ODT: 25 mg, 50 mg, 100 mg, 200 mg disintegrating mucous membrane tablet; Lamictal: 25 mg, 100 mg, 150 mg, 200 mg tablet; Lamictal XR: 25 mg, 50 mg, 100 mg, 200 mg, 300 mg tablet; generically available as 25 mg, 100 mg, 150 mg, 200 mg tablets and 5 mg and 25 mg chewable tablets	25 mg/day orally every other day for 2 weeks, then 25 mg/day for 2 weeks; may increase dosage by 25 mg to 50 mg/day orally every 1–2 weeks	Rx only	Slower titration is needed for patients who are also taking valproate
Levetiracetam (leh ve ti RA se tam)	Keppra, Keppra XR	IV, oral	Keppra: 100 mg/mL IV solution; 100 mg/mL oral solution; 250 mg, 500 mg, 750 mg, 1,000 mg tablet; Keppra XR: 500 mg, 750 mg tablet; Elepsia XR: 1,000 mg, 1,500 mg Generic immediate-release dosage forms available	500 mg orally or IV twice daily; up to 3,000 mg/day Children are dosed by age and weight	Rx only	Patients should report mood swings, agitation, hostile behavior, suicidal ideation, or unusual changes in behavior
Oxcarbazepine (ox car BAZ e peen)	Trileptal, Oxtellar XR	Oral	Trileptal: 300 mg/5 mL oral suspension; 150 mg, 300 mg, 600 mg tablet; all dosage forms available as generic	300 mg orally twice a day, then increase the dosage weekly up to 1200 mg–2400 mg/day	Rx only	
Perampanel (pe RAM pa nel)	Fycompa	Oral	Tablets 2 mg, 4 mg, 6 mg, 8 mg, 10 mg, 12 mg Suspension 0.5 mg/mL	2 mg at bedtime; titrate to 4–12 mg nightly	Schedule III controlled substance (CIII)	Monitor for serious psychiatric and behavior reactions

Continued next page

MEDICATION TABLE 6-4. Seizures/Epilepsy[3] (Continued)

CLASS Generic Name	Brand Name	Route	Forms	Dose	DEA Schedule/ Regulatory Status	Notes
Pregabalin (pre GAB a lin)	Lyrica	Oral	25 mg, 50 mg, 75 mg, 100 mg, 150 mg, 200 mg, 225 mg, 300 mg capsules	No greater than 75 mg orally 2 times daily or 50 mg orally 3 times daily and increased to a maximum dose of 600 mg/day in divided doses	CV, Rx only	Alcohol should be avoided with administration of pregabalin
Rufinamide (roo FIN a mide)	Banzel	Oral	40 mg/mL oral suspension; 200 mg, 400 mg tablets	400–800 mg/day orally in 2 equally divided doses; increase by 400–800 mg/day every 2 days to a maximum dose of 3,200 mg/day in 2 equally divided doses	Rx only	Abrupt discontinuation should be avoided; nonhormonal forms of contraception are recommended during use for female patients
Stiripentol (stir ee PEN tol)	Diacomit	Oral	Capsules 250 mg, 500 mg Powder for oral suspension packets 250 mg, 500 mg	Dose by weight, 50 mg/kg/day, in 2 or 3 divided doses; take with a meal	Rx only	For Dravet syndrome. monitor weight and growth
Tiagabine hydrochloride (ty AG a been)	Gabitril	Oral	2 mg, 4 mg, 12 mg, 16 mg tablet	Adjunct therapy for patients taking enzyme-inducing antiepileptics: 4 mg orally once a day; may increase dosage by 4–8 mg/day at weekly intervals to a maximum dose of 56 mg/day (given in 2–4 divided doses); lower doses are used in patients who are not taking enzyme-inducing drugs	Rx only	Modification of concomitant antiepilepsy drugs is not necessary, unless clinically indicated

Continued next page

MEDICATION TABLE 6-4. Seizures/Epilepsy[3] (Continued)

CLASS Generic Name	Brand Name	Route	Forms	Dose	DEA Schedule/ Regulatory Status	Notes
Topiramate (toe PYRE a mate)	Topamax, Eprotia, Trokendi XR	Oral	Topamax: 15 mg, 25 mg capsule; 25 mg, 50 mg, 100 mg, 200 mg tablet; Topiragen: 25 mg, 50 mg, 100 mg, 200 mg tablet (all forms also available generic)	Titrated over 6 weeks to maximum dose of 200 mg orally twice daily	Rx only	May decrease effectiveness of estrogen-containing oral contraceptives with concurrent use
Valproate (val PROE ate) sodium, valproic (val PROE ik) acid, divalproex (dye val PRO ex) sodium	Depakene, Depakote, Depakote ER, Depakote Sprinkles, Depakote DR	IV oral	Depakote ER: 250 mg, 500 mg extended-release tablets; Depakote: 125 mg, 250 mg, 500 mg delayed-release tablet; Depakote Sprinkles: 125 mg delayed-release capsule; generic: 100 mg/mL IV solution; Depakene: 250 mg liquid-filled capsule; 250 mg/5 mL oral syrup; Stavzor: 125 mg, 250 mg, 500 mg capsule; (many generic forms available)	15 mg/kg/day IV (maximum 60 mg/kg/day); 15 mg/kg/day orally in 2–3 divided doses	Rx only	May be administered with food to avoid gastrointestinal irritation
Vigabatrin (vye GA ba trin)	Sabril, Vigadrone	Oral	500 mg/packet oral powder for solution; 500 mg tablet	500 mg orally twice daily; titrate daily dose in 500 mg increment to a maximum dose of 1,500 mg twice daily	Rx only	Vigabitrin may cause permanent vision loss; only available through a special restricted distribution program called SHARE
Zonisamide (zoe NIS a mide)	Zonegran	Oral	25 mg, 50 mg, 100 mg capsule (also available in generic form)	100–600 mg/day in 1–2 divided doses	Rx only	No additional benefit has been demonstrated with dosages above 400 mg/day

CIII = Schedule III controlled substance; CIV = Schedule IV controlled substance; DEA = U.S. Food and Drug Administration; IM = intramuscular; IV = intravenous.

MEDICATION TABLE 6-5. Multiple Sclerosis (MS)[3]

Generic Name	Brand Name	Route	Forms	Dose	Notes
Glatiramer (gla TIR a mer)	Copaxone	SUBQ	20 mg/mL prefilled syringe, 40 mg/mL prefilled syringe	20 mg daily or 40 mg 3 times/week	Used to help relieve the severity and frequency of MS attacks
Interferon beta-1a (in ter FEER on)	Avonex Pen, generics	IM	Injection powder for reconstitution (containing albumin), single-use prefilled syringe, single-use autoinjector	Titrate to 30 mcg once weekly	Avonex must be given by IM injection
	Rebif	SUBQ	Injection solution (albumin free) 8.8 mcg, 22 mcg, and 44 mcg autoinjectors and prefilled syringes	Titrate to 22 mcg or 44 mcg 3 times/week	Rebif is to be administered SUBQ at the same time of day on the same 3 days each week, rotating injection sites; may premedicate with an analgesic
Peginterferon beta-1a	Plegridy	SUBQ	125 mcg/0.5 mg in single-dose pens or syringes; 63 mcg and 94 mcg prefilled pens	Titrate to 125 mcg every 14 days	May premedicate with an analgesic on treatment days
Interferon (in ter FEER on) beta-1b	Betaseron	SUBQ	Injection powder for reconstitution, with diluent (containing albumin)	0.25 mg every other day; titrate dose	Gradual dose titration, analgesics, and/or antipyretics may help decrease flu-like symptoms on treatment days
	Extavia	SUBQ	Injection powder for reconstitution, with diluent (containing albumin preservative free)	0.25 mg every other day; titrate dose	Patient should be well hydrated
Cladribine (KLAD ri been)	Mavenclad	Oral	Tablets 10 mg	Two yearly treatment courses; 2 cycles/course; cumulative dose 3.5 mg/kg	Do not use during pregnancy; dose should be given at least 3 hours before or after any other oral medication; hands must be dry when taking drug; wash hands well after taking
Mitoxantrone (mye toe ZAN trone)	Novantrone	IV	Injection solution: 2 mg/mL; add to D5W or NS for infusion	12 mg/m^2 every 3 months	Maximum lifetime cumulative dose: 140 mg/m^2
Dimethyl fumarate (dye METH il FU mar ate)	Tecfidera	Oral	Delayed-release capsules 120 mg, 240 mg	120 mg twice daily for 7 days, then 240 mg twice daily	Flushing is a common side effect; take with food, or take up to 325 mg non-enteric-coated aspirin 30 minutes before dose to reduce flushing
Diroximel fumarate (dir OX i mel FU mar ate)	Vumerity	Oral	Delayed-release capsules 231 mg	231 mg twice daily for 7 days, then 462 mg twice daily	Avoid administration with a high-fat, high-calorie meal, avoid co-administration with alcohol; flushing is a common side effect; take with food, or take up to 325 mg non-enteric-coated aspirin 30 minutes before dose to reduce flushing

Continued next page

MEDICATION TABLE 6-5. Multiple Sclerosis (MS)[3] (Continued)

Generic Name	Brand Name	Route	Forms	Dose	Notes
Fingolimod (fing GO li mod)	Gilenya	Oral	Capsules 0.25 mg, 0.5 mg	Adults: 0.5 mg daily Children under 10 years and less than 40 kg: 0.25 mg orally daily	Monitor patient for 6 hours after first dose for bradycardia, blood pressure, pulse; contraindicated with recent MI, unstable angina, stroke, TIA, Class III or IV heart failure
Siponimod (si PON i mod)	Mayzent	Oral	Tablets 0.25 mg and 2 mg	Genotype determines dose target; titrate from 0.25 mg daily to 1 mg or 2 mg daily dose	Contraindicated with MI, unstable angina, stroke, TIA, Class III or IV heart failure in last 6 months; contraindicated in CYP2C9*3/*3 genotype
Teriflunomide (te ri FLU no mid)	Aubagio	Oral	Tablets 7 mg and 14 mg	7 mg or 14 mg daily	Exclude pregnancy before starting therapy; use effective contraception during use; check liver function before and every month during treatment for 6 months
Alemtuzumab (al em TUZ you mab)	Lemtrada	IV	Injection solution 12 mg/1.2 mL (10 mg/mL); add 12 mg to 100 mL NS or D5W; gently mix, infuse over 4 hours	First course: 12 mg/day on 5 consecutive days Second: 12 mg/day on 3 consecutive days, 12 months after first course; repeat, if needed, 12 months later	Premedicate with corticosteroids before infusion for the first 3 days of each treatment course; administer antivirals for herpes prophylaxis and continue for 2 months after completion; monitor vital signs during infusion, watch patient for at least 2 hours after infusion
Natalizumab (na ta LIZ you mab)	Tysabri	IV	Injection solution: 300 mg/15 mL; add to 100 mL NS for infusion	300 mg infused over 1 hour every 4 weeks	Access to this medication is restricted; treatment must be reauthorized every 6 months; watch patient for 1 hour after infusion
Ocrelizumab (ok ri LIZ you mab)	Ocrevus	IV	Injection solution 300 mg/10 mL; add 300 mg to 250 mL NS for infusion; duration 2.5 hours or longer Add 600 mg to 500 mL NS for infusion; duration 3.5 hours or longer	Start: 300 mg IV infusion; repeat in 2 weeks; 600 mg IV infusion every 6 months thereafter	Only FDA-approved disease-modifying therapy for primary-progressive MS; premedicate with corticosteroid and antihistamine before infusion; observe patient for 1 hour after infusion
Dalfampridine (dal FAM pri deen)	Ampyra	Oral	Extended-release tablets 10 mg	10 mg twice daily	For improvement in walking for adults with MS; contraindicated in patients with history of seizures and CrCl ≤ 50 mL/min

D5W = dextrose 5% in water; FDA = U.S. Food and Drug Administration; IM = intramuscular; IV = intravenous; MI = myocardial infarction; NS = normal saline; SUBQ = subcutaneous; TIA = transient ischemic attack.

MEDICATION TABLE 6-6. Sleep Disorders[3]

CLASS Generic Name	Brand Name	Route	Forms	Dose	DEA Schedule/ Regulatory Status	Notes
Benzodiazepines						
Flurazepam (flure AZ e pam)	Dalmane	Oral	15 mg, 30 mg capsule	15–30 mg PO at bedtime	Schedule IV controlled substance (CIV)	Flurazepam is contraindicated in pregnancy; category X
Quazepam (KWAZ e pam)	Doral	Oral	15 mg tablet	7.5–15 mg at bedtime	CIV	Patient should avoid activities requiring mental alertness or coordination until drug effects are realized
Temazepam (te MAZ e pam)	Restoril	Oral	7.5 mg, 15 mg, 22.5 mg, 30 mg capsule	7.5–30 mg PO at bedtime	CIV	May cause the risk of "sleep-driving" and other complex behaviors when patient is not fully awake, especially when combined with alcohol
Triazolam (trye AY zoe lam)	Halcion	Oral	0.125 mg, 0.25 mg tablet	0.125–0.25 mg at bedtime	CIV	Although available in the United States, the United Kingdom's Committee on the Safety of Medicines (CSM) removed triazolam from the market in 1991
Sedative/Hypnotics						
Eszopiclone (es ZOE pi clone)	Lunesta	Oral	1 mg, 2 mg, 3 mg tablet	1 mg hs, may increase to 2–3 mg PO immediately before bedtime	CIV	Some fatal anaphylactic reactions have been reported with the administration of Lunesta
Ramelteon (ram EL tee on)	Rozerem	Oral	8 mg tablet	8 mg PO within 30 min of bedtime	Rx only	Alcohol should be avoided with the administration of sedatives such as ramelteon
Zaleplon (ZAL e plon)	Sonata	Oral	5 mg, 10 mg capsule	5–10 mg at bedtime, may increase to 20 mg	CIV	Zaleplon and other sedatives may cause impaired coordination

Continued next page

MEDICATION TABLE 6-6. Sleep Disorders[3] *(Continued)*

CLASS Generic Name	Brand Name	Route	Forms	Dose	DEA Schedule/ Regulatory Status	Notes
Zolpidem (ZOLE pi dem)	Ambien, Ambien CR, Edluar, Zolpimist	Oral	5 mg, 10 mg, 12.5 mg extended-release tablet (Ambien); 6.25 mg, 12.5 mg extended-release tablet (Ambien CR); 5 mg, 10 mg sublingual tablet (Edluar); 5 mg/0.1 mL mucous membrane spray (Zolpimist)	5–10 mg 6.25–12.5 mg for ER tablets PO immediately before bedtime	CIV	Tablet forms may cause visual disturbance and constipation
Antihistamines						
Diphenhydramine (dye fen HYE dra meen)	Benadryl, Nytol, and many others available OTC with diphenhydramine as sole active ingredient or in combination with others	Oral, IV, IM	25 mg, 50 mg (tablet and capsule); 12.5 mg/5 mL elixir and solution; 10 mg/mL, 50 mg/mL injection solution	25–50 mg PO at bedtime	Rx/OTC	Diphenhydramine is not to be taken concomitantly with MAO inhibitors or CNS depressants
Doxylamine (dox IL a meen)	Unisom, others	Oral	25 mg tablet; 5 mg chewable tablet (Aldex AN)	25–50 mg PO 30 min before bedtime	Rx/OTC	Doxylamine should not be taken for more than 2 weeks when used to treat insomnia

CNS = central nervous system; DEA = U.S. Drug Enforcement Administration; MAO = monoamine oxidase; OTC = over the counter; PO = by mouth.

Chapter 7
Psychiatric Diseases

Toy S. Biederman, PharmD

KEY TERMS AND DEFINITIONS

Addiction—the compulsive drive to use a substance in spite of the adverse consequences involved. Addiction meets at least one of the "five Cs" of drug using behavior: the drug is used chronically, compulsively, disregarding the consequences of use; the user craves the drug, and lacks control over use of the drug.

Delusion—a false, fixed belief (often an aspect of psychosis). Patients may believe that they are a historical figure, that someone is persecuting them, or that they have special powers, among other ideas.

Dependence—the condition of needing to take a medication to avoid symptoms of withdrawal. Although this is a common symptom in people who use drugs or alcohol recreationally, this may also be a feature of some drugs used for high blood pressure, depression, and pain. Dependence should not be confused with addiction, which involves psychological and motivational drives to use a drug.

Hallucination—a false sensory experience, such as hearing, seeing, smelling, or feeling something that is not really there. Hallucinations may be a symptom of a psychotic condition, such as schizophrenia, or a result from a drug reaction or medical condition, such as delirium.

Mania—the state of agitation associated with bipolar disorder, in which a patient may feel abnormally energetic, excited, creative, and irritable. Manic episodes can also include psychotic symptoms.

DOI 10.37573/9781585286638.007

Mood stabilizer—a medication that is prescribed to keep a patient with bipolar disorder from swinging into either mania or depression.

Phobia—the fear of an object, situation, or living thing, such as *arachnophobia* (the fear of spiders).

Psychosis—a condition in which a patient's experiences are not in agreement with objective reality (eg, hallucinations and delusions).

Suicide—the intentional taking of one's own life. Suicide and suicide attempts are more common in patients with psychiatric illnesses, such as depression, bipolar disease, and schizophrenia, than in the general population.

Tolerance—the phenomenon of requiring larger doses of a drug to get the same effect that was previously achieved by a lower dose. Tolerance can apply to both the desired and undesired effects of a medication. Although people who take drugs recreationally often become tolerant to the drug's effects, tolerance by itself is not the same as addiction.

LEARNING OBJECTIVES

After completing this chapter, you should be able to

1. Recall what is known of the causes and prevalence of mental illnesses.

2. List the symptoms and recall the expected course of the following illnesses:
   - Depression.
   - Anxiety disorders.
   - Schizophrenia.
   - Bipolar disorder.
   - Attention deficit hyperactivity disorder.
   - Substance use disorder.

3. Recognize the psychosocial consequences for patients and families of patients with psychiatric disorders.

4. State the generic and brand names of medications used to treat psychiatric disorders, along with dosage forms and available doses.

5. Discuss the mechanism of action, common adverse effects, and special precautions of medications used to treat psychiatric disorders.

Psychiatric disorders hold a special place in medicine. These disorders, for the most part, cannot be detected or monitored using blood tests, x-rays, or any number of diagnostic procedures in the way other medical problems are. Symptoms of these disorders are expressed in terms of emotions and behaviors. Patients with psychiatric conditions sometimes appear eccentric, disorderly, or peculiar. They are at a higher risk of early death due to violence and suicide. Along with patients with neurologic diseases, people with psychiatric diagnoses are burdened with stigma. Stigma is the condition of associating negative attitudes with a person due to a characteristic that person carries. The stigma of psychiatric disorders can cause delays in diagnosis and adherence to treatment. Psychiatric patients are sometimes blamed for their conditions, believed to be morally lacking, and told that they are weak. Patients are subjected to scrutiny and judgment that those with other medical conditions, such as diabetes and cancer, do not have to deal with.

These attitudes are unfortunate because psychiatric illnesses are caused by processes going wrong in the brain. These problems are usually caused by some abnormality in the chemical messengers that carry nerve signals around the brain and to other parts of the body. These chemical messengers, the neurotransmitters described in Chapters 4 and 5, are the targets of many of the medications used to treat mental illnesses. Neurotransmitters have different effects when their activity is either too high or too low. We know that neurotransmitters are involved in different psychiatric illnesses. In addition, other brain chemicals and chemical receptors have an effect on the way the brain processes information, moods, and perceptions. Often, a patient will have more than one psychiatric diagnosis at the same time. Due to the vast differences from one patient to another and the lack of a physical means of measuring brain chemical levels, doctors may need to try different medications to find the one that works best for a patient that is also well tolerated. For these reasons, treating psychiatric illnesses is often quite challenging.

Many psychiatric diseases tend to run in families, suggesting a genetic component. Some, such as schizophrenia, have genetic trends but may also occur in a family previously unaffected by the disease. Interestingly, many famous artists, musicians, writers, inventors, and scientists have suffered from psychiatric diseases. Although at times patients with psychiatric illnesses do not have the insight necessary to maintain good adherence to their therapy, members of their healthcare team need to apply empathy as well as good judgment in dealing with them. Patients need to know that their pharmacy team members are trustworthy, nonjudgmental, and concerned. With more openness and acceptance, individuals may find it easier to open up about concerns about themselves or family members. Psychiatric symptoms such as anxiety, depression, and delusions can also be side effects of medications and systemic medical problems. In addition, psychiatric conditions, such as depression and anxiety, can accompany many chronic medical problems.

Who treats patients with psychiatric illnesses? There are many practitioners who treat these patients. In most states, only physicians can prescribe medications for psychiatric illnesses. Of these physicians, the most commonly associated with these illnesses are psychiatrists. Psychiatrists are physicians who specialize in diagnosing and treating mental illnesses. Other practitioners include psychologists, psychiatric social workers, and various therapists, who provide counseling to help patients understand and manage their illnesses. However, most patients are treated by non-specialists, including family physicians, internists, and pediatricians. Nurse practitioners, physician's assistants, and psychiatric pharmacists also provide care under a physician's supervision.

Because psychiatric illnesses can't be detected or monitored with thermometers, stethoscopes, and x-rays, psychiatrists have developed diagnostic criteria for each illness that are gathered together in the *Diagnostic and Statistical Manual of Mental Disorders.*[1] This book is in its fifth edition and is referred to as the DSM-5. The DSM-5 lists characteristics and symptoms for each identified mental disorder and gives the criteria needed for diagnosing an illness. Many other diagnostic and assessment tools, such as the Mental Status Examination, the Hamilton Depression Inventory, and the Positive and Negative Symptom Scale are used to determine, measure, and monitor mental illnesses. During the interview with the patient, the practitioner will determine where the patient's symptoms fit among various potential diagnoses. The practitioner considers the patient's current symptoms, including mood, activity level, interests, behavior, appearance, and thought processes, and also the patient's personal and family history. The doctor will rate the patient's level of insight into the situation and whether the patient appears to have the potential to be dangerous to him- or herself or others. Some of the traits assessed are mood, affect, facial expressiveness, appearance, use of language, activity, thought disturbances, insight, and judgment. The practitioner will also consider whether the symptoms could be due to medication side effects or another illness. For example, when thyroid hormone levels are low, a patient will often feel tired and depressed, so when a person complains of depression, thyroid gland function will usually be checked.

When a diagnosis is made, a course of treatment will also be planned. This is frequently done in collaboration with the patient and sometimes with other family members. In some situations, there may be more than one reasonable alternative, such as medication or counseling. Medication is often necessary for the patient to be restored to a reasonable level of functioning. In most situations, counseling is also beneficial to help the patient learn to manage his or her illness.

DEPRESSION

CASE STUDY

Justine is a 36-year-old married woman who has gone to her doctor because she is having trouble sleeping and cannot concentrate on her work as a data entry technician. When the doctor questioned her, she also admitted that she and her husband have recently separated, her mother died 6 months ago, and she is having trouble with her 14-year-old daughter. Justine says that she has to make a lot of effort just to get out of bed and get ready for work, has frequent crying spells, and she does not have hope of her life getting better. She has stopped going to her quilting class and choir practice because, "I just don't feel up to it. I don't get anything out of it anymore." She denies any thoughts of suicide but says she thinks everyone would be happier if she disappeared. She describes waking up 2 to 3 hours before the alarm clock goes off and not being able to get back to sleep. She says she lies in bed thinking about her problems over and over. Justine is otherwise healthy, except for a history of two urinary tract infections in the past 4 years. She says she had "baby blues" after the birth of her second child but was not treated. She takes no medications except for occasional ibuprofen or acetaminophen for headache or menstrual cramps. She has two children: a 14-year-old daughter and a 9-year-old son.

Depression is a common psychiatric illness. It is more serious than just feeling "down," or having "the blues." It is deeper and more intense than sadness or mourning, although those conditions may be the beginning of depression and share some features. Depression can be a part of other diseases, especially chronic diseases, such as Alzheimer's and kidney failure. Sometimes depression can be caused or made worse by certain medications. Although certain groups are more likely to suffer from depression, it can affect young and old, as well as people of all genders and cultural groups. There are many treatments but no one-size-fits-all approach. Many people who have depression do not get treatment, and many self-medicate with alcohol or other drugs.

Pathophysiology

In the course of a lifetime, more than 10% of people experience depression.[2] The causes of depression are not known for certain, but depressive illnesses often run in families. About 8% of patients with major depression have a close relative who has also suffered from depression. Scientists believe that the feeling of depression is due to changes in brain neurotransmitters, especially norepinephrine, serotonin, and dopamine. What causes these changes is not known, but stress, lack of sunlight and exercise, chronic disease, and poor sleep are often associated with the development of depression. The medications used in treating depression work by increasing the levels of one or all of the neurotransmitters in order to raise the mood.

The symptoms of depression are not identical in every patient. Depression is diagnosed by assessing whether a patient's symptoms correlate with the definition of depression in the DSM-5, including number of symptoms and duration. (Depression is usually diagnosed only if a patient shows five or more signs over a period of at least 2 weeks.) All these symptoms are not necessary for a diagnosis of depression. The symptoms include pessimism and hopelessness, having much less interest and pleasure in doing usually enjoyable activities, sleeping problems (either too much or too little sleep nearly every day) often including waking up early in the morning and being unable to fall back to sleep, lack of energy, problems concentrating or making decisions, feeling worthless or excessively guilty, marked weight gain or loss, and thinking about death or suicide.[1] People who are depressed often look sad or expressionless and may be either agitated and irritable or slow and sluggish. Some people with depression will say that they want to die, but many will not. Asking a person if he or she has thought about suicide does not increase the likelihood that the person will actually attempt suicide. Asking may give the opportunity to offer help.

Nonpharmacologic Treatments

There are many treatments for depression that do not involve drugs. Some patients will respond to a nonpharmacologic method alone. Others have found that a nonpharmacologic method in addition to medication has more benefit. The type and severity of depression varies among patients, and often different medications and nonpharmacologic treatments must be tried.

One of the nonpharmacologic approaches is talking with a psychologist, psychiatrist, or other trained therapist. The therapist uses different approaches to help the patient understand their problem, stop the pattern of negative thinking about themselves, and discover ways to overcome or manage problems and stressors. Another form of treatment for depression is intensive light exposure for several minutes a day. This method may be especially helpful for patients who have seasonal affective disorder (SAD), a form of depression that sets in during late fall and winter in response to short periods of daylight. Exercise programs help many patients who are mildly or moderately depressed. Electroconvulsive shock therapy (ECT) is beneficial for many severely depressed patients and gives improvement quicker than most other methods. A good diet may be helpful; in addition, some physicians add a "medical food," such as methylfolate, to antidepressant regimens.

Pharmacologic Treatment

The medications used to treat depression are called antidepressants. They work to increase neurotransmitter levels by different mechanisms. (Some antidepressants are also used for other purposes, such as to treat pain conditions and to prevent migraine headaches. Antidepressants are also useful in treating anxiety, as we will discuss in the next section.) The class *antidepressants* is further subdivided based on how the agents work or their chemical structure. All antidepressants have one feature in common—they do not act immediately but must be taken for a few weeks to develop their full effect. Patients are often not aware of this characteristic and become discouraged with their medicine when they do not feel better right away. Patients need to be advised to give the medication a long enough trial and to check back with their doctor early in treatment to talk about their response.

CASE?

What symptoms does Justine have that are consistent with depression? Can her depression be causing problems with her family relationships and her job?

The most frequently used antidepressants are the selective serotonin reuptake inhibitors (SSRIs). They have been available since the late 1980s when fluoxetine (Prozac) was released onto the market. Since then, many other SSRIs have been marketed, including paroxetine (Paxil), sertraline (Zoloft), citalopram (Celexa), fluvoxamine, and escitalopram (Lexapro). They all work by reducing the uptake of serotonin into the presynaptic nerve ending, increasing the amount of serotonin available in the synapse between two nerves (Figure 7-1).

These medicines differ in how long they last in the body and in some of their side effects. Although their actions are similar, most of them (except citalopram and escitalopram) are very different from one another chemically and it is reasonable to try a different drug in this category if the first one does not have the desired effect.

ALERT!

LOOK-ALIKE/SOUND-ALIKE—Care must be exercised to prevent confusing the brand name Celexa (citalopram) with other drugs like Celebrex and Cerebyx.[3]

Patients treated with SSRIs seldom have an immediate response. A patient will begin to have some benefit in 1 or 2 weeks after beginning the medication, but it may take 4 weeks or more to have the maximum effect. In addition, patients who need to stop taking one of these medications should taper off the medication gradually by reducing the dose over a few weeks to avoid a withdrawal syndrome that can include anxiety, sleep problems, and shock-like sensations in the arms. Paroxetine is one of the worst for the withdrawal effects, because it is quickly removed from the body. Fluoxetine has the least potential for withdrawal, because it is removed very slowly. The others are somewhere in between these two.

CASE?

Justine has been prescribed Zoloft 25 mg, once daily, by her doctor. Can she expect to feel better right away?

Side effects of the SSRIs include sleep problems (less for paroxetine than the others). Many patients find that SSRI medications cause them to have trouble falling asleep. This is especially true of fluoxetine and sertraline. Dosing these medications in the morning (except for paroxetine) can help a patient avoid this problem. In addition, patients sometimes experience headaches, diarrhea, anxiety, or nausea due to SSRIs, especially when starting them. To lessen these

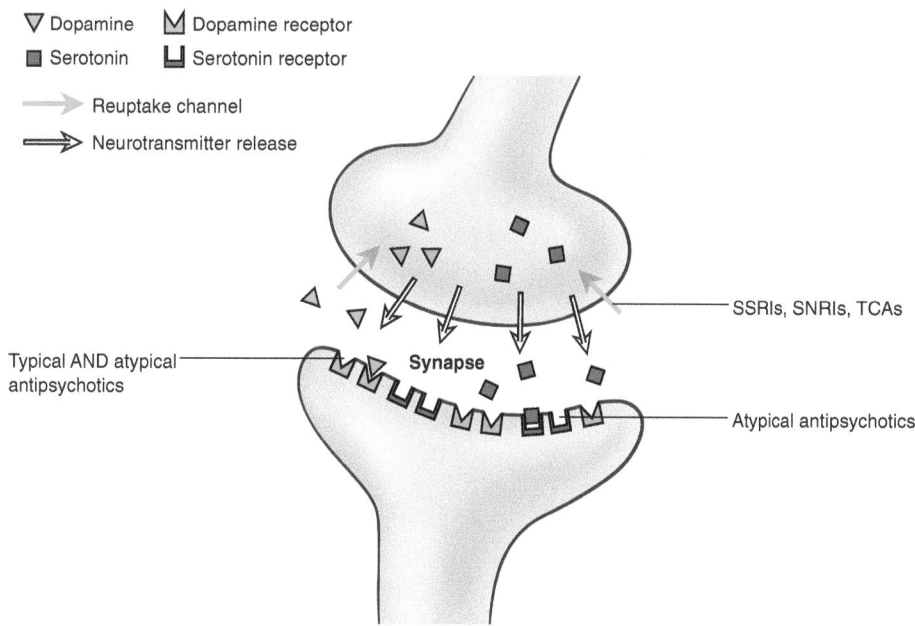

FIGURE 7-1. Neurotransmitters in the central nervous system.

effects, doctors will often start a patient on one-half the desired dose initially and increase to the full dosage in a few days to a week.

There is a rare but potentially dangerous side effect of SSRIs when used in combination with other medications that affect serotonin levels, called the serotonin syndrome. This syndrome can involve high or low blood pressure, confusion, diarrhea, and flushing of the skin. This is a potentially life-threatening reaction, and the patient needs to be treated in the hospital. Pharmacists monitor for other potentially interacting medications to avoid this situation.

Another class of antidepressants, the serotonin norepinephrine reuptake inhibitors (SNRIs), increases both serotonin and norepinephrine by inhibiting their reuptake. This class works similarly to the SSRIs and includes venlafaxine (Effexor XR), desvenlafaxine (Pristiq), and duloxetine (Cymbalta). This class may have a quicker onset in antidepressant effect. They are often second-line choices after the SSRIs due to side effects (especially withdrawal symptoms) and expense. The SSRIs and SNRIs are also useful in treating anxiety disorders, as we will discuss in the next section. SNRIs are often helpful in treating pain conditions, such as fibromyalgia, diabetic peripheral neuropathy, and chronic musculoskeletal pain. Some of these products (such as duloxetine) have formal indications for these conditions. Patients on SNRIs also can experience intense, distressing withdrawal symptoms when discontinuing them, or even after missing a few doses. As with the SSRIs and many other agents that act on the central nervous system (CNS), discontinuation should be gradual.

In addition to the SSRIs and SNRIs, there are medications that have additional activities. One is vilazodone (Viibryd), an SNRI that also acts as a partial agonist at one type of serotonin receptor, the 5-HT-1A receptor. Vortioxetine (Trintellix) acts as an SSRI, but has other activity at several serotonin receptors.

Selegiline, which is discussed in Chapter 6, is available as a transdermal patch (Emsam) for the treatment of depression. Another novel agent, esketamine (Spravato), is derived from ketamine (a medication used in anesthesia and, illegally, as a party drug). Esketamine is an N-methyl-D-aspartate (NMDA) antagonist (acting on some receptors that normally respond to the neurotransmitter glutamate), and is only available as a nasal spray for the treatment of depression that has not responded to other therapies. This product is administered in an office setting once or twice a week, and is only available through a restricted program. Because of a side effect called "dissociation," which is an eerie sensation that is distressing to many patients, patients must be monitored for at least two hours after receiving the drug.[4]

ALERT!

Esketamine is intended for patient administration under the direct observation of a healthcare provider, and there is a requirement that patients are monitored by a healthcare provider for at least 2 hours. Esketamine must never be dispensed directly to a patient for home use.[4]

PRACTICE POINT

U.S. pharmacies must be certified in the SPRAVATO® REMS (Risk Evaluation and Mitigation Strategy) Program to be able to receive and dispense esketamine (a DEA Schedule III controlled substance).

Several drugs known as "atypical antipsychotics," initially approved for the treatment of schizophrenia and other psychotic disorders (and discussed later in this chapter), have achieved approval for treatment of depression that is resistant to antidepressants alone. Some in this class are also approved for use in bipolar disorder.

CASE?

When Justine returns a week later with a new prescription for Zoloft 50 mg daily, she mentions that she has been having trouble sleeping since she started the Zoloft and is looking for something over-the-counter to help her. When the technician suggests pharmacist-counseling, what might be recommended?

There are two older categories of antidepressants: the tricyclic antidepressants (TCAs) and the monoamine oxidase inhibitors (MAOIs). Both medications increase the levels of norepinephrine and serotonin in the brain, although they do this by different mechanisms. MAOIs reduce an enzyme needed for the breakdown of neurotransmitters, causing their levels to rise. Unfortunately some medicines, such as decongestants, and foods, such as aged wines and cheeses, sardines, and fermented foods, can cause dramatic increases in the levels of norepinephrine in a patient who is taking an MAOI. This can lead to very high blood pressure with risk of stroke or other adverse event. For this reason, the MAOIs, including isocarboxazid, phenelzine, and tranylcypromine, are seldom used except for treatment of patients who have not responded well to other antidepressants. Patients who take MAOIs need to be cautioned about the risks of interactions with other medications and foods.

PRACTICE POINT

A medication guide must be provided to the patient with each dispensing of an MAOI.

The TCAs were the main drugs used for depression for many years but have taken a back seat to newer drugs, such as the SSRIs. TCAs work by reducing the reuptake of neurotransmitters from the small space between one nerve and another, the synapse. The higher levels of neurotransmitters in the synaptic space cause a neurotransmitter effect on the connecting nerve. The result is an increase of that neurotransmitter's activity in the brain, which improves the mood. There are many TCAs on the market. Because they have been around for so long, they are all available as generic medications, and doctors often order them using the generic name rather than the brand name. TCAs are still useful drugs for depression but have fallen from favor as first-line agents. If a patient deliberately takes an overdose of a TCA in an attempt at suicide, the TCA can cause rhythm problems in the heart, which are often fatal. The SSRIs are much safer in this regard. Since depressed patients are frequently suicidal, it is important to avoid giving them medications in amounts that can be used for a suicide attempt.

TCAs also have some other side effects that limit their use, and these side effects vary in severity from one drug to another. Anticholinergic side effects are common with the TCAs and include dry mouth, constipation, and urinary retention. Anticholinergic side effects can be especially troublesome in older patients and can even cause mental confusion. Among the TCAs, amitriptyline has the most anticholinergic activity, while desipramine has the least. Many TCAs also have some antihistamine activity, which can be useful but can also cause drowsiness. In fact, some doctors prescribe TCAs to help patients sleep. Doxepin has the most antihistamine activity of all the TCAs.

When TCAs are used to treat depression, they should be started at low doses and gradually increased over several weeks, depending on the response of the patient, side effects, and the expected effective dose of the medication. In addition to the anticholinergic side effects, TCAs can also cause orthostatic hypotension, in which the blood pressure falls when the patient gets up from a bed or chair. Patients should be advised to rise slowly from a sitting or lying position to avoid dizziness and falls.

All of the antidepressant classes discussed so far have the potential to cause sexual side effects, including decreased libido, orgasm, and erectile dysfunction. This side effect can be experienced by 20% or more of patients who use these medications, and it varies with the choice of medication and dosage. Depression itself can also cause sexual problems. Patients are often hesitant to mention sexual problems either as a symptom or a side effect. There are strategies that can be tried, and sometimes medication changes or additions will help with this problem. One class of antidepressants that does not usually cause this problem is aminoketones, of which bupropion is the only one. Bupropion (Wellbutrin) increases the levels of dopamine and norepinephrine in the brain but not serotonin levels. Bupropion is also particularly useful in treating SAD and in helping patients who wish to stop smoking. Bupropion has a less intense withdrawal syndrome than the SSRIs and SNRIs. Side effects of bupropion include sleep problems and headaches. Sometimes bupropion is added to an SSRI or SNRI if a patient is experiencing sexual problems due to the latter or to augment the antidepressant activity of another antidepressant.

CASE?

When she comes to the pharmacy to get her Zoloft refill, Justine mentions that her mother told her that people on antidepressants need to avoid wine and cheese and wonders why no one told her about this. What is the likely explanation?

Trazodone (Desyrel), nefazodone, and mirtazapine (Remeron) are antidepressants that also affect neurotransmitter levels but do not fall into the categories described earlier in this section. Trazodone is more frequently used for insomnia than for depression. Mirtazapine may also help with sleep and can increase appetite and weight. It may also cause dry mouth and orthostatic hypotension. Nefazodone has many drug interactions and can cause dangerous liver damage (although this is rare). It is reserved for patients who do not respond well to other antidepressants. Both mirtazapine and nefazodone cause fewer sexual side effects than other antidepressants. (See Medication Table 7-1; Medication Tables are located at the end of the chapter.)

ANXIETY

CASE STUDY

Victor is a 33-year-old stockbroker who, while at his doctor's office for a routine blood pressure follow-up, mentions that he has been having spells where he feels "like the walls are closing in and I can't escape. My gut tightens, I get sweaty, and my heart starts beating faster." He has had this feeling for several months before meetings, but he has also started feeling this way on airplanes and trains and recently after getting stuck on an elevator for a few minutes. He has declined some work assignments that have involved travel because of these spells. When he cannot avoid travel, he has begun using rituals, such as eating the same meal before each flight, circling the gate area seven times before boarding, and carrying a worry stone in his pocket. He denies any chest pain or shortness of breath on exertion. He says that he can't keep this up and is afraid that the problem will affect his work reviews. He says his company has been downsizing, and he is worried that he may be in the next round of layoffs. Victor is fidgeting with his keys while talking, and his fingernails show signs of chronic biting. He says he has always been a worrier "just like my dad." Victor is unmarried, owns his home, and is healthy except for hypertension for which he takes lisinopril 20 mg daily.

Pathophysiology

Anxiety is a common factor in our lives, but it is usually not so excessive as to be considered a disorder. Anxiety can be a normal response to certain medical conditions, such as hyperthyroidism or shortness of breath. There are several anxiety disorders, including generalized anxiety disorder (GAD), post-traumatic stress disorder (PTSD), obsessive-compulsive disorder (OCD), panic, social anxiety disorder, and phobias. A patient can experience more than one anxiety disorder and often has an anxiety disorder in addition to another psychiatric diagnosis such as depression or attention deficit hyperactivity disorder (ADHD). These disorders significantly interfere with the sufferers' lives—sometimes to the point of disability. Anxiety has been described as a feeling of fear that is disproportionate to the actual threat.[4] Anxiety disorders are the most common psychiatric disorder, with more than 20% of U.S. adults having this diagnosis every year.[2] Anxiety disorders are more common in women than men, often run in families, and usually develop before the age of 30.[2]

The reason for the development of anxiety is not well understood and probably includes several areas of the brain, including the most primitive areas, which are involved with the "fear, fight, or flight" response to a threat. Neurotransmitters believed to be involved with the anxiety response include norepinephrine, serotonin, and gamma-aminobutyric acid (GABA). GABA is the most important inhibitory (calming, suppressing) neurotransmitter in the brain. Drugs such as the benzodiazepines, which bind with GABA receptors in the brain, increase GABA activity and are one kind of medication used to treat anxiety.

The types of anxiety sound self-explanatory but deserve some elaboration. GAD is a condition in which the patient worries excessively and feels anxious most of the time. It is often accompanied by depression. OCD involves obsessions (intrusive, persistent thoughts) and compulsions (the driving need to act on those thoughts). People with OCD will ruminate on a certain idea, such as a fear of germs, and then feel compelled to try to control that fear through action, such as excessive hand washing or house cleaning. If thwarted in carrying out these compulsions, the patient will feel even more anxiety. Others will have a fear of intruders that will compel them to check the locks on their doors several times (often a specific number of times) before leaving the house. Still others will have a compulsion to pull the hairs of their eyebrows or eyelashes (trichotillomania) to ease their anxiety. Many types of OCD involve either safety or grooming issues. OCD should not be confused with obsessive-compulsive personality disorder, in which a person has a need to always be right and is excessively judgmental and controlling toward others.

PTSD is a response to a dangerous situation that the patient has experienced, such as a car wreck, house fire, rape, or battle. In addition to feelings of anxiety and depression, the patient will also often have a sleep disorder in which he or she re-experiences the traumatic event during dreaming. PTSD will sometimes appear years after the event, such as in retirement for a veteran of the battlefield.

Panic disorder is experienced as a feeling of sudden anxiety or impending doom, which can cause an overwhelming need to get out of a situation. The patient's heart may race or pound, or the patient may have difficulty breathing or may break out in a sweat. Panic disorder can cause a person to avoid the places or situations that he or she expects to cause the panic episode. Social anxiety disorder is a fear of dealing with people or being scrutinized and judged. Both panic disorder and social anxiety disorder can lead a person to withdraw from community life, sometimes to the point of confining themself to their home (agoraphobia).

CASE?

What symptoms does Victor have that suggest an anxiety disorder?

Nonpharmacologic Treatment

Nonpharmacologic treatment of anxiety disorders involves psychotherapy, including stress management techniques, cognitive behavioral therapy (CBT), and education on the disorder. OCD and PTSD often will not respond well to therapy alone and are among the more difficult types of anxiety to treat.

Pharmacologic Treatment

Because anxiety disorders are believed to involve the serotonin system in the brain, SSRIs and SNRIs are very useful in treating these disorders. All of the SSRI and SNRI medications can be used for anxiety disorders, although not all of them have formal Food and Drug Administration (FDA) indications for specific anxiety disorders. Clomipramine (Anafranil) is a TCA that has an FDA-approved indication for OCD. Since antidepressants can take several weeks to be effective in managing anxiety and sometimes make people feel jittery or anxious in the early phase of treatment, benzodiazepines may be used to quickly manage anxiety symptoms.[5]

Benzodiazepines are fast-acting medications that work by increasing the effects of GABA in the CNS. There are many benzodiazepines, which differ in onset of action, duration of action, how they are eliminated from the body, and the likelihood of interactions with other drugs. Alprazolam (Xanax) is the shortest-acting drug in this class and is usually dosed up to four times daily. Lorazepam (Ativan) is a little longer acting and is usually dosed three times a day. Diazepam (Valium) is longer acting than lorazepam and is dosed up to three times a day. Clonazepam (Klonopin) is the longest-acting drug in this class and is usually dosed once or twice a day. Other benzodiazepines—triazolam (Halcion), temazepam (Restoril), and flurazepam—are used specifically to treat insomnia. All benzodiazepines are sedating and have the potential to increase the respiratory depression caused by alcohol, barbiturates, and other sedating drugs. Patients who take benzodiazepines need to be warned that these medications can reduce alertness and make driving or operating machinery hazardous. Because benzodiazepines have the potential to become habit forming and are used illegally for recreational purposes, they are controlled substances.

Benzodiazepines have many uses beyond treating anxiety. They are used to calm an agitated or psychotic patient, relax muscle spasms, help with the management of nausea caused by chemotherapy, end seizures, manage withdrawal from alcohol and other sedating drugs of abuse, and to treat sleep disorders. Benzodiazepines used for anxiety disorders include alprazolam, diazepam, lorazepam, and clonazepam. Excessive sedation is an expected side effect, but some patients have paradoxical excitation or agitation when taking a particular benzodiazepine. In such patients, another benzodiazepine may be useful without causing that reaction. Many patients become tolerant to the sedating effects of benzodiazepines, especially after a few weeks of treatment. Diazepam and other long-acting benzodiazepines have more risk for elderly patients, especially for causing falls.

Buspirone is a medication that modifies the effects of serotonin at the serotonin 1A receptors. Buspirone affects serotonin in a manner different from the SSRIs. It is used to treat anxiety but is not habit forming and is much less sedating than the benzodiazepines. Buspirone takes 3 to 4 weeks to have its full effect in treating anxiety, so it is not useful for acute episodes. Side effects are usually mild and include dizziness, headache, and nausea. Other drugs sometimes used to treat anxiety disorders include TCAs and MAOIs, discussed in the section on depression (see Medication Table 7-2).

CASE?

What medication(s) might you expect to see prescribed for Victor?

SCHIZOPHRENIA

Perry is a 20-year-old man who until recently worked at a gardening store. He began working there after dropping out of the local community college, where he was enrolled for one semester. After working for about 6 months, Perry began to hear voices that told him he was no good. He also began to believe that his boss was planting small video cameras in the potted plants to catch him making mistakes. Perry became increasingly agitated at work and began talking strangely to customers (about how the other workers had it in for him and were trying to get him arrested, that he used to work for the FBI as an espionage specialist, and insisting that his name is Dirk Storm).

Perry lives with his parents. He quit his job one night after an argument with his boss about the cameras and has stayed in his room most of the time since. He will only give his parents brief comments about the people who are trying to get him in trouble. His room is a mess with clothes and food containers strewn about and several blankets covering the window. He has refused to let either parent in to help clean it up because they might interfere with a project he is working on to protect himself against people on TV who are stealing his thoughts. Perry has also neglected to bathe and frequently forgets to eat. One evening he started yelling at his mother because "she has turned against" him. His father persuaded him to take a ride in the car and took him to the hospital emergency room where he was admitted. Perry is 5'11" tall and weighs 245 lb. He denies alcohol and other drug use but smokes 1½ pack of cigarettes per day.

Pathophysiology

Schizophrenia is truly among the most tragic of medical diagnoses. Schizophrenia literally means *divided mind* and describes the split between the world as it really is and the way the schizophrenic patient perceives it. Schizophrenia usually develops in late adolescence or early adulthood. It occurs equally among men and women, although it often develops later in women and sometimes has a milder course. Schizophrenia affects up to 0.6% of the population in almost every culture in the world.[6] It is believed to be influenced by genetic factors, and severe physical or emotional stress of the mother during pregnancy is also associated with higher incidence of schizophrenia.[7] Abuse of marijuana and other drugs may also increase the risk that a person may develop a psychotic break from reality. People with schizophrenia often have abnormalities in brain structures, but exactly how these changes cause the symptoms is not known. The positive symptoms (see below) are associated with excessive activity of dopamine in the brain. There are many types of dopamine receptors in the brain, and the excessive activity at the dopamine-2 (D2) receptors are thought to drive the positive symptoms of hallucinations and delusions. Abnormalities in serotonin function are believed to influence the negative symptoms. Schizophrenia should not be confused with having multiple personalities (a dissociative disorder).

Schizophrenia often has an initial phase, when the patient is not yet diagnosed but begins to exhibit unusual behavior, such as becoming socially withdrawn, having difficulties with family members, friends, and coworkers, and becoming unusually suspicious or eccentric. The symptoms of schizophrenia are of three main types: positive symptoms, negative symptoms, and cognitive symptoms.[7] Positive does not mean that the symptoms are good; it means that symptoms are present that should not be there, such as hallucinations and delusions. Delusions may be the idea that someone is persecuting the patient. This is known as *paranoia*. Other delusions include beliefs that someone is trying to control or steal the patient's thoughts, beliefs that the patient is someone whom he or she is not (e.g., Moses, Jesus, Queen Elizabeth), or that simple gestures or greetings from strangers are code expressions. With schizophrenia, hallucinations are usually auditory—patients hear voices in their head, often telling them that they are evil or worthless, or telling them to do something bad or to harm themselves. Negative symptoms include a flattening in emotional response or expression, a withdrawal from social contacts, and a lack of interest in previous pleasurable activities. Cognitive symptoms include problems with memory, organization, logic, and insight into the patient's own problem.[8] People with schizophrenia are usually of normal intelligence but can have a decline in abilities as the disease progresses.

Schizophrenia is a disease that is lifelong and has no cure. It is one of the main causes of disability worldwide. Early treatment and control of symptoms is important for the long-term management of the disease, but there are many obstacles to management, including poor adherence to therapy due to poor insight into the disease or side effects of medication. Treatment of schizophrenia typically involves trials of many different medications, with relapses in which the patient has a psychotic break from reality and ends up in the hospital. People with schizophrenia are more likely to be withdrawn than to be violent but sometimes will become violent in response to their delusions and hallucinations. They are also at risk for homelessness, becoming victims of crime, substance abuse, and suicide. Interestingly, a high percentage (50% to 60%) of people with schizophrenia are also smokers, adding smoking-related illnesses to the problems faced by these patients.[9]

CASE?

What symptoms of schizophrenia does Perry have?

Nonpharmacologic Treatment

Nonpharmacologic treatment can be used in addition to treatment with medication to improve the patient's understanding of his or her disease, improve socialization, and help the patient deal with stress, substance abuse, and housing issues. Psychotherapy often includes the patient's family, to improve understanding of the disease and family dynamics. Schizophrenia is primarily managed with medication.

Pharmacologic Treatment

Pharmacologic treatment rests most heavily on drugs called antipsychotics. Older antipsychotic drugs treat schizophrenia by blocking D2 receptors, while the newer agents (atypical antipsychotics) affect both dopamine and serotonin. Both types of antipsychotics are employed in treating schizophrenia. These drugs have been invaluable for patients with schizophrenia, helping many to normalize their lives and avoid living in institutions, but even with these medications about one-third of patients are not well managed and will have a downhill course with their disease. In addition, antipsychotics have many short- and long-term side effects that can also impair the patient's health. Managing schizophrenia is a challenging undertaking.

Antipsychotics are categorized as *typical*, the older drugs that work by blocking dopamine activity, and *atypical*, newer drugs that antagonize (block) the serotonin 2A receptor in addition to antagonizing the D2 receptor. The atypical agents also disassociate from (let go of) the D2 receptor more quickly than the typical agents, and that is thought to reduce the risk of extrapyramidal side effects, which involve muscles

and movement.[8] Because of the long-term side effects of the typical antipsychotics, atypical agents are the most commonly used class now, although they have some different long-term challenges. Typical antipsychotics are further divided into low-potency and high-potency drugs, which also helps to sort out expected side effects. With low-potency drugs, higher doses are needed to provide the antipsychotic effects. Low-potency antipsychotics include chlorpromazine and thioridazine. High-potency drugs have antipsychotic activity at low doses. There are many high-potency medications on the market, including haloperidol (Haldol), fluphenazine, thiothixene, trifluoperazine, and others. Both classes have approximately equal antipsychotic activity if given at equipotent doses. For example, 300 mg of the low-potency drug chlorpromazine is equivalent to 5 mg of the high-potency drug haloperidol. This is because haloperidol is much more active at the D2 receptor than is chlorpromazine. It takes much more chlorpromazine to have the same effect as a little bit of haloperidol. Low-potency antipsychotics have more anticholinergic side effects (dry mouth, constipation, urinary retention, confusion) and cause more orthostatic hypotension than high-potency antipsychotics. Both classes can cause extrapyramidal side effects, but these side effects are more likely with low-potency antipsychotics.

ALERT!

When antipsychotic drugs are ordered as injections, it is important to distinguish between long-acting and immediate-acting dosage forms and dispense the correct product. Long-acting haloperidol decanoate is usually administered only once every 4 weeks (while haloperidol lactate is sometimes ordered as often as hourly) and fluphenazine decanoate is usually dosed on a 3-week schedule (while fluphenazine hydrochloride is repeated every 6 to 8 hours). Individual doses of the long-acting injections are much higher than the doses of the immediate-acting forms. Substituting an immediate-acting injection in the dose of a long-acting one can cause serious harm to the patient.

Antipsychotic drugs are available in oral dosages forms, immediate-release injectable products, and long-acting injectable (intramuscular [IM]) forms. Immediate-release injectable antipsychotics are used when a patient is agitated due to delusions and hallucinations, such as in the emergency room setting. Oral antipsychotics can be used for long-term maintenance. Long-acting injectable products called depot injections, in which the antipsychotic is added to an oil base for IM injection, are used when a patient cannot adhere to oral regimens.

Extrapyramidal side effects occur due to the effects of blocking dopamine receptors. There are several kinds of extrapyramidal reactions, but they all involve muscles and movement. Some extrapyramidal symptoms occur soon after an antipsychotic is begun, while others do not occur until after months or years of use. An early reaction that sometimes occurs is dystonia, which is a sudden, severe muscle spasm often in the neck, jaw, tongue, or eyes. Dystonic reactions usually occur within a few days of starting an antipsychotic, and it can be resolved by giving the patient an anticholinergic drug, such as benztropine, trihexyphenidyl, or diphenhydramine. Anticholinergic medications can also help with symptoms of pseudoparkinsonism, which can include slow movement, tremor, balance problems, and a mask-like face.[7] Amantadine is another medication that can help with pseudoparkinsonism symptoms. Akathisia is a condition in which the patient feels restless and has the need to move in order to relieve this symptom. People with akathisia may squirm constantly when sitting, pace or tap their feet, and generally feel uncomfortable with this jittery sensation. Anticholinergics can be used for this condition also, but they do not always work. Alternative useful medications include benzodiazepines and beta blockers (such as propranolol and nadolol).

An extrapyramidal effect that is often a consequence of long-term use of typical antipsychotics is tardive dyskinesia (TD). TD is a syndrome of abnormal, involuntary body movements. It usually begins in the facial area, such as the mouth and tongue, but can include the upper body, arms, and legs. The patient will pucker, grimace, smack the lips, move the tongue around, and eventually the whole body will writhe around in a peculiar dance-like pattern. The only way to stop TD is to prevent it in the first place by monitoring the patient for abnormal movements and usually changing medications if the movements are detected.

Atypical antipsychotics cause a lower incidence of extrapyramidal side effects than the typical agents, and this is a major reason for choosing them. In addition, atypical agents are believed to help with negative symptoms, which is not the case with typical agents. Atypical antipsychotics include risperidone (Risperdal), olanzapine (Zyprexa), quetiapine (Seroquel), aripiprazole (Abilify), ziprasidone (Geodon), paliperidone (Invega), iloperidone (Fanapt), and clozapine (Clozaril). Clozapine is a special type of atypical antipsychotic. It is actually an old drug that is limited in its use due to the potential for several dangerous adverse effects,

including blood cell production problems, seizures, orthostatic hypotension, and heart rhythm problems. Clozapine is still a very useful drug, especially in patients who have not responded well to other antipsychotics and in those who are suicidal, but its use must be carefully monitored with frequent blood tests to detect changes in blood cell production.

Agranulocytosis—loss of production of white blood cells (WBCs)—has been a dangerous adverse effect of clozapine therapy. WBCs are necessary to fight infection, and when their numbers are low the body can become overwhelmed by infectious agents and the patient often dies. When patients are treated with clozapine, their absolute neutrophil (a type of white blood cell) counts (ANC) must be monitored. The ANC is the combined number of both mature and immature neutrophils.

ALERT!

All patients who take clozapine must be recorded in a national registry of patients taking that drug to ensure that the ANC is being properly monitored. The WBC/ANC must be checked weekly for the first 6 months, every 2 weeks for the next 6 months, then monthly for as long as the patient is on the drug, if the WBC/ANC are within desirable limits. If these values are below a certain threshold, the drug must be interrupted or discontinued.[10]

Other side effects that may occur with antipsychotic drugs as a class include sedation, seizures, heart rhythm disturbances, blood and skin reactions, deposits in the eyes, and neuroleptic malignant syndrome—a life-threatening reaction in which the muscles become rigid and the body temperature rises dangerously. The risks of these reactions vary with the medication. Antipsychotics—including related drugs used for nausea, such as promethazine, chlorpromazine, and metoclopramide—should be avoided in patients who have Parkinson's disease (PD). Patients with PD are already severely depleted of CNS dopamine. Using dopamine blockers such as antipsychotics will impair movement and balance. At low doses, quetiapine and clozapine have less of this effect on PD patients than the other antipsychotics.

The atypical antipsychotics have some side effects that are not usually seen in the older antipsychotics. Treatment with atypical antipsychotics is often associated with weight gain, glucose intolerance, and lipid abnormalities. These effects may lead to diabetes and cardiovascular problems. Patients who take atypical antipsychotics should be monitored for weight, waist circumference, blood glucose levels, and lipid levels. Some atypical antipsychotics, such as olanzapine and clozapine, carry a higher risk of weight gain than others (see Medication Table 7-3).

BIPOLAR DISORDER

CASE STUDY

Doris is a 44-year-old woman with a 20-year history of bipolar disorder. She was brought to the emergency department of the local hospital by the police after becoming agitated and striking the assistant manager in a local restaurant. She is accompanied by her husband, Albert, who says his wife has been excitable and sleeping very little for the past 2 weeks and blamed it on the fact that last month she began stopping at the new convenience store for a large cup of coffee every day after work. She has recently started several home improvement projects and has been going on shopping sprees for expensive new clothes and jewelry and even a new car. Doris was in the hospital 3 years ago for a manic episode, which had followed several months of depression. Her moods have been controlled until now with lithium carbonate and ziprasidone. While out to dinner tonight, Doris became upset, yelling that she needed to go to Washington to help the president. While Albert and the staff were trying to calm her, she became angry and hit the manager with her purse. Albert tells the staff that he has never seen her like this, as he has only known her for 2 years. He says that he is her fourth husband and that she attempted suicide in her 20s. Doris has one daughter with depression and two uncles who are alcoholics. When she is feeling well, Doris is a peppy, friendly, and creative person, but she is prone to long bouts of depression. She works as the manager of a local theater company and drinks two to three cocktails and smokes one pack of cigarettes daily.

Pathophysiology

Bipolar disorder is a condition that affects up to 4.5% of the U.S. population.[11] The exact cause is unknown, but most people with bipolar disorder have had a family member (sibling, parents, grandparents, cousins) with some psychiatric illness, including depression and substance abuse disorder, so a genetic link is strongly suggested. Bipolar disorder is characterized by mood fluctuations between depression, normal mood, and manic or hypomanic moods. A manic mood is one in which a person is extremely excited, energetic, creative, talkative, loud, distractible, and agitated. In addition, the manic patient may have wild flights of ideas, speak very rapidly and dart from subject to subject, act in an uncharacteristically promiscuous manner, spend money wildly and carelessly, and go without sleep or with little sleep for days or weeks. A manic person may also experience psychosis, including delusions of power and importance, and hallucinations. If the patient does not go all the way into out-of-control mania but still feels unusually excited, energetic, creative, or irritable, the mood is described as *hypomanic*, meaning less than manic.

Most patients with bipolar disorder spend the majority of their lives with either depression or normal moods, with manic and hypomanic episodes occurring infrequently. In fact, many bipolar patients are initially diagnosed with depression and may be treated for depression for years with less-than-adequate success before getting a diagnosis of bipolar disorder. Bipolar disorder is usually diagnosed between the ages of 15 and 35 and occurs in both men and women. Bipolar disorder is a major cause of disability and is also a factor in accidents, divorces, arrests, substance abuse, and suicide.

CASE?

In which phase of bipolar disorder is Doris? What characteristics support this conclusion?

Nonpharmacologic Treatment

Bipolar disorder is primarily managed with medication, but nonpharmacologic treatments can improve the patient's understanding of the disease and help the patient to be alert to swings into depression or mania. Psychotherapy can help with negative thinking, just as in depressed patients. Patients are also counseled to monitor their moods and sleep habits with a calendar or diary, in order to detect the beginnings of a mood change. Patients are also taught to avoid certain triggers, such as excess stress, and medications that can cause stimulation, such as decongestants and corticosteroids. In some patients, ECT is beneficial for bipolar depression.

Pharmacologic Treatment

Unfortunately, for people for whom depression can be so debilitating, the SSRI and SNRI antidepressants must be used cautiously in bipolar patients. Serotonin is believed to have an activating effect on bipolar disorder, and SSRIs and SNRIs will sometimes cause a patient in a depressed phase to switch rapidly into mania. In fact, many patients who were originally diagnosed as depressed have been shown to have bipolar disorder when treatment with an antidepressant caused a manic reaction. Many doctors recommend that patients with bipolar disorder not take SSRI or SNRI antidepressants unless they are also taking a mood stabilizer or antipsychotic drug.

The mainstay of treatment for bipolar disorder is mood stabilizers. Mood stabilizers include forms of lithium such as lithium carbonate and lithium citrate and certain antiepilepsy drugs. Among the antiepilepsy drugs, valproate, lamotrigine, and carbamazepine have been studied the most and shown effective in forms of bipolar disorder. These drugs are discussed in Chapter 6. In addition, antipsychotics, especially atypicals, are also useful in stabilizing the mood and in managing depression without promoting mania. Antipsychotics are also used to treat the acute agitation and psychosis of mania, as are benzodiazepines such as lorazepam and diazepam.

Lithium is the oldest and best-studied mood stabilizer. Lithium is a metal, similar to sodium, which exists in nature as a salt called lithium carbonate. Lithium has effects on neurotransmitters but exactly how is not known with certainty. Lithium enhances the effects of norepinephrine and serotonin in the CNS, which explains how it helps with depression, but it also has effects on the sleep cycle, body temperature, and the endocrine system. Lithium can be used to help stabilize a patient in acute mania, lifts the mood of those who are depressed, and helps to prevent the swinging from one mood to another. Some studies show that the use of lithium lowers the likelihood that a patient with bipolar disorder will commit suicide. However, lithium has several drawbacks, and therapy with this drug must be regulated by keeping blood levels within a desired range, as well as monitoring for side effects. Lithium can cause sedation, gastrointestinal side effects such as diarrhea, tremor, weight gain, and may reduce the function of the thyroid. Lithium levels can be affected by the patient's salt and caffeine intake, dehydration, and the use of other medications, such as ibuprofen, naproxen, and diuretics.

CASE?

Doris has been controlled on lithium for 2 years. Why might it suddenly have stopped working?

Of the other drugs used as mood stabilizers, valproate is especially useful for patients who cycle rapidly between depression and mania or hypomania, and lamotrigine is particularly useful in bipolar depression. Atypical antipsychotics are also useful in bipolar depression. As with patients with schizophrenia, nonadherence to treatment is common with patients with bipolar disorder. Patients often say that they enjoy the hypomanic and manic phases of their illness and feel that medications inhibit their creativity. The long-term outcome for patients with bipolar disorder is better if they can be kept stable, so that they avoid the physical and psychosocial risks associated with their mood fluctuations.

ALERT!

Lithium is available as two salt forms: lithium carbonate, which is used in solid dosage forms, and lithium citrate, which is available as an oral solution. Lithium citrate is labeled as 8 mEq/5 mL. Each 5 mL of lithium citrate provides the same amount of lithium that is available in the 300 mg lithium carbonate tablets. Lithium carbonate is marketed as both immediate-release (IR) products and extended-release (ER) products. Extended-release products offer less frequent dosing and may reduce gastrointestinal side effects. It is important to distinguish between the various lithium products to be sure the patient receives the dosage form and strength the physician ordered.

ATTENTION DEFICIT HYPERACTIVITY DISORDER

CASE STUDY

Duncan is a 9-year-old boy repeating the second grade because of his poor progress in reading. Duncan's mother says that he has always been "very wound up, even when he was little." He also likes to stare out the window or open the classroom door while the teacher is giving instructions. He likes recess but has been in fights on the playground. He has trouble finishing his work and even starting it. At home, he likes to play video games and will have tantrums when told to do his homework or to go to bed. In his Sunday school class, he has often been disruptive, yelling out answers or telling stories not connected to the lesson. In the school conference about his behavior and learning problems, his dad says, "He's just like my brother."

Pathophysiology

The causes of ADHD are not known, but, as with many other psychiatric illnesses, genetics plays a part, with ADHD patients often having a relative with similar symptoms, even if undiagnosed. Some brain scans have shown small differences in the brain structure in patients with ADHD. Other studies suggest that patients with ADHD have a defect in the activity of dopamine and norepinephrine in the brain. ADHD affects about 5% to 10% of children in the United States, and it is more common in males than in females. More than half of these children will continue to have symptoms of ADHD into adulthood. The symptoms of ADHD revolve around problems in maintaining focus on a task. Children with ADHD are usually disorganized and easily distracted. They are often fidgety and have problems sitting still, and sometimes they are extremely energetic, as if they were propelled by a motor, darting from one brief interest to another. Some children are not as hyperactive but mostly have problems organizing and maintaining focus

on their tasks. Patients who are suspected of having ADHD must display these symptoms before the age of 7 years, and in at least two areas of their lives—not just in school. In addition, children with ADHD frequently have comorbidities, which are other diagnoses, such as oppositional-defiant disorder, conduct disorder, depression, Tourette syndrome (tics), autism spectrum disorders, learning disabilities, and enuresis, which is bedwetting. Children who do not receive adequate treatment for ADHD are at risk for poor school and work performance, reckless behavior, accidents, substance abuse, and relationship problems.

CASE?

What symptoms of ADHD does Duncan have? What parts of his life is this affecting?

Nonpharmacologic Treatment

Nonpharmacologic treatment for ADHD is centered on detecting and managing learning disorders and giving the child a structured environment with clear rules, with incentives and rewards for good performance. Nonpharmacologic treatment by itself is usually not adequate for managing the attention problems associated with ADHD, but it is beneficial when used along with medication.

Pharmacologic Treatment

Pharmacologic management of ADHD centers on CNS stimulants. In addition, other medications are also used, including antidepressants, antipsychotics, mood stabilizers, and certain medicines originally used to control blood pressure, such as clonidine and guanfacine. It often takes trial and error to find the optimal medication for a child or adult with ADHD. Doctors will usually focus on the most distressing or problematic symptoms and aim medication at controlling those symptoms.

The drug of choice for patients with ADHD is one of the CNS stimulants. Stimulants enhance the effects of norepinephrine and dopamine in the CNS, improving the ability to focus and tune out distractions. (In a weaker manner, this function is also accomplished by caffeine and nicotine use.) Either methylphenidate or an amphetamine compound is used as the first choice. All of the stimulant medications are variations methylphenidate and amphetamines. Some of the variations are chemical—such as dexmethylphenidate and dextroamphetamine—and others are variations in the dosage form—such as several types of sustained action preparations and transdermal patches. The particular choice usually depends on patient factors (such as age of the patient), whether the patient's schedule will allow for drug administration, and prescriber preference. If the patient does not do well with the first stimulant choice, due to less-than-optimal response or side effects, another stimulant is chosen. Side effects of stimulants include jitteriness, sleep disturbances, loss of appetite, gastrointestinal upset, tics, and possible increases in heart rate and blood pressure. To reduce side effects, doses should begin low and be titrated to the most effective and tolerated dosage.

ALERT!

Children are often unable or unwilling to take solid tablets and capsules, so parents should inquire about options that are easier to administer. Only immediate-release tablet forms (Ritalin, Adderall) may be crushed and mixed with food for administration. Only scored tablets may be cut in half. Some extended-release capsules, including Adderall XR and Aptensio XRs, may be opened and sprinkled on applesauce for children who cannot swallow the intact capsule. Vyvanse capsules may be opened and mixed with water, yogurt, or orange juice. It is important to consult product literature for information on proper and safe administration of each product, as there are many differences between them.

The various stimulant products are designed to meet the focus, duration, and tolerance needs of the patient. Immediate-release products work quickly but must be dosed both in the morning and in the middle of the day to provide coverage throughout the school or work day. Extended-release products take longer to start working in the morning but have sustained activity throughout the day. Some products, such as Aptensio XR, Ritalin LA, Focalin XR (dexmethylphenidate), and Adderall XR (a mixture of amphetamine and dextroamphetamine), combine both immediate-release and extended-release forms of the stimulant drug. Methylphenidate patches (Daytrana) also provide sustained activity. The patches are worn for 9 hours

and provide therapeutic activity for 12 hours. Vyvanse (lisdexamfetamine) is a prodrug that is converted in the body to dexamphetamine. It, too, has sustained activity and is dosed once daily in the morning. Jornay PM is an extended-release methylphenidate product that is dosed in the evening but is delayed in its action until the following day.

PRACTICE POINT

All stimulants currently available in the United States for the treatment of ADHD are Drug Enforcement Administration (DEA) Schedule II controlled substances. Prescriptions for them are subject to all the rules for such medications and can never be refilled or renewed via telephone.

If the stimulant class does not benefit the patient or is not tolerated, drugs from the antidepressant class are tried. Other reasons for choosing this class is if the patient is also depressed or if someone in the patient's household abuses drugs. Drugs in this class—bupropion; the tricyclic antidepressants imipramine, desipramine, and nortriptyline; and atomoxetine—also enhance the effects of norepinephrine and dopamine in the CNS by mechanisms different than those of the stimulants. Atomoxetine is a selective norepinephrine reuptake inhibitor, which was specifically approved by the FDA for the treatment of ADHD.[12] Side effects are similar to those of the stimulants, although this class usually has less effect on sleep.

CASE?

While Duncan's mother understands that he will not become addicted to stimulant medications, she is uncomfortable with having controlled substances in her home. She is also concerned that she may be unable to travel to Duncan's physician's office every month for a new prescription. What are some other options for his treatment?

Clonidine and guanfacine are alpha-2 adrenergic agonists. They were originally developed to treat high blood pressure, but they have the effect in the CNS to improve blood flow to the prefrontal cortex, which is the "thinking" part of the brain behind the forehead. The effect is to enhance memory and decision making. These drugs also have effects on norepinephrine activity. Both clonidine and guanfacine can be used alone for ADHD but are more commonly used as adjuncts to stimulants to improve sleep and to reduce disruptive behavior.[5] Clonidine and guanfacine can cause sedation, dry mouth, dizziness, reduced blood pressure, and constipation. These drugs are especially useful in patients with ADHD who also have Tourette syndrome, since they also help to control tics.

Antipsychotics, especially atypical agents, are also employed to treat ADHD. As with clonidine and guanfacine, they are also useful in treating comorbid Tourette syndrome. In addition, antipsychotics and mood stabilizers help with aggressive behavior and conduct disorder (see Medication Table 7-4).

SUBSTANCE USE DISORDERS

CASE STUDY

Joel is a 26-year-old man who has been arrested for public intoxication after a football game. Joel had a previous arrest 3 years ago for trying to pass an altered prescription. He started drinking beer and smoking marijuana at a friend's house in the ninth grade. While Joel had been a good student in middle school, he barely managed to graduate from high school. His mother admitted him to a teen rehabilitation program during his senior year. He stayed off alcohol and drugs for 18 months but has had several relapses since. He was admitted to the hospital 1 year ago for pancreatitis due to excessive alcohol use. After this arrest, Joel was taken to the hospital for detoxification. His toxicology screen tested positive for alcohol, hydrocodone, and cocaine.

Pathophysiology

Substance use disorder is a problem an individual experiences that has serious consequences for families and communities—even internationally. It is a common comorbidity in patients with other psychiatric disorders and is a cause of crime, broken relationships, physical ailments, and

child neglect. Substance use disorder can be relatively mild, such as the jitteriness that comes from overuse of coffee and other caffeinated drinks, or deadly, due to respiratory depression from opioid or other overdoses or seizures and heart rhythm problems due to cocaine. Alcohol use disorder alone is a cause of liver disease, pancreatitis (inflammation of the pancreas), cognitive decline, cancer, homelessness, and disabling and fatal accidents. While the use of some substances such as tobacco mostly affects the user and his or her family, the use of others, such as methamphetamine, are a major societal problem. Each year, the United States spends more than $400 billion on problems related to substance use disorders, which are the biggest preventable source of illness, death, and disability in the country.[13]

Substance use disorder is a maladaptive use of a drug with repeated negative consequences to the user due to that use. It is important to remember that many drugs implicated in substance use disorders are also legal medications with legitimate uses.

Addiction refers to a chronic, compulsive craving of a drug, which will cause a person to lose control of his or her behavior and use the drug in spite of the consequences. In contrast, a patient may become tolerant to the therapeutic effects or side effects of a drug, meaning that the dose would need to be increased to give the same effect. Physical dependence means that a patient may experience withdrawal symptoms if a drug is suddenly stopped. Tolerance and physical dependence are normal conditions that develop with many drugs. Merely experiencing tolerance or physical dependence does not make a person addicted to a drug. For example, a patient with cancer or some other debilitating painful disease may need high doses of opioids in addition to benzodiazepines for anxiety or muscle spasms. The patient is not considered to have a substance use disorder, but a person who steals those same medications to use them recreationally is. Similarly, many drugs, such as antidepressants, beta blockers, proton pump inhibitors, and antiepileptics, can cause physical dependence or tolerance; however, these patients are not addicted because they are using the medications for legitimate purposes, under supervision, and without the craving, compulsive drive associated with addiction. Drugs used by people with substance use disorders have many effects on the CNS. Depending on the drug, it may cause stimulation (as with cocaine and methamphetamine), sedation (as with benzodiazepines, barbiturates, alcohol, and marijuana), or some other effect (such as the hallucinations associated with LSD). Some non-drug products (eg, inhalants [spray paint], airplane glue, dry erase markers) are used by individuals with substance use disorders. Even some OTC medications, such as pseudoephedrine and dextromethorphan, have abuse potential. The withdrawal pattern with these medications varies with the drug, dosage, length of time it has been taken, and patient individual factors.

PRACTICE POINT

We must also be careful of the terms we use in describing the use of drugs with abuse potential, distinguishing addiction from tolerance and dependence.

CASE?

Which of Joel's characteristics are consistent with substance use disorder?

Nonpharmacologic Treatment

The nonpharmacologic treatment of substance use disorder includes individual psychotherapy and 12-step support groups, such as Alcoholics Anonymous. There are many inpatient and outpatient programs that specialize in the treatment of substance use disorders. Relapses are common though, and it often takes many attempts over several years before a person manages to recover from substance use disorder.

Pharmacologic Treatment

Not all abused substances are physically habit forming or addictive. Substances such as marijuana, inhalants, and hallucinogens are often psychologically habit forming, but there is little or no withdrawal syndrome when their use is abruptly stopped. This section will focus on those physically addictive drugs for which there are medicinal approaches to manage dependency and withdrawal (see Medication Table 7-5). There are two main goals of managing substance use disorder: 1) managing the acute withdrawal symptoms and avoiding the consequences of acute withdrawal (such as seizures, agitation, and sleep disturbances in withdrawal from alcohol and other sedatives), and 2) managing the craving and compulsive desire for the drug in the long term.

For nicotine users, the most intense phase of withdrawal is in the first hours, days, and weeks. Nicotine has an intense but brief effect, and withdrawal from it is also intense and usually brief although the habits accompanying smoking—smoking when eating, smoking when with smokers, smoking

when driving—and the craving for nicotine can take months or even years to dissipate. Patients who are withdrawing from nicotine experience a physical withdrawal, such as feeling tired, anxious, agitated, less mentally focused, and constipated. The physical withdrawal intensity is closely related to the daily intake of nicotine. There are two approaches to managing nicotine withdrawal. For nicotine replacement therapy, gums (Nicorette), patches (Nicoderm CQ), lozenges (Commit), nasal sprays (Nicotrol NS), or nasal inhalers (Nicotrol inhaler) containing nicotine are used to manage the acute withdrawal and then gradually tapered off. Oral medications, bupropion (Wellbutrin) and varenicline may manage the withdrawal symptoms by actions on neurotransmitter activity in the CNS. Nicotine gums, patches, and lozenges are available over the counter (OTC). A prescription is required for Nicotrol inhaler and Nicotrol NS (nasal spray), as well as bupropion and varenicline.

PRACTICE POINT

Bupropion is indicated and prescribed for psychiatric disorders as well as for smoking cessation and has specific dosage ranges depending on its use. This may affect insurance coverage. Most plans, for instance, cover bupropion for depression but may not cover bupropion for smoking cessation. Some plans require prior authorization before filling a prescription for bupropion, so that only prescriptions used for depression are covered.

With alcohol withdrawal, the acute phase bears the risk of seizures due to the sudden decrease in the sedating power of alcohol. In addition, patients with alcohol use disorder are often deficient in vitamins, especially thiamine, which is necessary for good functioning of the CNS. The management of alcohol withdrawal focuses on replacing vitamins and replacing the sedative effects of alcohol by using a benzodiazepine, such as diazepam or lorazepam, and then gradually withdrawing the benzodiazepine. After the acute withdrawal, the goal is to prevent the patient from relapsing. This can be aided medically by using disulfiram (sometimes still called by its former brand name, Antabuse), naltrexone (Vivitrol), or acamprosate. They work by entirely different mechanisms. Disulfiram tablets cause intense nausea and vomiting, headaches, and flushing when someone drinks alcohol while taking this medicine. This is a negative feedback to discourage alcohol use. The reaction to disulfiram can also cause seizures and serious cardiac effects, so this drug should not be used in patients already at risk of these events.

ALERT!

Patients taking disulfiram must be warned to avoid all alcohol, including that found in cough medicines, sauces, and even skin products such as aftershave lotions. A serious reaction to alcohol can occur up to 14 days after disulfiram is discontinued.

Naltrexone and acamprosate reduce the cravings for alcohol. Both medications commonly cause nausea.[14]

Opioid withdrawal can be managed with supportive therapy during the early phase, which is not life-threatening but can cause intense muscle cramping, gastrointestinal distress, and agitation. Many opioid-addicted patients benefit from enrollment in a methadone maintenance program. Methadone is an opioid that has a very long duration in the body. The peak effect does not give the intense high of shorter-acting opioids, and the cravings are suppressed by the long-acting effects of methadone. This program does replace one dependency with another but allows the patient to return to a productive place in society while learning to manage life without opioids. When methadone is used to manage opioid addiction, it must be done in a licensed methadone clinic according to federal law. (Methadone used to treat pain does not have this requirement.)

ALERT!

LOOK-ALIKE/SOUND-ALIKE—Psychiatric medications involved in look-alike/sound-alike errors include alprazolam and lorazepam (both for anxiety); Celexa (citalopram, depression) and Celebrex (celecoxib, arthritis); Klonopin (clonazepam, seizures) and clonidine (ADHD, hypertension); clozapine (for schizophrenia) and trazodone (sleep, depression) and tramadol (pain).

Another option for managing patients who wish to stop abusing opioids is to employ buprenorphine, a drug that both has some of the effects of opioids and blocks other effects. Two drugs containing buprenorphine are used in an acute and long-term manner to reduce the drug-craving urges of the patient. Buprenorphine alone is used at the beginning of treatment, when the patient's withdrawal symptoms are most intense. Later, a combination buprenorphine/naloxone sublingual or buccal preparation (Suboxone, Zubsolv) is used in the maintenance phase of management. Naloxone, a narcotic antagonist (discussed in detail in chapter 5), is added to buprenorphine to block the effects of buprenorphine if the user tries to dissolve and inject the drug. Doctors who prescribe buprenorphine preparations for substance abuse must have the proper credentials and be trained in the use of these products.

ALERT!

LOOK-ALIKE/SOUND-ALIKE: Buprenorphine has been confused with hydromorphone.[3]

Like naloxone, naltrexone blocks the effects of opioids, but it is not used to counteract acute opioid overdoses, as naloxone is. Naltrexone is used in a 50 mg daily oral dose and a 380 mg once monthly intramuscular injection (Vivitrol) to block the effects of opioids and assist the maintenance of sobriety. As mentioned earlier, naltrexone is also used to reduce the urge to drink alcohol.

SUMMARY

Because psychiatric disorders are often expressed by behavioral rather than physical signs, patients suffering from them are sometimes incorrectly considered to be at fault for their own symptoms and judged in a negative manner. It is important for the pharmacy technician to remember that these conditions, across the spectrum from depression and psychosis, through attention deficit hyperactivity disorder (ADHD) and substance use disorders, are real illnesses and that patients receiving treatment for them deserve just as much consideration and care as is extended to those who have asthma or heart disease. Many of the medications used in the therapy of psychiatric disorders affect the neurotransmitters detailed in Chapter 4 and Chapter 5 and have side effects often throughout the body related to the actions of these neurological messengers. Some patients have short-term therapy, but many must be treated for a lifetime for conditions that can only be controlled and not cured.

REFERENCES

1. American Psychiatric Association. *Diagnostic and Statistical Manual of Mental Disorders*. 5th ed. Arlington, VA: American Psychiatric Association; 2013.

2. VandenBerg AM. Major depressive disorder. In: DiPiro JT, Yee GC, Posey L, et al., eds. *Pharmacotherapy: A Pathophysiologic Approach. 11th ed*. New York, NY: McGraw Hill; 2020.

3. Institute for Safe Medication Practices. List of Confused Drug Names. https://www.ismp.org/recommendations/confused-drug-names-list. Accessed July 11, 2022.

4. Janssen Neuroscience. SPRAVATO® REMS (Risk Evaluation and Mitigation Strategy). https://www.spravatorems.com/. Accessed July 10, 2022.

5. Melton ST, Kirkwood CK. Anxiety disorders: Generalized anxiety, panic, and social anxiety disorders. In: DiPiro JT, Yee GC, Posey L, et al., eds. *Pharmacotherapy: A Pathophysiologic Approach. 11th ed*. New York, NY: McGraw Hill; 2020.

6. Charlson FJ, Ferrari AJ, Santomauro DF, et al. Global epidemiology and burden of schizophrenia: Findings from the Global Burden of Disease Study 2016. *Schizophr Bull.* 2018;44:1195-1203.

7. Crismon M, Smith T, Buckley PF. Schizophrenia. In: DiPiro JT, Yee GC, Posey L, et al., eds. *Pharmacotherapy: A Pathophysiologic Approach. 11th ed.* New York, NY: McGraw Hill; 2020.

8. Stahl SM. Antipsychotic agents. In: Stahl SM, ed. *Stahl's Essential Psychopharmacology: Neuroscientific Basis and Practical Applications.* 3rd ed. Cambridge, UK: Cambridge University Press; 2008.

9. Šagud M, Vuksan-Ćusa B, Jakšić N, et al. Smoking in schizophrenia: An updated review. *Psychiatr Danub.* 2018;30(Suppl 4):216-223.

10. Clozapine REMS. https://www.newclozapinerems.com/. Accessed July 11, 2022.

11. Drayton SJ, Fields CS. Bipolar disorder. In: DiPiro JT, Yee GC, Posey L, et al., eds. *Pharmacotherapy: A Pathophysiologic Approach. 11th ed*. New York, NY: McGraw-Hill; 2020.

12. Dopheide JA, Stutzmann DL, Pliszka SR. Attention deficit/hyperactivity disorder. In: DiPiro JT, Yee GC, Posey L, et al., eds. *Pharmacotherapy: A Pathophysiologic Approach. 11th ed*. New York, NY: McGraw-Hill; 2020.

13. U.S. Department of Health and Human Services, Office of the Surgeon General. *Facing Addiction in America: The Surgeon General's Report on Alcohol, Drugs, and Health.* Washington, DC: U.S. Department of Health and Human Services; 2016.

14. Lexi-Drugs. Lexicomp [Database]. Hudson, OH: Wolters Kluwer. http://online.lexi.com.

REVIEW QUESTIONS

1. Why are SSRIs preferred to MAOIs and tricyclic antidepressants for the initial treatment of depression?

2. What side effects should be anticipated in a patient who is taking olanzapine for schizophrenia?

3. Why are bupropion and varenicline started ahead of time (before the last cigarette is smoked) in a patient who wants to quit smoking?

4. What are the advantages of using an SSRI or buspirone for anxiety rather than a benzodiazepine?

5. Why are antiepilepsy drugs, such as valproate, used to treat bipolar disorder?

MEDICATION TABLES

MEDICATION TABLE 7-1. Antidepressants[14]

CLASS Generic Name	Brand Name	Route	Forms	Dose
Selective Serotonin Reuptake Inhibitors (SSRIs)				
Citalopram (sye TAL oh pram)	Celexa	Oral	Tablet: 10 mg, 20 mg, 40 mg; oral solution: 10 mg/5 mL (generic)	20–60 mg/day
Escitalopram (es sye TAL oh pram)	Lexapro	Oral	Tablet: 5 mg, 10 mg, 20 mg; oral solution: 5 mg/5 mL	10–20 mg/day
Fluoxetine (floo OX e teen)	Prozac, Sarafem	Oral	Capsule: 10 mg, 20 mg, 40 mg Tablet 10 mg, 20 mg Solution: 20 mg/5 ml Delayed-release tablet: 90 mg	20–60 mg/day or (delayed release) 90 mg once a week
Fluvoxamine (floo VOX a meen)	Generics	Oral	Tablet: 25 mg, 50 mg, 100 mg; extended-release capsule (Luvox CR): 100 mg, 150 mg	50–300 mg/day
Paroxetine (pa ROX e teen)	Paxil, Paxil CR, Pexeva	Oral	Tablet (Paxil and Pexeva): 10 mg, 20 mg, 30 mg, 40 mg; controlled-release tablet (Paxil CR): 12.5 mg, 25 mg, 37.5 mg; oral suspension: 10 mg/5 mL	20–60 mg/day
Sertraline (SER tra leen)	Zoloft	Oral	Tablet: 25 mg, 50 mg, 100 mg; oral solution: 20 mg/mL	25–200 mg/day
Vilazodone (SSRI + 5HT-1A receptor partial agonist)	Viibryd	Oral	Tablet: 10 mg, 20 mg, 40 mg	20–40 mg/day; begin titration with 10 mg
Serotonin Norepinephrine Reuptake Inhibitors (SNRIs)				
Desvenlafaxine (des VEN la FAX een)	Pristiq	Oral	Extended-release tablet: 50 mg, 100 mg	50–100 mg/day
Duloxetine (doo LOX e teen)	Cymbalta, Drizalma	Oral	Delayed-release capsule or delayed-release sprinkle capsule: 20 mg, 30 mg, 40 mg, 60 mg	30–120 mg/day or in divided doses twice daily
Levomilnacipran (lee vo mil NAH sih pran)	Fetzima	Oral	Extended-release capsule: 20 mg, 40 mg, 80 mg, 120 mg	40–120 mg/day; begin titration with 20 mg/day
Venlafaxine (VEN la fax een)	Effexor XR	Oral	Tablet: 25 mg, 37.5 mg, 50 mg, 75 mg, 100 mg; extended-release capsule: 37.5 mg, 75 mg, 150 mg; extended-release tablet: 37.5 mg, 75 mg, 150 mg, 225 mg	75–225 mg/day

Continued next page

MEDICATION TABLE 7-1. Antidepressants[14] *(Continued)*

CLASS Generic Name	Brand Name	Route	Forms	Dose
Tricyclics				
Amitriptyline (a mee TRIP ti leen)	Generics	Oral	Tablet: 10 mg, 25 mg, 50 mg, 75 mg, 100 mg, 150 mg	100–300 mg/day
Amoxapine (a MOX a peen)	Generics	Oral	Tablet: 25 mg, 50 mg, 100 mg, 150 mg	200–300 mg/day
Clomipramine (kloe MI pra meen)	Anafranil	Oral	Capsule: 25 mg, 50 mg, 75 mg	100–250 mg/day
Desipramine (des IP ra meen)	Norpramin	Oral	Tablet: 10 mg, 25 mg, 50 mg, 75 mg, 100 mg, 150 mg	100–300 mg/day
Doxepin (DOX e pin)	Silenor	Oral	Tablet: 3 mg, 6 mg; capsule: 10 mg, 25 mg, 50 mg, 75 mg, 100 mg, 150 mg; oral concentrate: 10 mg/mL	100–300 mg/day
Nortriptyline (nor TRIP ti leen)	Pamelor	Oral	Capsule: 10 mg, 25 mg, 50 mg, 75 mg; solution: 10 mg/5 mL	50–200 mg/day
Monoamine Oxidase Inhibitors (MAOIs)				
Phenelzine (FEN el zeen)	Nardil	Oral	Tablet: 15 mg	30–90 mg/day
Selegiline (se LE ji leen)	Emsam, Zelapar	Oral, transdermal	Capsule, tablet / Orally disintegrating tablet / Transderm patch	5 mg–10 m/day / 1.25–2.5 mg/day / 6–12 mg/day
Tranylcypromine (tran il SIP roe meen)	Parnate	Oral	Tablet: 10 mg	20–60 mg/day
Miscellaneous				
Bupropion HCl (byoo PROE pee on)	Generics	Oral	Immediate-release tablet: 75 mg, 100 mg	75–100 mg 3 times/day
	Wellbutrin SR		12-hr extended-release tablet: 100 mg, 150 mg, 200 mg	100–200 mg 2 times/day
	Wellbutrin XL		24-hr extended-release tablet: 150 mg, 300 mg	150–300 mg daily
Bupropion HBr (byoo PROE pee on)	Aplenzin	Oral	24-hr extended-release tablet: 174 mg, 348 mg, 522 mg	174–522 mg daily in the morning
Mirtazapine (mir TAZ a peen)	Remeron, Remeron SolTab	Oral	Tablet: 7.5 mg, 15 mg, 30 mg, 45 mg; disintegrating tablet (Remeron SolTab): 15 mg, 30 mg, 45 mg	15–45 mg/day
Nefazodone (nef AY zoe done)	Serzone	Oral	Tablet: 50 mg, 100 mg, 150 mg, 200 mg, 250 mg	200–600 mg/day
Trazodone (TRAZ oh done)	Generics	Oral	Tablet: 50 mg, 100 mg, 150 mg, 300 mg; extended-release tablet (Oleptro): 150 mg, 300 mg	150–300 mg/day

MEDICATION TABLE 7-2. Anxiolytics[14]

CLASS Generic Name	Brand Name	Route	Forms	Dose
Benzodiazepines				
Alprazolam (al PRAY zoe lam)	Xanax	Oral	Tablet	0.75–4 mg/day
Clonazepam (kloe NA ze pam)	Klonopin	Oral	Tablet, disintegrating tablet	0.25–4 mg/day
Diazepam (dye AZ e pam)	Valium	Oral, IV	Tablet, injection	6–40 mg/day
Lorazepam (lor A ze pam)	Ativan	Oral, IV	Tablet, injection	1.5–8 mg/day
Oxazepam (ox A ze pam)	Generics	Oral	Capsule	7.5–60 mg/day
Others				
Buspirone (byoo SPYE rone)	Generics	Oral	Tablet	15–60 mg/day

IV = intravenous.

MEDICATION TABLE 7-3. Antipsychotics[14]

CLASS Generic Name	Brand Name	Route	Forms	Dose
First Generation				
Chlorpromazine (klor PROE ma zeen)	Generics	Oral, IM	Injection solution: 25 mg/mL; tablet: 10 mg, 50 mg, 100 mg, 200 mg	100–800 mg/day
Fluphenazine (floo FEN a zeen)	Generics	Oral, IM	IM solution: 2.5 mg/mL; elixir: 2.5 mg/5 mL; oral solution: 5 mg/mL; tablet: 1 mg, 2.5 mg, 5 mg, 10 mg	2.5–10 mg/day in divided doses
Haloperidol (ha loe PER i dole)	Haldol	Oral, IM	Tablet: 1 mg, 2 mg, 5 mg, 10 mg, 20 mg; oral solution: 2 mg/mL; injection solution: 5 mg/mL; extended-release injection oil: 50 mg/mL, 100 mg/mL	0.5–5 mg 2–3 times daily
Loxapine (LOX a peen)	Generics	Oral	Tablet: 5 mg, 10 mg, 25 mg, 50 mg	10–100 mg/day
Trifluoperazine (trye floo oh PER a zeen)	Stelazine	Oral	Tablet: 1 mg, 2 mg, 5 mg, 10 mg	2–40 mg/day
Second Generation				
Aripiprazole (ay ri PIP ray zole)	Abilify Aristada Aristada Initio	Oral, IM	Abilify: 9.75 mg/1.3 mL IM solution; 1 mg/mL oral solution: 2 mg, 5 mg, 10 mg, 15 mg, 20 mg, 30 mg tablet; Abilify Discmelt: 10 mg, 15 mg disintegrating tablet Abilify MyCite contains a sensor in tablets and a patch to detect ingestion Aristada: IM extended-release injectable suspension 441 mg, 662 mg, 882 mg, 1,064 mg prefilled syringes	15–30 mg/day Aristada Initio: one-time 675 mg IM Aristada: 441–882 mg monthly; 882 mg every 6 weeks; 1,064 mg every 2 months
Asenapine (ah SEN ah peen)	Saphris Secuado	Oral Transdermal	SL tablets 2.5 mg, 5 mg, 10 mg Daily patch: 3.8 mg, 5.7 mg, 7.6 mg	2.5–10 mg/day
Brexpiprazole (brex PIH prah zole)	Rexulti	Oral	Tablets 0.25 mg, 0.5 mg, 1 mg, 2 mg, 3 mg, 4 mg	1–4 mg/day
Clozapine (KLOE za peen)	Clozaril, Versacloz	Oral	Generic: 25 mg, 50 mg, 100 mg, 200 mg tablet; Clozaril: 25 mg, 100 mg tablet Versacloz: Oral suspension 50 mg/ml	50–500 mg/day
Iloperidone (eye loe PER i done)	Fanapt	Oral	Tablet: 1 mg, 2 mg, 4 mg, 6 mg, 8 mg, 10 mg, 12 mg	2–24 mg/day
Lumateperone (loo ma TEH per one)	Caplyta	Oral	Capsule: 42 mg	42 mg daily, with food

Continued next page

MEDICATION TABLE 7-3. Antipsychotics[14] *(Continued)*

CLASS Generic Name	Brand Name	Route	Forms	Dose
Lurasidone (lu RAZ ih done)	Latuda	Oral	Tablet: 20 mg, 40 mg, 60 mg, 80 mg, 120 mg	20–160 mg/day
Olanzapine (oh LAN za peen)	Zyprexa, Zyprexa Zydis Zyprexa Relprevv	Oral, IM	Tablet: 2.5 mg, 5 mg, 7.5 mg, 10 mg, 15 mg, 20 mg Zyprexa Zydis: 5 mg, 10 mg, 15 mg, 20 mg disintegrating tablet Zyprexa IntraMuscular: 10 mg powder for injection after reconstitution	5–20 mg/day Zyprexa Relprevv: 100–300 mg every 2 weeks or 300–405 mg every 4 weeks IM
Paliperidone (pal ee PER i done)	Invega Invega Sustenna Invega Trinza	Oral IM IM	Extended-release tablet: 1.5 mg, 3 mg, 6 mg, 9 mg Extended-release prefilled syringes: 39 mg, 78 mg, 117 mg, 156 mg, 234 mg Extended-release prefilled syringes: 273 mg, 410 mg, 546 mg, 819 mg	3–9 mg/day 39–234 mg/ month IM 273–819 mg IM every 3 months
Quetiapine (kwe TYE a peen)	Seroquel, Seroquel XR	Oral	Generic: 25 mg, 100 mg, 200 mg; Seroquel: 25 mg, 50 mg, 100 mg, 200 mg, 300 mg, 400 mg tablet; Seroquel XR: 50 mg, 150 mg, 200 mg, 300 mg, 400 mg tablet	250–500 mg/day
Risperidone (ris PER i done)	Risperdal, Risperdal M-Tab Risperdal Consta Perseris	Oral IM SUBQ	Immediate-release tablet: 0.25 mg, 0.5 mg, 1 mg, 2 mg, 3 mg, 4 mg Risperdal M-Tab: 0.5 mg, 1 mg, 2 mg oral disintegrating tablet; Risperdal: 1 mg/mL oral solution Risperdal Consta:12.5 mg, 25 mg, 37.5 mg, 50 mg IM powder for suspension Perseris extended-release SUBQ suspension 90 mg, 120 mg	2–8 mg/day Risperdal Consta 12.5–50 mg IM every 2 weeks Perseris: 90–120 mg monthly
Ziprasidone (zi PRAY si done)	Geodon	Oral, IM	Capsule: 20 mg, 40 mg, 60 mg, 80 mg Powder for reconstituted injection solution: 20 mg/ml	20–100 mg twice a day 10 mg IM every 2 hours, up to 40 mg/day

IM = intramuscular; SUBQ = subcutaneous.

MEDICATION TABLE 7-4. Attention Deficit Hyperactivity Disorder Agents[14]

CLASS Generic Name	Brand Name	Route	Forms	DEA Schedule/ Regulatory Status	Dose
Short-Acting Stimulants					
Methylphenidate (meth il FEN i date)	Ritalin	Oral	Tablet: 5 mg, 10 mg, 20 mg	Schedule II controlled substance (CII)	10–60 mg/day
Dextroamphetamine (DEX tro am FET ah meen)	Zenzedi	Oral	Tablet: 2.5 mg, 5 mg, 7.5 mg, 10 mg, 15 mg, 20 mg, 30 mg	CII	2.5–40 mg/day, in divided doses
Dexmethylphenidate (dex meth ill FEN i date)	Focalin, Focalin XR	Oral	Focalin: 2.5 mg, 5 mg, 10 mg; Focalin XR: 5 mg, 10 mg, 15 mg, 20 mg, 30 mg	CII	5–20 mg/day
Mixed amphetamine salts (am FET a meen)	Adderall	Oral	Tablet: 5 mg, 7.5 mg, 10 mg, 12.5 mg, 15 mg, 20 mg, 30 mg	CII	10–40 mg/day, in divided doses; Adderall XR used for once daily dosing
Intermediate-Acting Stimulants					
Methylphenidate (meth il FEN i date)	Metadate ER	Oral	Extended-release tablet: 20 mg	CII	10–60 mg/day
Long-Acting Stimulants					
Methylphenidate (meth il FEN i date)	Aptensio XR	Oral	Extended-release capsule: 10 mg, 15 mg, 20 mg, 30 mg, 40 mg, 50 mg, 60 mg	CII	10–60 mg/day
	Ritalin LA	Oral	Extended-release capsule: 10 mg, 20 mg, 30 mg, 40 mg	CII	20–60 mg/day
	Concerta	Oral	Extended-release tablet: 18 mg, 27 mg, 36 mg, 54 mg	CII	18–72 mg/day
	Daytrana	Transdermal	Transdermal patch: 10 mg, 15 mg, 20 mg, 30 mg	CII	10–30 mg (12.5–37.5 cm2/day)
	Quillivant XR QuilliChew ER	Oral	Suspension reconstituted to 25 mg/5 ml Chewable tablets: 20 mg, 30 mg, 40 mg	CII	6 years and up: 20–60 mg/day
	Jornay PM	Oral	Extended-release capsule: 20 mg, 40 mg, 60 mg, 80 mg, 100 mg	CII	20–100 mg every evening
Mixed amphetamine salts (am FET a meen)	Adderall XR	Oral	Capsule: 4 mg, 10 mg, 15 mg, 20 mg, 25 mg, 30 mg	CII	10–30 mg/day
Lisdexamfetamine (lis dex am FET a meen)	Vyvanse	Oral	Capsule: 20 mg, 30 mg, 40 mg, 50 mg, 60 mg, 70 mg	CII	20–70 mg/day

Continued next page

MEDICATION TABLE 7-4. Attention Deficit Hyperactivity Disorder Agents[14] *(Continued)*

CLASS Generic Name	Brand Name	Route	Forms	DEA Schedule/ Regulatory Status	Dose
Nonstimulants					
Atomoxetine (AT oh mox e teen)	Strattera	Oral	Capsule: 10 mg, 18 mg, 25 mg, 40 mg, 60 mg, 80 mg, 100 mg	Rx	10–100 mg/day
Clonidine (KLOE ni deen)	Kapvay	Oral	Extended-release tablet: 0.1 mg, 0.2 mg	Rx	0.1–0.4 mg/day
	Generics	Oral	Tablet: 0.1 mg, 0.2 mg, 0.3 mg	Rx	0.1–1.6 mg/day in divided doses
	Catapres-TTS	Transdermal	Extended-release patch: 0.1 mg/24 hr, 0.2 mg/24 hr, 0.3 mg/24 hr	Rx	0.1–0.3 mg/day; Change patch weekly
Guanfacine (GWAHN fa seen)	Generics	Oral	Tablet: 1 mg, 2 mg	Rx	1–4 mg/day
	Intuniv	Oral	Extended-release tablet: 1 mg, 2 mg, 3 mg, 4 mg	Rx	1–4 mg/day

DEA = U.S. Drug Enforcement Administration.

MEDICATION TABLE 7-5. Substance Use Disorder Medications[14]

CLASS Generic Name	Brand Name	Route	Forms	DEA Schedule/ Regulatory Status	Dose
Alcohol/Opioid Abstinence Managers					
Acamprosate (a KAM pro sate)	Generics	Oral	Delayed-release tablet: 333 mg	Rx	999–1,998 mg/day
Buprenorphine (byoo pre NOR feen)	Belbuca, Sublocade	Oral, SUBQ extended-release	SL tablet: 2 mg, 8 mg Sublocade: 100 mg/0.5 mL, 300 mg/1.5 mL prefilled syringes	Schedule III controlled substance (CIII)	6*24 mg/day 100–300 mg monthly
Buprenorphine plus naloxone (byoo pre NOR feen)	Suboxone, Zubsolv	SL	SL tablet: (buprenorphine/ naloxone) 2 mg/0.5 mg, 8 mg/2 mg Sublingual film: (buprenorphine/naloxone) 2 mg/0.5 mg, 8 mg/2 mg	CIII	6–24 mg/day buprenorphine
Disulfiram (dye SUL fi ram)	Generics	Oral	Tablet: 250 mg	Rx	250–500 mg/day
Lofexidine (lo FEX ih deen)	Lucemyra	Oral	Tablet: 0.18 mg	Rx	0.54 mg 4 times daily for up to 14 days
Naltrexone (nal TREX one)	Vivitrol	Oral, IM	Tablet: 50 mg; IM suspension: 380 mg	Rx	50–100 mg/day
Smoking Cessation					
Nicotine (NIK oh teen)	Nicorette	Transmucosal	Gum: 2 mg, 4 mg	OTC	Up to 24 pieces/day
	Commit	Transmucosal	Lozenge: 2 mg	OTC	Up to 20 lozenges/day
	Nicotrol	Inhalation	Inhaler: 4 mg delivered (10 mg/cartridge)	Rx	24–64 mg/day
	Nicotrol NS	Nasal inhalation	Nasal spray: 0.5 mg nicotine/ actuation (10 mg/mL)	Rx	8–40 mg/day
	Nicoderm	Transdermal	Nicotine transdermal system: (step 1: 21 mg/day; step 2: 14 mg/day; step 3: 7 mg/day); Nicoderm CQ: (step 1: 21 mg/ day; step 2: 14 mg/day; step 3: 7 mg/day); Nicotrol (step 1: 15 mg/day; step 2: 10 mg/day; step 3: 5 mg/day)	OTC	7–21 mg/day
Bupropion (byoo PROE pee on)	Wellbutrin SR	Oral	Extended-release tablet: 150 mg	Rx	Target: 300 mg/day
Varenicline (var EN i kleen)	Generics	Oral	Tablet: 0.5 mg, 1 mg	Rx	Target: 2 mg/day

DEA = U.S. Drug Enforcement Administration; OTC = over the counter; SL = sublingual; SUBQ = subcutaneous.

Part 3

THE ENDOCRINE SYSTEM

Chapter 8

Overview of the Endocrine System and Agents

Sherrill J. Brown, DVM, PharmD, BCPS |
Kendra Keeley Procacci, PharmD, BCPS, AE–C |
Katherine S. Hale, PharmD, BCPS

KEY TERMS AND DEFINITIONS

Acromegaly—overproduction of growth hormone.

Feedback system—method of regulation of hormone levels where the target hormone affects the production of the stimulating hormone, either negatively (inhibits production) or positively (stimulates production).

Hyperparathyroidism—overactive parathyroid glands, classified as primary, secondary, or tertiary depending on the cause of parathyroid hyperactivity and the presence of hyper- or hypocalcemia.

Hypoparathyroidism—a disorder related to inadequate secretion of parathyroid hormone by the parathyroid glands resulting in abnormally low levels of calcium in the blood.

Hypopituitarism—deficiency of pituitary hormones.

Hypothyroidism—a condition in which the body does not produce enough thyroid hormone.

Osteomalacia—bone disease characterized by softening of the bones due to inadequate deposits of calcium and vitamin D.

Primary hyperparathyroidism (PHPT)—a disorder resulting from one or more overactive parathyroid glands, resulting in high levels of calcium in the blood.

DOI 10.37573/9781585286638.008

Pseudohypoparathyroidism (PHP)—a collection of disorders resulting from genetic mutations where patients exhibit clinical symptoms of hypoparathyroidism, but are resistant to the actions of parathyroid hormone versus inadequate secretion.

Renal osteodystrophy—bone disease characterized by defective bone development and softening of the bones due to chronic kidney disease.

Secondary hyperparathyroidism (SHPT)—a disorder resulting from chronic, long-term states of hypocalcemia and resistance to the actions of parathyroid hormone; the parathyroid glands become overactive and the glands become enlarged.

Serum—the clear fluid obtained from blood when it has been separated into its solid and liquid components after clotting has occurred.

Tertiary hyperparathyroidism (THPT)—severe secondary hyperparathyroidism despite efforts to correct the condition; patients are in a chronic state of hypercalcemia due to constant overproduction of parathyroid hormone.

Trophic hormones—hormones released by the pituitary gland that regulate other endocrine glands.

LEARNING OBJECTIVES

After completing this chapter, you should be able to

1. Describe the negative feedback system used to regulate levels of many of the body's hormones.

2. Define the following:
   - Acromegaly
   - Hyperparathyroidism
   - Hyperthyroidism
   - Hypoparathyroidism
   - Hypopituitarism
   - Hypothyroidism

3. State the brand and generic names of the most widely prescribed medications for pituitary disorders, thyroid disorders, and parathyroid disorders.

4. Be familiar with the routes of administration and dosage forms, and the most common adverse effects of medications used to treat pituitary disorders, thyroid disorders, and parathyroid disorders.

5. Describe the therapeutic effects of medications used to treat pituitary disorders, thyroid disorders, and parathyroid disorders.

The endocrine system consists of glands located throughout the body, which release hormones into the blood. Hormones are chemicals released from one cell in the body that affect other cells in other parts of the body. Endocrine hormones are released or secreted directly into the bloodstream.[1]

The release of many hormones is regulated by a feedback system. Positive feedback in the form of low levels of the target hormone results in an increase in the release of the stimulating pathway. Negative feedback in the form of high levels of the target hormone decreases the release of the stimulating pathway. For example, the hypothalamus produces thyrotropin-releasing hormone (TRH), which stimulates the production and secretion of thyroid-stimulating hormone (TSH) by the pituitary gland. TSH then signals the thyroid gland to produce thyroid hormones. The presence of thyroid hormones in the blood provides negative feedback, which inhibits the production and secretion of more TRH by the hypothalamus. This negative feedback ensures that thyroid hormones do not exceed normal levels and cause toxic effects (Figure 8-1).[1]

PITUITARY GLAND

CASE STUDY

Traumatic hypopituitarism

Amy Bird is a 47-year-old female who fractured her skull in an automobile accident 10 months ago. She was unconscious for 4 days but appeared to recover completely from her injuries. Since the accident, Ms. Bird has lost weight, becomes dizzy when she stands up, and says that she is tired "all the time." Her doctor told her that the blood supply to her pituitary gland was damaged in the accident and that she would need to take several different medications to treat this problem.

Overview of Pituitary Gland

The pituitary gland is located in the brain and consists of two lobes: the anterior lobe and the posterior lobe (Figure 8-2). Most hormones released from the pituitary gland regulate other endocrine glands and are called trophic hormones. The trophic hormones secreted by the anterior pituitary gland are listed below:[1,2]

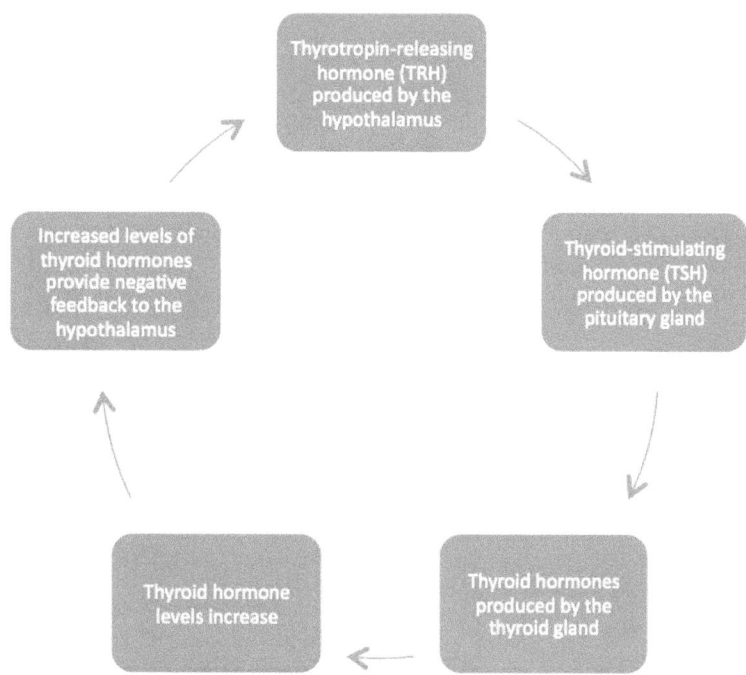

FIGURE 8-1. Example of feedback system for hormone regulation.

- Luteinizing hormone (LH) and follicle-stimulating hormone (FSH) control the production of sex hormones by the ovaries and testicles.

- Corticotropin, also called adrenocorticotropic hormone or ACTH, acts on the adrenal gland (the adrenal gland is covered in more detail in Chapter 9).

- Thyroid-stimulating hormone (TSH) stimulates the production of thyroid hormones.

Nontrophic hormones produced by the anterior pituitary gland are growth hormone (GH) and prolactin. GH induces growth in children, and prolactin stimulates milk production and secretion in lactating women. The hypothalamus releases hormones that stimulate the release of hormones from the anterior pituitary gland. These releasing hormones are part of the negative feedback system described above. Gonadotropin-releasing hormone (GnRH) stimulates the release of LH and FSH. TRH stimulates the release of TSH, and corticotropin-releasing hormone stimulates the release of ACTH. Growth hormone-releasing hormone (GHRH) stimulates the release of GH, while somatostatin from the hypothalamus inhibits the release of GH. The hypothalamus does not produce a hormone to stimulate the secretion of prolactin, but it does inhibit the release of prolactin by releasing dopamine.[1,2]

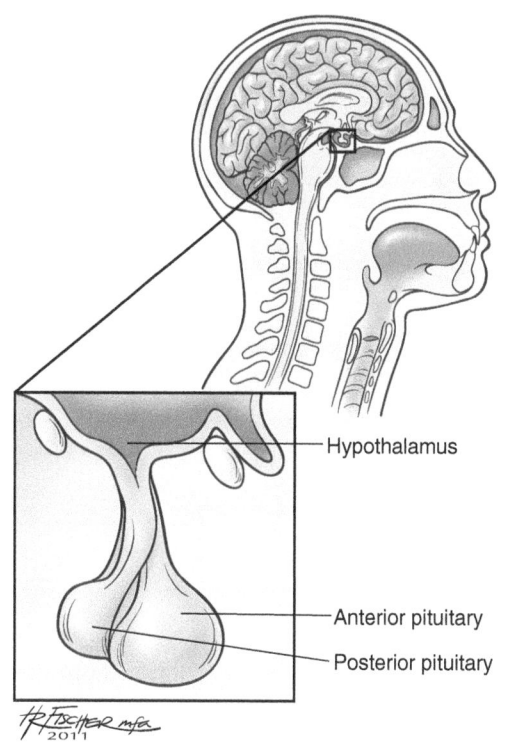

FIGURE 8-2. Location and structure of pituitary gland.

The posterior pituitary produces two hormones: vasopressin (also known as antidiuretic hormone or ADH) and oxytocin. Vasopressin helps the body control blood pressure. When hypotension or low blood pressure occurs, vasopressin causes the blood vessels to constrict and the kidney to reabsorb water in order to maintain normal blood pressure.[2] Oxytocin induces uterine contractions in pregnant women and promotes milk letdown in women who are breastfeeding.[1,2]

CASE?

Ms. Bird has come into the pharmacy today with prescriptions for levothyroxine (thyroid medication), prednisone (a glucocorticoid), and Prempro (a combination estrogen and progesterone product). If Ms. Bird's problem is her pituitary gland, why does she need to take thyroid medication, estrogen, progesterone, and prednisone?

Overview of Pituitary Gland Disorders

Hypopituitarism

Hypopituitarism, or a deficiency in pituitary hormones, is rare. Common causes are pituitary surgery or radiation therapy for pituitary tumors or a tumor that blocks blood flow to the pituitary gland. When blood flow to the pituitary gland is decreased, hormones from the hypothalamus cannot reach the pituitary to stimulate the production and release of pituitary hormones. Other causes of hypopituitarism include genetic disorders, head injuries, and other diseases affecting the blood flow to the pituitary gland and hypothalamus.[3]

Signs and symptoms of hypopituitarism are those seen with deficiencies of the target glands. For example, the patient will display signs and symptoms of thyroid hormone deficiency (hypothyroidism) since the thyroid is not stimulated to produce thyroid hormone due to the lack of TSH from the pituitary.[2,3] However, patients may have an excess of prolactin because of the disruption of inhibition from the hypothalamus.[2]

Treatment of hypopituitarism depends on the cause of the pituitary deficiency. For causes that cannot be treated, replacement of either the pituitary hormone or the target hormone is essential. Patients are most often treated with glucocorticoids, such as prednisone or hydrocortisone (for ACTH deficiency), thyroid hormones (for TSH deficiency), and sex hormones (for LH and FSH deficiency).[2,3] GH and vasopressin replacement may also be required.[3] Hormone replacement for hypopituitarism will often be lifelong, and patients will require monitoring for the various hormones.[2]

CASE?

How long will Ms. Bird need to take these medications? What symptoms might she have if she does not take them?

Excessive Growth Hormone (Acromegaly)

Acromegaly is caused by excessive GH production, usually from a tumor in the anterior pituitary. Sometimes, a tumor located outside the pituitary can secrete GH, also resulting in acromegaly. Overproduction of GHRH by the hypothalamus can cause overproduction of GH, which will also lead to acromegaly.[2,3]

Patients with acromegaly have overgrowth of soft tissues. They may have large hands and fingers, large feet, an enlarged tongue, and coarse facial features. Many patients will have heart disease and high blood pressure. Osteoarthritis and joint problems are common in patients with acromegaly. These patients may also have type 2 diabetes mellitus, sleep apnea, or respiratory disorders.[2,3] Diagnosis of acromegaly is made based on the blood levels of certain chemicals and markers, as well as glucose tolerance tests (see Chapter 10, Diabetes Mellitus).[2]

Treatment of acromegaly depends on the cause for the excessive GH. If acromegaly is caused by a tumor outside the pituitary, then removal of the tumor will usually cure the acromegaly. If the patient has a pituitary tumor that cannot be removed with surgery, the patient can be treated with radiation therapy or pharmacological therapy. Pharmacologic therapies include dopamine agonists, somatostatin analogs, and GH receptor antagonists.[2,3]

Bromocriptine and cabergoline are the dopamine agonists used to treat acromegaly.[2,3] Bromocriptine will decrease GH levels within 1–2 hours after an oral dose, and the GH levels will remain low for 4–5 hours.[2] Most patients will see a benefit within 4–8 weeks of bromocriptine therapy.[2,4] The initial dose is 1.25 or 2.5 mg daily.[4] The dose may be increased in 1.25 or 2.5 mg increments every 3–7 days as needed to suppress GH levels. The maximum dose is 100 mg daily, although most patients with acromegaly can be controlled with doses of 20–30 mg daily.[2,4] For acromegaly, the daily bromocriptine dose should be divided into three or four doses.[2]

ALERT!

Drugs that inhibit liver metabolism, especially verapamil, some antibiotics (eg, erythromycin, clarithromycin, doxycycline), some antifungal medications, and some HIV treatments, may increase levels of bromocriptine, while metoclopramide and some antipsychotic medications may decrease the drug's effectiveness.[4] Be sure the pharmacist is aware if such combinations are prescribed for a patient, particularly if more than one physician is involved.

Cabergoline is a long-acting dopamine agonist that is dosed twice a week and is used off-label to treat acromegaly.[2,4] Cabergoline is usually begun with a dose of 0.25 mg twice weekly and may be increased as needed.[4] Cabergoline doses for acromegaly are much higher than those used for hyperprolactinemia (up to 0.5 mg/day).[3]

Dopamine agonists often cause nausea, constipation, and headache. Other common side effects include orthostatic hypotension (a decrease in blood pressure upon standing), dry mouth, drowsiness, and vomiting. Cold-sensitive digital vasospasm (constriction of the blood vessels in the fingers as a response to cold temperatures) may occur with high doses of bromocriptine.[2,4] Administration with food is recommended to decrease the likelihood of gastrointestinal side effects.[2]

PRACTICE POINT

Keeping fingers and body warm will help prevent cold-sensitive digital vasospasm, although sometimes the bromocriptine dose must be reduced. Patients reporting or commenting about such a reaction should be referred to the pharmacist and/or physician for advice.

ALERT!

Dopamine agonists should be discontinued during pregnancy and lactation.[4]

Somatostatin is naturally produced by the body and has many functions, including inhibition of the secretion of GH, insulin, and TSH. Because somatostatin has a short half-life and must be given by continuous intravenous (IV) infusion, somatostatin analogs have been developed that have a longer duration of action and more specific activity.[5] Somatostatin analogs used to treat acromegaly are octreotide, lanreotide, and pasireotide.[2,3]

Octreotide is a somatostatin analog often prescribed to prevent the secretion of GH by the pituitary gland. Octreotide is an injection available in two different formulations: a subcutaneous (SUBQ) solution used as initial treatment and a depot suspension used for maintenance therapy. The SUBQ solution is injected 3 times daily, and the dose is adjusted as needed to maintain the appropriate GH and insulin-like growth factor-1 (IGF-1) levels in the body.[2,4] The target GH blood level is <1 ng/mL.[2,4,6] The target IGF-1 level is based on the age-normalized IGF-1 level.[6] Once a patient is on a stable dose of SUBQ octreotide for at least 2 weeks, the drug can be switched to the depot formulation. The depot suspension is injected intramuscularly every 4 weeks.[4]

PRACTICE POINT

Octreotide injections should be refrigerated and protected from light. They should be allowed to come to room temperature for 30–60 minutes prior to preparation but never warmed artificially. Octreotide suspension must be administered immediately and should not be stored after reconstitution. Once opened, the multiple dose vials of the solution must be discarded after 14 days.[7]

The initial dose of octreotide depot injection is 20 mg every 4 weeks. After 3 months, the dose can be adjusted based on response. The maximum dose of octreotide depot injections is 40 mg every 4 weeks, and doses greater than 40 mg are not recommended for acromegaly. Patients receiving octreotide injections commonly develop diarrhea, nausea, and dyspnea (breathing difficulties). Octreotide injections may also cause injection-site pain, dizziness, fatigue, malaise, gallbladder problems, joint pain, and hyperglycemia (high glucose levels). Octreotide may alter heart rate and the conduction of the electrical signal through the heart muscle. Because of this, octreotide may slow the heart rate and enhance the effect of other medications that affect the conduction in the heart.[2,4]

Lanreotide is another somatostatin analog indicated for the treatment of acromegaly. Lanreotide is an SUBQ depot injection that is given every 4 weeks. The initial dose is 90 mg every 4 weeks. After the first 3 months, the dose is adjusted based on GH and IGF-1 levels.[2,4] The lanreotide dose is decreased to 60 mg every 4 weeks if the GH and IGF-1 levels are normal and the patient's symptoms are controlled.[4] Patients receiving lanreotide injections have reported constipation, diarrhea, nausea, abdominal pain, and injection-site reactions. Lanreotide may decrease the heart rate, cause gallstones, and alter blood glucose levels.[2,4]

PRACTICE POINT

Lanreotide is a prefilled syringe packaged in a sealed pouch; it must be refrigerated and protected from light. The package should be removed from the refrigerator 30 minutes prior to administration and allowed to come to room temperature. The sealed pouch should not be opened until just before injection of lanreotide.[8]

Pasireotide is the third somatostatin analog. It is available as a long-acting release (LAR) intramuscular formulation for treatment of acromegaly and as a short-acting SUBQ formulation used only as treatment for Cushing's disease.[2,9,10] Pasireotide LAR intramuscular injection should be initiated at 40 mg every 4 weeks. After 3 months, the dose is titrated based on GH and IGF-1 levels.[2] Hyperglycemia is more common with pasireotide LAR than with octreotide or lanreotide, and patients may require treatment for diabetes. Other adverse effects include diarrhea, headache, decreased heart rate, and gallstones.[2,9]

Somatostatin analogs may decrease the secretion of TSH by the pituitary gland. This will decrease the production of thyroid hormones and may lead to hypothyroidism. Thyroid function should be monitored regularly in patients receiving octreotide, lanreotide, or pasireotide.[4]

ALERT!

Octreotide and other somatostatin analogs, as well as pegvisomant, can affect blood glucose levels. In patients with type 1 diabetes mellitus, extremely low glucose levels can occur. In patients with type 2 diabetes mellitus and in patients who do not have diabetes mellitus, glucose levels may greatly increase. As a result, patients may have to adjust doses of insulin and other antidiabetic medications.[2,4]

Pegvisomant is a GH receptor antagonist used to lower IGF-1 levels without affecting GH secretion. It is administered daily as an SUBQ injection.[2] A loading dose of 40 mg is given under physician supervision then followed by a daily dose of 10 mg. The dose may be adjusted by 5 mg every 4–6 weeks based on IGF-1 levels. Pegvisomant treatment may not be appropriate for patients with elevated liver enzymes at baseline. If liver enzymes become elevated during treatment, the medication may have to be discontinued.[2,4] Common adverse effects are injection-site reactions, nausea, diarrhea, and flu-like symptoms.[2] Growth hormone deficiency (GHD) symptoms may occur, even in patients with elevated GH concentrations.[4]

PRACTICE POINT

Pegvisomant is stored in the refrigerator. After the powder has been reconstituted, the solution should be used within 6 hours. The vial should not be reused, and any remaining solution should be discarded after the dose has been administered. The vial should not be shaken, and the solution should not be used if foam or cloudiness occurs.[11]

Growth Hormone Deficiency

GHD usually occurs with hypopituitarism, and patients may have signs of other pituitary hormone deficiencies. GHD without hypopituitarism is usually due to a genetic defect. Regardless of the cause, patients with GHD are often short or have delayed growth.[2,12] They may be obese, with excessive fat deposits around the abdomen. Adults may have more bone fractures due to weaker bones. High cholesterol and insulin resistance are also common in adults with GHD.[3,12]

ALERT!

Medication doses for GHD are different for children and adults, and doses and frequency differ between products. It is important to note the age of the patient and to be sure that the correct product is being dispensed.

GHD is treated with hormone replacement. Somatropin is a GH produced using recombinant DNA technology; it is identical to that secreted by the human pituitary gland.[2,5] Somatropin is usually administered daily as an SUBQ injection, although some products can be given intramuscularly. In children, therapy is usually continued until the desired height is reached or until after the pubertal growth spurt.[2] In adults, GH replacement decreases body fat, increases lean body mass, and improves cholesterol levels.[3] Recombinant GH is also used to treat children with short stature not related to GHD.[2]

PRACTICE POINT

Not all recombinant GH products have the same directions for proper storage. Be sure to refer to the packaging to determine storage temperatures, light protection requirements, and reconstitution instructions.

In children, adverse effects from GH are uncommon, although injection-site reactions and joint pain have been reported. Some patients experience headache, blurred vision, nausea, and vomiting. This usually resolves when the somatropin is discontinued.[2] Hyperglycemia and diabetes mellitus can occur in both adults and children; patients already being treated for diabetes may need therapy adjustments.[3,13] Because GH can stimulate the growth and recurrence of tumors, patients with a malignant tumor or history of recurrent tumors should not be treated with GH.[5] (See Medication Table 8-1; Medication Tables are located at the end of the chapter).

THYROID GLAND

CASE STUDY

Hypothyroidism
Cindy Clark is a 41-year-old female who went to see her family doctor because she was always really tired, gaining weight, and feeling "sluggish." Her doctor diagnosed her with a thyroid disorder and said her thyroid function tests showed a thyroid-stimulating hormone (TSH) level of 14.2 milli-International Units/L and a free thyroxine (T4) level of 0.71 ng/dL.

Overview of Thyroid Function

The thyroid gland is a butterfly-shaped gland composed of two lobes located in the anterior (front) of the neck (Figure 8-3). The thyroid gland uses iodine from food and

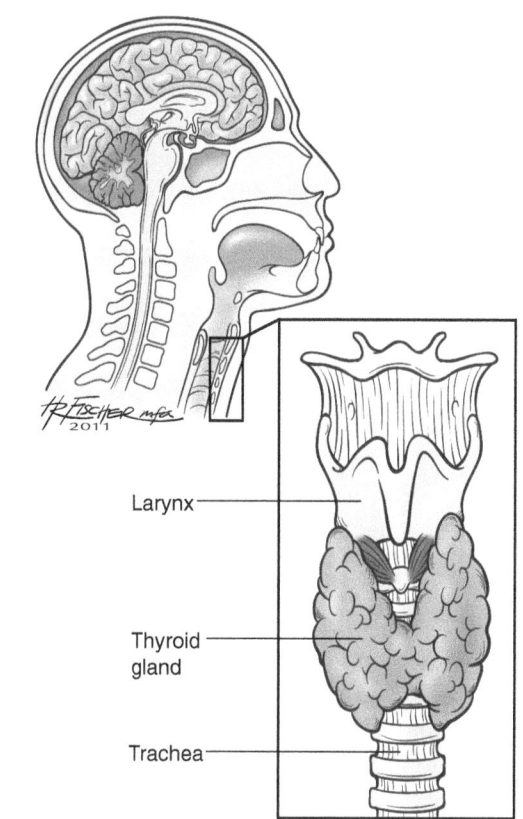

FIGURE 8-3. Thyroid gland.

water to make the thyroid hormones triiodothyronine (T3) and thyroxine (T4), which are then released into the bloodstream. T3 is more biologically active than T4 (which is converted by many body tissues to T3). Most of the T4 and T3 circulating in the bloodstream are bound to blood proteins, and only the unbound (free) hormones are able to exert effects on the body. Thyroid hormones work in every organ system to regulate the body's metabolism (ie, how the body uses and stores energy). Thyroid hormones affect consumption of oxygen, production of heat, and cardiac (heart) function, and they are required for normal growth and development.[2,3,14]

Regulation of the thyroid hormones is through a complex negative feedback system, which involves the hypothalamus, the pituitary, and the thyroid gland. When levels of thyroid hormones are low, TRH is released from the hypothalamus and stimulates the production of TSH from the pituitary, which tells the thyroid gland to produce more thyroid hormones. When increased levels of thyroid hormones are circulating, further release of TRH and TSH is inhibited, thus decreasing further release of T3 and T4 from the thyroid gland.[3,14]

Hypothyroidism

Hypothyroidism is a condition in which the body is not producing enough thyroid hormone. In the United States, the most common cause of hypothyroidism is a condition called Hashimoto's thyroiditis, an autoimmune disorder, which causes the body to produce antibodies that destroy the thyroid gland.[2,3,14] Other causes may be radioactive iodine therapy, surgical removal of the thyroid gland, side effects of medications such as amiodarone or lithium, pregnancy, and iodine deficiency (more common in underdeveloped countries). Clinical features of hypothyroidism are due to the body's decreased metabolic state and include weight gain, fatigue, cold intolerance, dry skin, brittle hair, constipation, and depression.[2,14]

CASE?

Which of Cindy Clark's symptoms are consistent with hypothyroidism?

Diagnosis of thyroid disorders can be done through blood tests called thyroid function tests, which measure the amounts of TSH, free T4, and T3 circulating in the bloodstream.[2,3,14] The level of TSH in the body is the best indicator of how the thyroid gland is working. In hypothyroidism, TSH is elevated and the amounts of free T4 and T3 are low, because the pituitary gland detects low T3 and T4 and releases more TSH in an attempt to stimulate more thyroid hormone production.[3,14]

Treatment of hypothyroidism is through thyroid replacement therapy. The treatment of choice is levothyroxine, T4, a synthetic hormone that replenishes the body's low thyroid hormone levels.[15] Just as the body's endogenous thyroid hormones work, levothyroxine is converted into the more active hormone, T3, in the liver and other body tissues. Levothyroxine is available in oral and IV formulations. The oral formulation has an onset of action of 3–5 days and has a slow elimination half-life (6–7 days), which makes the levels of medication more constant and predictable in a patient. Oral doses are started at 12.5–50 mcg and may be titrated up every 4–6 weeks to maintain normal TSH levels. The medication should be taken on an empty stomach, at least 30 minutes before eating.[2,4,15]

ALERT!

LOOK-ALIKE/SOUND-ALIKE—Levothyroxine may be confused with levofloxacin or liothyronine. Brand name or generic levothyroxine (Levoxyl) may be confused with Lanoxin, lamotrigine, or levofloxacin.

Liothyronine, T3, has a rapid onset of action (2–3 hours) and is more rapidly cleared from the body than levothyroxine (elimination half-life 2.5 days). This can make the levels of medication in the body fluctuate. Because the body converts T4 to T3, there is no clear benefit of liothyronine over levothyroxine. Liothyronine is available in oral and IV formulations. Oral doses are initiated at 25 mcg/day and are titrated by 12.5–25 mcg/day. A typical maintenance dose is 25–75 mcg/day.[4]

Liotrix, a combination of synthetic T4 and T3, is less commonly prescribed due to cost and difficulty of monitoring. The dose is typically initiated at 25 mcg daily and titrated up to a maintenance dose of 60–120 mcg/day. Thyroid USP, also known as desiccated thyroid, is a natural hormone derived from the thyroid of beef and pork. Natural thyroid hormone products are less commonly prescribed because the potency and amount of drug absorbed by the patient can vary.[2,4]

PRACTICE POINT

It is recommended that patients do not switch between brand name and generic formulations of thyroid replacement medications.

The dose of thyroid replacement therapy is typically based on factors such as patient age, weight, and other disease states. Although symptoms may improve after 2–3 weeks, steady-state TSH concentrations are not achieved for 6–8 weeks. Once steady state is reached, TSH levels are assessed to determine how the patient is responding to the medication and if the dosage is appropriate.[2] Once the patient is maintained on an appropriate replacement dose, TSH levels are typically measured annually. Adverse effects are unusual if the patient is receiving the correct dosage of medication. If patients are receiving too much medication they may experience symptoms of hyperthyroidism. Thyroid replacement hormones can interact with other medications, including warfarin, digoxin, rifampin, and carbamazepine.[4] Patients who are also taking antacids, cholestyramine, orlistat, sucralfate, or iron must separate the time of administration of thyroid replacement by at least 4 hours.[4] Thyroid replacement medications may be safely used during pregnancy. Hypothyroidism caused by pregnancy or medications may resolve after delivery or when the medications are discontinued.[4] Autoimmune hypothyroidism, caused by Hashimoto's thyroiditis, is permanent and patients are treated lifelong with hormone therapy.[2,3]

CASE?

Why were Cindy Clark's TSH levels elevated when she has an underactive thyroid?

Myxedema coma is a rare consequence of severe hypothyroidism, which leads to hypothermia and decreased mental status, which may progress to coma. Myxedema coma has a high mortality rate and is considered a medical emergency. Treatment of myxedema coma is with IV levothyroxine or liothyronine. The medications may be used together or individually.[2]

PRACTICE POINT

IV levothyroxine must be stored at room temperature. The medication must be reconstituted immediately prior to administration. IV solutions containing this drug should not be mixed with other IV solutions. Vials of injectable liothyronine must be refrigerated.

Hyperthyroidism

Hyperthyroidism is a condition in which the body produces too much thyroid hormone. The most common cause of hyperthyroidism is Grave's disease, a genetic autoimmune disorder in which the body produces antibodies that attack the thyroid gland and causes the thyroid gland to make too much thyroid hormone. Hyperthyroidism can also be caused by tumors, nodules, or too much medication for treatment of hypothyroidism.[2,3,14]

Clinical features of hyperthyroidism are due to the body's increased metabolic state and include heat intolerance, weight loss, increased sweating, heart palpitations, increased pulse and systolic pressure, nervousness, irritability, emotional liability, and insomnia. Thyroid function tests of patients with hyperthyroidism will show decreased TSH and increased T4 and T3 because the thyroid gland is overproducing T4 and T3, which in turn inhibits the production of TSH.[2,3,14]

Hyperthyroidism can be treated with radioactive iodine, antithyroid medications, or surgery if a nodule is causing the problem. Radioactive iodine is taken orally and works by damaging the thyroid cells. Radioactive iodine is a cure of hyperthyroidism but may lead to hypothyroidism. There are two antithyroid medications that are approved by the Food and Drug Administration (FDA) for the treatment of hyperthyroidism: propylthiouracil and methimazole.[2] These medications work by blocking the body's productions of thyroid hormones. Patients often require high initial doses and notice improvement in 4–8 weeks. Dose changes may be made on a monthly basis. Methimazole is initiated at 15–30 mg/day in three divided doses and gradually reduced to a maintenance dose of 5–15 mg/day given in three divided doses. Prophylthiouracil is initiated at 300 mg daily in three divided doses and decreased to a maintenance dose of 50–300 mg/day in three divided doses. Occasionally patients may require 600–900 mg daily.[4]

ALERT!

LOOK-ALIKE/SOUND-ALIKE—Methimazole may be confused with metolazone or methazolamide.

Propylthiouracil can interact with other medications, including warfarin and lithium. Methimazole may interact with medications that cause bone marrow suppression. Patients are usually treated with antithyroid medications for 1–2 years and 40% to 50% are cured.[14] If patients are cured by medications they still need to continue to be monitored because hyperthyroidism may recur. The medications are usually tolerated well. Adverse effects of the medications include rash, joint aches, and fever.[4] (See Medication Table 8-2.)

PARATHYROID GLAND

CASE STUDY

Mr. Smith's Parathyroid Disorder
John Smith is a 64-year-old male who saw his physician a few days ago because his fingers and toes were tingling. He had also been feeling anxious and irritable for weeks prior to his visit to the doctor's office.

Overview of the Parathyroid Glands

Despite the name, the parathyroid glands have no relation to the thyroid other than their location. These four, small oval-shaped glands are located behind the thyroid (Figure 8-4) and produce parathyroid hormone (PTH), which regulates calcium concentrations in the blood.[3] Control of calcium concentrations is especially important because disorders affecting calcium homeostasis affect cell membranes, neuromuscular activity, endocrine function, anticoagulation, platelet adhesion, bone metabolism, and cardiac and smooth muscle tissues.

Production of PTH is tightly controlled via a rapid negative feedback mechanism that provides minute-to-minute control of calcium concentrations. PTH acts directly on the bone and kidneys and indirectly on the gut. For example, if a person has low blood calcium levels, known as hypocalcemia, then more PTH is produced. Bones break down at a faster rate, resulting in a flow of calcium from bone to blood. In the kidneys, less calcium is cleared and it returns to the extracellular fluid and blood. Additionally, PTH stimulates the conversion of calcidiol (25-hydroxyvitamin D) to calcitriol (1α,25-dihydroxyvitamin D), the active form of vitamin D. Traveling to the intestinal tract, calcitriol binds to vitamin D receptors and increases levels of calcium binding protein, thus increasing intestinal absorption of calcium and phosphorus. In contrast, high calcium levels (hypercalcemia) lead to a decrease in PTH production and the process reverses itself.[2,3,16-18]

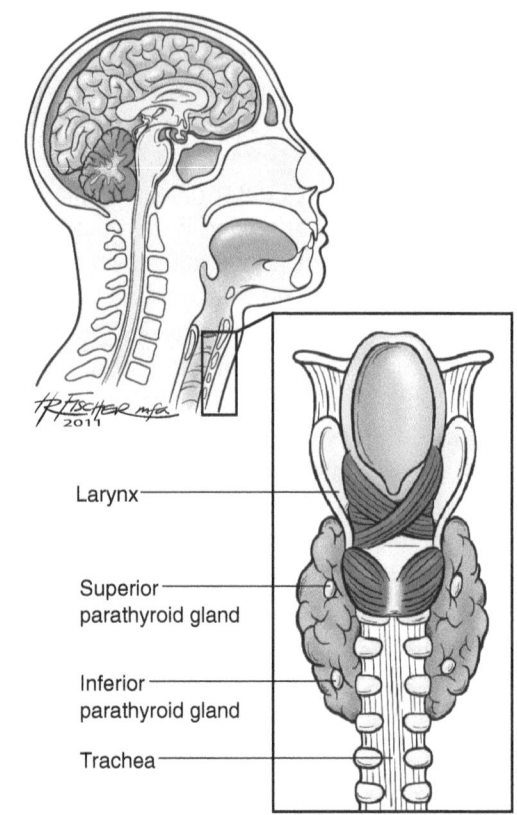

FIGURE 8-4. Parathyroid gland.

CASE?

Mr. Smith's physician contacted him regarding the results of his blood work, including a low calcium level and a high phosphorus level. What type of parathyroid disorder does he probably have?

Hypoparathyroidism

Individuals who lack available or functioning PTH have a disorder known as hypoparathyroidism. This disorder may be hereditary, often occurring with no known cause (idiopathic), or it may be the result of surgical procedures that damage the parathyroid glands, autoimmune disorders, radiation-induced damage (from cancer treatments), and severe, chronically low magnesium. If the parathyroid glands functioned normally, PTH would be secreted in response to low calcium levels causing decreased calcium clearance in the kidneys and an increased rate of bone breakdown, leading to a flow of calcium into the blood. Because PTH is absent in hypoparathyroidism, the body's response to low calcium levels does not occur and other physiologic systems are affected. Symptoms of hypoparathyroidism include burning and tingling of the extremities, seizures, anxiety, calcium deposits in vital organs, tremors, ataxia, nystagmus, vertigo, apathy, depression, irritability, delirium, and psychosis. These symptoms are associated with abnormally low blood levels of calcium and magnesium and high phosphate levels, which often disappear once these electrolyte abnormalities are corrected. Individuals are diagnosed with hypoparathyroidism if they present with low calcium and magnesium levels, high phosphate levels, and little to no PTH present. Past medical and family history, kidney function, and the potential for vitamin D deficiency are also taken into account.[3,19]

CASE?

What medications might his physician order for Mr. Smith?

The primary treatment for hypoparathyroidism is long-term calcium and vitamin D replacement to correct and maintain calcium levels slightly below the normal.[2,3,19] Treatment with oral calcium supplements includes the use of calcium carbonate and calcium citrate. Typical dosing is 500–1,000 mg elemental calcium 3 times daily with meals. Calcium supplements will be discussed in more detail in Chapter 14.

Vitamin D therapy is used to correct vitamin D deficiency. Available therapies include ergocalciferol—vitamin D_2, calcifediol—vitamin D_3, calcitriol, and dihydrotachysterol. The vitamin D analogs paricalcitol and doxercalciferol will be discussed later in this section.

CASE?

Mr. Smith brings a prescription to the pharmacy for calcitriol capsules. What are these expected to do to help his condition?

PRACTICE POINT

Vitamin D is a fat-soluble vitamin, stored in body fat, so it may take weeks to see the full effects of oral vitamin D supplementation.

Calcitriol, the active metabolite of vitamin D, is a widely used alternative to fat-soluble formulations of vitamin D. Calcitriol has a rapid onset of action, rapid turnover, and is not fat soluble. The initial dose is 0.25 mcg daily, with maintenance dosages ranging from 0.5–2 mcg oral or IV per day. Doses may be increased every 2–4 weeks.

ALERT!

Because of differences in absorption, strength, and dosing, vitamin D supplements cannot be substituted for one another without consulting the pharmacist or physician.

Treatment with oral calcium and vitamin D, however, does not reverse the decrease in calcium reabsorption from the urinary tract that is typical of hypoparathyroidism. While taking calcium and vitamin D replacements, patients are at risk of developing kidney stones. Thiazide diuretics (discussed in Chapter 13) can be used to reduce urinary calcium levels and lower the risk of kidney stones.

Pseudohypoparathyroidism (PHP) is a collection of disorders resulting from genetic mutations. Patients exhibit symptoms of hypoparathyroidism but have normal kidney function and normal levels of vitamin D. PTH levels are also elevated, but patients don't respond due to resistance to the hormone.[3,17,18]

As in the treatment of hypoparathyroidism, calcium and vitamin D supplementation is also the mainstay for treatment of PHP. The goals of treatment are to bring calcium and PTH levels back to normal and to avoid high calcium levels in the urine (hypercalciuria). A total daily dose of 1–3 grams elemental calcium is recommended to normalize and maintain calcium levels. Calcitriol is the vitamin D supplement of choice because individuals with PHP often require less vitamin D supplementation than individuals with hypoparathyroidism. Additionally, calcitriol is not fat soluble. The effective dose of calcitriol ranges from 0.25 mcg twice daily to 0.5 mcg 4 times daily.

Hyperparathyroidism

Overactive parathyroid glands are the cause of hyperparathyroidism. This condition is classified as primary, secondary, or tertiary depending on the cause of parathyroid hyperactivity and the presence of hyper- or hypocalcemia.[3]

Primary hyperparathyroidism (PHPT) is a response to one or more enlarged glands causing overproduction of

PTH resulting in hypercalcemia. Women are three times more likely than men to develop PHPT, and the condition is more common after menopause, with an estimated prevalence of 1%.[16,20] PHPT is typically the result of growth or a tumor and is independent of other organs. Overgrowth of the gland(s) is considered irreversible. Other potential causes of PHPT include external neck irradiation, genetic mutations, and lithium therapy.[3,16,20]

Unlike primary hyperparathyroidism, secondary hyperparathyroidism (SHPT) occurs in response to long-term states of hypocalcemia and is associated with resistance to PTH. The result, however, is similar with enlarged glands and overproduction of PTH. Most notably SHPT occurs in the presence of chronic kidney disease and decreased renal function, but it is also frequently due to other causes of bone softening (eg, deficiency of vitamin D action and pseudohypoparathyroidism).[2,16] Unlike PHPT, overgrowth of the gland(s) can be reversed if the underlying condition is corrected. In the early stages of chronic renal failure, PTH secretion is consistently elevated in order to correct calcium and phosphate levels. As kidney function worsens, less phosphorus is eliminated leading to high phosphate levels and plummeting calcium levels. Another complication of worsening kidney function is severe vitamin D deficiency because there is less conversion of vitamin D to its active metabolite. Because PTH is produced continuously, resistance to the effects of calcium and vitamin D therapy develops because fewer vitamin D and calcium-sensing receptors are available. Over time renal osteodystrophy (bone disease) develops.[2]

When patients with secondary hyperparathyroidism are no longer responsive to medical treatment, a chronic state of hypercalcemia develops due to constant overproduction of PTH. The term tertiary hyperparathyroidism (THPT) originated to describe these patients exhibiting severe manifestations of secondary hyperparathyroidism despite aggressive medical efforts to correct the condition.[3] The treatment of choice for PHPT and THPT in symptomatic patients is surgery to remove one or more of the affected parathyroid glands. Surgical management is also recommended for asymptomatic PHPT patients who are less than 50 years old; are not able to participate in adequate medical follow-up; have serum calcium more than 1 mg/dL (0.25 mmol/L); have a T-score less than or equal to –2.5 at the lumbar spine, total hip, femoral neck, or distal one-third radius; have significant bone mineral density decrease; and/or have creatinine clearance <60 mL/min.[21]

Because SHPT is considered reversible if electrolyte imbalances are corrected, SHPT can be managed with medication instead of surgery. The goals for managing SHPT include the management of PTH, phosphate, and calcium balances, while minimizing aluminum exposure. These activities are important in slowing or preventing the progression of SHPT, renal osteodystrophy, and calcifications in the cardiovascular system or soft tissues. Phosphate-binding medications, calcium supplements, vitamin D, and calcimimetics are all therapies utilized to meet these goals.[2,3,16]

> ## PRACTICE POINT
>
> *Because medications for hyperparathyroidism are dependent on and may also affect gastric pH and the bioavailability of other drugs, it is important for the physician and pharmacist to evaluate potential drug interactions prior to choosing an appropriate treatment.*

Phosphate-binding agents are medications that work in the gastrointestinal tract, combining dietary phosphates with other molecules to form insoluble salts. This prevents the phosphate from being absorbed into the bloodstream; instead, it is excreted in the feces, resulting in an overall lowering of circulating phosphates.

Available phosphate-binding agents include calcium-, lanthanum-, aluminum-, and magnesium-containing compounds, sevelamer hydrochloride, and sevelamer carbonate. Newer agents include sucroferric oxyhydroxide and ferric citrate.[22] Sevelamer HCl is a nonabsorbable hydrogel phosphate-binding agent that does not contain aluminum, calcium, or magnesium. The dose is determined based on the patient's current serum phosphate level and is adjusted as needed. Doses typically range from 800–1,600 mg 3 times daily. Common side effects include nausea and vomiting, indigestion, flatulence, and diarrhea. It also has the potential to cause a drop or increase in blood pressure. Sevelamer carbonate is an agent similar to sevelamer hydrochloride but contains a carbonate buffer instead. The carbonate component was added to maintain bicarbonate levels and reduce gastrointestinal (GI) side effects. Dosing strategies and side effects are the same as for sevelamer HCl and may affect the bioavailability of antiarrhythmic and anticonvulsant medications. The sevelamer agents should be given at least 1 hour before or 3 hours after antiarrhythmic or anticonvulsant drugs to reduce the potential for drug interactions.

CASE?

Mr. Smith, who was diagnosed with hypoparathyroidism, had a high phosphate level. What type of medication, other than calcitriol, is his physician likely to prescribe?

Lanthanum carbonate is a phosphate-binding agent that complexes with phosphates in meals and prevents their absorption. The initial dose is 1,500 mg daily, administered in divided doses. The dose may be titrated up every 2–3 weeks to a maximum recommended dose of 3,000 mg per day. Common side effects include diarrhea, nausea, and vomiting.

Aluminum carbonate and aluminum hydroxide are used if phosphorus levels are particularly high. Aluminum salts are considered third-line agents in the treatment of higher-than-normal phosphate levels, known as hyperphosphatemia, and may be prescribed alone or in combination with calcium-containing binding agents or sevelamer for patients who do not respond to one agent alone. Long-term use can lead to aluminum toxicity and could result in the development of the bone disease osteomalacia, anemia, joint disease, and encephalopathy. Dosing ranges from 300–600 mg 3 times daily with meals, depending on the agent used. Typical side effects include constipation, nausea and vomiting, and a chalky taste.

Antacids containing magnesium carbonate or magnesium hydroxide can also be used as phosphate binders, which may decrease the need for calcium-based phosphate-binding agents; however, use of these agents may be limited because of magnesium accumulation and resulting toxicity. The typical dose is given 3 times daily and ranges from 70 mg (magnesium carbonate) to 300–400 mg (magnesium hydroxide). Common side effects include diarrhea, GI distress, and elevated magnesium and potassium levels.

ALERT!

Aluminum salts should not be taken with calcium citrate preparations, even those available over the counter, due to significant increases in aluminum absorption and the potential for aluminum toxicity.

Calcium supplements, such as calcium carbonate and calcium acetate, are considered first-line therapy in the treatment of hyperphosphatemia associated with low calcium levels. Calcium supplements are especially useful in the early stages of chronic kidney disease (CKD) to treat and prevent the hypocalcemia that leads to an overproduction of PTH. Calcium acetate is more potent and binds twice as much phosphorus in comparison to calcium carbonate when given in similar doses. Because of the higher binding capacity for phosphorus there is less calcium absorption in the GI tract. Doses of calcium agents range from 500–667 mg per meal, or 168–200 mg elemental calcium per meal, depending on which calcium agent is used. Individuals taking a calcium supplement should take no more than 1,500 mg daily, with a 2,000-mg daily limit that includes all sources of calcium.

Sucroferric oxyhydroxide and ferric citrate are oral iron-based phosphate binders indicated for patients on dialysis with CKD and hyperphosphatemia.[22] The iron in these agents binds strongly to phosphorus and the resulting iron-phosphorus compound is not soluble and therefore precipitates out. Sucroferric oxyhydroxide binds to phosphate ions in the GI tract by ligand exchange between hydroxyl groups or water in the dietary phosphate and sucroferric oxyhydroxide. Tablets of sucroferric oxyhydroxide are chewable and are available in a strength of 2,500 mg, which is equivalent to 500 mg of iron. It is recommended to take one tablet prior to each meal 3 times daily. Titration up or down in increments of 500 mg of iron per day (2,500 mg sucroferric oxyhydroxide) may occur after the first week to achieve recommended serum phosphorus levels $\leq$5.5 mg/dL. Ferric citrate creates the precipitate ferric phosphate when it binds to dietary phosphate in the GI tract. Ferric citrate comes in a 1-g chewable tablet, which is equivalent to 210 mg of ferric iron. The recommended starting dose of ferric citrate is 2 tablets (420 mg ferric iron) taken with meals orally 3 times daily. The dose may be increased weekly by 1 to 2 tablets to a maximum of 12 tablets daily (2,520 mg ferric iron) to achieve serum phosphorus levels $\leq$5.5 mg/dL. Common side effects of iron-based phosphate binders include nausea, vomiting, diarrhea or constipation, and discolored stool. Ferric citrate has the potential to increase aluminum absorption, so it is important to watch for aluminum toxicity.[22]

Because sucroferric oxyhydroxide and ferric citrate are iron based, potential drug interactions may occur. Therefore, it is important to review the timing of medication administration. Ferric citrate has the potential to reduce the absorption of medications that bind to polyvalent cations. Examples include levothyroxine, quinolone antibiotics (eg, ciprofloxacin), some antivirals (eg, dolutegravir), and levodopa preparations. Sucroferric oxyhydroxide may reduce absorption of levothyroxine, cephalexin, tetracyclines, and aspirin.

Vitamin D therapy is often necessary because patients with CKD cannot convert vitamin D to its active form in the kidneys; therefore, the active form of vitamin D, calcitriol, is used in the treatment of SHPT in addition to the vitamin D analogs paricalcitol and doxercalciferol. Oral formulations may be used in earlier stages, but IV treatment is given to those who are on dialysis. For patients who are not on dialysis, oral calcitriol is initiated at a dose of 0.25 mcg daily. For dialysis patients who require the IV formulation, the dose is initiated at 0.5 mcg 3 times weekly at dialysis (about every other day). Doses are adjusted based on PTH levels and may be increased every 2–4 weeks. Potential side effects include edema, nausea and vomiting, itching, dizziness, and headache.

Paricalcitol is a synthetic analog of vitamin D_2. If PTH levels are very low, paricalcitol may be administered orally in doses of 1 mcg daily or 2 mcg 3 times a week given every other day. For patients whose PTH level is nearer the normal range, paricalcitol may be given orally as 2 mcg daily or 4 mcg 3 times per week given every other day. The IV form of paricalcitol is given at dialysis (before, during, or after) with an initial dose of 2.8–7 mcg. Dose increases may be done every 2–4 weeks. Common side effects of paricalcitol include nausea, diarrhea, skin rash, and edema.

ALERT!

Unlike other vitamin D therapies, doxercalciferol should not be given with magnesium antacids because the combination could result in high magnesium levels (hypermagnesemia), especially in patients who are on dialysis.

Doxercalciferol is also a synthetic analog of vitamin D_2 and is available in oral and IV dosage forms. For patients not yet on dialysis, doxercalciferol may be given in doses of 1 mcg by mouth daily with the dose adjustments based on PTH levels. For those patients who are on dialysis, doxercalciferol may be given at the time of dialysis. Common side effects of doxercalciferol include nausea and vomiting, dizziness, itching, headache, general malaise, cough, dyspnea, and edema.

Potential drug interactions are important to consider when vitamin D therapy is prescribed. Bile acid sequestrants (eg, cholestyramine) and drugs affecting lipid absorption (eg, orlistat) can decrease the oral absorption of calcitriol, paricalcitol, and doxercalciferol. Paricalcitol and doxercalciferol have also shown interactions with drugs such as ketoconazole that inhibit certain liver enzymes. This inhibition can lead to dangerously elevated levels of vitamin D analogues and other medications.

Cinacalcet is a calcimimetic agent approved to treat patients with SHPT on dialysis. Cinacalcet is not a source of calcium, but it binds to calcium-sensing receptors on parathyroid cells and mimics the action of extracellular ionized calcium. The result is an increase in sensitivity of the calcium receptors to extracellular calcium levels, which reduces the release of PTH and decreases blood calcium levels. For patients on dialysis, the starting dose is 30 mg orally once daily and may be titrated up every 2–4 weeks to a maximum dose of 180 mg daily. Side effects most often reported with cinacalcet use include nausea and vomiting, hypocalcemia, cramping, myalgias, tetany, and convulsions. Because cinacalcet is processed in the liver and is a potent inhibitor of at least one liver enzyme, drug interactions may be an issue. If cinacalcet is added to a regimen including drugs metabolized by the liver, dose adjustments may be required. Concentrations of cinacalcet may also be significantly increased if given with some liver enzyme inhibitors such as erythromycin and ketoconazole.

For patients taking cinacalcet, serum calcium levels must be monitored. If a patient's serum calcium rises above the normal range or PTH decreases, cinacalcet use should be discontinued or avoided.

Cinacalcet is also effective in treating the hypercalcemia associated with parathyroid carcinoma, a type of cancer. Dosing of cinacalcet in this situation is different compared to SHPT. The initial dose is 30 mg orally twice daily, with titration every 2–4 weeks in sequential doses of 60 mg twice daily, 90 mg twice daily, to 90 mg 3–4 times daily, up to a maximum of 360 mg per day. At these doses, nausea and vomiting are the most common side effects and may require a reduction in the dose or even discontinuing cinacalcet. (See Medication Table 8-3.)

SUMMARY

The pituitary, thyroid, and parathyroid glands are just a few of the endocrine glands located throughout the body that release hormones directly into the bloodstream. Action and release of these hormones is regulated by positive and negative feedback systems. When these systems are disrupted, a variety of disorders occur. Often these disruptions are due to glandular over- or underactivity leading to excessive amounts of hormone, decreased amounts or complete lack of hormone, or resistance to hormone action. Disruption of these feedback systems may also be the result of other disease states whose symptoms affect these endocrine glands.

Endocrine disorders may affect males and females of all ages. Hypopituitarism, acromegaly, and growth hormone deficiency (GHD) are disorders of the pituitary gland treated with a variety of medications, including somatostatin analogs, dopamine agonists, recombinant growth hormone (GH), and GH receptor antagonists. Use of these agents depends on the specific disorder treated. Hypothyroidism and hyperthyroidism are thyroid gland disorders treated with thyroid hormone supplementation or antithyroid medications. Disorders of the parathyroid include hypoparathyroidism, pseudohypoparathyroidism, and hyperparathyroidism. Parathyroid disorders are also treated with a variety of medications, among them calcium supplements, vitamin D therapies, phosphate-binding agents, thiazide diuretics, and calcimimetics. While treatment of these disorders may appear drastically different from each other, the common goal is to treat the overabundance, lack of, or resistance to hormones produced by the pituitary, thyroid, and parathyroid glands.

REFERENCES

1. Rhoades RA, Bell DR, eds. *Medical Physiology: Principles for Clinical Medicine*. 5th ed. Philadelphia, PA: Wolters Kluwer; 2018.
2. DiPiro JT, Yee GC, Posey L, et al., eds. *Pharmacotherapy: A Pathophysiologic Approach*. 11th ed. New York, NY: McGraw-Hill; 2020.
3. Jameson J, Fauci AS, Kasper DL, et al., eds. *Harrison's Principles of Internal Medicine*. 20th ed. New York, NY: McGraw-Hill; 2018.
4. Lexicomp Online, AHFS DI (Adult and Pediatric), Hudson, OH: Wolters Kluwer Clinical Drug Information; 2021.
5. Katzung BG, ed. *Basic & Clinical Pharmacology*. 14th ed. New York, NY: McGraw-Hill; 2018.
6. Katznelson L, Laws ER Jr, Melmed S, et al. Acromegaly: An Endocrine Society clinical practice guideline. *J Clin Endocrinol Metab*. 2014;99(11):3933–3951.
7. Octreotide acetate [package insert]. Berkeley Heights, NJ: Hikma Pharmaceuticals; June 2020.
8. Somatuline Depot [package insert]. Cambridge, MA: Ipsen Biopharmaceuticals; June 2019.
9. Signifor LAR [package insert]. East Hanover, NJ: Novartis Pharmaceuticals; April 2019.
10. Signafor [package insert]. East Hanover, NJ: Novartis Pharmaceuticals; January 2020.
11. Somavert [package insert]. New York, NY: Pharmacia and Upjohn Company; September 2019.
12. Porth CM, Gaspard KJ, eds. *Essentials of Pathophysiology Concepts of Altered Health States*. 4th ed. Philadelphia, PA: Wolters Kluwer; 2015.
13. Genotropin [package insert]. New York, NY: Pharmacia and Upjohn Company; April 2019.
14. Crees Z, Fritz C, Heudebert A, et al., eds. *The Washington Manual® of Medical Therapeutics*. 36th ed. Philadelphia, PA: Wolters Kluwer; 2016.
15. Jonklass J, Bianco AC, Bauer AJ, et al. Guidelines for the treatment of hypothyroidism: Prepared by the American Thyroid Association task force on thyroid hormone replacement. *Thyroid*. 2014;24(12)16:1670–1751.
16. Michels TC, Kelly KM. Parathyroid disorders. *Am Fam Physician*. 2013;88(4):249–257.
17. Molina PE. ed. *Endocrine Physiology*. 5th ed. New York, NY: McGraw-Hill; 2018.
18. Jameson JL, De Groot LJ, de Kretser DM, et al., eds. *Endocrinology: Adult and Pediatric*. 7th ed. Philadelphia, PA: Elsevier Saunders; 2016.
19. Brandi ML, Bilezikian JP, Shoback D, et al. Management of hypoparathyroidism: Summary statement and guidelines. *J Clin Endocrinol Metab*. 2016;101(6):22732283.
20. Wilhelm SM, Wang TS, Lee JA, et al. The American Association of Endocrine Surgeons guidelines for definitive management of primary hyperparathyroidism. *JAMA Surg*. 2016;151(10):959–968.
21. Bilezikian JP, Brandi ML, Eastell R, et al. Guidelines for the management of asymptomatic primary hyperparathyroidism: Summary statement from the Fourth In-

ternational Workshop. *J Clin Endocrinol Metab*. 2014; 99(10):3561–3569.

22. Pai AB, Jang SM, Wegrzyn N. Iron-based phosphate binders: A new element in management of hyperphosphatemia. *Expert Opin Drug Metab Toxicol*. 2016;1: 115–127.

23. Cinacalcet [package insert]. Pennington, NJ: Zydus Pharmaceuticals; March 2018.

REVIEW QUESTIONS

1. What is a negative feedback system and how does it regulate the release of hormones from the pituitary gland?

2. How does dopamine normally affect the pituitary gland? Which pituitary disorders are treated with dopamine agonists?

3. What symptoms may a person with hyperthyroidism experience and why?

4. Why is control of calcium concentrations in the blood so important? What systems are affected by a disruption in calcium homeostasis?

5. What is hypoparathyroidism? Describe how calcium homeostasis is affected by this disorder.

MEDICATION TABLES

MEDICATION TABLE 8-1. Medications for Pituitary Disorders[4,7-11,13,a]

CLASS Generic Name	Brand Name	Route	Dosage Forms	Dose	Notes
Somatostatin Analogs					
Octreotide (ok TREE oh tide)	Sandostatin	SUBQ	Solution for injection	50 mcg 3 times daily, titrated to maintain GH levels <2.5 ng/mL, normal IGF-1 levels, and clinical symptoms; usual dose 100–200 mcg 3 times daily	Acromegaly; store in refrigerator and protect from light; may allow to come to room temperature before administration; multiple-dose vials must be discarded after 14 days
	Sandostatin LAR	IM	Depot suspension	After patient is stabilized on octreotide for at least 2 wk, inject 20 mg in the gluteal muscle q 4 wk for 3 mo, then titrate dose based on response; maximum dose is >40 mg q 4 wk; doses <40 mg are not recommended per the package insert	Acromegaly; store in refrigerator and protect from light; allow kit to come to room temperature for 30–60 min prior to reconstitution; use immediately
Lanreotide (lan REE oh tide)	Somatuline Depot	SUBQ	Depot suspension in prefilled syringes	Initial dose is 90 mg q 4 wk for 3 mo, then adjust dose based on response; maximum dose 120 mg q 4 wk	Acromegaly; store in refrigerator and protect from light; remove the sealed pouch containing lanreotide prefilled syringe from the refrigerator 30 min prior to administration and allow it to come to room temperature; do not open sealed pouch until injection
Dopamine Agonists					
Bromocriptine (broe moe KRIP teen)	Parlodel	Oral	Capsule, tablet	For acromegaly: 1.25 or 2.5 mg daily, titrate by 1.25–2.5 mg/day q 3–7 days to a maximum dose of 100 mg/day; for hyperprolactinemia: 1.25–2.5 mg/day, titrated by 2.5 mg/day q 3–7 days based on response	Acromegaly; hyperprolactinemia
Cabergoline (kA BER goe leen)	Dostinex	Oral	Tablet	0.25 mg twice weekly; if needed, adjust dose q 4 wk; increase by 0.25 mg twice weekly up to maximum dose of 1 mg twice weekly	Acromegaly (off-label); hyperprolactinemia
Growth Hormone Receptor Antagonists					
Pegvisomant (peg VI soe mant)	Somavert	SUBQ	Powder for injection	Initial loading dose of 40 mg followed by 10 mg daily; doses may be adjusted by 5 mg q 4–6 wk based on IGF-1 levels; maximum dose is 30 mg/day	Acromegaly; store in the refrigerator; use solution within 6 hr after reconstituting; single-use vials: discard after dose has been administered

Continued next page

MEDICATION TABLE 8-1. Medications for Pituitary Disorders[4,7-11,13,a] *(Continued)*

CLASS Generic Name	Brand Name	Route	Dosage Forms	Dose	Notes
Recombinant Growth Hormone					
Somatropin (soe ma TROE pin)	Genotropin, Omnitrope	SUBQ	Powder for injection	For adults: 0.04 mg/kg/wk; adjust dose q 4–8 wk up to maximum 0.08 mg/kg/wk; for children: 0.16–0.24 mg/kg/wk divided into 6–7 doses	Growth hormone deficiency; prescribers encouraged to strictly follow the indications for use and approved doses; store in refrigerator; do not freeze; Omnitrope vials should be stored in carton to protect from light
	Humatrope	SUBQ	Powder for injection	For adults: ≤0.006 mg/kg daily; adjust dose to a maximum of 0.0125 mg/kg daily; for children, 0.18–0.3 mg/kg/wk divided into 6–7 doses	Growth hormone deficiency; store in refrigerator; do not freeze; protect from light during storage
	Norditropin	SUBQ	Solution for injection	For adults: 0.004 mg/kg daily; maximum 0.016 mg/kg/day; for children: 0.024–0.034 mg/kg/day 6–7 times/wk	Growth hormone deficiency; store unused pens in refrigerator; do not freeze; avoid direct light
	Nutropin AQ	SUBQ	Powder for injection	For adults: ≤0.006 mg/kg daily; maximum dose for patients ≤35 yr: 0.025 mg/kg/day; maximum dose for patients >35 yr: 0.0125 mg/kg/day; for children: 0.3 mg/kg/wk, divided into daily doses; for pubertal patients: 0.7 mg/kg/wk divided into daily doses	Growth hormone deficiency; store in refrigerator; do not freeze; protect from light
	Saizen	SUBQ	Powder for injection	For adults: ≤0.005 mg/kg daily; may increase to maximum ≤0.01 mg/kg/day after 4 wk; for children: 0.18 mg/kg/wk divided into daily doses or 0.06 mg/kg administered 3 times/wk or 0.03 mg/kg administered 6 times/wk	Growth hormone deficiency; store at room temperature before reconstitution; refrigerate after reconstitution; do not freeze
	Zomacton	SUBQ	Powder for injection	For adults: 0.006 mg/kg daily; maximum 0.0125 mg/kg/day; For children: 0.18–0.3 mg/kg/week in equal doses given either 3, 6, or 7 days/wk	Growth hormone deficiency; refrigerate before and after reconstitution; do not freeze

yr = years old.
[a]Pronunciations have been adapted with permission from USP Dictionary of USAN and International Drug Names (USP Dictionary) © 2022.

MEDICATION TABLE 8-2. Medications for Thyroid Disorders[4,a]

CLASS Generic Name	Brand Name	Route	Forms	Dose	Notes
Thyroid Supplement					
Levothyroxine (lee voe thye ROX een)	Levothroid, Levoxyl, Synthroid, Tirosint, Unithroid	IM, IV, oral	Injection, tablet	Dosing individualized based on clinical response and lab values Oral: 1.6 mcg/kg/day, usually less than 200 mcg/day. Dose adjusted by approximately 25 mcg/day as needed every 4–6 wk IM, IV: 50% of the oral dose	Used to treat hypothyroidism; store at room temperature; protect from light; IV formulation must be reconstituted immediately before use
Liothyronine (lye oh THYE roe neen)	Cytomel	Oral	Tablet	Dose varies from 5 mcg – 75 mcg depending on indication and co-therapy	Used to treat hypothyroidism
	Triostat	IV	IV solution	Maintenance dose 25–75 mcg/day in divided doses 4–12 h apart	Store IV formulation in refrigerator; used for myxedema coma
Liotrix (LYE oh trix)	Thyrolar	Oral	Tablet	Initial: Levothyroxine 25 mcg/liothyronine 6.25 mcg/day. Dose may be increased by 12.5 mcg levothyroxine/liothyronine 3.1 mcg every 2–3 wk.	Used to treat hypothyroidism
Thyroid USP (THYE roid)	Armour Thyroid	Oral	Tablet	Initial: 30–32.5 mg; increase with 15 mg increments q 2–3 wk Maintenance: 60–130 mg/day	Used to treat hypothyroidism
Antithyroid					
Propylthiouracil (PTU) (proe pill thye oh YOOR a sill)	None	Oral	Tablet	Usual maintenance dose 100–150 mg/day in divided doses	Used to treat hyperthyroidism
Methimazole (MMI) (meth IM a zole)	Tapazole	Oral	Tablet	Initial: 15–60 mg/day based on clinical status and gland size Maintenance: 5–15 mg/day	Used to treat hyperthyroidism
Radioactive iodine (EYE oh dine)	None	Oral	Capsule, oral solution	Initial: 10–50 mCi Subsequent dosing: 100–150 mCi	Used to treat hypothyroidism

[a]Pronunciations have been adapted with permission from USP Dictionary of USAN and International Drug Names (USP Dictionary) © 2022.

MEDICATION TABLE 8-3. Medications Used to Treat Parathyroid Disorders[4,23,a]

CLASS Generic Name	Brand Name	Route	Forms	Dose	Notes
Calcium Supplement					
Calcium carbonate (KAL see um) (KAR bon ate)	Calcium carbonate, Tums, Os-Cal, Caltrate, VIACTIV	Oral	Tablet, oral suspension, soft chew	500–2,000 mg 3 times daily	Used for HP, PHP, and SHPT; OTC; take with food; may also be found in combination with magnesium and aluminum salts and with vitamin D
Calcium citrate (KAL see um) (SIH trate)	Calcium Citrate, Cal-C-Caps, Cal-Cee, Cal-citrate 225, Citracal, Calcitrate	Oral	Tablet	500–1,000 mg of elemental calcium 2–3 times daily	Used for HP and PHP; OTC; supplement of choice for those who routinely take H2-blockers or proton pump inhibitors; may be found in combination with vitamin D
Calcium acetate (KAL see um) (AH seh tate)	PhosLo, Eliphos	Oral	Tablet	Initial: 1,334 mg with each meal Usual dose: 2,001–2,668 mg with each meal	Used for SHPT; RX only; 1 tablet = 667 mg; no additional calcium supplements should be taken
Vitamin D therapies					
Calcitriol (kal si TRYE ole)	Rocaltrol, Calcitriol oral solution, Calcijex	Oral, IV	Capsule, solution, solution for injection	Oral for hypocalcemia in HP/PHP: ranges from 0.25 to 2 mcg daily Oral for CKD patients on dialysis with SHPT: ranges from 0.25 to 1 mcg daily IV: Start at 0.25 to 0.5 mcg 3 times weekly. May adjust dose in 0.5 to 1 mcg increments in 2 to 4 week intervals to maximum of 4 mcg 3 times weekly	Used for HP, PHP, and SHPT; RX only
Dihydrotachysterol (dy hy dro tak is TER ol)	DHT, DHT Intensol, Hytakerol	Oral	Tablet, solution, capsule	Initial dose: 0.8 mg to 2.4 mg daily for several days. Maintenance dose: 0.2 mg to 1.0 mg daily as required for normal serum calcium levels. The average maintenance dose is 0.6 mg daily.	Used for HP and PHP; RX only; contraindicated with cytochrome P450 3A4 enzyme inhibitors
Doxercalciferol (dox ehr kal SIFF eh role)	Hectorol	Oral, IV	Capsule, solution for injection	Non-dialysis patients: 1 mcg orally daily; dialysis patients 4–6 mcg IV 3 × weekly or 10–20 mcg orally 3 × weekly	Used for SHPT; RX only; capsules made with coconut oil; may be given with or without food *IV formulation is administered during dialysis as an IV bolus.*

Continued next page

MEDICATION TABLE 8-3. Medications Used to Treat Parathyroid Disorders[4,23,a] *(Continued)*

CLASS Generic Name	Brand Name	Route	Forms	Dose	Notes
Ergocalciferol (er goe kal SIF e role)	Drisdol, Calciferol	Oral, IM	Capsule, solution for injection	25,000 to 200,000 units daily	Used for HP and PHP; RX/OTC
Paricalcitol (PAR i kal si tol)	Zemplar	Oral, IV	Capsule, solution for injection	Oral: 1 mcg daily or 2 mcg 3 times/wk for PTH <500 pg/mL; 2 mcg daily or 4 mcg 3 times/wk for PTH > 500 pg/mL IV: Initial: 0.04–0.1 mcg/kg (2.8–7 mcg) at dialysis (no more than every other day) Maintenance: adjusted individually based on PTH levels	Used for SHPT; RX only; used in patients who are already on dialysis
Phosphate-Binding Agents					
Sevelamer HCl (se VEL a mer)	Renagel	Oral	Capsule, tablet	Dose based on serum phosphorus concentrations: 5.5–7.5 mg/dL: 800 mg 3 times daily 7.5–9 mg/dL: 1,600 mg 3 times daily ≥9 mg/dL: 1,600 mg 3 times daily	Used for SHPT; RX only; administer with meals; dose may be increased or decreased by 1 tablet/capsule per each meal at 2-wk intervals
Sevelamer carbonate (se VEL a mer) (KAR boh nate)	Renvela	Oral	Tablet	For patients not taking a phosphate binder, the initial dose is based on serum phosphorus concentrations: Dose based on serum phosphorus concentrations: 5.5–7.5 mg/dL: 800 mg 3 times daily 7.5–9 mg/dL: 1,600 mg 3 times daily ≥9 mg/dL: 1,600 mg 3 times daily Maintenance dosing is guided by ongoing monitoring of serum phosphorus concentrations. The maximum studied dose of sevelamer carbonate was 14 g/day.	Used for SHPT; RX only; administer with meals; dose may be increased or decreased by 1 tablet/capsule per each meal at 2-wk intervals
Lanthanum carbonate (LAN tha num) (KAR boh nate)	Fosrenol	Oral	Chewable, tablet	Initial: 1,500 mg/day in divided doses Maintenance: 1,500–3,000 mg	Used for SHPT; RX only; administer with meals

Continued next page

MEDICATION TABLE 8-3. Medications Used to Treat Parathyroid Disorders[4,23,a] (Continued)

CLASS Generic Name	Brand Name	Route	Forms	Dose	Notes
Aluminum carbonate (a LOO mi num) (KAR boh nate)	AlternaGel	Oral	Capsule, tablet, oral liquid	300–600 mg 3 times daily	Used for SHPT; OTC; therapy should be limited to 4 wk or less due to potential for aluminum toxicity; 1 tablet/capsule = 608 mg; 1 tsp suspension = 400 mg
Aluminum hydroxide (a LOO mi num) (hye DROX ide)	Alu-Cap, Amphojel, Alu-Tab, Gaviscon, Maalox, Mylanta	Oral	Capsule, tablet (chewable), suspension	300–600 mg 3 times daily	Used for SHPT; OTC; most commonly found in combination with magnesium salts
Magnesium carbonate (mag NEE zee um) (KAR boh nate)	Gaviscon	Oral	Suspension, tablet	80 mg **elemental** magnesium 3 times daily Per the Gaviscon labels: Tablets – 2 to 4 tablets up to 4 times daily (1 tablet contains 105mg magnesium carbonate which is equal to 35 mg elemental magnesium) Suspension – 2 to 4 teaspoons up to 4 times daily (1 teaspoon contains magnesium carbonate 237.5mg which is equivalent to 80mg elemental magnesium)	Used for SHPT; OTC; only available in combination with aluminum hydroxide
Magnesium hydroxide (mag NEE zee um) (hye DROX ide)	Milk of Magnesia, Maalox, Mylanta	Oral	Suspension, tablet	300–400 mg 3 times daily	Used for SHPT; OTC; commonly found in combination with aluminum hydroxide
Calcimimetic					
Cinacalcet (sin a CAL set)	Sensipar	Oral	Tablet	Initial dose 30 mg daily. Titrate dose up as needed every 2 to 4 weeks in 30 mg increments to maximum dose of 180 mg daily to maintain intact PTH levels between 150 to 300 pg/mL. Carcinoma: 30 mg twice daily to 90 mg 3–4 times daily	Used for SHPT, parathyroid carcinoma, and PHPT ineligible for surgery; RX only; take with food

CYP3A4 =; HP = hypoparathyroidism; IM = intramuscular; IV = intravenous; OTC = over the counter; PHP = pseudohypoparathyroidism; PHPT = primary hyperparathyroidism; RX = prescription only; SHPT = secondary hyperparathyroidism; SUBQ = subcutaneous.
[a]Pronunciations have been adapted with permission from USP Dictionary of USAN and International Drug Names (USP Dictionary) © 2022.

Chapter 9

Adrenal Gland Hormones

Devra Dang, PharmD, CDCES, FNAP |
Jayden Lee, PharmD, BCACP

KEY TERMS AND DEFINITIONS

Addison disease—a disorder in which the adrenal glands do not produce enough steroid hormones.

Adenoma—a benign (noncancerous) tumor of glandular origin.

Adrenal insufficiency—a term referring to a deficiency in the levels of adrenal hormones.

Adrenocorticotropic hormone (ACTH)—a hormone produced by the pituitary gland that stimulates the adrenal cortex to produce glucocorticoids, mineralocorticoids, and androgens.

Aldosterone—a hormone produced by the adrenal glands that regulates the balance of sodium, water, and potassium concentrations in the body.

Androgen—any of the male sex hormones that regulate the development and maintenance of male characteristics.

Corticotropin-releasing hormone (CRH)—a hormone released by the hypothalamus that regulates the release of ACTH from the pituitary gland.

Corticosteroid—any of the steroid hormones made by the cortex of the adrenal gland.

Cortisol—the primary glucocorticoid produced by the adrenal cortex.

Cushing's syndrome—a hormonal disorder caused by prolonged exposure of the body to a higher cortisol concentration than the body normally requires.

Endogenous—produced or synthesized from within an organism.

DOI 10.37573/9781585286638.009

Exogenous—originating from outside an organism.

Glucocorticoid—a steroid hormone that has anti-inflammatory and immunosuppressive properties.

Hyperaldosteronism—an excess amount of aldosterone.

Hypoaldosteronism—an insufficient amount or impaired function of aldosterone.

Hypercortisolism—an excess amount of circulating cortisol.

Hypocortisolism—an insufficient amount of circulating cortisol.

Mineralocorticoid—a steroid hormone that affects fluid and electrolyte balance in the body.

Steroidogenesis—a synthetic process that produces steroids (glucocorticoids and mineralocorticoids).

LEARNING OBJECTIVES

After completing this chapter, you should be able to

1. Identify the hormones produced by the adrenal glands.

2. Describe the functions of mineralocorticoids and glucocorticoids in the body.

3. Recognize the signs and symptoms of adrenal insufficiency.

4. List the pharmacological treatment of patients with acute and chronic adrenal insufficiency.

5. Recognize the signs and symptoms of Cushing's syndrome and the result of too much cortisol.

6. List the pharmacologic and nonpharmacologic management of patients with Cushing's syndrome.

7. List the pharmacologic management of primary aldosteronism.

8. List management strategies for the administration of glucocorticoid and mineralocorticoid therapy to avoid the development of adrenal disorders.

The adrenal glands are an integral part of the endocrine system, secreting hormones that act throughout the body to regulate functions and promote homeostasis. In addition to the neurotransmitters epinephrine and norepinephrine, the corticosteroids secreted by the adrenal glands are vital to

various physiological processes. Pharmacologic agents that resemble the adrenal hormones in chemistry and action are essential in treating many conditions.

CASE STUDY

Adrenal Insufficiency

Mrs. Smith is a 30-year-old woman who presents to the emergency department with complaints of fatigue, muscle weakness, anorexia, and dizziness for the last few days. She also states that she has a bad cold, has been coughing, and had a fever of 101°F. She has a history of autoimmune disease and has been treated for it with prednisone 10 mg daily and hydroxychloroquine 400 mg daily for the past 5 years.

Her vital signs include blood pressure 108/64 mm Hg and pulse 96 beats per minute (bpm) lying down, blood pressure 80/45 mm Hg and pulse 110 bpm sitting, respiration rate of 26 breaths per minute, and temperature of 99.8°F. Laboratory data show low serum sodium and blood glucose (sugar) levels along with high calcium and potassium levels.

ANATOMY AND PHYSIOLOGY OF THE ADRENAL GLANDS

The adrenal glands are small triangular-shaped organs located on top of both kidneys (Figure 9-1). Each adrenal gland consists of two main regions: the adrenal cortex, which makes up the outer region of the gland, and the adrenal medulla, which makes up the inner region of the gland. The inner medulla is responsible for secreting the hormones epinephrine and norepinephrine (also known as adrenaline and noradrenaline, respectively). These hormones are involved in the activities of the sympathetic nervous system, which regulates the body's responses to stress (eg, the fight-or-flight response). See Chapter 4 for a more detailed discussion of epinephrine and norepinephrine. The outer adrenal cortex secretes three major classes of hormones: glucocorticoids, mineralocorticoids, and androgens.[1] These three major classes of hormones control many important functions in the body. This chapter focuses on the actions and pharmacologic uses of glucocorticoids and mineralocorticoids.

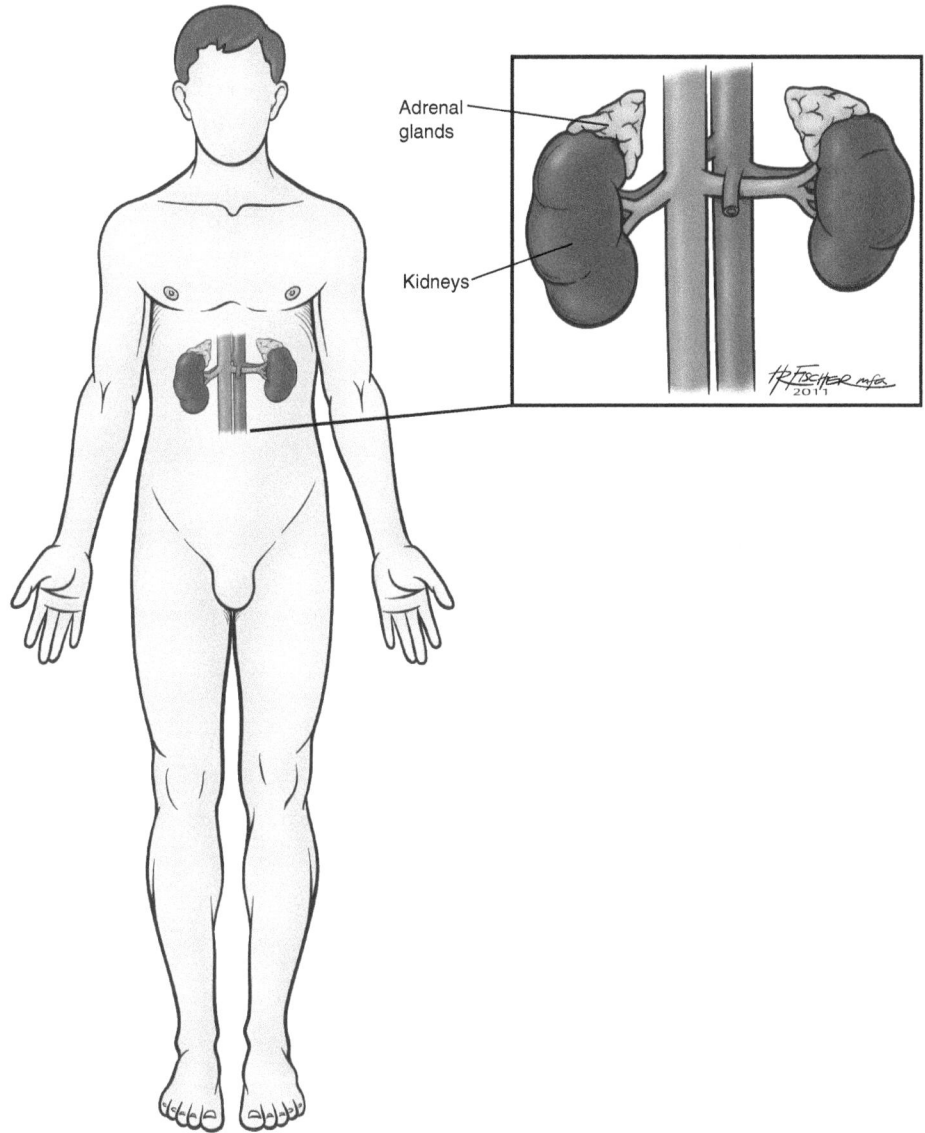

FIGURE 9-1. Structure and location of the adrenal glands.
Anatomy of the adrenal gland. There are two adrenal glands, one on top of each kidney. The outer part of each gland is the adrenal cortex; the inner part is the adrenal medulla.

The adrenal glands work interactively with the hypothalamus and pituitary gland, and this is referred to as the hypothalamic-pituitary-adrenal (HPA) axis. The hypothalamus releases corticotropin-releasing hormone (CRH), which in turn stimulates the pituitary gland to release adrenocorticotropic hormone (ACTH). ACTH then stimulates the adrenal cortex, which is made up of three distinct zones: the outer zona glomerulosa, the middle zona fasciculata, and the inner zona reticularis. When stimulated, these zones produce and release mineralocorticoids (from the zona glomerulosa), glucocorticoids (from the zona fasciculata), and androgens (from the zona reticularis).[1]

Cortisol is the primary glucocorticoid and its main functions are to regulate blood glucose concentrations, maintain normal blood pressure, promote protein and lipid (fat) breakdown while preventing protein synthesis, and regulate inflammation. Cortisol also affects wound healing and normal immune activity. Aldosterone is the primary mineralocorticoid and is responsible for maintaining the balance of sodium (salt), potassium, and water in the body. Adrenal androgens control sexual maturation during childhood and puberty.

A disorder of the adrenal cortex may result in decreased production of glucocorticoids. This is known as hypocortisolism or adrenal insufficiency. When the adrenal cortex produces too much cortisol, hypercortisolism results. This can lead to the development of a condition called Cushing's syndrome. These are the two most common disorders of the adrenal glands and are discussed in detail later in this chapter.

Abnormal aldosterone concentration can reveal disorders of the adrenal glands. Hyperaldosteronism results from the overproduction of aldosterone, whereas the shortage or impaired function of aldosterone results in hypoaldosteronism. These conditions may occur together with the cortisol abnormalities or by themselves as primary disorders.

PHARMACOLOGIC USES OF CORTICOSTEROIDS

Corticosteroids are steroid hormones that are further classified as glucocorticoids (eg, cortisol) or mineralocorticoids (eg, aldosterone) based on their biologic activity. Glucocorticoids bind to receptors in the body to suppress the immune response and provide anti-inflammatory effects. Mineralocorticoids also bind to receptors but cause sodium and water retention and potassium depletion.

Corticosteroids may be produced and secreted naturally by the body (endogenous) or administered to the body (exogenous). Exogenous glucocorticoid medications, such as prednisone, can be prescribed for a multitude of indications, such as adrenal insufficiency, inflammatory conditions (eg, skin conditions, asthma, allergic rhinitis), and autoimmune diseases (eg, rheumatoid arthritis). Corticosteroids are commonly prescribed for their glucocorticoid activity, but some patients require medications with mineralocorticoid effects.

Mineralocorticoids may be prescribed for conditions such as primary adrenal insufficiency or low blood pressure. Fludrocortisone is a synthetic mineralocorticoid, which is available as an oral tablet. It is typically administered once daily in the morning. Adequacy of the mineralocorticoid dose is dependent on blood levels of sodium and potassium, symptoms of dizziness upon standing, and blood pressure in the sitting, standing, and lying down positions.[2,3]

CASE?

What steroid medication has Mrs. Smith been taking? Besides suppressing her autoimmune disease what else might you expect this medication to do?

Exogenous corticosteroids are differentiated on the basis of their half-life, glucocorticoid potency, and mineralocorticoid activity (see Table 9-1).[3] Hydrocortisone has fairly significant mineralocorticoid activity and is closely related to endogenous cortisol. Prednisone and prednisolone have minimal mineralocorticoid activity. For situations in which mineralocorticoid activity is to be avoided, methylprednisolone and dexamethasone are good alternatives.[4]

PRACTICE POINT

While glucocorticoid medications are commonly (and properly) referred to as steroids, they are not to be confused with the anabolic steroids (similar in chemical structure), which have been the subject of abuse by athletes seeking to build muscle mass and enhance athletic performance. This type of steroid is discussed in Chapter 11.

Prednisone is the most commonly prescribed oral corticosteroid due to its widespread availability, many dosage strengths, and low cost. In general, selecting a glucocorticoid medication for a medical condition depends on its half-life, glucocorticoid potency, and mineralocorticoid activity.

Inhaled corticosteroids are typically used for respiratory disorders (such as asthma, bronchitis, and emphysema) and are available as single-ingredient products or in combination with other medications. These treatments are discussed extensively in Chapter 19. (See Medication Table 19-1 for information about inhaled corticosteroids.)

Since corticosteroids can be prescribed for a vast number of conditions, a variety of different formulations are available to facilitate optimal drug delivery (eg, oral, inhaled, nasal, topical, intravenous [IV], intramuscular [IM], intra-articular, or intravitreal injections). Oral and IV corticosteroids are usually prescribed in situations where systemic (throughout the body) anti-inflammatory effects are desired, such as severe asthma attacks and severe allergic reactions. IV administration of corticosteroids results in the highest concentration of the medication in the blood. IM and intra-articular

TABLE 9-1. Characteristics of Corticosteroids[3,22]

Corticosteroid	Glucocorticoid (Anti-inflammatory) Activity	Mineralocorticoid (Sodium and Water-Retaining) Activity	Equivalent Dose (mg)
Short-acting (duration 8–12 hr)			
Cortisone	0.8	0.8	25
Hydrocortisone	1	1	20
Intermediate-acting (duration 12–36 hr)			
Methylprednisolone	5	0	4
Prednisolone	4	0.8	5
Prednisone	4	0.8	5
Triamcinolone	5	0	4
Fludrocortisone	15	150	Irrelevant
Long-acting (duration 36–72 hours)			
Betamethasone	25	0	0.6
Dexamethasone	30–40	0	0.75

Source: Data adapted from Liu D, Ward AA, Krishnamoorthy P, et al. A practical guide to the monitoring and management of the complications of systemic corticosteroid therapy. *Allergy Asthma Clin Immunol.* 2013;9(1):30.

preparations have lower systemic absorption and, therefore, fewer systemic side effects.[5] They can be used in patients with musculoskeletal disorders or inflammatory joint disorders, such as arthritis, to provide localized relief of pain and inflammation at the site of administration. For example, an intra-articular injection to the knee can provide pain relief for a patient with osteoarthritis in this joint. Medication Table 9-1 lists the corticosteroids that are available in oral and injectable formulations. (Medication Tables are located at the end of the chapter).

Intranasal corticosteroids (covered in Chapter 36) are typically prescribed for patients with allergic rhinitis (hay fever). Their effects are localized in the nasal pathway, and the side effects can include nasal dryness and crusting, nosebleeds, sneezing bouts, and irritation of the nose and throat. In some instances, intranasal administration may lead to systemic absorption of the drug if a large portion of the dose is swallowed.[6]

Dermatologic corticosteroids are used for a variety of skin conditions, including allergic reactions, and are available as creams, ointments, lotions, gels, and aerosols. Creams can be used on most body surfaces, while ointments may be beneficial for dry or scaly lesions because of their occlusive properties. Other dosage forms, such as lotions, gels, and aerosols, can be applied to areas with hair. Local side effects

include drying and cracking of the skin, thinning of the skin, and pinkish or purplish scar-like lesions on the skin. Systemic side effects with topical administration can occur when large skin areas are involved, prolonged use occurs, occlusive dressings are used, or if the skin is broken.[7]

ALERT!

Topical corticosteroids are often available in a variety of salts (propionate, diacetate, etc.) and dosage forms (creams, ointments, gels), as well as different strengths. These are not interchangeable, and it is important to recognize the appropriate salt, strength, and dosage form from the prescription or medication order.

Topical corticosteroids vary in potency and are listed in Medication Table 9-2.[8] High-potency agents are reserved for resistant conditions or for use on areas of the skin that are harder to penetrate (eg, palms or soles). Medium-potency agents can be used on the trunk, arms, and legs. Low-potency agents are recommended for use in children or for patients requiring that the medication be applied over large areas of the body. They are preferred for use on the face, genitals, armpits, and skin folds.[7,8]

Ophthalmic corticosteroids are used to treat inflammatory eye conditions. They are also available in combination with an ophthalmic antibiotic to treat eye infections. These preparations are covered in Chapter 34.

SIDE EFFECTS OF CORTICOSTEROID THERAPY

Regardless of the formulation used, corticosteroids can result in a multitude of systemic effects if absorbed into the circulation (see Table 9-2).[4] While some of the effects are related to therapeutic effectiveness of the medications, they may also become unwanted side effects that may limit the use of these drugs. For example, immunosuppressant, anti-inflammatory, and antiproliferative effects of corticosteroids are beneficial for conditions such as psoriasis, atopic dermatitis, and arthritis but potentially harmful in patients with serious infections.

In general, side effects may be minimized by using localized formulations (eg, inhalers, nasal sprays, creams, ointments, lotions, gels, intra-articular injections), but overuse of these medications in any formulation can lead to an increased risk of side effects. Corticosteroids administered in routes that lead to the highest blood concentration (eg, IV, oral) pose the greatest risk for side effects.[6] The dose and duration of corticosteroid use can also affect the risk for systemic side effects. The most common side effects related to corticosteroid therapy are osteoporosis, high blood glucose, weight gain, anxiety, and insomnia.[4] Two serious complications associated with exogenous corticosteroid administration are adrenal insufficiency and Cushing's syndrome.

In contrast to those associated with other corticosteroids, side effects from fludrocortisone are mainly related to its powerful mineralocorticoid activity and typically result from overtreatment. These side effects include high blood pressure, low potassium level, and fluid retention. If any of these occur, the fludrocortisone dose is usually reduced, and the patient is monitored for resolution of symptoms.[3]

ADRENAL INSUFFICIENCY OR HYPOCORTISOLISM

Adrenal insufficiency (AI) occurs when the adrenal glands are unable to produce enough cortisol to satisfy the needs of the body. AI is classified as primary, secondary, or tertiary. Primary AI occurs as a result of the destruction of the adrenal glands. Secondary AI occurs when there is dysfunction of the pituitary gland, while tertiary AI is the result of dysfunction in the hypothalamus.[9]

Primary AI (also known as Addison disease) occurs infrequently in Western populations. It is more common in women than men and peaks in the fourth decade of life.[9] Primary AI occurs as a consequence of destruction of greater than 90% of the adrenal glands. The majority of primary AI cases are caused by the patient's own immune system (autoimmune disease) destroying the adrenal glands. Infections, such as tuberculosis, human immunodeficiency virus (HIV), and acquired immunodeficiency syndrome (AIDS), can also cause primary AI. Other less-common causes include bleeding or a decrease in blood supply to the adrenal glands, cancers that may have spread to the adrenal glands, and side effects from some medications.[10] In primary AI, there is a decrease in production of both glucocorticoids and mineralocorticoids.[9]

In secondary AI, dysfunction of the pituitary gland causes a decrease in the production of ACTH. This results in less stimulation of the adrenal gland to produce its hormones by ACTH. Cancers, infection, head trauma, or radiation of the pituitary gland can cause secondary AI.[10] Secondary AI occurs more frequently than primary AI but is still rare. It is also more common in women and peaks in the sixth decade of life.[9]

TABLE 9-2. Major Systemic Side Effects Associated with Corticosteroid Therapy[4]

Musculoskeletal	
Thinning of the bones (osteopenia or osteoporosis)	Death of a bone or part of a bone (avascular necrosis)
Growth retardation of long bones	Muscle weakness and pain
Ophthalmologic	
Cataracts	Glaucoma
Infection	Hemorrhage
Bulging of one or both eyes	
Gastrointestinal	
Nausea, vomiting	Ulcers in the lining of the stomach
Intestinal perforation	Inflammation of the pancreas
Inflammation of the esophagus	
Metabolic	
High blood sugars	High cholesterol
Weight gain due to increased appetite and/or fluid retention	Low blood calcium
Low blood potassium	
Cardiovascular	
High blood pressure	Atherosclerosis
Fluid and sodium retention	
Gynecologic/Obstetric	
Amenorrhea	Fetal effects
Hypothalamic-Pituitary-Adrenal Axis	
Chronic adrenal insufficiency	Glucocorticoid withdrawal syndrome
Acute adrenal insufficiency (adrenal crisis)	
Hematologic	
Abnormal numbers of red blood cells	Abnormal numbers of white blood cells
Suppression of the immune system	Infections
Nervous System	
Psychiatric problems: mood changes, nervousness, psychosis	Insomnia
Seizures	Pseudotumor cerebri
Peripheral neuropathy	
Cutaneous	
Thinning of the skin	Purplish discoloration of the skin
Hirsutism	Hyperpigmentation
Acne	Infections

Source: Data adapted from Jackson S, Gilchrist H, Nesbitt LT, Jr. Update on the dermatologic use of systemic glucocorticosteroids. Dermatol Ther. 2007;20:187-205.

Drug therapy with corticosteroids for various medical conditions is a common contributor to the development of both secondary and tertiary AI.[10] Administration of exogenous corticosteroids can suppress the HPA axis by inhibiting the secretion of CRH from the hypothalamus and ACTH from the pituitary gland. As a result, secretion of endogenous corticosteroids by the adrenal gland is suppressed, resulting in AI.[4] In secondary and tertiary AI, mineralocorticoid function is preserved, and only the glucocorticoid production is decreased.

The clinical manifestations of AI depend on multiple factors. The onset of *chronic* AI is slow and gradual over time with nonspecific symptoms, including persistent fatigue, weakness, lethargy, loss of appetite, weight loss, postural hypotension (sudden drop in blood pressure upon standing, which may result in dizziness or feeling faint), and gastrointestinal complaints, such as nausea, vomiting, and abdominal pain. Hyperpigmentation or development of dark spots, especially in skin areas unexposed to sunlight, is another characteristic symptom of chronic AI.[11] *Acute* AI (also known as adrenal crisis) is mainly caused by glucocorticoid deficiency and is dramatic in onset.[11] In adrenal crisis, patients usually have a combination of the following signs or symptoms: low sodium level (hyponatremia), high potassium level (hyperkalemia), high calcium level (hypercalcemia), low fasting blood glucose level (hypoglycemia), fever, abdominal pain, and hypotensive shock that does not correct with fluid supplementation.[10,11] Adrenal crisis can be the end result of chronic AI, where the overwhelmed adrenal glands are not able to meet the increased glucocorticoid demand in physiologic stress situations, such as severe infections, trauma, or surgical procedures.[10] Adrenal crisis can also result from abrupt withdrawal of chronic corticosteroid medication use, which is the most common cause of adrenal crisis.[10]

Diagnosis of Adrenal Insufficiency

A number of tests are used to diagnose AI. The most widely used is the ACTH (cosyntropin) stimulation test. This test evaluates the ability of the adrenal glands to secrete cortisol after administration of cosyntropin, a synthetic form of ACTH. In patients with AI, the blood concentration of cortisol measured during the test is low since their adrenal glands are unable to respond to ACTH stimulation. Several other blood tests, including the insulin tolerance test, overnight metyrapone test, plasma aldosterone concentration, and plasma renin concentration, can be used to determine whether the patient has the primary, secondary, or tertiary form of AI.

Treatment of Chronic Adrenal Insufficiency

Supplementation with glucocorticoids and mineralocorticoids is the treatment of choice for AI. The healthy body produces cortisol in the amount approximately equivalent to 20–30 mg/day of oral hydrocortisone or 5–7.5 mg/day of oral prednisone. Corticosteroid supplementation is available in tablet and injectable formulations, where the IV formulation is given only when patients are not able to swallow or are critically ill. Therapy for chronic AI is individualized for each patient and usually requires oral hydrocortisone dosed at 20–30 mg in two to three divided doses a day to maintain normal glucocorticoid balance, with the last dose no later than 4–6 hours before bedtime. Patients are treated to normalize their blood pressure, heart rate, and temperature. Treatment with corticosteroid can also achieve improvement in sense of well-being and eliminate other symptoms. In primary AI, supplementation with a mineralocorticoid, such as fludrocortisone at 0.05–0.1 mg/day, is also required to correct the low sodium concentration and prevent orthostatic hypotension.

CASE?

The pharmacy has received an order to send a stat dose of 100 mg IV hydrocortisone for Mrs. Smith in the emergency room. For what condition do you think they are treating her?

Prevention and Treatment of Acute Adrenal Insufficiency

Patients with chronic AI require supplemental doses of corticosteroid in addition to their normal corticosteroid doses in situations of severe physiologic stress, such as acute severe illness, surgery, or trauma, to prevent adrenal crisis. The supplemental corticosteroid stress dose depends on the severity of the stress situation. For example, during a major surgery or for diseases that require intensive care, doses of IV hydrocortisone will be approximately 100–200 mg/day, plus fludrocortisone if needed.[12]

ALERT!

After a patient has recovered from the physiologic stress, the dose of supplemental corticosteroid should be gradually tapered off and not abruptly discontinued.

Therapy for adrenal crisis is intended to stabilize the patient as quickly as possible and consists of IV fluid and hydrocortisone replacement as soon as the diagnosis is made.[11] IV hydrocortisone at 100–400 mg/day should be administered immediately and continued for at least 2–3 days or until full recovery. Once the patient is stable, the hydrocortisone dose is tapered over 1–4 days and converted to oral maintenance therapy. Fluid replacement with 0.9% sodium chloride injection solution ("normal saline") may be administered at rates of up to 1 liter/hr to treat the hypotension. Patients with low blood glucose may also receive supplemental dextrose solution.[11,12]

Since the most common cause of adrenal crisis is the abrupt withdrawal of corticosteroid therapy, patient education is an important way to prevent adrenal crisis in patients who are on a long-term corticosteroid therapy. The pharmacist should educate these patients about the importance of adherence to glucocorticoid therapy and advise them to contact their providers if they become ill as they may need higher doses of glucocorticoids.

ALERT!

Patients who are on long-term systemic glucocorticoids or frequently placed on high-dose, short courses of systemic glucocorticoids (eg, for recurrent asthma exacerbation) are at risk for adrenal crisis if they experience an acute episode of physiologic stress, such as surgery, trauma, or severe illness. They should be advised to carry documentation (eg, medical bracelet, wallet card) that they take glucocorticoid medications regularly.

CUSHING'S SYNDROME OR HYPERCORTISOLISM

Hypercortisolism, also known as Cushing's syndrome, is a consequence of long-term exposure to excessive amounts of glucocorticoids circulating in the body. The source of the glucocorticoid may be exogenous or endogenous. Endogenous Cushing's syndrome is classified as ACTH-dependent or ACTH-independent. In ACTH-dependent Cushing's syndrome, the rise in glucocorticoid concentrations is either due to pituitary adenomas that produce excess amounts of ACTH or from the ectopic (located away from the normal location) of ACTH from outside the pituitary gland, such as in small cell lung cancer or cancers of various endocrine glands.[13] ACTH-independent Cushing's syndrome is the result of abnormalities with the adrenal gland. Adenoma of the adrenal gland accounts for approximately 60% of ACTH-independent Cushing's syndrome, and the remaining 40% is due to cancer of the adrenal glands. The most common cause of exogenous Cushing's syndrome is the long-term administration of glucocorticoids in doses that are higher than is normally needed in the healthy body.[13] Note that occasionally the terms Cushing's syndrome and Cushing's disease may be used interchangeably but Cushing's syndrome is a more general term, while Cushing's disease refers specifically to hypercortisolism due to an ACTH-secreting pituitary adenoma.

Cushing's syndrome involves multiple organs and systems in the body. The classic cutaneous (skin) presentation of Cushing's syndrome is facial plethora (swollen and red face), oily skin and acne, purpura (patches of purplish discoloration on the skin), hirsutism (excessive hair growth), and wide purplish striae (stretch marks) over the abdomen, flanks, and upper arms. The skin is thin, bruises easily, and heals slowly from wounds or abrasions. Women with adrenal tumors may develop male pattern baldness and/or excess hair on the face, upper lip, chin, or abdomen. Hyperpigmentation occurs in some patients. Weight gain is common in Cushing's syndrome. The pattern of weight gain is described as *central,* with fat deposits in the abdomen, chest, face, and neck that leads to the description of *moon face* and *buffalo hump.* Muscle weakness in the legs and arms and low blood potassium levels can occur. There is an increased risk of bone fractures (breaks) because of low bone density. Emotional status may range from depression to mania, and some patients experience mood swings, decreased concentration, and impaired memory. There are also dysfunctions of the reproductive system, loss of sexual drive, and menstrual abnormalities in women. High blood glucose levels can occur in Cushing's syndrome. Patients with Cushing's syndrome are also at higher risk of developing hypertension (high blood pressure) and cardiovascular disease (diseases that involve the heart and blood vessels). Thromboembolism (the blockage of a blood vessel from a blood clot) and increased risk of infections, especially with fungal or opportunistic microorganisms may also occur. The diagnosis of Cushing's syndrome is made by evaluating the signs and symptoms, with confirmation by laboratory values. An endocrinologist is usually consulted to make a definitive diagnosis of Cushing's syndrome.

Treatment of Cushing's Syndrome

Therapy for Cushing's syndrome is intended to reduce the cortisol concentration in the body to normal levels and avoid causing pituitary or adrenal insufficiency. Treating the hypercortisolism will also prevent or delay complications and deaths from hypercortisol-related disorders, such as diabetes, cardiovascular abnormalities, thromboembolism, and infections. The treatment method selected depends on the reason for the hypercortisolism. Surgical removal of the benign or malignant tumor in the pituitary or adrenal gland is the treatment of choice for patients with pituitary or adrenal adenomas or cancers. If removal is incomplete, radiation or chemotherapy may be required. In extreme cases, one or both adrenal glands must be removed.

Pharmacologic therapy is not indicated as the primary therapy for Cushing's syndrome but instead is used while a patient is preparing for surgery or as additive therapy after surgery or radiation. Pharmacologic therapy is also selected for patients who are unable or unwilling to undergo surgery.[13] Several classes of medications are used in the pharmacologic management of Cushing's syndrome: steroidogenesis inhibitors, somatostatin agonist (pasireotide, subcutaneous injection), peripheral glucocorticoid antagonist (mifepristone,

ALERT!

Ketoconazole administration may increase the concentration of other drugs in the body and may result in drug toxicities due to this drug–drug interaction. Whenever a drug–drug interaction warning occurs upon ketoconazole being entered in a patient's medication profile, a technician must be sure to notify the pharmacist. Examples of drug–drug interactions with ketoconazole include alprazolam, midazolam, triazolam, simvastatin, apixaban, dabigatran, certain HIV medications, dasatinib, fluticasone, and sirolimus, along with many others.

oral), dopamine agonist (cabergoline, oral). Most of these medications are used off-label for the management of Cushing's syndrome. The most commonly prescribed medications are the steroidogenesis inhibitors, which prevent glucocorticoid production in the adrenal glands. Metyrapone, ketoconazole, etomidate, mitotane, and osilodrostat are steroidogenesis inhibitors. Osilodrostat is a recently available medication approved by the Food and Drug Administration for adults with Cushing's disease who are not candidates for pituitary surgery or who still have hypercortisolism after undergoing the surgery. Metyrapone and ketoconazole inhibit enzymes that are involved with cortisol synthesis. Metyrapone is also used as a diagnostic test for hypothalamic-pituitary ACTH function. Etomidate is a general anesthetic agent that also inhibits enzymes involved in cortisol synthesis. Etomidate (the only steroidogenesis inhibitor that is available as an injectable formulation) is used in situations where

PRACTICE POINT

Metyrapone has drug interactions with phenytoin and acetaminophen. Phenytoin increases the inactivation of metyrapone, resulting in a lower concentration of metyrapone in the body. The metabolism of acetaminophen may be decreased by metyrapone, leading to an increased risk of acetaminophen toxicity. Notify the pharmacist if the patient is taking either of these drugs and is prescribed metyrapone.

rapid control of cortisol levels is necessary or the patient is not able to take medications by mouth. Mitotane inhibits the production of cortisol by destroying the adrenal gland.[14,15] See Medication Table 9-3 for common dosing, side effects, and preparations of these drugs.[16,17]

ALERT!

LOOK-ALIKE/SOUND-ALIKE—Do not confuse etomidate with edetate disodium.

PRACTICE POINT

Mitotane is an anticancer drug and is considered a biohazard. Gloves should be worn not only when handling the tablets, but during receiving, unpacking, and placing the item in storage. The manufacturer cautions that these tablets should not be crushed.

ALERT!

Mitotane may increase the metabolism of many medications, including glucocorticoids such as prednisone and dexamethasone. Notify the pharmacist when a drug–drug interaction alert appears when mitotane is added to a patient's medication regimen that contains these drugs.

PREVENTION OF DRUG-INDUCED ADRENAL INSUFFICIENCY AND CUSHING'S SYNDROME

Several strategies have been employed to minimize the risk for AI and Cushing's syndrome associated with corticosteroid administration. To mimic the physiologic release of cortisol in the body, corticosteroid preparations with intermediate-acting duration, such as prednisone, are typically preferred and administered as a single dose after waking in the morning. This regimen causes less profound and shorter-lived adrenal suppression than divided doses or doses given at other times of the day.[4,18] When patients take systemic corticosteroids for more than 7–14 days, slowly decreasing the dose (dosage tapering) can minimize the risk for adrenal suppression. In practice, most physicians develop their own withdrawal regimens based on previous experience. Pharmacy personnel must be careful with dosage calculations for these situations. Alternate-day dosing can minimize the risk for adrenal suppression by allowing the HPA axis to recover during the off days.[18] Minimizing the corticosteroid dose to 7.5 mg or less and for the shortest duration of time needed for clinical benefit can help to prevent the development of drug-induced Cushing's syndrome.

PRACTICE POINT

Some oral glucocorticoids (methylprednisolone and dexamethasone) are available in a "dose pack" package, which allows for ease of tapering the dose.

HYPERALDOSTERONISM

An excess amount of aldosterone in the blood is termed hyperaldosteronism, which can be classified as primary or secondary. Primary hyperaldosteronism, also known as primary aldosteronism (PA), is a result of overproduction of aldosterone due to stimulation within the adrenal glands, whereas secondary hyperaldosteronism results from stimulation coming from outside the adrenal glands.

The most common causes of PA are bilateral adrenal hyperplasia (enlargement of both adrenal glands) and aldosterone-producing adenoma. The diagnosis of PA involves evaluation of the aldosterone-to-renin ratio, aldosterone suppression test, genetic testing, computed tomography (CT) scan of the adrenal glands, and adrenal vein sampling (measurement of aldosterone from both adrenal veins). It is important that these tests are utilized to identify the exact cause of PA because treatment options are different depending on the cause. Bilateral adrenal hyperplasia is generally treated with drugs that inhibit aldosterone receptors, whereas aldosterone-producing adenoma needs surgical removal.[19]

PA is a common cause of resistant hypertension (high blood pressure despite being adherent on three or more blood pressure drugs at maximum doses). Patients with PA typically present with high blood pressure, as well as low potassium level and water retention. Additional signs and symptoms of PA include muscle weakness, fatigue, headache, and increased thirst. Additionally, patients with hypertension and sleep apnea, a family history of early onset of hypertension or stroke (at an age less than 40 years), and a first-degree family member diagnosed with PA are at higher risk for PA. If patients with PA are left untreated for a long time, they are at increased risk of cardiovascular disease and cerebrovascular disease (diseases that involve the blood vessels of the brain).[20]

Treatment of Hyperaldosteronism

The aldosterone receptor inhibitors spironolactone and eplerenone are the treatment of choice in patients with PA due to bilateral adrenal hyperplasia. They bind to aldosterone receptor to block the effects of endogenous aldosterone. Their effects also include an increase in blood potassium level and a decrease in blood pressure. Unlike eplerenone, which only binds to aldosterone receptors, spironolactone also binds to androgen and progesterone (a sex hormone involved in the menstrual cycle and pregnancy) receptors as well, causing additional side effects, such as gynecomastia (enlarged male breasts) and menstrual irregularities. The alternative to aldosterone receptor inhibitors is the potassium-sparing diuretic amiloride. Amiloride is reserved for patients who cannot tolerate either spironolactone or eplerenone because it is less effective than the aldosterone receptor inhibitors. These medications are discussed in detail in Chapter 15 and included in Medication Table 15-4.

As mentioned earlier, hyperaldosteronism due to aldosterone-producing adenomas requires surgical removal of the affected adrenal gland. The surgical removal improves blood pressure control and cures the disease in the majority of patients. If a patient is not a candidate for the surgery, an aldosterone receptor inhibitor is recommended as medical management.

HYPOALDOSTERONISM

Low aldosterone production causes hypoaldosteronism, which is a rare condition, seen more in patients with diabetes, postural hypotension, or a surgical history of adrenal gland removal. As noted earlier in this chapter, hypoaldosteronism can be part of an overall insufficiency of the adrenal gland (Addison disease) or a stand-alone disorder. Patients typically present with low sodium and high potassium concentrations in the body. Because the disorder is mainly due to deficiency in mineralocorticoid production, replacement with fludrocortisone is the treatment of choice.[21]

SUMMARY

Disorders of the adrenal gland result in decreased or increased production of glucocorticoids or mineralocorticoids, and the clinical presentations differ significantly depending on the production level and the type of steroid hormones involved. Treatment for disorders of hypocortisolism involves administering glucocorticoids such as hydrocortisone, prednisone, or dexamethasone, and in some instances, also the mineralocorticoid fludrocortisone. In situations of physiologic stress, such as during surgery or severe illness, giving supplemental glucocorticoids is necessary to prevent adrenal crisis. Treatment for hypercortisolism involves eliminating the source of excessive cortisol. Long-term administration of glucocorticoid at higher doses than the body needs is the most common cause of AI and Cushing's syndrome. Therefore, patient education and monitoring are needed when these medications are dispensed.

Aldosterone abnormalities can also occur together with disorders of glucocorticoids or by themselves as primary disorders. Treatment options for hyperaldosteronism depend on the cause, and aldosterone receptor inhibitors are the main pharmacological therapy for PA. Fludrocortisone is an effective therapy for hypoaldosteronism.

ACKNOWLEDGMENTS

The authors wish to acknowledge and thank Jennifer Lee, PharmD, and Trinh Pham, PharmD, coauthors of this chapter in the first edition of this book.

REFERENCES

1. Carroll TB, Aron DC, Findling JW, Tyrrell JB. Glucocorticoids and adrenal androgens. In: Gardner DG, Shoback D, eds. *Greenspan's Basic & Clinical Endocrinology*. 10th ed. New York, NY: McGraw-Hill; 2018:299–342.

2. Lovas K, Husebye ES. Replacement therapy for Addison's disease: Recent developments. *Expert Opin Investig Drugs*. 2008;17:497–509.

3. Liu D, Ward AA, Krishnamoorthy P, et al. A practical guide to the monitoring and management of the complications of systemic corticosteroid therapy. *Allergy Asthma Clin Immunol*. 2013;9(1):30.

4. Jackson S, Gilchrist H, Nesbitt LT, Jr. Update on the dermatologic use of systemic glucocorticosteroids. *Dermatol Ther*. 2007;20:187–205.

5. Cardone DA, Tallia AF. Joint and soft tissue injection. *Am Fam Physician*. 2002;66:283–289.

6. Mortimer KJ, Tattersfield AE. Benefit versus risk for oral, inhaled, and nasal glucocorticosteroids. *Immunol Allergy Clin North Am*. 2005;25:523–539.

7. Del Rosso J, Friedlander SF. Corticosteroids: Options in the era of steroid-sparing therapy. *J Am Acad Dermatol*. 2005;53:S50–S58.

8. Comparison table: Some topical corticosteroids. *Med Lett Drugs Ther*. 2017;59(1520)e91-e95. Updated June 5, 2019.

9. Arlt W, Allolio B. Adrenal insufficiency. *Lancet*. 2003;361: 1881–1893.

10. Munver R, Volfson IA. Adrenal insufficiency: Diagnosis and management. *Curr Urol Rep*. 2006;7:80–85.

11. Bouillon R. Acute adrenal insufficiency. *Endocrinol Metab Clin North Am*. 2006;35:767–775, ix.

12. Carroll TB, Aron DC, Findling JW, Tyrrell J. Glucocorticoids and Adrenal Androgens. In: Gardner DG, Shoback D. eds. *Greenspan's Basic & Clinical Endocrinology*, 10e. McGraw Hill; 2017. https://accessmedicine.mhmedical.com/content.aspx?bookid=2178&sectionid=166246461

13. Pivonello R, De Martino MC, De Leo M, et al. Cushing's syndrome. *Endocrinol Metab Clin North Am*. 2008;37: 135–149, ix.

14. Diez JJ, Iglesias P. Pharmacological therapy of Cushing's syndrome: Drugs and indications. *Mini Rev Med Chem*. 2007;7:467–480.

15. Labeur M, Arzt E, Stalla GK, et al. New perspectives in the treatment of Cushing's syndrome. *Curr Drug Targets Immune Endocr Metabol Disord*. 2004;4:335–342.

16. Dang DK, Polomoff C, Chen JT. Adrenal gland disorders. In: Chisholm MA, Schwinghammer TL, Wells BG, et al., eds. *Pharmacotherapy Principles and Practice*. 5th ed. New York, NY: McGraw-Hill; 2019:703–718.

17. Nieman LK, Biller BM, Findling JW, et al. Treatment of Cushing's syndrome: An Endocrine Society Clinical Practice Guideline. *J Clin Endocrinol Metab*. 2015;100:2807–2831.

18. Alves C, Robazzi TC, Mendonca M. Withdrawal from glucocorticosteroid therapy: Clinical practice recommendations. *J Pediatr (Rio J)*. 2008;84:192–202.

19. Monticone S, Burrello J, Tizzani D, et al. Prevalence and clinical manifestations of primary aldosteronism encountered in primary care practice. *J Am Coll Cardiol*. 2017;69:1811–1820.

20. Catena C, Colussi G, Nadalini E, et al. Cardiovascular outcomes in patients with primary aldosteronism after treatment. *Arch Intern Med*. 2008;168:80–85.

21. Tan SY, Burton M. Hyporeninemic hypoaldosteronism: An overlooked cause of hyperkalemia. *Arch Intern Med*. 1981;141:30–33.

22. Lexicomp. Hudson, OH. http://online.lexi.com.

REVIEW QUESTIONS

1. What are the three major types of hormones that the adrenal glands secrete? What are the characteristics of each?

2. Catherine Jones is a 76-year-old female with rheumatoid arthritis who comes to your pharmacy every month to pick up her prescription for prednisone. You know that long-term corticosteroid use can increase the risk for osteoporosis. What counseling should the pharmacist provide to Mrs. Jones to minimize this risk?

3. Which route of administration of glucocorticoid can lead to the highest blood concentration?

4. What is the most common cause of adrenal insufficiency and Cushing's syndrome? How can this be avoided?

5. Nancy Smith is a 40-year-old female with newly diagnosed Cushing's syndrome based upon high blood cortisol level and a low-dose dexamethasone suppression test (LD-DST). She is prescribed ketoconazole for treatment of her hypercortisolism. The patient also has a diagnosis of anxiety and is on alprazolam. What should you do if a drug–drug interaction alert appears when you type ketoconazole into the patient's medication profile?

MEDICATION TABLES

MEDICATION TABLE 9-1. Systemic Corticosteroid Preparations[22,a]

Glucocorticoid	Brand Name	How Supplied	Comments
Budesonide (byoo DES oh nide)	Entocort EC	Capsule, enteric pellets: 3 mg	May be opened and sprinkled onto 1 tablespoonful of applesauce; do not chew or crush granules
	Ortikos	Capsule ER 24-hour therapy pack: 6 mg, 9 mg	Swallow whole; do not crush or chew
	Uceris	24-hour tablet: 9 mg	Swallow whole; do not crush, chew, or break
Betamethasone (bay ta METH a sone)	Celestone Soluspan	Suspension for injection: 6 mg/mL	Dosages expressed as combined amount of betamethasone sodium phosphate and betamethasone acetate
	BSP 0820, Pod-Care 100C, ReadySharp Betamethasone	Injection kit: 30 mg/5 mL	
Cortisone (KOR ti sone)	Generic only	Tablet: 25 mg	
Dexamethasone (deks a METH a sone)	Generic only	Elixir: 0.5 mg/5 mL	Raspberry-flavored; contains 5.1% ethanol; contains propylene glycol and sugar; store at room temp; avoid freezing
	Generic only	Oral solution: 0.5 mg/5 mL	Cherry-flavored; store at room temp
	Decadron, Hemady	Tablets: 0.5 mg, 0.75 mg, 1 mg, 1.5 mg, 2 mg, 4 mg, 6 mg, 20 mg	Hemady only available as 20-mg tablets
	Dexamethasone Intensol	Oral concentrate: 1 mg/mL	Contains 30% alcohol; contains propylene glycol; dye-free and sugar-free; can be mixed with liquids or semisolid foods; use only the calibrated dropper provided with the product; do not store for future use; do not freeze
	Dxevo, HiDex, TaperDex	Tablet therapy pack: 1.5 mg	21, 27, 35, 49, or 51 scored tablets on a taper dose card
	Generic only	Injectable solution: 4 mg/mL, 10 mg/mL	May need further dilution; prefilled syringe available at 10 mg/mL; protect from light, heat, and freezing
	TopiDex, Active Injection D, DoubleDex, MAS Care-Pak, ReadySharp Dexamethasone	Injection kit: 10 mg/mL	
Fludrocortisone (floo droe KOR ti sone)	Generic only	Tablet: 0.1 mg	

Continued next page

MEDICATION TABLE 9-1. Systemic Corticosteroid Preparations[22,a] *(Continued)*

Glucocorticoid	Brand Name	How Supplied	Comments
Hydrocortisone (hye droe KOR ti sone)	Solu-CORTEF	Injection powder: 100 mg, 250 mg, 500 mg, 1,000 mg	Reconstitution required
	Cortef	Tablets: 5 mg, 10 mg, 20 mg	
	Alkindi Sprinkle	Capsule, sprinkles: 0.5 mg, 1 mg, 2 mg, 5 mg	For pediatrics; only available through a specialty pharmacy; do not swallow whole
Methylprednisolone (meth il pred NIS oh lone)	Solu-Medrol	Injection powder: 40 mg, 125 mg, 500 mg, 1,000 mg, 2,000 mg	Reconstitution required
	Depo-Medrol	Injection suspension: 20 mg/mL, 40 mg/mL, 80 mg/mL	Preservative-free formulation available
	Medrol	Tablets: 2 mg, 4 mg, 8 mg, 16 mg, 32 mg	Scored
	Medrol Dose Pack	Tablets: 4 mg	21 tablets on a taper dose card
Prednisolone (pred NISS oh lone)	PediaPred	Oral solution: 5 mg/5 mL, 10 mg/5 mL, 15 mg/5 mL, 20 mg/5 mL, 25 mg/5 mL	Grape-flavored; store at room temp; contains corn syrup; no alcohol or sorbitol; dye-free
	Millipred	Tablets: 5 mg	
	OraPred ODT	Orally disintegrating tablets: 10 mg, 15 mg, 30 mg	Grape-flavored; store at room temp; orally disintegrating tablets (do not break or use partial tablets)
Prednisone (PRED ni sone)	Generic only	Tablets: 1 mg, 2.5 mg, 5 mg, 10 mg, 20 mg, 50 mg Oral solution: 5 mg/5 mL Therapy Pack: 5 mg, 10 mg	Therapy pack contains 21 tablets
	Prednisone Intensol	Oral concentrate: 5 mg/mL	Vanilla-flavored; contains alcohol 30%; contains fructose; use only the calibrated dropper provided with the product
	Rayos	Tablets: 1 mg, 2 mg, 5 mg	Delayed-release formulation
Triamcinolone (trye am SIN oh lone)	Kenalog	Injection suspension: 10 mg/mL, 40 mg/mL, 80 mg/mL	
	P-Care K40, P-Care K80, Pod-Care 100K, Pro-C-Dure 5, Pro-C-Dure 6	Injection kit: 40 mg/mL	

[a]Pronunciations have been adapted with permission from USP Dictionary of USAN and International Drug Names (USP Dictionary) © 2022.

MEDICATION TABLE 9-2. Topical Corticosteroids[22,a]

Glucocorticoid	Brand Name	Strength/Formulation	Comments
Very High Potency			
Augmented betamethasone dipropionate (bay ta METH a sone)	Diprolene, generics	0.05% cream 0.05% gel 0.05% lotion 0.05% ointment	Not to exceed 2-wk use; avoid occlusive dressings; avoid use on face, groin, armpits, skin folds; higher risk for systemic absorption
Clobetasol propionate (kloe BAY ta sol)	Clobex, Cormax, Olux-E, Temovate, Temovate E, Tovet, generics	0.05% cream 0.05% emollient cream 0.05% ointment 0.05% gel 0.05% foam 0.05% lotion 0.05% shampoo 0.05% solution for scalp application 0.05% spray	
Fluocinonide (floo oh SIN oh nide)	Vanos	0.1% cream	
Halobetasol propionate (hal oh BAY ta sol)	Ultravate, generics	0.05% cream 0.05% ointment 0.05% lotion	
High Potency			
Amcinonide (am SIN oh nide)	Generics only	0.1% cream 0.1% ointment 0.1% lotion	Use occlusive dressings with caution; avoid use of occlusive dressings with augmented betamethasone dipropionate or betamethasone dipropionate; may use on scalp, trunk, hands, and feet; avoid use on face and skin folds
Betamethasone dipropionate (bay ta METH a sone)	Diprolene AF, generics	0.05% cream (augmented formulation) 0.05% ointment	
Desoximetasone (des ox i MET a sone)	Topicort	0.25% cream 0.25% ointment 0.25% spray 0.05% gel	
Diflorasone diacetate (dye FLOR a sone)	ApexiCon E, generics	0.05% cream 0.05% ointment	
Fluocinonide (floo oh SIN oh nide)	Generics only	0.05% cream 0.05% ointment 0.05% gel 0.05% solution	
Halcinonide (hal SIN oh nide)	Halog	0.1% cream 0.1% ointment 0.1% solution	
Triamcinolone acetonide (trye am SIN oh lone)	Generics	0.5% ointment	

Continued next page

MEDICATION TABLE 9-2. Topical Corticosteroids[22,a] *(Continued)*

Glucocorticoid	Brand Name	Strength/Formulation	Comments
Medium Potency			
Betamethasone dipropionate (bay ta METH a sone)	Sernivo, generics	0.05% cream 0.05% ointment 0.05% lotion 0.05% spray	May be used on scalp, trunk, or extremities; do not use occlusive dressings with mometasone
Betamethasone valerate (bay ta METH a sone)	Beta-Val, Luxiq, generics	0.1% cream 0.1% ointment 0.12% foam	
Clocortolone pivalate (kloe KOR toe lone)	Cloderm	0.1% cream	
Desoximetasone (des ox i MET a sone)	Generics only	0.05% cream 0.05% ointment	
Fluocinolone acetonide (floo oh SIN oh lone)	Synalar, Derma-Smoothe/FS	0.025% cream 0.025% ointment 0.01% body oil 0.01% scalp oil	
Flurandrenolide (flure an DREN oh lide)	Cordran	0.05% cream 0.05% lotion 0.05% ointment	
Fluticasone propionate (floo TIK a sone)	Cutivate, generics	0.05% cream 0.05% lotion 0.005% ointment	
Hydrocortisone butyrate (hye droe KOR ti sone)	Locoid, generics	0.1% cream 0.1% lotion 0.1% ointment 0.1% solution	
Hydrocortisone probutate (hye droe KOR ti sone)	Pandel®	0.1% cream	
Hydrocortisone valerate (hye droe KOR ti sone)	Westcort®, generics	0.2% cream 0.2% ointment	
Mometasone furoate (moe MET a sone)	Generics only	0.1% cream 0.1% ointment 0.1% lotion 0.1% solution	
Prednicarbate (pred ni KAR bate)	Dermatop, generics	0.1% cream 0.1% ointment	
Triamcinolone acetonide (trye am SIN oh lone)	Kenalog®, Triderm®, Trianex®, generics	0.1% cream 0.1% ointment 0.1% lotion 0.025% cream 0.025% ointment 0.025% lotion 0.147 mg/g spray	

Continued next page

MEDICATION TABLE 9-2. Topical Corticosteroids[22,a] *(Continued)*

Glucocorticoid	Brand Name	Strength/Formulation	Comments
Low Potency			
Alclometasone dipropionate (al kloe MET a sone)	Aclovate, generics	0.05% cream 0.05% ointment	Low potency agents preferred in children; low potency agents preferred when large areas are to be covered; low potency agents preferred on the face and skin folds; hydrocortisone is available by prescription or over the counter (nonprescription) based on strength and formulation; maximum strength of nonprescription hydrocortisone available is 1%
Desonide (DES oh nide)	DesOwen, LoKara, Verdeso, generics	0.05% cream 0.05% ointment 0.05% lotion 0.05% gel 0.05% foam	
Fluocinolone acetonide (floo oh SIN oh lone)	Synalar®, Capex®, generics	0.01% cream 0.01% solution 0.01% shampoo	
Hydrocortisone acetate (hye droe KOR ti sone)	Vanicream HC Maximum Strength, MiCort HC	1%, 2.5% cream	
	NuCort	2% lotion	
	Cortifoam	10% rectal foam	
	Anusol-HC, Anucort-HC, Proctocort	25 mg, 30 mg suppository	
Hydrocortisone base (hye droe KOR ti sone)	Ala-Cort, Anusol-HC, Cortaid, Hydroskin, Preparation-H, Procto-Med, Procto-Pak, Proctocort, ProctoCream® - HC, Proctosol HC, Protozone-HC, Recort Plus, generics	0.5%, 1%, 2.5% cream	
	Corticool	1% gel	
	Aquanil HC, Beta-HC, Hydroskin, generics	1%, 2% lotion	
	Cortizone-10, generics	0.5%, 1%, 2.5% ointment	
	Cortizone-10, generics	1% spray	
	Scalpicin Maximum Strength, Texacort	1%, 2.5% solution	
	Cortenema, generic	100 mg/60 mL rectal suspension	
Hydrocortisone butyrate (hye droe KOR ti sone)	Generics	0.1% ointment, 0.1% solution	
Hydrocortisone valerate (hye droe KOR ti sone)	Generics	0.2% ointment	

[a]Pronunciations have been adapted with permission from USP Dictionary of USAN and International Drug Names (USP Dictionary) © 2022.

MEDICATION TABLE 9-3. Steroidogenesis Inhibitors for Cushing's Syndrome[22,a]

Generic Name (brand name)	Usual Dose in Adults	Common and/or Major Side Effects	How Supplied	Comments
Etomidate (e TOE mi date) (Amidate®)	Bolus based on mg/kg and titrate	Nausea, vomiting, hypotension, injection site pain	IV solution: 2 mg/mL	Do not confuse with edetate disodium; only for IV administration; discard unused portion; store at room temperature
Ketoconazole (KEE toe KON a zole) (Nizoral®, generic formulations available)	400-1,600 mg/day as every 6- to 8-hour dosing	Gynecomastia (breast enlargement in men), nausea, vomiting, headache, sedation, liver toxicity, impotence, decreased sexual drive, adrenal insufficiency at high doses	Tablet: 200 mg	Also available in cream, shampoo, gel, and foam formulations but only the tablets are used in the treatment of Cushing's syndrome; store at room temperature
Metyrapone (me TEER a pone) (Metopirone®)	500 mg/day to 6 g/day as every 6- to 8-hour dosing	Nausea and abdominal discomfort, skin rash, sedation, headache, dizziness, hypertension, adrenal insufficiency	Capsule: 250 mg	Available only for compassionate use for treatment of Cushing's syndrome; store at room temperature
Mitotane (MYE toe tane) (Lysodren®)	500 mg/day to 8 g/d (as 3 times/day dosing)	Nausea, vomiting, anorexia, diarrhea, lethargy, drowsiness, dizziness, rash, gynecomastia (breast enlargement in men), elevation of serum cholesterol, adrenal insufficiency	Tablets: 500 mg	Wear gloves when handling bottles of mitotane tablets; do not crush tablets; wash area immediately and thoroughly if in contact with broken tablets; store at room temperature
Osilodrostat (oh sil oh droe stat) (Isturisa®)	Start at 2 mg twice daily and titrate up as clinically indicated; usual range 2-7 mg twice daily, maximum 30 mg twice daily	Adrenal insufficiency, headache, vomiting, nauseas, fatigue, edema, QTc prolongation (heart rhythm disturbance), hypertension, hypokalemia, increased androgens	Tablet: 1, 5, 10 mg	FDA-approved for Cushing's disease

Source: Lexicomp. Hudson, OH. http://online.lexi.com.
FDA = United States Food and Drug Administration.
[a]Pronunciations have been adapted with permission from USP Dictionary of USAN and International Drug Names (USP Dictionary) © 2022.

Chapter 10

Diabetes Mellitus

Mary Ann Stuhan, PharmD, RPh

KEY TERMS AND DEFINITIONS

Antihyperglycemic medications—agents that cause reductions in circulating blood glucose.

Diabetes mellitus (DM)—a disorder of metabolism that results in elevated blood glucose levels, most often related to insufficient insulin production, inability of the cells to react to circulating insulin, or a combination of both. (Diabetes mellitus—"sugar" diabetes—is not to be confused with diabetes insipidus, a condition associated with lack of the pituitary hormone vasopressin.)

Estimated average glucose (eAG)—an estimate of blood glucose levels over an 8–12-week period that is calculated from the percentage value of hemoglobin A1C, but reported in the same units (mg/dL) as most regularly recorded blood glucose readings.

Fasting plasma glucose level (FPG)—concentration of glucose (sugar) in the bloodstream 8 or more hours after the last meal or snack. Levels <100 mg/dL are considered "normal," while two recorded levels >126 support a diagnosis of diabetes mellitus.

Gestational diabetes—impaired glucose metabolism related to pregnancy.

Glycemic—related to blood glucose levels.

Hemoglobin A1C—blood protein used as an indicator of average blood sugar levels over the preceding 8–12 weeks. Frequently referred to simply as "A1C," levels are reported as a percent.

Hyperglycemia—higher than normal levels of circulating glucose (sugar) in the bloodstream.

Hypoglycemia—lower than normal levels of circulating glucose (sugar) in the bloodstream.

DOI 10.37573/9781585286638.010

Insulin resistance—decrease in the ability of cells to react to circulating insulin.

Type 1 diabetes—disease resulting from the cessation of insulin production, most often caused by the destruction of the pancreatic beta cells by a process in which the patient's own immune system reacts against them.

Type 2 diabetes—form of diabetes in which patients generally still produce some insulin, but it is insufficient to regulate their blood sugar levels, either because they are producing smaller amounts, or because their cells have developed an insensitivity to this hormone (or even a combination of reduced production and reduced sensitivity).

LEARNING OBJECTIVES

After completing this chapter, you should be able to

1. Define the following:
   - Diabetes mellitus, type 1 and type 2
   - Hemoglobin A1C
   - Hyperglycemia

2. Outline the physiology of normal carbohydrate metabolism and the role of pancreatic hormones.

3. List the causes and results of diabetes mellitus.

4. Describe nonpharmacologic treatments for diabetes mellitus.

5. Review the therapeutic effects of insulin and other medications used in the treatment of diabetes and list their most common side effects and adverse reactions.

6. State the brand and generic names of the medications most widely used to treat diabetes, along with their routes of administration and dosage forms.

7. Recognize common regimens for the treatment of diabetes mellitus.

All human body processes require energy. Most of the energy used in these processes comes from the metabolism of glucose, a sugar. To function properly, the human body requires a constant level of glucose in the tissues and bloodstream—high enough to provide for the energy needs of the cells but below the level where unwanted effects will occur.

CASE STUDY

Ms. Parker's Insulin
Karen Parker is a 32-year-old female who is 5 feet tall and weighs 110 lb. Her type 1 diabetes was diagnosed while she was still in high school, and since she moved to town for a new job last year, she has been coming to the pharmacy counter every month to purchase NPH and regular human insulin, along with supplies for self-monitoring of blood glucose (SMBG) and insulin syringes. Today she has a prescription for an insulin glargine pen injector and has asked to speak to the pharmacist.

The pancreas, illustrated in Figure 10-1, is a body organ with endocrine (hormone-secreting) functions. Among its major hormones are insulin and glucagon, both of which are important in glucose metabolism. Insulin, produced by the beta cells in sections of the pancreas known as the islets of Langerhans, is the hormone that allows glucose to enter body cells to be used for the energy to power cell processes. When levels of circulating glucose are too high, insulin promotes storage of the excess as glycogen. Insulin also promotes the synthesis of proteins, the building blocks of many body tissues. Glucagon is produced in the alpha cells of the islets of Langerhans. In contrast to insulin, glucagon promotes the *release* of glucose from stored glycogen and enables the body to produce energy from other resources. Together, these two pancreatic hormones (insulin and glucagon) are responsible for normal carbohydrate metabolism and blood glucose levels, and the body depends on the balance and interaction between them. Another pancreatic hormone, amylin, also affects blood glucose levels by inhibiting the release of glucagon, slowing stomach emptying (delaying the absorption of dietary carbohydrates) and causing feelings of fullness (inhibiting additional food intake).

DIABETES MELLITUS: A GROUP OF METABOLIC DISORDERS

Diabetes mellitus (often abbreviated DM) is a disorder of metabolism that results in elevated blood glucose levels, usually related to insufficient insulin production, inability of the cells to react to circulating insulin, or a combination of both. It results in abnormal metabolism not only of carbohydrates but fats and proteins as well, and its most

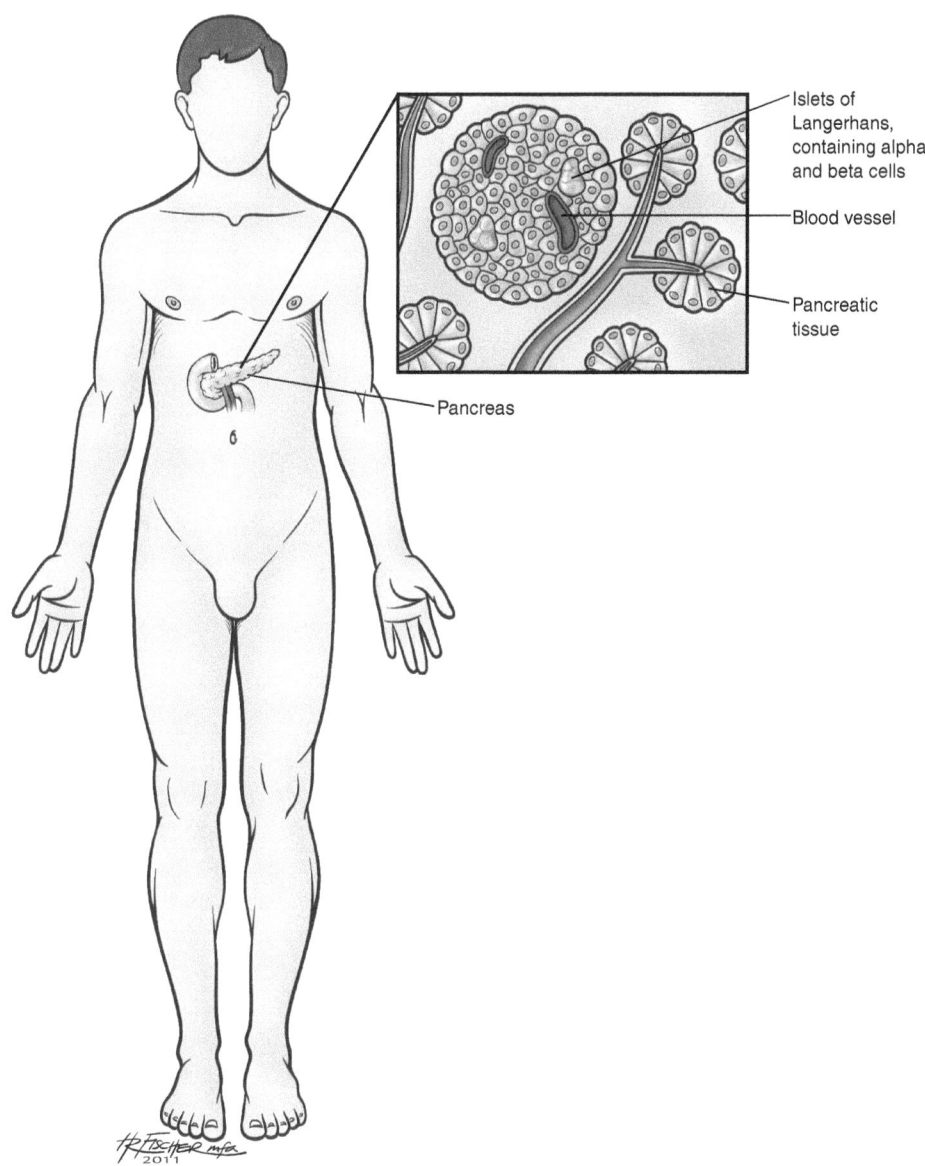

Islets of
Langerhans,
containing alpha
and beta cells

Blood vessel

Pancreatic
tissue

Pancreas

FIGURE 10-1. The pancreas is located in the abdominal cavity. Within it, specialized regions known as islets of Langerhans have specialized alpha and beta cells that produce the hormones glucagon and insulin.

characteristic sign is increased levels of circulating glucose (sugar), known as hyperglycemia.

The defects of metabolism associated with diabetes mellitus can lead to serious, chronic complications if not controlled. These are grouped in two main categories: *microvascular* (affecting the small blood vessels) and *macrovascular* (affecting the major blood vessels). Damage to the eye is a major microvascular complication. The Centers for Disease Control and Prevention reports that diabetic retinopathy (damage to the retina, a major structure of the eye) is "the leading cause of blindness among U.S. working-aged adults aged 20–74 years."[1] Another serious microvascular complication is nephropathy, or kidney damage. About one in three adults with diabetes in the United States may have chronic kidney disease, which can lead to end-stage renal disease (ESRD) requiring chronic dialysis or kidney transplant for survival.[2] A third microvascular complication is neuropathy (nerve damage), which can result in pain or defective sensation, especially in the hands and feet, as well as digestive problems. These nerve problems can even lead to more serious conditions requiring amputation, especially of the lower extremities (feet and legs).

Macrovascular complications of diabetes can be life threatening. These include hypertension, coronary heart disease, and stroke, the primary causes of death in patients with diabetes. (These conditions are addressed in detail in Chapters 15 and 16.) The progression of many complications of diabetes, especially those classified as microvascular, is very closely linked to blood sugar control and can be avoided or slowed by careful regulation of the levels of glucose in the blood. Patients with diabetes are frequently instructed to monitor blood sugar levels before and after meals, which, when tracked over time, can provide an idea of how well their therapy is working. An even better indicator of this, however, is the level of a blood protein, hemoglobin A1C (usually abbreviated A1C). Levels of A1C indicate average blood sugar levels over the preceding 8–12 weeks and have been correlated with both the control and the level of complications of diabetes.

CASE?

If Ms. Parker's diabetes is not treated adequately, what kinds of health problems might she encounter as a result?

Most cases of diabetes mellitus are classified as either type 1 or type 2. About 5%–10% of patients with diabetes have type 1 (once known as *juvenile diabetes*), which is characterized by a complete lack of insulin production.[3] It is thought to be caused by the destruction of the pancreatic beta cells by a process in which the patient's own immune system reacts against them. Although it generally develops in children and young adults, type 1 diabetes can occur at any age, and may develop over several years. Hyperglycemia does not become evident until more than 80% of the beta cells are destroyed. Because their bodies are unable to produce any insulin of their own, people with type 1 diabetes must be treated with external insulin preparations to avoid or delay the complications associated with their disease.

Type 2 diabetes is the most common form of diabetes and its incidence rises with age. It is, however, increasingly being diagnosed in adolescents and younger adults.[3] Patients with this form of disease generally still produce some insulin, but it is insufficient to regulate their blood sugar levels, either because they are producing smaller amounts or because their cells have developed an insensitivity to this hormone (or even a combination of reduced production and reduced sensitivity). Insulin therapy may still be useful or even necessary in type 2 diabetes, but many patients are helped by

lifestyle modifications such as diet and exercise. Frequently, patients with type 2 diabetes are treated with agents to either increase insulin production or help the body respond appropriately to circulating insulin. Often, a combination of therapies is used, reflecting the combination of factors contributing to the processes involved in this disorder.

Less-common forms of diabetes account for fewer than 2% of patients diagnosed. Gestational diabetes (sometimes abbreviated GDM) is a complication of pregnancy, and the initial therapy is generally a dietary adjustment. Insulin may be used if necessary, but the oral drugs used in type 2 diabetes are not currently approved for use during pregnancy. There are other types of diabetes, caused by hormone abnormalities and imbalances, adverse drug reactions, pancreatitis, and rare genetic defects, but they are encountered even less often than gestational diabetes.

TREATMENT OF DIABETES

While diabetes has different causes (eg, autoimmune disease, insulin resistance, pregnancy), the treatment goals for all types are a decrease in the dangerous complications described earlier and a reduction in symptoms. Macrovascular complications (hypertension, coronary heart disease, and stroke) are best addressed by managing risk factors for these conditions and treating them with both drug and nondrug therapies (see Chapters 14 and 15). The development of microvascular complications (damage to the eye, kidneys, and nerves), however, can be diminished or slowed by regulating blood sugar to keep levels consistently within normal range. These are the therapies that will be discussed in this chapter.

Glycemic Goals

The term glycemic refers to the level of glucose (sugar) in the blood. Blood glucose is normally lowest in the fasting state, 8–12 hours after the most recent meal, generally 70–110 mg/dL. Higher levels can be expected after meals. Hypoglycemia refers to blood glucose below the normal level, and hyperglycemia is a blood glucose level higher than would be expected. Glycemic goals are based on the fact that maintaining blood glucose levels within the normal range has been shown to reduce microvascular complications. Various groups of medical practitioners have established slightly different definitions of what "normal" should be, but most agree that fasting levels of glucose should be below 125 mg/dL and that the levels obtained after meals (postprandial blood glucose) should not rise higher than 199 mg/dL.[4] Most patients with diabetes engage in regimens of self-monitoring of blood glucose (SMBG) with varying frequency, as prescribed by their physicians. There is a wide array of SMBG equipment available for these patients, with choices in cost, features, and size. Most blood glucose meters produce readings on a digital display, and some have a memory to keep track of several consecutive levels. Some may be connected to a personal computer for detailed recordkeeping and printouts. Meters require various supplies (testing strips or solutions, etc.) and, as of this writing, SMBG generally involves testing an actual blood sample obtained by using a lancet (a small, sharp blade) to prick a finger or other place on the skin. A meter must be calibrated with a standard sample on a regular basis to ensure its accuracy. Researchers are studying less invasive ways to measure blood glucose without breaching the skin, and, while some devices to do this already exist, most are not yet considered reliable enough for exclusive use in an SMBG regimen.

While SMBG is a valuable tool for tracking day-to-day (and even hour-to-hour) blood glucose levels and is used to adjust insulin dosing for immediate regulation, the best indicator of overall long-term glycemic control is the blood protein known as hemoglobin A1C. As noted earlier, levels of A1C indicate average blood sugar levels over the preceding 8–12 weeks. A1C is measured as a percentage of overall hemoglobin, and the American Diabetes Association recommends a glycemic goal of less than 7% for most nonpregnant adults.[5] Some physicians may set an even lower target, as may the guidelines from other organizations. Because SMBG readings are reported as a specific amount of blood glucose in a specific sample size (mg/dL) and A1C is reported as a percentage, it is sometimes difficult for patients and even clinicians to see the relationship between them. An additional measurement, estimated average glucose (eAG), correlates with A1C but uses the same units (mg/dL) as SMBG readings. While it is an "average," it is NOT the average of the readings from the SMBG meter, but just a translation of A1C into a different type of unit that represents an average of glucose levels 24 hours per day over a longer period. Overall, A1C and eAG have the same meaning, and an A1C of 7% is equal to an eAG of 154 mg/dL.[5]

Nonpharmacologic (Nondrug) Therapy

Regardless of type, all patients diagnosed with diabetes mellitus should receive medical nutrition therapy. An individual diet plan formulated by a healthcare professional (preferably a licensed dietitian) will facilitate intake of balanced amounts of protein, fat, and carbohydrate, help the person reach or maintain a healthy weight, and contribute to reaching the glycemic goals described above. A planned activity regimen is also a vital tool in the treatment of diabetes. The goals of the activity regimen are weight loss, a healthy blood sugar level, and cardiovascular health, but the individual's age, weight, current level of fitness, and other health conditions must be taken into account.

In some cases of type 2 diabetes or gestational diabetes, nonpharmacologic therapy may be the only initial treatment indicated. For others, it may be part of a treatment plan that also involves medications. For patients diagnosed with type 1 diabetes, nutrition and activity will always be coordinated with an insulin regimen to optimize health and promote glycemic control.

Pharmacologic Therapy: Insulin

Insulin is a hormone that governs the body's use of nutrients. Diabetes mellitus is, primarily, a condition in which there is a deficiency of insulin production or a resistance to its actions, or a combination of these two factors. It is not surprising, therefore, that insulin therapy has been a major component of the therapy for DM. Originally, insulin was derived from beef or pork. Both types of animal-derived insulin are very similar to the insulin produced by the human body. Recombinant DNA (rDNA) technology now allows pharmaceutical manufacturers to engineer microorganisms (usually bacterial species) so that they can produce insulin identical to that secreted by the human pancreas. They can also produce insulins that differ slightly from that normally secreted in the human body and have characteristics (either longer or shorter in onset or duration of action) that make them advantageous in diabetes therapy. Because insulin is a protein that would be digested (and thus inactivated) in the gastrointestinal tract, it cannot be administered by the oral route. Currently, most insulin products are given by injection, but an inhalation is also available. (See Medication Table 10-1; Medication Tables are located at the end of the chapter).

Types of Insulin

The standard insulin product is regular human insulin (Humulin R, Novolin R, Afrezza), a hormone identical to that produced by the healthy human pancreas. It can be administered by the subcutaneous (SUBQ), intravenous (IV), or inhaled routes of administration. It is considered a short-acting insulin, with an onset of effect 30–60 minutes after SUBQ injection and a duration of around 3–6 hours.

For many years, a large number of patients with DM have "covered" their carbohydrate intake with injections of regular insulin 30 minutes before meals.

A person who does not have diabetes, however, does not have insulin secreted only around mealtime. To maintain a constant level of circulating insulin in patients with DM, formulations with a longer duration of action have been developed over the years. While you may still hear of Lente and Ultralente insulins in this context, these have not been available since 2006. One older formulation that *is* still available is isophane insulin suspension (Humulin N), commonly known as NPH insulin, made by complexing insulin with zinc and protamine to form an insoluble compound. It is considered intermediate acting, with an onset of 2–4 hours after SUBQ injection (the only route by which it may be administered) and a duration of 10–24 hours. Also included in the intermediate-acting classification is regular human insulin 500 units/mL (Humulin R 500).[4]

PRACTICE POINT

No prescription is required for regular or isophane human insulin injections in the U-100 (100 units/mL) strength. The concentrated (U-500) injection and the inhalation, however, are available only when prescribed by a licensed practitioner.

With rDNA technology, pharmaceutical companies have been able to engineer insulins with slight changes in the amino acid sequences that make up the insulin molecule to give them properties that make them especially useful in the treatment of DM. Because these products are similar to insulin (but slightly different), they are known as insulin analogs.

PRACTICE POINT

At the time of this writing, all analog insulins, alone or in combination, require a physician's prescription.

One set of analogs is a group of rapid-acting insulins. Unlike short-acting regular insulin, which must be administered at least 20–30 minutes before a meal, these insulins begin working within 15–30 minutes of SUBQ administration and continue for only 3–4 hours. The three rapid-acting analogs

are insulin lispro (Humalog), insulin aspart (Fiasp, NovoLog), and insulin glulisine (Apidra). Inhaled regular human insulin (Afrezza) is also considered rapid-acting.[4]

CASE?

Ms. Parker has been giving herself injections of NPH insulin twice every day. The pharmacist reminds her that she will no longer be needing the NPH insulin and notes she is only to inject the insulin glargine once daily. What is the difference between the two types of insulin?

ALERT!

LOOK-ALIKE/SOUND-ALIKE—Care must be *exercised to avoid confusing Humalog with Humulin and NovoLog with Novolin.*

The other set of analogs are long-acting insulins, which only begin to act hours after injection but may continue their effect for up to a full day and reduce the hazards of hyperglycemia (between doses) or hypoglycemia (soon after doses). Some preparations of insulin glargine (Lantus, Basaglar) have an onset 2–4 hours after administration and last for 20–24 hours, and the U-300 insulin glargine formulation (Toujeo) begins acting about 6 hours after administration, lasting up to 36 hours.[4] Insulin detemir (Levemir) begins working in about 90 minutes to 4 hours and has been shown to last 16–20 hours, depending on the dose (with higher doses having a longer action). Insulin degludec (Tresiba) starts to act about an hour after injection; its effects can last up to 42 hours. Unlike the intermediate-acting NPH insulin, which requires at least two injections daily, these analogs may be injected only once a day by many patients.

CASE?

The insulin glargine is considerably more expensive than the NPH Ms. Parker has been using in the past and, unlike the NPH she has been purchasing, it requires a prescription from her physician. Does it have any advantages that might justify the price and inconvenience?

Dosing of insulin is highly individualized, depending on the type of diabetes being treated, the size and health of the patient, the daily caloric needs and exercise patterns, and patient variables like insulin sensitivity and daily schedule. All patients with type 1 diabetes and some with type 2 require a *basal* dose of intermediate- or long-acting insulin scheduled once or twice a day, with additional doses of short- or rapid-acting insulin to control the glycemic *spikes* that occur with meals and snacks. This pattern is thought to mimic the natural pattern of insulin secretion. Patients whose SMBG records show a regular pattern can often use premixed combination products containing 50%–75% (50–75 units/mL) intermediate- or long-acting insulin with 25%–50% (25–50 units/mL) short- or rapid-acting insulin. These products may be NPH/regular insulin combinations (eg, Humulin 50/50, Humulin 70/30, and Novolin 70/30). Others are insulin analog combinations, including protamine lispro with unbound lispro (eg, Humalog Mix 75/25 and Humalog Mix 50/50) and protamine aspart suspension with unbound insulin aspart (eg, NovoLog Mix 70/30) (see Medication Table 10-1).

Regardless of the type or mixture, the most commonly used injectable insulin products in the United States, including all those available without prescription, have a concentration of 100 units/mL. For patients who require large doses of insulin, there are a concentrated regular human insulin product of 500 units/mL, insulin degludec injectors of 200 units/mL, and insulin glargine injectors with a 300 unit/mL strength.

Another option for maintaining insulin levels is continuous insulin therapy. For outpatients, this is generally accomplished by the use of an insulin pump (Figure 10-2), which delivers a continuous SUBQ infusion of a short- or rapid-acting insulin. The rate of infusion can be varied by patient adjustment to account for meals, snacks, and exercise as they occur and also adjusted based on SMBG readings to give an immediate remedy for any high or low values encountered. At one time, only regular insulin was used in these pumps, but insulin lispro and aspart are becoming the agents of choice for insulin pumps. The other situation in which continuous insulin therapy is indicated is for hospital inpatients who have been admitted with diabetic ketoacidosis, a life-threatening condition in which blood glucose levels are extremely high and the body's electrolyte chemistry becomes altered as well. These patients will be treated with an IV infusion of regular insulin, which can be regulated in rate depending on regularly obtained blood glucose readings until the condition has been resolved. Only insulin *solutions* may be administered intravenously (because the insoluble particles in NPH insulin suspensions would endanger the patient if given through a vein), and regular insulin is usually chosen (rather than lispro, aspart, or glulisine) because, when directly infused, its action is nearly as rapid and the product itself costs much less.

ALERT!

NPH insulin is a suspension and must never be chosen for IV administration.

A rapid-acting, noninjectable human insulin inhalation for use at mealtimes, Afrezza, can relieve patients dependent on insulin from the need for injections to control the glycemic spikes often experienced after eating. This preparation must be supplemented by a basal or long-acting insulin dose in the treatment of type 1 diabetes, but, in some cases, may be the only insulin needed for type 2 diabetes therapy.

The primary adverse effect observed with insulin therapy is hypoglycemia (low blood sugar). This can result from

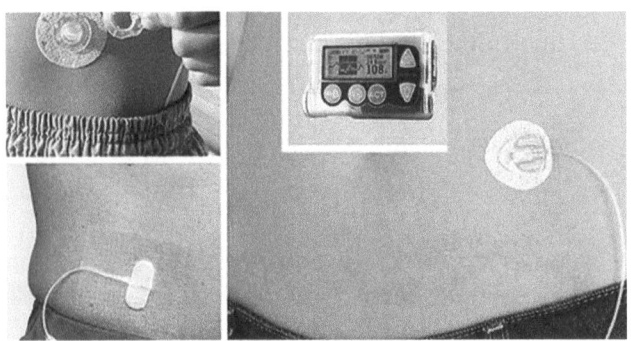

FIGURE 10-2. Insulin infusion sets and pump.

PRACTICE POINT

Afrezza is supplied as single-dose cartridges with strengths of 4, 8, or 12 units of powder each, in perforated blister strips. The dose must be specified by the prescriber. Opened strips must be used within 3 days. The Afrezza inhaler is packaged and dispensed separately, and must be discarded and replaced with a new unit every 15 days (so patients will require at least two inhalers for a one-month supply).[4]

improper dosing, fluctuations in patient meal or exercise patterns (e.g., skipping a meal or particularly heavy workouts), or poor adherence to the prescribed SMBG regimen. Hypoglycemia symptoms may include fatigue, weakness, hunger, irritability, shaking, and/or sweats, and, if untreated, may progress to unconsciousness. Hypoglycemia in conscious patients is treated by administration of a readily available source of sugar—either a dextrose gel or solution specially designed for this circumstance or a high-sugar food like nondiet soda or sugary candy. The unconscious patient must receive a remedy via injection, which may be a concentrated dextrose injection or glucagon (the hormone that causes the release of the body's stored glucose into the bloodstream). Glucagon kits that include an easy-to-reconstitute vial of glucagon with a syringe for administration should be carried by patients who receive insulin injections because hypoglycemia can be a life-threatening emergency.

The other adverse effect of insulin administration, seen much less often today than in the past when insulin products

CASE STUDY

Mr. Robinson's Diabetes Medications

Stanley Robinson is a 56-year-old male who is 6 feet tall and weighs 240 lb. After a physical examination and blood tests 6 months ago, his doctor told him he has diabetes and gave him a plan for diet and exercise, along with a prescription for metformin, which he has been taking twice daily. He has lost 5 lb and today he got another blood test result showing that his A1C is 8%. He has returned to the pharmacy with a prescription for sitagliptin.

were of animal origin and not as well purified as those available today, is lipodystrophy, a change in the subcutaneous fat at sites of injection. One type, lipohypertrophy, is a raised mass of fat at an injection site where too many injections have been given. It is generally advised that injection sites be rotated, so that a variety of different sites are used and the same one is not repeated too often. This both prevents lipodystrophy and contributes to consistent insulin absorption (Figure 10-3). The other type sometimes seen is lipoatrophy, the destruction of fat at the injection site, probably caused by antibodies to the insulin product.

While insulin products do not appear to be involved in any direct drug–drug interactions, many medications are known to affect glycemic control, and patients taking these medications or changing their doses may need to adjust their insulin dosing as well.

Pharmacologic Therapy: Oral Agents

While injected insulin is necessary for all patients with type 1 diabetes, many people with type 2 diabetes can be treated with noninsulin medications taken by mouth if

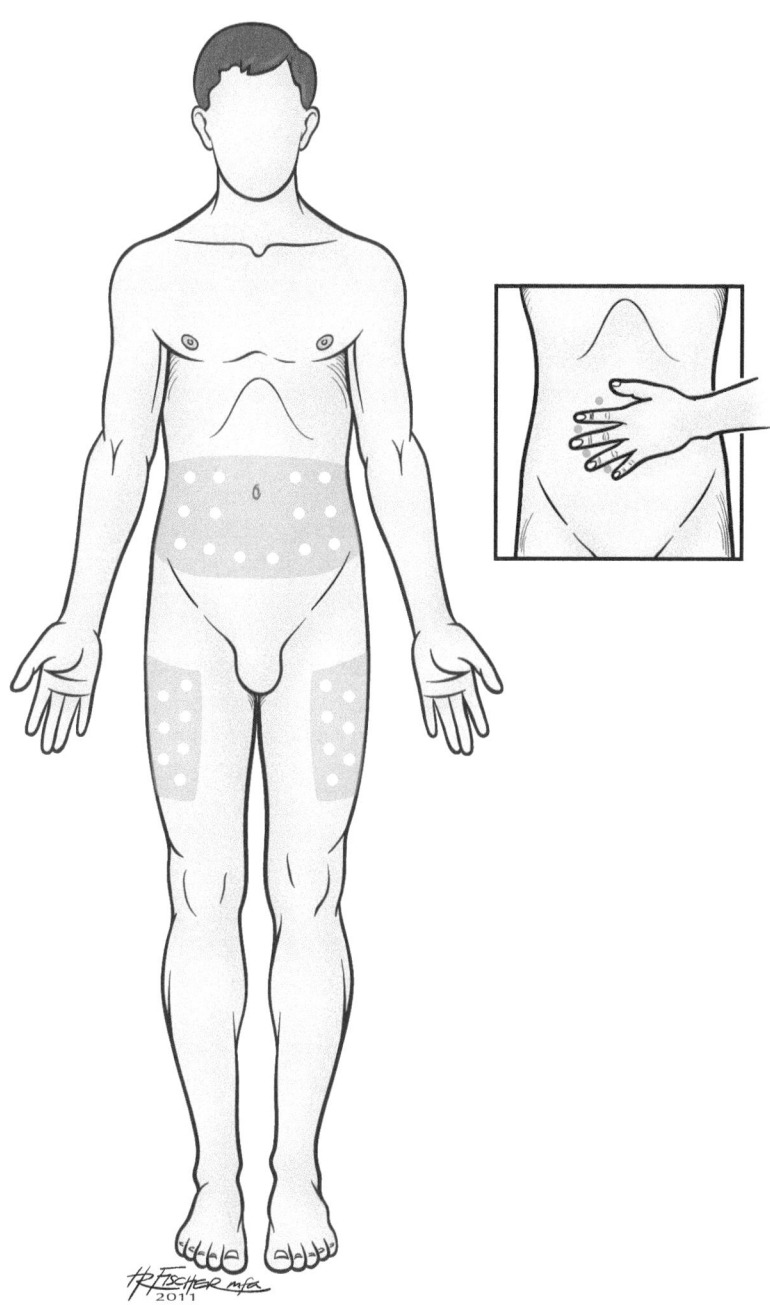

FIGURE 10-3. Insulin injection sites and rotation schemes.

nonpharmacologic therapies (diet and exercise) are ineffective in meeting their glycemic goals. Oral diabetes medications currently available work in a variety of ways but fall into five basic categories, distinguishable by their actions, time course, and side effects.

CASE?

What type of diabetes has Mr. Robinson's physician diagnosed?

Biguanides

Recall that an issue for many patients diagnosed with type 2 diabetes is insulin resistance, a condition in which their cells no longer respond to normal levels of circulating insulin. Biguanides have several actions, including increasing the insulin sensitivity of cells in the peripheral muscle tissues, allowing effective uptake and use of blood glucose, thus decreasing glucose levels. They have no direct effect on the pancreatic beta cells and may actually decrease levels of circulating insulin because lower levels of insulin become sufficient for the needs of treated patients. The only biguanide currently marketed in the United States is metformin, available as both brand and generic products. Dosage forms, all oral, include immediate-release (tablet, solution, suspension) and extended-release (tablet) preparations, as well as fixed-dose combination products with other agents. The immediate-release products are generally dosed twice daily, and the dose can be increased weekly until either the glycemic goal or the maximum dose (850 mg three times daily with meals) is reached. Extended-release metformin (Glucophage XR and generics) is generally begun once daily and can be increased up to a single dose of 2,000 mg/day or divided doses up to 750 mg 3 times/day.

The most common side effects of metformin involve the gastrointestinal system. Up to 30% of patients treated experience diarrhea, stomach upset, and/or abdominal discomfort, but it is usually mild and can be minimized by beginning with a low dose and slowly increasing it, taking the drug with or immediately after meals and/or using the extended-release form. Less common adverse effects include a metallic taste and vitamin B-12 deficiency. Rare, but more dangerous, is a condition called lactic acidosis, a serious electrolyte disturbance that can occur with the accumulation of metformin in the bloodstream, particularly the sustained-release dosage form. The most significant interactions reported have been with medications that may increase serum concentrations of metformin and could result in lactic acidosis. These include cimetidine and dolutegravir.

PRACTICE POINT

While not approved by the Food and Drug Administration for any indication other than type 2 diabetes, metformin is sometimes prescribed off-label for DM type 2 prevention, gestational diabetes, and to reduce the weight gain associated with some antipsychotic agents (see Chapter 7). Its use in the treatment of women diagnosed with polycystic ovary syndrome is discussed in Chapter 11.

ALERT!

Risk factors for lactic acidosis include renal impairment, interacting drugs, age over 65 years, radiological study with contrast, surgery, hypoxic states (e.g., acute congestive heart failure), excessive alcohol intake, and hepatic impairment.

Metformin therapy can lower A1C by 1.5%–2% and fasting glucose by 60–80 mg/dL (even if they are extremely high). It has also been shown to reduce triglycerides and low density lipoprotein (LDL) cholesterol, and therapy often leads to modest weight reduction. For these reasons, along with its relatively low cost and usually tolerable side effects, metformin is usually the first medication prescribed in the treatment of type 2 diabetes.[6] If glycemic targets (A1C and fasting blood glucose) have not been met in 3 months, another agent (sulfonylurea and insulin have the best validation) may be added to the treatment regimen. Sometimes metformin is added as the second drug when treatment with a sulfonylurea or thiazolidinedione (next sections) alone has been unsuccessful in meeting the target goals. For patients taking common fixed dosages of metformin with other diabetes therapies, products containing two drugs in the same tablet may be convenient. Some of these combinations are included in Medication Table 10-2.

CASE?

What might be the meaning of Mr. Robinson's A1C level of 8% after being treated with metformin for 6 months?

Sulfonylureas

Medications in this group were the earliest agents devised for the oral treatment of type 2 diabetes (see Medication Table 10-2). They work mainly by increasing pancreatic insulin secretion. (They are, thus, ineffective for type 1 diabetes, a condition in which the pancreatic cells responsible for insulin production have been destroyed by an autoimmune reaction.) Sometimes these drugs are subclassified as *first-generation* and *second-generation* sulfonylureas, reflecting both the order in which they were brought to market and the increased potency (and corresponding lower dosage) of the newer agents. The first-generation agents are chlorpropamide, tolazamide, and tolbutamide. Seldom prescribed in the United States, they are generic products, and all are oral tablets. Second-generation agents include glipizide (Glucotrol), glyburide (Glynase), and glimepiride (Amaryl). These are available as both brand name and generic oral tablets, although not all products can be interchanged, especially those in extended-release (glipizide) or micronized (low-dose glyburide) forms.

> ## ALERT!
> LOOK-ALIKE/SOUND-ALIKE—Glipizide and glyburide are similar names for noninterchangeable drugs with similar dosing, and glimepiride may also be confused with these.

Most patients treated with these drugs are able to take the full daily dose in the morning with breakfast or the first main meal of the day (although glipizide is almost always scheduled before breakfast). Doses are started low and then titrated upward every 1–2 weeks based on patient response, until either the glycemic goal or the maximum effective dose is reached. Older patients and those with decreased liver or kidney function generally receive lower doses.

As with insulin, the most common adverse effect of the sulfonylureas is hypoglycemia. This occurs more frequently in patients whose initial fasting plasma glucose is lower and in patients who lose weight, skip meals, or exercise heavily. Treatment for sulfonylurea-induced hypoglycemia is the same as that for hypoglycemia related to insulin use. Another common side effect of sulfonylurea therapy is weight gain in patients who are treated without reducing their dietary intake. The enhanced blood glucose control resulting from therapy comes from the body storing the excess glucose, and weight gain can result. Other less-common side effects of sulfonylureas include hyponatremia (decreased sodium), skin rash, hemolytic anemia (destruction of red blood cells), and gastrointestinal upset. A *disulfiram reaction,* resulting in nausea, vomiting, and flushing, may occur if alcohol is consumed, especially in patients taking first-generation sulfonylureas.

In general, when dosed at equivalent levels (higher doses for less potent drugs), all the drugs in the sulfonylurea class can have an equal effect on blood glucose levels, lowering A1C by 1.5%–2% and fasting glucose by 60–70 mg/dL.[6] (Remember, the goals for sulfonylureas are A1C <7 and fasting glucose <130 mg/dL.) Because this is not usually enough of a reduction for most patients (who may start with an A1C of 10% or more and fasting glucose levels >250 mg/dL), few will be controlled sufficiently on a sulfonylurea alone. The drugs in this class, however, all act in the same way, so there is no reason to add an additional sulfonylurea if the patient is already taking one; instead, a drug from a different class will be added. The second-generation sulfonylureas are also available in fixed-dose combinations with other types of antihyperglycemic agents (metformin or a thiazolidinedione) for patient convenience in a multi-drug treatment regimen. (See Medication Table 10-2.)

Meglitinides

Also known as short-acting insulin secretagogues, drugs in this class are similar to sulfonylureas as they work by stimulating pancreatic insulin production, although their actions are both faster in onset and shorter in duration. Like the sulfonylureas, they are ineffective in the treatment of type 1 diabetes, where pancreatic insulin production has ceased. Currently available agents in this class include nateglinide (Starlix and generics) and repaglinide (generics only, alone or with metformin) in tablet dosage form (see Medication Table 10-2).

Meglitinides are rapidly absorbed from the gastrointestinal tract and also rapidly cleared from the body. Because of this, they must be taken just before (within 30 minutes of) each meal. If a meal is low in carbohydrates or is skipped, the dose is skipped as well. Repaglinide therapy is generally begun at a low dose and may be titrated upward toward the maximum effective dose. Nateglinide is usually ordered as 120 mg before each meal with no dosage adjustments indicated.

The most common side effect of the meglitinides is hypoglycemia, but it is less of an issue than with the sulfonylureas because, when glucose levels decrease, so do the actions of the drugs. Weight gain has also been noted in patients taking these drugs, although more significantly with repaglinide. Because meglitinides are metabolized in the liver, there is a possibility of interactions with other liver-metabolized drugs, which could result in changes in the actions of either the meglitinides or of the other drugs.

When used alone, the meglitinides do not produce as much of a reduction in A1C as the sulfonylureas. Their main use is in treating patients who are near (within 1%) their glycemic goals. While the need for multiple daily doses may be a problem for many patients, meglitinides could be advantageous for those with irregular eating patterns, since they are taken immediately prior to a meal rather than on a fixed schedule. They are not used in addition to sulfonylureas when another drug must be added to the regimen because the similarity in their mechanism of action (increased insulin production) means that there will be little likelihood of additional benefit.

Thiazolidinediones

This group of drugs causes an increase in the insulin sensitivity of muscle, liver, and fat tissues (see Medication Table 10-2). Significantly, they accomplish this by an indirect action (unlike the biguanides) and require the presence of significant amounts of circulating insulin to be effective. Drugs in this class are sometimes known as glitazones. The two thiazolidinediones marketed in the United States are pioglitazone (Actos and generics) and rosiglitazone (generics only), both oral tablets. Both drugs are begun on a once-daily schedule—pioglitazone at 15–30 mg and rosiglitazone at 4 mg—and doses can be increased slowly, balancing therapeutic goals against side effects until the target goals or the maximum doses are reached. Some studies have shown a greater benefit for rosiglitazone if the maximum dose of 8 mg is divided and given as 4 mg twice daily.

ALERT!

LOOK-ALIKE/SOUND-ALIKE—Actos looks and sounds like Actonel, a drug used for the treatment and prevention of osteoporosis.

The most common adverse effects associated with the thiazolidinediones are upper respiratory tract infection, headache, sinusitis, fluid retention, and hyperglycemia. Many patients treated with these drugs experience a modest weight gain. When used with another agent (such as metformin or a sulfonylurea), they may also be associated with hypoglycemia. While much less common, the fluid retention associated with pioglitazone and rosiglitazone can aggravate or even cause congestive heart failure. For this reason, these drugs are contraindicated in patients with symptomatic or advanced stages of

heart failure and should be initiated at a lower dose for patients with cardiac problems less serious than advanced heart failure.

ALERT!

Rosiglitazone and pioglitazone both carry boxed warnings for congestive heart failure; rosiglitazone has as boxed warning for myocardial infarction as well. A medication guide approved by the Food and Drug Administration (FDA) must be dispensed with these medications.

Thiazolidinediones therapy can lower A1C by 1.5% and fasting glucose by as much as 70 mg/dL.[6] These effects, however, are not immediate, and the full benefit may not be seen for as long as 3–4 months after treatment begins. These medications cause increases in high density lipoprotein (HDL—"good cholesterol") and pioglitazone usually causes beneficial decreases in plasma triglyceride levels.

PRACTICE POINT

Patients who are self-monitoring blood glucose levels may be disappointed in their initial response to pioglitazone or rosiglitazone. If they mention the possibility of discontinuing the medication "because it is not working," it is important to refer them to the pharmacist, their physician, or a diabetes educator for counseling on the delayed effects of these drugs.

Thiazolidinediones may be used alone in the treatment of type 2 diabetes, but they are seldom considered first-line therapy and are usually used in combination with metformin or a sulfonylurea for patients who have been unable to meet their glycemic goals on a single agent.[6]

PRACTICE POINT

For patients who are stabilized on fixed doses of two agents, combination products may be convenient. Table 10-2 lists some of these combination products.

CASE?

Mr. Robinson notes that the sitagliptin is more expensive than the metformin, and asks, "Is this a better drug than the one I used to take?" What should the pharmacy technician say?

DPP-4 Inhibitors

Research has shown that, in addition to producing too little insulin and/or having insulin-resistant cells, patients with type 2 diabetes have lower than expected levels of a substance called *glucagon-like peptide-1 (GLP-1)*. Dipeptidyl peptidase 4 (DPP-4) is an enzyme related to the natural degradation of GLP-1, so a substance that inhibits DPP-4 should cause an increase in the amount of circulating GLP-1, and, ultimately, result in an increase in insulin secretion after meals. That is the theory underlying the DPP-4 inhibitors, and, since it is specific to type 2 diabetes, these drugs should be used only to treat patients with this form of the disease. DPP-4 inhibitors available in the United States are alogliptin, linagliptin, saxagliptin, and sitagliptin (see Medication Table 10-2). As of this writing, alogliptin is the only DPP-4 inhibitor available as a generic product, so therapy with this group may be expensive for some patients.

DPP-4 inhibitors are usually taken once daily without regard to meals. Drugs from this class may be used alone (in conjunction with diet and exercise therapy), but, because by themselves they produce A1C reductions of less than 1%, they are usually prescribed in combination with another agent. Fixed-dose combination products containing DPP-4 inhibitors along with another agent are available for patient convenience (see examples in Medication Table 10-2).

Few patients experience adverse effects from DPP-4 inhibitors, with the most common being nasal congestion, upper respiratory tract infection, and occasional headaches. Severe joint pain and heart failure have been reported in some patients as well. Treatment with DPP-4 inhibitors has been associated with some cases of rare but severe (even fatal) pancreatitis and hypersensitivity reactions.

CASE?

The following month Mr. Robinson returns for his refills. He mentions that it is inconvenient for him to carry around "all those tablets" and asks if there is an easier way to get his therapy. What might the pharmacist suggest in a phone call to the doctor?

SGLT-2 Inhibitors

Sodium-glucose cotransporter-2 (SGLT-2) inhibitors reduce circulating glucose by increasing urinary glucose excretion. While they are approved as single-agent therapy (in conjunction with diet and exercise) for improved glycemic control in type 2 diabetes, they are usually prescribed in combination with metformin or one of the other oral medications already discussed. There are four agents in this category currently available in the United States: canaglifozin, dapaglifozin, empagliflozin, and ertuglifozin; each is available alone and in combination with one or more other type 2 diabetes therapies. All of these products are brand-name only (no generics available as of this writing), so may be quite expensive for many patients.

SGLT-2 inhibitors as add-on therapy have advantages in several patient populations with conditions often seen along with type 2 diabetes. The increase in glucose excretion can contribute to weight loss and even some blood pressure reduction. Empagliflozin and canagliflozin have both been shown to reduce the risk of cardiovascular events, including myocardial infarction, stroke, and other related fatalities. They can be beneficial in patients unable to tolerate the first-line therapies described in earlier parts of this chapter.

Because SGLT-2 inhibitors act at the level of the kidney, they may be less effective in lowering plasma glucose for patients with significant renal impairment (although their cardiovascular benefits may still apply). The most common adverse effects are related to the increase in urinary glucose, including genital fungal infections and urinary tract infections, so patients receiving these agents must be alert to symptoms of these conditions, which are best treated early in their course. Other side effects, also related to the mechanism of action, include increased urinary frequency, dizziness, dehydration, or even hypotension.[6]

PRACTICE POINT

An FDA-approved medication guide must be provided to all patients to whom SGLT-2 inhibitors are dispensed, whether alone or as part of a combination product. This guide describes the signs, symptoms, and dangers of dehydration and yeast infections (and, for canagliflozin, the increased risk for lower-limb amputations) associated with these products.

CASE?

If Mr. Robinson's A1C is still high after a few months of metformin and sitagliptin therapy, what changes might his physician make in his medication regimen? Might any of these be appropriate for Ms. Parker? Why or why not?

Alpha-Glucosidase Inhibitors

Medications in this group act in the small intestine by inhibiting the enzymes responsible for breaking complex sugars and carbohydrates down into glucose. This delays absorption of the glucose into the bloodstream and lowers the peak glucose level after meals of patients with diets high in complex carbohydrates (starches and sucrose). They have little effect on fasting glucose levels. Alpha-glucosidase inhibitors currently in use in the United States include acarbose (Precose

and generics) and miglitol (generic only), both available as oral tablets (see Medication Table 10-2).

Medications in this class are begun at low doses with only one meal per day (to avoid side effects) and gradually increased to higher doses (based on patient weight) taken with every meal, ideally with the first bite of food. The most common adverse effects are gastrointestinal (bloating, flatulence, diarrhea), so alpha-glucosidase inhibitors is contraindicated in patients with gastrointestinal conditions such as inflammatory bowel disease. Because they depend on the kidneys for excretion, drugs from this class should not be administered to patients with more than mild renal dysfunction, either.

Alpha-glucosidase inhibitors are used only in type 2 diabetes, since they delay, rather than prevent, the absorption of glucose. This class of medications is of benefit mainly to patients who are near their glycemic goals (within 1% of their target A1C) with acceptable fasting blood sugar levels but higher than desirable levels after meals. They may be used alone, or to supplement other diabetes therapy.

CASE?

If the oral medications are the right treatment for Mr. Robinson, why does Ms. Parker have to continue with her injections?

ALERT!

Patients who have taken an alpha-glucosidase inhibitor and then become hypoglycemic must be treated with pure glucose either orally or by injection because the drug will prevent rapid absorption of more complex sugars like the ones found in candy or beverages.

Noninsulin Injectable Therapies
Amylin Analog

Pramlintide (Symlin) is a synthetic form of the natural human hormone amylin, normally secreted by the same pancreatic cells that produce insulin. It affects blood glucose levels by inhibiting the release of glucagon, slowing stomach emptying (delaying the absorption of dietary carbohydrates), and causing feelings of fullness. Pramlintide is used only in the treatment of patients who are using insulin (for either type 1 or type 2 diabetes) and is helpful in controlling glucose levels after meals. It has been shown to produce decreases in A1C when added to insulin therapy, and it often produces weight loss (advantageous for patients seeking this effect) probably because of a reduction in food intake (due to the feelings of fullness). Pramlintide is administered by SUBQ injection just prior to each meal, and dosages vary from 15 mcg as a beginning dose for people with type 1 diabetes to a maximum of 120 mcg before each meal for type 2 diabetes. It does not replace the premeal insulin dose, although this dose may sometimes require adjustment, especially for patients whose after-meal blood glucose was near normal on insulin alone.

The most common adverse effects of pramlintide are related to its action on the gastrointestinal tract, mainly nausea in type 2 diabetes patients and vomiting and/or loss of appetite in both type 1 and type 2 patients. Usually, these effects diminish over time and can be minimized by starting with a low dose. As with many other treatments for diabetes, hypoglycemia can also occur. Because of its effects on stomach emptying, pramlintide can delay the absorption, and, thus, action, of orally administered medications. This can be avoided by scheduling other medications 1 hour before or 2 hours after a dose.

PRACTICE POINT

Pramlintide is available as a prefilled multi-dose pen injector specific to the dose a patient is prescribed. The medication must be discarded 30 days after first use, whether refrigerated or kept at room temperature.

ALERT!

Pramlintide carries a boxed warning for the risk of severe hypoglycemia, which can result in serious injury. An FDA-approved medication guide emphasizing this warning must be dispensed with this medication.

GLP-1 Receptor Agonists

Recall from the section on DPP-4 inhibitors that patients with type 2 diabetes have lower than expected levels of a substance called *glucagon-like peptide-1 (GLP-1)*. Naturally produced (endogenous) GLP-1 stimulates insulin secretion in response to plasma glucose levels (usually in relation to meals), limits hepatic glucose output, slows gastric emptying, and increases feelings of fullness. The synthetic GLP-1 receptor agonists (GLP1-RAs) exhibit these same actions in patients to whom they are administered, ultimately resulting in the reduction of circulating plasma glucose and body weight. They may even have a protective effect on pancreatic beta cell function,[6] potentially delaying disease progression in type 2 diabetes. Pharmaceutical GLP1-RAs are more resistant to the actions of the DPP-4 enzymes (described in the earlier section of this chapter on DPP-4 inhibitors) than endogenous GLP-1, so they offer sustained blood levels and therapeutic action.

There are currently five GLP1-RAs available in the United States in seven different dosage forms (see Medication Table 10-2): dulaglutide, exenatide (regular and XR), lixisenatide, liraglutide, and semaglutide (injectable and oral). Except for the oral semaglutide (Rybelsus) tablet, they are administered as subcutaneous injections. While they all act at the body's GLP-1 receptors, the properties of these agents vary, causing differences in dose, dosing interval, actions, and side effects. Prescribers tailor treatment to individual patient needs and responses, sometimes adapting the treatment to match affordability and insurance considerations. As of this writing, the GLP1-RAs are marketed in the United States only as brand name products, with no available generics.

Exenatide (Byetta) was the first agent of this class to be approved. Its action is relatively short, and it is administered twice daily before breakfast and dinner. Exenatide XR (Bydureon) is a longer-acting formulation dosed once weekly. They cannot be interchanged for one another.

GLP1-RAs with once daily dosing are lixisenatide (Adlyxin), and liraglutide (Victoza), administered by subcutaneous injection, and oral semaglutide (Rybelsus) tablets. Weekly dosing (by subcutaneous injection) is indicated for dulaglutide (Trulicity) and injectable semaglutide (Ozempic), in addition to exenatide XR.

ALERT!

Liraglutide is FDA approved for use in chronic weight management (see Chapter 24), but only under the Saxenda brand name. Liraglutide for the treatment of diabetes is marketed as Victoza.

GLP1-RAs used in diabetes management are seldom the sole therapy for patients being treated. The once-daily agents are also available as combination injections with long-acting insulin to reduce the number of injections patients must receive. (See Medication Table 10-2.) GLP1-RAs are not used with DPP-4 inhibitors, however, as both target increased action at the GLP-1 receptor (by increasing the agonists acting there).

Some of the GLP1-RAs have been demonstrated to reduce the risk of cardiovascular events (including myocardial infarction, stroke, and related fatalities) in patients treated with them. Ongoing research may yield additional details in this area.

The most common side effects associated with agents in this class are nausea, vomiting, and diarrhea. For many patients, these tend to be more noticeable at the start of treatment, and dose adjustment reduces them. They are contraindicated in patients with chronic pancreatitis, and in those with a history of certain types of thyroid cancer.

All of the agents in this class are supplied in proprietary injectors, some single-dose and some multiple dose. Patients must receive instructions specific to the medication and dosage form prescribed.

ALERT!

An FDA-approved medication guide must be dispensed with all GLP1-RAs. Several of these agents (dulaglutide, exenatide XR, liraglutide, semaglutide) carry a boxed warning regarding thyroid T cell tumors.

PRACTICE POINT

While all of these agents are refrigerated before dispensing, storage conditions that must be followed by patients (before and after packages are opened for use) are specific to each product and must be followed carefully. It is important to call this information to patients' attention at the time of dispensing.

SUMMARY

Diabetes mellitus is a disorder related to insufficient insulin production, the inability of the cells to react to circulating insulin, or a combination of both, and results in abnormal metabolism of dietary nutrients. Its most characteristic sign is increased levels of circulating glucose, which can lead to serious and life-threatening complications. The most common types of diabetes mellitus are type 1, usually diagnosed in children and young adults and characterized by the complete lack of insulin production, and type 2, most often diagnosed in adults and characterized by lower than necessary insulin production and/or decreased sensitivity to the effects of insulin. Other types of diabetes include gestational diabetes, as well as a few even less-common forms.

Type 1 diabetes must be treated with insulin, although there are a few other medications that may be added to therapy. Type 2 diabetes can be treated with diet and exercise, oral medication, insulin, some novel injections, or, more commonly, a combination of therapies. For both types of diabetes, blood glucose levels are monitored both in the short term (with blood glucose meters) and the long term (via A1C levels), and doses are adjusted to achieve glycemic control.

REFERENCES

1. Centers for Disease Control and Prevention. Vision Health Initiative. Common eye disorders and diseases. https://www.cdc.gov/visionhealth/basics/ced/. Accessed February 24, 2021.

2. Centers for Disease Control and Prevention. Chronic Kidney Disease Initiative. Chronic Kidney Disease in the United States, 2019. https://www.cdc.gov/kidneydisease/. Accessed March 22, 2022.

3. Centers for Disease Control and Prevention. Diabetes. What is diabetes? https://www.cdc.gov/diabetes/basics/diabetes.html. Accessed February 24, 2021.

4. Mannkind Corporation. AFREZZA prescribing information. https://www.afrezza.com. Accessed April 15, 2021.

5. American Diabetes Association. Understanding A1C. A1C and eAG. https://www.diabetes.org/diabetes/a1c-test-meaning/a1c-and-eag. Accessed February 24, 2021.

6. Trujillo J, Haines S. Diabetes mellitus. In: DiPiro JT, Yee GC, Posey L, et al., eds. *Pharmacotherapy: A Pathophysiologic Approach.* 11th ed. New York, NY: McGraw-Hill; 2020.

7. Lexicomp. Hudson, OH. http://online.lexi.com.

REVIEW QUESTIONS

1. What is diabetes mellitus, and what are its most serious effects?

2. List and describe differences between type 1 and type 2 diabetes.

3. Describe at least two types of insulin regimens that may be used by patients with type 1 diabetes.

4. What are glycemic goals, and how are they measured? What are considered *target* measurements?

5. Why might a patient with type 2 diabetes use multiple medications from different drug classes to reach his or her glycemic goals?

MEDICATION TABLES

MEDICATION TABLE 10-1. Insulins[a]

Insulin Type	Brand Name	Dosage Form	Route	Action	Note
Human Insulin (rDNA)					
Regular	Humulin R, Novolin R	Solution	SUBQ	Short	OTC
Regular concentrate	Humulin R U500 concentrated	Solution	SUBQ, IV	Short	Rx Only
Isophane or NPH	Humulin N, Novolin N	Suspension	SUBQ	Intermediate	OTC
Analog					
Insulin (rDNA origin) aspart (IN su lin) (AS part)	NovoLog	Solution	SUBQ	Rapid	Rx Only
Insulin (rDNA origin) lispro (IN su lin) (LYE sproe)	Humalog	Solution	SUBQ	Rapid	Rx Only
Insulin glulisine (IN su lin) (GLOO lis een)	Apidra	Solution	SUBQ, IV	Rapid	Rx Only
Insulin detemir (IN su lin) (DE te mir)	Levemir	Solution	SUBQ	Long	Rx Only
Insulin glargine (IN su lin) (GLAR geen)	Lantus	Solution	SUBQ	Long	Rx Only
Premixed					
Human insulin/isophane 70 units/mL with regular 30 units/mL	Humulin 70/30, Novolin 70/30	Suspension	SUBQ		
Insulin aspart protamine/insulin aspart (IN su lin) (AS part) (PROE ta meen)	Novolog Mix 70/30	Suspension	SUBQ		Rx Only
Insulin lispro protamine/insulin lispro (IN su lin) (LYE sproe) (PROE ta meen)	Humalog Mix 75/25, Humalog Mix 50/50	Suspension	SUBQ		Rx Only

IV = intravenous; OTC = over the counter; SUBQ = subcutaneous.
[a]Pronunciations have been adapted with permission from USP Dictionary of USAN and International Drug Names (USP Dictionary) © 2022.

MEDICATION TABLE 10-2. Representative Noninsulin Agents for Diabetes Therapy[7,a]

CLASS Generic Name	Brand Name	Route	Forms	Dose	Notes
α-GLUCOSIDASE INHIBITORS					
Acarbose (AY car bose)	Precose	Oral	Tablet	25–100 mg 1–3 times daily at start of meal	Type 2 diabetes only
Miglitol (MIG li tol)		Oral	Tablet	25–100 mg 1–3 times daily at start of meal	Type 2 diabetes only
AMYLIN ANALOG					
Pramlintide (PRAM lin tide)	SymlinPen	SUBQ	Pen injector	15–120 mcg immediately before major meals	Type 1 and Type 2 diabetes, as adjunct to other therapies
BIGUANIDES					
Metformin (met FOR min)	Glucophage	Oral	Tablet	500 mg twice daily up to 850 mg 3 times daily	Type 2 diabetes only
	Riomet	Oral	Solution	500 mg twice daily—850 mg 3 times daily	
	Fortamet, Glucophage XR, Glumetza	Oral	Extended-release tablet	500–2,000 mg daily with evening meal (or dose may be divided and administered twice daily)	
DPP-4 INHIBITORS					
Alogliptin (al oh GLIP tin)	Nesina	Oral	Tablet	25 mg daily	Alogliptin (al oh GLIP tin) Type 2 diabetes only
Linagliptin (lin a GLIP tin)	Tradjenta	Oral	Tablet	5 mg daily	
Saxagliptin (sax a GLIP tin)	Onglyza	Oral	Tablet	2.5–5 mg daily	
Sitagliptin (sit a GLIP tin)	Januvia	Oral	Tablet	100 mg daily (less in renal impairment)	
GLP-1 Receptor Agonists					
Dulaglutide (doo la GLOO tide)	Trulicity	SUBQ	Pen injector	0.75–4 mg once weekly	Not currently indicated for Type 1 diabetes

Continued next page

MEDICATION TABLE 10-2. Representative Noninsulin Agents for Diabetes Therapy[7,a] *(Continued)*

CLASS Generic Name	Brand Name	Route	Forms	Dose	Notes
Exenatide (ex EN a tide)	Byetta	SUBQ, immediate release	Pen injector	5–10 mcg twice daily within 60 min of breakfast and dinner	
	Bydureon	SUBQ, extended release	Auto-injector; pen injector	2 mg weekly without regard to meals	
Liraglutide (lir a GLOO tide)	Victoza	SUBQ	Pen injector	0.6–1.8 mg daily	Type 2 diabetes only; with insulin or oral agents
	Saxenda	SUBQ	Pen injector	3 mg once daily (titrated at weekly intervals)	Chronic weight management (NOT indicated for diabetes)
Lixisenatide (lix i SEN a tide)	Adlyxin	SUBQ	Pen injector	10–20 mcg once daily	
Semaglutide (sem a GLOO tide)	Ozempic	SUBQ	Pen injector	0.25 mg weekly for first 4 weeks; increased to 0.5–1 mg once weekly	
	Rybelsus	Oral	Tablet	3 mg daily for the first 30 days, then 7–14 mg once daily	Must be taken at least 30 minutes or more before the first food, beverage, or other medications of the day
MEGLITINIDES					Type 2 diabetes only
Nateglinide (na te GLYE nide)	Starlix	Oral	Tablet	60–120 mg 3 times daily	1–30 min before meals
Repaglinide (re PAG li nide)		Oral	Tablet	0.5–4 mg up to 4 times daily	With meals or snacks
SULFONYLUREAS					Type 2 diabetes only
Glimepiride (GLYE me pye ride)	Amaryl	Oral	Tablet	1–8 mg daily	With breakfast or first main meal
Glipizide (GLIP i zide)	Glucotrol	Oral	Tablet	5 mg daily–20 mg twice daily	
	Glucotrol XL	Oral	Extended-release tablet	5–20 mg daily	
Glyburide (GLYE byoor ide)		Oral	Tablet	1.25–20 mg daily	Single or divided doses
	Glynase	Oral	Micronized tablet	0.75–12 mg daily	Single or divided doses

Continued next page

MEDICATION TABLE 10-2. Representative Noninsulin Agents for Diabetes Therapy[7,a] *(Continued)*

CLASS Generic Name	Brand Name	Route	Forms	Dose	Notes
SGLT-2 INHIBITORS					
Canagliflozin (kan a gli FLOE zin)	Invokana	Oral	Tablet	100–300 mg once daily	Type 2 diabetes
Dapagliflozin (dap a gli FLOE zin)	Farxiga	Oral	Tablet	5–10 mg once daily	Also indicated for chronic kidney disease, heart failure
Empagliflozin (em pa gli FLOE zin)	Jardiance	Oral	Tablet	10–25 mg once daily	Also indicated for heart failure
Ertugliflozin (er too gli FLOE zin)	Steglatro	Oral	Tablet	5–15 mg daily	
THIAZOLIDINEDIONES					
Pioglitazone (pye oh GLI ta zone)	Actos	Oral	Tablet	15–30 mg daily	Type 2 diabetes only
COMBINATIONS					
Glipizide/metformin	Metaglip	Oral	Tablet		Type 2 diabetes only
Glyburide/metformin	Glucovance	Oral	Tablet		Type 2 diabetes only
Pioglitazone/glimepiride	Duetact	Oral	Tablet		Type 2 diabetes only
Pioglitazone/metformin	ActoPlus Met	Oral	Tablet		Type 2 diabetes only
Repaglinide/metformin	Prandimet	Oral	Tablet		Type 2 diabetes only
Saxagliptin/metformin	Kombiglyze XR	Oral	Extended-release tablet		Type 2 diabetes only
Sitagliptin/metformin	Janumet	Oral	Tablet		Type 2 diabetes only
Liraglutide/insulin degludec	Xultrophy	SUBQ	Pen injector	Once daily	Type 2 diabetes only
Lixisenatide/insulin glargine	Soliqua	SUBQ	Pen injector	Once daily	Type 2 diabetes only

[a]Pronunciations have been adapted with permission from USP Dictionary of USAN and International Drug Names (USP Dictionary) © 2022.

Chapter 11

Reproductive Hormones

Kathleen K. Adams, PharmD, BCPS |
Devra Dang, PharmD, CDCES, FNAP

KEY TERMS AND DEFINITIONS

Amenorrhea—the absence of menstrual periods.

Androgen—a predominantly male sex hormone that promotes the development and maintenance of male sex characteristics; testosterone is the major androgen found naturally in the body.

Benign prostatic hyperplasia (BPH)—an abnormal enlargement of the prostate gland that may cause lower urinary tract symptoms.

Contraception—the use of medications, devices, methods, or procedures to prevent or decrease the likelihood of pregnancy.

Contraindicated—should not be used due to known risk of harm.

Dysmenorrhea—menstrual cramps.

Dyspareunia—painful intercourse.

Endometriosis—a condition in which tissue similar to that normally lining the uterus is found outside of the uterus (usually on the ovaries, fallopian tubes, and other pelvic structures).

Endometrium—tissue that lines the uterus.

Estrogen—primary female sex hormone responsible for normal female sexual development and reproduction.

Follicle-stimulating hormone (FSH)—a hormone released by the pituitary gland that is important for sperm and egg maturation, as well as maintaining normal human reproduction.

DOI 10.37573/9781585286638.011

Gonadotropins—compounds made by the body or made synthetically, used to stimulate the ovaries (eg, follicle-stimulating hormone and luteinizing hormone).

Gonadotropin-releasing hormone (GnRH)—a hormone released by the hypothalamus that stimulates the pituitary gland to release luteinizing hormone and follicle-stimulating hormone.

Gonads—the primary sex organs responsible for release of the reproductive hormones.

Gynecomastia—noncancerous enlargement of the breast tissue.

Hypogonadism—a condition resulting in not enough secretion of the sex hormones from the male or female gonads.

Intrauterine—administration of a substance in the uterus.

Intravaginal—administration of a substance in the vaginal canal.

Luteinizing hormone (LH)—a hormone released by the pituitary gland that stimulates release of the primary sex hormones and helps to maintain normal human reproduction.

Menopause—the permanent cessation of menses.

Menorrhagia—abnormally heavy and prolonged menstrual period at regular intervals.

Menstruation/menses—the monthly flow of blood from the uterus of nonpregnant women from puberty to menopause.

Ovaries—the primary female reproductive organs.

Ovulation—the part of the menstrual cycle when the egg is released from the ovaries.

Postmenopausal—the time after which a woman has experienced 12 consecutive months without a menstrual period.

Progesterone—the female sex hormone important for normal ovulation and maintaining healthy pregnancies.

Progestin—a general term for synthetic progesterone.

Testes—the primary male reproductive organs.

Testosterone—the primary sex hormone important for maintaining normal sexual development and reproduction in males.

Urethra—the tube connected to the bladder that carries urine from the bladder to be eliminated from the body.

Urinary incontinence—a loss of voluntary control over urination.

Uterus—a hollow muscular organ located in the female pelvis between the bladder and rectum; its main function is to nourish the developing fetus prior to birth.

Vasomotor symptoms—hot flashes or night sweats that can occur due to hormonal fluctuations during perimenopause or menopause.

Virilization—the development of secondary male sexual characteristics.

LEARNING OBJECTIVES

After completing this chapter, you should be able to

1. List the basic physiologic roles for each of the major reproductive hormones.

2. Recognize common therapeutic indications for the use of reproductive hormones.

3. Recognize available dosage forms and describe common and serious adverse effects, administration, storage, and handling techniques for the available estrogen and progestin preparations.

4. Recognize available dosage forms and describe common and serious adverse effects, administration, storage, and handling techniques for the available testosterone preparations.

5. Recognize available dosage forms and describe common and serious adverse effects, administration, storage, and handling techniques for the available preparations to treat benign prostatic hyperplasia.

The primary sex organs in the human reproductive system are called gonads. In males the gonads are the testes, and in females the gonads are the ovaries. The male and female reproductive systems are carefully regulated by numerous hormones that are secreted by various organs in the human body. These specific hormones must be released in appropriate amounts and at the right time for the reproductive organs of each sex to function properly. The hypothalamus is located in the brain and is responsible for secreting many hormones. Gonadotropin-releasing hormone (GnRH) is one hormone released by the hypothalamus that is important for maintaining normal functioning of the human reproductive system in both males and females. In response to the release of GnRH, the pituitary gland, another organ located in the brain responsible for hormone release, secretes luteinizing hormone (LH) and follicle-stimulating hormone (FSH). LH and FSH are responsible for controlling the production and release of the primary sex hormones, estrogen, progesterone, and testosterone, from the gonads.[1,2] Figure 11-1 illustrates how hormones involved in the human reproductive system work together.

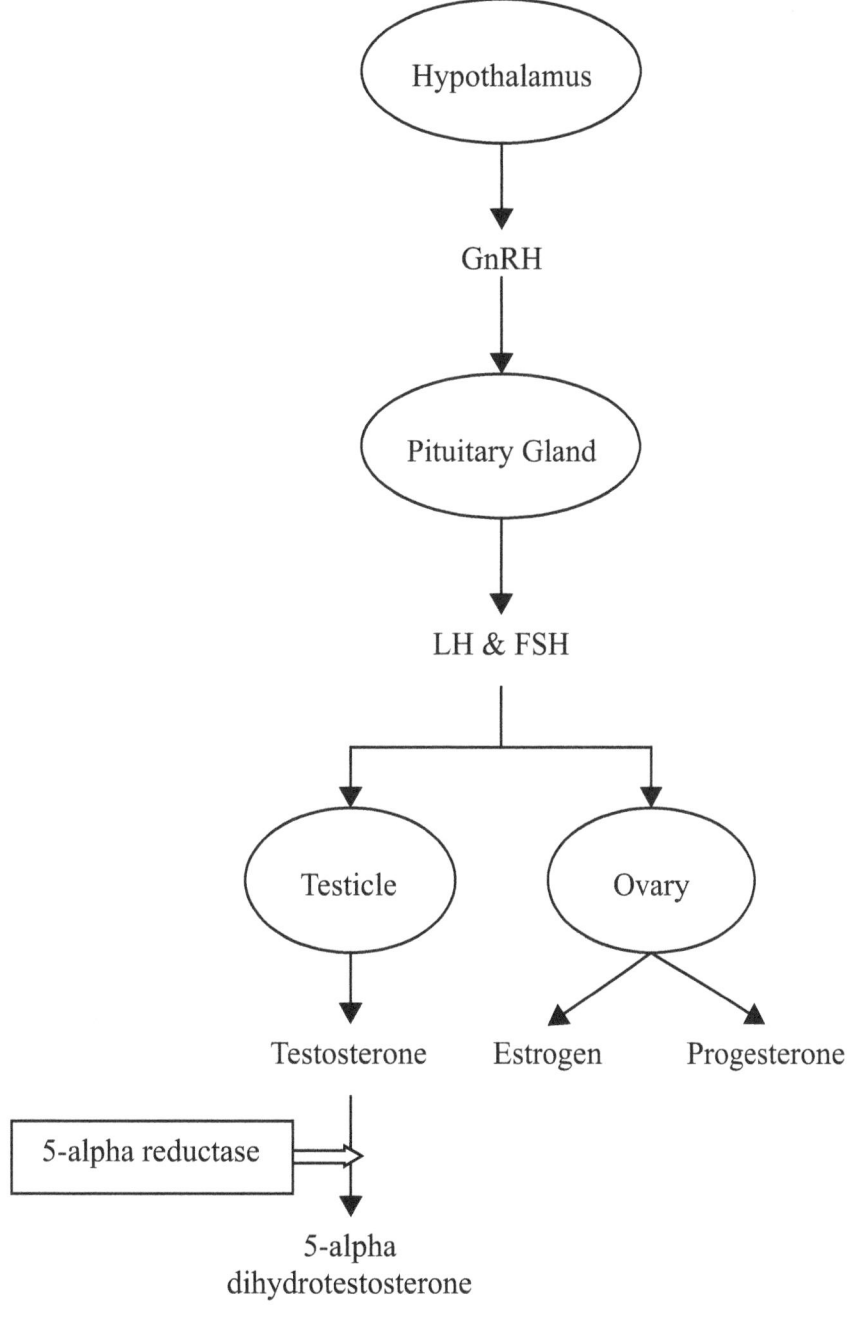

FIGURE 11-1. Hormones of the human reproductive system. The hypothalamus, located in the brain, releases gonadotropin-releasing hormone (GnRH), which signals the pituitary gland. In response to GnRH, the pituitary gland releases luteinizing hormone (LH) and follicle-stimulating hormone (FSH). In the male body, LH and FSH signal the testes to release testosterone. Once released, testosterone can be converted into 5-alpha dihydrotestosterone by the enzyme 5-alpha reductase. In females, LH and FSH signal the ovaries to release estrogen and/or progesterone.

The testes, the main sex organs of the male reproductive system, are responsible for producing male sex hormones called androgens (Figure 11-2). The main androgen is the hormone testosterone. The testes are also responsible for the production of sperm cells. In normal male reproduction, LH and FSH are released by the pituitary gland to stimulate the cells inside of the testes to produce testosterone. In response to the increase in testosterone levels, sperm formation and maturation begins after puberty. In males, this process of hormone release and sperm production can continue until death. Another important part of the male reproductive system is the prostate gland. The prostate itself is donut shaped and surrounds a portion of the urethra. It is responsible for making fluids that will be secreted into the semen to help activate sperm movement.

The ovaries are the main sex organs of the female reproductive system. Figure 11-3 illustrates the major parts of the female reproductive system, including the ovaries. Similar to the testes in males that produce sperm, in females, the main function of the ovaries is to produce eggs for fertilization. The ovaries are also responsible for secreting the main female sex hormones, estrogens and progesterone. When GnRH is released by the hypothalamus in the female body, it triggers the release of LH and FSH by the pituitary gland as well. LH and FSH are released in different amounts at various times in the female body to regulate the release of estrogens and progesterone from the ovaries, stimulate ovulation, and to control other parts of the female reproductive system.

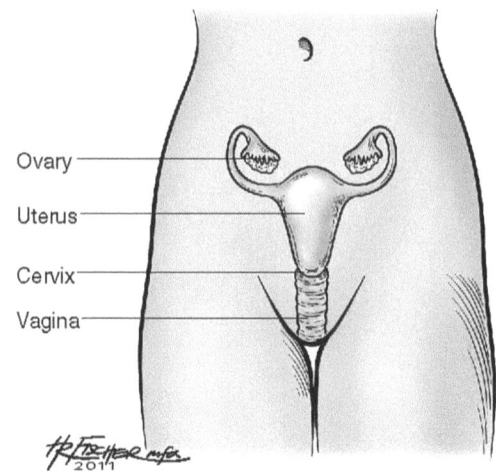

FIGURE 11-3. Female reproductive anatomy. The major parts of the female reproductive system.

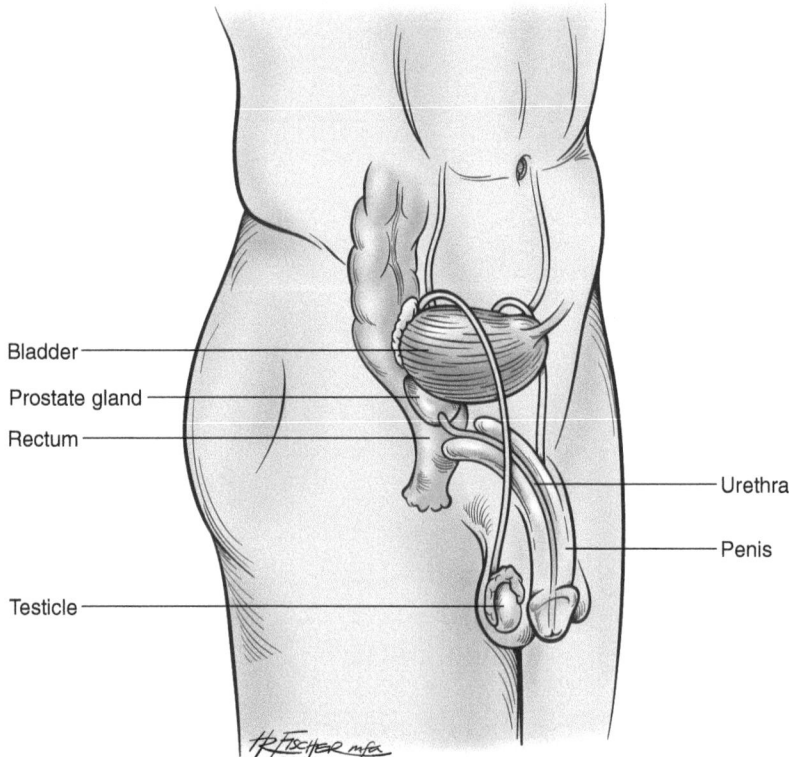

FIGURE 11-2. Male reproductive anatomy. The major parts of the male reproductive anatomy and also neighboring parts such as the bladder and rectum.

This repeating cycle of hormonal changes and egg release in the female is also known as menstruation or the menstrual cycle. In females, each menstrual cycle is approximately 28 days and will continue to repeat itself from puberty until menopause. It is during this period of a female's life, when menstruation occurs, that a pregnancy can be maintained.[1,2]

PHYSIOLOGIC EFFECTS OF THE REPRODUCTIVE HORMONES

The major sex hormones in the human body are estrogens, progesterone, and androgens. Each of these hormones plays a crucial role in either the male or female body to maintain a healthy reproductive system. To understand why medications are prescribed to affect the reproductive system, it is important to know the function of each of these hormones in the human body.

Estrogens

Estrogens are a group of hormones that act as the primary sex hormones involved in the female reproductive system. There are three main estrogens naturally produced by the female body. The most common estrogen produced is estradiol and the other two important estrogens are estrone and estriol. The estrogens' main function is to maintain normal development of the female internal and external reproductive parts. They are also responsible for the development and maintenance of female sex characteristics. Estrogens are needed for proper breast development, growth of pubic and underarm hair, and fat distribution. They also have nonreproductive effects on bone health, blood clotting, and cholesterol levels.[2]

Progesterone

Progesterone is another major hormone that is important for the female reproductive system. In the female body, progesterone is important for maintaining normal ovulation and plays an important role in maintaining a healthy pregnancy until full term. Progesterone levels are highest when a female is pregnant. Outside of the reproductive system, progesterone can also affect metabolism and body temperature.[2]

Androgens

Androgens are the main male sex hormones. The main active androgen produced is testosterone. Testosterone can be broken down in the body into inactive products that are eliminated by the body or converted into other active hormones that play a role in the human reproductive system. For example, testosterone can be converted by the liver into estrogens. 5-alpha dihydrotestosterone is another important androgen found in the male body that is created from testosterone by an enzyme called 5-alpha reductase. Testosterone and 5-alpha dihydrotestosterone are predominately involved in male reproduction and the development of male sex characteristics. They have many functions in the male body, such as maintaining proper growth and development of the male sex organs. Throughout adolescence and adulthood, testosterone regulates bone and muscle development and growth, sperm cell maturation, deepening of the voice, body hair growth patterns, sexual drive and performance, and aggressive behavior. In addition, testosterone also has effects on red blood cell production and cholesterol levels.[1,2]

CASE STUDY

Samantha Jones is a 16-year-old female who comes to the pharmacy with her first prescription for Tri-Sprintec®. She went to her gynecologist with complaints of heavy menstrual periods, menstrual cramps, and migraines every month related to menses. In addition, she is in a relationship and interested in an effective form of contraception. She has no medical conditions and is not currently taking any medications.

CONTRACEPTION

Based on the known physiologic effects of both estrogen and progesterone, a combination product of both hormones was initially approved by the Food and Drug Administration (FDA) in 1960 for the treatment of menstrual disorders and infertility. This combination, Enovid®, was found to prevent unplanned pregnancy by inhibiting normal mechanisms for menstrual cycle control and ovulation. Since then, Enovid® has been withdrawn from the market and newer contraceptives have been developed. Newer contraceptives are intended to improve efficacy, minimize side effects, facilitate adherence, and decrease the frequency of menstrual periods. Pharmaceutical contraceptives are now available as transdermal, intravaginal, injectable, implantable, and intrauterine, as well as oral dosage forms. In addition to providing an effective means of contraception, hormonal contraceptive agents also provide noncontraceptive benefits, including regulation of the menstrual cycle, reduction of menstrual symptoms, protection against endometrial and ovarian cancers, and improvement of acne.[3,4]

Combined Hormonal Contraceptives

Combined hormonal contraceptives (COCs) contain two hormones: estrogen and progesterone (see Medication Table 11-1 for examples; Medication Tables are located at the end of the chapter). Estrogen exerts its contraceptive effects by inhibiting the release of FSH from the pituitary gland (discussed at length in Chapter 8), resulting in the inhibition of egg formation and maturation. This leads to subsequent prevention of ovulation. Estrogen also improves menstrual cycle control by stabilizing the endometrium and minimizing breakthrough bleeding. The progesterone component of hormonal contraceptives provides contraceptive activity through several mechanisms. Progesterone blocks the activity of LH to inhibit ovulation, thickens cervical mucus to decrease sperm motility, and thins the endometrium making it a less suitable environment for implantation.[4]

CASE?

What phasic formulation is Samantha's COC?

COCs are the most widely used form of hormonal contraception in the United States. Although some COCs contain the estrogen named mestranol or estradiol valerate, most COCs contain a synthetic estrogen named ethinyl estradiol, which varies in dose based on the product. Standard doses of ethinyl estradiol range from 30–35 mcg and are considered low dose, while COCs that contain 20–25 mcg of ethinyl estradiol are considered very low dose. The progesterone (also referred to as progestins) component of COCs can vary greatly according to dose and type. The various progestins used in COCs differ in their estrogenic, androgenic, and progestogenic effects.

COC regimens can be categorized as monophasic, biphasic, triphasic, or four-phasic. Monophasic COCs contain the same amount of estrogen and progesterone in each active pill. Biphasic pills contain the same amount of estrogen but two different doses of progestin depending where in the cycle they are to be taken. Triphasic pills provide escalating estrogen and/or progestin doses weekly for 3 consecutive

---

ALERT!

Because many pill packs contain placebo pills during the last week of the regimen and even varying amounts of hormone in the initial weeks, it is important for patients to take contraceptive pills sequentially. Active pills of different strengths and placebo pills can usually be distinguished by a difference in color.

---

weeks, with the goal of decreasing breakthrough bleeding and amenorrhea. At the time of writing, there is only one 4-phasic contraceptive available, which contains four different dose combinations over a 28-day cycle. Studies have shown no difference in contraceptive efficacy between these regimens, but a possible reduction in dose-dependent adverse effects may be achieved.

The standard cycle for COCs is 28 days (21 days of active pills and 7 days of placebo pills). This regimen was devised to mimic the average natural menstrual cycle of a nonpregnant female. Using this regimen, women experience a monthly menstrual period during the placebo week.

Some COCs have been designed to alter the frequency and/or duration of menses. These agents are also referred to as extended- or continuous-cycle oral contraceptive regimens. Extended- and continuous-cycle regimens typically shorten the menstrual cycle, decrease the frequency of menses to four times per year, or eliminate menses altogether. As a result, these regimens may be beneficial for patients with menstrual-related conditions such as menstrual migraines, cramps, or endometriosis.[4]

ALERT!

LOOK-ALIKE/SOUND-ALIKE—Although several similarities exist between Seasonale®, Seasonique®, and LoSeasonique®, they are not interchangeable and should not be substituted for one another without contacting the prescribing physician.

Seasonale®, Seasonique®, and LoSeasonique® are examples of extended-cycle regimens. Seasonale® contains 84 days of active pills and 7 days of placebo pills (84/7), while Seasonique® contains 84 days of active pills and 7 days of low-dose ethinyl estradiol. LoSeasonique® contains 84 active tablets but with lower doses of both the estrogen and progesterone components compared to Seasonale® and Seasonique®. Similar to Seasonique®, LoSeasonique® also contains 7 days of low-dose ethinyl estradiol in place of placebo. Using either of these regimens, women reduce the frequency of menses to four times per year.[5]

Yaz®, Minastrin 24 Fe®, and Lo Loestrin Fe® are also considered extended-cycle regimens because they have more than 21 days of active hormone. Yaz® contains 24 days of active pills and 4 days of placebo pills (24/4), while Minastrin 24 Fe® contains 24 days of active pills and 4 days of an iron supplement called ferrous fumarate. Lo Loestrin Fe® contains a lower dose of estrogen compared to Minastrin 24 Fe® and has 26 active pills. Using these regimens, women experience a monthly menstrual period but with a lighter flow and shorter duration.[4,6]

ALERT!

Caution should be taken not to confuse Yaz® *with* Yasmin 28® or Loestrin 21 1/20® *with* Loestrin 21 1.5/30®, Loestrin FE 1/20®, or Loestrin FE 1.5/30.® Yasmin 28®, Loestrin 21 1/20®, and Loestrin 21 1.5/30® are not considered extended-cycle regimens and contain different doses of estrogen and/or progestin.

Amethyst® is a continuous-cycle contraceptive. This product is packaged as a 28-day pill pack, but each package contains 28 days of active pills to be taken continuously for 1 year without a placebo. Although women using Amethyst® do not get a scheduled menstrual bleed, women may experience breakthrough bleeding or spotting during the first 3–6 months of use.[7]

Common side effects associated with COCs are related to the dose of estrogen and the activity of the progestin. Estrogenic effects include nausea, breast tenderness, increased blood pressure, and headache. Progestogenic effects include breast tenderness, headache, fatigue, and mood changes. Androgenic effects, due to the progestin component, include increased appetite, weight gain, acne, oily skin, hirsutism, and cholesterol abnormalities. In addition to these common side effects, patients should be counseled regarding the possibility for more serious adverse effects. Although not common in younger women, estrogen and progestin can increase a woman's risk for blood clots,

heart attacks, and strokes. These risks are further increased in older women, smokers, women who are genetically more prone to forming blood clots, those with existing high blood pressure or cholesterol, or those with certain migraine syndromes.[4]

CASE?

Based on Samantha's symptoms of heavy menstrual periods, menstrual cramps, and monthly migraines related to menses, do you think some physicians might prescribe a different COC for her? Why or why not?

PRACTICE POINT

The acronym ACHES can be used to help patients remember what symptoms may indicate a more serious side effect (A = abdominal pain— severe; C = chest pain—severe; H = headaches— severe; E = eye problems; S = severe leg pains).[4] Patients experiencing any of these symptoms should be advised to seek medical attention.

Initiation of COCs can occur a few different ways: Day 1 Start, Sunday Start, and Quick Start. Using the Day 1 Start, patients take the first pill of the COC on the first day of their menstrual period. The Sunday Start method involves starting COCs on the first Sunday after the start of their menstrual period. Using this method of initiation, women may avoid having their menstrual period on the weekends. More recently, the Quick Start regimen has been recommended. Using this regimen, women begin taking their first pill the same day they see their physician, which may help improve adherence. For women initiating COCs using the Sunday Start or Quick Start regimens, 7 days of backup contraception is recommended.

Examples of non-oral combined hormonal contraceptives include the patch and the intravaginal ring. Both of these products offer alternatives for patients who have difficulty remembering to take COCs on a regular basis. The two intravaginal rings available are NuvaRing® and Annovera®. NuvaRing® is a flexible vaginal ring that releases 15 mcg of ethinyl estradiol and 120 mcg of etonogestrel per day.

It is available in a single size that can easily be inserted and removed at home and does not require fitting. NuvaRing® should be inserted between days 1 and 5 of the menstrual cycle. Each contraceptive ring is worn for 3 consecutive weeks followed by a 1-week, ring-free period. A new contraceptive ring is inserted 1 week after the previous ring was removed. If the user forgets to remove the ring on time, the NuvaRing® has the ability to provide protection for up to four weeks. A new ring should be inserted after a 1-week, ring-free period. Adverse effects are similar to that of COCs; however, NuvaRing® is associated with more vaginal complaints (inflammation, discomfort, and infections).[4] Prior to dispensing, NuvaRing® should be stored in the refrigerator (2°C to 8°C). Once dispensed to a patient, NuvaRing® can be kept at room temperature for up to 4 months.[8] Annovera® is a silicone vaginal ring that releases 13 mcg of ethinyl estradiol and 150 mcg of segesterone acetate per day. Annovera® is unique because it can be used for 13 cycles, unlike the NuvaRing®, which is discarded after one use. Annovera® should be stored in a black container during the 1-week, ring-free period. The black container is provided when the drug is dispensed to the patient.[9]

PRACTICE POINT

Caution should be taken if either of the rings slip out. If the NuvaRing® slips out or is left out for 3 hours or less, it can be rinsed with cool or lukewarm water and reinserted without losing effectiveness. Similar handling instructions apply to Annovera®; however, the maximum time is 2 hours. If the ring is left out for longer or if the duration is unknown, patients should rinse the ring, reinsert, and use a backup form of contraception for 1 week.[8,9]

Xulane® is a contraceptive patch that releases 150 mcg per day of norelgestromin and 35 mcg per day of ethinyl estradiol. Xulane® is dispensed in a package of three patches. The patch can be started using the Day 1 Start or Sunday Start methods. If therapy starts after the first day of the menstrual cycle, a backup form of contraception is recommended for the first 7 days of the first treatment cycle. Women should apply one patch every week and replace it with a new patch for 3 consecutive weeks. Each patch is removed and replaced on the same day of the week, also referred to as the Patch Change Day. A 1-week, patch-free interval allows for a menstrual period.

If a patch is partially or completely detached for less than 24 hours, a patient can use the same patch if it still contains adhesive. The Patch Change Day will remain the same. If the patch is partially or completely detached for more than 24 hours, a new patch should be applied immediately and 7 days of backup contraception is recommended. As a result, there is a new Patch Change Day. Side effects are similar to COCs, with the exception of increased breast tenderness during the first 2 months of use and skin irritation at the application site. Xulane® may be less effective in women weighing more than 90 kg (198 lb). Therefore, an alternative form of contraception may be preferred in these women.[10]

ALERT!

Although an estrogen patch is worn for 7 consecutive days, active hormone is still present after the patch is removed. Therefore, women should be reminded to fold the patch in half when discarding to minimize the potential for ingestion by or exposure to children, pets, or anyone else. Women should avoid the use of lotions or occlusive dressings at the patch application site.

Patient education is extremely important for patients initiating combined hormonal contraception. Written and verbal information regarding proper use of the medications, common and serious side effects, management of side effects, and when to seek medical attention must be provided, and the FDA requires a medication guide for these. While combined hormonal contraceptives provide an effective form of contraception, some women must be reminded that they do not protect against transmission of sexually transmitted diseases (STDs), including human immunodeficiency virus (HIV). Information about how to initiate the various combined hormonal products (oral, intravaginal, transdermal) should be provided, as well as potential drug interactions (discussed below), which may decrease contraceptive efficacy. The importance of routine daily administration should be stressed, including suggestions on how to improve adherence (ie, alarms, calendars, associating medication administration with a daily routine, etc.). For patients interested in getting pregnant, return to fertility after discontinuing combined hormonal contraceptives is immediate, with an average delay to ovulation of 1–2 weeks.

PRACTICE POINT

Patients taking combined hormonal contraceptives can expect their menses to start 1–3 days after their last hormone exposure. Subsequent cycles of combined hormonal contraceptives should start every 28 days even if menses is not completed. Spotting is common during the first 1–3 months of starting a hormonal contraceptive.

Progestin-Only Contraceptives

Progestin-only products may be prescribed for women who are not good candidates for COCs or those who are breastfeeding. Similar to COCs, several formulations of progestin-only products exist, including oral, injectable, intrauterine, and subdermal.

Oral progestin-only products are referred to as progestin-only pills (POPs) or "mini-pills." They contain lower progestin doses compared to progestins contained in COCs and no estrogen. When taken correctly, POPs are as effective as COCs in protecting against pregnancy. Examples include Ortho Micronor® and Norlyroc®. Like COCs, POPs are packaged as 28-day pill packs; however, each pill contains active hormone and none may be skipped or discarded. POPs can be initiated anytime during the menstrual cycle. Although women taking POPs experience less menstrual bleeding overall, side effects include irregular menses that range from amenorrhea to increased days of spotting and bleeding.

Depo-Provera® is an injectable progestin-only contraceptive agent. It is a good option for women who are not candidates for COCs, have difficulty remembering to take pills on a daily basis, or want a contraceptive agent that is convenient and discrete. Depo-Provera® may be administered by patients themselves or in a physician's office every 3 months. Since this form of contraception relies little on patient cooperation, it is highly effective. Depo-Provera® is injected either intramuscularly (IM) in the gluteal or deltoid muscles or subcutaneously (SUBQ) in the thigh or abdomen. Side effects include irregular bleeding with eventual amenorrhea, breast tenderness, weight gain (average 1 kg annually), and decrease in bone mass. Return to fertility after discontinuation of Depo-Provera® may be delayed for approximately 9 months.[11]

PRACTICE POINT

Women using Depo-Provera® are often advised to consume 1,200–1,500 mg of calcium and 400 International Units of vitamin D daily through diet and/or supplementation to minimize risks for decreased bone mineral density and osteoporosis.

Mirena®, Kyleena®, Liletta®, and Skyla® are examples of intrauterine progestin-only contraceptive agents that provide another alternative for women who cannot take pills on a regular basis. It is a T-shaped contraceptive device that requires an office visit for physician insertion and removal from the uterine cavity. Mirena®, Kyleena®, and Liletta® are effective forms of contraception that last up to 5 years. Skyla® is effective for up to 3 years. In addition to being a highly effective contraceptive agent, Mirena® can also be beneficial in patients with dysmenorrhea, menorrhagia, anemia related to heavy menses, or endometriosis. The other agents have not been formally evaluated for these indications. Bleeding abnormalities are common during the first 3 months of use; however, with continued use patients experience amenorrhea. Side effects include headaches, acne, breast tenderness, and moodiness. Complications associated with the use of intrauterine devices include an increased risk for pelvic inflammatory disease, uterine perforations (incidence of 0–1.3 per 1,000 insertions), and expulsion (about 5% of users).[12-15]

PRACTICE POINT

Women using intrauterine devices should receive information about possible complications. The acronym PAINS is often used (P = period late— abnormal spotting or bleeding; A = abdominal pain—pain after intercourse; I = infection exposure (sexually transmitted infections)—abnormal vaginal discharge; N = not feeling well—fever, chills; S = string missing—shorter or longer).

Nexplanon® is the only subdermal contraceptive available on the U.S. market. It is a single implantable rod that is made of a nonbiodegradable solid composed of ethylene vinyl acetate that is just over 1.5 inches long and less than 1/10 inch in diameter. Each implantable rod contains 68 mg of etonogestrel and is effective for 3 years. Initially, Nexplanon® releases 60–70 mcg etonogestrel daily and decreases to 25–30 mcg etonogestrel daily by the end of 3 years. Nexplanon® is inserted just under the skin above the elbow of the nondominant arm. Both insertion and removal must occur in the physician's office. Although Nexplanon® is associated with unpredictable and irregular bleeding initially, many patients transition to amenorrhea. As a result, Nexplanon® may be beneficial for patients with dysmenorrhea and anemia related to menorrhagia. Nexplanon® is associated with an immediate return to fertility after removal. Depo-Provera®, intrauterine devices, and Nexplanon® are sometimes prescribed for patients who are nonadherent as these methods of contraception require little patient effort.[16]

PRACTICE POINT

The use of reminder systems should be highly encouraged in patients using POPs to maximize compliance and contraceptive efficacy.

Drug-Drug Interactions

To preserve contraceptive efficacy, women should be made aware of the potential for drug-drug interactions. Medications have the potential to minimize contraceptive efficacy by interfering with gastrointestinal absorption, reducing intestinal reabsorption by altering gut bacteria, and increasing breakdown of the estrogens and progestins contained in hormonal contraceptives. In general, the lower the dose of hormones contained in the contraceptive agent, the greater the risk for compromised efficacy.

CASE?

Samantha is picking up a 10-day prescription for amoxicillin, an antibiotic, and is concerned about possible contraceptive failure. What might the pharmacist advise her to do?

Medications that have been shown to interact with contraceptives include some HIV medications, anticonvulsants, and certain antibiotics. Anticonvulsants that have been implicated include carbamazepine (Tegretol®), phenytoin (Dilantin®), primidone (Mysoline®), and phenobarbital. The interaction between antibiotics and hormonal contraceptives can vary based on the antibiotic and on the individual patient. The interactions with rifampin (Rifadin®) and griseofulvin are most significant. It is recommended that women using either of these medications use an additional form of contraception during the course of treatment and for 4 weeks afterward.[17] Studies of other antibiotics have shown less of an impact on contraceptive efficacy. Despite the potential lower risk for contraceptive failure, it is generally recommended that women use a backup form of contraception during the course of antibiotic treatment and for 1 week afterward as a precaution in patients receiving less than 30 mcg of ethinyl estradiol or 150 mcg of levonorgestrel.[18]

Hormone-Free Contraceptives

Paragard® is a copper intrauterine device that can be used for the prevention of pregnancy or emergency contraception. Paragard® releases copper ions, which cause inflammation to prevent the movement of sperm to the egg. Like the other intrauterine devices, Paragard® is inserted by a trained healthcare professional in a clinic. Paragard® has similar warnings to the other intrauterine devices. One main difference is that Paragard® is contraindicated in patients with Wilson's disease, a disorder in which copper builds up in the body. Paragard® can be inserted for up to 10 years.[19]

Nonoxynol 9 is an over-the-counter medication that is available as a vaginal gel, suppository, sponge, film, and foam. Nonoxynol 9 works as a spermicide to stop sperm from moving. Spermicide can be irritating and may cause urinary tract infections. Patients should be counseled to review the individual instructions on the packaging since there are many different products available.[20]

CASE?

Samantha comes to the pharmacy frantically on a Saturday morning and says she has been forgetting to take her birth control and she had unprotected intercourse. She would like to purchase Plan B One Step®. What might the pharmacist tell her?

Emergency Contraception

Emergency contraception (EC) can be used to prevent pregnancy after a known or suspected failure of contraception or unprotected intercourse. It can be up to 90% effective in reducing the pregnancy rate when used within 72 hours of unprotected intercourse. Studies suggest that the primary mechanism of action of EC is the inhibition or delay of ovulation, or inhibition of fertilization and/or implantation. The Yuzpe method, Plan B One Step®, Ella®, and insertion of an intrauterine copper contraceptive are all FDA-approved methods of emergency contraception.

The Yuzpe method allows women to take their regular oral contraceptive pills as an emergency contraceptive regimen. This method requires patients to take multiple pills to equal 100 mcg of ethinyl estradiol and 0.5 mg of levonorgestrel per dose, administered as two doses 12 hours apart. Depending on the product they take at home, patients may have to take 4 to 6 pills with each dose. The Yuzpe method is approximately 75% effective in reducing the incidence of unplanned pregnancies. The most common adverse effect associated with the Yuzpe method is nausea. Many patients are counseled to take an antiemetic 1 hour before the EC dose is taken.[21]

Plan B One-Step® is a common EC agent. Plan B One-Step® is associated with nausea and vomiting but at a much lower rate compared to the Yuzpe method. Other side effects associated with Plan B One-Step® use include irregular bleeding and, less frequently, dizziness, fatigue, breast tenderness, headache, and abdominal pain. In 2014, the FDA announced that Plan B One-Step® and its generic products would be available over the counter without age limitations.

These products no longer need to be kept behind the pharmacy counter and can be stocked in the family planning section of the pharmacy.[21,22]

Ella® is a prescription-only medication. While it may be more effective than Plan B One-Step®, it is often harder for patients to get since it is not stocked as routinely as Plan B One-Step® and its generics.[23] Ella® should be taken within 5 days of unprotected sex. Adverse effects associated with Ella® are similar to other products and include headache, nausea, abnormal bleeding, and dizziness.[24]

ALERT!

If the patient vomits within 2 or 3 hours of taking a dose of the EC (Yuzpe or any Plan B®) the dose should be repeated.[22]

PRACTICE POINT

It is not required that Plan B One-Step® be purchased by the patient herself; it can be purchased by men and women.

Yuzpe, Plan B One-Step®, and Ella® should not be used as a regular form of contraception. They are also not effective for women who are pregnant.[21]

POSTMENOPAUSAL HORMONE THERAPY

CASE STUDY

Paula Smith is a 52-year-old female who is picking up her blood pressure medications. She is complaining of several episodes of feeling hot and flushed throughout the day and waking up sweating at night and tells you a few of her friends are also "going through the change."

As women age, their ovaries become less active and production of estrogen decreases. The changes are associated with alterations in the menstrual cycle, including a change in cycle length or skipped menstrual periods, known as perimenopause. Perimenopause typically lasts 1 to 2 years during which time menstrual periods become further apart and finally cease. After 12 consecutive months of amenorrhea, a woman is considered to be experiencing menopause. Most women experience menopause between the ages of 44 and 55, the average age is 50 to 52.[25] Women who have had a hysterectomy are likely to have an earlier menopause. Symptoms associated with menopause and perimenopause are similar and can be categorized as vasomotor, psychological, or sexual.

Vasomotor symptoms, including hot flashes and night sweats, are commonly associated with low estrogen levels. Hot flashes occur spontaneously and can manifest as a sensation of warmth, which is accompanied by skin flushing and perspiration. A chill may follow afterward as the body temperature drops. When occurring at night hot flashes can cause insomnia, which may result in daytime sedation and difficulty concentrating. The frequency and severity of symptoms can vary, with some women experiencing occasional symptoms while other women may experience multiple hot flashes throughout the day. Vasomotor symptoms can have a profound impact on quality of life and can have a psychological impact, including depression, irritability, and anxiety. For most women, vasomotor symptoms are most pronounced during the first two postmenopausal years and will resolve spontaneously within 5 years of onset. However, some women will continue to experience symptoms beyond 5 years.

CASE?

What is likely causing the symptoms Paula is experiencing?

In addition to vasomotor symptoms and subsequent psychological manifestations, women may also have vaginal changes. Dryness, atrophic vaginitis, a vaginal inflammation related to thinning tissues, and dyspareunia, painful intercourse, are common for postmenopausal women.

Treatment of menopausal issues focuses on symptomatic relief, improvement in quality of life, and minimizing the risk of side effects and complications relating to therapy. For some women, lifestyle modifications such as exercise, weight control, smoking cessation, and a healthy diet can effectively manage postmenopausal symptoms. Complementary and alternative therapies such as black cohosh should not be recommended to patients. They have not been shown to reduce hot flashes and some carry a risk of hepatotoxicity.

For many women, estrogen therapy is needed to restore low hormone levels and provide postmenopausal symptomatic relief.[26]

CASE?

Paula mentions that she has read a lot of "scary stuff" about hormone replacement therapy, and she does not currently want to even discuss it with her doctor. What remedies might she be able to try on her own? Should she still be directed to see her physician?

Hormone therapy (HT), including estrogen-only and estrogen–progestin combinations, has been the mainstay of menopausal and postmenopausal management for more than 50 years (Medication Table 11-2 lists examples). Estrogen is FDA approved for the treatment of moderate to severe vasomotor symptoms, moderate to severe symptoms of vulvar and vaginal atrophy (such as dryness, itching, and burning), and the prevention of postmenopausal osteoporosis. Several products, formulations, and routes of administration are available for estrogen, including oral; transdermal; intravaginal tablets, rings, gels, and creams; and sprays. The oral and transdermal routes are the most frequently used form of estrogen administration by women whose major complaints are vasomotor symptoms. Local products such as intravaginal tablets, rings, gels, and creams are reserved for women with vaginal complaints such as dryness and pain. The decision regarding the product, route, and method of delivery of estrogen should be made with the patient and her physician to ensure optimal acceptability and adherence.

Oral estrogen replacement products include conjugated equine estrogens (prepared from the urine of pregnant mares), synthetic conjugated estrogens, esterified estrogens, estropipate, and estradiol. When administered via the oral route, estrogens are absorbed into the circulatory system and broken down by the liver. Transdermal administration and use of some intravaginal rings may yield a slightly better side effect profile as less estrogen reaches the systemic circulation.[26]

CASE?

Paula Smith has not had a menstrual period in more than 12 months. Is she a candidate for estrogen therapy?

Dosage requirements for estrogen depend on the individual and therapy is usually started with the lowest dose that provides effective relief of symptoms. Vasomotor symptoms may begin to improve within 1 to 2 weeks. Side effects of estrogen therapy include nausea, headache, breast tenderness, and heavy bleeding. Serious side effects include increased risk for coronary heart disease, stroke, venous thromboembolism, breast cancer, and cholecystitis.[26]

> ## ALERT!
>
> For women prescribed HT, estrogen and progesterone may be prescribed as separate medications or combination products. These products may have similar names so caution must be used to avoid dispensing the wrong product. Premarin® is an estrogen-only product available in several doses. Prempro® and Premphase® are both estrogen–progestin combination oral products. However, Prempro® contains a continuous dose of progesterone while Premphase® contains an intermittent dose of progesterone. They must not be interchanged unless authorized by the physician.

HT is usually considered to be contraindicated in women with the following conditions: current, past, or suspected breast cancer; known or suspected progesterone- or estrogen-dependent cancers; undiagnosed vaginal bleeding; untreated endometrial hyperplasia; previous or current clotting disorders; coronary heart disease, stroke, untreated high blood pressure; and active liver disease. When HT is dispensed, women must receive information about the potential risks and benefits associated with HT and when to seek medical attention.

In women with a uterus, progesterone should be added to the estrogen regimen to reduce the risk for endometrial cancer. Progesterone may be given intermittently or continuously. Intermittent dosing usually involves progesterone administration for 12–14 days every month or every 2–6 months and may be preferred to minimize overall hormone exposure. Continuous dosing involves daily administration of progesterone. Progesterone is typically given orally, although some combination products (with estrogen) are available in other formulations and contain various types of progesterone. Examples of progestin-only products include medroxyprogesterone (Provera®) and micronized progesterone (Prometrium®). Side effects may vary depending on the agent prescribed and the most common include irritability, depression, and mood swings. Other side effects are bloating, fluid retention, and sleep disturbance. Switching from an intermittent to a continuous regimen or from one progestin to another may reduce the incidence or severity of symptoms.

Vaginal creams, gels, rings, or tablets are available for intravaginal (local) administration of HT. These are often effective for patients with complaints of vaginal dryness, atrophic vaginitis, and dyspareunia. Although this route of administration results in some systemic absorption, significant systemic exposure is limited. Progesterone is generally not needed when estrogen is prescribed at low doses and administered vaginally. An exception is the vaginal ring, Femring®, which delivers high levels of estrogen to the body. Improvement in vaginal symptoms may take months of estrogen therapy. Nonhormonal vaginal moisturizers and lubricants can also be used to provide symptomatic relief of postmenopausal vaginal complaints of mild intensity. These products can be used alone or in combination with local administration of HT.

> ## ALERT!
>
> Some intravaginal estrogen products contain oils that can weaken latex condoms. The patient should check with the pharmacist or their prescriber if this precaution applies to the product they are prescribed.

Although controversial, the use of testosterone in women is becoming more widespread. In addition to estrogen and progesterone deficiency commonly seen in postmenopausal women, androgen deficiency has also been proposed. Symptoms that may be associated with androgen deficiency include a diminished sense of well-being, persistent or unexplained fatigue, decreased libido, decreased sexual receptivity, and decreased sexual pleasure. The use of testosterone therapy in women will be discussed in a later section of this chapter, "Testosterone Therapy in Females."[26]

INFERTILITY

Infertility is typically defined as a failure to achieve pregnancy after 1 year of frequent, unprotected intercourse and affects about 10% to 15% of couples in the United States. Factors that can influence fertility include a history of previous fertility problems for the couple and each partner individually, frequency and timing of intercourse, impaired sperm quality or quantity, hypogonadism, ovulation disorders, disorders that affect the fallopian tubes, and uterine or cervical factors. This section focuses on the management of infertility of the female partner, specifically ovulation disorders.[27,28]

For more than 40 years, clomiphene citrate has been the first-line treatment for infertility due to ovulatory disorders. Although clomiphene citrate is very effective in inducing ovulation, pregnancy rates are only 10% to 40%. In women who conceive after a course of clomiphene citrate, there is a 10% to 20% chance of a multiple pregnancy. Clomiphene citrate is taken orally and is easy to use. The starting dose is typically 50 mg daily (one tablet) for 5 days starting on the fifth day of the menstrual cycle. If ovulation does not occur, the dose is increased to 100 mg daily (two 50-mg tablets given as a single dose) and may be started as early as 30 days after the previous dose. Increasing the dose or the duration of therapy beyond 100 mg/day for 5 days is not recommended.

For pregnancies associated with clomiphene citrate use, the risk for birth defects is reported to be the same as for the general population. The most common side effects are ovarian enlargement, flushing, abdominal problems (pelvic discomfort/distention/bloating, nausea, vomiting) breast discomfort, and visual disturbances. These side effects are mild and temporary and usually disappear after therapy is discontinued.

Women should be counseled about the possibility for ovarian hyperstimulation syndrome (OHHS), which has been reported with clomiphene citrate therapy. OHSS is an exaggerated response to fertility medications. It is a self-limiting disorder that usually resolves spontaneously within several days. Signs and symptoms associated with OHSS can range from mild illness requiring careful observation to severe disease requiring hospitalization and intensive care. Early warning signs include abdominal pain and distention, nausea, vomiting, diarrhea, and weight gain. Women who experience these symptoms should be instructed to seek medical care.[29]

Some women seeking treatment for infertility have a condition known as polycystic ovarian syndrome (PCOS). These patients have developed small cysts on their ovaries and frequently have testosterone levels that are considered above normal. They are usually affected by menstrual irregularities and may also have problems with their heart and blood vessels. Some complain of excessive facial and body hair. In women with PCOS, clomiphene citrate alone may be ineffective for the management of infertility.

Exogenous gonadotropins, such as FSH and LH, can also be used for the management of infertility. These agents are given by injection. Gonadotropins are more effective than clomiphene citrate but are more expensive and are associated with a higher risk for OHSS and multiple pregnancies. Three main types of gonadotropins are available for the management of infertility: human chorionic gonadotropin (hCG), which is similar to LH; human menopausal gonadotropin (hMG), which contains natural FSH and LH purified from the urine of postmenopausal women; and recombinant human follicle-stimulating hormone (rFSH), which is synthesized in a laboratory. Multiple pregnancy is a common complication associated with gonadotropins. Compared to clomiphene citrate, gonadotropins are also associated with a higher risk for OHSS. Although the risk can be minimized by using a lower dose of hCG or a GnRH agonist, the risk cannot be completely eliminated.

Aromatase inhibitors are emerging as a potential replacement for clomiphene citrate as the first-line treatment for ovulation disorders. They are not FDA approved for ovulation stimulation. These agents are orally administered, easy to use, and relatively inexpensive. Traditionally used for the treatment of breast cancer, aromatase inhibitors exert their effect of inducing ovulation by inhibiting the production of estrogen, thus increasing the release of FSH and stimulating the production of eggs from the ovaries. Anastrozole (Arimidex®) and letrozole (Femara®) are examples of aromatase inhibitors. The rate of multiple pregnancies is lower with aromatase inhibitors than with clomiphene citrate. Aromatase inhibitors may also be used in combination with gonadotropins. Side effects are mild (gastrointestinal disturbances, weakness, hot flashes, headache, and back pain).[30]

HYPOGONADISM

Hypogonadism is a condition in which the primary sex organs, or gonads, are not functioning at all or are functioning at an inadequate level. As a result, the gonads fail to produce the reproductive hormones or produce inadequate amounts and cannot maintain development of either sperm or eggs. There are two major types of hypogonadism: primary and secondary. In primary hypogonadism, there is a defect with the gonads themselves, affecting their ability to produce and secrete appropriate amounts of reproductive hormones. Primary hypogonadism can occur due to a genetic or developmental defect. It can also occur when the gonads are damaged in any manner, such as after surgery, radiation exposure, infection, or an autoimmune disorder.

Unlike primary hypogonadism, secondary hypogonadism is not caused by a defect with the gonads themselves but with the glands that help to regulate normal functioning of the gonads. This can occur at the level of the hypothalamus, which is responsible for the release of GnRH, or at the level of the pituitary gland, which releases LH and FSH. Secondary hypogonadism can be caused by cancerous tumors, damage from surgery, radiation exposure, infection, trauma, genetic problems, or nutritional deficiency.

Female Hypogonadism

In females, hypogonadism results in low levels of estrogen. In younger females, this can cause delays in growth and sexual development. Adult females with this condition cannot maintain normal reproductive cycles and experience either irregular menstrual cycles or amenorrhea, and may experience infertility. They are more likely to experience symptoms similar to female menopause, such as hot flashes or painful intercourse. Hormone replacement therapy is the main treatment for female hypogonadism. Both estrogen alone and estrogen–progesterone combination products may be used in females with hypogonadism. Estrogen is also available in combination with testosterone. The regular-strength tablets contain 1.25 mg of esterified estrogens and 2.5 mg of methyltestosterone; there is also a half-strength (H.S.) tablet containing 0.625 mg of esterified estrogens and 1.25 mg of methyltestosterone. Combination therapy with oral estrogen and methyltestosterone carry the same adverse effects and risk as use of either agent alone.

Male Hypogonadism

In males, hypogonadism results when the testes do not produce or release enough testosterone to maintain normal bodily functions that are dependent on testosterone. Besides primary (a problem within the testes) and secondary forms of male hypogonadism (eg, when the pituitary gland does not signal the testes to produce enough testosterone), more recently there has been evidence that points toward hypogonadism occurring as a result of male menopause, also known as andropause. Similar to female menopause, it is thought that during the natural course of aging in males, the level of testosterone produced by the testes decreases dramatically, leading to the same symptoms as hypogonadism. With this condition, there is no defect in the gonads or the hypothalamus or pituitary glands but just the natural decline in hormone production.

The signs and symptoms of low testosterone levels can include depressed mood, decreased muscle mass and/or strength, decreased energy, poor concentration, and sexual dysfunction, including decreased libido or impotence. Health complications that can result from untreated hypogonadism are anemia or low red blood cells, decreased bone density or bone loss that puts patients at increased risk of fractures, and infertility. If hypogonadism occurs in a child before he has completed puberty, the patient may experience a delay or impairment in development. This includes poor pubic or underarm hair growth, small testes and prostate size, decreased muscle development, and a high-pitched voice that fails to deepen. In adult males, particularly older men, with hypogonadism, the condition will be slower to develop and signs and symptoms are less noticeable. For example, adult men may experience decreased prostate size, decrease in muscle mass, sexual dysfunction, and low sperm production and secretion.

Testosterone Therapy in Males

Since the root of the problems associated with hypogonadism are related to the decrease in testosterone production and release, supplementing these patients with testosterone is the primary method of treatment. It is the same concept as HT to treat postmenopausal symptoms in women. In this case, the patient is supplied with an exogenous source of the hormone testosterone to provide what the body is deficient in. Testosterone supplementation is effective at restoring and keeping a patient's testosterone levels within the normal range when given as continuous long-term therapy. Improvement in these symptoms may be noticed by the patient as quickly as a few days after initiation of testosterone supplementation.[31]

Testosterone replacement products are currently available in varying dosage formulations, including oral tablet, intranasal gel, IM injection, SUBQ injection, transdermal patch, transdermal gel, transdermal solution, implantable pellet, and buccal formulation (Medication Table 11-3). Testosterone products are also prescribed off label for many other conditions. One of the more common off-label uses for testosterone products is for sexual dysfunction in men with normal testosterone levels. It is still controversial whether men without hypogonadism who experience sexual dysfunction could benefit from testosterone replacement therapy. In addition, supplementing with testosterone in men with already-normal levels of the hormone may put patients at increased risk for side effects. For this reason, testosterone replacement therapy is not recommended for off-label use in these patients.[31,32]

As with all other drug treatment, testosterone replacement therapy is not without risks or side effects. Adverse effects when used in males can include headache, acne, gynecomastia, abnormal cholesterol levels, fluid retention, and weight gain. Major side effects that may be of concern are liver disease, benign prostatic hyperplasia (BPH), and polycythemia (increase in red blood cell mass). Some of the testosterone formulations carry an FDA black box warning on the increased risk of heart attack, stroke, and cardiovascular death due to blood pressure increases. The intramuscular testosterone undecanoate has an FDA black box warning for serious pulmonary oil microembolism reaction and the product is only available through the Aveed REMS program. All of the testosterone-only replacement products are indicated only for use in males. The use of testosterone replacement therapy is contraindicated in men diagnosed with cancers of the prostate and/or breast, because it may stimulate further growth of the cancer.[32] Each of the various testosterone preparations is unique in its cost, adherence considerations, and application site.

ALERT!

Testosterone preparations are contraindicated in patients who are pregnant or expecting to become pregnant because they have the potential to cause abnormalities in the fetus if administered at any time during pregnancy.

Oral Testosterone Products

Unmodified or natural testosterone is very poorly absorbed in the gut when given orally. Once natural testosterone is absorbed in the gastrointestinal tract, most of it is metabolized by the liver into its inactive forms. Oral formulations

are seldom preferred because they are less effective and are associated with more toxicity than injectable therapies. Besides causing abnormal cholesterol levels, oral formulations are associated with serious liver toxicity that does not typically occur with the other testosterone dosage forms. Damage to the liver can be as severe as the development of liver cancer.

Intramuscular Injection

IM injections have traditionally been the preferred route of administration for testosterone replacement therapy. They are inexpensive and they can be dosed at longer time intervals. Testosterone cypionate (Depo-Testosterone®) and testosterone enanthate are two available testosterone preparations available in the United States for IM injection. Testosterone undecanoate (Aveed®), which is even longer acting, is more expensive. The injections are formulated as oil solutions to help prolong the time of absorption and are considered long-acting preparations. Testosterone enanthate and testosterone cypionate are typically dosed every 1 to 2 weeks. Testosterone undecanoate can be dosed every 10 weeks. The injectable testosterone products are only formulated to be given as deep IM injections

ALERT!

Injectable testosterone vials should be stored at room temperature (between 68°F and 77°F). Multiple-dose vials should always be visually inspected before dispensing and prior to administration for discoloration and contaminates. When stored at temperatures lower than 68°F, crystals may form in the solution. Warming the vial by gently rolling it in the palm of the hands may help to dissolve these crystals prior to administration.

to the buttock muscle. They should not be administered at alternate (nonrecommended) sites and should never be administered SUBQ or intravenously. The disadvantage to IM injections is that administration can be painful and the dosage form may be poorly accepted by patients who fear injections and find them to be invasive.[32]

Transdermal Patches

The transdermal patch (Androderm®) allows delivery of testosterone through normal skin layers into the bloodstream. It is recommended that this patch be applied to the skin on the upper arms, abdomen, back, or thighs, once daily in the evening. The most common side effect with the transdermal patch is local skin irritation at the site of patch application, specifically itching and redness. Although the testosterone patches are much less invasive then the injections, the disadvantage with this type of testosterone therapy is that it is also much more expensive.[33,34]

> ### PRACTICE POINT
>
> *Patients using the transdermal testosterone patch should be reminded to apply the patch to a clean, dry area of skin. Application sites should be rotated daily, without repeating use of the same site for at least 1 week to minimize skin irritation.*

> ### ALERT!
>
> Although transdermal testosterone patches should be changed daily, discarded patches may still contain active medication. Patients should be advised to discard patches in a manner that minimizes the potential for ingestion by or exposure to children, pets, or anyone else. The best method of disposal is to fold the patch in half over the adhesive portion before discarding in an enclosed waste bin. Patients should wash their hands after handling the patch.

Transdermal Gels

Transdermal testosterone gel formulations are intended for once-daily application to the skin areas on the shoulders, upper arms, or abdomen. Although it is usually recommended that the transdermal testosterone gel be administered in the morning to a clean, dry skin area, it is more important that the medication be applied around the same time every day (whether morning or evening). The gels were originally supplied in unit-dose packets for convenience and ease of administration. More recently, transdermal testosterone gel was also made available in a multidose gel pump that delivers a metered dose per actuation of the pump. Like the transdermal patches, the gels can also cause local skin irritation but to a much lesser extent than the transdermal patches.[35]

> ### PRACTICE POINT
>
> *Occasionally, multiple actuations of the pump or multiple packets are required to obtain the dose prescribed. Patients may be advised that the total dose may be applied to the skin area in multiple steps, one actuation or one gel packet at a time, or as a single application with the full amount of gel required combined together.*

> ### ALERT!
>
> The transdermal gel formulations are not designed to be applied to the genital area.

Once applied, transdermal testosterone gel takes approximately 30 minutes for absorption, but complete absorption of the medication may take as long as several hours. To ensure maximum absorption of the product and for the best results, patients should be advised to apply the gel after showering. Patients should be advised to avoid showering, bathing, or swimming for at least 5 hours after application of the medication for those using AndroGel® and at least 2 hours for those using Testim®. Once the testosterone gel is applied to the skin, the drug can be transferred from person to person through direct contact with the skin area where the medication was applied. Studies have shown that people who come into direct skin contact with patients using testosterone gel are at risk for absorbing testosterone from the areas the gel was applied to. Cases of inappropriate virilization (development of adult male characteristics) in children have been reported to the FDA.

Transdermal testosterone gels are alcohol-based preparations and the alcohol in the gel is considered to be flammable until the gel is completely dried from the skin. Patients should avoid smoking or coming into close proximity with flames to avoid the potential for burns.[35,36]

Implantable Pellet

An implantable testosterone pellet, marketed under the trade name Testopel®, is a small cylinder-shaped pellet that contains 75 mg of testosterone in each pellet. Multiple pellets can be inserted SUBQ at the same time through a minor surgical procedure to achieve the desired dose of testosterone. Patients who have testosterone administered by insertion of the pellet implant may experience pain and inflammation at the site of insertion. In addition, there is a risk for infection at the site of implantation.[37]

The most important drug interactions that are of concern with testosterone supplementation are when it is prescribed to a patient on warfarin or insulin therapy. There is potential for testosterone preparations to enhance the effects of warfarin and put patients at increased risk for bleeding. Testosterone also has the potential to affect glucose metabolism and possibly decrease blood glucose levels or increase insulin sensitivity. Dose changes may be required in patients with diabetes who are being treated with insulin.

Testosterone Therapy in Females

Although testosterone is predominantly a male reproductive hormone, it is also found in the female body and serves some very important roles. In the female body, testosterone is also made in the ovaries and is converted by the human body into estrogen. As women age, the level of testosterone in the body slowly decreases over time as they reach menopause. Low testosterone levels in women have been found to be associated with decreased sexual drive. For this reason, testosterone replacement therapy is sometimes prescribed off label for use by women to treat decreased sexual drive and performance. However, this practice is not recommended due to unknown long-term effects of testosterone supplementation in women and the potential for undesirable side effects. When used in females, side effects may include acne, hirsutism, male-patterned hair loss, and deepening of the voice. Currently, testosterone-only products are not recommended for use in females for any reason until there are more long-term studies to support its safety.

BENIGN PROSTATIC HYPERPLASIA

Benign prostatic hyperplasia (BPH) is an abnormal but noncancerous enlargement of the prostate gland. It is one of the most common conditions affecting the older adult male population, affecting approximately 60% of men who are

60 years of age.[38] In the earlier stages of BPH, patients may not be aware that they have prostate enlargement because it does not cause any noticeable signs or symptoms. As the prostate grows in size, it can push on the urethra, leading to problems with urination. Figure 11-4 shows how these urination problems can occur in a patient with BPH. The most common symptoms associated with BPH are lower urinary tract symptoms (which may include weak urine stream), dribbling of urine when trying to urinate, incomplete bladder emptying, urinating frequently especially during the night, and urinary incontinence.

CASE?

Why might the pharmacist advise Mr. Johnson to schedule an appointment with his physician?

For most patients, BPH is a slowly progressing disease and, if treated, many can experience a reversal in symptoms. If left untreated, complications such as bladder stones, urinary tract infections, hematuria, or problems with kidney

function can occur. Although not all patients require medication treatment to manage their BPH, many will be prescribed medications to help control their symptoms. The two main classes of medication therapy prescribed to treat BPH are alpha$_1$-receptor blockers and 5-alpha reductase inhibitors. A brief summary of these medications can be found in Medication Table 11-4. Both classes of medications can be prescribed either as a single drug or in combination with each other (ie, an alpha$_1$-receptor blocker plus a 5-alpha reductase inhibitor).

Alpha$_1$-receptor Blockers

Alpha$_1$-receptor blockers are commonly used to treat the urinary symptoms associated with BPH. They are typically used to treat patients with moderate to severe symptoms. These medications can cause the muscles in the urinary tract and the prostate gland to relax. This muscle relaxation helps to improve patients' ability to urinate normally. Doxazosin (Cardura®), terazosin (Hytrin®), and prazosin (Minipress®) are the three older alpha$_1$ blockers used in BPH that are also prescribed for the treatment of high blood pressure. This is because they also work to relax the muscles of the

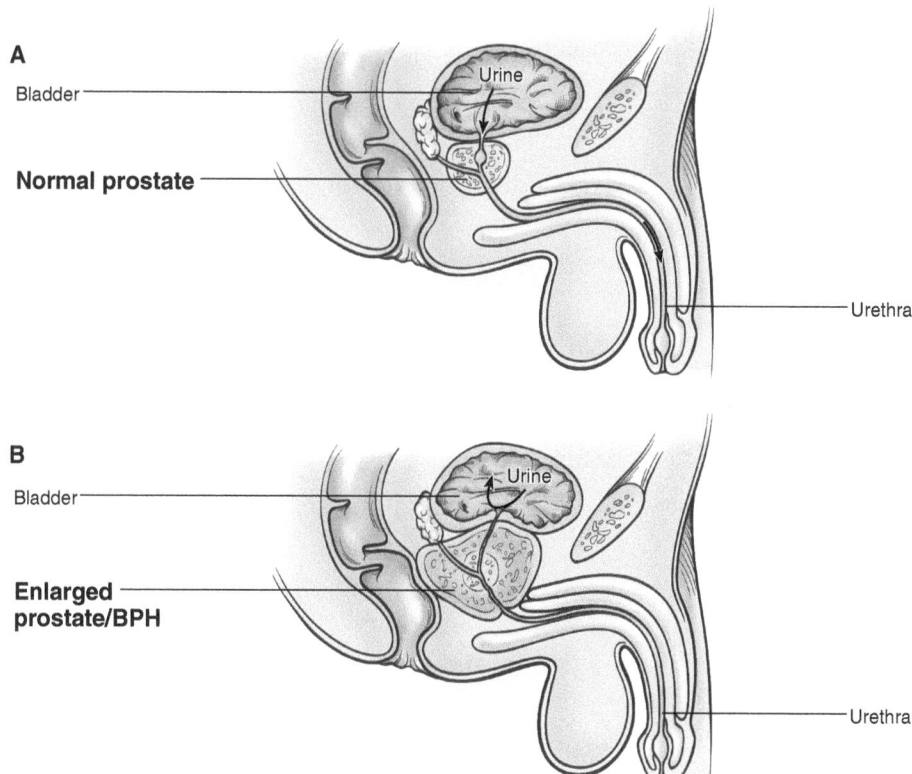

FIGURE 11-4. Benign prostatic hyperplasia. A, normal urine flow when the prostate is not enlarged; B, obstructed urine flow when the prostate is enlarged and pushing on both the bladder and the urethra.

blood vessels in other areas of the body, which can lower blood pressure. Refer to Chapter 15 for detailed information regarding the three alpha$_1$ blockers and their use for the treatment of high blood pressure.

CASE?

Mr. Johnson saw his doctor, who told him he has developed an enlarged prostate but that medication might control his symptoms. Along with his other medications, Mr. Johnson presents a new prescription for tamsulosin. He asks what kind of medication this is and if there is any important information he should know before taking it. What would you expect the pharmacist to tell him?

There are three relatively newer alpha$_1$-receptor blockers currently available that have unique properties compared to ones mentioned earlier that make them especially useful for treating BPH symptoms. Tamsulosin (Flomax®), alfuzosin (Uroxatral®), and silodosin (Rapaflo®) are alpha$_1$-receptor blockers that work only on the receptors in the human prostate when prescribed at their normal doses. These medications are currently FDA approved only for the treatment of BPH. In patients with BPH and normal blood pressure, the use of the older alpha$_1$-receptor blockers can cause unwanted side effects, such as low blood pressure. Unlike the older alpha$_1$-receptor blockers, the newer medications are not as effective in lowering blood pressure because they work more specifically on the prostate itself. This selectivity for the prostate is the advantage to using these newer drugs. All are available in a generic equivalent.[38]

ALERT!

Patients who are prescribed the newer alpha$_1$-receptor blockers for their BPH should not be taking the older alpha$_1$-receptor blockers at the same time, even if these are being used to treat their high blood pressure. The pharmacist should be alerted to such duplication of therapy.

Tamsulosin is available as a 0.4-mg capsule, dosed once a day. It is recommended that tamsulosin be taken approximately 30 minutes after the same meal each day to achieve steady levels of the drug in the body. Even though tamsulosin is not effective at treating hypertension compared to the older alpha$_1$-blockers, a drop in the blood pressure with positional changes (eg, from sitting to standing) may occur, especially after the first dose or when the dose is increased. Patients would need to use caution and watch for dizziness when first starting on the drug or when there is a dose increase, especially if they are taking blood pressure medications. Other side effects that may occur with tamsulosin treatment include runny nose and abnormal ejaculation. There have been reports of a rare condition called intraoperative floppy iris syndrome (IFIS) occurring in patients undergoing cataract surgery who are using, or have taken in the past, alpha$_1$-receptor blockers, including tamsulosin. Patients who are on tamsulosin considering cataract surgery should inform their eye doctor that they are on this medication. Patients on tamsulosin should also be counseled that, although extremely rare, there may be a risk of developing priapism with the use of tamsulosin. Tamsulosin dosing does not require adjustment in patients with kidney or liver problems. The medication is broken down by liver enzymes in the cytochrome P450 system and should be used cautiously in patients on medications that inhibit these enzymes, such as cimetidine, ketoconazole, or paroxetine (Paxil®).[39]

ALERT!

LOOK-ALIKE/SOUND-ALIKE—Flomax (tamsulosin) can be confused with the medication Fosamax® (alendronate) that is used for the treatment of osteoporosis. When receiving prescriptions with poor handwriting and/or without any medication strength indicated, the medication prescribed should always be verified with the prescriber. When taking a verbal order, the drug names may sound similar.

Alfuzosin is also a selective alpha$_1$-receptor blocker. It is available as a 10-mg extended-release tablet and is dosed once daily given after the same meal each day. Although alfuzosin can be used in patients with poor kidney function, it should not be prescribed to patients with moderate to severe liver dysfunction. Alfuzosin seems to be well tolerated, with the common side effects being dizziness, headache, and tiredness. In addition, it is associated with less abnormal ejaculation problems than tamsulosin. Similar to tamsulosin, patients on alfuzosin should also be counseled on the risk of IFIS if they will be undergoing cataract surgery. Alfuzosin is primarily broken down by the cytochrome

P450 liver enzyme system. As a result, it should not be used together with medications that specifically block alfuzosin breakdown through these enzymes, including ketoconazole, itraconazole (Sporanox®), and ritonavir (Norvir®).[40]

The newest selective alpha$_1$-receptor blocker is silodosin, which is available in two strengths: a 4- or 8-mg capsule. The usual dose for silodosin is 8 mg once daily with a meal, but it can also be dosed lower at 4 mg once daily in patients with moderate kidney impairment. Like tamsulosin and alfuzosin, the most common side effects of silodosin include abnormal ejaculation, dizziness, drops in blood pressure with positional changes, and headache. Some patients may also experience diarrhea. Silodosin has similar drug-drug interactions as alfuzosin and should not be prescribed with medications such as ketoconazole, itraconazole (Sporanox®), and ritonavir (Norvir®).[41]

CASE?

Mr. Johnson returns to the pharmacy months later and now has a prescription for finasteride. He says the doctor thinks this medicine will help his urinary symptoms even more than the tamsulosin alone. Should he be taking both these medications at the same time?

5-alpha Reductase Inhibitors

In the male body, testosterone is converted into another active hormone known as dihydrotestosterone (DHT) by an enzyme called 5-alpha reductase. DHT is a testosterone-like hormone that is responsible for causing the abnormal enlargement of the prostate gland in BPH. 5-alpha reductase inhibitors are a class of medications that lower the levels of DHT circulating in the body to reduce overgrowth of prostate tissue. Therefore, this particular class of medications works best to relieve BPH symptoms for patients who

have larger prostates by shrinking the prostate gland. In the United States, there are currently only two medications in this class available: finasteride (Proscar®) and dutasteride (Avodart®). Both of these medications work the same way by reducing the testosterone responsible for enlarging the prostate. These agents can reduce the size of the prostate gland by an estimated 25%, which in turn leads to a reduction in urinary symptoms. However, they do not provide quick relief. Patients who are prescribed finasteride or dutasteride for their BPH should be made aware that the medication takes 6–12 months of continuous treatment to reach its full effect. Patients should keep taking their medication even if they do not feel any symptom relief initially. If the medication is discontinued, the effects of the medication will likely reverse over time and the patient may experience a return of his original symptoms.[38]

CASE?

Mr. Johnson has been taking finasteride in addition to his tamsulosin for 2 months now, and he comes back for a refill of the tamsulosin but says he doesn't think he wants to refill the finasteride because it doesn't seem to be helping. Should the technician put in only the tamsulosin refill, or should something additional be considered?

Finasteride and dutasteride are both available as generics. Finasteride is only dosed as 5 mg given once a day with or without food. Common side effects are related to sexual function and include decreased sex drive, erectile dysfunction, or ejaculation problems. Recent data suggest that patients using finasteride for long-term therapy of BPH had a lower risk of developing prostate cancer, but those who did get prostate cancer while taking finasteride were more likely to be diagnosed with a more advanced form. Although the information regarding the use of finasteride and risk for prostate cancer is still unclear, patients should discuss these risks with their doctors. No dosing adjustments for poor kidney function is needed, but since it is broken down in the liver, finasteride should be used carefully in patients with poor liver function.[38]

Dutasteride is the newer of the two 5-alpha reductase inhibitors. It is only available in one strength, 0.5 mg, and is dosed as one capsule (0.5 mg) given once daily. Patients taking dutasteride most commonly complain of the same sexual side effects as patients taking finasteride. Also similar to finasteride, dutasteride does not need to be adjusted for poor kidney function and should be used cautiously in liver disease. Although dutasteride does not appear to have any significant drug-drug interactions, it is broken down extensively by the liver cytochrome P450 enzymes. Patients taking dutasteride should be monitored carefully by their physicians for increased side effects if they will be taking medications, such as ritonavir, that can block the breakdown of dutasteride by these enzymes. Dutasteride is also available in a capsule formulation in combination with tamsulosin under the brand name Jalyn® for the convenience of patients on both medications for their BPH.[42,43]

ANDROGEN RECEPTOR BLOCKERS AND GnRH ANALOGUES

Antiandrogens and GnRH analogues are medications that are designed to block the effects of testosterone in the body. The main type of antiandrogen medications is androgen receptor blockers. The second group of medications is the GnRH analogues, which work indirectly to suppress the effects of testosterone. These two groups of medications are not very widely prescribed because they are used to treat conditions that are uncommon. One of the main medical conditions that both of these classes of medications are used to treat is prostate cancer in males. In prostate cancer, the sex hormones testosterone and 5-alpha dihydrotestosterone are responsible for stimulating growth of the prostate and causing further advancement of the cancer. Medication therapy with the antiandrogens and GnRH analogues is typically reserved for more advanced stages of prostate cancer.[44]

Androgen Receptor Blockers

The androgen receptor blockers (antiandrogens) directly block the effects of testosterone in the body by competing with natural androgens at their sites of action. These medications do not allow androgens such as testosterone to bind to their receptors to cause changes in the body. There are a number of androgen receptor blockers available in the United States. They are apalutamide (Erleada®), darolutamide (NUBEQUA®), enzalutamide (Xtandi®), flutamide (Eulexin®), nilutamide (Nilandron®), and bicalutamide (Casodex®). Apalutamide (Erleada®), darolutamide (NUBEQUA®), enzalutamide (Xtandi®) are all brand name only. Bicalutamide, nilutamide, and flutamide are available as generics. Darolutamide (NUBEQUA®) is dosed twice daily, while flutamide is dosed every 8 hours. All the others within the class are dosed once daily at the same time every day. Darolutamide (NUBEQUA®) should be taken with food, while the other medications in the class can be taken with or without food. Side effects associated with this class of medications include nausea, diarrhea or constipation, gynecomastia, hot flushes, and potential liver toxicity. Flutamide appears to be associated with more diarrhea than bicalutamide. Nilutamide also appears to be associated with visual disturbances and intolerance to alcohol. Enzalutamide increases the risk of patients having a seizure. Medication Table 11-5 lists these medications.[44-50]

ALERT!

LOOK-ALIKE/SOUND-ALIKE—Thalidomide (Thalomid®) and flutamide have been confused as sound-alike drugs when taken as verbal prescriptions. Thalidomide is only available through a restricted program, which helps to avoid this confusion. However, verbal orders for these two medications should be avoided whenever possible.

Androgen Synthesis Blocker

Abiraterone is an antiandrogen that acts in a different way from the androgen receptor blockers described above. It works by blocking an enzyme needed for the production of testosterone, thereby decreasing the amount of testosterone available at the receptor sites. The usual dose is 1,000 mg once daily. Abiraterone is available as Zytiga®, which must be taken on an empty stomach. It is also available as Yonsa®, which can be taken without regard to meals. This dose may be reduced for patients with liver impairment. The most common adverse reactions associated with abiraterone are swelling or discomfort, hypokalemia, edema, muscle discomfort, hot flushes, diarrhea, urinary and upper respiratory tract infection, cough, hypertension, cardiac arrhythmia, and urinary frequency.[51,52]

Gonadotropin-Releasing Hormone Analogues

GnRH analogues work indirectly to suppress the actions of the androgens in the body. They are sometimes also called luteinizing hormone-releasing hormone (LHRH) agonists. When given as continuous therapy, GnRH analogues mimic natural GnRH that is usually released by the hypothalamus. In the first few weeks of treatment, this leads to stimulation of the pituitary gland to secrete more LH and FSH, which stimulates the testes to make and release more androgens. However, after this initial period, there is a drop off of LH, FSH, and testosterone production and release. Available GnRH analogues are leuprolide (Lupron®), goserelin (Zoladex®), and histrelin (Vantas®). Goserelin (Zoladex®) and leuprolide (Lupron®) are also FDA approved to be used for other conditions besides prostate cancer, such as endometriosis in females. Histrelin (Vantas®) is only FDA approved for prostate cancer. Goserelin is available as two different long-acting SUBQ implants, one lasts for 28 days while the other lasts for 12 weeks. Leuprolide is available as a daily injection or as long-acting formulations for SUBQ or IM injection. A list of available formulations for use in prostate cancer can be found in Medication Table 11-5. Common side effects that may occur with GnRH analogues include injection or insertion site reactions, hot flashes, and sexual dysfunction. In the first 2 weeks of starting treatment, patients should be made aware that they may experience an initial worsening of

ALERT!

Leuprolide is available in multiple dosage formulations for use in prostate cancer under the brand names of Lupron Depot® and Eligard®. The short-acting version is the only one available generically. Prescriptions received for leuprolide should be verified and dispensed with extra caution to avoid confusing these formulations as they are all dosed and administered differently.

their condition due to the initial increase in androgen release. Combination therapy with an androgen receptor blocker may help to avoid this initial disease flare-up.[53-55]

SUMMARY

Hormones involved in the human reproductive system include gonadotropin-releasing hormone (GnRH), luteinizing hormone (LH), follicle-stimulating hormone (FSH), estrogens, progesterone, and androgens. The estrogens and progesterone are the primary sex hormones released by the ovaries that are involved in the female reproductive system. Androgens, specifically testosterone, are the primary sex hormones released by the testes that are involved in the male reproductive system. Medications containing both natural and manmade forms of the primary sex hormones are available for the treatment of disorders related to the human reproductive systems. Estrogens and progestins are used either alone or in combination with one another for planned or emergency contraception (EC) as well as hormone therapy (HT) in postmenopausal women. Testosterone is most commonly seen prescribed as hormone replacement in males with hypogonadism. In addition to these, there are other medication classes on the market that can affect levels of the major sex hormones and how the male or female reproductive system functions. These medications may include gonadotropins and aromatase inhibitors used for female infertility, alpha-blockers and 5-alpha reductase inhibitors used in benign prostatic hyperplasia (BPH), and androgen receptor blockers or GnRH analogues prescribed for the treatment of prostate cancer.

ACKNOWLEDGMENT

The authors wish to acknowledge and thank Jennifer Lee, PharmD, and Nina Yen, PharmD, coauthors of this chapter in the first edition of this book.

REFERENCES

1. Rizzo D. The reproductive system. In: Rizzo D, ed. *Fundamentals of Anatomy and Physiology*. 4th ed. Boston, MA: Delmar Cengage Learning; 2015:452-488.

2. Chrousos GP. The gonadal hormones and inhibitors. In: Katzung BG, ed. *Basic & Clinical Pharmacology*. 14th ed. New York, NY: McGraw-Hill; 2018:720-746.

3. Christin-Maitre S. History of oral contraceptive drugs and their use worldwide. *Best Pract Res Clin Endocrinol Metab*. 2013;27(1):3-12.

4. El-Ibiary SY, Shrader SP, Ragucci KR. Contraception. In: Dipiro JT, Yee GC, Posey L, et al., eds. *Pharmacotherapy: A Pathophysiologic Approach*. 11th ed. New York, NY: McGraw-Hill; 2020:41-60.

5. Bonnema RA, Spencer AL. The new extended-cycle levonorgestrel-ethinyl estradiol oral contraceptives. *Clin Med Insights Reprod Health*. 2011;5:49-54.

6. Levin ER, Vitek WS, Hammes SR. Estrogens, progestins, and the female reproductive tract. In: Bruton LL, Hilal-Dandan R, Knollmann BC, eds. *Goodman & Gilman's: The Pharmacological Basis of Therapeutics*. 13th ed. New York, NY: McGraw-Hill; 2018:803-832.

7. Sulak PJ, Smith V, Coffee A, et al. Frequency and management of breakthrough bleeding with continuous use of the transvaginal contraceptive ring: A randomized controlled trial. *Obstet Gynecol*. 2008;112(3):563-571.

8. Nuvaring [package insert]. Whitehouse Station, NJ: Merck & Co., Inc.; 2019.

9. Annovera [package insert]. New York, NY: Population Council; 2018.

10. Xulane [package insert]. Morgantown, WV: Mylan Pharmaceuticals Inc.; 2014.

11. Depo-Provera [package insert]. New York, NY: Pfizer Inc.; 2020.

12. Mirena [package insert]. Wayne, NJ: Bayer HealthCare Pharmaceuticals Inc.; 2020.

13. Kyleena [package insert]. Whippany, NJ: Bayer HealthCare Pharmaceuticals Inc.; 2016.

14. Skyla [package insert]. Whippany, NJ: Bayer HealthCare Pharmaceuticals Inc.; 2018.

15. Liletta [package insert]. Odyssea Pharma, Belgium: Actavis Pharma, Inc.; 2015.

16. Nexplanon [package insert]. Whitehouse Station, NJ: Merck & Co., Inc.; 2019.

17. Mansour V, Murdico AT, Fundin J. Oral contraceptives are susceptible to several interactions. *Pharmacy Times*. https://www.pharmacytimes.com/publications/issue/2019/may2019/oral-contraceptives-are-susceptible-to-several-interactions. Updated May 22, 2019. Accessed December 12, 2019.

18. Simmons KB, Haddad LB, Nanda K, Curtis KM. Drug interactions between non-rifamycin antibiotics and hormonal contraception: A systematic review. *Am J Obstet Gynecol*. 2018;218(1):88-97.

19. Paragard [package insert]. Trumbull, CT: CooperSurgical, Inc.; 2019.

20. Spermicide. HHS.gov: Office of Population Affairs. https://www.hhs.gov/opa/pregnancy-prevention/birth-control-methods/spermicide/index.html. Updated May 20, 2019. Accessed December 12, 2019.

21. Bosworth MC, Olusola PL, Low SB. An update on emergency contraception. *Am Fam Physician*. 2014;89(7):545-550.

22. Cleland K, Raymond EG, Westley E, Trussell J. Emergency contraception review: Evidence-based recommendations for clinicians. *Clin Obstet Gynecol*. 2014;57(4):741-750.

23. Cleland K, Bass J, Doci F, Foster AM. Access to emergency contraception in the over-the-counter era. *Women's Health Issues*. 2016;26(6):622-627.

24. Ella [package insert]. Osny, France: Cenexi; 2015.

25. Lund KJ. Menopause and the menopausal transition. *Med Clin North Am*. 2008;92(5):1253-1271.

26. Dang DK, Wheeler KE, Chen JT. Hormone therapy in women. In: Dipiro JT, Yee GC, Posey L, et al., eds. *Pharmacotherapy: A Pathophysiologic Approach*. 11th ed. New York, NY: McGraw-Hill; 2020:1363-1382.

27. American Pregnancy Association. What is infertility? https://americanpregnancy.org/getting-pregnant/what-is-infertility/. Accessed December 23, 2019.

28. Cheang KI, Umland EM. Menstruation-related disorders. In: Dipiro JT, Yee GC, Posey L, et al., eds. *Pharmacotherapy: A Pathophysiologic Approach*. 11th edition. New York, NY: McGraw-Hill; 2020:1335-1352.

29. Clomiphene citrate [package insert]. Chestnut Ridge, NY: Par Pharmaceutical; 2019.

30. Pavone ME, Bulun SE. Clinical review: The use of aromatase inhibitors for ovulation induction and superovulation. *J Clin Endocrinol Metab*. 2013;98(5):1838-1844.

31. Richard-Eaglin A. Male and female hypogonadism. *Nurs Clin North Am*. 2018;53(3):395-405.

32. Mulhall JP, Trost LW, Brannigan RE, et al. Evaluation and management of testosterone deficiency: AUA Guideline. *J Urol*. 2018;200(2):423-432.

33. Luthy KE, Williams C, Freeborn DS, Cook A. Comparison of testosterone replacement therapy medications in the treatment of hypogonadism. *JNP*. 2017;13(4):241-249.

34. Androderm [package insert]. Markham, Ontario: Allergan Inc; 2018.

35. Androgel [package insert]. North Chicago, IL: AbbVie Inc.; 2019.

36. Testim [package insert]. Malvern, PA: Endo Pharmaceuticals Inc.; 2020.

37. Testopel [package insert]. Malvern, PA: Endo Pharmaceuticals, Inc.; 2018.

38. Lee M, Sharifi R. Benign prostatic hyperplasia. In: Dipiro JT, Yee GC, Posey L, et al., eds. *Pharmacotherapy: A Pathophysiologic Approach*. 11th ed. New York, NY: McGraw-Hill; 2020:1411-1430.

39. Tamsulosin [package insert]. Parsippany, NJ: Actavis Pharma, Inc.; 2015.

40. Alfuzosin [package insert]. Warren, NJ: Cipla USA Inc.; 2020.

41. Silodosin [package insert]. Markham, Ontario: Allergan Inc.; 2018.

42. Dutasteride [package insert]. Research Triangle Park, NC: GlaxoSmithKline; 2014.

43. Jalyn [package insert]. Research Triangle Park, NC: GlaxoSmithKline; 2020.

44. Norris LB. Prostate cancer. In: Dipiro JT, Yee GC, Posey L, et al., eds. *Pharmacotherapy: A Pathophysiologic Approach*. 11th ed. New York, NY: McGraw-Hill; 2020:2301-2318.

45. Erleada [package insert]. Gurabo, PR: Janssen Ortho LLC; 2018.

46. Nubequa [package insert]. Espoo, Finland: Orion Corporation; 2019.

47. Xtandi [package insert]. St. Petersburg, FL: Catalent Pharma Solutions, LLC; 2012.

48. Eulexin [package insert]. Toronto, Canada: Teva Canada Limited; 2014.

49. Nilandron [package insert]. St. Michael, Barbados: Concordia Pharmaceuticals Inc.; 2015.

50. Casodex [package insert]. Wilmington, DE: AstraZeneca Pharmaceuticals; 2017.

51. Zytiga [package insert]. Horsham, PA: Janssen Biotech; 2018.

52. Yonsa [package insert]. Cranbury, NJ: Sun Pharma Global FZE; 2018.

53. Lupron Depot [package insert]. North Chicago, IL: AbbVie Inc.; 2014.

54. Zoladex [package insert]. Wilmington, DE: AstraZeneca Pharmaceuticals; 2015.

55. Supprelin LA [package insert]. Chadds Ford, PA: Endo Pharmaceuticals Solutions Inc.; 2011.

REVIEW QUESTIONS

1. What contraceptive agents would the pharmacist recommend for a patient who frequently forgets to take her daily oral contraceptive?

2. Sandy Nichols is a 55-year-old postmenopausal female who had a hysterectomy at the age of 32. She presents to your pharmacy counter to pick up her prescription for oral Estrace. However, she tells you her friends who are also taking postmenopausal hormone therapy are also taking progesterone. She wonders if she should also be taking progesterone. What information should the pharmacist tell her?

3. What are the primary reproductive hormones in the male and female body and what are their main functions?

4. What is hypogonadism and what classes of medications are available to treat male and/or female hypogonadism?

5. What are common symptoms of benign prostatic hyperplasia? Explain two types of medications to treat this condition.

MEDICATION TABLES

MEDICATION TABLE 11-1. Representative Contraceptive Products

	Contraceptive[®]	Estrogen	Progestin	Route	Phase
Combined Oral Contraceptives	Nextstellis	Estetrol 14.2 mg	Drosperinone 3 mg	Oral	M
	Yasmin 28	EE 30 mcg	Drosperinone 3 mg	Oral	M
	Loestrin 1.5/30, Loestrin Fe 1.5/30[a]	EE 30 mcg	Norethindrone acetate 1.5 mg	Oral	M
	Seasonique	EE 30 mcg × 84 days EE 10 mcg × 7 days	Levonorgestrel 0.15 mg	Oral	M
	Loestrin 1/20, Loestrin Fe 1/20,[a] Minastrin 24 Fe[a]	EE 20 mcg	Norethindrone acetate 1 mg	Oral	M
	Lo Loestrin Fe[a]	EE 10 mcg	Norethindrone acetate 1 mg	Oral	M
	Yaz	EE 20 mcg	Drosperinone 3 mg	Oral	M
	LoSeasonique	EE 20 mcg × 84 days EE 10 mcg × 7 days	Levonorgestrel 0.1 mg	Oral	M
	Mircette, Kariva, Azurette	EE 20 mcg days 1–21 EE 10 mcg days 24–28	Desogestrel 0.15 mg days 1–21	Oral	B
	Tri-sprintec	EE 35 mcg days 1–7	Norgestimate 0.18 mg days 1–7	Oral	T
		EE 35 mcg days 8–14	Norgestimate 0.215 mg days 8–14		
		EE 35 mcg days 15–21	Norgestimate 0.25 mg days 15–21		
	Natazia	EV 3 mg days 1–2	Dienogest 0 mg days 1–2	Oral	F
		EV 2 mg days 3–7	Dienogest 2 mg days 3–7		
		EV 2 mg days 8–24 EV 1 mg days 25–26	Dienogest 3 mg days 8–24 Dienogest 0 mg days 25–26		
Combined Hormonal Contraceptives (alternatives)	NuvaRing	EE 15 mcg/d	Etonogestrel (0.12 mg/d)	Vaginal	M
	Annovera	EE 13 mcg/d	Segesterone acetate (0.15 mg/d)	Vaginal	M
	Xulane	EE 35mcg/d	Norelgestromin (0.15 mg/d)	Transdermal	M
Progestin-Only Contraceptives	"Camila": Slynd	N/A	Drosperinone 4 mg	Oral	M
	Camila, Ortho Micronor, Norlyroc	N/A	Norethindrone 0.35 mg	Oral	M
	Depo-Provera	N/A	Medroxyprogesterone 150 mg (IM)	Injectable	M
	Depo-SubQ Provera 104	N/A	Medroxyprogesterone 104 mg (SUBQ)	Injection	M
	Nexplanon	N/A	Etonogestrel 68 mg	Implant	M
	Mirena	N/A	Levonorgestrel 20 mcg/day	Intrauterine	M
	Kyleena	N/A	Levonorgestrel 17.5 mcg/day	Intrauterine	M

Continued next page

MEDICATION TABLE 11-1. Representative Contraceptive Products *(Continued)*

	Contraceptive[®]	Estrogen	Progestin	Route	Phase
	Liletta	N/A	Levonorgestrel 20 mcg/day	Intrauterine	M
	Skyla	N/A	Levonorgestrel 14 mcg/day	Intrauterine	M
Non-Hormonal Contraceptives	Paragard[b]	N/A	N/A	Intrauterine	N/A
	Nonoxynol 9	N/A	N/A	Intravaginal	N/A
Emergency Contraceptives	Plan B One Step	N/A	Levonorgestrel 1.5 mg	Oral	N/A
	Ella	N/A	Ulipristal 30 mg	Oral	N/A

Source: Lexicomp® Online.
List is not all inclusive. B = biphasic; EE = ethinyl estradiol; EV = estradiol valerate; F = four-phasic; IM = intramuscular; M = monophasic; SUBQ = subcutaneous; T = triphasic.
[a] Products with Fe in the name contain iron in place of placebo pills.
[b] Products are additionally FDA approved for emergency contraception.

MEDICATION TABLE 11-2. Representative Female Hormone Therapy

Preparations	Brands[®]	Route	Dose
Estrogen Preparations			
Conjugated equine estrogen	Premarin	Oral	Initial 0.3 mg/day; adjust based on response
Transdermal 17ß estradiol	Alora, Vivelle-Dot	Transdermal	0.025–0.1 mg/24-hr patch 2×/wk
Estradiol transdermal spray	Evamist	Transdermal	1–3 sprays/day
Conjugated equine estrogen	Premarin	Vaginal	0.5–2 g intravaginally daily (3 wk on and 1 wk off)
	Femring	Vaginal	1 ring q 3 mo (0.05–0.1 mg/24 hr)
Estradiol vaginal tablet	Vagifem	Vaginal	1 vaginal tablet (10 mcg) once daily for 2 wk, then 1 tab vaginally 2–3/wk
Progesterone Preparations			
Medroxyprogesterone acetate	Provera	Oral	5 or 10 mg/day for12–14 consecutive days each month
Micronized progesterone	Prometrium	Oral	200 mg/day on days 1–12 every 28–day cycle
Combined Hormone Therapy Preparations			
Conjugated estrogens/ medroxyprogesterone acetate tablets	Prempro	Oral	0.3-0.625 mg/1.5–5 mg tablets (conjugated estrogens/ medroxyprogesterone tablets, respectively) 1 tablet daily
Conjugated estrogens and conjugated estrogens/ medroxyprogesterone acetate tablets	Premphase	Oral	#14 conjugated estrogens 0.625 mg tablets & #14 conjugated estrogens 0.625 mg/MPA 5 mg tablets 1 tablet daily
Estradiol and norethindrone acetate transdermal system	CombiPatch	Transdermal	0.05/0.14 mg & 0.05/0.25 mg (estradiol/norethindrone acetate, respectively) 1 patch 2×/wk

Continued next page

MEDICATION TABLE 11-2. Representative Female Hormone Therapy *(Continued)*

Preparations	Brands(®)	Route	Dose
Estrogen/Testosterone Preparations			
Oral esterified estrogens/oral methyltestosterone	Covaryx	Oral	1.25 mg/2.5 mg tablets 1 tablet daily (esterified estrogens/methyltestosterone, respectively) (3 wk on and 1 wk off)
	Covaryx H.S.	Oral	0.625 mg/1.25 mg tablets (esterified estrogens/methyltestosterone, respectively) 1–2 tablets at bedtime (3 wk on and 1 wk off)

Source: Lexicomp® Online.

MEDICATION TABLE 11-3. Testosterone Replacement Therapy for Males

Generic Name	Brand Name(®)	How Supplied	Usual Dosing	Administration Site
Oral Preparation				
Testosterone undecanoate	Jatenzo	158 mg, 198 mg, 237 mg tablets	158–396 mg twice daily	N/A
Intranasal				
Testosterone gel	Natesto	11 mg gel (60 metered pump actuations)	11 mg (2 pump actuations, 1 per nostril 3 times/day; 6–8 hours apart)	Nostrils
Intramuscular Injection				
Testosterone cypionate	Depo-Testosterone	100 mg/mL, 200 mg/mL vials	50–400 mg q 2–4 wk or 75-100 mg/week or 150–200 mg/q 2 weeks	Gluteal muscle
Testosterone enanthate	N/A (generic)	200 mg/mL vials	50–400 mg q 2–4 wk or 75–100 mg/week or 150–200 mg/q 2 weeks	
Testosterone undecanoate	Aveed	750 mg/3 mL vials	750 mg followed by 750 mg 4 weeks later; then 750 mg administered every 10 weeks thereafter	
Subcutaneous (SUBQ) Injection				
	Xyosted	50 mg/0.5 ml, 75 mg/0.5 ml, 100 mg/0.5 ml of solution in auto-injector	50–100 mg once a week	Abdomen
Transdermal Patch				
Testosterone	Androderm	2 mg/24 hr, 4 mg/24 hr patches	2–6 mg/day	Skin on back, abdomen, upper arms, or thighs

Continued next page

MEDICATION TABLE 11-3. Testosterone Replacement Therapy for Males *(Continued)*

Generic Name	Brand Name(®)	How Supplied	Usual Dosing	Administration Site
Transdermal Gel				
Testosterone	Androgel 1%	25 mg/2.5 g, 50 mg/5 g	50–100 mg/day	Shoulders, upper arms, abdomen (AndroGel); thigh (Fortesta); shoulders, upper arms (Vogelxo)
	Androgel 1.62%	20.25 mg/1.25 g, 40.5 mg/2.5 g	20.25–81 mg/day	
	Fortesta	10 mg/actuation	10–70 mg once daily in the morning	
	Testim 1%	50 mg/5g tube	1–2 tubes once daily	
	Vogelxo	50 mg (unit-dose tube), 50 mg (unit-dose packet), 12.5 mg/one pump actuation in metered-dose pump	50–100 mg once daily	
Transdermal Solution				
	Testosterone solution (generic only)	30 mg/actuation	30–120 mg to axilla once daily each morning	Axilla
Implantable Pellet				
Testosterone	Testopel	75 mg pellets	150–450 mg implanted q 3–6 mo	SUBQ implantation

Source: Lexicomp® Online.

MEDICATION TABLE 11-4. Treatment of Benign Prostatic Hyperplasia

Generic Name	Brand Name(®)	How Supplied	Usual Dosing
Nonselective Alpha$_1$-Receptor Blockers			
Doxazosin	Cardura	1 mg, 2 mg, 4 mg, 8 mg tablets	1–8 mg once daily
Terazosin	N/A (generic)	1 mg, 2 mg, 5 mg, 10 mg capsules	1–20 mg once daily
Selective Alpha$_1$-Receptor Blockers			
Tamsulosin	Flomax	0.4 mg capsule	1 capsule once daily
Silodosin	Rapaflo	4 mg, 8 mg capsule	1 capsule once daily
Alfuzosin	Uroxatral	10 mg extended-release tablet	1 tablet once daily
5-alpha Reductase Inhibitors			
Finasteride	Proscar	5 mg tablet	1 tablet once daily
Dutasteride	Avodart	0.5 mg capsule	1 capsule once daily
Combination Products			
Dutasteride/Tamsulosin	Jalyn	0.5 mg/0.4 mg capsule	1 tablet once daily

Source: Lexicomp® Online.

TABLE 11-5. Antiandrogen Medications for Prostate Cancer

Generic Name	Brand Name(®)	How Supplied
Antiandrogens		
Androgen Receptor Blockers		
Flutamide	N/A (generic)	125 mg capsules
Nilutamide	Nilandron	150 mg tablets
Bicalutamide	Casodex	50 mg tablets
Apalutamide	Erleada	60 mg tablets
Darolutamide	Nubequa	300 mg tablets
Enzalutamide	Xtandi	40 mg capsules
Androgen Synthesis Inhibitor		
Abiraterone	Zytiga	250 mg, 500 mg tablets
	Yonsa	125 mg tablets (micronized)
GnRH Analogues		
Leuprolide acetate	Lupron Depot	3.75 mg, 7.5 mg, 11.25 mg, 22.5 mg, 30 mg depot IM injection syringe kit
	Eligard	7.5 mg, 22.5 mg, 30 mg, 45 mg SUBQ injection syringe kit
Goserelin acetate	Zoladex	3.6 mg, 10.8 mg SUBQ implant
	Vantas	50 mg SUBQ injection syringe kit

Source: Lexicomp® Online.
This table is not all inclusive and does not include other formulations of the medications that are not made to be used for the treatment of prostate cancer.
IM = intramuscular; SUBQ = subcutaneous.

Part 4

THE MUSCULOSKELETAL SYSTEM AND RELATED TOPICS

Chapter 12

Overview of the Musculoskeletal System

Karen A. Newell, MMSc, PA-C, DFAAPA

KEY TERMS AND DEFINITIONS

Antispasmodic—an agent that prevents or relieves spasms (chronic conditions).

Asthenia—weakness.

Excitation—causes a response.

Inhibition—prevents a response.

Spasm—an involuntary contraction of a muscle due to injury or overuse.

Spasmolytic—an agent that relieves or relaxes acute spasms.

Spasticity—a state of increased tone of a muscle (and an increase in the deep tendon reflexes). For example, with spasticity of the legs (spastic paraplegia) there is an increase in tone of the leg muscles so they feel tight and rigid and the knee jerk reflex is exaggerated.

LEARNING OBJECTIVES

After completing this chapter, you should be able to

1. Describe the basic anatomy and physiology of the musculoskeletal system and its relationship to the central and peripheral nervous systems.

2. List common conditions causing musculoskeletal pain.

DOI 10.37573/9781585286638.012

3. Discuss the different categories of skeletal muscle relaxants and state their common uses.

4. Recognize neuromuscular blocking agents used in surgery or procedures.

5. State the generic names of widely used skeletal muscle relaxants used to treat muscle pain in the acute setting.

6. List the general mechanisms of action, therapeutic benefit, and adverse effects of some of the most common skeletal muscle relaxants.

The musculoskeletal system is quite complicated because it consists of so many moving parts—the bones, muscles, joints, and connecting tissues. To begin with the fundamentals, the human body consists of 206 bones that form the skeleton. The skeleton is what gives our body a shape and form. Musculoskeletal pain is one of the most common medical complaints among adult patients. This chapter introduces the basic structure and function of the musculoskeletal system and examines medications that are used to modify its actions and treat some of the conditions that affect it (Figure 12-1).

Just by holding this book, you are using 27 bones in each hand! Bones are connected to each other by ligaments, a dense fibrous band that helps to hold the two structures together and can control or limit movement. Joints are the areas where bones are connected to one another and allow certain movement to occur. This is also an area of the skeleton where injuries frequently occur. Consider the last time you twisted your ankle, which is an example of a common sports injury that happens at a joint.

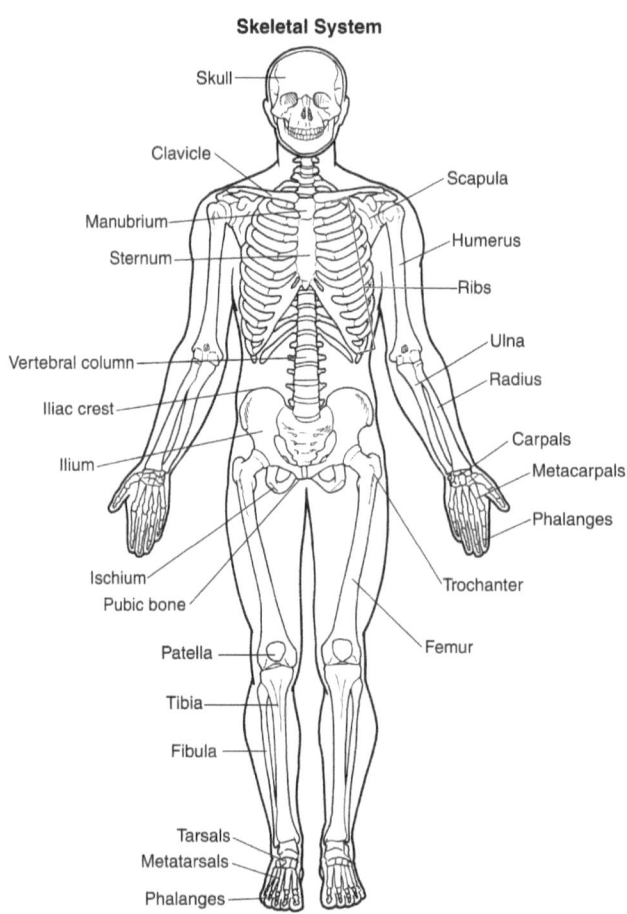

FIGURE 12-1. The skeletal system anterior view. The skeletal system is an extensive system of large and small bones that supports the muscle and protects the internal organs.

BASIC ANATOMY AND PHYSIOLOGY

As noted, the human skeleton is made up of 206 bones in varying sizes and shapes. Some, like the bones of the skull and rib cage, are fixed in position to protect the organs they surround and maintain the body's shape. Others are movable to different extents, ranging from the flexibility of the spinal column to the full motion possible with joints (such as the knee, hip, or elbow). Overlying the bones of the skeleton are more than 600 skeletal muscles (Figure 12-2). There are two other types of muscle, cardiac and smooth muscle, which are not covered in this chapter. Muscles are often attached to the bones of the skeleton by tendons, which are elastic tissue that allow for stretching and contracting. In normal muscle movement, these tendons stretch out like a rubber band, and then can return to their original size and shape. Movement that is sudden or extreme may cause these elastic tendons to be injured, which can result in pain.

Muscle is regulated by the nervous system. Recall from Chapters 4 and 5 that the nervous system of the human body can be broadly divided into two main categories: the central nervous system (CNS—the brain, brainstem, and spinal cord) and the peripheral nervous system (PNS). The PNS can be further subdivided into a somatic component (voluntary control) and an autonomic component (involuntary control). The somatic component consists of sensory and motor neurons that affect primarily skeletal muscle. Nerve impulses transmitted by the somatic nervous system cause muscles to contract and relax; the result affects the movement of the part of the body controlled by that muscle, whether it is the flexing of a joint or the maintenance of a position or posture. When muscles are injured, overused, underused, affected by disease, or when the nerve impulses controlling them are abnormal, difficulty in moving or pain can result.

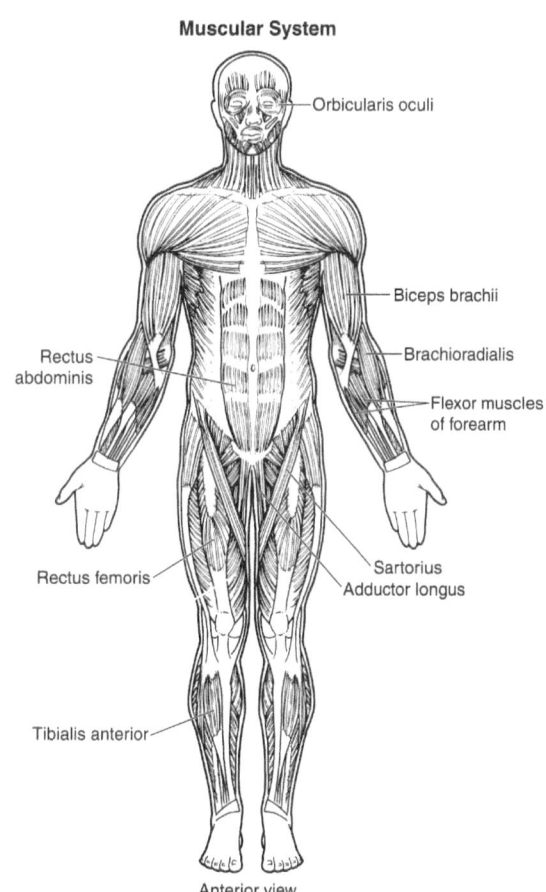

Muscular System

Orbicularis oculi

Biceps brachii

Brachioradialis

Flexor muscles of forearm

Rectus abdominis

Rectus femoris

Sartorius
Adductor longus

Tibialis anterior

Anterior view

FIGURE 12-2. The skeletal muscles of the body. The skeletal muscles of the body attach to the skeleton via ligaments and tendons. When they contract, they can move or restrain parts of the body.

CASE STUDY

Mr. P is a 32-year-old pizza delivery man who hurt his low back yesterday while lifting heavy drinks out of his car. He noticed a "pull" on the lower right side of his back after lifting the box, but he now describes his pain as all over and worse when he tries to bend forward. He complains of difficulty sleeping due to his back pain, and when he woke up this morning, he was stiff.

Muscle pain is a common complaint. The most frequent cause of this type of pain is trauma or an injury, such as a sprain or strain. A sprain is an abnormal stretching or tear of a ligament that can result in swelling, pain, and even bruising. A common example of this is a twisted ankle that can result in the sprain of the ligament(s) and may cause pain and swelling of the area on the outside of the ankle. Sometimes it can even cause some bruising, which is evidence of very small tears in the ligament(s) from being overstretched. A strain is an overstretched muscle or tendon that is often twisted, pulled, or even slightly torn. Overuse of a muscle or repetitive use can also cause a muscle strain. Muscle strains can result in pain of the injured muscle as well as the surrounding muscles. Strains may also cause swelling, cramping, or even a muscle spasm. A muscle spasm is a cramp, tightness, or involuntary contraction of muscle. A spasm can occur following a strain, overuse of that muscle, or may occur due to lack of certain nutrients the muscle needs to function.

CASE?

After a thorough history and physical exam, the physician assistant determines Mr. P has an acute low back muscle strain with a moderate amount of muscle spasm. An NSAID is prescribed along with cyclobenzaprine 10 mg by mouth three times a day. What are the possible adverse reactions to these drugs? Could these affect his work in any way?

Low back pain caused by a muscle strain is an example of a common musculoskeletal complaint. Due to the predominant symptom of pain, the first-line treatment of choice for a muscle strain is usually acetaminophen or a nonsteroidal anti-inflammatory drug (NSAID). The NSAID may be used in a high dose or prescription form or in lower doses readily available in over-the-counter medications, such as ibuprofen. For more serious injuries or for patients whose pain is not relieved by analgesics or anti-inflammatory drugs, short-term use of skeletal muscle relaxants can also be prescribed alone or used as an adjunct to the first-line treatment. The types of muscle relaxants used can vary, but most beneficial are the drugs commonly called spasmolytics due to their effects on the pain–spasm cycle of the injured muscle. If the spasm is decreased, the pain should also be lessened. There is some controversy in the use of muscle relaxants in the setting of low back pain due to their numerous side effects and potential for abuse and dependency. Drowsiness and dizziness are the most common adverse effects in this class of medication.

SKELETAL MUSCLE RELAXANTS

The category of skeletal muscle relaxants is a broad term and includes drugs from several specific categories. They are grouped based on their mechanism of action or the distribution of medication. For purposes of understanding how they work, these medications can be broken down into two general areas of use: spasmolytics and antispasmodic medications. In acute painful conditions, spasmolytic drugs are often used for the relief of muscle spasm. Antispasmodic medications have antispasticity effects and are usually prescribed to treat chronic conditions causing generalized muscle cramping, increased muscle tone, or spasticity. The final category, neuromuscular blocking agents, contains drugs primarily used for anesthesia in the hospital or operating room setting.

Spasmolytics

Spasmolytic is a term used to denote the type of medications that are routinely used for the relief of muscle spasm and pain in the setting of acute musculoskeletal injury. This includes two categories of the muscle relaxant medicines: the centrally acting drugs and the miscellaneous skeletal muscle relaxants. Both categories are used mainly in the outpatient setting for the treatment of acute musculoskeletal pain and spasm but may also be ordered for hospitalized patients.

Centrally acting drugs are so called because they exert their effects on the CNS (brain, brainstem, or spinal cord). Not every medication has the exact same mechanism of action, but many of these drugs act at the level of the brainstem and have sedative properties. Specifically, these drugs can affect the motor neuron signal, either by increasing the level of inhibition or reducing the level of excitation. The results of these actions are to decrease the muscle tone and the involuntary movement of the muscles. Most commonly, spasmolytics are used in conjunction with other medicines for the relief of pain and spasm associated with muscle strain or injury. These medicines may be recommended for short-term use in acute musculoskeletal injury. The medications in this category are similar in their effectiveness, and provider preference and medication safety are usually considered when choosing the preferred treatment.

Methocarbamol (brand name Robaxin) is an example of a centrally acting skeletal muscle relaxant. When given orally it begins to take effect in about 30 minutes. Its mechanism of action is not completely known, but it may decrease the number of impulses that get from the spinal cord to the muscle. It also may have some CNS depression, which would account for some of its adverse reactions. Common side effects include dizziness, drowsiness, lightheadedness, headache, and nausea. Methocarbamol is also available as an injectable product, but the other medications in this category are always administered by mouth (see Medication Table 12-1; Medication Tables are located at the end of the chapter).

ALERT!

LOOK-ALIKE/SOUND-ALIKE—The centrally acting muscle relaxant tizanidine has been confused with tiagabine, an anticonvulsant.

The difficulty with centrally acting spasmolytics is twofold: first, they can cause some unpleasant side effects and second, there is potential for abuse or dependency. Most commonly, this class of medication may cause dizziness, drowsiness, lightheadedness, fatigue, dry mouth, or nausea. For this reason, patients should not drive or operate heavy machinery while using these medications. Pharmacologically, several of the individual medicines are similar to other common drug classes such as tricyclic antidepressants and antihistamines, which are also known to cause drowsiness, dry mouth, and dizziness.

PRACTICE POINT

Caution is advised when a centrally acting skeletal muscle relaxant is used to treat an older patient (potential for sedation and falls), or a patient with liver or kidney disease (reduced drug clearance and increased drug action/side effects).

Other Skeletal Muscle Relaxants

Medication Table 12-2 lists skeletal muscle relaxants that differ from the centrally acting ones described above in some important ways, including their uses. Of these, only orphenadrine is used for the short-term treatment of musculoskeletal pain. Orphenadrine is in a category by itself. It is a unique medication among skeletal muscle relaxants because it also has an analgesic effect along with its muscle relaxing effect. Its mechanism of action is not fully known, but it is thought to be centrally acting like the medications in the category above. Chemically this medication is very similar to diphenhydramine (Benadryl), which also has many anticholinergic properties. The side effects of this medication are also very similar to the antihistamines, including dry mouth, blurred vision, and urinary retention. It can be given orally or injected.

CASE?

Mr. P asks if there is anything else he can do to help his back get better. He is anxious about getting back to work as soon as he can.

Because muscle relaxants and analgesics (pain relievers) are frequently used together, several are available as combination products to increase compliance and patient convenience. These are listed in Medication Table 12-3.

Alternative Treatments

Most acute musculoskeletal injuries are self-limiting and resolve on their own. There is some benefit to the application of heat and/or ice to the injured area for 20 to 30 minutes at a time. Patients should be told to use heating pads for limited periods only and cautioned not to fall asleep with a heating pad due to the risk of burns and other injury. Over-the-counter analgesics may also provide temporary relief of the pain associated with injury. Acetaminophen at recommended doses is an appropriate first-line treatment, especially in the setting of gastrointestinal issues. Ibuprofen or naproxen (and other NSAIDs) offer pain relief as well as some additional anti-inflammatory properties, but they must be taken with food to avoid gastric irritation.

Patients are often given a list of stretches or other exercises to help the injured muscles. These exercises usually start out gently and gradually increase in intensity as recovery occurs over days and weeks. Instruction in proper lifting techniques (bending at the knees and keeping the back straight, avoiding twisting and turning while lifting) as well as proper sleeping positions (on the side, with knees flexed) may help reduce the risk of future injury and pain. Patients may benefit from massage to the area. Some providers recommend using ice to massage over painful muscles (holding the ice with a cloth or glove for application). Similar in principle to the application of heat, ice should only be used for 15 to 20 minutes every few hours while awake to avoid the possibility of skin or other tissue damage. Additionally, physical therapists can offer several treatment modalities to aid in the healing of a muscle strain, as well as teach exercises for stretching of the area and prevention of reinjury. Some patients may prefer complementary and alternative treatments for relief of their symptoms—such as herbal remedies for pain, or nontraditional approaches to musculoskeletal problems, such as acupuncture or Rolfing (a form of deep tissue manipulation). Bed rest is not recommended for the treatment of acute low back pain related to a muscle strain.

ALERT!

Use of herbal remedies may sometimes introduce the possibility of drug interactions; they should be documented in the patient's pharmacy profile. Additionally, it should be noted that patients are increasingly experimenting with CBD (cannabidiol) products for relief of musculoskeletal pain. These preparations also have many potential drug interactions.

Antispasmodics

Skeletal muscle relaxants that decrease muscle tone and help relieve chronic muscle contraction and spasm are often called antispasmodics. Chronic conditions causing generalized muscle spasticity can be found in many diseases. Following a cerebrovascular accident (CVA or stroke), some patients develop weakness, or asthenia, in one or more extremities and may also have increased muscle tone that can cause the arm (or leg) to contract or be held in flexion. Skeletal muscle relaxants can offer these patients some relief by decreasing the tone and spasm and allowing them to have improved function and possibly less pain.

Cerebral palsy (CP) is a motor disorder that is usually accompanied by some type of spasticity or involuntary movement. The spasticity is related to a malfunction of the upper motor neurons and may have various effects on motor function. Besides spasticity, muscles can be underdeveloped, weak, and have increased muscle tone and reflexes. Spasticity may be a complication of spinal cord injury or

multiple sclerosis (MS). Muscle relaxants can be helpful when used properly in the setting of chronic muscle spasm and increased muscle tone.

There are two main medications that fall into this group of antispasmodics. The first medication is dantrolene (brand name Dantrium), which is a direct-acting skeletal muscle relaxant. Essentially, it blocks the release of calcium in the cells of the skeletal muscle. This medication does not have an effect on the CNS but acts at the level of the muscle fibers to weaken the contraction of the muscle. In its oral form it can be used to help decrease muscle spasm in chronic conditions such as CP, MS, and spinal cord injury.

PRACTICE POINT

Oral dantrolene is available only as a capsule, but some patients with the chronic conditions described above may have difficulty swallowing a solid dosage form. An appropriate number of capsules may be emptied into an acidic vehicle that has suspending properties, such as Syrup NF or methylcellulose syrup.

A life-threatening condition known as malignant hyperthermia is the result of heightened metabolic activity in the skeletal muscle of susceptible patients exposed to certain anesthetic agents. This is a rare, inherited condition and dantrolene is used for its treatment and prevention. In patients suspected to be at risk, dantrolene may be given by mouth or injection prior to the surgery. When malignant hyperthermia crisis occurs during surgery, an intravenous (IV) dose based on the patient's body weight is prepared and administered immediately. This is usually followed by additional oral dantrolene doses over the next 3 days.

PRACTICE POINT

IV dantrolene doses must be reconstituted immediately before dosing only with sterile water for injection (never dextrose or saline solutions or bacteriostatic water). Reconstituted solutions may be transferred to plastic bags but never to large-volume glass containers and should not be used if they show particulate matter, cloudiness, or discoloration.[1]

There is a black box warning (the strongest possible requirement of the Food and Drug Administration (FDA) indicating possible serious or life-threatening adverse effects) for this medication due to the incidence of hepatotoxicity. Side effects of this medicine include hepatic impairment, diarrhea, weakness, and somnolence.

The second type of antispasmodic is baclofen (brand names Lioresal, Ozobax) and is considered to be in a separate category called GABA-derivative skeletal muscle relaxant. This drug acts by causing hyperpolarization of the neurons. The activity is mostly focused on the CNS by inhibiting the transmission at the spinal level. In severe cases of spasticity and pain, baclofen can be delivered via an implanted pump that delivers the drug directly into the spinal fluid; this is called intrathecal (IT) administration. Common side effects of baclofen include drowsiness, dizziness, weakness, nausea, and confusion. Caution is used when this medication is prescribed for patients who have seizures or renal disease (Medication Table 12-2).

Neuromuscular Blockers

Neuromuscular blocking agents are given intravenously for a variety of clinical situations, such as surgery or an emergency procedure in which muscle relaxation is desirable. In surgery it is used with anesthesia so that less anesthetic agent is required, which helps to minimize serious side effects. It also helps to lessen a muscle spasm when the breathing tube is inserted into the airway (endotracheal intubation). Because these drugs help muscles relax, the muscle tissue itself can be cut more easily during surgery. Additionally, because they have a quick onset and resolution of action, they are safe and aid in rapid recovery.

Neuromuscular blocking agents can be classified into two main groups: depolarizing blocking agents and the nondepolarizing blocking agents, depending on their activity with respect to the neurotransmitter acetylcholine. The prototype depolarizing blocking agent is succinylcholine, which is commonly utilized as a brief paralyzing agent in emergency departments and operating rooms to assist in rapid-induction endotracheal intubation (placing a breathing tube through a patient's mouth and into their airway). The mechanism of action begins when succinylcholine occupies the nicotinic receptor and produces a flaccid (relaxed) paralysis. Additionally, because succinylcholine is not broken down by the enzyme that normally breaks down acetylcholine, it remains at the site longer, exhibiting its action of inducing flaccid paralysis. A second phase occurs when the receptor becomes so desensitized that it no longer responds to acetylcholine. Adverse reactions to succinylcholine can include bronchiole constriction, decreased blood pressure,

cardiac arrhythmias, and malignant hyperthermia. Another serious adverse reaction can occur in those few individuals who lack the degrading enzyme for succinylcholine as it can take several hours to reverse the response during which time they require mechanical assisted ventilation. Most individuals successfully degrade the drug rapidly, in a matter of several minutes.

The prototype nondepolarizing blocking agent is tubocurarine, which also produces muscle relaxation and decreased muscle tone. It is generally used for longer periods of paralysis and functions by blocking acetylcholine from gaining access to the nicotinic receptor. Adverse effects once again can include bronchiole constriction and decreased blood pressure. Other neuromuscular blocking agents and their characteristics are listed in Medication Table 12-4.

PRACTICE POINT

Reversal of neuromuscular blockade induced by rocuronium or vecuronium can be achieved using sugammadex (Bridion).

SUMMARY

Skeletal muscle relaxants are helpful in many unique medical settings. The neuromuscular blockers are used in surgery and with procedures, while the other categories of medications may be used in the outpatient setting. Centrally acting skeletal muscle relaxants and orphenadrine can be used effectively in the setting of acute muscle strain. Dantrolene and baclofen are distinctive in that they are more often used with chronic conditions that cause spasticity, such as cerebral palsy (CP) or after a stroke.

REFERENCES

1. AHFS. Clinical Drug Information: Dantrolene. https://www.ahfscdi.com/drugs/382576. Accessed 2011.
2. Lexicomp. Lexi-Drugs. Hudson, Ohio: Wolters Kluwer. https://online.lexi.com/lco/action/home/. Accessed April 8, 2022.
3. U.S. Department of Justice. Office of Diversion Control. Drugs and Chemicals of Concern: Carisoprodol. https://www.deadiversion.usdoj.gov/fed_regs/rules/2011/fr1212_10.htm;https://www.deadiversion.usdoj.gov/drug_chem_info/cyclobenzaprine.pdf#search=cyclobenzaprine. Accessed June 17, 2022.

ADDITIONAL RESOURCES FOR MUSCULOSKELETAL PHARMACOLOGY

For additional information, consider the sources below

Kruidering-Hall M, Campbell L. Skeletal muscle relaxants. In: Katzung B ed. *Basic and Clinical Pharmacology*. 14th ed. New York, NY: McGraw-Hill Education/Lange; 2018:474.

Luke A, Ma C. Sports Medicine and Outpatient Orthopedics. In: Papadakis MA, McPhee SJ, Rabow MW. eds. Current Medical Diagnosis and Treatment 2020. McGraw Hill; 2020

Sports Medicine and outpatient orthopedics. In: Papadakis M, McPhee S, Rabow M, eds. *Current Medical Diagnosis & Treatment 2020*. New York, NY: McGraw-Hill Education/ Lange; 2020:1708.

Trevor AJ, Katzung BG, Kruiderling-Hall M. Skeletal muscle relaxants. General anesthetics. In: *Katzung & Trevor's Pharmacology: Examination & Board Review*. 12th ed. New York, NY: McGraw-Hill Education/Lange; 2019.

Whalen K., Drugs affecting the central nervous system. In: *Lippincott Illustrated Reviews: Pharmacology*.7th ed. Philadelphia: Wolters Kluwer; 2019.

REVIEW QUESTIONS

1. Name the categories of skeletal muscle relaxants and list one example drug for each.

2. Why are skeletal muscle relaxants used in the setting of acute low back pain, and what precautions should be taken?

3. What are five common side effects of centrally acting skeletal muscle relaxants?

4. List the components of the musculoskeletal system and their functions.

5. Why are neuromuscular blocking agents commonly used in the operating room or in emergency situations?

MEDICATION TABLES

MEDICATION TABLE 12-1. Centrally Acting Skeletal Muscle Relaxants*

Generic Name	Brand Name	Route	Dose[2]	Notes
Carisoprodol (kar eye soe PROE dole)	Soma	Oral	250–350 mg PO TID and nightly	Carisoprodol is subject to control under the Federal Controlled Substances Act of 1970 as a schedule IV (C-IV) drug. Preparations containing the drug in combination with codeine phosphate are subject to control under the Federal Controlled Substances Act of 1970 as schedule III (C-III) drugs.[3]
Chlorzoxazone (klor ZOX a zone)	Lorzone	Oral	250–500 mg PO TID to QID	Can discolor urine orange to red
Cyclobenzaprine hydrochloride (sye kloe BEN za preen)	Fexmid (7.5 mg tablets) Amrix (15 mg, 30 mg extended-release caplets)	Oral	5–10 mg PO TID 15–30 mg PO daily	Drowsiness is common While not (as of this writing) a controlled substance, cyclobenzaprine has been the subject of many reports of intentional abuse or misuse[3]
Metaxalone (me TAX a lone)	Skelaxin	Oral	800 mg PO TID to QID	Taken on empty stomach; causes less sedation than other agents in this class
Methocarbamol (meth oh KAR ba mole)	Robaxin (750 mg Oral) or 100 mg per mL (IM/IV) Generic methocarbamol is available in 500 mg or 750 mg for oral use	Oral IM/IV	1,000 mg PO QID 1,000–3000 mg/day IM/IV	May discolor urine black, brown, or green
Tizanidine hydrochloride (tye ZAN i deen)	Zanaflex (2 mg, 4 mg, 6 mg caplet or 4 mg tablet)	Oral	8 mg PO q 6–8 hr PRN	May cause hypotension; initial dose is 2 mg PO ×1 carefully titrated upward

*Pronunciations have been adapted with permission from USP Dictionary of USAN and International Drug Names (USP Dictionary) © 2022.
IM = intramuscular; IV = intravenous; PO = by mouth; PRN = as needed; QID = 4 times daily; TID = 3 times daily.

MEDICATION TABLE 12-2. Other Skeletal Muscle Relaxants*

Category	Generic Name	Brand Name	Route	Dose[2]	Notes
Skeletal muscle relaxants, miscellaneous	Orphenadrine (or FEN a dreen)		Oral, IM, IV	Oral: 100 mg PO BID; IM/IV: 60 mg q 12 hr	Also analgesic effect; rare side effect: aplastic anemia
Direct-acting skeletal muscle relaxants/ Antispasmodic	Dantrolene sodium (DAN troe leen)	Dantrium Ryanodex (injection) and Revonto (injection)	Oral, IV	Oral: 100 mg PO TID to QID; IV titrated based on body weight and patient condition	Commonly used in IV form to treat malignant hyperthermia, potential for hepatotoxicity
GABA-derivative skeletal muscle relaxants/ Antispasmodic	Baclofen (BAK loe fen)	Ozobax (solution) Fleqsuvy (suspension) Lioresal (inj-see dosing) Gablofen (inj-see dosing)	Oral, IT	Oral: 20–80 mg/day PO divided TID to QID; IT: titrated up to a maintenance dose of 90–700 mcg/day infusion via implanted pump	Should be tapered gradually rather than abruptly discontinued

*Pronunciations have been adapted with permission from USP Dictionary of USAN and International Drug Names (USP Dictionary) © 2022.
BID = 2 times daily; IM = intramuscular; IT = intrathecal; IV = intravenous; PO = by mouth; QID = 4 times daily; TID = 3 times daily.

MEDICATION TABLE 12-3. Oral Combination Products (Muscle Relaxant with Analgesic)*

Brand Name	Muscle Relaxant/tablet strength	Analgesic(s)/tablet strength	Dose	Notes
Norgesic	Orphenadrine citrate/25 mg (or FEN a dreen)	Aspirin/385 mg and (AS pir in)	½ to 1 tablet PO TID to QID	Also contains caffeine 30 mg (KAF een)
Norgesic, Orphengesic	Orphenadrine citrate/50 mg (or FEN a dreen)	Aspirin/770 mg and (AS pir in)	½ to 1 tablet PO TID to QID	Also contains caffeine 60 mg (KAF een)
(Various generics)	Carisoprodol/200 mg) (kar eye soe PROE dole)	Aspirin 325 mg and Codeine/16 mg	1–2 PO QID	Addiction, abuse, Misuse potential. DEA Schedule IV

*Pronunciations have been adapted with permission from USP Dictionary of USAN and International Drug Names (USP Dictionary) © 2022.
PO = orally; QID = 4 times daily; TID = 3 times daily.

MEDICATION TABLE 12-4. Neuromuscular Blocking Agents[2]*

Neuromuscular Blocking Agents (type)	Generic Name	Brand Name	Notes	Adverse Effects
Depolarizing	Succinylcholine chloride "Sux" (SUX i nil KOE leen) (KLOR ide)	Anectine, Quelicin	Ultrashort-acting, less than 5 min	May increase intraocular pressure; may cause malignant hyperthermia; may increase potassium levels; may cause cardiac arrhythmias, use in pediatric patients is strictly used for emergency situations only
Nondepolarizing	Atracurium besylate (a tra KURE ree um) (BES i late)		May need higher doses in burn patients	Flushing is a common dermatologic effect; may also cause hives, rash, and bronchospasm
	Cisatracurium besylate (sis at ra KURE ee um) (BES i late)	Nimbex	May cause prolonged relaxation, which may be useful in a critical care situation with a patient on mechanical ventilation	May cause prolonged apnea
	Pancuronium bromide (pan kure OH nee um) (BROE mide)		Black box warning: this drug should be administered by adequately trained individuals familiar with its actions, characteristics, and hazards	Avoid in renal impairment
	Rocuronium bromide (roe kure OH nee um) (BROE mide)		Compatible in solution with N5, D5W, D5NS, LR, or sterile water for injection	Anaphylaxis is a serious immunologic adverse effect; common adverse effects also include hypertension, hypotension, tachycardia, and increased pulmonary vascular resistance
	Vecuronium bromide (VEK ue ROE nee um) (BROE mide)			Black box warning: this drug should be administered by adequately trained individuals familiar with its actions, characteristics, and hazards

*Pronunciations have been adapted with permission from USP Dictionary of USAN and International Drug Names (USP Dictionary) © 2022.
D5W = 5% Dextrose in Water; D5NS = 5% Dextrose in Normal Saline; LR = lactated Ringer's solution; NS = Normal Saline.

Chapter 13

Disorders of the Musculoskeletal System

Bianca Harris, PharmD |
Amanda R. Margolis, PharmD, MS, BCACP

KEY TERMS AND DEFINITIONS

Autoimmune—characterization of diseases caused by the body's immune system attacking its own tissues.

Cytokines—proteins that help to mediate the immune system. They are cell signaling proteins, which in the case of rheumatoid arthritis increase inflammation.

Gouty arthritis—a painful joint condition caused by increased levels of uric acid.

Osteoarthritis (OA)—a painful joint condition primarily found in older adult patients and characterized by decreased cartilage.

Osteoporosis—a bone condition with decreased bone density that leaves patients at increased risk for bone fractures.

Rheumatoid arthritis (RA)—a painful joint condition caused by autoimmune mechanisms that can lead to joint deformity and disability.

Systemic lupus erythematosus (SLE)—a systemic autoimmune condition that can lead to multiple organ system failure.

Uric acid—a natural byproduct the body produces from metabolism of purines. It has no known physiologic function.

DOI 10.37573/9781585286638.013

LEARNING OBJECTIVES

After completing this chapter, you should be able to

1. Recognize the cause of gouty arthritis and list the therapies to prevent an attack.

2. Describe prescription and supplemental therapies for osteoporosis.

3. Calculate the amount of elemental calcium in a calcium supplement.

4. Describe prescription and supplemental therapies for osteoarthritis.

5. Recognize common regimens for rheumatoid arthritis and their adverse effects.

6. Recognize common symptoms of and organs affected by systemic lupus erythematosus.

7. State the brand and generic names of widely used medications for musculoskeletal conditions, along with their routes of administrations and dosage forms available.

As we learned in Chapter 12, the musculoskeletal system is a complex set of moving parts. Disorders of this system can make movement difficult and result in acute or chronic pain for the patients affected. Gout, arthritis, and osteoporosis are widespread conditions, and, while less common, auto-immune disorders such as lupus can be life threatening. In this chapter, we will discuss the causes of and treatments for several musculoskeletal disorders.

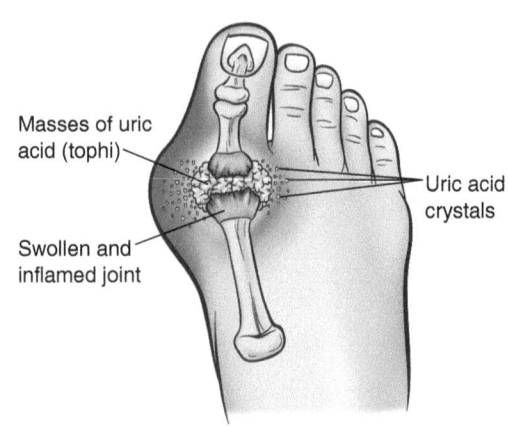

FIGURE 13-1. Tophus.

dietary sources or be made by the body as building blocks for nucleotides. High levels of uric acid are attributed to either the overproduction or underexcretion of uric acid. When the uric acid level becomes too high, it causes uric acid crystals to form in the joints and other organs, such as the kidney, and under the skin. These crystals cause inflammation in the joints, which leads to a gouty attack (also referred to as "gout flare").

The primary symptoms of a gouty attack include joint pain and swelling, which often presents in the great toe. Other joints that can be affected include the instep of the foot, ankles, heels, knees, wrists, fingers, and elbows. High uric acid levels may precipitate in the kidneys, causing renal stones, and under the skin, forming nodules called a tophus (plural = tophi). The incidence of gout increases with age, male gender, high blood pressure, increased body weight, and increased alcohol consumption (Figure 13-1).

CASE STUDY

Mr. Bob is a 58-year-old male who currently is not overweight but does report joint pain in his knees and hips to his pharmacist. He does not drink alcohol on a regular basis.

CASE?

Mr. Bob visits his physician for his yearly physical and receives a blood test that shows his uric acid is high. Would you expect him to need a prescription for this?

GOUT

High levels of uric acid are directly correlated with gouty arthritis. Uric acid is considered an unusable byproduct of degraded purines. Purines are chemicals that can come from

High levels of uric acid do not always lead to the occurrence of gout and should only be treated when there is an acute attack or to prevent recurrent attacks. While gouty arthritis attacks resolve spontaneously within a few weeks, medications are often used to speed the resolution. Some patients may be candidates for prophylactic medications to prevent attacks depending on certain factors, including frequency of gouty attacks or if the attacks are very severe. Medications for gout can be divided into two groups: medications used to speed the resolution of an acute attack and medications used to prevent future attacks. See Medication Table 13-1 for details on doses and dosage forms of antigout medications. (Medication Tables are located at the end of the chapter.)

CASE?

Mr. Bob comes to the pharmacy to ask for the strongest pain reliever he can get without a prescription because he developed a terrible pain in his big toe 3 days ago and it has still not gone away. He mentions that his doctor had told him he had a high uric acid level. What do you expect the pharmacist might recommend?

Medications to Stop an Acute Attack

Colchicine, nonsteroidal anti-inflammatory drugs (NSAIDs), or corticosteroids are appropriate therapies for an acute gouty attack. Short courses of high-dose NSAIDs are the most frequently used treatment for an acute attack of gout. Treatment is usually prescribed for 1 to 2 weeks and is usually most effective when started soon after the onset of symptoms. Gastrointestinal (GI) side effects are the most common problems encountered with NSAIDs, including serious GI bleeding, ulceration, and perforation. They should be avoided in patients with renal failure as they can worsen this condition. In patients with heart failure, salt and water retention from NSAIDs may lead to worsening of this condition. NSAIDs can also increase the risk of serious and possibly fatal cardiovascular thrombotic events.

Colchicine reduces the body's inflammatory reaction to uric acid crystals, which decreases inflammation and pain. However, colchicine is not an analgesic. It can be very effective if initiated early after the onset of symptoms. Dose-related GI toxicity (nausea, vomiting, and diarrhea) are common. For an acute gouty attack, patients are directed to take two tablets (0.6 mg) at the first sign of a gout flare, followed by 0.6 mg 1 hour later (max 1.8 mg per total dose/course). For some patients, colchicine can also be used to prevent future acute attacks with a dose of 0.6 mg once or twice daily. Some patients may need a dose adjustment depending on renal function and/or drug-drug interactions.

Short treatment courses of corticosteroids are also useful to treat acute gout. They are preferred drugs for patients with contraindications to NSAIDs and colchicine (eg, renal failure) or when patients are unresponsive to these drugs. Dosing regimens vary, but most patients are treated initially with prednisone 20–60 mg daily and the dose is then tapered over 1 to 2 weeks. Injectable triamcinolone acetonide may also be administered directly into an inflamed joint or by intramuscular (IM) injection if the oral route is not desired or multiple joints are affected.

CASE?

Mr. Bob took the pharmacist's advice and got in touch with his physician, and returns with two prescriptions, one for enough ibuprofen 800 mg tablets to last 2 weeks and one for colchicine 0.6 mg tablets. There are no refills ordered for the ibuprofen, but for colchicine there is a 90-day supply with three refills. Why do you think the prescriptions were written this way?

Medications to Prevent Acute Attacks

Although colchicine alone may be effective for prophylaxis given chronically in low doses, it does not lower uric acid levels in the blood. Lowering uric acid is warranted in some patients, for example, patients who form renal stones or develop tophi. Many of the pharmacologic therapies to prevent attacks either work to increase the excretion or decrease the production of uric acid.

Probenecid is a uricosuric agent, meaning it prevents the kidneys from reabsorbing uric acid and thus increases its excretion. This decreases uric acid levels in the blood, which prevents the formation of uric acid crystals in joints. Probenecid is slowly titrated to a therapeutic dose (see Medication Table 13-1). Common adverse events associated with uricosuric agents include nausea, rash, occurrence of an acute gouty attack, and formation of uric acid stones. Probenecid should be avoided in patients with poor renal function and in those with a history of renal stones. Probenecid is not effective in patients who have high uric acid levels due to overproduction. Patients who are overproducers of uric acid should receive a medication to block the formation of uric acid.

Allopurinol, which decreases the blood uric acid level by preventing its formation, is used to prevent gout attacks.

A very rare but serious rash can occur with allopurinol and any signs of rash should be reported to the patient's physician as soon as possible. Allopurinol, if used alone, may actually induce an acute gout attack when therapy is initiated. That is the reason medications to minimize gout attack, such as colchicine, are usually given concurrently with the allopurinol when it is started. This helps prevent gout attacks while uric acid levels are being adjusted. Colchicine may be discontinued 3 months after patients achieve their target uric acid level in the blood if they do not have tophi. In a patient with tophi, colchicine is typically continued for 6 months after the patient achieves the target uric acid level in the blood. A lower dose of allopurinol and colchicine may be prescribed for patients with poor renal function.

Febuxostat is also used to prevent uric acid formation and decrease uric acid levels in the blood. It can be taken by some patients who develop side effects to allopurinol or those with an inadequate response to allopurinol. The recommended dose is 40–80 mg once daily. As with allopurinol, the maximum dose of febuxostat is decreased in patients with poor renal function. Febuxostat has been associated with an increased risk of cardiovascular-related deaths in patients with a history of cardiovascular disease compared with allopurinol.

PRACTICE POINT

Alcohol can exacerbate a gouty attack. Patients with gout should be encouraged to minimize or abstain from alcohol.

Some patients suffer from chronic gout and do not respond to any of the therapies listed above; they are said to have treatment-resistant gout. There is an injectable enzyme preparation, pegloticase, which can be used in their care. Pegloticase reduces serum uric acid by promoting a chemical reaction that changes it to allantoin, a metabolite that is excreted by the kidney. Use of pegloticase is limited by the fact that it must be administered intravenously every 2 weeks and it has been associated with severe and potentially fatal reactions, such as anaphylaxis and congestive heart failure. It has also been associated with infusion reactions and blood disorders such as hemolysis, a breakdown of red blood cells in certain patients. It is, thus, reserved for patients whose gout is severe and cannot be treated otherwise. It is not used to reduce uric acid levels in patients without symptoms.

ALERT!

Pegloticase is administered intravenously over at least 2 hours and only in a healthcare setting by healthcare providers who are prepared to manage severe reactions.

PRACTICE POINT

Pegloticase infusions are prepared by diluting the dose in 250 mL of 0.9% or 0.45% sodium chloride injection, and no other drug or solution may be added to the admixture. This infusion is stable for 4 hours and should be protected from light. Pegloticase preparations may be gently inverted, but should never be shaken.

OSTEOPOROSIS

Bones are constantly being remodeled by osteoclasts and osteoblasts. Osteoclasts are cells that resorb the bone and osteoblasts rebuild the bone. Osteoporosis is the consequence of decreased bone density that occurs when the osteoclasts are more effective than the osteoblasts; over time, more bone is removed than rebuilt. In osteoporosis bone density is declining. This leaves bones frail, brittle, and easily broken.

Osteoporosis is a health threat that puts older adult patients at a much higher risk for fractures after a fall. Fractures can be very painful and debilitating. It is not uncommon for a patient to spend time at a rehabilitation facility after a hip fracture, and many patients never regain their baseline level of function. Mortality is increased for patients who have hip fractures. Women are at risk, particularly postmenopause, but osteoporosis also occurs in males. Vitamin D deficiency, cigarette smoking, low calcium intake, low physical activity, and corticosteroid therapy all increase the risk for osteoporosis.

Osteoporosis is a silent disease as patients do not feel the decrease in their bone density unless a fracture occurs. Osteoporosis is diagnosed through a bone density test. The test used to measure bone density is a dual energy x-ray

TABLE 13-1. Percent Elemental Calcium in Various Calcium Salts

Calcium Salt	Percent Elemental Calcium
Calcium gluconate	9
Calcium citrate	21
Calcium carbonate	40

Source: LexiComp Online. Hudson, OH: Wolters Kluwer.

in a supplement will often be included in the Supplemental Facts Panel of a product.

absorptiometry (DXA). It uses x-rays to take images of the thickness of the bones in specific areas, which are then interpreted as T-scores. A T-score assesses bone density, comparing a patient's bone density to that of a young healthy sex-matched reference value. As people age, their bone density and T-scores decrease. A diagnosis of osteoporosis is usually made following a low-impact fracture or when the T-score is less than 2.5 but other circumstances in special populations may also meet the definition of osteoporosis. Treatment of osteoporosis includes nondrug and drug therapy. Lifestyle changes include a healthy diet, limiting alcohol intake, stopping smoking, weight-bearing exercise, and prevention of falls.

Osteomalacia is another silent bone disease resulting from improper mineralization of the bones. In children this is called rickets. Osteomalacia occurs when a patient has deficiencies of calcium, phosphorus, or vitamin D. Treatment for osteomalacia varies based on the underlying cause. For some patients, vitamin D supplementation is appropriate while others may require the help of a specialist.

Calcium

Proper calcium supplementation is crucial to maintaining healthy bones. Appropriate levels of calcium help to prevent osteoclasts from over-resorbing bone. Women over the age of 50 years and men over the age of 70 years are advised to take 1,200 mg of elemental calcium daily. Calcium from dietary sources is preferred but supplementation can be used if needed. When a patient asks which calcium to choose it is important to take the salt form of the calcium into account. Different forms of calcium have different percentages of elemental calcium, which is the amount available for absorption (Table 13-1). The amount of elemental calcium found

Calcium from food should also be considered when choosing an appropriate amount of calcium supplementation. As a general rule, a serving of dairy (eg, milk, yogurt, cheese) can be considered 300 mg of elemental calcium. Calcium supplements may cause upset stomach and can be taken with food to minimize nausea. Constipation can also be a problem for some patients taking calcium supplements.

Vitamin D

Vitamin D must also be supplemented to help calcium be absorbed. An appropriate daily dose for an adult with osteoporosis is 1,000–2,000 units of vitamin D, but some patients will need higher doses. Often patients are prescribed a daily dose. Some patients take vitamin D in a 50,000-unit capsule if their vitamin D level is deficient. Patients will start with one capsule once or twice a week until their level is normalized and then take one 50,000-unit capsule monthly. It is frequently necessary for patients to take supplemental vitamin D in addition to the vitamin D they may get from their diet and the vitamin D they produce from sunlight exposure. Clinicians can measure vitamin D levels and adjust the vitamin D dose as needed.

Bisphosphonates

Bisphosphonates are a first-line medication option for the prevention and treatment of osteoporosis (see Medication Table 13-2). They work by inhibiting osteoclasts from resorbing bone. Bisphosphonates attach to bone and are taken up by the osteoclasts. They then prevent the osteoclast from functioning. Bisphosphonates can be administered on varying schedules. Some people prefer to take them daily so they will not forget a dose, but they are commonly dosed weekly or monthly. Bisphosphonates can also be given intravenously and dosed every 3 months to yearly.

ALERT!

There is a LOOK-ALIKE SOUND-ALIKE warning for Actonel, a commonly used bisphosphonate, and Actos, a medication to lower blood glucose in patients with diabetes.

ALERT!

Bisphosphonates are not interchangeable and must be administered on the dosing schedule appropriate for each medication and preparation.

Oral bisphosphonates are not absorbed very well. Patients should take them first thing in the morning on an empty stomach with a large glass of water. After taking the tablet they should refrain from eating and remain upright for an additional 30 minutes. The common adverse effects of bisphosphonates include bone pain, heartburn, and upset stomach. Irritation and ulceration of the esophagus may occur with oral bisphosphonates. Patients with a history of esophageal reflux or swallowing disorders are at increased risk. Patients should report new or worsening heartburn symptoms to a healthcare provider. A serious but rare adverse

effect of bisphosphonates is osteonecrosis of the jaw (ONJ). ONJ results in exposure of jaw bone, with severe pain due to the death of bone tissue, and a high risk of infection. While still rare, it is more common in patients using intravenous (IV) bisphosphonates in an oncology setting. Patients should alert their dentists if they take bisphosphonates since ONJ is more likely to occur after dental procedures. See Medication Table 13-2 to review specific bisphosphonates and their dosing schedules.

CASE?

Mrs. Roberts was told she had a T-score of -3 and had to start a prescription for weekly alendronate. She doesn't like having to take the tablet and wait another 30 minutes until she can have her breakfast. What are possible alternatives that the pharmacist can recommend to her doctor to minimize the number of bisphosphonate tablets she takes?

Denosumab

Denosumab is a monoclonal antibody RANK ligand inhibitor that prevents the formation of functional osteoclasts. In addition to osteoporosis, denosumab is used in several other populations of patients at high risk for fracture, such as men with prostate cancer undergoing androgen deprivation therapy. Denosumab is administered subcutaneously (SUBQ) by a healthcare professional every 6 months using a prefilled syringe. While denosumab is generally well tolerated, the most common adverse effects include skin rashes and other dermatologic reactions unrelated to injection site reactions. Severe but rare side effects include skin infections, back and joint pain, ONJ, and severe hypocalcemia (ie, very low blood calcium). Hypocalcemia is more likely in individuals with poor kidney function.

Romosozumab

Romosozumab is a monoclonal antibody that inhibits the formation of sclerostin. Sclerostin helps to regulate bone metabolism. This in turn increases bone formation and is associated with a small reduction in bone resorption. Romosozumab is administered by a health professional once a month for up to 1 year. Each dose is 210 mg of romosozumab SUBQ, but this requires the use of two 105-mg prefilled syringes per dose. The prefilled syringe should be stored in the refrigerator but can be at room temperature up to 30 days. The most common adverse effect is joint pain. More serious adverse effects include headache and injection site reactions. Romosozumab has a black box warning for increased risk of stroke, heart attack, and cardiovascular death. Like other medications for osteoporosis, there is a slight risk for ONJ.

Selective Estrogen Receptor Modulators

There are two approved selective estrogen receptor modulators (SERMs), raloxifene and bazedoxifene. Estrogen has a positive impact on bone. It binds to receptors on the bone and decreases the activity of osteoclasts while increasing the activity of osteoblasts. This is why bone density significantly decreases in postmenopausal women. However, the benefits do not outweigh the risk of using hormone replacement therapy in postmenopausal women for osteoporosis due to the high risk of heart attack and stroke. Raloxifene stimulates estrogen receptors at the bone but blocks estrogen in breast and uterine tissue. Raloxifene is approved both as an agent to prevent bone loss and also for breast cancer prevention. Raloxifene is only indicated for use in postmenopausal women because before menopause women create enough estrogen naturally to maintain an adequate bone density. Bazedoxifene comes in combination with conjugated equine estrogens and is also useful for women experiencing menopausal symptoms, but is not approved for breast cancer prevention.

The common side effects of SERMs include leg cramps, swelling of the extremities, joint pain, and sweating. Raloxifene can also cause hot flashes, which is reduced with bazedoxifene. SERMs also make women more likely to experience blood clots. Patients taking SERMs should be educated on the signs and symptoms of a blood clot and to take precautions, such as moving legs regularly while traveling, to help prevent clots.

ALERT!

Be aware of a LOOK-ALIKE SOUND-ALIKE potential for Evista (raloxifene) and Avinza. Avinza is a brand name for morphine sulfate.

Parathyroid Hormone Analogs

Parathyroid hormone (often called PTH) regulates the activity of osteoclasts and osteoblasts so that osteoblasts are more active than osteoclasts. This generates the formation of bone and a higher bone density. Teriparatide and abaloparatide are both analogs of PTH, meaning they act similarly in the body. PTH therapy is usually used if bisphosphonate therapy fails in a patient. PTH analogs are given SUBQ once daily. Both teriparatide and abaloparatide comes as a multi-dose, autoinjector pen. Both teriparatide and abaloparatide pens must be stored in the refrigerator before use. While abaloparatide can be stored at room temperature after the first use, the teriparatide pen must stay in the refrigerator, even between uses. There is no specific time of the day PTH analog therapy should be used; however, it is best if the patient has a consistent time to use the medication. It is currently suggested not to use these agents for longer than 2 years.

Patients are cautioned to give themselves the teriparatide injection in an environment where they can sit or lie down if they become lightheaded. PTH analogs can cause injection site reactions, leg cramps, headache, dizziness, and nausea. Lastly, as PTH analogs have increased the risk of osteomalacia in animal studies, patients are cautioned there is a potential for increased risk in humans, but this has not yet been confirmed.

ALERT!

The teriparatide pens contain enough medication for 28 days and should be discarded at 28 days even if there is medication remaining in the pen. The abaloparatide pen contains enough medication for 30 days and should be discarded at 30 days even if there is medication remaining in the pen.

PRACTICE POINT

Patients who receive teriparatide pens will also need pen needles to inject the medication.

Calcitonin

Calcitonin also prevents further bone loss. It is not as effective as bisphosphonates and is more expensive so it is reserved for patients who cannot tolerate bisphosphonate therapy or when bisphosphonate therapy fails. Calcitonin is only approved for women 5 years postmenopause, but it is also used for men. Salmon calcitonin is used because it is more potent and works longer than human calcitonin. Most patients administer the calcitonin nasally but it can also be given SUBQ.

PRACTICE POINT

Like other prescription nasal sprays, patients using the calcitonin nasal spray should be reminded to prime the device before giving themselves the first dose. The usual dose is one spray in one nostril alternating daily. Some patients may experience some irritation of the nostrils but the nasal spray is otherwise well tolerated.

OSTEOARTHRITIS

There are two main forms of arthritis: osteoarthritis (OA), is localized to the joints while rheumatoid arthritis (RA) is a more systemic condition. OA is characterized by loss of joint cartilage. Cartilage is the connective tissue between joints that minimizes friction between bones. Reasons for decreased cartilage in OA is multifactorial and include joint injury (possibly from trauma or stress from obesity), decreased ability to repair joint damage, and inflammation. Over time the balance between the formation and destruction of cartilage is lost and the cushion between joints diminishes. The incidence of OA increases with age. Risk factors for OA include obesity, joint trauma, gender, and race.

OA is characterized by pain in the joints, morning stiffness lasting less than 30 minutes, crepitus (crackling sound with joint movement), and instability of weight-bearing joints. The joints most often affected are the hands, knees, and hips, but the neck and spine can also be affected. In the late stages of OA there are abnormal alignment of the joints and severe debilitation from pain. OA is diagnosed based primarily on physical exam and history; however, x-ray and specific lab tests can be used to determine the severity of OA and rule out other forms of arthritis. Patients with OA may have radiographic changes characteristic of the condition.

All patients with OA should be educated about nonpharmacologic options such as exercise, weight loss, and assistive devices. See Medication Table 13-3 for medications used for OA.

CASE?

Mr. Bob, first introduced in the section on gout, is found by his physician to have OA. He has been told to try an over-the-counter (OTC) acetaminophen product to help with his knee and hip pain. He also has Tylenol PM on his medication list. What should be reviewed with Mr. Bob regarding his Tylenol OTC with the suggested acetaminophen?

Acetaminophen

Acetaminophen is often the first-line pharmacologic agent for patients with OA. Acetaminophen is an analgesic. It has fewer adverse effects within the older adult population than NSAIDs and is the preferred agent for patients with kidney failure. The usual range of doses is 325–650 mg every 4–6 hours or 1 gram three to four times daily. Patients should be reminded not to exceed 4,000 mg per day of acetaminophen to prevent liver damage. In some cases, the medical provider may choose a lower maximum dose for a patient. For example, some suggest a maximum dose of 2,000 mg acetaminophen daily for older adults. Acetaminophen comes in many dosage forms, strengths, and combinations. Patients should be cautioned to verify the amount of acetaminophen they are taking to stay under the maximum amount. Patients with existing liver failure or high alcohol usage should not use acetaminophen.

Nonsteroidal Anti-Inflammatory Drugs

NSAIDs are commonly used medications. NSAIDs can be first line for OA, or if acetaminophen is ineffective in a patient with OA, NSAIDs are often the next choice for pharmacotherapy. Ibuprofen and naproxen are available OTC at low doses, but all remaining NSAIDs are available by prescription only. NSAIDs work by inhibiting an enzyme called cyclooxygenase (COX). This decreases the production of prostaglandins, which reduces inflammation and relieves pain. See Medication Table 13-4.

ALERT!

LOOK-ALIKE/SOUND-ALIKE—Watch for a common mistake of confusing Celexa, an antidepressant, with Celebrex, a COX-2-selective NSAID.

PRACTICE POINT

Not all NSAIDs and products containing them are appropriate for treating arthritis. An NSAID combination NOT used for arthritis is Treximet, which contains sumatriptan, a triptan used for migraines, and naproxen.

There are two different COX enzymes: COX-1 and COX-2. COX-1 is found in the GI system, kidneys, and platelets. COX-2 is found in macrophages, epithelial cells, the central nervous system, bone, kidney, the reproductive tract, and other areas. Most NSAIDs block both COX-1 and COX-2. Celecoxib is a COX-2-selective NSAID. Since it only blocks COX-2 and does not block cyclooxygenase in the stomach, it is thought to lower the incidence of GI symptoms associated with NSAIDs. Celecoxib is not more potent than other NSAIDs but may have a lower incidence of epigastric pain in the first 3 to 6 months of use. However, following that initial use the incidence of GI adverse effects is similar to nonselect NSAIDs and there is little convincing evidence that celecoxib reduces the risk of serious GI bleeding.

ALERT!

Patients who have an allergy to sulfa-containing medications should refrain from using celecoxib because of a potential cross reaction.

A common adverse effect of NSAIDs is nausea. Nausea can be minimized by taking the medication with food or milk.

Some patients may also notice mild dizziness or fatigue; however, these are not common effects. NSAIDs can increase blood pressure in patients and when possible should be avoided in patients who already have hypertension. Patients who have asthma are at higher risk of having sensitivity to aspirin and other NSAIDs and should contact their physician immediately with any signs of difficulty breathing after using the medications.

There can be serious adverse effects with the use of NSAIDs. They increase the risk of GI bleeding or a stomach ulcer. Approximately 20% to 30% of all serious GI bleeds that cause death or require hospitalization are attributed to NSAIDs in patients over 65 years old. For patients with other risk factors for a GI bleed or a previous GI bleed, NSAIDs should be avoided or other medications, such as a proton pump inhibitor, can be used to lower the risk of stomach ulcers. All patients who take NSAIDs should be taught the warning signs of GI bleeding. This includes dark tarry stools or vomit that looks like coffee grounds.

NSAIDs can also induce renal failure in patients and are contraindicated in patients with kidney failure. This is especially true for patients who are over 65 years old with comorbid conditions like hypertension or heart failure. NSAIDs can also increase the risk for heart attack (also known as myocardial infarction) and stroke and may worsen congestive heart failure. To reduce the risk of these toxicities, the lowest possible effective dosage should be used for the shortest time. Only a single NSAID should be taken by a patient at a time.

Diclofenac is an NSAID that can also be used topically and has similar evidence to oral NSAID use. However, topical diclofenac has decreased adverse effects and may be used in some patients with contraindications to oral NSAIDs. Topical diclofenac is especially beneficial for knee OA but can also be considered for hand OA; it is not advised for hip OA as the medication does not reach the joint. There is an increase in local adverse effects where the product is administered on the skin, including itching and rash. Different topical preparations, such as a gel or a solution, have different application instructions, which the patient needs to be educated on.

PRACTICE POINT

All NSAIDs are associated with increased cardiovascular risk and should be used with caution in patients with cardiovascular disease and older adults.

Tramadol

Tramadol is approved for moderate to severe pain and can be used in patients with contraindications to NSAIDs. It can also be used in patients with poor kidney function or if other oral medications fail. Doses range from 200–300 mg in four divided doses. Tramadol is generally well tolerated, with fewer adverse effects than NSAIDs; notably there is not an increased risk for GI bleeding or cardiovascular events. Side effects are similar to opioids and include nausea, dizziness, drowsiness, and constipation. Tramadol also has the potential for withdrawal symptoms when stopped abruptly following chronic use. Additionally, tramadol does have the potential to cause seizures and caution should be used in deciding to start another medication that can lower the seizure threshold. Tramadol is a scheduled medication due to the potential for dependence and diversion.

Duloxetine

Patients in whom first-line agents for OA fail or who have contraindications to NSAIDs may find duloxetine beneficial. Duloxetine is a serotonin/norepinephrine reuptake inhibitor (SNRI) and is thought to minimize pain by blocking pain receptors. As duloxetine is effective for central pain, it is especially useful for patients who have neuropathic pain, or nerve pain, in addition to OA. Duloxetine is taken once daily and it can take up to 4 weeks before an improvement in pain is seen. Common adverse effects include dry mouth,

drowsiness, headache, nausea, vomiting, and constipation. Rare but severe adverse effects include severe rash, called Stevens-Johnson syndrome, and liver damage.

Capsaicin

Capsaicin cream is made from the ingredient in chili peppers that makes them hot. Capsaicin can be used in combination with oral medications for knee OA and is directly applied to painful joints. Capsaicin is not recommended for use with hand OA. Capsaicin is thought to work by dulling the nerves in the immediate area where the cream is applied, minimizing the pain from OA. When the cream is applied to the skin it creates a warming feeling, which some patients are not able to tolerate. This warming sensation does diminish over time with continued use.

Capsaicin cream should be applied four times a day. However, some individuals still experience benefit using it twice a day with better adherence. The onset of action is typically several weeks to a month of using the cream until there is relief from OA.

Intraarticular Hyaluronan Injection

There is limited evidence of efficacy, but some patients with knee OA may benefit from intraarticular hyaluronan injections. The doses used vary from 16–30 mg injected into the knee once weekly for 3–5 weeks. One product (Synvisc-One) contains 48 mg and is intended to be given as a single injection. It may take 1–2 weeks for patients to feel improvement. Given the lack of evidence supporting its effectiveness, the risk versus benefit of hyaluronan injections must be considered and it should only be offered to patients who have contraindications to other therapies or when other therapies have failed.

Patients with avian (bird) allergies should refrain from using hyaluronan. The most common adverse effects of intraarticular hyaluronan injections are injection site pain and swelling. Patients should be cautioned to avoid excessive or strenuous activity on the knee for 48 hours.

Opioids

Opioids are generally not recommended for the treatment of OA, but they may be considered when patients have exhausted other options or have contraindications to recommended therapies. They should be used in the lowest possible dose for the shortest period of time possible. The risk-to-benefit ratio must be considered carefully before deciding to try an opioid for a patient with OA. All opioids can cause dizziness and drowsiness. Patients will require counseling on the increased risk of falls and may benefit from having their home evaluated to decrease their fall potential. All patients who are prescribed opioids must also be counseled on the risk for dependence, tolerance, and diversion.

Glucosamine and Chondroitin

Glucosamine and chondroitin are OTC nutritional supplements with very limited efficacy and only for OA of the hand. There is no evidence to support the use of glucosamine and chondroitin in hip or knee OA and guidelines recommend against the use of these agents in those patients. The potential mechanism of action of glucosamine and chondroitin is unclear. The usual dose is a total of 1,500 mg glucosamine and 1,200 mg chondroitin daily. Many people split this into three doses a day. Patients can take the medication with food if they experience stomach upset, but it is usually well tolerated. Patients with shellfish allergies should be cautioned not to take glucosamine as there may be cross reactions.

PRACTICE POINT

Patients who have a history of bleeding problems, asthma, diabetes, cancer, or liver disease should consult their primary care providers before using glucosamine.

RHEUMATOID ARTHRITIS

Rheumatoid arthritis (RA) is a systemic form of arthritis that primarily affects the small joints of the hands, wrists, and feet in a symmetrical manner. RA is a progressive autoimmune disorder where the body's immune system attacks itself. RA is characterized by prolonged joint stiffness in the morning

(usually greater than 30 minutes) and inflamed joints, which are usually painful. If inadequately treated it leads to joint deformity, disability, and early mortality. The factors that stimulate the autoimmune process in RA are unknown, but in RA the immune system can no longer distinguish between a foreign substance that needs to be removed and natural joint tissues. This causes antibodies called rheumatoid factors to attack the joints, causing inflammation and degradation of cartilage and bone. B cells and T cells are also activated in RA; activated T cells produce cytokines. The cytokines contribute to joint inflammation and are directly toxic to joint tissue.

CASE STUDY

Ms. Jones is a 45-year-old woman who comes to the pharmacy wondering what she can try for her joint pain. She reports pain in her fingers and toes in the morning and feels like it takes several hours for her to "loosen up" every morning.

Nonpharmacologic measures for treating RA include physical therapy, specific exercise classes, and assistive devices to make it easier to maintain activities of daily living. Pharmacologic intervention is needed to prevent disease progression.

CASE?

Is there anything the pharmacist can recommend for Ms. Jones's pain?

Pharmacologic therapy consists of NSAIDs, corticosteroids, and disease-modifying antirheumatic drugs (DMARDs). While NSAIDs can be used to help with some of the pain associated with RA, they do not slow disease progression. Corticosteroids are not considered DMARDs, but they can help with pain and inflammation until the DMARD is efficacious. This is called bridging. Specific dosage forms and schedules of medications used in RA can be found in Medication Table 13-5.

Disease-Modifying Antirheumatic Drugs

All patients should be prescribed a DMARD within 3 months of being diagnosed with RA. Baseline evaluation of the renal and hepatic system should be conducted at diagnosis because many DMARDs have adverse effects on the kidneys and liver. DMARDs are classified as *conventional* and *biologic*. All work by decreasing different inflammatory mediators within the body to reduce RA disease activity. It is not unusual for triple therapy with conventional DMARDs to be used as first line or in the case that monotherapy or double DMARD therapy fails. Conventional DMARDs can be used in combination with a biologic DMARD; however, a biologic agent should never be used in combination with another biologic DMARD.

Conventional DMARDs

Conventional DMARDs are older drugs that reduce inflammation. Most conventional DMARDs are effective when taken orally.

Hydroxychloroquine

The exact mechanism of action of hydroxychloroquine is unknown. The usual dose is 200–400 mg daily. It may take up to 6 weeks before hydroxychloroquine is efficacious; however, a course of 6 months should be tried before discontinuing the medication. Short-term adverse effects include nausea, vomiting, and diarrhea. This is often minimized by taking the medication with food. Hydroxychloroquine does not cause liver or bone marrow toxicity, which is an advantage to using the medication. Hydroxychloroquine can cause macular damage, which can lead to blurry vision, decreased peripheral vision, and night blindness. Patients who take hydroxychloroquine should report any changes in vision. An eye exam is recommended at baseline, then yearly if the patient has significant risk factors for ocular toxicity, otherwise yearly eye exams can be started after 5 years of therapy with hydroxychloroquine. Patients should also report any signs of rash while taking the medication. Hydroxychloroquine can also cause an increase in pigmentation of the skin. This is a cosmetic effect and not considered a serious adverse effect.

CASE?

Ms. Jones had an appointment with her physician and was diagnosed with RA. She has a prescription for hydroxychloroquine and she is concerned about adverse effects. What might the pharmacist review with her when the prescription is dispensed?

Leflunomide

Leflunomide decreases lymphocyte proliferation. This means lymphocytes do not divide into new cells. The lymphocytes are white blood cells responsible for protecting the body from invading cells. Decreasing the number of lymphocytes in a patient with an autoimmune disease means there are fewer cells targeting the body as foreign. Since leflunomide interferes with the immune system, live vaccinations may not work properly for patients taking it. Leflunomide has a loading dose of 100 mg three times daily for 3 days. The maintenance dose is then 10–20 mg once daily. Some clinicians do not use loading doses because of the increased side effects associated with the higher doses. The onset of action ranges from 4–12 weeks.

Common adverse effects of leflunomide include hair loss and diarrhea. Leflunomide is teratogenic (ie, can cause birth defects in the children of pregnant women taking the medication). Women on leflunomide who wish to have children should speak with their physicians. The half-life of leflunomide is long (14 days) and it takes several months after discontinuation of the medication before it is out of the patient's system and it is safe for her to become pregnant.

Leflunomide rarely causes liver damage and liver failure. Liver function tests should be checked regularly in patients taking leflunomide. Any signs of rash should be reported to the physician as it may become life threatening. Cholestyramine may be used to eliminate leflunomide more rapidly in planned pregnancy or if severe side effects with leflunomide occur.

Methotrexate

The mechanism of action of methotrexate is believed to be related to decreasing cytokines or other inflammatory mediators. The dose of methotrexate can vary based on response and severity but the usual dosage is 7.5–25 mg once weekly. This can be taken orally, SUBQ, or by IM injection. Using a weekly dose helps to minimize adverse effects. Onset of action may be seen as soon as 2–3 weeks but may take up to 2 months. Methotrexate may be first-line therapy for some patients if their RA is more active, but for other patients it may be second line after a different conventional DMARD fails. Methotrexate may also be used in combination with another conventional DMARD or biologic DMARD.

ALERT!

Use caution in processing methotrexate prescriptions. Unlike other oral DMARDs, methotrexate dosing is once weekly. Taking methotrexate daily markedly increases the risk for toxicity and is never used this way for RA treatment (although daily doses are indicated for some other conditions).

Methotrexate can cause birth defects, and if pregnancy is desired by a woman taking methotrexate she should consult her physician. Less severe adverse effects include nausea, vomiting, and diarrhea. There can also be hair loss and photosensitivity. More severe adverse effects include very low platelet count, liver damage, kidney failure, and pulmonary damage. Patients should have their blood counts and liver function tests checked periodically. They should also be educated to report any signs of rash, problems breathing, or jaundice. Patients who take methotrexate should also take a daily folic acid supplement (1 mg/day) because methotrexate can cause folate deficiency. There is an antidote available for methotrexate toxicity, glucarpidase. It can be administered IV within 48–60 hours from the start of a high-dose methotrexate infusion to prevent methotrexate toxicities. However, given that the doses of methotrexate used for RA treatment are generally oral, SUBQ, or IM and significantly lower than those used for other indications, the antidote is generally not utilized in this setting.

Sulfasalazine

The exact mechanism of action of sulfasalazine in RA is unknown. It is not readily absorbed from the GI system, and bacteria in the colon cleave (divide) sulfasalazine into sulfapyridine and 5-aminosalicylic acid. The components are then absorbed systemically from the colon. The initial dose of sulfasalazine is 500 mg orally twice daily. This can be increased to 1–1.5 g twice daily if tolerated. Onset of action is seen in 1–3 months after starting sulfasalazine.

The dose-limiting toxicities of sulfasalazine include nausea, vomiting, diarrhea, and anorexia. This can be lessened by starting at a lower dose and slowly titrating up to the maintenance dose or using an enteric coated product. A rare but serious adverse effect is leukopenia, or decreased white blood cells, and patients should have their complete blood count monitored every 2–3 months. Patients should also have their liver function monitored as sulfasalazine can cause liver damage. Patients should be instructed to report any rashes to their physicians.

> ## ALERT!
>
> Patients who have an allergy to sulfa-containing medications should refrain from using sulfasalazine because of a potential cross reaction.

Other less used DMARDs include azathioprine, cyclosporine, cyclophosphamide, gold salts, d-penicillamine, and minocycline.

Biologic DMARDs

Biologic DMARDs are used when methotrexate or another conventional DMARD have failed to control the symptoms and disease progression or initially in patients with more severe disease. Biologic DMARDs are genetically engineered proteins that block pro-inflammatory mediators. They are all SUBQ or IV agents because, if taken orally, they are destroyed in the stomach. Their primary adverse effect is injection site reactions. Patients taking SUBQ biologics should be reminded to rotate injection sites to prevent scarring.

Biologic DMARDs require much less laboratory monitoring than conventional DMARDs; however, they put patients at risk for serious life-threatening infections. Biologic DMARDs carry a black box warning about the risk of tuberculosis and invasive fungal infections. In most cases patients will complete a tuberculosis skin test before starting, to assess their risk of latent tuberculosis, which could be reactivated while on a biologic DMARD. Hepatitis B (HBV) screening should also be completed prior to treatment with a biologic because therapy should not be initiated in acutely infected patients. In patients who are HBV carriers, there is a risk for reactivation and consideration for HBV prophylaxis may be needed.

Tumor Necrosis Factor-Alpha Inhibitors (TNF-α Blockers) Biologics

Tumor necrosis factor-alpha (TNF-α) is a key cytokine in the inflammation cascade for patients with RA. TNF-α blockers bind to TNF-α and prevent the TNF-α from interacting with the T-lymphocytes and other cells, which decreases inflammation. TNF-α may play a role in cancer prevention in the body. It has been suggested that TNF-α blockers may increase the risk of cancer; however, long-term data is lacking. Other serious adverse effects include worsening of heart failure and, very rarely, patients experience symptoms similar to multiple sclerosis. Patients taking TNF-α blockers should avoid live vaccines due to a decreased response to the vaccine and lack of safety data for this use. Methotrexate is often given with TNF-α inhibitors as it increases the efficacy of these drugs.

> ## ALERT!
>
> All currently available TNF-α blockers are stored in the refrigerator. Patients will need a sharps container as all biologic DMARDs are injected and the autoinjector and prefilled syringes will require proper disposal.

Etanercept is a fusion TNF-α blocker. It has two TNF receptors fused onto an IgG antibody. Etanercept comes as a syringe or an autoinjector and is given by SUBQ injection either 25 mg twice weekly or 50 mg once weekly.

CASE?

Approximately 2 years after starting hydroxychloroquine, Ms. Jones notes that it is no longer relieving her RA symptoms. She brings a new prescription for Humira (adalimumab) to the pharmacy and isn't sure where to store it when she goes home. What does the package insert advise?

Infliximab is also a TNF-α blocker and is only indicated for use in RA when used in combination with methotrexate. Infliximab is a chimeric IgG antibody to TNF-α. This means the antibody is part human and part mouse. The antibody was created by injecting human TNF-α into mice. The part of the mouse antigen that binds to TNF-α is fused to a human IgG antibody. This reduces the chance that patients react to the mouse part of the antibody.

Infliximab is administered IV in a clinic and the dose is 3 mg/kg at weeks 0, 2, and 6, and then every 8 weeks. Benefits may begin within 2 weeks of administration. Since infliximab incorporates mouse proteins, patients who use it may form antibodies to the medication. These antibodies may cause infusion reactions or loss of response, requiring higher doses or less time between treatments. To prevent this, methotrexate is continued for the duration of treatment with infliximab.

Adalimumab is an IgG antibody for TNF-α. It is fully humanized, but antibodies to the medication can still form. Adalimumab comes as a pen and a prefilled syringe. The usual dose is 40 mg SUBQ every other week. There is also a citrate-free formulation available that has several benefits, including reduced injection volume and decreased pain at the injection site.

Golimumab is a TNF-α blocker requiring once-monthly administration. It is available as an autoinjector and prefilled syringe for patients to use at home. It is suggested that, when used to treat RA, golimumab should be prescribed in combination with methotrexate.

Certolizumab is a pegylated TNF-α blocker. It is given as two SUBQ injections of 200 mg for a 400 mg dose. The 400 mg dose is given every 2 weeks for a total of three doses. Then it can be given as either 200 mg every 2 weeks or 400 mg every 4 weeks. Most patients will use it as a prefilled syringe.

Non-Tumor Necrosis Factor-Alpha Inhibitor Biologics

Anakinra

Interleukins are a type of cytokine that signals and stimulates other inflammatory cells to the site of inflammation. Some patients with RA produce excess interleukin-1. Anakinra is an interleukin-1-receptor antagonist (IL-1ra). It binds to the interleukin-1 receptor and prevents the interleukin from binding and interacting with the cell. This stops the activity of interleukin-1 and decreases inflammation in the joints.

Anakinra is used infrequently in RA. The recommended dose is 100 mg SUBQ daily. Anakinra is packaged in single-use, prefilled glass syringes. If a syringe has been dropped or has been left at room temperature for 24 hours, it should be discarded, even if there is no noticeable damage.

ALERT!

The needle cover for anakinra is made of a latex-based material and should not be handled by patients with latex sensitivities.

Abatacept

Abatacept is indicated for use in patients with moderate or severe RA. Abatacept inhibits T cell activity by binding to receptors responsible for cell activation. Activated T-lymphocytes have been found in the joint fluid of patients with RA and a decrease in their activity decreases inflammation and slows disease progression. Abatacept can be given as a 30-minute IV infusion by a healthcare professional and is also available in a prefilled syringe or autoinjector. For the IV formulation, dosing is based on the patient's weight. If the patient's weight is less than 60 kg, a 500-mg dose is used, 750 mg if a patient's weight is 60–100 kg, and 1,000 mg if the patient's weight is more than 100 kg. The dosing interval is week 0, 2, and 4, then every 4 weeks. For the subcutaneous route, the dose is 125 mg weekly. A patient may be started on the subcutaneous route at the initiation of therapy or may be started on the IV formulation (at weight-based dosing) and then switched to the subcutaneous route.

Patients with chronic obstructive pulmonary disease who take abatacept are more likely to experience acute exacerbations and should be monitored closely while taking the medication. Abatacept also makes patients more prone to headaches, upper respiratory infections, and urinary tract infections. There have been very rare cases of hypersensitivity or anaphylaxis while infusing the medication.

Rituximab

B-lymphocytes are blood cells that have a role in promoting inflammation associated with RA. Rituximab binds to B-lymphocytes, causing the death of these cells. The decreased activity of B-lymphocytes causes the inflammation to lessen and slows disease progression. Rituximab is an antibody against B-lymphocytes. It should only be used in patients in whom a TNF-α blocker has failed or in patients with contraindications to TNF-α blockers. Rituximab is usually prescribed in combination with methotrexate. The initial dose is 1,000 mg IV. A second dose is given 2 weeks later. The course may be repeated every 16–24 weeks and redosing is typically based on the patient's symptoms and disease control.

While receiving rituximab some patients have experienced severe infusion reactions, which rarely can result in death. To minimize the risk of infusion reaction patients are generally premedicated with a corticosteroid (such as prednisone), an antihistamine (often diphenhydramine), and acetaminophen 30 minutes prior to administration. Common adverse effects include itching, nausea, vomiting, and headache. Rare but serious adverse effects include low white blood cell counts, cardiac toxicity, and increased risk of infection. Patients should report any rashes to

their physician after receiving rituximab. The risk of HBV reactivation is high in patients who are HBV carriers starting rituximab; therefore, screening prior to treatment is important.

Tocilizumab

Tocilizumab is a recombinant humanized antihuman IL-6 receptor monoclonal antibody. It binds to IL-6 receptors, a proinflammatory cytokine, and inhibits cell signaling of T cells, B cells, lymphocytes, and monocytes. This helps to decrease the inflammatory process in RA. It is available as an IV formulation, an autoinjector, or a prefilled syringe to be administered subcutaneously. The IV formulation can be dosed at 4 mg/kg every 4 weeks and the dose may be increased to 8 mg/kg every 4 weeks, with a maximum of 800 mg per dose. The SUBQ formulation is dosed at 162 mg weekly; however, if a patient's weight is less than 100 kg, the dose should be started at 162 mg every other week and may be increased to weekly if needed. Tocilizumab can be used with or without methotrexate but should not be used in combination with another biologic DMARD. Common adverse effects of tocilizumab include headache, elevated blood pressure, increased liver enzymes, and increased cholesterol levels. Like other biologic DMARDs, the most serious adverse effect is infection, which can be life threatening. Other serious adverse reactions include GI perforation, low white blood cell count, and low platelet count.

Sarilumab

Sarilumab is a monoclonal antibody that binds to IL-6 receptors, which reduces inflammation and alters immune response. Sarilumab can be used alone or with methotrexate or other conventional DMARDs. It is available as a pen and prefilled syringe and is given as a 200-mg dose every 2 weeks. Sarilumab has been associated with serious infections, blood disorders, liver enzyme elevations, GI perforation, and increases in cholesterol.

Biosimilars

A biosimilar is a biologic product that is very similar in structure and function to an already-FDA-approved biologic medication. A biosimilar has no clinically meaningful differences compared to the existing biologic medication. Due to the high-cost nature of most biologic medications, there is an abbreviated approval pathway for the approval of a biosimilar medication to avoid duplication of clinical trial costs and to provide more affordable options to patients. Biosimilars are different than generics in that they are very similar but not identical to the original medication. Examples of biosimilar products that are available referencing infliximab for the treatment of RA include infliximab-abda, infliximab-dyyb.

Janus-Associated Kinase (JAK) Inhibitors

> **ALERT!**
>
> JAK Inhibitors are labeled with warnings for increased infection risk, mortality, cardiovascular events, thrombosis, and malignancies.

Tofacitinib

Tofacitinib is an oral synthetic small molecule that inhibits janus-associated kinases (JAK) 1, 2, and 3. This mechanism of action leads to the disruption of cytokine and growth factor signaling pathways. Tofacitinib can be used alone or with methotrexate or other conventional DMARDs but should not be used with biologic DMARDs. It is available as an extended-release tablet for a dose of 11 mg daily or an immediate-release tablet for a dose of 5 mg twice daily. Tofacitinib has been associated with an increased risk of serious infections, including tuberculosis and fungal infections. It is important to screen for tuberculosis before starting this medication. Tofacitinib has also been associated with increased cancer risk; however, long-term data is lacking. Common side effects include increased cholesterol, rash, diarrhea, elevated blood pressure, liver enzyme elevations, and infections. Tofacitinib can also lead to blood disorders, including anemia, neutropenia (a decrease in the type of white blood cells called neutrophils), or lymphopenia (a decrease in the type of blood cells called lymphocytes). Tofacitinib may require dose adjustment in hepatic and renal impairment or for drug-drug interactions.

Baricitinib

Baricitinib is a JAK inhibitor similar to tofacitinib. It is also administered by mouth and is available in a 1-mg and 2-mg tablet. It can be used alone or with methotrexate or other conventional DMARDs. Typical dosing is 2 mg daily, but lower doses (1 mg daily) may be used in patients with renal impairment and baracitinib may need to be avoided with certain degrees of renal impairment. Baricitinib also carries a risk for serious infections and cancer. It has also been associated with thrombosis. It has similar side effects as tofacitinib, including blood disorders, GI perforation, liver enzyme elevations, and cholesterol increases.

Upadacitinib

Upadacitinib is also a JAK inhibitor for the treatment of RA. It is available in an extended-release tablet dosed as 15 mg daily. It can also be used with methotrexate or other conventional DMARDs. Possible side effects are similar to baricitinib and tofacitinib and include serious infections, blood disorders, cancer, GI perforation, liver enzyme increases, thrombosis, and cholesterol increases.

Corticosteroids

Corticosteroids work by decreasing the levels and actions of inflammatory mediators such as cytokines, prostaglandins, and leukotrienes. Decreasing the mediators reduces the number and activation of inflammatory cells, diminishing inflammation. In cases of autoimmune diseases where the body is attacking itself with these inflammatory cells, corticosteroids can stop the cells from attacking the body. This decreases the inflammation and pain associated with RA. Corticosteroids have minimal disease-modifying activity and are not considered DMARDs. They are primarily used for bridging with a DMARD, because it often takes several weeks to months for the full efficacy of DMARD treatment to be established. They may also be given by injection directly into sites of inflammation in joints, tendons, or bursa. Intraarticular glucocorticoid injections are corticosteroid injections given in the joints and are used in both OA and RA.

Corticosteroid therapy is associated with many adverse effects. As with NSAIDs, practitioners try to limit the corticosteroid use to the lowest dose for the shortest period of time that is necessary. There are both long- and short-term effects to take into account. Short-term effects include upset stomach, restlessness, and trouble sleeping. Upset stomach is greatly reduced by taking the medication with food and trouble sleeping is minimized by taking steroids earlier in the day. Short courses of use under 2 weeks are generally well tolerated.

Patients may also experience an increased appetite while taking corticosteroids. This can begin with the first dose and last until the patient discontinues the medication. Long-term effects include increased risk of osteoporosis, cataracts, dermatologic changes, high blood pressure, and metabolic changes. The metabolic changes cause fat redistribution or a Cushing's appearance (increased fat at the face and back with less fat in the extremities). Metabolic changes also include hyperglycemia, which makes it harder to control blood glucose levels in diabetes, and hyperlipidemia. The dermatologic changes include thinning of the skin, bruising, and acne.

There are also a number of adverse effects that are dose related. At doses higher than 10 mg daily patients may experience hypertension from increased sodium and fluid retention. High-dose corticosteroids may increase the risk of infection. At very high doses, even for a short period of time, some patients experience mood changes. When patients take corticosteroids for a long time, the body's natural production of steroids is suppressed. In this case, patients need to be slowly tapered off the medication over the course of several months.

SYSTEMIC LUPUS ERYTHEMATOSUS

Systemic lupus erythematosus (SLE) is a chronic autoimmune condition. While many patients experience arthritis and joint pain as part of their illness, multiple other organ systems are involved. Other organ systems that can be damaged include the skin, central nervous system, lungs, heart, kidneys, and the hematologic system. A butterfly-shaped rash covering the bridge of the nose and cheekbones is a classic symptom of SLE. Fatigue can also cause quality of life concerns for many patients. The primary form of therapy consists of medications to suppress the immune system from attacking the body. Treatments chosen are dependent on disease severity and organ systems involved. Ultraviolet light from the sun can trigger flairs in SLE and patients should be cautioned to wear sunscreen and protective clothing when spending time outside.

During an SLE flair, NSAIDs are used to treat fever, joint pain, and inflammation. The same toxicities must be monitored as in other arthritic conditions. Renal toxicity especially must be monitored as decreased renal function is present in many patients with SLE. Hydroxychloroquine, described in the section on RA, is used for long-term management of SLE. It is particularly useful for skin and musculoskeletal manifestations not controlled by NSAIDs. Corticosteroids are also used, especially for SLE flares. However, the lowest dose possible for the shortest amount of time should be used to minimize toxicity. Topical corticosteroids are used to help control topical symptoms.

Immunosuppressive Drugs

Belimumab is used for the treatment of SLE. It is an IgG1-lambda monoclonal antibody that prevents the survival of B-lymphocytes, thus reducing the activity of B cell–mediated immunity and the autoimmune response. It is available to be given IV or SUBQ. Initial IV dosing is 10 mg/kg every 2 weeks for three doses, then 10 mg/kg every 4 weeks. The SUBQ formulation is given as a 200-mg dose weekly. Side effects include infusion reactions with the IV formulation, GI side effects, depression and suicidality, as well as increased cancer and infection risk.

For patients with severe or refractory SLE, immunosuppressive drugs such as azathioprine (1.5–2 mg/kg every day), methotrexate (7.5–20 mg/wk with folic acid), cyclophosphamide regimens (0.5–1 g/m^2 IV monthly), mycophenolate mofetil (0.5–3 g every day), and/or rituximab (1 g IV) are used. Cyclophosphamide is used in combination with corticosteroids as an immunosuppressant, especially in patients with potentially life-threatening disease complications. Cyclophosphamide therapy can decrease the likelihood that dialysis or a kidney transplant will be needed for patients with renal involvement. Cyclophosphamide can be given orally or by IV. The preferred dosing is once a month for 6 months, then every 3 months by IV. The intermittent dosing reduces adverse effects.

The adverse effects of cyclophosphamide include suppression of the immune system, which leaves patients at risk for opportunistic infections. Signs and symptoms of infection require immediate attention. The drug may suppress the bone marrow's ability to produce blood cells and complete blood counts are needed periodically during treatment. Cyclophosphamide is teratogenic and should not be used during pregnancy. Patients with childbearing potential should use birth control measures to prevent pregnancy. The drug may cause infertility. At high doses patients are at risk from hemorrhagic cystitis, which is inflammation of the bladder that can lead to bleeding. Cyclophosphamide increases the risk of cancer. Rituximab has been found to be effective in reducing disease activity in SLE as it reduces B-lymphocytes that are responsible for the production of antibodies, which promote the inflammatory response.

MANAGEMENT OF OTHER CONDITIONS

Raynaud's phenomenon is excess vasoconstriction resulting from the body's overreaction to cold temperature. This lessens the blood flow to extremities and can cause tingling and pain in the hands and feet and can induce white and blue skin coloring. Raynaud's phenomenon can occur on its own, but is more likely to be observed in patients with SLE or other autoimmune conditions. Primary prevention of Raynaud's phenomenon involves wearing appropriate clothing in cold weather to prevent reactions. In severe cases calcium channel blockers (eg, nifedipine, amlodipine), losartan, sildenafil, or fluoxetine can be used to minimize the severity and number of reactions.

Another condition commonly seen in conjunction with SLE and autoimmune diseases is antiphospholipid syndrome. Phospholipids are part of the cell membrane, and when antibodies against them are formed this puts patients into a hypercoagulable state where they are at a higher risk for thrombosis or clots. Therapy for antiphospholipid syndrome revolves around proper anticoagulation with warfarin and aspirin.

SUMMARY

Some musculoskeletal conditions, such as gout and osteoporosis, are related to metabolic or hormonal disorders; others, such as osteoarthritis (OA), may be related to injury and overuse. Rheumatoid arthritis (RA) and systemic lupus erythematosus (SLE) are autoimmune disorders in which the body's defenses mistakenly attack its own tissues. Treatments for these conditions often require a combination of drug therapies to manage not only the diseases but also the associated pain. Because patients often use a combination of over-the-counter and prescription medications to manage their pain, patient education is important to reduce the risk of toxicities and other adverse reactions. Technicians play an important role in this education, but to do this successfully they must be able to recognize the causes and symptoms of the disease, understand the treatments, and work with the pharmacist to ensure accuracy and safety during the process.

CHAPTER RESOURCES

Fanouriakis A, Kostopoulou M, Alunno A, et al. EULAR recommendations for the management of systemic lupus erythematosus [2019 update]. *Ann Rheum Dis.* 2019;78(6): 736-745. doi: 10.1136/annrheumdis-2019-215089.

Singh JA, Saag KG, Bridges Jr SL, et al; American College of Rheumatology. 2015 American College of Rheumatology guidelines for the treatment of rheumatoid arthritis. *Arthritis Care Res.* 2016;68(1):1-25. doi: 10.1002/acr.22783.

Khanna D, Fitzgerald JD, Khanna PP, et al; American College of Rheumatology. Guidelines for management of gout. part 1: systematic nonpharmacologic and pharmacologic therapeutic approaches to hyperuricemia. *Arthritis Care Res.* 2012;64(10):1431-1446. doi: 10.1002/acr.21772.

Khanna D, Khanna P, Fitzgerald JD, et al; American College of Rheumatology. Guidelines for management of gout. part 2: therapy and antiinflammatory prophylaxis of acute gouty arthritis. *Arthritis Care Res.* 2012;64(10):1447-1461. doi: 10.1002/acr.21773.

Camacho PM, Petak SM, Binkley N, et al. American Association of Clinical Endocrinologists and American College of Endocrinology clinical practice guidelines for the diagnosis and treatment of postmenopausal osteoporosis–2016. *Endocr Pract.* 2016;22(suppl 4):1-42. doi: 10.4158/EP161435.GL.

Kolasinski SL, Neogi T, Hochberg MC, et al. 2019 American College of Rheumatology/Arthritis Foundation guideline for the management of osteoarthritis of the hand, hip, and knee. *Arthritis Care Res.* 2020;72(2):149-162. doi: 10.1002/art.41142.

REVIEW QUESTIONS

1. How much elemental calcium is in a 1,500-mg tablet of calcium carbonate?

2. What is the maximum daily dose for acetaminophen?

3. What is included in the black box warning on all NSAIDs?

4. What class of medications is used to slow the disease progression of rheumatoid arthritis?

5. In patients with chronic obstructive pulmonary disease, which biologic can increase the risk of an exacerbation?

MEDICATION TABLES

MEDICATION TABLE 13-1. Antigout Medications[a]

Class Generic Name	Brand Name	Route	Forms	Dose	Notes
Xanthine Oxidase Inhibitor					
Allopurinol (al oh PURE i nole)	Zyloprim	Oral, IV	Tablet: 100 mg, 300 mg	100-600 mg/day in single or divided doses	Take with meals
Febuxostat (feb UX oh stat)	Uloric	Oral	Tablet: 40 mg, 80 mg	40–80 mg once daily	CrCl 15–29 ml/min; max 40 mg/day
Antigout					
Colchicine (KOL chi seen)	Colcrys, Colsalide	Oral	Tablet: 0.6 mg	Treatment: 0.6–1.2 mg initially then 0.6 mg every hr until symptoms resolve or diarrhea occurs Max: 1.8 mg total dose/course and a 3-day colchicine-free interval postattack Prophylaxis: 0.6 mg 1–2 times daily	Requires dose adjustment based on renal function and drug-drug interactions
Uricosuric					
Probenecid (proe BEN e sid)	Benemid, Probalan	Oral	Tablet: 500 mg	500 mg twice daily; if needed can increase up to 2,000–3,000 mg/day	Ineffective for patients with CrCl <50 ml/min
Combination Product					
500 mg probenecid, 0.5 mg colchicine (proe BEN e sid) (KOL chi seen)	Generics	Oral	Tablet	1 tablet/day for 1 wk followed by 1 tablet twice/day	If necessary, the daily dosage may be increased by 1 tablet at 4-wk intervals as tolerated (usually not more than 4 tablets/day)
Enzyme					
Pegloticase (peg LOE ti kase)	Krystexxa	IV	Injection solution concentrate: 8 mg/mL	8 mg q 2 wk	Must be diluted before use; diluted solution is stable only 4 hr and must be administered in a healthcare setting

Source: LexiComp Online, 2021.
CrCl = creatinine clearance; IV = intravenous.
[a] Pronunciations have been adapted with permission from USP Dictionary of USAN and International Drug Names (USP Dictionary) © 2022.

MEDICATION TABLE 13-2. Representative Prescription Medications for Osteoporosis [a]

Class Generic Name	Brand Name	Route	Forms	Dose	Notes
Parathyroid Hormone Analog					
Teriparatide (terr ih PAR a tyd)	Forteo	SUBQ	2.4 mL prefilled pen: 250 mcg/mL	20 mcg SUBQ once daily	Need needles for pen injector
Abaloparatide (a bal oh PAR a tide)	Tymlos	SUBQ	1.56 mL prefilled pen: 2,000 mcg/mL	80 mcg SUBQ once daily	Need needles for pen injector
Calcitonin					
Calcitonin (kal si TOE nin)	Miacalcin, Fortical	SUBQ, IM, and nasal	Nasal spray: 200 International Units/ actuation Injection solution: 200 International Units/mL	100 units SUBQ or IM every other day; 200 units (1 spray) intranasal every day alternating nostrils	Must prime the nasal spray
Selective Estrogen Receptor Modulators					
Raloxifene (ral OX i feen)	Evista	Oral	Tablet: 60 mg	60 mg once daily	Black box warning: increased risk of deep vein thrombosis and pulmonary embolism have been reported
Estrogens (conjugated/equine) and Bazedoxifene (ES troe jenz, KON joo gate ed/EE kwine and ba ze DOX i feen)	Duavee	Oral	Tablet: Conjugated estrogens 0.45 mg and bazedoxifene 20 mg	Conjugated estrogens 0.45 mg and bazedoxifene 20 mg once daily	Black box warning: increased risk of deep vein thrombosis and pulmonary embolism have been reported Black box warning: Estrogens (conjugated/ equine) can increase the risk of dementia and endometrial cancer
Bisphosphonates					
Alendronate (a LEN droe nate)	Fosamax	Oral	Tablet: 5 mg, 10 mg, 35 mg, 40 mg, 70 mg Solution: 70 mg/75 mL	5 or 10 mg once daily; 35 or 70 mg once weekly	Indicated for male osteoporosis, osteoporosis due to corticosteroids, and postmenopausal osteoporosis treatment and prophylaxis
Ibandronate (i BAN droh nate)	Boniva	Oral, IV	Tablet: 150 mg IV solution: 1 mg/mL	2.5 mg once daily; 150 mg once monthly; 3 mg IV once q 3 mo	Serious GI adverse effects include duodenal ulcer disease and various esophageal pathologies

Continued next page

MEDICATION TABLE 13-2. Representative Prescription Medications for Osteoporosis [a] *(Continued)*

Class Generic Name	Brand Name	Route	Forms	Dose	Notes
Risedronate (ris ED roe nate)	Actonel, Atelvia	Oral	Actonel: 5 mg, 30 mg, 35 mg, 150 mg tablet Atelvia: 35 mg delayed-release tablet	5 mg once daily; 35 mg once weekly; 75 mg once for 2 consecutive days once monthly; 150 mg once monthly	Delayed-release form for the treatment of osteoporosis in postmenopausal women
Zoledronic acid (ZOE le dron ik)	Reclast, Zometa	IV	Reclast: 5 mg/100 mL IV solution Zometa: 4 mg/5 mL IV solution	5 mg/yr	Calcium and vitamin D must be adequately supplemented
Monoclonal Antibodies					
Denosumab (den OH sue mab)	Prolia	SUBQ	Prefilled syringe: 100 mg/0.67 mL	60 mg SUBQ once q 6 mo	Patients should receive adequate calcium and vitamin D supplementation
Romosozumab (ROE moe SOZ ue mab)	Evenity	SUBQ	Prefilled syringe: 105 mg/1.17 mL	210 mg SUBQ once monthly	Two injections are needed to administer one dose; patients should receive adequate calcium and vitamin D supplementation

Source: LexiComp Online, 2021

GI = gastrointestinal; IM= intramuscular; IV = intravenous; SUBQ = subcutaneous.

[a] Pronunciations have been adapted with permission from USP Dictionary of USAN and International Drug Names (USP Dictionary) © 2022.

MEDICATION TABLE 13-3. Representative Medications for Osteoarthritis [a]

Class / Generic Name	Brand Name	Route	Forms	Dose	DEA Schedule/ Regulatory Status	Notes
Analgesic						
Tramadol (TRA ma dole)	Ultram, Ultram ER, Ryzolt, Rybix ODT	Oral	Tablet: 50 mg oral disintegrating tablet (Rybix): 50 mg Extended-release tablet: 100 mg, 200 mg, 300 mg	50–100 mg q 4–6 hr as needed; max 400 mg/day		
Acetaminophen (a set a MEE noe fen)	Tylenol	Oral	Tablet: various (325 mg and 500 mg common) Capsule: extra strength (500 mg common) Oral liquid: various (500 mg/15 mL common)	Dosing schedules vary; max dose of 4,000 mg daily	OTC	Increased risk of hepatic and renal impairment; do not take with alcohol
Serotonin Norepinephrine Reuptake Inhibitor						
Duloxetine (doo LOX e teen)	Cymbalta, Drizalma Sprinkle	Oral	Capsule: 20 mg, 30 mg, 4 mg, 60 mg Sprinkle: 20 mg, 30 mg, 40 mg, 60 mg	30 mg once daily for 1 week then 60 mg daily; max of 120 mg daily	Rx	
Supplement						
Glucosamine/chondroitin (gloo KOE sah meen) (kon DROI tin)	Osteo Bi-Flex	Oral	Tablet, capsule	500/400 mg 3 times daily	OTC	Take with meals
Capsaicin (cap SAY ih sin)	Zostrix, Icy Hot Arthritis Therapy, and others	Topical	Cream, lotion, gel, stick	Use topically 3–4 times daily	OTC	Wash hands after use

Source: LexiComp Online, 2021.

DEA = U.S. Drug Enforcement Administration; OTC = over the counter.

[a] Pronunciations have been adapted with permission from USP Dictionary of USAN and International Drug Names (USP Dictionary) © 2022.

MEDICATION TABLE 13-4. Nonsteroidal Anti-Inflammatory Drugs [a]

Generic Name	Brand Name	Route	Forms	Dose	Regulatory Status	Notes
Aspirin (AS pir in)	Various	Oral	Tablet: (common) 81 mg, 325 mg, 500 mg	325–650 mg q 4 hr; max 3.9 g daily	OTC	Risk of Reye's syndrome in children
Celecoxib (sell a KOX ib)	Celebrex	Oral	Capsule: 50 mg, 100 mg, 200 mg	100 mg twice daily or 200 mg once daily	Rx	COX-2 inhibitor
Diclofenac (dye KLOE fen ak)	Cataflam, Flector patch, Pennsaid, Solaraze, Voltaren, Voltaren-XR, Zipsor	Oral, topical patch	Tablet: 50 mg Extended-release tablet: 75 mg, 100 mg Topical solution: 1.5% Powder for solution: 50 mg Flector: topical patch 1.3%; also available as topical gel 1%, 3%	100–150 mg in 3–4 divided doses OR 100 mg ER 1–2 times daily; one patch (180 mg) twice daily	Rx	Can come in combination with misoprostol to help prevent stomach ulcers
Diflunisal (dye FLOO ni sal)	Dolobid	Oral	Tablet: 500 mg; also generically available in 250-mg tablet	500–1,000 mg in 2 divided doses	Rx	
Etodolac (ee toe DOE lak)	Lodine, Lodine XL	Oral	Capsule: 200 mg, 300 mg Tablet: 400 mg, 500 mg Extended-release tablet: 400 mg, 500 mg, 600 mg	200–1,200 mg in 2–4 divided doses	Rx	
Fenoprofen (fen oh PROE fen)	Nalfon	Oral	Capsule: 200 mg, 300 mg, 400 mg Tablet: 600 mg	300–600 mg 3–4 times daily	Rx	
Ibuprofen (eye byoo PROE fen)	Motrin, Advil, and combination products	Oral	Tablet: 200 mg, 400 mg, 600 mg, 800 mg Suspension: 100 mg/5 mL, 50 mg/1.25 mL Chewable tablet: 100 mg	OTC: 200-400 mg q 4–6 hr (max 1,200 mg/day)	Rx/OTC	Rx: max 3,200 mg/day divided in 3–4 doses
Indomethacin (in doe METH a sin)	Indocin, Indocin SR	Oral, rectal	Capsule: 25 mg, 50 mg Extended-release capsule: 75 mg Rectal suppository: 50 mg	IR and rectal: 25–50 mg 2–3 times daily; max 200 mg daily SR: 75 mg 1–2 times daily	Rx	

Continued next page

MEDICATION TABLE 13-4. Nonsteroidal Anti-Inflammatory Drugs [a] *(Continued)*

Generic Name	Brand Name	Route	Forms	Dose	Regulatory Status	Notes
Ketoprofen (kee toe PROE fen)	Orudis, Orudis KT, Oruvail	Oral	Orudis: 75 mg capsule Orudis KT: 12.5 mg tablet Oruvail extended-release capsule: 150 mg, 200 mg	IR: 150–300 mg divided 3–4 times daily ER: 100–200 mg once daily	Rx	Formerly available OTC
Meloxicam (mel OX i cam)	Mobic	Oral	Tablet: 5 mg, 7.5 mg, 15 mg Oral disintegrating tablet: 7.5 mg, 15 mg Suspension: 7.5 mg/5 mL	5–15 mg once daily	Rx	
Nabumetone (na BYOO me tone)	Relafen	Oral	Tablet: 500 mg, 750 mg	1,000 mg orally once a day	Rx	
Naproxen (na PROK sen)	Naprosyn, EC Naprosyn, Aleve (OTC), Naprelan	Oral	Tablet (controlled release, delayed release, and enteric coated): 250 mg, 375 mg, 500 mg Suspension: 25 mg/mL	OTC: 220 mg naproxen sodium tablets (200 mg naproxen) Rx: 250–500 mg twice daily	Rx and OTC	Do not crush, break, or chew enteric coated tablets; comes in combination with both sumatriptan (for migraine) and lansoprazole
Oxaprozin (ox a PROE zin)	Daypro	Oral	Tablet: 600 mg	0.6–1.8 g in 1–3 divided doses daily	Rx	Max 26 mg/kg/day
Piroxicam (peer OX i kam)	Feldene	Oral	Capsule: 10 mg, 20 mg	20 mg daily in 1–2 doses	Rx	
Sulindac (sul IN dak)	Clinoril	Oral	Tablet: 150 mg, 200 mg	150 mg twice daily	Rx	
Tolmetin (TOLE met in)	Tolectin 600, Tolectin DS	Oral	Tablet: 200 mg, 600 mg Capsule: 400 mg	0.6–1.8 g in 3 divided doses	Rx	

Source: LexiComp Online, 2021.
ER = extended release; IR = immediate release; OTC = over the counter; SR = sustained release.
[a] Pronunciations have been adapted with permission from USP Dictionary of USAN and International Drug Names (USP Dictionary) © 2022.

TABLE 13-5. Medications for Rheumatoid Arthritis [a]

Class Generic Name	Brand Name	Route	Forms	Dose	Notes
Conventional Disease-Modifying Antirheumatic Drugs					
Hydroxychloroquine (hye drox ee KLOR oh kwin)	Plaquenil	Oral	Tablet: 200 mg	200–400 mg daily	Also used as an antimalarial agent
Leflunomide (le FLOO na mide)	Arava	Oral	Tablet: 10 mg, 20 mg	10–20 mg once daily	Contraindicated in pregnant women
Methotrexate (meth oh TREX ate)	Trexall, Rheumatrex	Oral, SUBQ, IM	Trexall: 5 mg, 7.5 mg, 10 mg, 15 mg tablet Rheumatrex dose pack: 2.5 mg tablet Solution for injection: 25 mg/mL; 1 g powder for solution	7.5–25 mg once weekly	Contraindicated in pregnant women and nursing mothers; taken with a daily folic acid supplement
Sulfasalazine (sul fa SAL a zeen)	Azulfidine	Oral	Tablet: 500 mg	500 mg twice daily; may increase to 1,000 mg – 1,500 mg twice daily	Also comes as enteric coated
Tumor Necrosis Factor-Alpha Inhibitor Biologics					
Etanercept (et a NER set)	Enbrel	SUBQ	Prefilled syringe: 25 mg/0.5 mL, 50 mg/1 mL; autoinjector: 50 mg; powder for solution: 25 mg/1 mL	50 mg weekly	
Infliximab (in FLIX i mab)	Remicade	IV	Powder for solution: 100 mg	3 mg/kg IV over 2 hr given at weeks 0, 2, 6, then q 8 wk	
Adalimumab (a dal AYE mu mab)	Humira	SUBQ	Prefilled syringe and pen: 40 mg/0.8 mL, 40 mg/0.4 mL (citrate-free)	40 mg every other week	
Golimumab (goe LIM ue mab)	Simponi	SUBQ	Autoinjector: 50 mg; prefilled syringe: 50 mg/0.5 mL	50 mg once monthly	
Certolizumab (SER toe LIZ oo mab)	Cimzia	SUBQ	Prefilled syringe: 200 mg/mL	400 mg × 1 on weeks 0, 2, 4, then 200 mg q 2 wk or 400 mg q 4 wk	

Continued next page

TABLE 13-5. Medications for Rheumatoid Arthritis [a] *(Continued)*

Class Generic Name	Brand Name	Route	Forms	Dose	Notes
Non-Tumor Necrosis Factor-Alpha Inhibitor Biologics					
Anakinra (an a KIN ra)	Kineret	SUBQ	Prefilled syringe: 100 mg/0.67 mL	100 mg daily	Patient should report a rubber or latex sensitivity prior to administration due to composition of prefilled syringe needle cover
Abatacept (a ba TA sept)	Orencia	IV, SUBQ	Powder for IV solution: 250 mg; autoinjector and prefilled syringe: 125 mg/mL	IV: Dosed by weight q 4 wk: 500 mg if <60 kg; 750 mg if 60–100 kg; 1,000 mg if >100 kg SUBQ: 125 mg weekly	May cause nausea, headache, urinary tract infections, nasopharyngitis, or upper respiratory infection
Rituximab (ri TUX i mab)	Rituxan	IV	IV solution: 10 mg/mL	1,000 mg with a second 1,000-mg dose 2 wk later; max of 2 doses not more often than q 16 wk	Premedicate with corticosteroid 30 min prior to administration
Tocilizumab (toe si LIZ oo mab)	Actemra	IV, SUBQ	Concentrated solution for injection: 20 mg/mL; autoinjector: 162 mg; prefilled syringe: 162 mg/0.9 mL	IV: 4 mg/kg q 4 wk, may increase to 8 mg/kg q 4 wk SUBQ: 162 mg weekly, if <100 kg, start 162 mg q 2 wk, then may increase to 162 mg weekly	Maximum dose of 800 mg/infusion
Sarilumab (sar IL ue mab)	Kevzara	Oral	Pen: 200 mg; prefilled syringe: 200 mg/1.14 mL	200 mg q 2 wk	Avoid use with active hepatic disease
Janus-Associated Kinase (JAK) Inhibitors					
Tofacitinib (toe-fa-SYE-ti-nib)	Xeljanz, Xeljanz XR	Oral	ER tab: 11 mg IR tab: 5 mg	ER: 11 mg daily; IR: 5 mg twice daily	Dose adjustment based on renal and hepatic impairment, drug-drug interactions
Baricitinib (bar-i-SYE-ti-nib)	Olumiant	Oral	Tab: 1 mg, 2 mg	2 mg daily	Dose adjustment for renal impairment
Upadacitinib (ue-PAD-a-SYTE-ti-nib)	Rinvoq	Oral	ER tab: 15 mg	15 mg daily	Do not cut, crush, chew tablet

Continued next page

TABLE 13-5. Medications for Rheumatoid Arthritis [a] *(Continued)*

Class Generic Name	Brand Name	Route	Forms	Dose	Notes
Corticosteroid					
Prednisone (PRED ni sone)	Deltasone, Prednisone Intensol	Oral	Tablet: 1 mg, 2.5 mg, 5 mg, 10 mg, 20 mg, 50 mg Oral solution: 5 mg/5 mL	Dose varies	Patient should not suddenly discontinue
Cytotoxic					
Cyclophosphamide (sye kloe FOSS fa mide)	Cytoxan	IV	Powder for IV solution: 1 g, 2 g, 500 mg Tablet: 25 mg, 50 mg	Usual dose for SLE is 0.5-1 gm/m²/month	Typically combined with corticosteroid
Immunosuppressives					
Belimumab (be-LIM-yoo-mab)	Benlysta	IV, SUBQ	Autoinjector: 200 mg; prefilled syringe: 200mg/mL Powder for injection: 120 mg, 400 mg	IV: Start 10 mg/kg q 2 wk × 3 doses, then 10 mg/kg q 4 wk SUBQ: 200 mg every week	
Azathioprine (ay zah THYE oh preen)	Azasan, Imuran	Oral	Tablet: 50 mg, 75 mg, 100 mg	2 mg/kg/day	
Cyclosporine (SYE kloe spor een)	Neoral, Gengraf (others not indicated for RA)	Oral	Oral capsule: 25 mg, 100 mg Oral solution: 100 mg/mL	2.5 mg/kg/day orally divided into 2 doses	Neoral and Gengraf are indicated for the treatment of patients with severe, active RA where the disease has not adequately responded to methotrexate
Gold Compound					
Auranofin (au RANE oh fin)	Ridaura	Oral	Capsule: 3 mg	6 mg daily	Watch for signs of gold toxicity
Heavy Metal Antagonist					
Penicillamine (pen i SILL a meen)	Cuprimine, Depen	Oral	Cuprimine: 250 mg capsule Depen: 250 mg tablet	125–250 mg/day orally; increase dose at 1–3 mo intervals by 25 mg or 250 mg/day	Indicated for severe RA that has failed to respond to conventional therapy

Source: LexiComp Online, 2021.

ER = extended release; IM = intramuscular; IR = immediate release; IV = intravenous; RA = rheumatoid arthritis; SLE = systemic lupus erythematosus; SUBQ = subcutaneous.

[a] Pronunciations have been adapted with permission from USP Dictionary of USAN and International Drug Names (USP Dictionary) © 2022.

Part 5

THE CARDIOVASCULAR AND RENAL SYSTEMS

Chapter 14

Overview of the Cardiovascular and Renal Systems

Mate M. Soric, PharmD, BCPS, FCCP

KEY TERMS AND DEFINITIONS

Antidiuretic hormone (ADH)—also known as vasopressin, a hormone that controls the insertion of aquaporins into the collecting ducts, regulating the reabsorption of water.

Aquaporins—channels inserted into the collecting ducts in response to antidiuretic hormone, allow for reabsorption of free water.

Arrhythmias—abnormal heartbeats.

Arteries—blood vessels that carry blood away from the heart.

Arterioles—nearly microscopic blood vessels delivering blood to the capillary bed.

Atrium—a small, upper chamber of the heart.

Bladder—the organ that stores urine before excretion.

Capillaries—the smallest blood vessels where cellular exchange occurs.

Cardiovascular system—the body system, made up of the heart, arteries, and veins, responsible for transporting blood throughout the body.

Coronary arteries—blood vessels surrounding the heart.

Coronary artery disease—a condition that causes a narrowing of coronary arteries and a decrease in oxygen supply to the heart.

DOI 10.37573/9781585286638.014

Creatinine clearance—a measure of kidney function based on the volume of plasma cleared by the kidneys of the metabolic byproduct creatinine (and, presumably, other wastes) in a given period of time.

Diabetes insipidus—a condition involving a lack of production of or response to antidiuretic hormone.

Dialysis—the process of using a machine to artificially perform the functions of the kidney.

Diuretics—medications that increase the excretion of water in the urine.

Electrolyte—a substance that, when dissolved in water, has an electrical charge, such as sodium, potassium, or calcium.

Glomerular filtration rate (GFR)—a measure of the amount of blood filtered in the kidneys in 1 minute.

Glomerulus—a tightly tangled mass of capillaries located within the kidneys.

Kidneys—the pair of bean-shaped organs responsible for urine production and electrolyte, pH, and water balance.

Nephron—the functional unit of the kidney where blood is filtered and urine is created.

Nephropathy—renal disease.

pH—a measure of acidity or alkalinity of a solution on a scale of 0 to 14, with 0 being the most acidic and 14 the most alkaline (basic). pH 7 is neutral and body fluid pH is about 7.4 (slightly alkaline).

Renal—pertaining to the kidneys.

Renal corpuscle—a component of the nephron made of a **glomerulus** and Bowman's capsule.

Renal tubule—a component of the nephron made of the proximal tubule, loop of Henle, distal tubule, and collecting duct.

Systemic vascular resistance (SVR)—the sum of all forces opposing the flow of blood.

Tubular reabsorption—the transportation of filtered substances from the renal tubule back into the blood stream.

Tubular secretion—the transportation of substances from the peritubular capillaries into the renal tubule.

Urine—a filtrate of the blood containing waste and excess materials that is eventually excreted.

Vasculature—the blood vessels.

Veins—blood vessels that carry blood towards the heart.

Ventricles—the large, lower chambers of the heart.

Venules—nearly microscopic vessels of the venous system emerging from capillary beds.

LEARNING OBJECTIVES

After completing this chapter, you should be able to

1. Describe the structure of the heart, including the chambers, valves, and conduction systems.

2. Review the course of blood flow around the body from the arterial system to capillaries to the venous system.

3. Describe the gross anatomy of the kidney and its functional unit, the nephron.

4. List the major classes of diuretics and their sites of action in the nephron.

5. Explain the pathophysiology of kidney stones, diabetes insipidus, and nephropathy and the common strategies used to treat them.

In order for the human body to maintain the delicate balance of homeostasis, it is important for oxygen, nutrients, waste, and many other important substances to have an efficient way to travel from one place to another within it. Without such transport, even the simplest processes would be difficult to perform. The winding courses of arteries and veins act as the vast highway of the body, while the pumping of the heart provides the driving force. Together, the heart, arteries, and veins make up the cardiovascular system.

Without a way to remove ever-accumulating waste, however, the body's highway system would soon become bogged down with the byproducts of cellular metabolism. Roughly one-fourth of the blood leaving the heart is sent to the kidneys, where it is filtered of unwanted substances. In addition to filtering the blood, the kidneys also play a role in keeping water, electrolytes, and pH balanced while regulating blood pressure. In this chapter, the anatomy and function of the cardiovascular and renal systems are reviewed, followed by a discussion of selected kidney disorders and their treatment.

ANATOMY AND PHYSIOLOGY OF THE CARDIOVASCULAR SYSTEM

The Heart

The heart is located in the chest, behind the sternum (breastbone), slightly to the left of the center of the body. Surrounding and protecting the heart is a membrane called the pericardium (literally meaning "around the heart"). Though the heart muscle tirelessly pumps blood around the body for a lifetime, the size of the organ is relatively small. A normal heart is approximately the size of a closed fist. A cross-section reveals four chambers, two upper chambers known as atria, and two lower chambers called ventricles.

The right atrium is attached to the vena cava, a vein that returns deoxygenated blood to the heart and is the largest vein in the body. The right atrium is a relatively small chamber with limited muscle mass that serves largely as a holding chamber for blood returning to the heart. Separating it from the right ventricle is the tricuspid valve. This three-leafed valve, like the other valves of the heart, is made of strong connective tissue to hold up against the heart's powerful beats. When the right ventricle is contracting, the tricuspid valve is tightly closed. After the contraction is complete, the pressure in the right ventricle decreases, allowing the tricuspid valve to open and the blood in the atrium to flow to the ventricle. Just before the tricuspid valve closes once more, the atrium contracts to force extra blood into the right ventricle.

The right ventricle, located below the right atrium, is responsible for pumping blood out of the heart and into the lungs, where it can become oxygenated. It is the second-largest chamber of the heart but is considerably smaller than the left ventricle because it only pumps blood a relatively short distance. Separating the left and right ventricles is the septum, a thick wall of cardiac muscle. When the right ventricle contracts, the rising pressures force open the pulmonary valve and drive the blood into the pulmonary artery system, toward the lungs. Oxygenated blood returning to the heart via the pulmonary veins enters the left atrium. Like the right atrium, blood flows freely into the ventricle while the valve between the two is open. The mitral valve, also known as the bicuspid valve for its two leaflets, allows blood to enter the left ventricle. Just before its closure, the left atrium contracts to ensure the left ventricle is at capacity.

The true powerhouse of the heart is the left ventricle. This is the largest of the heart's chambers and makes up the pointed end of the heart known as the apex. The muscles around the chamber need to be bulky and powerful enough to pump blood around the entire body. When a contraction begins, the mitral valve is slammed closed and the blood is pushed through the aortic valve.

> ### PRACTICE POINT
>
> *The characteristic "lub-dub" sound of a beating heart is actually made by the various valves slamming shut. The closing of the tricuspid and mitral valves makes up the "lub" while the "dub" is the result of the pulmonary and aortic valves closing.*

These four chambers of the heart work in harmony to pump blood to the body; however, without a functioning pacemaker to keep each chamber in sync, the pump would quickly fail. Beneath the mighty cardiac muscles is a complex electrical system that ensures each chamber contracts on time (Figure 14-1). The origin of each beat is in the sino-atrial (SA) node. This is a collection of specialized cells in the right atrium that are autorhythmic, which are able to initiate electrical impulses themselves (without external input) and stimulate heart muscle contraction. Once the cells of the SA node start the contraction, a wave is set off in neighboring cells, allowing them to contract, as well. The wave of contraction first moves across the right atrium and, next, enters the left atrium, causing it to contract soon after the right.

When the wave reaches the bottom of the atria, it encounters a second area of autorhythmic cells called the atrioventricular (AV) node. This is the gateway to the electrical system of the ventricles. If the wave of depolarization that started in the SA node were simply allowed to spread across the entire heart, the beats would be slow, out of sync, and ineffective. Instead, the heart contains a system of nerves that quickly move the wave from the AV node down to the bottom of the ventricles. The electrical charge passes through the AV node to the Bundle of His (HISS), a group of nerve fibers in the septum that distributes it between the left and right bundle branches in the septum and down to another nerve group, the Purkinje fibers, that quickly spreads the depolarization from the bottom of the ventricular muscles upward. The resulting ventricular contraction can be compared to squeezing toothpaste from the bottom of the tube rather than from the top.

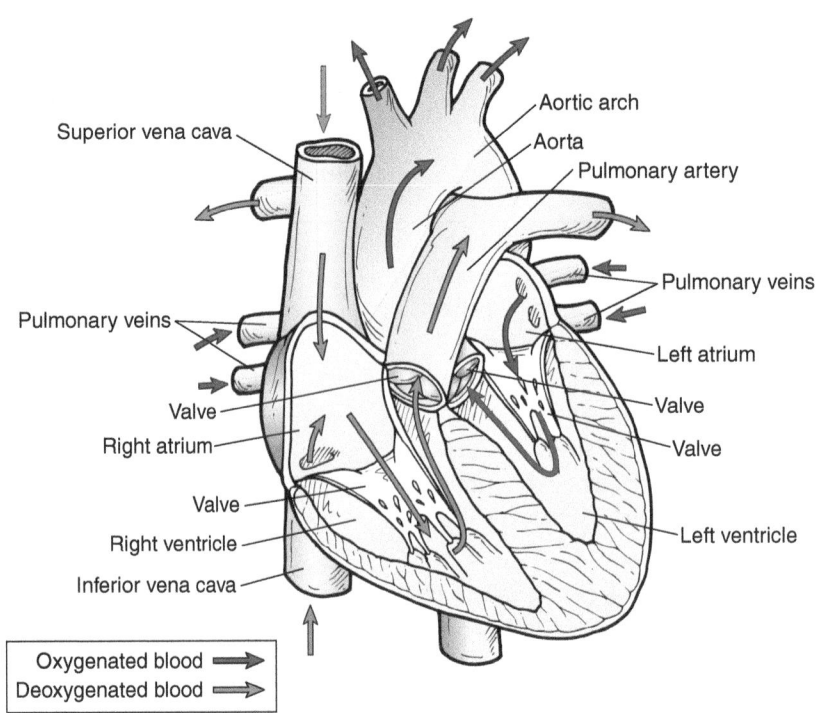

Superior vena cava

Aortic arch

Aorta

Pulmonary artery

Pulmonary veins

Pulmonary veins

Left atrium

Valve

Valve

Valve

Right atrium

Valve

Right ventricle

Left ventricle

Inferior vena cava

Oxygenated blood ➡
Deoxygenated blood ➡

FIGURE 14-1. Anatomy of the heart.

> ## PRACTICE POINT
>
> *When the electrical system of the heart malfunctions, arrhythmias may take place. These are abnormal heartbeats that often originate from places other than the SA node.*

Without any outside input, the regular depolarization of the SA node can keep a steady heartbeat around 100 beats per minute. There are, however, certain events that can alter the rate of the heart's natural pacemaker. The sympathetic nervous system (SANS), responsible for the so-called "fight or flight response," can raise the heart rate in order

> ## PRACTICE POINT
>
> *In addition to hormones, medications, such as beta blockers, calcium channel blockers, and digoxin, can block the AV node and slow the heart rate. These agents will be discussed in greater detail in Chapter 16.*

to increase the amount of oxygen-rich blood circulating the body, while the parasympathetic nervous system (PANS) can slow the heart rate down. A number of hormones, such as epinephrine, can also influence the rate at which the SA node depolarizes.

The Vasculature

The contraction of the left ventricle ejects approximately 70 mL (just over 2 ounces) of blood through the aortic valve into the aorta, the largest artery in the vasculature (Figure 14-2). Most of the blood ejected from the heart follows this large artery out to the rest of the body, but a small amount enters the coronary arteries that surround the heart and supply the oxygen needed to keep the heart pumping. Arteries are large vessels surrounded by layers of elastic fibers, smooth muscle, and endothelial cells. The arteries closest to the heart play an important role in helping the heart push blood around the body and are often called elastic arteries. The beat of the left ventricle causes a sharp increase in pressure in the arteries, resulting in a stretching of the vessel walls. As the heart relaxes, the artery constricts to its normal size and advances blood further along. These larger arteries branch off into smaller arteries that tend to have less-elastic fibers and thicker muscular layers. Often called muscular arteries, they play a role in regulating blood

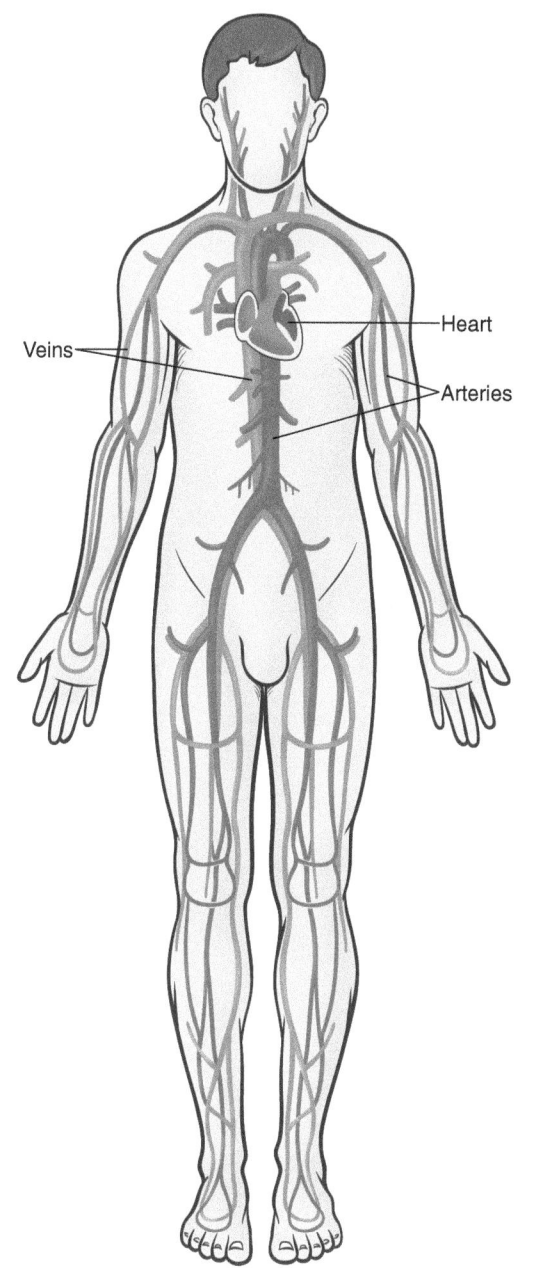

FIGURE 14-2. Vasculature.

important factor in determining blood pressure. Arterioles also contain precapillary sphincters, small rings of smooth muscle that control the flow of blood into the capillary beds. Signals from surrounding tissues help to regulate the opening and closing of the sphincters and which capillary beds receive blood flow.

The smallest of all blood vessels are the capillaries, bridging the gap between the arterial and venous sides of the circulatory system. These microscopic blood vessels fan outward from arterioles and come into contact with nearly every cell in the body. Some capillaries are so small that red blood cells must move in single file at their narrowest point. It is at the level of the capillary that cellular exchange can occur, trading oxygen, nutrients, and hormones from the blood for cellular debris, carbon dioxide, and other waste products from the cells. The capillaries next begin to converge, each smaller vessel joining with another, to form the beginnings of the venous system. As capillaries come together, they create venules, small vessels that eventually flow into full-sized veins. While veins, like arteries, contain layers of elastic fibers, smooth muscle, and endothelial cells, there are a number of important differences. Due to their distance from the heart, veins are not designed to withstand high pressures; therefore, all the layers are thinner on the venous side of the vasculature. The veins of the extremities (hands, feet) contain one-way valves to help encourage the flow of blood, even against the force of gravity. Without these valves, blood could flow backward or pool in the feet, delaying its return to the heart. Since the beating of the heart only minimally affects venous blood flow, veins rely on the help of surrounding skeletal muscle to keep blood moving. As we move about, muscles contract, putting pressure

pressure. Signals from the ANS, hormones, or other substances can interact with the smooth muscle to cause vasoconstriction or vasodilation.

As the blood moves throughout the body, it next encounters arterioles, which are nearly microscopic blood vessels that eventually connect to the capillaries. Like the muscular arteries, arterioles play an important role in regulating blood pressure. As blood vessels become smaller, the friction of the blood against the vessel wall increases and contributes to systemic vascular resistance (SVR), an

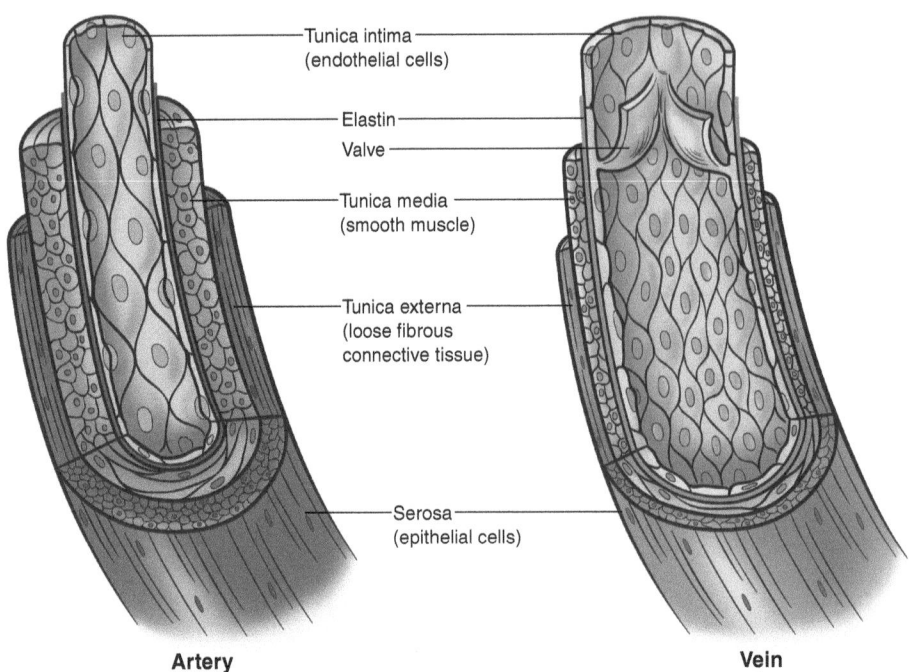

Tunica intima (endothelial cells)

Elastin

Valve

Tunica media (smooth muscle)

Tunica externa (loose fibrous connective tissue)

Serosa (epithelial cells)

Artery

Vein

FIGURE 14-3. Arteries versus veins.

on nearby veins. Blood is then forced upward through sets of valves, one step closer to returning to the heart. As the veins approach the heart, many of them converge to form the vena cava, the largest vein in the vasculature, which returns the deoxygenated blood to the right atrium where the cycle can begin once more (Figure 14-3).

ANATOMY AND PHYSIOLOGY OF THE RENAL SYSTEM

The Kidneys

The kidneys are the pair of bean-shaped organs responsible for filtering blood and regulating a number of important processes. Located near the lower back, the kidneys are often described as retroperitoneal organs because they can be found behind (retro to) the peritoneal cavity (Figure 14-4). A number of important features can be identified in a cross-section view of a kidney. First, blood is delivered via the renal artery. The renal artery enters the kidney through the renal hilus, the concave area in the middle of the organ. The blood vessels spread outward, reaching the outermost area of the kidney, called the renal cortex. Just beneath the renal cortex lies the renal medulla. Embedded between these two areas are roughly 1 million nephrons, specialized units that filter

the blood, working together to regulate blood pressure and create urine, among other important tasks. Once filtered, the blood and urine leave the kidney through the renal hilus in renal veins and the ureter, respectively.

The Nephron

To understand the kidney's vital role in homeostasis and the creation of urine, we must understand its functional unit, the nephron. Each nephron contains two main components: the renal corpuscle and the renal tubule (Figure 14-5). Blood entering the kidney travels along arterioles until it reaches a glomerulus, a tightly tangled mass of capillary vessels. A membrane known as Bowman's capsule surrounds each glomerulus. Here, nearly all of the blood's water and solutes pass out of the bloodstream and into the renal tubule. The rate at which these substances are filtered into the renal tubule is called the glomerular filtration rate (GFR), an important estimate of overall renal function. This value is used to classify patients into various stages of kidney disease. See Table 14-1 for more details. The remaining blood flows out of the glomerulus and enters the peritubular capillaries. These small vessels closely follow along the route of the renal tubule so that additional solutes and water can be exchanged between the bloodstream and the nephron in processes called tubular reabsorption and tubular secretion.

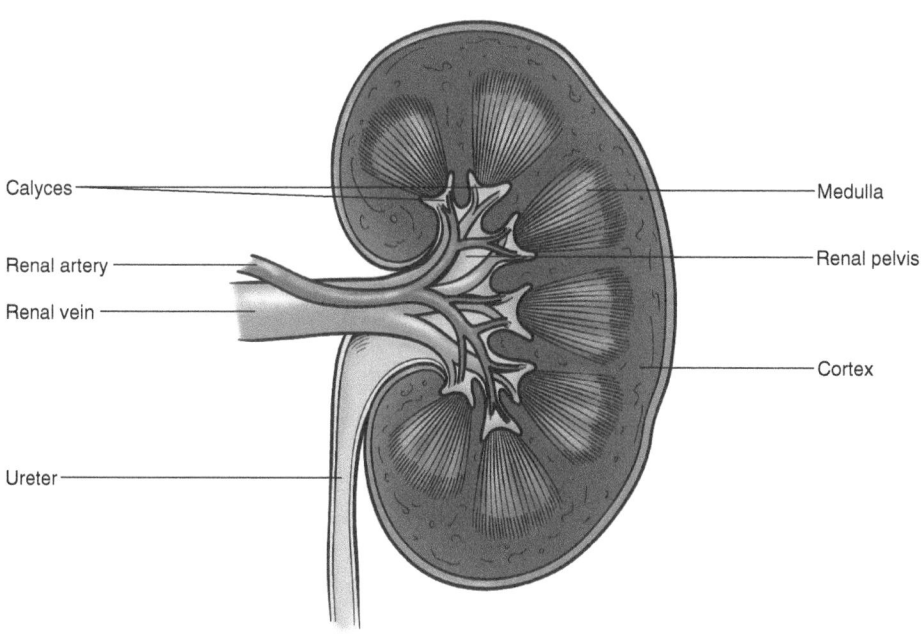

FIGURE 14-4. Anatomy of the kidney.

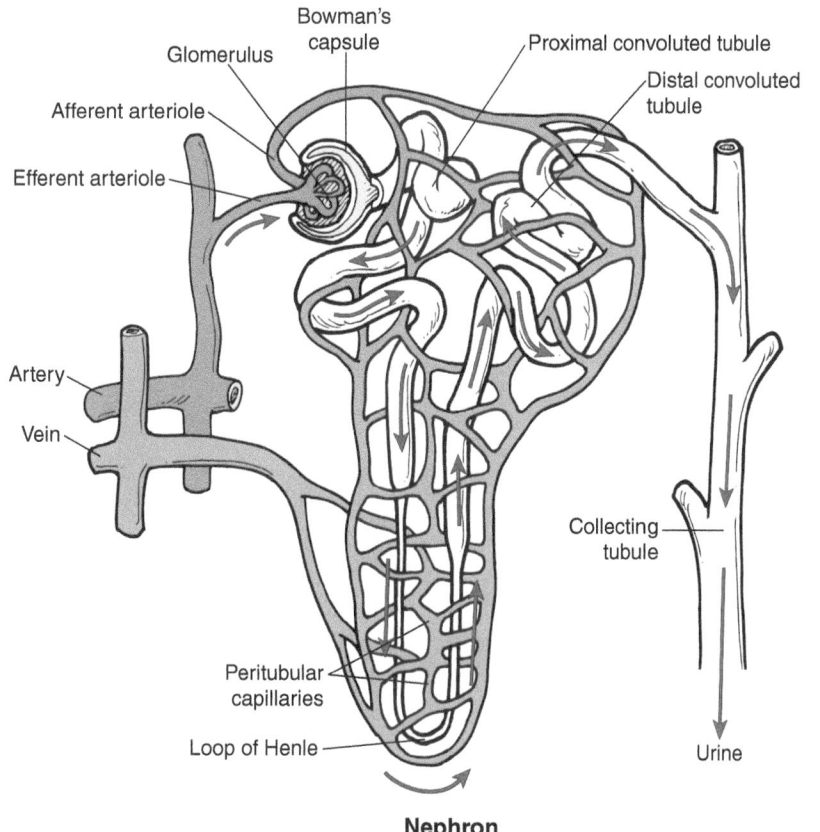

FIGURE 14-5. Structure of the nephron.

TABLE 14-1. Staging of Chronic Kidney Disease[2]

Stage	Description	GFR (mL/min)
1	Kidney damage with normal or increased GFR	≥90
2	Kidney damage with mildly decreased GFR	60–89
3	Moderately decreased GFR	30–59
4	Severely decreased GFR	15–20
5	Kidney failure	<15 or on dialysis

PRACTICE POINT

In a clinical setting, it is very difficult to get an accurate measurement of the GFR. Instead, physicians often check the amount of creatinine in the blood. Creatinine is a metabolic waste product that is filtered in the glomerulus and minimally reabsorbed. The creatinine level can be converted (by an equation) to an estimated GFR (eGFR) or creatinine clearance, giving an estimate of the patient's kidney function.

The first segment of the tubule, known as the proximal convoluted tubule, performs the bulk of the reabsorption. Most of the usable solutes, such as glucose, amino acids, and nutrients, are transported back into the blood from the renal tubule. In the reverse direction, tubular secretion causes unfiltered waste products in the blood to move into the renal tubule for excretion.

Thus far, the filtered materials in the renal corpuscle and proximal tubule have been located in the renal cortex, the outermost layer of the kidney. The next segment of the renal tubule, called the loop of Henle, takes the filtrate deep into the medulla of the kidney before making a sharp turn and returning to the renal cortex. Here, the body can perform important adjustments to both the concentration and the composition of the urine being formed. In the descending loop, additional water can be reabsorbed into the blood, while, in the ascending loop, electrolytes can be independently reabsorbed. Depending on signals from the body, the loop of Henle can help to create either dilute or concentrated urine by reabsorbing more or less water.

Next, the filtrate enters the distal convoluted tubule. Since a great deal of the filtered water has already been absorbed in previous areas of the tubule, very little reabsorption takes place here. The urine in a number of distal tubules drains into a single shared collecting duct. Like the loop of Henle, the collecting ducts play a major role in regulating urine concentration. Usually, the collecting ducts are impermeable to water, meaning nearly all of the water delivered to them is excreted in the urine. An important hormone, called vasopressin or antidiuretic hormone (ADH), can drastically alter the way a collecting duct works. As its name implies, the body releases ADH when it needs to hold onto extra fluid. ADH, discussed in detail later in this chapter, acts at the level of the collecting duct, causing the opening of aquaporins. These small channels allow the body to reabsorb large amounts of water that typically would be excreted, to create very concentrated urine.

The composition of the urine draining through the numerous collecting ducts will remain largely unchanged throughout the rest of its journey. A number of collecting ducts converge to drain into minor and major calyces, which are cup-like containers that eventually lead to the ureter and bladder before being excreted as urine.

CASE STUDY

Mr. Turner, a 67-year-old male, is well known to the hospital staff because he was recently hospitalized with a diagnosis of chronic kidney disease and high blood pressure. Today he has presented to the emergency department complaining of fatigue and heart palpitations.

Electrolyte Balance and Diuretics

The term electrolyte refers to a substance that has an electrical charge when dissolved in water. Also known as ions, these substances are further divided into two groups, cations and anions, depending on the type of charge they have. When a cation comes into contact with an anion, the opposite charges lead to a strong attraction. Once dissolved in water, however, the two halves are separated and surrounded by water molecules. In their dissolved form, the body can use electrolytes in a number of ways to perform the various functions needed to maintain homeostasis. It is important that the body have a sufficient amount of each of these electrolytes stored but having excessive amounts can also lead to serious dysfunctions. The kidneys are responsible for maintaining the proper electrolyte balance, holding on to the electrolytes the body needs while excreting those it has in excess.

The cations are positively charged ions and include substances like sodium (Na^+), potassium (K^+), calcium (Ca^{2+}), and magnesium (Mg^{2+}). Sodium is the most abundant cation in the body and is found primarily outside of the cells. Levels of this electrolyte can be reduced if a patient has vomiting, diarrhea, or does not take in enough sodium in the diet. The resulting condition is known as hyponatremia and can be remedied with intravenous (IV) administration of normal saline.

PRACTICE POINT

Normal saline is a solution of 0.9% sodium chloride (9 mg/mL) that approximates the concentration of dissolved substances in plasma and body fluids.

Hypernatremia, or elevated sodium levels, is typically caused by dehydration. The body's natural thirst mechanism is usually sufficient to replace lost fluids and bring the sodium concentration into the normal range, though some patients may require IV rehydration. When sodium levels are outside of the normal range, the central nervous system is the primary organ system affected, causing symptoms such as dizziness, confusion, or seizures.

CASE?

At his last doctor's appointment, Mr. Turner was given a new prescription for lisinopril, an angiotensin-converting enzyme (ACE) inhibitor. He also reports that he has been using a potassium-containing salt substitute. How would these two changes affect his potassium levels?

Potassium is primarily found inside of the cells, with only small amounts measurable in the blood. When potassium levels are either elevated or depleted, patients are at risk for developing life-threatening arrhythmias or muscle paralysis. Potassium levels are often decreased, a condition known as hypokalemia, when a patient is taking diuretics, a group of medications that will be discussed below. Potassium

supplements can be prescribed to help patients maintain appropriate levels in the body. Potassium supplements are available in a variety of *salts* (potassium chloride, potassium gluconate, etc.) and oral dosage forms (liquids, long-acting tablets, effervescent tablets) that are listed in Medication Table 14-1 (Medication Tables are located at the end of the chapter). Potassium may also be administered intravenously for patients who are unable to take oral doses or who need a fast-acting dose.

ALERT!

Concentrated potassium solutions must never be injected intravenously; the potassium dose must be diluted in a suitable fluid for infusion. Administration of a concentrated potassium solution can be fatal to the patient. Many pharmacists recommend limiting the concentration to 10 mEq/100 mL and infusing it no faster than 10 mEq/hr.

PRACTICE POINT

Oral potassium supplementation can be used for mild to moderate hypokalemia. Though they can be irritating to the gastrointestinal tract, taking the supplement with food will usually decrease this side effect.

PRACTICE POINT

IV potassium supplementation is notorious for causing burning and pain at the site of injection.

Hyperkalemia, on the other hand, is an increased level of potassium usually caused by decreased kidney function. If the kidneys cannot filter properly, potassium can accumulate in the blood stream, and patients may require medications or dialysis to bring these levels down. Some medications also predispose patients to hyperkalemia, including the potassium-sparing diuretics (discussed later in the chapter) and the ACE inhibitors (covered in Chapter 15). Potassium supplements and salt substitutes may also increase potassium levels.

The most common pharmacological treatment for hyperkalemia is sodium polystyrene sulfonate (SPS or Kayexalate). This medication, available as a suspension or powder, is a resin that contains sodium ions. When administered orally or rectally, the sodium is exchanged for potassium ions in the large intestine before being excreted in the feces. Doses of 15 g can be given by mouth as compared to 30–50 g given rectally up to four times per day. If not monitored carefully, patients may experience hypokalemia or hypernatremia, though the most common side effects are nausea, vomiting, diarrhea, and constipation.

Anions have a negative charge and include chloride (Cl^-), phosphate (PO_4^{3-}), and bicarbonate (HCO_3^-). The most common anion, chloride, works to balance the positively charged sodium in the body. Like its counterpart, chloride is primarily found outside of cells and helps regulate the balance of water. Phosphate is important in many of the body's metabolic processes.

Bicarbonate is an important component of the body's acid–base balancing system. The kidney and respiratory system regulate acid–base balance, measured as pH. Reported on a scale of 0 to 14, with 0 being the most acidic and 14 the most alkaline (basic), pH 7 is *neutral* and body fluid pH is about 7.4 (slightly alkaline). Often called a buffer, bicarbonate helps to neutralize acid and keep pH at appropriate levels.

Clinicians frequently order laboratory tests to check the precise amount of each electrolyte in the serum. For a detailed list of *normal* serum electrolyte concentrations, see Table 14-2.

Diuretics are medications that increase the excretion of water in the urine by various actions on the kidney. For many patients who have hypertension or retain water, diuretics are an important treatment. By creating more dilute urine, diuretics cause a decrease in the blood volume and pressure but can also have a significant impact on the concentration of electrolytes in the body. There are many different classes of diuretics and each tends to affect a different segment of the nephron.

Some of the most potent diuretics available work at the loop of Henle. These so-called loop diuretics, such as bumetanide, furosemide, and torsemide, stop the reabsorption of sodium and water into the bloodstream, leaving them in the urine. Compared to other diuretics, the loop diuretics cause a profound diuresis that is often dose-related, meaning the effect can be intensified as the dose is increased. The effect is so strong that care must be taken not to cause an over-diuresis and dehydration. As is the case with nearly all diuretics, the effect on electrolyte balance must be closely monitored to avoid deficiencies in sodium, potassium, magnesium, and calcium.

The thiazide diuretics work at the distal convoluted tubule. This commonly used class of diuretics includes hydrochlorothiazide, chlorthalidone, and metolazone. As their mechanism is very similar to the loop diuretics, thiazides cause many of the same electrolyte-related side effects when used at higher doses. Fortunately, when they are used to treat hypertension, low doses are typically sufficient and the electrolyte depletion is often avoided. One of the unique

TABLE 14-2. Serum Electrolytes*

Electrolyte	Abbreviation	Adult Reference Range[a] (mEq/L)
Sodium (SOE dee um)	Na^+	134–149
Potassium (poe TASS i um)	K^+	3.5–5.2
Magnesium (mag NEE zhum)	Mg^{2+}	1.6–2.5
Calcium (KAL see um)	Ca^{2+}	8.6–10.3
Chloride (klor ide)	Cl^-	95–108
Phosphate (FOS fate)	PO_4^{3-}	2.8–4.2
Bicarbonate (bye KAR bon ate)	HCO_3^-	23–30

[a]Reference ranges may vary depending on individual lab techniques used.
*Pronunciations have been adapted with permission from USP Dictionary of USAN and International Drug Names (USP Dictionary) © 2022.

side effects of the thiazides is hyperglycemia, necessitating cautious use in patients with type 2 diabetes (Medication Table 14-2).

While diuretics act on the renal tubules and loop of Henle, other agents cause diuresis by interfering with the action of ADH. One of the most common substances hindering the ADH effect is alcohol. When consumed, it decreases the production of ADH and, consequently, causes a decrease in the number of aquaporins in the collecting duct. Spironolactone and eplerenone, the potassium-sparing diuretics, are examples of medications that interfere with aldosterone to cause diuresis. They are called potassium-sparing because, unlike the other diuretics described above, these cause a loss of sodium and water in exchange for potassium. By blocking the receptors that aldosterone normally acts upon, aquaporin insertion is limited. Without these important channels, water cannot be reabsorbed into the blood and is excreted in the urine. Other potassium-sparing diuretics are available, including amiloride and triamterene, but their mechanism of action is poorly understood. It is thought that they block the reabsorption of sodium in the distal tubule and collecting duct.

SELECTED KIDNEY DISORDERS

Kidney Stones

In a functioning nephron, numerous minerals are successfully filtered out of the bloodstream and into the renal tubule. If conditions are optimal, these dissolved substances can be effectively transported without causing harm, either being reabsorbed or excreted in the urine. Under certain circumstances, however, kidney stones, or renal calculi, can form when dissolved substances bind together to create a solid precipitate. Though the composition of a stone can vary, the most common is a combination of calcium and oxalate. About 80% of all kidney stones are made of this combination. Since the renal tubules and the ureters are not designed to transport solid masses, patients experience intense, sharp flank pain as the stones travel down the urinary system. Left untreated, most small stones can be passed without significant damage to the body. If the stones exceed 1–2 mm in size, however, an obstruction may occur. Without an open passage to the bladder, urine backs up into the kidney, potentially causing permanent damage and renal failure.

ALERT!

Though controversial, some studies show that high-dose supplementation of vitamin C may increase the risk of calcium oxalate kidney stone formation.

A number of strategies can be used to treat kidney stones, though the most effective treatment is to prevent the formation of the stone in the first place. Patients experiencing dehydration are at an increased risk of stone formation, and adequate hydration can ensure that enough fluid is filtered into the tubule to keep stone-forming substances dissolved. Another approach to preventing kidney stones is to decrease the concentration of the ingredients necessary to create a stone. Dietary sources of oxalate, such as chocolate, rhubarb, and spinach, should be avoided and medications, such as hydrochlorothiazide, can be used to increase the reabsorption of calcium out of the kidney.

Once a kidney stone has formed, medications can, once again, play a large role in treatment. To treat the intense pain associated with stone formation, nonsteroidal anti-inflammatory drugs (NSAIDs) and opioids are commonly used to improve a patient's quality of life. In the most severe cases, however, medications may not be sufficient to treat large stones. In a noninvasive procedure known as litho-tripsy, physicians can attempt to break apart a stone using sound waves. For the rare case where noninvasive methods fail, surgical removal of a calculus is also an option.[3]

Diabetes Insipidus

Diabetes insipidus is a disorder involving ADH. As described earlier, ADH is responsible for the insertion of aquaporins into the collecting ducts of the kidneys. Released in response to dehydration, ADH allows the body to reabsorb extra water that would otherwise be excreted in the urine. Diabetes insipidus disrupts the body's ability to produce or use this important hormone.

ADH is typically produced in the hypothalamus and stored in the pituitary gland of the brain. In cases of central diabetes insipidus, this function is lost, due to trauma, infection, cancer, or other reasons. For some patients, the dysfunction lies not with the ability of the brain to produce the hormone, but with the kidney's ability to respond to it. Nephrogenic (originating in the kidneys) diabetes insipidus, which may be caused by certain medicines or genetics, does not affect the ability to produce ADH, but disrupts the body's ability to use it.

The symptoms of diabetes insipidus are uniform, regardless of the cause of the disease. Because these patients cannot concentrate their urine, excessive amounts of water are lost. In severe cases, patients can have increased urine output, up to 10 times that of a healthy individual. The brain responds to this dehydration with extreme thirst in an attempt to replace fluid losses.

The treatment of central diabetes insipidus relies on the replacement of ADH. Desmopressin (DDAVP), a synthetic version of the hormone that can be administered orally or as a nasal spray, can restore the body's ability to concentrate urine and relieve the symptoms of extreme thirst. Orally, desmopressin is initially dosed as 0.05 mg twice daily or one spray (10 mcg) 1–3 times per day intranasally and is titrated to the desired effect. Typically, the medication is well tolerated but may cause low sodium levels or water retention if patients do not follow strict fluid restrictions.[4]

> ### PRACTICE POINT
> *Desmopressin may also be used to treat bedwetting or nocturnal enuresis in some patients.*

> ### ALERT!
> Certain formulations of desmopressin, including some nasal sprays and IV solutions, must be refrigerated.

As nephrogenic diabetes insipidus decreases the kidney's ability to respond to ADH, a different approach must be used in its treatment. If caused by a medication, the symptoms may resolve after the offending agent is discontinued. For those patients with genetic defects, treatment focuses on maintaining adequate hydration and limiting sodium intake.

Nephropathy

Renal disease, also known as nephropathy, is a process in which damage occurs to the kidney, resulting in a decreased functionality of the organ. Many conditions can lead to a nephropathy, and the most common include hypertension, diabetes, and analgesic use. If left unchecked, the damage done to the kidney can become extensive, leaving the patient without a way to filter the blood of waste products and maintain electrolyte balance. In such cases, patients must rely on dialysis.

Hypertensive nephropathy takes place in patients who have longstanding hypertension. While high blood pressure can negatively affect a number of body systems, the kidneys are especially at risk. The tiny capillaries of the glomerulus and the larger arterioles become thickened under the increased pressure, leading to a condition known as glomerulosclerosis, or scarring of the glomerulus. As the vessel walls become thicker, it becomes more difficult for blood to flow freely to the kidney and oxygen supply dwindles. Without oxygen, the cells of the nephron begin to die off and cannot continue to filter the blood. If left untreated, the glomerulosclerosis can become so widespread that the kidney may cease to function all together, ending in complete renal failure and dialysis. To avoid these dire results, it is important to treat the underlying cause: uncontrolled hypertension. Refer to Chapter 15 for a detailed explanation of the treatment of hypertension.

Diabetic nephropathy refers to a progressive decline in renal function that can be attributed to uncontrolled diabetes mellitus. Though the root cause of this kidney dysfunction differs from hypertensive nephropathy, the type of damage seen at the level of the nephron is very similar. Chronically elevated blood sugar leads to a glomerulosclerosis and decreased functioning of the nephron. If blood sugars remain elevated, the disease can progress to complete renal failure and a dependence on dialysis. In the United States, diabetic nephropathy is the leading cause of dialysis dependence. As seen in hypertensive nephropathy, the best treatment for diabetic nephropathy is to control its underlying cause. By keeping blood sugars at acceptable levels, the risk of glomerulosclerosis is greatly reduced and progression of kidney disease becomes less likely. In addition to preventative measures, many patients diagnosed with diabetes are prescribed medications from the class known as ACE inhibitors, such as lisinopril, enalapril, or ramipril, or angiotensin receptor blockers (ARBs), such as candesartan, irbesartan, or valsartan. These agents help to protect the kidneys from damage by increasing the blood flow in renal arteries. For more information regarding the treatment of diabetes mellitus, see Chapter 10.

PRACTICE POINT

To monitor the effects of elevated blood sugar on the kidney, clinicians can monitor the amount of protein in the urine. As glomerulosclerosis worsens, increasing amounts of proteins are spilled into the urine because the kidney can no longer reabsorb them properly.

In some cases, medications may be the primary cause of nephropathy. The most commonly used class of medications that cause kidney damage is NSAIDs, such as ibuprofen, naproxen, or indomethacin. Though generally safe if taken for short periods of time, chronic use of these medications can cause serious damage to the kidneys. In a normally functioning glomerulus, many different substances help regulate blood pressure. One such compound is prostaglandin E2 (PGE2), which acts as a vasodilator on renal arterioles and helps maintain adequate blood supply. In the presence of NSAIDs, the production of PGE2 is inhibited and the blood pressure balance is tipped in favor of vasoconstriction. With blood supply decreased, glomerulosclerosis can set in and lead to decreased GFR and, eventually, all-out renal failure.

To avoid the consequences of analgesic nephropathy, the use of NSAIDs should be limited to the lowest dose and shortest duration possible.

PRACTICE POINT

In addition to NSAIDs, there are a number of other medications that can cause direct damage to the kidney. These include the aminoglycosides, amphotericin B, lithium, and vancomycin.

SUMMARY

The cardiovascular system serves as the transport system for the body. At its center, the heart provides the driving force that propels blood to the farthest reaches of the vasculature. Blood enters the heart via the vena cava into the right atrium and quickly moves to the right ventricle before being sent to the lungs for oxygenation. After its return from the pulmonary system, blood travels through the left atrium to the left ventricle. Since this chamber is responsible for pumping blood to the rest of the body via the aorta, it is the largest of the four chambers.

Keeping all four chambers in sync is the responsibility of the electrical system of the heart. Each beat originates in the sinoatrial (SA) node, a collection of autorhythmic cells in the right atrium. The wave of depolarization travels across the right and left atria before reaching the atrioventricular (AV) node. Once here, the electrical impulse quickly travels along specialized nerves to the bottom of the ventricle.

Once blood is ejected from the left ventricle, it enters the vascular system. The vessels nearest the heart are large arteries, designed to hold up against the high pressures of each heartbeat and help the heart move blood outward to the rest of the body. As the blood travels further from the heart, it enters arterioles and capillaries. In these smallest vessels, an exchange occurs between the blood stream and nearby cells, trading oxygen, nutrients, and hormones for carbon dioxide and waste products. On the return trip to the heart, blood vessels pass through venules and, eventually, large veins.

Roughly 25% of the blood ejected from the heart enters the renal system for filtration. In the functional unit of the kidney, the nephron, blood crosses from the vasculature into the renal tubule. In a long, winding journey through the proximal tubule, loop of Henle, and distal tubule, numerous substances are reabsorbed into the blood stream or secreted into the tubules. Along the way, electrolytes, pH, and water balance are finely adjusted to meet the body's needs. The newly formed urine then travels through the collecting ducts, calyces, and ureter to the bladder before being excreted from the body.

Though they are of vital importance, the kidneys can be affected by a number of medications and conditions that alter their ability to perform key functions. The use of various diuretics can inhibit the reabsorption of electrolytes and free water, increasing their presence in the urine. Antidiuretic hormone (ADH) allows the body to reabsorb extra water when the body is at risk for dehydration, but some patients suffer from diabetes insipidus, where the hormone cannot be produced or is not recognized by its receptors in the kidney. If certain conditions are met, it is possible for some of the dissolved components of the filtrate to come together to form insoluble precipitates. These kidney stones can become lodged in the urinary system and cause serious damage to the nephron, much like the effect of longstanding hypertension, diabetes, or chronic NSAID (nonsteroidal anti-inflammatory drug) use.

REFERENCES

1. American Heart Association. Heart disease and stroke statistics - 2022 update. https://professional.heart.org/en/science-news/heart-disease-and-stroke-statistics-2022-update. Accessed March 23, 2022.

2. Kidney Disease: Improving Global Outcomes (KDIGO) CKD Work Group. KDIGO 2012 Clinical Practice Guideline for the Evaluation and Management of Chronic Kidney Disease. *Kidney Inter Suppl.* 2013;3:1-150.

3. Portis AJ, Sundaram CP. Diagnosis and initial management of kidney stones. *Am Fam Physician.* 2001;63:1329-1339.

4. Singer I, Oster JR, Fishman LM. The management of diabetes insipidus in adults. *Arch Intern Med.* 1997;157:1293-1301.

5. Lexi-Drugs. Lexicomp. Hudson, OH. http://online.lexi.com. Accessed April 1, 2021.

CHAPTER RESOURCES

Barrett KE, Barman SM, Brooks HL, et al. *Ganong's Review of Medical Physiology.* 26th ed. New York, NY: McGraw-Hill; 2019.

DiPiro JT, Yee GC, Posey M, et al. *Pharmacotherapy: A Pathophysiological Approach.* 11th ed. New York, NY: McGraw-Hill; 2020.

REVIEW QUESTIONS

1. Describe the flow of blood through the heart, starting as it arrives from the body in the vena cava.

2. Describe the sequence of blood vessels used to deliver blood to the body and return it to the heart.

3. List the components of the nephron in the order in which the filtrate passes through it.

4. Outline the mechanism of action of sodium polystyrene sulfonate.

5. Describe the actions of antidiuretic hormone and the disease that results when it is deficient. What treatments are available?

MEDICATION TABLES

MEDICATION TABLE 14-1. Oral Potassium Preparations[5,a]

Salt	Brand Name	Dosage Form
Potassium chloride (KCl) (poe TASS i um)	Kaon Cl, Klor-Con, Klotrix, K-Tab, K Dur	Tablets, controlled release
	Klor-Con M	Tablets, extended release
	Micro-K Extencaps, generics	Capsules, controlled release
	Cena-K, Kaon-Cl, generics	Liquid
	K-Lor, Gen-K, K-Lyte/Cl, K-Vescent various generics	Powder (to be dissolved), tablets
Potassium gluconate (poe TASS i um)	Various generics	Tablets
	Kaon, Kaylixir	Liquid
Potassium citrate (poe TASS i um)	Cytra-3	Syrup
	Cytra-LC, Cytra-K, Oracit, Naturalyte	Solution
	Taron-Crystals	Powder (to be dissolved)

[a]Pronunciations have been adapted with permission from USP Dictionary of USAN and International Drug Names (USP Dictionary) © 2022.

MEDICATION TABLE 14-2. Diuretics[5,a]

CLASS Generic Name	Brand Name	Dosage Form	Usual Dose	Notes
Loop Diuretics				
Bumetanide (byoo MET a nide)	Formerly Bumex, now various generics	Oral tablet	0.5–2 mg daily	
		IV/IM injection	0.5–1 mg	May be repeated for second or third dose
Ethacrynic acid, ethacrynate sodium (eth a KRIN ik)	Edecrin	Oral tablet	50–100 mg daily	
		IV injection	0.5–1 mg/kg	Usually one dose only
Furosemide (fyoor OH se mide)	Lasix	Oral tablet and solution	20–80 mg daily	
		IV/IM injection	20–40 mg	IV doses should be administered slowly (1–2 min for usual doses; infusion for high doses)
Torsemide (TORE se mide)	Demadex	Oral tablet, IV injection	10–20 mg daily	

Continued next page

MEDICATION TABLE 14-2. Diuretics[5,a] *(Continued)*

CLASS Generic Name	Brand Name	Dosage Form	Usual Dose	Notes
Potassium-Sparing Diuretics				
Amiloride hydrochloride (a MIL oh ride)	Midamor	Oral tablet	5 mg daily	
Eplerenone (e PLER en one)	Inspra	Oral tablet	50 mg daily	
Triamterene (trye AM ter een)	Dyrenium	Oral capsule	100 mg BID	
Spironolactone (speer on oh LAK tone)	Aldactone	Oral tablet	25–200 mg daily	
Thiazide Diuretics				
Chlorothiazide, chlorothiazide sodium (KLOR oh THYE a zide)	Diuril	Oral tablet, oral suspension, IV injection	0.5–2 g/day (500–2000 mg/day)	
Hydrochlorothiazide (HCTZ) (hye droe klor oh THYE a zide)	Microzide, various generics	Oral capsule, oral tablet	12.5–50 mg/day	
Thiazide-Like Diuretics				
Chlorthalidone (klor THAL i done)	Thalitone (also Hygroton, now discontinued)	Oral tablet	15–200 mg/day	
Indapamide (in DAP a mide)	Lozol	Oral tablet	1.5–5 mg/day	
Metolazone (me TOLE a zone)	Mykrox, Zaroxolyn	Oral tablet	5–20 mg daily	
Combination Products				
Hydrochlorothiazide/spironolactone (hye droe klor oh THYE a zide) (speer on oh LAK tone)	Aldactazide	Oral tablet	100 mg (of each hydrochlorothiazide and spironolactone) daily	
Hydrochlorothiazide/triamterene (hye droe klor oh THYE a zide) (trye AM ter een)	Dyazide, Maxzide	Oral capsule, oral tablet	1 to 2 tablets or capsules once daily	

IM = intramuscular; IV = intravenous.

[a]Pronunciations have been adapted with permission from USP Dictionary of USAN and International Drug Names (USP Dictionary) © 2022.

Chapter 15

Hypertension

Mate M. Soric, PharmD, BCPS, FCCP

KEY TERMS AND DEFINITIONS

Aldosterone—a hormone released in response to angiotensin II that causes excretion of potassium and retention of water and sodium.

Angiotensin—proteins of the renin-angiotensin-aldosterone system. Angiotensin I is produced by the actions of renin on angiotensinogen, and angiotensin II is produced by the actions of angiotensin-converting enzyme on angiotensin I.

Angiotensin-converting enzyme—an enzyme responsible for the production of angiotensin II.

Baroreceptors—receptors of the nervous system that detect changes in the stretching of arterial walls.

Blood pressure—the force exerted on vessel walls by the blood within, reported in the units mm Hg (millimeters of mercury).

Cardioselective beta blockers—agents that act primarily on $beta_1$ receptors and avoid the noncardiac issues associated with $beta_2$ blockade in the respiratory and other body systems.

Chemoreceptors—receptors of the nervous system that detect changes in levels of oxygen, carbon dioxide, or other chemicals.

Contractility—the force of a heartbeat.

DOI 10.37573/9781585286638.015

Diastolic blood pressure—the pressure of the blood against the vessel walls when the heart is at rest.

Edema—swelling.

Hypertension—a state of persistently elevated blood pressure.

Hypertrophy—enlargement of a tissue or organ.

Orthostatic hypotension—a sudden drop in blood pressure that occurs when a patient stands.

Primary hypertension—also known as essential hypertension, this form of hypertension does not have a single identifiable cause.

Reflex tachycardia—an increase in heart rate in response to sudden vasodilation.

Renin—an enzyme released by the kidney that initiates a cascade of events that lead to the production of angiotensin II and increases in blood pressure.

Renin-angiotensin-aldosterone system (RAAS)—a series of proteins and enzymes that help to regulate blood pressure and is a target of numerous antihypertensive agents.

Secondary hypertension—a form of hypertension with an identifiable cause, such as a disease or medication.

Sphygmomanometer—a device used to measure blood pressure.

Systolic blood pressure—the force of the blood against the vessel walls during a heartbeat.

Vasoconstriction—narrowing of the blood vessels as a result of contraction of the smooth muscles in the vessel walls.

LEARNING OBJECTIVES

After completing this chapter, you should be able to

1. Define the terms blood pressure and hypertension.

2. Describe the various mechanisms used by the body to regulate blood pressure.

3. List the blood pressure values associated with each blood pressure classification.

4. Identify the consequences of untreated hypertension.

5. Explain nonpharmacological strategies used to treat hypertension.

6. Describe the mechanism of action, typical dosing, and side effects of the commonly used antihypertensive agents.

7. State the brand and generic names and pharmacological classes of the most commonly used antihypertensive agents and combinations.

Hypertension, defined as a persistently high blood pressure, is one of the most common disorders affecting the cardiovascular system. It affects as many as 72 million Americans, nearly a quarter of the population.[1] If left unchecked, the damage can affect nearly every organ system in the body, and lead to severe heart disease, the leading cause of death in the United States. What makes this disorder particularly dangerous is the utter lack of symptoms in the vast majority of cases. Earning it the nickname "The Silent Killer," only the most severe high blood pressure provides patients with a hint of its presence, allowing for years of organ damage to take place before a patient is diagnosed. Even when caught early through blood pressure screening, it is often difficult to convince patients to take medications with obvious side effects to treat a disease they never knew was present. With proper treatment, however, hypertension can be brought under control and the risks of organ damage can be effectively reduced. In this chapter, the basics of blood pressure will be introduced, including its measurement and the body's natural mechanisms of regulation, followed by a review of the causes of hypertension and its treatment.

CASE STUDY

Mr. Anderson, a 52-year-old male, went to his doctor's office for a checkup. His blood pressure was measured at 153/98 mm Hg.

PATHOPHYSIOLOGY OF HYPERTENSION

The Basics of Blood Pressure

Blood pressure is a term used to describe the force that blood exerts on the vessel walls around it. One component of this pressure comes from the force of each heartbeat. As the left ventricle contracts, blood is forced through the aortic valve and into the systemic vasculature, increasing the amount of pressure in the arteries. The other component of blood pressure is the friction of blood against the walls of the arteries, also known as systemic vascular resistance (SVR). This friction opposes blood flow, making it more difficult for the heart to circulate blood around the body.

Like many other body systems, blood pressure must be kept in a delicate balance, high enough to adequately supply the body with oxygen but not excessively high where it may lead to organ damage. Though the contraction of the heart and the SVR are its two main components, the body employs a number of other factors to influence blood pressure and keep it in a desirable range. One such mechanism comes from the nervous system, with the sympathetic autonomic nervous system (SANS) acting to increase blood pressure and the parasympathetic autonomic nervous system (PANS) working to reduce it. Special receptors called baroreceptors and chemoreceptors can detect changes in arterial stretching and concentrations of oxygen, respectively. They then send signals to the brain to either increase or decrease the blood pressure, accordingly.

Hormones also play a large role in regulating blood pressure and are often targets of antihypertensive medications. In response to signals from the SANS, the hormones epinephrine and norepinephrine, also known as catecholamines, are released from the adrenal glands. When these hormones interact with the heart, they cause an increase in contractility, raising blood pressure by raising cardiac output. In the vasculature, epinephrine and norepinephrine cause the blood vessels to constrict, increasing SVR.

If the kidneys sense a decline in blood pressure, they release a substance called renin. When renin interacts with angiotensinogen, angiotensin I is produced. This protein further interacts with angiotensin-converting enzyme to release an active protein called angiotensin II. Angiotensin II acts on the vasculature to cause a profound vasoconstriction, increasing blood pressure. In addition to its direct effects on blood vessels, angiotensin II signals for the release of a hormone called aldosterone. This hormone causes the kidneys to reabsorb extra water in exchange for potassium, increasing the total volume circulating in the bloodstream and further raising blood pressure. This regulatory mechanism is referred to as the renin-angiotensin-aldosterone system (RAAS) and is a target of many antihypertensive medications. See Figure 15-1 for a depiction of the RAAS. These and a number of other hormones all work together to help maintain an appropriate blood pressure.

Since blood pressure reflects two different forces, it must be measured with two different values: the systolic and diastolic blood pressures. Systolic blood pressure refers to the pressure in the arteries during a contraction of the heart, or systole. It is the larger of the two values as it includes both the pressure of the SVR and the added pressure of a heartbeat. Diastolic blood pressure is the term used to describe the pressure in the arteries when the heart is at rest, or diastole. It is mainly a measure of SVR, alone.

Clinicians screen for hypertension by measuring the blood pressure. This is done using a device, commonly called a blood pressure cuff, but professionally known as a sphygmomanometer, made up of an inflatable cuff and a pressure gauge that gives a blood pressure reading in mm Hg (Hg is the chemical symbol for mercury, the liquid metal long

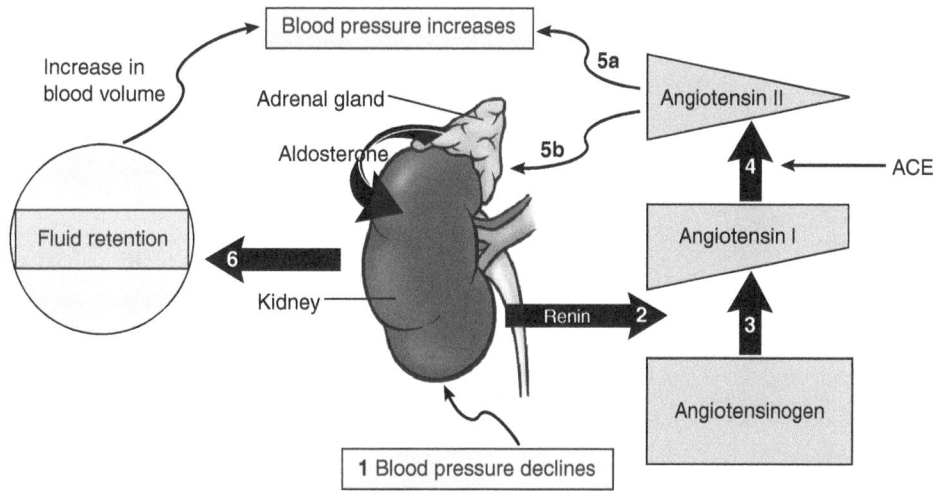

FIGURE 15-1. The renin-angiotensin-aldosterone system (RAAS) is a hormone system that regulates blood pressure and water (fluid) balance.

used in the hollow column of devices for measuring many kinds of pressure, including that of the atmosphere). The cuff is fitted snugly around a patient's upper arm and inflated to a pressure well above the expected blood pressure value, effectively stopping the flow of blood through the artery. Next, the pressure is slowly released from the cuff. When the pressure of the cuff is reduced to the point where the artery opens, blood will begin to flow through the artery once more, making a sound that can be heard using a stethoscope. The pressure reading on the cuff at the instant the sound is heard corresponds to the patient's systolic blood pressure. To detect the diastolic pressure, the cuff is deflated until the sounds of the blood flow become very faint or disappear. The pressure on the gauge at this point corresponds to the patient's diastolic blood pressure. A normal blood pressure is a systolic pressure less than 120 mm Hg and a diastolic pressure less than 80 mm Hg. These two values are usually documented as the systolic blood pressure over the diastolic pressure, such as 120/80 (Figure 15-2).

CASE?

What was Mr. Anderson's systolic blood pressure? What was his diastolic blood pressure?

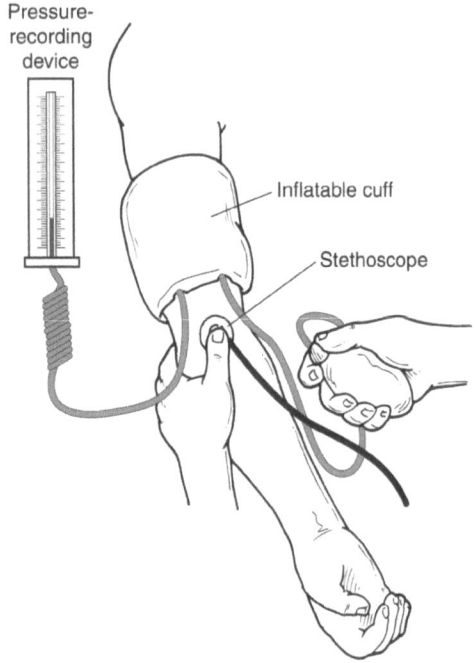

FIGURE 15-2. The sphygmomanometer. This instrument accurately measures arterial blood pressure.

Classification and Causes of Hypertension

The American College of Cardiology and American Heart Association have released a classification scheme to help clinicians diagnose patients with hypertension.[2] Table 15-1 lists the blood pressure values and their corresponding diagnoses. Since blood pressure can be temporarily elevated, the average of two different blood pressures obtained at separate office visits is used to diagnose hypertension. Patients with Stage I hypertension are those with mild disease and are often treated with only one medication, as opposed to patients with stage II hypertension, who have moderate to severe disease and often require at least two agents for control.

CASE?

At his previous office visit, Mr. Anderson's blood pressure was 148/88. How would his blood pressure status be classified? How many agents will he likely be started on to bring his pressure under control?

The most common type of hypertension is known as primary (or essential) hypertension, occurring in more than 90% of all patients with hypertension. In these cases, the exact cause of the elevated blood pressure is difficult to identify since many different factors play a role in its development.

TABLE 15-1. Blood Pressure Classifications[2]

Classifications	Systolic Blood Pressure (mm Hg)	Diastolic Blood Pressure (mm Hg)
Normal	Less than 120	Less than 80
Elevated blood pressure	120–139	Less than 80
Stage I hypertension	130–139	80–89
Stage II hypertension	140 or higher	90 or higher

One such factor is genetics. It has been shown that patients with hypertensive family members are at an increased risk of developing the condition. This is likely due to inheritable dysfunctions in one of the many regulatory systems such as the RAAS or adrenal hormones. A patient's lifestyle also can have a large influence on the risk of developing high blood pressure. Diets high in sodium and limited physical activity have been shown to be important risk factors. Because of its varying causes, primary hypertension cannot be cured. The goal of therapy is control of the condition, reducing blood pressure to less than 140/90 mm Hg in higher-risk patients.

For the fewer than 10% of patients with secondary hypertension, the high blood pressure is caused by an underlying condition or medication. The list of possible secondary causes is long, but some of the most common culprits are kidney disease, cancers of the adrenal gland, hyperthyroidism, and sleep apnea. In addition to diseases, medications and supplements such as nonsteroidal anti-inflammatory drugs (NSAIDs), corticosteroids, nasal decongestants, and cocaine can also cause elevations in blood pressure. In many cases of secondary hypertension, a cure is possible if the underlying disease can be found and treated or the causative medication is stopped.

CASE?

Mr. Anderson currently has no other health conditions and is not taking any medications. What type of hypertension does he likely have?

PRACTICE POINT

The stress of a doctor's appointment is sometimes enough to increase a patient's blood pressure temporarily. This is known as white coat hypertension. To verify that a patient has hypertension, clinicians may have patients check their own blood pressure at home for a comparison with in-office values.

Implications of Uncontrolled Hypertension

Because blood flow is a crucial requirement for the proper functioning of nearly every body system, hypertension has the potential to cause damage in many different areas of the body.

The systems most at risk include the kidneys, brain, heart, vasculature, and eyes. The higher a patient's blood pressure, the greater the risk of developing serious complications or death.

Perhaps the largest impact of hypertension can be seen in the cardiovascular system, where it is a major risk factor for the development of a heart attack or stroke. Elevated pressures accelerate the development of atherosclerotic plaques, accumulations of cholesterol and cellular debris that can block the flow of blood through a vessel. When these plaques rupture, small pieces can travel downstream and become lodged in smaller arterioles or capillaries, blocking blood flow. Without a supply of oxygen, the areas around the blockage begin to die. When these events happen in a coronary artery, the result is a heart attack, or myocardial infarction; if the ruptured plaque travels to the brain, the result is a stroke. Longstanding hypertension can also cause significant changes to the structure of the heart and blood vessels. After many years of pumping against high pressures, the heart can become enlarged, or hypertrophied, and the blood vessels can become less elastic (hardened). At their most severe, these changes can cause a patient to develop heart failure or arrhythmias. For a detailed discussion of heart disease, see Chapter 16.

As described in Chapter 14, the consequence of hypertension in the kidney is nephropathy. Under pressure, the small capillaries of the glomerulus become thickened and sclerosis, or scarring, reduces the nephron's ability to filter blood. This condition can progress to renal failure, in which case the kidneys can no longer filter blood on their own. These patients require dialysis to remove cellular waste from the blood.

CASE?

Mr. Anderson doesn't have any symptoms and is concerned about the inconveniences involved in lowering his blood pressure. What types of health risks does Mr. Anderson face if his hypertension is not controlled?

Just as in the kidneys, it is the smallest blood vessels in the eyes that bear the brunt of the effects of elevated blood pressure. Though it usually requires extremely high pressures, the capillaries in the retina, the inner surface of the eye, can become damaged or even rupture. This condition, known as hypertensive retinopathy, causes swelling behind the eye and may lead to blindness.

TREATMENT OF HYPERTENSION

As the consequences of uncontrolled hypertension are numerous, the goal of treatment is to reduce the risk of developing hypertension-related complications and death. By keeping blood pressure less than 130/80 mm Hg, the chances of developing sclerosis and other vascular changes are reduced. To keep blood pressure below dangerous levels, clinicians rely on lifestyle changes and pharmacological treatments to decrease the chance of developing negative outcomes.

Nonpharmacological Treatment

No treatment regimen for hypertension would be complete without paying attention to a patient's lifestyle choices. Without making changes to lifestyle, controlling hypertension becomes difficult and often requires the addition of many drugs, each with its own side effects. To minimize the need for medications, clinicians focus on improving a number of important areas, including diet, exercise, weight, salt intake, and alcohol and tobacco exposure.

Diet

The types of foods a patient eats can have a direct impact on their overall hypertension control. By following a diet that is high in fruits, vegetables, whole grains, and fish and low in saturated fats, cholesterol, and salt, patients can lower their systolic blood pressure by 5–15 mm Hg. The Dietary Approaches to Stop Hypertension (DASH) diet is one example of a proper blood pressure–reducing diet. In addition to increasing fruits and vegetables while limiting saturated fats, the DASH diet recommends limiting sodium intake to less than 2.4 g daily.[3] Excess salt in the diet causes the body to retain water. This extra volume in the blood vessels can increase blood pressure dramatically. To reach this goal, patients must be educated on the many hidden sources of sodium in the typical Western diet, such as processed foods and canned goods, in addition to table salt. Reducing sodium intake can often lower systolic blood pressure by an additional 2–8 mm Hg. Finally, the amount of alcohol a patient drinks can also negatively affect blood pressure. The DASH diet sets limits on daily alcohol ingestion to no more than two drinks for men and one drink for women.

Physical Activity

An appropriate level of physical activity each day is important, not only for blood pressure control but for the overall health of all patients. Though most patients can safely include physical activity in their treatment regimens, patients who have signs of organ damage may need to consult their physician first. In general, experts recommend 30 minutes of aerobic exercise, such as brisk walking, jogging, bicycling, or swimming, most days of the week. If this goal is met, patients can expect an additional 4–9 mm Hg reduction in blood pressure.

CASE?

In addition to any pharmacological treatments, list three lifestyle modifications that might improve Mr. Anderson's blood pressure.

Weight Loss

Though lifestyle modifications are often difficult to achieve, usually requiring intense follow-up and monitoring, those patients who manage to incorporate diet and exercise into their daily routines typically see significant weight loss. Even small reductions can have far-reaching effects, reducing the risk of developing a wide variety of medical conditions. Regarding hypertension, every 10 kg of weight that is lost equates to an estimated 5–20 mm Hg drop in blood pressure in patients who are overweight.

Pharmacological Treatment

Diuretics

Diuretics, covered at length in Chapter 14, are a class of medications that cause water to be removed from the body. When extra volume is removed from the vasculature, blood pressure is reduced. Though there are a number of different types of diuretics, the classes most commonly used to treat hypertension are the thiazide, loop, and potassium-sparing diuretics. As a group, diuretics can cause electrolyte imbalances, as potassium, magnesium, and other electrolytes are lost along with extra water in the urine. To avoid the possibility of nocturia (the need to waken at night to urinate), they are usually dosed in the morning.

CASE?

Mr. Anderson gets a prescription for hydrochlorothiazide 25 mg daily in addition to his lifestyle modifications. What lab tests may be ordered to check for side effects?

Thiazide and related diuretics are usually considered the first-line agents to treat hypertension in otherwise healthy patients. In addition to inhibiting the reabsorption of water at the distal convoluted tubule, thiazides have an additional antihypertensive effect: vasodilation. Because they relax the smooth muscle surrounding arteries and veins, thiazides are more effective than other diuretics at lowering blood pressure. Medications in this class are usually available in a generic form and are dosed once daily. Thiazide diuretics are generally well-tolerated antihypertensive medications. When being used for hypertension, lower doses of the thiazide diuretics are used, minimizing their potential to cause electrolyte disturbances. Thiazides may also cause hyperglycemia and increased uric acid levels, known as hyperuricemia—side effects not seen with other diuretics. These side effects could increase a patient's risk of developing or worsening diabetes and gout.

For patients who develop kidney disease, the effectiveness of the thiazides can be drastically reduced and a switch to another medication is recommended if the glomerular filtration rate falls below 30 mL/min. Though they are not as effective at lowering blood pressure, loop diuretics retain much of their effectiveness when kidney function declines. Most are available generically. When used to control hypertension, bumetanide and furosemide require twice daily dosing, while torsemide and ethacrynic acid are dosed once daily. In addition to being useful for patients with kidney disease, loop diuretics play a large role in treating hypertension and edema in patients with congestive heart failure. Because of their increased potency, patients prescribed loop diuretics must be monitored closely for low electrolyte levels and orthostatic hypotension, a sudden drop in blood pressure upon rising from a lying or seated position to standing.

PRACTICE POINT

If renal function is very poor, metolazone, a thiazide-related diuretic, can be administered with a loop diuretic. When these agents are used together, they cause much more diuresis than either agent can cause alone.

The potassium-sparing diuretics allow the body to excrete sodium instead of potassium when causing a diuretic effect. If used alone, these medications are much less potent then other diuretics. They are most often ordered for an additive effect or to counteract the potassium loss seen with other diuretics. Spironolactone (Aldactone) and eplerenone (Inspra) are aldosterone antagonists, primarily used in patients with congestive heart failure. They lower blood pressure by blocking the ability of aldosterone to cause the body to retain water and sodium. Both are available in a generic form and are dosed once daily. Spironolactone's unique side effect is gynecomastia, or a painful enlargement of the breasts in male patients. If it develops, patients can often be safely switched to eplerenone. The other potassium-sparing diuretics are available as individual ingredients or in combination with hydrochlorothiazide and include amiloride (Midamor, Moduretic) and triamterene (Dyrenium, Dyazide). Like thiazides, potassium-sparing diuretics should be avoided in patients with reduced kidney function and are typically dosed once daily. Table 14-4 (in Chapter 14) provides a summary of the available diuretics.

Calcium Channel Blockers

Calcium is an important cation necessary for vasoconstriction of blood vessels and quickening of the heart rate. In the arteries and veins, calcium must be transported from the extracellular fluid and into smooth muscle cells before vasoconstriction can occur. Using a similar transport mechanism, calcium must move into the autorhythmic cells of the sinoatrial node to raise the heart rate. These are important targets in the treatment of hypertension. The calcium channel blockers can inhibit the ability of cells to transport this important ion, causing vasodilation, slowing of the heart rate, and a drop in blood pressure. This class of medications can be divided into two subgroups: the dihydropyridines and the nondihydropyridines. Though they both inhibit calcium transport and lower blood pressure, these two subgroups are very different from one another. Dihydropyridines act primarily in the vasculature, causing vasodilation with very little effect on heart rate, whereas the nondihydropyridines inhibit calcium transport in the cardiac tissue, mainly decreasing heart rate and contractility.

The larger of the two subgroups is the dihypropyridines. Medications in this group include amlodipine (Norvasc), felodipine (Plendil), isradipine (DynaCirc), nicardipine (Cardene SR), and nifedipine (Adalat CC, Procardia XL). Nearly all of the agents in this subgroup are dosed once daily, with the exception of the immediate-release formulations of isradipine and nicardipine, which are dosed twice daily. As described above, the effect of dihydropyridines on the vasculature is far greater than their effect on the cardiac tissue. If the vasodilation is too great, the heart rate may suddenly increase in an attempt to maintain adequate blood pressure. This phenomenon is known as reflex tachycardia and is much less common in the longer-acting agents. Other common side effects of the dihydropyridines include orthostatic hypotension, dizziness, headache, and edema. Because these agents cause dilation of the coronary arteries, dihydropyridine calcium channel blockers are very effective in treating chest pain and increasing oxygen supply to the heart.

The nondihydropyridine subgroup contains only two agents: diltiazem (Cardizem CD, Cardizem LA, Tiazac) and verapamil (Calan, Covera, Verelan), though they are available in a number of different formulations. In general, they are dosed once to twice daily, depending on which formulation is chosen. Because they slow the heart rate and decrease its contractility, the nondihydropyridines have side-effect profiles very similar to beta blockers, including bradycardia, hypotension, congestive heart failure, and dizziness. Like other calcium channel blockers, they may also cause edema. Constipation is another frequently reported side effect with diltiazem and verapamil, but it is particularly common with verapamil therapy. The ability of these agents to slow the heart rate makes them very useful in the treatment of arrhythmias, such as atrial fibrillation.

ALERT!

Be careful when dispensing verapamil and diltiazem. There are many different formulations of these drugs that are not interchangeable because of different release mechanisms. For example, Cardizem CD and Tiazac, both extended-release diltiazem capsules, cannot be interchanged with one another or with some generic diltiazem ER capsules (see Medication Table 15-2.)

PRACTICE POINT

The nondihydropyridine calcium channel blockers are broken down by the liver. Patients are often warned to limit their intake of grapefruit juice if they are taking these agents, as it interferes with the liver enzymes and can cause an increase in verapamil and diltiazem concentrations.

Angiotensin-Converting Enzyme Inhibitors

One of the most widely used classes of antihypertensive agents is the angiotensin-converting enzyme (ACE) inhibitors. As described above, angiotensin-converting enzyme

is responsible for the formation of angiotensin II, a protein that causes vasoconstriction and signals for the release of aldosterone. At the same time, ACE is responsible for the breakdown of a number of substances that cause vasodilation. The overall effect of its release is vasoconstriction, an increase in plasma volume, and, consequently, an increase in blood pressure. As their name implies, the ACE inhibitors bind to angiotensin-converting enzyme, blocking its ability to create angiotensin II. When it is inhibited, the balance between vasodilation and vasoconstriction is tipped in favor of vasodilation and blood pressure is reduced. The medications in this class, including benazepril (Lotensin), enalapril (Vasotec), lisinopril (Prinivil, Zestril), and ramipril (Altace), among others, are available as generics. Nearly every agent in the class is typically dosed once daily, with the exception of captopril, which is dosed 2–3 times/day. In certain populations, however, ACE inhibitors may require twice daily dosing to get a full 24-hour antihypertensive effect.

ALERT!

ACE inhibitors are contraindicated in pregnancy.

Like other blood pressure medications, ACE inhibitors are initiated at lower doses and slowly titrated toward an effective dose. This is done to avoid possible side effects. If doses are increased too suddenly, blood pressure may drop quickly, causing dizziness, orthostatic hypotension, or palpitations. Other ACE inhibitor–specific side effects also must be carefully monitored. Angioedema is a possibly life-threatening reaction that causes swelling of the lips, tongue, and throat that has been associated with ACE inhibitors. In most cases, stopping the ACE inhibitor causes a reversal of the symptoms, but, when severe, patients may need to be put on a ventilator to support their breathing. Fortunately, this side effect is rare, but if it does occur these patients should never be exposed to ACE inhibitors again. Another rare consequence of ACE inhibitor use is kidney failure, though it usually only presents in patients with preexisting kidney disease or on other medications that damage the kidney. Because inhibiting angiotensin-converting enzyme also inhibits the release of aldosterone, patients taking these medicines need to have their potassium levels monitored closely. Without aldosterone, the body can retain potassium, leading to dangerous arrhythmias if potassium levels increase significantly. Finally, one of the most common side effects of ACE inhibitor use is a dry cough. Over time, using an ACE inhibitor causes an accumulation of the substances that are normally broken down by the angiotensin-converting enzyme. It is theorized that some of these substances can cause a patient to develop a dry cough that is unrelated to any infectious or allergic origin. Though this is not a sign of any physiological illness, it can be a significant annoyance for patients. To reverse the effect, the ACE inhibitor can be discontinued and therapy switched to another class of antihypertensive agent. Though a number of side effects have been outlined here, it should be noted that these agents are generally well tolerated.

ALERT!

Combining ACE inhibitors with potassium-sparing diuretics or potassium supplements significantly increases the risk of hyperkalemia, especially in patients with poor kidney function.

The ACE inhibitors have been studied in a number of clinical trials and have been found to be very effective agents in controlling hypertension, especially in a number of populations at increased risk of developing serious complications. Because this class of blood pressure agents causes a dilation of the renal arteries, they can be used in patients with kidney disease or diabetes to delay the onset or progression to renal failure. In patients with heart failure or who have had a heart attack, ACE inhibitors have been shown to protect the heart from the damaging effects of angiotensin II and aldosterone, increasing survival and decreasing the risk of additional cardiovascular events. In patients who have had a stroke, the combination of an ACE inhibitor and a diuretic has been shown to significantly reduce the risk of having a second stroke. For these reasons, ACE inhibitors are considered a very close second-line agent in the treatment of hypertension behind the thiazide diuretics.

Angiotensin II Receptor Blockers

The angiotensin II receptor blockers (ARBs, but sometimes called AIIRAs) are a class of medications that are closely related to the ACE inhibitors. Instead of preventing the production of angiotensin II, the ARBs interact with the angiotensin II receptor, interfering with the ability of the protein to carry out its functions. Candesartan (Atacand), losartan (Cozaar), olmesartan (Benicar), valsartan (Diovan), and the other ARBs are typically dosed once daily, though they may require twice daily dosing in some cases for a full 24-hour

effect. Nearly all ARBs are available as generics. Because their mechanism of action is similar to the ACE inhibitors, there is a great deal of overlap in side effects. Like the ACE inhibitors, the ARBs are started at lower doses and increased slowly to avoid the side effects associated with large drops in blood pressure, such as dizziness, hypotension, and palpitations. Patients taking ARBs must also have their potassium levels and kidney function monitored closely to screen for hyperkalemia and kidney failure. Unlike the ACE inhibitors, the ARBs do not cause a dry cough, as the angiotensin-converting enzyme is not being inhibited. In patients who develop angioedema after ACE inhibitor use, the ARBs may be used cautiously since cross-reactivity is rare. The ACE inhibitors and the ARBs also differ in that the ARBs are not quite as well studied. Though the ARBs have proven benefit in preventing kidney damage, they have not yet been shown to be as effective as the ACE inhibitors in patients with cardiovascular disease or stroke. Therefore, ARBs are generally reserved for use as an alternative in patients who develop side effects to ACE inhibitor therapy (see Medication Table 15-3).

Direct Renin Inhibitors

The newest class of antihypertensive agents is the direct renin inhibitors (DRIs). The mechanism of action of this class involves blocking the ability of renin to initiate the cascade of events that lead to angiotensin II production. Currently, the only agent in the class approved by the Food and Drug Administration is aliskiren (Tekturna). This is a generic medication that is dosed once daily. Though aliskiren acts much earlier in the RAAS, many of the side effects and cautions are similar to those for ACE inhibitors and ARBs. Hyperkalemia, decreases in renal function, and angioedema are all possible side effects of DRI therapy. Because aliskiren is a newer agent, its exact role in treating hypertension has not been established. Its antihypertensive effectiveness is comparable to ACE inhibitors and ARBs, but studies are still underway to characterize its effect on nephropathy, cardiovascular disease, and stroke.

Alpha₁ Antagonists

If blood pressure falls, the systemic vasculature can respond to signals from the autonomic nervous system (ANS) to increase blood pressure levels. To accomplish this, epinephrine and norepinephrine are released so they can interact with alpha₁ (α_1) receptors on the vessel walls. When these receptors are activated, the smooth muscle surrounding the vasculature is constricted, raising SVR and blood pressure. In patients with hypertension, medications can be administered that interfere with this interaction between the ANS and blood vessels. The alpha$_1$ antagonists, also known as alpha blockers, are a class of medicines that inhibit the ability of the catecholamines to activate alpha$_1$ receptors. This causes a vasodilation and lowering of blood pressure. Agents in this class include doxazosin (Cardura), prazosin (Minipress), and terazosin (Hytrin). All of the medications in this class are available generically. Doxazosin and terazosin are typically dosed once daily, whereas prazosin is dosed 2–3 times daily. The most common side effects of alpha$_1$ antagonist administration are dizziness, palpitations, and orthostatic hypotension, all due to rapid drops in blood pressure. These effects usually happen after the first dose or with a dose increase. To avoid these side effects, these medicines can be taken at bedtime. A number of studies have shown that this class of medications, though excellent at lowering blood pressure, does not lower the risk of cardiovascular events or death. For this reason, alpha blockers are only used as adjuncts for patients not at goal on other antihypertensives. (Alpha$_1$ receptors are also located in the prostate, and administering alpha$_1$ blockers causes a relaxation of the smooth muscles and relief of urinary symptoms for men with benign prostatic hyperplasia, discussed in Chapter 11).

Beta Antagonists

In addition to alpha receptors in the periphery, the ANS can also activate beta receptors located throughout the body. Beta$_1$ (β_1) receptors are found in the heart and the kidney and, when stimulated, cause an increase in heart rate, contractility, and renin release. Beta$_2$ (β_2) receptors are located in many tissues and help regulate a wide variety of systems, such as bronchodilation in the lungs. The beta antagonists, also known as beta blockers, interfere with the interaction of the catecholamines with these beta receptors. When these receptors are inhibited, hypertension is reduced as the heart rate and force of contraction are diminished and the release of renin is blocked. These medications are started at lower doses and slowly increased or decreased (titrated) based on their effect. Clinicians must be careful, however, to avoid the side effects associated with too much beta$_1$ or unwanted beta$_2$ blockade, including dizziness, hypotension, sexual dysfunction, bronchospasm, and exercise intolerance. This class of antihypertensive medications is further divided into subgroups, which include cardioselective, nonselective, and mixed α- and β-blockers.

> ## ALERT!
>
> Patients should receive a warning not to stop taking beta blockers abruptly. When beta blockers are discontinued, the dose must be decreased gradually over time to reduce the likelihood of rebound hypertension and withdrawal side effects. In some patients, abrupt discontinuation can lead to chest pain, heart attack, or death.

At their typical doses, the cardioselective beta blockers act primarily on beta$_1$ receptors and avoid the noncardiac issues associated with beta$_2$ blockade. This feature makes them the preferred subgroup of beta blockers for treatment of hypertension. The cardioselective beta blockers include atenolol (Tenormin), bisoprolol (Zebeta), and metoprolol (Lopressor, Toprol XL). Atenolol, bisoprolol, and the extended-release form of metoprolol, the succinate salt, can be dosed once daily but the immediate-release form of metoprolol, the tartrate salt, is dosed twice a day. The most common side effects of these agents are bradycardia, hypotension, congestive heart failure, dizziness, and impotence. If higher doses are used, cardioselectivity can be lost, allowing these agents to block beta$_2$ receptors along with the beta$_1$ receptors, possibly worsening asthma or diabetes symptoms.

The nonselective beta blockers, such as nadolol (Corgard), propranolol (Inderal), and timolol (Blocadren), interact with both the beta$_1$ and beta$_2$ receptors, blocking the actions of epinephrine and norepinephrine. Nadolol, timolol, and the extended-release versions of propranolol are dosed once daily, and the immediate-release form of propranolol is dosed twice daily. Like the selective beta blockers, their antihypertensive effects come from reducing the rate and force of the heart's contractions while inhibiting the release of renin from the kidneys. The main difference with these agents, the fact that they also block beta$_2$ receptors, allows them to have additional uses and side effects. Blockade of the beta$_2$ receptors in the lungs may decrease the ability of the bronchioles to dilate, putting asthmatic patients at higher risk of asthma attacks. While their unique side effects often limit their use in hypertension, the nonselective beta blockade is desirable in a number of other disease states, such as glaucoma, tremors, and migraine headaches.

Carvedilol (Coreg) and labetalol (Normodyne, Trandate) are classified as mixed alpha and beta antagonists. These medications block alpha$_1$, beta$_1$, and beta$_2$ receptors, lowering blood pressure by causing vasodilation, slowing the heart rate and decreasing contractility. Both of these agents are dosed twice daily, with the exception of extended-release carvedilol, which is only dosed once daily. Though most side effects are similar to those described for the alpha and beta antagonists, the addition of the alpha antagonist to the beta blockade further increases the risk of orthostatic hypotension.

Central Alpha$_2$ Agonists

While blocking alpha$_1$ receptors in the vasculature is one way blood pressure can be reduced, the alpha$_2$ receptors in the brain have a very different function. The receptors in the central nervous system cause a decrease in blood pressure when they are activated. They do this by increasing the activity of the PANS, the part of the nervous system that counteracts the SANS, lowering heart rate, contractility, and causing vasodilation. Clonidine (Catapres), guanfacine (Tenex), guanabenz (Wytensin), and methyldopa (Aldomet) are agents designed to activate alpha$_2$ receptors in the brain to lower blood pressure. All of the medications in this class are available generically. The oral formulations of these medications are typically administered twice daily, though guanfacine may be dosed once daily. (Note: because of their central activity, guanfacine and clonidine are also used in the treatment of attention deficit hyperactivity disorder; see Chapter 7 for more information.)

In addition to the typical oral preparations, clonidine is also available as a once weekly transdermal patch. Started at 0.1 mg/24 hr, the patch's dose can be increased every 1–2 weeks to a typical maximum of 0.3 mg/24 hr. It is recommended to apply new patches at bedtime to a hairless portion of the upper arm or chest, reducing the risk of the patch falling off. To minimize redness at the site of application, patients should rotate the location of the patch each week.

When the alpha$_2$ agonists are discontinued, the dose must be decreased slowly over time to reduce the risk of developing rebound hypertension. Though the alpha$_2$ agonists are very effective blood pressure lowering agents, several important side effects limit their use. Because these agents are centrally acting, there is an increased risk of developing depression. Long-term use has also been shown to cause an increase in water and sodium retention. Their potent reduction of blood pressure also equates to much higher rates of orthostatic hypotension and dizziness than is seen with other blood pressure agents. If higher doses are necessary, alpha$_2$ selectivity may be lost, leading to activation of peripheral alpha$_1$ receptors and vasoconstriction. Though the side effects are numerous, there are specific situations where an alpha$_2$ agonist may be a good choice.

Direct Arterial Vasodilators

The direct arterial vasodilators are a class of hypertension medications that cause a relaxation of the smooth muscles surrounding arteries. This can result in profound decreases in blood pressure. Medications in this class include hydralazine (Apresoline) and minoxidil (Loniten). Both agents are generic. Hydralazine is typically dosed 2–4 times each day, and minoxidil is dosed 1–2 times each day. Like the $alpha_2$ agonists, these agents are very effective at reducing blood pressure, but side effects tend to limit their use. When the arteries are suddenly dilated, the baroreceptors detect a drop in blood pressure and attempt to maintain adequate profusion. Signals are sent from the ANS to increase heart rate and retain fluid to keep blood pressure high. Over time, the body's compensation leads to a drastic decrease in the efficacy of the direct arterial vasodilators, a phenomenon known as tachyphylaxis or tolerance. To avoid this result, hydralazine and minoxidil are usually prescribed in conjunction with beta blockers and diuretics to blunt the body's compensatory mechanisms. Each agent also has unique side effects. Hydralazine has been shown to cause a drug-induced lupus. This is a disorder in which the body's immune system begins to attack itself, causing joint pain, fatigue, and possible damage to the heart and lungs. The incidence of this side effect increases as the dose of the drug is increased, and, if it occurs, hydralazine must be discontinued. Minoxidil use may lead to hypertrichosis, or unwanted hair growth of the face, chest, arms, and back. To stop this hair growth, the minoxidil must be discontinued (see Medication Table 15-4).

PRACTICE POINT

Minoxidil is a common ingredient in many topical hair growth products used to treat baldness. Oral minoxidil, however, is indicated only for hypertension.

Combination Products

In addition to the single products discussed above, many antihypertensive medications are available in combination forms. The most common pairings include ACE inhibitors, angiotensin receptor blockers, direct renin inhibitors, or beta blockers in combination with thiazide diuretics; however, many different couplings exist. As most hypertensive patients require more than two agents to control the disease, incorporating multiple ingredients in a single tablet or capsule can significantly reduce the pill burden, giving patients greater convenience and potentially improving adherence. However, the practice of combining blood pressure medications can also have considerable drawbacks. Healthcare practitioners who choose to use these products sacrifice a great deal of flexibility in dose adjustments when only certain options exist as combinations. If a patient experiences side effects and requires a dose reduction of one ingredient, a suitable combination product may not exist. Also, many combination products are available as brand name agents, leading to higher costs when compared with generic alternatives (see Medication Table 15-5).

Choosing an Agent

As described above, the options available to treat hypertension are numerous. To help decide among the multitude of classes, clinicians consider individual patient issues, including severity of hypertension, cost and insurance coverage, tolerability, and concurrent disease states. For otherwise-healthy patients with stage I hypertension, current guidelines recommend the use of thiazide diuretics, ACE inhibitors, and dihydropyridine calcium channel blockers as first-line agents. These affordable, well-tolerated agents have proven mortality reduction, even when compared to newer antihypertensive therapies.[2] For patients with stage II hypertension, it is recommended to start two medications. There may be other clinical scenarios that call for specific agents. For patients with congestive heart failure, a history of heart attacks, or coronary artery disease, beta blockers, ACE inhibitors, and aldosterone antagonists have added benefit. Calcium channel blockers work well for patients with chest pain and older adults. For patients with diabetes, ACE inhibitors and ARBs have been shown to decrease the risk of cardiovascular events and the progression of kidney disease. An individualized drug regimen can make it possible for therapeutic goals to be reached while limiting the potential for side effects.

CASE?

Mr. Anderson is back in the physician's office 1 year after starting hydrochlorothiazide. His blood pressure has averaged 165/99 at his last two visits. He has also been diagnosed with type 2 diabetes. What additional antihypertensive therapy might help him reach his blood pressure goals and also may have added benefit in his new medical condition?

HYPERTENSIVE CRISIS

If hypertension is not adequately controlled, some patients may develop a hypertensive crisis, or a blood pressure elevated to a point greater than 180/120 mm Hg. Overall, there are two main categories of hypertensive crises: hypertensive urgencies and emergencies. A hypertensive urgency is defined as a blood pressure higher than 180/120 mm Hg in a patient who has no signs of organ damage or failure. In these cases, fast-acting oral therapies, such as captopril, labetalol, or clonidine, can be used to slowly bring the blood pressure to safer values. In hypertensive emergencies, however, patients have both an elevated blood pressure and show signs of organ damage or failure, such as blurred vision, kidney failure, or confusion. Healthcare practitioners must act quickly to start intravenous (IV) therapies to protect the patient's organs and prevent further damage.

A number of IV treatment options exist to counter the effects of a hypertensive crisis. One of the most commonly used IV agents is sodium nitroprusside (Nitropress). Dosed initially at 0.3–0.5 mcg/kg/min, this vasodilator is titrated upward to meet blood pressure reduction goals. For a full discussion of sodium nitroprusside, see Chapter 16. Clevidipine (Cleviprex), a fast-acting IV nondihydropyridine calcium channel blocker, is typically started at 1–2 mg/hr. The most rapid-acting beta blocker, esmolol (Brevibloc), is another common choice. Patients usually receive a loading dose

followed by a weight-based continuous infusion. Finally, fenoldopam (Corlopam) is an agent with a unique mechanism of action, targeting dopamine receptors to cause vasodilation. Its starting dose is 0.1–0.3 mcg/kg/min. In addition to these agents, a number of the classes described in the sections above contain agents available in an IV formulation. Dosing guidelines for IV hydralazine, enalapril, nicardipine, nitroglycerin, and labetalol are included in the Medication Tables in this chapter. Though they may have varying mechanisms, all of the above agents have similar characteristics, a rapid onset of action and a short duration allowing for careful control of a patient's blood pressure. For these same reasons, similar side effects must be monitored, including hypotension and reflex tachycardia.

SUMMARY

Hypertension is a very common disease state in the United States. In most cases, the cause is difficult to identify but is likely made up of genetic and environmental factors. This silent killer can be present for many years before the signs of its presence are made known. If left unchecked, it causes damage across numerous body systems and increases the risk of serious complications and death. Fortunately, the risks associated with hypertension can be greatly reduced if caught early through blood pressure screenings and treated with appropriate therapy. To ensure blood pressure goals are met, every treatment regimen must include both pharmacological and nonpharmacological treatment. Patients must be educated on the benefits of physical activity and dietary changes, while clinicians evaluate each patient carefully to determine which agents will help decrease blood pressure, reduce the risk of complications, and avoid unwanted side effects.

REFERENCES

1. American Heart Association. The facts about high blood pressure. Available at: https://www.heart.org/en/health-topics/high-blood-pressure/the-facts-about-high-blood-pressure. Accessed March 23, 2022.

2. 2017 ACC/AHA/AAPA/ABC/ACPM/AGS/APhA/ASH/ASPC/NMA/PCNA Guideline for the Prevention, Detection, Evaluation, and Management of High Blood Pressure in Adults: A Report of the American College of Cardiology/American Heart Association Task Force on Clinical Practice Guidelines. *J Am Coll Cardiol*. 2018;71:e127-e248.

3. National Institutes of Health. Your guide to lowering your blood pressure with DASH. Available at http://www.nhlbi.nih.gov/health/public/heart/hbp/dash/new_dash.pdf. Accessed March 23, 2022.
4. Lexi-Drugs. Lexicomp. Hudson, OH. Accessed April 1, 2021. http://online.lexi.com.

CHAPTER RESOURCES

Barrett KE, Barman SM, Brooks HL, et al. *Ganong's Review of Medical Physiology*. 26th ed. New York, NY: McGraw-Hill; 2019.

DiPiro JT, Yee GC, Posey M, et al. *Pharmacotherapy: A Pathophysiological Approach*. 11th ed. New York: NY: McGraw-Hill; 2020.

REVIEW QUESTIONS

1. Define the terms blood pressure and hypertension.

2. Every blood pressure reading is made up of two values. What are the names of these two numbers that make up a blood pressure reading? What does each signify?

3. Describe the mechanism of the renin-angiotensin-aldosterone system (RAAS).

4. Describe the differences in the mechanism of action of the four types of beta-receptor antagonists.

5. Inhibiting the release or response of aldosterone may cause increased blood levels of what substance? Which classes of drugs are sometimes implicated in this problem?

MEDICATION TABLES

MEDICATION TABLE 15-1. Sympathetic Receptor Antagonists[4a]

CLASS Generic Name (pronunciation)	Brand Name	Route	Forms	Dose	Notes
Alpha₁ Antagonists					
Doxazosin (dox AY zoe sin)	Cardura, Cardura XL	Oral	Tablet	1–16 mg daily	No proven mortality or cardiovascular benefit; also used for benign prostatic hyperplasia
Prazosin (PRA zoe sin)	Minipress	Oral	Capsule	2–20 mg 2–3 times daily	
Terazosin (ter AY zoe sin)	Hytrin	Oral	Capsule	1–20 mg 1–2 times daily	
Beta Adrenergic Blockers					
Cardioselective					
Atenolol (a TEN oh lole)	Tenormin	Oral	Tablet	25–100 mg 1–2 times daily	Proven cardiovascular risk reduction; added benefit in heart failure, coronary artery disease, and atrial fibrillation
Betaxolol (be TAX oh lol)	Kerlone and generics	Oral	Tablet	5–20 mg once daily	
Bisoprolol (bis OH proe lol)	Zebeta	Oral	Tablet	2.5–10 mg once daily	
Esmolol (ES moh lol)	Brevibloc	IV	Solution	500–1,000 mcg/kg × 1 then 150 mcg/kg/min	
Metoprolol tartrate (me TOE proe lole)	Lopressor	Oral	Tablet	50–100 mg twice daily, maximum dose 400 mg/day	
Metoprolol succinate (me TOE proe lole)	Toprol XL	Oral	Tablet	50–200 mg once daily, maximum dose 400 mg/day	
Nonselective					
Nadolol (nay DOE lole)	Corgard	Oral	Tablet	40–120 mg once daily	Not often used for hypertension; added benefit in tremors and migraine
Propranolol (proe PRAN oh lole)	Inderal	Oral	Tablet	40–120 mg 2–3 times daily	
	Inderal LA, InnoPran XL, Inderal XL	Oral	Capsule	80–160 mg once daily	
Timolol (TYE moe lole)	Generic only	Oral	Tablet	10–30 mg twice daily	
Mixed Alpha and Beta Blockers					
Carvedilol (KAR ve dil ol)	Coreg	Oral	Tablet	6.25–25 mg twice daily	Increased risk of orthostatic hypotension; carvedilol has added benefit in heart failure
	Coreg CR	Oral	Capsule	20–80 mg once daily	
Labetalol (la BET a lole)	Trandate brand no longer available in US	Oral	Tablet	200–800 mg twice daily	
	Trandate brand no longer available in US	IV	Solution	10–20 mg × 1 then 20–80 mg q 10 min	

[a]Pronunciations have been adapted with permission from USP Dictionary of USAN and International Drug Names (USP Dictionary) © 2022.

MEDICATION TABLE 15-2. Calcium Channel Blockers[4a]

CLASS Generic Name (pronunciation)	Brand Name	Route	Forms	Dose	Notes
Dihydropyridine Calcium Channel Blockers					
Amlodipine (am LOE di peen)	Norvasc	Oral	Tablet	2.5–10 mg once daily	Proven cardiovascular risk reduction; added benefit in angina
Clevidipine (kle VID a peen)	Cleviprex	IV	Solution	1–2 mg/hr titrated to effect	
Felodipine (fe LOE di peen)	Plendil	Oral	Tablet	2.5–10 mg once daily	
Isradipine (iz RA di peen)	Generic only	Oral	Capsule	2.5–5 mg twice daily	
Nicardipine (nye KAR de peen)	Generic only	Oral	Capsule	20–40 mg 3 times daily	
	Cardene	IV	Solution	5–15 mg/hr	
Nifedipine (nye FED i peen)	Adalat CC, Procardia, Procardia XL	Oral	Capsule, extended-release tablet	30–90 mg once daily	
Nondihydropyridine Calcium Channel Blockers					
Diltiazem (dil TYE a zem)	Generics only	Oral	Capsule, Extended-release, 12-hour	60–180 mg twice daily	Only oral extended-release dosage forms are indicated for treatment of hypertension (added benefit in atrial fibrillation)
	Cardizem CD, Cartia-XT, Dilt-XR, Taztia XT, Tiadylt ER, Tiazac, Generics	Oral	Capsule Extended-release, 24-hour	120–360 mg daily	
	Cardizem LA, Matzim LA, Generics	Oral	Tablet Extended-release, 24-hour	120–360 mg daily	
	Cardizem	Oral	Tablet	Not indicated for hypertension	
	Generics only	IV	Solution		
Verapamil (ver AP a mil)	Calan SR, Isoptin SR	Oral	Tablet	180–480 mg 1–2 daily	
	Verelan PM	Oral	Capsule	100–400 mg at bedtime	

[a]Pronunciations have been adapted with permission from USP Dictionary of USAN and International Drug Names (USP Dictionary) © 2022.

MEDICATION TABLE 15-3. Representative Angiotensin-Converting Enzyme Inhibitors and Angiotensin II Receptor Blockers[4a]

CLASS Generic Name (pronunciation)	Brand Name	Route	Forms	Dose	Notes
Angiotensin-Converting Enzyme (ACE) Inhibitors					
Benazepril (ben AY ze pril)	Lotensin	Oral	Tablet	10–40 mg 1–2 times daily	Proven cardiovascular risk reduction; added benefit in diabetes and kidney disease
Captopril (KAP toe pril)	Brand name no longer available; generics only	Oral	Tablet	6.25–25 mg 2–3 times daily	
Enalapril (e NAL a pril)	Vasotec, Epaned	Oral	Tablet, Solution	5–20 mg 1–2 times daily	
Enalaprilat (e NAL a pril at)	Generic only	IV	Solution	1.25–5 mg 4 times daily	
Fosinopril (foe SIN oh pril)	Brand no longer available in US; generics only	Oral	Tablet	10–40 mg once daily	
Lisinopril (lyse IN oh pril)	Prinivil, Zestril	Oral	Tablet	10–40 mg once daily	
Perindopril (per IN DOE pril)	Aceon	Oral	Tablet	4–16 mg once daily	
Quinapril (KWIN a pril)	Accupril	Oral	Tablet	5–40 mg 1–2 times daily	
Ramipril (ra MI pril)	Altace	Oral	Capsule	2.5–10 mg 1–2 times daily	
Angiotensin II Receptor Blockers (ARBs)					
Azilsartan (ay zil SAR tan)	Edarbi	Oral	Tablet	40–80 mg once daily	Proven cardiovascular risk reduction useful in patients who have experienced an ACE inhibitor-induced cough
Candesartan (kan des AR tan)	Atacand	Oral	Tablet	8–32 mg 1–2 times daily	
Eprosartan (ep roe SAR tan)	Teveten	Oral	Tablet	600–800 mg once daily	
Irbesartan (ir be SAR tan)	Avapro	Oral	Tablet	150–300 mg once daily	
Losartan (loe SAR tan)	Cozaar	Oral	Tablet	50–100 mg once daily	
Olmesartan (all mi SAR tan)	Benicar	Oral	Tablet	20–40 mg once daily	
Valsartan (val SAR tan)	Diovan	Oral	Tablet	80–320 mg once daily	

[a]Pronunciations have been adapted with permission from USP Dictionary of USAN and International Drug Names (USP Dictionary) © 2022.

MEDICATION TABLE 15-4. Additional Antihypertensive Agents[4a]

CLASS Generic Name (pronunciation)	Brand Name	Route	Forms	Dose	Notes
Aldosterone Antagonists					
Eplerenone (e PLER en one)	Inspra	Oral	Tablet	50 mg 1–2 times daily	Proven cardiovascular risk reduction; added benefit in heart failure
Spironolactone (speer on oh LAK tone)	Aldactone	Oral	Tablet	25–50 mg 1–2 times daily	
Representative Central Alpha$_2$ Agonists					
Clonidine (KLON i deen)	Brands not available in US; generics only	Oral	Tablet, extended-release tablet	0.1–0.8 mg twice daily	No proven mortality or cardiovascular benefit; methyldopa is drug of choice in pregnancy
	Catapres TTS	Topical	Patch	0.1–0.3 mg once weekly	
Guanfacine (GWAHN fa seen)	Tenex, Intuniv	Oral	Tablet, extended-release tablet	0.5–2 mg at bedtime	
Methyldopa (meth il DOE pa)	Brand not available in US; generics only	Oral	Tablet	250–1000 mg twice daily	
Direct Arterial Vasodilators					
Hydralazine (hye DRAL a zeen)	Generic only	Oral	Tablet	10–50 mg 2–4 times daily	No proven cardiovascular risk reduction
		IV	Solution	10–20 mg 4–6 times daily	
Minoxidil (mi NOX i dill)	Generic only	Oral	Tablet	5–20 mg 1–2 times daily	
Direct Renin Inhibitors					
Aliskiren (a lis KYE ren)	Tekturna	Oral	Tablet	150–300 mg once daily	No proven cardiovascular risk reduction
Dopamine Agonist					
Fenoldopam (fe NOL doe pam)	Corlopam	IV	Solution	0.1–0.3 mcg/kg/min titrated to effect	Unique mechanism of action
Vasodilators					
Nitroglycerin (nye troe GLI ser in)	Generic only	IV	Solution	5–20 mcg/min titrated to effect	For use in hypertensive urgency or emergency
Nitroprusside (nye troe PRUS ide)	Nitropress	IV	Solution	0.3–0.5 mcg/kg/min titrated to effect	

[a]Pronunciations have been adapted with permission from USP Dictionary of USAN and International Drug Names (USP Dictionary) © 2022.

MEDICATION TABLE 15-5. Selected Combination Antihypertensive Products[4a]

CLASS Generic Name (pronunciation)	Brand Name
Angiotensin-Converting Enzyme (ACE) Inhibitor + Thiazide	
Benazepril/hydrochlorothiazide (HCTZ) (ben AY ze pril) (hye droe klor oh THYE a zide)	Lotensin HCT
Captopril/HCTZ (KAP toe pril) (hye droe klor oh THYE a zide)	Capozide
Enalapril/HCTZ (e NAL a pril) (hye droe klor oh THYE a zide)	Vaseretic
Fosinopril/HCTZ (foe SIN oh pril) (hye droe klor oh THYE a zide)	Generic only
Lisinopril/HCTZ (lyse IN oh pril) (hye droe klor oh THYE a zide)	Prinzide, Zestoretic
Quinapril/HCTZ (KWIN a pril) (hye droe klor oh THYE a zide)	Accuretic, Quinaretic
ACE inhibitor + Calcium Channel Blocker	
Benazepril/amlodipine (ben AY ze pril) (am LOE di peen)	Lotrel
Angiotensin Receptor Blocker (ARB) + Thiazide	
Candesartan/HCTZ (kan des AR tan) (hye droe klor oh THYE a zide)	Atacand HCT
Irbesartan/HCTZ (ir be SAR tan) (hye droe klor oh THYE a zide)	Avalide
Losartan/HCTZ (loe SAR tan) (hye droe klor oh THYE a zide)	Hyzaar
Olmesartan/HCTZ (all mi SAR tan) (hye droe klor oh THYE a zide)	Benicar HCT
Valsartan/HCTZ (val SAR tan) (hye droe klor oh THYE a zide)	Diovan HCT
ARB + Calcium Channel Blocker	
Olmesartan/amlodipine (all mi SAR tan) (am LOE di peen)	Azor
Valsartan/amlodipine (val SAR tan) (am LOE di peen)	Exforge
Amlodipine/telmisartan (am LOE di peen) (tel mi SAR tan)	Twynsta
Beta Blockers + Thiazide	
Atenolol/chlorthalidone (a TEN oh lole) (klor THAL i done)	Tenoretic

Continued next page

MEDICATION TABLE 15-5. Selected Combination Antihypertensive Products[4a] *(Continued)*

CLASS Generic Name (pronunciation)	Brand Name
Beta Blockers + Thiazide	
Bisoprolol/HCTZ (bis OH proe lol) (hye droe klor oh THYE a zide)	Ziac
Metoprolol/HCTZ (me TOE proe lole) (hye droe klor oh me THYE a zide)	Lopressor HCT
Propranolol/HCTZ (proe PRAN oh lole) (hye droe klor oh THYE a zide)	Inderide, Inderide LA
Direct Renin Inhibitor + ARB	
Aliskiren/valsartan (a lis KYE ren) (val SAR tan)	Valturna
Direct Renin Inhibitor + Calcium Channel Blocker	
Aliskiren/amlodipine (a lis KYE ren) (am LOE di peen)	Tekamlo
Direct Renin Inhibitor + Thiazide	
Aliskiren/HCTZ (a lis KYE ren) (hye droe klor oh THYE a zide)	Tekturna HCT
Thiazide + Central Alpha$_2$ Agonists	
Chlorthalidone/clonidine (klor THAL i done) (KLOE ni deen)	Clorpres
Thiazide + Potassium-Sparing Diuretic	
Amiloride/HCTZ (a MIL oh ride) (hye droe klor oh THYE a zide)	Generic only
Spironolactone/HCTZ (speer on oh LAK tone) (hye droe klor oh THYE a zide)	Aldactazide
Triamterene/HCTZ (trye AM ter een) (hye droe klor oh THYE a zide)	Dyazide, Maxzide, Maxzide-25
Triple Therapy	
Amlodipine/HCTZ/olmesartan (am LOE di peen) (hye droe klor oh THYE a zide) (all mi SAR tan)	Tribenzor
Amlodipine/HCTZ/valsartan (am LOE di peen) (hye droe klor oh THYE a zide) (val SAR tan)	Exforge HCT
Amlodipine/aliskiren/HCTZ (am LOE di peen) (a lis KYE ren) (hye droe klor oh THYE a zide)	Amturnide

[a]Pronunciations have been adapted with permission from USP Dictionary of USAN and International Drug Names (USP Dictionary) © 2022.

Chapter 16

Heart Disease

Mate M. Soric, PharmD, BCPS, FCCP

KEY TERMS AND DEFINITIONS

Acute coronary syndrome—a collection of heart conditions caused by an acutely blocked coronary artery, including myocardial infarction and unstable angina.

Angina—chest pain or pressure. Stable angina is experienced by patients with ischemic heart disease. Unstable angina is the mildest form of acute coronary syndrome caused by temporary blockages of coronary arteries.

Bradycardia—slower than normal heart rate, usually considered lower than 60 beats per minute. Seldom symptomatic until heart rate decreases below 50 beats per minute.

Cardiac catheterization—a diagnostic and/or therapeutic procedure in which a catheter is inserted into the heart and used to administer a dye to visualize the coronary arteries. If blockages are present, stents may be inserted to open blocked arteries.

Contractility—the ability of the cardiac muscle to undergo the changes needed to cause a contraction.

Depolarization—movement of ions within a cell that leads to a change in the electrical charge of the cell.

Electrocardiogram (ECG or EKG)—a graphic representation of the electrical activity of the heart. The device used for this test is an electrocardiograph.

DOI 10.37573/9781585286638.016

Heart failure—a condition in which cardiac output is reduced to the point where the blood supply can no longer meet the metabolic demands of the body.

Inotropic—related to cardiac contractility. Positive inotropic effects result in increased contractility while negative ones produce decreased contractility.

Ischemia—an imbalance between oxygen supply and demand.

Ischemic heart disease—a condition of lowered oxygen supply or increased oxygen demand of the heart, often caused by chronically blocked coronary arteries.

Myocardial—referring to the heart muscle.

Myocardial infarction—an emergency caused by an acutely blocked coronary artery, leading to decreased oxygen supply to the heart and myocardial cell death.

Refractory period—a brief period of time after a depolarization during which a new depolarization cannot occur.

Shock—a state in which the body cannot provide the necessary materials to support metabolic function. Shock is characterized by its cause and may be

- Anaphylactic—severe allergic reaction.
- Cardiogenic—damage to the cardiovascular system.
- Hemorrhagic—blood loss.
- Hypovolemic—loss of fluid from the vascular space.
- Neurogenic—traumatic brain injury.
- Septic—infection.

LEARNING OBJECTIVES

After completing this chapter, you should be able to

1. Define ischemic heart disease, acute coronary syndrome, heart failure, arrhythmia, and shock and identify their causes, symptoms, and consequences.

2. List the nonpharmacologic treatments for the heart diseases above.

3. Identify the various pharmacological treatments used to treat heart diseases and their basic mechanisms of action.

4. Describe the common side effects caused by each of the medication classes used to treat heart diseases.

The heart lies at the center of the cardiovascular system, providing the force that circulates blood around the body. As discussed in Chapter 14, the heart is divided into four chambers, each separated by valves. Deoxygenated blood arriving at the right atrium passes into the right ventricle, which pumps it into the lungs. Upon its return to the heart, the blood enters the left side of the heart, passing through the left atrium before being pumped to the rest of the body by the left ventricle. Keeping the system pumping in synchrony is a complex electrical system and a continuous supply of oxygen delivered via the coronary arteries. These areas of the heart are vital to its proper function but are also vulnerable to a number of dysfunctions. If the coronary arteries are blocked, oxygen supply to the heart can be reduced, leading to ischemic heart disease. This condition may progress to an emergency known as an acute coronary syndrome, including myocardial infarctions, commonly known as heart attacks. In the long term, patients with decreased oxygen supply to the heart may develop a condition known as heart failure, a decreased ability of the heart to pump blood around the body. Finally, if the heart's electrical systems are damaged, patients may develop life-threatening arrhythmias or abnormal heartbeats. Diseases of the heart can be particularly devastating, causing nearly 1 million deaths in the United States each year.[1]

A number of common heart diseases are discussed in this chapter, including ischemic heart disease, acute coronary syndromes, heart failure, arrhythmias, and shock. The causes, signs, symptoms, and diagnosis of each condition are reviewed, followed by a discussion of the most widely used pharmacological and nonpharmacological treatments.

ISCHEMIC HEART DISEASE

The coronary arteries that surround the heart are responsible for delivering a constant supply of oxygen. This oxygen is used by the myocardial (heart muscle) cells, allowing the heart to pump ceaselessly throughout a lifetime. When there is an imbalance between oxygen supplied from the blood stream and demand of the cardiac cells, a patient is said to have ischemic heart disease.

CASE STUDY

G. S. is a 59-year-old man with a history of coronary artery disease. During a visit to his doctor's office, he mentions that he has occasionally felt short of breath and a feeling "like something was sitting on my chest." The symptoms tend to occur when he is shoveling snow from his driveway. His doctor explains that he is likely experiencing angina due to his ischemic heart disease.

Pathophysiology

Ischemia, or an imbalance between oxygen supply and demand, may be caused by a number of circumstances. In most cases, one underlying factor of ischemic heart disease is coronary artery disease. The process of developing coronary artery disease, or atherosclerosis, begins decades before symptoms or an acute event. Starting in small areas of vascular damage, deposits of cholesterol, called fatty streaks, begin lining the walls of a vessel. These deposits continue to grow over time and eventually spread into the layers beneath the vessel wall. Once the cholesterol has infiltrated these lower layers, white blood cells enter the area. In an effort to remove the cholesterol, the immune cells become activated, causing more irritation in the area and attracting additional white blood cells. This collection of cholesterol, white blood cells, and cellular debris, known as an atherosclerotic plaque, causes narrowing of the blood vessel, leading to a sharp drop in blood flow to the heart and a decline in oxygen supply. (This problem, and its treatment, is discussed extensively in Chapter 17.)

In addition to atherosclerosis, other factors can also affect myocardial oxygen balance. Some patients' oxygen supply may be reduced as a result of vasospasms—an uncontrollable and unintended constriction of blood vessels that cause significant constriction of coronary arteries. Oxygen demand is determined by heart rate and contractility. Demand is higher when both are increased, such as during exercise. Typically, both supply and demand issues must occur to tip the oxygen balance in an unfavorable direction.

When oxygen concentration dwindles, the first signs of dysfunction are a decrease in the cardiac cell's ability to cause a contraction. If the oxygen-depleted state lasts, the ischemic area widens. The larger the ischemic zone, the more

likely the patient will experience the most common symptom of ischemic heart disease: angina or chest pain. Though descriptions of angina may vary from patient to patient, the typical presentation is a sensation of chest pressure or burning. This sensation may be coupled with radiation of the pain to the left arm, neck, and jaw. Patients may also complain of nausea, shortness of breath, and diaphoresis (sweating). It is important for clinicians to collect information about what the patient was doing at the time the angina began. This information can aid in the diagnosis of ischemic heart disease. Activities that cause increases in oxygen demand or decreases in oxygen supply can give rise to an anginal attack. These activities include exercise, cold temperatures, emotional upset, and eating a large meal, among others. It is also important to note that some patients, especially those with diabetes or certain nervous system disorders, may have ischemic heart disease and experience no symptoms whatsoever.

CASE?

What situations led to G. S.'s angina symptoms? What other activities besides shoveling snow should G. S. avoid?

Diagnosis

Since ischemic heart disease is a serious condition that indicates increased cardiovascular risk (the risk of having a cardiovascular event such as a heart attack or stroke), it is important that it is appropriately differentiated from other conditions that may present with similar symptoms. Anxiety, gastroesophageal reflux disease (GERD), and acute coronary syndromes can all present similarly, and a number of diagnostic tests can help clinicians obtain the correct diagnosis. One of the earliest tests ordered is the EKG, or electrocardiogram. This measures the electrical activity of the heart, producing a graphic record that can help clinicians decide if a patient is having angina or a myocardial infarction. For patients who have intermittent angina, a stress test, or exercise tolerance test, can be ordered to reproduce the conditions that caused the chest pain. In this test, patients are asked to run on a treadmill while attached to an EKG machine. If a patient has ischemic heart disease, the increased demand of exercising should cause a recurrence of chest pain. For patients who cannot exercise, agents such as adenosine (Adenoscan) and regadenoson (Lexi-Scan) can be administered to mimic the effect of exercise. The most invasive of tests is cardiac catheterization. In this procedure, a catheter (thin tube) is inserted into an artery and guided into the coronary arteries. A dye, such as iodixanol (Visipaque) or iohexol (Omnipaque), is injected and images are taken to give clinicians a clear view of the coronary arteries to aid in diagnosis. If extensive coronary artery disease is discovered, this procedure can also be used therapeutically, allowing physicians to insert stents to open clogged arteries. It is also possible to combine the exercise tolerance test with the imaging techniques of a catheterization to directly observe the effect of exercise on the coronary arteries. See Medication Table 16-1 for more information on diagnostic agents (Medication Tables are located at the end of the chapter).

ALERT!

The dyes that are commonly used during cardiac catheterizations can lead to serious side effects, such as anaphylactic reactions, drug interactions, and kidney failure, especially among patients sensitive to iodine-containing agents.

PRACTICE POINT

When used for cardiac catheterization, adenosine is dosed as a 140-mcg/kg/min infusion over 6 minutes, while regadenoson is given as a single 0.4-mg dose via intravenous (IV) push.

Treatment

For patients who develop ischemic heart disease, the goal of treatment is to both relieve symptoms of angina and reduce the risk of future cardiac events. A number of medications, lifestyle modifications, and procedures can be used to reach these goals.

CASE?

G. S.'s doctor would like to investigate his symptoms further. What noninvasive test can be used to help differentiate true ischemic heart disease from other conditions with similar symptoms?

Lifestyle Modifications

Though some risk factors for the development of ischemic heart disease cannot be changed or avoided, such as male sex, family history, and genetics, there are a number of lifestyle modifications that can reduce the risk of cardiovascular events. Perhaps of the highest importance is the control of underlying conditions that increase cardiovascular risk, including hypertension and hyperlipidemia. Refer to Chapters 14 and 17, respectively, for discussions of these conditions and their treatment. Cigarette smoking is another important modifiable risk factor. Smoke exposure, both first and second hand, causes decreases in oxygen supply via vasoconstriction and increases in oxygen demand as the heart pumps against higher blood pressure. If a patient can quit smoking, cardiovascular risk falls significantly within 5 years of quitting.[2] Finally, obesity significantly increases cardiovascular risks. Clinicians frequently recommend calorie-restricted diets and physical activity to bring patients down to normal weight.

Beta Antagonists

The most commonly used agents in the treatment of ischemic heart disease are the beta antagonists (beta blockers), especially in patients who have more than one episode of chest pain per day. As discussed in Chapter 15, these medications block the ability of the catecholamines to cause increases in heart rate, contractility, and blood pressure. The resulting decreased oxygen demand helps restore oxygen balance, reducing the risk of angina attacks. In addition to decreasing the risk of developing angina, beta blockers have additional benefits in patients with coronary artery disease, such as blood pressure reduction, cutting the risk of heart attack, and protecting against arrhythmias.

Of the four subgroups of beta antagonists, the cardioselective agents are typically the drugs of choice in the treatment of angina. By selectively inhibiting the beta$_1$ receptor, side effects, such as sexual dysfunction, hyperglycemia, and bronchospasm that are common with nonselective agents, can be minimized. Though certain side effects are reduced, the cardioselective beta blockers still have a number of troublesome effects. Bradycardia, dizziness, hypotension, and decreased exercise tolerance are common reactions that warrant a slow titration of these medications. For a complete discussion of the various beta antagonists and their typical dosing, refer to Chapter 15.

Calcium Channel Blockers

Calcium channel blockers, also discussed in Chapter 15, can improve the symptoms of ischemic heart disease by both decreasing oxygen demand and increasing supply. The dihydropyridines (eg, amlodipine, nifedipine) act primarily on the vasculature, causing vasodilation that can improve coronary blood flow and allow the heart to pump against lower levels of systemic vascular resistance. The nondihydropyridines (eg, diltiazem, verapamil), on the other hand, target the heart and cause a reduction in contractility and heart rate. Like the beta blockers, normalizing the oxygen balance improves chest pain and reduces the likelihood of future episodes of angina. Unlike the beta blockers, however, the calcium channel blockers may not have as many additional cardiovascular benefits. For this reason, the beta blockers remain the first-line therapy in ischemic heart disease. For patients with contraindications to beta blocker therapy or those who develop significant side effects, however, calcium channel blockers are appropriate alternatives. One exception to this rule is in patients who experience angina that is related to vasospasm. Studies have shown that calcium channel blockers are among the most efficacious medications in the treatment of this form of angina and should be used as first-line therapy in these cases.

Clinicians choosing between the two types of calcium channel blockers must take individual patient characteristics into consideration. For patients with concurrent atrial fibrillation or rapid heart rates, the mechanism of action of the nondihydropyridines may give added benefits beyond regulation of oxygen balance. For those patients with slow heart rates or heart failure, the dihydropyridines may be better agents. Regardless of the agent chosen, side effects must be closely monitored, with the nondihydropyridines likely to cause constipation and bradycardia, the dihydropyridines causing tachycardia and edema, and both groups likely to cause hypotension and dizziness. Chapter 15 contains an in-depth review of the calcium channel blockers, including agent names, dosing, and interactions.

Nitrates

Nitric oxide is a substance produced by the body that causes vasodilation. This effect can be mimicked with the administration of nitrates, medications that are broken down into nitric oxide–like compounds that cause a direct vasodilation. In ischemic heart disease, the vasodilation throughout the body produced by nitrates decreases oxygen demand of the heart while increasing oxygen supply by dilating coronary arteries. Many of the adverse effects experienced by patients taking nitrates are directly related to their mechanism of action. Headache, orthostatic hypotension, and reflex tachycardia are the most common side effects. In addition to the setting of acute ischemic heart disease, nitrates can be used alone to treat infrequent, predictable angina or in addition to

beta blockers or calcium channel blockers to reduce the risk of future attacks.

For patients with acute chest pain, the most rapid-acting and widely used treatment is sublingual nitroglycerin (Nitro-Stat). Patients are typically instructed to place one nitroglycerin tablet (most often 0.4 mg) under the tongue at the onset of chest pain. Another dose may be administered every 5 minutes if the chest pain persists, up to a maximum of three tablets. Nearly 90% of patients with ischemic heart disease will have resolution of the acute symptoms with proper administration of nitroglycerin. If the symptoms are not relieved after two doses, the patient should seek immediate medical attention for the possibility of an acute coronary syndrome. In addition to the sublingual tablets, a number of other formulations of nitroglycerin are available. The lingual spray (Nitrolingual) is an alternative to the sublingual tablets in the treatment of acute angina attacks. It has a longer shelf life but higher cost. Intravenous (IV) nitroglycerin is available for use in a hospital setting.

PRACTICE POINT

Sublingual nitroglycerin tablets must be dispensed only in their original, amber glass container. They should be protected from light and heat to retain their effectiveness. Patients may need regular refill reminders, especially those with infrequent symptoms whose supply may go out of date before it is all used.

ALERT!

IV nitroglycerin interacts with many of the polyvinyl chloride (PVC) infusion sets routinely used in hospitals. Nonabsorbing tubing is available, and pharmacy technicians, as well as other personnel involved, must be aware that the dose administered through the nonabsorbing sets (5 mcg/min) is only 20% of that commonly given (25 mcg/min) if a regular PVC set is used. Be aware of your institution's supplies and policies.

A number of nitrate medications are available for prophylaxis of ischemic heart disease symptoms, with a goal of reducing the number of angina attacks that patients experience. Nitroglycerin is available in a transdermal patch formulation (Minitran, Nitro-Dur) that can be applied once daily. Nitroglycerin ointment (Nitro-Bid) and oral capsules (Nitro-Time) can also be used for long-term prophylaxis of angina but are rarely used due to difficulty of administration, sometimes requiring as many as four doses per day.

PRACTICE POINT

While the chest is the preferred application site for transdermal nitroglycerin patches, any area of clean, dry, hairless skin will suffice as long as it is not below the knee or elbow. Hair that interferes with patch placement may be trimmed with scissors but not shaved.

Isosorbide mononitrate (Monoket) and dinitrate (Isordil) are oral nitrate therapies that are used solely for prophylaxis. These agents are available in sustained-release formulations that have longer half-lives and require dosing only one to three times daily. Refer to Medication Table 16-2 for available products and dosage forms.

ALERT!

Combining nitrates with erectile dysfunction drugs like sildenafil (Viagra) can cause a profound drop in blood pressure. Because patients may be seeing more than one physician, it is especially important to be alert to the patient's medication history and profile when prescriptions are filled for medications in either of these classes (nitrates or erectile dysfunction drugs).

PRACTICE POINT

One important reminder for any patient on long-acting nitrate medications is the need for an 8–12-hour, nitrate-free interval. Without this interval, patients quickly develop a tolerance to the nitrate effect, losing all the benefit this type of therapy has to offer.

Other Treatments

A number of other important therapies are initiated in patients with ischemic heart disease that will be discussed in later sections of this chapter. Aspirin or clopidogrel are antiplatelet therapies that have been proven to reduce mortality and the risk of heart attack and stroke. If a patient has an elevated cholesterol level or is otherwise at high risk of heart attack or stroke, treatment with statin medications (discussed in Chapter 17) is indicated, and the angiotensin-converting enzyme (ACE) inhibitors (Chapter 15) are another class of medications with proven benefit for reducing mortality in patients with coronary artery disease.

CASE?

It is determined that G. S. is suffering from angina. Choose one possible pharmacological treatment and describe how it would help to relieve his symptoms.

For patients with advanced disease, physicians may decide to aggressively treat coronary artery disease with revascularization procedures to restore blood flow to an area of the heart with a blocked vessel. In percutaneous coronary intervention (PCI), a stent (small tube) is inserted into blocked arteries. Coronary artery bypass grafting (CABG) is the attachment of arteries from the patient's arms or legs to the heart to allow blood to flow around blockages.

ACUTE CORONARY SYNDROMES

For patients with ischemic heart disease, symptoms of angina are the result of chronic changes in oxygen supply and demand. When these changes are acute in nature, the risks are much greater, warranting a diagnosis of acute coronary syndrome. For the past 100 years, this life-threatening cardiovascular emergency has claimed more lives than any other heart disease in the United States.[3]

CASE STUDY

V. O. is a 76-year-old female brought to the emergency department by emergency medical services. She experienced sudden, severe chest pain that radiated to her neck and left arm. Her husband called 911 immediately.

Pathophysiology

As seen in ischemic heart disease, the most important risk factor for the development of acute coronary syndrome is underlying coronary artery disease. When associated with acute coronary syndromes, symptoms of angina are not due to progressive changes in blood vessels but to an acute event known as a plaque rupture. This occurs when an unstable atherosclerotic plaque is damaged and breaks open. The body sees the ruptured plaque as an area of damage and attempts to form a blood clot at the site. Unfortunately, this attempt to remedy the situation only makes conditions worse. The clot that is formed ultimately causes either partial or complete blockage of the coronary artery, quickly diminishing blood flow to the heart. With the oxygen supply severely reduced or completely cut off, heart cells in the area begin to die. At this stage of cell death, a patient is said to be having a heart attack, or myocardial infarction, and typically experiences sudden, crushing chest pain, diaphoresis, nausea, and shortness of breath. Other patients, however, may be susceptible to a *silent* (without severe pain) myocardial infarction. This particularly dangerous form of heart attack, seen commonly in patients with diabetes and nerve disorders, may cause a patient to delay seeking medical attention until it is too late.

Diagnosis

Acute coronary syndromes can be classified into three groups, depending on the extent of damage to the heart and the types of changes seen on an EKG. The mildest form is known as unstable angina in which cell death is minimal and most likely due to temporary interruptions in blood flow. Unstable angina differs from the chest pain seen in ischemic heart disease, often called stable angina, in that it occurs at rest, is more severe, has an uncharacteristic duration, or is not relieved with nitrate therapy. EKG strips of patients with unstable angina typically will not reveal any evidence of changes in the electrical conduction of the heart.

The second classification of acute coronary syndrome is called a non-ST-segment-elevation myocardial infarction, or NSTEMI. In these patients, coronary blood flow is obstructed to a degree that causes considerable cell death to occur. These effects are evident when clinicians obtain levels of troponin, an enzyme that is leaked from dying heart cells. However, because the area of damage seen in an NSTEMI does not traverse the entire thickness of the heart, EKGs obtained in these patients do not show an elevation in the ST segment of the tracing, a sign of cell death across the entire organ wall.

The most-deadly form of acute coronary syndrome is known as an ST-segment-elevation myocardial infarction, or STEMI. When the damage caused by an occluded coronary artery is severe enough to kill heart cells across the entire chamber wall, the electrical conduction is affected. This type of myocardial infarction gets its name from the characteristic changes in the EKG reading of the heart's electrical activity, a rise in the ST segment of the tracing. In addition to these EKG changes, patients will also have high levels of troponins leaking from damaged cardiac cells. When both of these telltale signs are present, clinicians must work quickly to restore blood flow to the heart and minimize the long-term effects of ischemia.

CASE?

Upon her arrival to the emergency department, V. O.'s blood sample has high levels of troponin and her EKG shows evidence of abnormal conduction. What type of acute coronary syndrome is V. O. likely having?

Early Treatment of Acute Coronary Syndromes

The first goal that must be reached in patients suffering from an acute coronary syndrome is to return blood flow to the area of the heart being damaged by ischemia. The earlier the revascularization, the less likely the patient will develop lasting consequences of a myocardial infarction, such as arrhythmias and congestive heart failure. Both pharmacological and nonpharmacological treatments play important roles in restoring oxygen supply to an area of infarction.

Nonpharmacological Treatment

It has been established that the best way to restore circulation to occluded (blocked) vessels is to perform PCI or CABG. PCI is usually the preferred therapy for patients with coronary artery disease that is less extensive and contained to areas that can be reopened with stents. CABG, on the other hand, is reserved for the most severe cases of coronary artery disease, as the procedure is much more invasive and carries higher risks.

Glycoprotein IIB/IIIA Inhibitors

In both STEMI and NSTEMI patients who undergo PCI revascularization, glycoprotein IIB/IIIA (GP IIB/IIIA) inhibitors are important medications that lower the risk of occlusion of stents and the need to have additional PCI procedures. Agents in this class of medications, including abciximab (ReoPro), eptifibatide (Integrilin), and tirofiban (Aggrastat), are administered intravenously and bind to a receptor that is responsible for platelet adhesion, or the ability of platelets to stick together. With the function of platelets reduced, patients are less likely to develop blood clots that re-occlude stented vessels. Because they decrease platelet function, the major side effect of these agents is unwanted bleeding, especially when they are combined with other agents that interfere with platelet function or the body's ability to form clots. If a patient has received fibrinolytic therapy (medication to dissolve blood clots, described next), has active bleeding, or has low numbers of platelets, these agents should be avoided. Dosing of GP IIB/IIIA inhibitors is based on a patient's weight. See Medication Table 16-3 for dosing and adjustment information.

Fibrinolytics

In some areas, access to life-saving PCI and CABG is limited. In these cases, patients with STEMI may receive fibrinolytic therapy to help restore blood supply to the heart. These IV agents, including alteplase (Activase), reteplase (Retavase), and tenecteplase (TNKase), bind to fibrin, an important component of blood clots. Once bound, the fibrinolytics begin to break down the clot and open the occluded coronary artery. Because of their mechanism of action, the fibrinolytics will dissolve clots throughout the body, not only those present in coronary arteries. For this reason, these agents should not be used in patients with active bleeding, a history of hemorrhagic stroke, extremely high blood pressure (higher than 180/110 mm Hg), or recent internal bleeding, among other contraindications. Finally, the use of fibrinolytics is also controversial in patients older than 75 years of age. Some studies suggest that patients treated may have higher mortality rates when compared to those who did not receive these agents. The dosing regimens for fibrinolytic therapies are complex and are listed in Medication Table 16-3.

ALERT!

Because the effectiveness of fibrinolytics decreases as time elapses after the onset of a cardiovascular event, it is important that therapy be initiated as soon as possible. When used to treat stroke, the window is only 3 hours from the onset of symptoms. Many emergency departments stock a fibrinolytic for ready use upon admission of a patient with suspected stroke or acute coronary syndrome.

Unfractionated and Low Molecular Weight Heparins

Unfractionated heparin and the low molecular weight heparins, enoxaparin (Lovenox) and dalteparin (Fragmin), are important anticoagulant medications that are typically administered in the early stages of an acute coronary syndrome. Unlike GP IIB/IIIA inhibitors, aspirin, and clopidogrel, which work on platelet function, these anticoagulants interfere with the body's clotting cascade to inhibit clot formation. For a full discussion of their mechanism of action and dosing, refer to Chapter 27. Regardless of whether the patient has suffered a STEMI or NSTEMI, undergoing PCI or fibrinolytic therapy, heparins are typically administered for the first 24–48 hours of hospitalization to decrease the risk of additional clot formation. Like other agents that affect the body's ability to form blood clots, these agents must be used cautiously in patients who have active bleeding, are taking other medications that interfere with the body's clotting ability, or have a high risk of developing a bleed.

CASE?

V. O. is taken to a community hospital emergency department that does not have the facilities to perform revascularization procedures, but she has a history of hemorrhagic stroke. Should she receive fibrinolytic therapy? Why or why not?

Other Treatments

In addition to these important early treatments for STEMI and NSTEMI, a number of other supportive measures are also initiated. For some patients with oxygen saturation less than 90%, intranasal oxygen should be started. Nitroglycerin and morphine can be used together to control chest pain. Other therapies that are often started in the early treatment phase of an acute coronary syndrome, such as aspirin, beta blockers, and clopidogrel, are continued into the long-term treatment phase and are discussed below.

Long-term Treatment of Acute Coronary Syndromes

Once a patient is stabilized and revascularization is complete, the clinician's primary focus is shifted to avoiding future cardiovascular events and preventing ventricular remodeling, or the stiffening of the chamber wall at the site of ischemia. A number of pharmacological agents have proven benefits for reducing mortality when used in the aftermath of a myocardial infarction and are typically initiated before a patient's discharge from the hospital.

Beta Antagonists

Beta antagonists are typically initiated via the IV route in the early phase of treatment and later switched to an oral formulation and continued indefinitely. After a myocardial infarction, beta blockers have a proven survival benefit, reduce the risk of having a second event, and prevent ventricular remodeling. Their antihypertensive effects also help to control another important cardiovascular risk factor, elevated blood pressure. Similar to the agents chosen to treat ischemic heart disease, the cardioselective beta antagonists are the most commonly used subgroup. Clinicians must carefully monitor the side effects of hypotension and bradycardia as they can induce additional ischemic events or stoke. To avoid these issues, the beta blockers are initiated at lower doses and slowly increased toward target levels.

Aspirin

Aspirin is another agent that is typically initiated in the early stages of an acute coronary syndrome, regardless of the type of event. The primary benefit of this agent is platelet inhibition. Within 10 minutes of administration, aspirin irreversibly binds to cyclooxygenase-1 (COX1), the enzyme responsible for the production of thromboxane A2, an important factor in platelet aggregation and adhesion. It is also theorized that aspirin's anti-inflammatory effects may play a role in risk reduction. With platelet function diminished and the immune system tempered, the risk of forming additional clots, occluding a stent, and having future cardiovascular events is reduced. Like other antiplatelet therapies, the major side effect of aspirin therapy is a risk of bleeding, particularly of the gastrointestinal tract. To help reduce this risk, the lowest effective dose of aspirin is used. In the early phase of treatment, an initial 162-mg dose is administered followed by 81 mg daily, thereafter.

Platelet Aggregation Inhibitors

Another type of antiplatelet therapy that may be considered in acute coronary syndrome are the platelet aggregation inhibitors. These agents (clopidogrel, prasugrel, and ticagrelor) inhibit platelet function by binding to receptors that normally play a role in platelet aggregation. For patients who have undergone PCI with stenting, they can help to prevent stent occlusion. Depending on the type of stent inserted, patients may be treated with platelet aggregation inhibitors daily for several months up to an indefinite period of time. Clopidogrel is also used as an alternative to aspirin in patients with contraindications to its use. Because of bleeding risk, clopidogrel and prasugrel are not administered to patients who may require CABG. If CABG is needed in patients who have received this medication, a 5-day wash-out period must pass before the procedure can be performed. (This appears to be less of an issue with ticagrelor.) When these agents are used in combination with aspirin, bleeding risk is increased. To reduce this risk, only low-dose aspirin (100 mg or less) is usually used in combination with platelet aggregation inhibitors.

CASE?

After being transported to another institution for revascularization, V. O. is being discharged on clopidogrel and aspirin. What is an appropriate dose of aspirin for this patient?

Angiotensin-Converting Enzyme Inhibitors and Angiotensin II Receptor Blockers

In the first 24 hours following a myocardial infarction, treatment with an oral angiotensin-converting enzyme (ACE) inhibitor is usually started and continued indefinitely. Many studies have shown improved survival and reduced re-infarctions when these agents are initiated in the early phase of treatment. The body releases angiotensin II and aldosterone after ischemic events in an attempt to maintain appropriate blood pressure. In the long term, however, these substances are actually harmful to the heart, increasing the rate and degree of cardiac remodeling. An ACE inhibitor can reduce the levels of these substances. If a patient exhibits symptoms of heart failure, which are discussed below, ACE inhibitor therapy has been shown to be even more beneficial. For patients with contraindications or side effects while on ACE inhibitor therapy, angiotensin II receptor blockers (ARBs) may be a good alternative option. The common side effects of ACE inhibitor and ARB therapy include elevations of potassium levels, decreases in kidney function, and low blood pressure. For a complete discussion of ACE inhibitor and ARB medications, refer to Chapter 15.

Statins

The statins are a group of medications used to reduce cholesterol levels in the blood. As described above, high levels of cholesterol increase a patient's risk of developing atherosclerotic plaques and coronary artery disease. Statin therapy can reduce cholesterol levels significantly and, in turn, reduce the risk of cardiovascular disease. In patients with existing coronary artery disease or a myocardial infarction, it is theorized that statins have additional benefits, called pleiotropic effects, that go beyond their cholesterol-lowering effects. One hypothesis is that statins help to stabilize plaques,

making unstable plaques less likely to rupture and cause future myocardial infarctions. The anti-inflammatory effects of statins may decrease cardiovascular risks, as well. For a full discussion of statins and other lipid-lowering medications, see Chapter 17.

HEART FAILURE

One of the most devastating long-term consequences of an acute coronary syndrome is known as heart failure. When a significant area of the heart becomes ischemic and dies off, its pumping ability can be reduced. When the heart can no longer pump blood at a rate sufficient to meet the oxygen demands of the body, a diagnosis of heart failure is made.

CASE STUDY

B. R. is a 52-year-old male with a history of myocardial infarction. Ever since his acute coronary syndrome incident, B. R. has been excessively tired performing tasks that were previously easy for him. He has also noticed that it is difficult to put on his shoes due to swelling in his legs. His physician fears he has developed heart failure.

Pathophysiology

In a normally functioning heart, the amount of blood ejected during each heartbeat, called the stroke volume, is determined by three factors: preload, afterload, and contractility. Preload is defined as the amount of blood in the ventricle before the contraction begins. As more blood is forced into the ventricle, the preload increases and allows for a greater stroke volume. This effect, however, only improves stroke volume to a point. Beyond it, additional fluid in the ventricle is no longer beneficial. Afterload is described as the forces that impede the ejection of blood out of the ventricle. These include systemic vascular resistance and the physical shape of the ventricle wall. As afterload increases, it becomes more difficult for the heart to pump blood, decreasing the stroke volume. Finally, contractility is defined simply as the ability of the heart's cells to cause a contraction. If myocardial cells are replaced by scar tissue after an event such as a myocardial infarction, contractility and, as a result, stroke volume are decreased.

To upset the natural balance among the three factors that make up stroke volume, one or more inciting events must take place. As discussed earlier in the chapter, the most common of these events is an acute coronary syndrome; however, other causes of heart failure include longstanding hypertension, heart valve diseases, arrhythmias, fluid overload, or certain medications. After one of these events initially reduces stroke volume, the body attempts to compensate. Increased levels of aldosterone and vasopressin cause retention of sodium and water. The additional fluid in the vasculature allows for extra blood to fill the ventricle, increasing preload. As a result of declines in stroke volume, blood pressure is also reduced. In an effort to maintain tissue perfusion, the body activates the renin-angiotensin-aldosterone system and the autonomic nervous system, resulting in vasoconstriction, increased blood pressure, and increases in afterload. Finally, the increased workload on the heart and the numerous hormones released in an attempt to compensate cause changes to the heart tissue called ventricular hypertrophy, or a thickening of the ventricular walls.

Taken as a whole, these compensatory changes help the heart maintain adequate circulation in the short term, all while leading to heart failure in the future. To review, decreased stroke volume and blood pressure lead to the release of a number of hormones that temporarily improve stroke volume and tissue perfusion. To truly compensate, however, these hormones must increase systemic vascular resistance and afterload, making it harder for the heart to eject blood. These conditions cause remodeling that further reduces stroke volume and restarts the cycle.

The types of symptoms a patient experiences depend largely on what areas of the heart are damaged. If the left side of the heart is affected, decreases in cardiac output cause a backing up of blood into the lungs. In these patients, many of the resulting symptoms are lung-related, including wheezing, cough, pulmonary edema, and tachypnea, or rapid breathing. When the right side of the heart is damaged, blood backs up into the systemic circulation and patients suffer from symptoms such as lower leg edema, bloating, cold extremities, and liver damage. All patients with heart failure, regardless of the side of the heart affected, can expect to have symptoms of fatigue, weakness, fluid overload, and decreased quality of life due to decreased cardiac output.

CASE?

If B. R.'s symptoms are primarily lower-leg edema and cold extremities, what side of the heart is likely compromised?

Treatment of Chronic Heart Failure

The goals of treating heart failure include relief of symptoms and improving quality of life in the short term, but focus on improving survival and slowing progression of the disease in the long term. To accomplish these goals, treatment focuses on halting and reversing the harmful compensatory mechanisms. Medications and lifestyle changes are started that reduce preload to near-normal levels, decrease afterload, and disrupt the barrage of harmful hormones and proteins that eventually worsen the condition.

Nonpharmacological Treatment

The body's normal response to decreased stroke volume is to retain sodium and water. This harmful response to heart failure is made even worse if a patient consumes large quantities of salt in the diet. Most experts recommend a sodium restriction to less than 2 g each day. This lifestyle modification can significantly decrease the risk of heart failure exacerbations and reduce the doses of medicines needed to control the disease. It is also important for heart failure patients to remain active. Though overexertion can worsen heart function, mild to moderate exercise has been proven to be an important piece of many treatment regimens. Finally, clinicians focus heavily on improving patient adherence to the medication regimen. It has been shown that nonadherence is the most common cause of hospitalization for heart failure exacerbation. Educating patients about pillboxes, simplifying drug regimens, and reducing other barriers to adherence are of utmost importance.

PRACTICE POINT

One teaspoon of table salt contains more than the 2 g daily allowance in the sodium-restricted diet described above.

Beta Antagonists

In the past, the beta antagonists were a class of medications avoided in patients with heart failure. It was not until a number of recent trials showed a significant improvement in patient mortality and decreases in hospitalizations for heart failure that these agents became routinely used components of heart failure treatment regimens. It is theorized that the benefit of beta blockers lies in their ability to stop the effects of catecholamines on the heart, decrease oxygen demand, or stop ventricular remodeling.

Because of their tendency to reduce contractility and cause heart failure symptoms, however, these agents are only started in patients with stable heart failure and at very low doses. Dose increases are performed in 2-week intervals and monitored closely. If a patient experiences worsening heart failure, the dose is immediately reduced to previously tolerated levels and only increased after another 2-week interval has passed.

PRACTICE POINT

It is important to note that not all beta blockers are approved for use in heart failure. To date, three beta blockers have proven benefit. These are bisoprolol (Zebeta), carvedilol (Coreg), and metoprolol succinate (Toprol XL).

Angiotensin-Converting Enzyme Inhibitors and Angiotensin Receptor Blockers

The ACE inhibitors are considered the cornerstone of heart failure treatment. By inhibiting the renin-angiotensin-aldosterone system, these medications have numerous benefits. Preload is reduced when aldosterone release is inhibited, afterload is decreased when angiotensin II production declines, and ventricular remodeling can be halted or reversed. Studies have shown that the ACE inhibitors not only reduce the risk of heart failure exacerbations, but they also improve survival. For those patients who develop a cough due to ACE inhibitor exposure, the ARBs can be substituted. Though they are not as well studied as the ACE inhibitors, these medications do have some evidence to support their use. The ARB valsartan may be used in combination with sacubitril, a neprilysin inhibitor, to further reduce the risk of death in patients with heart failure (Medication Table 16-4).

Hydralazine and Isosorbide Dinitrate

Before renin-angiotensin-aldosterone system–mediating medications were widely available, another combination of vasodilators was commonly used to treat heart failure. Studies predating the ACE inhibitors and ARBs shed light on the favorable effects of the combination of hydralazine (Apresoline) and isosorbide dinitrate (Isordil) on both mortality and hospitalizations due to worsening heart failure. Hydralazine is a potent direct arterial vasodilator that reduces afterload, while the isosorbide dilates veins and reduces preload. Today, ACE inhibitors and ARBs are first- and second-line agents with considerably better efficacy and safety evidence. However, for some populations, especially African Americans, the combination of hydralazine and isosorbide dinitrate can still be an important treatment option. Though both agents are available generically, a name brand combination tablet (BiDil) is available combining 37.5 mg of hydralazine and 20 mg of isosorbide dinitrate, dosed one to two tablets three times daily. Despite their efficacy in select patients, side effects still limit the overall use of this combination. Headaches, rebound tachycardia, and the potential to cause drug-induced lupus require close monitoring.

Aldosterone Antagonists

Another group of medications that have proven risk reduction and mortality benefits is the aldosterone antagonists. Though these agents fall under the class of potassium-sparing diuretics, it is their antialdosterone effects that are responsible for their benefit in heart failure. As described in Chapter 14, aldosterone causes retention of water and sodium, increasing preload initially, but worsening symptoms of pulmonary and lower-extremity edema in the long term. Aldosterone may also have a direct effect on heart tissue, increasing the rate of ventricular remodeling. Spironolactone (Aldactone) has been studied extensively in heart failure and shows the greatest benefit in patients with severe heart failure. Eplerenone (Inspra) is an alternative in male patients who experience spironolactone-induced gynecomastia (painful breast enlargement).

Diuretics

Accumulating fluid and edema are a constant concern for heart failure patients. To help treat these symptoms, patients are usually prescribed a diuretic. Though these medications have no mortality benefit, they are used to improve quality of life. Thiazide diuretics are considered too weak to adequately control edema related to heart failure. For this reason, loop diuretics, including bumetanide (Bumex), furosemide (Lasix), and torsemide (Demadex) are the drugs of choice. Close attention must be paid to ensure proper dosing, as over-diuresis may be harmful. Clinicians often instruct patients to use their body weight as a guide for diuretic dosing, increasing the dose if weight increases and vice versa.

Digoxin

Digoxin (Lanoxin) comes from a class of medications known as the cardiac glycosides. In the past, it was theorized that the main benefit of adding this medication was a positive inotropic effect, meaning an increase in contractility. Today, it is thought that low doses of digoxin actually improve heart failure symptoms by blocking a number of the harmful proteins and hormones that cause ventricular remodeling. This agent is available in two doses, 0.125 mg and 0.25 mg, is available generically, and is dosed once daily. Over the years, a number of conflicting studies caused debate about whether digoxin should be used in heart failure, at all. The evidence suggests that digoxin may reduce heart failure symptoms and the risk for hospitalization, but it does not improve survival. Experts generally agree that the lack of a mortality benefit and serious side effects such as nausea, dizziness, bradycardia, or other arrhythmias make this drug difficult to use. What was once a first-line therapy for heart failure has now become the last-line agent, only used when all other treatments are maximized and a patient is still having exacerbations.

PRACTICE POINT

A blood test can be performed to monitor digoxin levels. If a patient overdoses, a dose of IV digoxin antibodies, digoxin immune fab (Digibind), can be given to neutralize the drug and reduce the concentration to nontoxic levels. Digoxin antibodies are dosed based on the amount of digoxin ingested or a measurement of the amount of digoxin in the blood.

Treatment of Acute Exacerbations of Heart Failure

When heart failure symptoms become suddenly worse, a patient is said to be having an exacerbation. The usual cause of an exacerbation is nonadherence to lifestyle changes or medications, but it may also be caused by progression of the underlying disease. The end result is usually worsening edema, decreased profusion, and hospitalization. The following agents are used to help bring these worsening symptoms under control.

Diuretics

To help reduce pulmonary and lower-extremity edema, high doses of diuretics are started upon hospital admission. IV loop diuretic therapy is usually initiated. If the loop diuretic is not sufficient on its own to improve symptoms, a thiazide-like diuretic, such as metolazone, can be

added for a synergistic effect. When the acute exacerbation has resolved, the patient can be returned to oral loop diuretics.

ALERT!

When drugs are dosed on the basis of mg/kg/min or mcg/kg/min, care must be taken to be sure that patient weights expressed in pounds are converted to their kg equivalent and that infusion rates in mL/hr have been adjusted for the factor of 60 minutes per hour.

Positive Inotropes

The positive inotropes are medications that increase heart contractility. These agents are used temporarily to boost stroke volume until the exacerbation can be controlled. One mechanism by which this action is accomplished is by activation of cardiac beta$_1$ receptors. Dobutamine, an IV synthetic catecholamine, is the most commonly used beta$_1$ agonist in the treatment of acute exacerbations of heart failure. This agent is relatively selective for the beta$_1$ receptors, leading to minimal side effects through alpha$_1$ and beta$_2$ activation. Doses are typically started at 2.5–5 mcg/kg/min and slowly increased to a maximum of 20 mcg/kg/min.

PRACTICE POINT

Long-term, beta blocker use may decrease the effectiveness of dobutamine and some patients may require higher than normal doses.

Another mechanism by which contractility is increased is inhibition of an enzyme called phosphodiesterase III (PDE3). Under normal conditions, this enzyme plays a role in regulating calcium concentration in heart cells. When it is inhibited, calcium levels rise and contractility is increased. The effect, however, is not limited to cardiac tissue. PDE3 inhibition in the vasculature causes vasodilation and reductions in preload and afterload, effects that contribute to improved stroke volume. Milrinone is the most commonly used PDE3 inhibitor. It is dosed intravenously at a rate of 0.5 mcg/kg/min but must be adjusted if patients have renal failure. Because it does not act on beta receptors, patients on beta blocker therapy will not have a reduction in effect, but side effects such as hypotension, arrhythmias, and headache are still a possibility.

Regardless of which positive inotrope is chosen, two important factors must be considered. With long-term use, both of these medications, and others with similar mechanisms of action, cause an increase in mortality. They must be used for the shortest time possible, and, when they are discontinued, it must be done carefully to avoid a return of heart failure symptoms. The doses must be slowly decreased to ensure the patient can tolerate their withdrawal.

Vasodilators

In acutely ill heart failure patients, fluid retention causes large increases in preload and afterload. Clinicians use potent IV vasodilators to return these factors to normal levels. They are categorized by their predominant effect: arterial or venous vasodilation.

Nitroglycerin in its IV formulation is an important heart failure treatment. It acts primarily on the venous side of the vasculature, with only minimal dilation of arteries. Preload reductions with a subsequent improvement in pulmonary edema are its main benefit. Doses of 0.5–3 mcg/kg/min are administered via continuous infusion, starting at the lower end of the range and titrated upward to effect and tolerability. The most commonly reported side effects in this setting are headache and hypotension due to excessive vasodilation. As seen when it is used in ischemic heart disease, tolerance to these effects may develop when nitroglycerin is used for extended periods.

Nitroprusside (Nitropress) is a mixed vasodilator, affecting both the arterial and venous systems. It causes dilation by increasing production of nitric oxide, one of the body's natural vasodilators. The result is a decrease in both preload and afterload. Doses of 0.5–3 mcg/kg/min are administered as continuous infusions starting at lower doses that are increased every 5–10 minutes. Beside the expected side effects of hypotension, dizziness, and headache, nitroprusside has a unique adverse event: cyanide and thiocyanate toxicity. High levels of cyanide affect the body's ability to transport oxygen, leading to confusion, weakness, and syncope (feeling faint or passing out). Though this effect is rare at typical doses, patients with kidney failure are at higher risk.

ARRHYTHMIAS

When damage is done to the electrical system of the heart, the potential for arrhythmias, or abnormal heartbeats, increases. Though ischemia is only one cause among many, including longstanding hypertension, heart failure, certain medications, and structural defects of the heart, it is one of the most common. The consequences of these abnormal heartbeats are as varied as the number of arrhythmias possible, ranging from asymptomatic to life threatening, and the treatments are just as numerous.

CASE STUDY

T. B. is a 46-year-old female having a routine checkup with her family physician. She does not have any worrisome symptoms at this time; however, the nurse notices an irregular pulse when checking her heart rate. The physician orders an EKG to help diagnose T. B.'s arrhythmia.

Review of Normal Conduction

As described in Chapter 14, a normal heartbeat originates from the sinoatrial (SA) node, located near the right atrium. This group of cells, often called the heart's pacemaker, has leaky membranes that allow electrolytes to cross freely, causing depolarization and the start of a contraction. The depolarization spreads outward from the SA node, leading to contraction of the atria. When the depolarization reaches the junction between the atria and ventricles, another important group of cells, called the atrioventricular (AV) node, allow the depolarization to cross over into the lower half of the heart. To ensure the ventricles contract from the bottom up, the depolarization travels from the AV node down the left and right bundle branches to the Purkinje fibers at the bottom of the heart. From there, the depolarization can move upward, allowing efficient contractions of the ventricles. When the cycle is complete, the leaky cells of the SA node are ready to depolarize once more and start another contraction.

When the heart undergoes normal depolarization, the EKG tracing will have a predictable pattern for each beat of the heart, going from a small P wave to a large QRS complex and finishing with a T wave, as shown in Figure 16-1. The small P wave is a representation of the depolarization and contraction of the atria. The large QRS complex corresponds to the electrical charge moving toward the AV node and passing into the ventricles, causing ventricular contraction. Finally, as the ventricles repolarize after contraction, the T wave appears on the EKG tracing. Figure 16-2 illustrates a *normal sinus rhythm,* which would be expected in a patient without heart abnormalities. Figure 16-3 shows the ST segment *elevation* (raised above the baseline), which alerts physicians to a STEMI acute coronary syndrome.

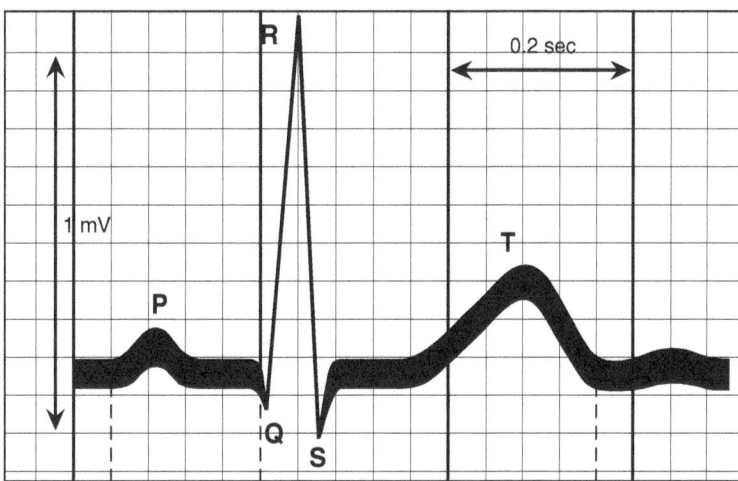

FIGURE 16-1. When the heart undergoes normal depolarization, the EKG tracing will have a predictable pattern for each beat of the heart, going from a small P wave to a large QRS complex and finishing with a T wave. The small P wave is a representation of the depolarization and contraction of the atria. The large QRS complex corresponds to the electrical charge moving toward the AV node and passing into the ventricles, causing ventricular contraction. Finally, as the ventricles repolarize after contraction, the T wave appears on the EKG tracing.

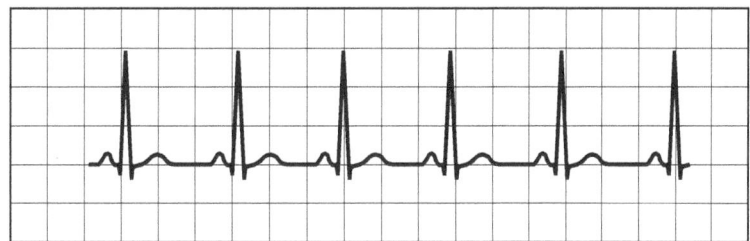

FIGURE 16-2. Illustrates a normal sinus rhythm, which would be expected in a patient without heart abnormalities.

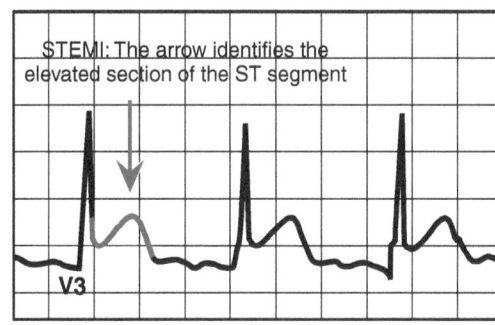

FIGURE 16-3. Shows the ST segment elevation (raised above the baseline), which alerts physicians to a STEMI acute coronary syndrome.

Selected Arrhythmias

Overall, the various arrhythmias that have the potential to occur can be divided into two groups. The first are those caused when cells outside of the SA node take over as the pacemaker of the heart. The second type of arrhythmia begins when a pathway is opened up to allow the wave of depolarization to travel along an abnormal route. The most common types of arrhythmias are discussed below.

Atrial Fibrillation

Atrial fibrillation is characterized by rapidly beating atria. It is thought that this abnormal heartbeat occurs when an extra pathway opens to allow depolarization to reenter the atria and restart an unneeded contraction. If this dysfunction occurs, the atria will contract at a rate of 400–600 beats per minute, well above the normal rate of 60–100 beats per minute. Though this is extremely fast, many patients have no symptoms and can be in atrial fibrillation for years before a clinician discovers it. The lack of symptoms is due to regulation by the AV node, the gateway to the ventricles. When it is functioning properly, the AV node will not allow all of the

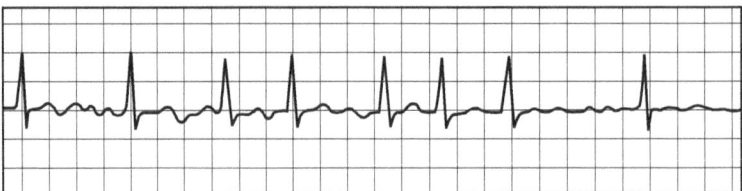

FIGURE 16-4. An example of an EKG tracing of atrial fibrillation.

400–600 depolarizations to be transmitted to the lower half of the heart. If this ability is lost, however, patients will often begin to complain of "skipped heartbeats" or palpitations. When clinicians listen to the patient's heart with a stethoscope, they will discover an *irregularly irregular heartbeat* as the atria and ventricles beat out of sync.

EKG tracings performed on patients with atrial fibrillation will display one major difference when compared to a normal EKG. In these cases, the typical P wave is replaced with many jagged, erratic waves or no P wave, at all. For an example of an EKG tracing of atrial fibrillation, see Figure 16-4.

CASE?

The EKG performed on T. B. reveals atrial fibrillation. Why has T. B. felt no symptoms?

The consequences of atrial fibrillation can vary greatly. Some patients may have the condition for many years and not develop serious complications. In other cases, however, the outcome may be the onset of heart failure, atrial enlargement, or, the most worrisome result, a stroke. When the atria beat at a very high rate, blood cannot be pumped effectively. If it is allowed to pool, clots will begin to form in the atrium. A dislodged blood clot may travel to the brain and cause a stroke, an event that happens in 5% to 7% of atrial fibrillation patients each year.[4] To reduce this risk, these patients are often started on warfarin (Coumadin), dabigatran (Pradaxa), rivaroxaban (Xarelto), apixaban (Eliquis), or edoxaban (Savaysa). These medications interfere with the production of important clotting factors, inhibiting the formation of a clot. For a full discussion of these agents and the clotting cascade, refer to Chapters 26 and 27.

Ventricular Tachycardia and Fibrillation

Often the result of ischemic damage to the heart after an acute coronary syndrome, ventricular tachycardia and fibrillation are very dangerous rhythms with dire consequences.

Ventricular tachycardia is defined as heartbeats originating in the ventricle that occur at a rate faster than 100 beats per minute. When large areas of the heart die, the electrical system can become badly damaged. This leads to the formation of reentry pathways in the ventricles that allow depolarization to occur chaotically along abnormal routes. The result is a rapidly beating ventricle, unguided by the timely depolarization of the SA node. In contrast to atrial fibrillation, fast heart rates in the ventricle are considered life threatening, as blood cannot be pumped to the body effectively.

If it is allowed to progress, ventricular tachycardia may lead to ventricular fibrillation, or complete disarray of the electrical system of the heart. This lethal condition is the cause of death in 50% of myocardial infarctions. When the ventricle is in fibrillation, no coherent heartbeats occur, only minor quivering of the chamber. Unless it is rapidly treated, all blood flow stops and the risk of death is extremely high.

EKG tracings of ventricular tachycardia and fibrillation lose all resemblance to the normal EKG tracing discussed above, due to the extreme disarray of the electrical system of the heart. In ventricular tachycardia, the disorganized, rapid contraction of the ventricles appears as a series of repetitive narrow or wide spikes, completely lacking P waves, QRS complexes, or T waves. If this condition progresses to ventricular fibrillation, this repetitive pattern is lost to a chaotic, jagged tracing that mirrors the quivering of the fibrillating ventricle. See Figures 16-5 and 16-6 for examples of ventricular tachycardia and fibrillation tracings.

Torsades de Pointes

Torsades de pointes is translated to mean *twisting of the points,* a description of what this arrhythmia looks like on an EKG (as seen in Figure 16-7). Like ventricular fibrillation, torsades de pointes is a life-threatening abnormal heartbeat. It arises during the phase of rest after each depolarization, called the refractory period, when electrical conduction is limited. In normally functioning hearts, this resting phase is in place to help avoid having a new contraction begin before the heart has fully recovered from the previous one. After this period is over, repolarization is complete and the heart

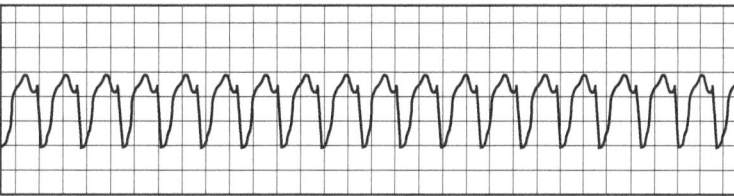

FIGURE 16-5. An example of ventricular tachycardia tracing.

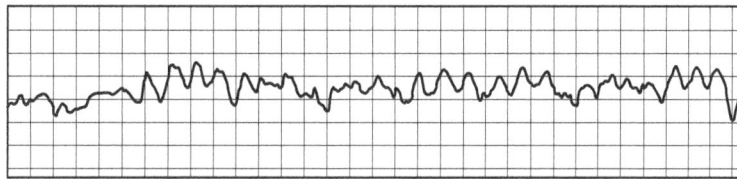

FIGURE 16-6. An example of ventricular fibrillation tracing.

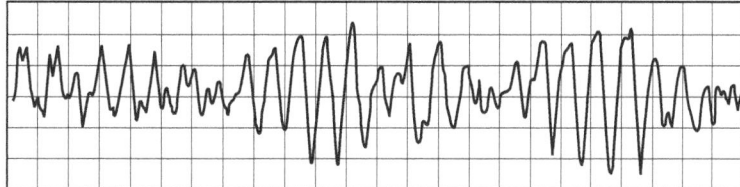

FIGURE 16-7. Torsades de pointes.

cells are ready for another contraction. Certain medical conditions, electrolyte imbalances, genetic defects, or medications can delay repolarization. This weakens the ability of the myocardial cells in the refractory period to ward off early contractions. If a new wave of depolarization happens during this weakened refractory period, the patient can develop torsades. Clinicians monitor the chance for developing torsades by examining the section of an EKG called the QT interval. If this segment of the tracing is prolonged, there is an increased risk of developing this life-threatening arrhythmia. Much like ventricular fibrillation, torsades causes an ineffective heartbeat, leading to impaired circulation of blood. If left untreated, death is a very common result. For a list of the common medications that can cause or contribute to torsades, see Table 16-1.

Bradyarrhythmias

In addition to rapid heart rates, arrhythmias can also come in the form of abnormally slow heartbeats. Called bradyarrhythmias, these slowed rhythms come in many types and range from the common sinus bradycardia, a slow heartbeat seen in athletes, to troubling AV blocks and escape rhythms.

AV block is the result of a malfunctioning AV node. Though the atria contract normally, the wave of depolarization occasionally is not transmitted past the AV node, meaning the ventricles miss a beat. In its mildest form, no treatment is necessary, but symptoms can develop as the dropped beats become more frequent.

Escape rhythms are the heart's way of replacing a damaged pacemaker. If the SA node is unable to perform its functions, the responsibility of initiating each heartbeat falls to the surrounding atrial tissue. When this happens, however, the heart rate is slightly slower. If the atrial tissue is also damaged, the responsibility falls to the AV node and the resting heart rate is even slower. If even the AV node cannot fulfill the duties of the pacemaker, the ventricular tissue itself can depolarize spontaneously, though the rate is as low as 30 beats per minute.

Treatment

The treatment of the various arrhythmias has changed significantly in recent years, as most clinicians move away from antiarrhythmic drugs that have troublesome side effects

TABLE 16-1. Selected Medications That May Cause Torsades de Pointes

Antiarrhythmics
Amiodarone
Disopyramide
Dofetilide
Ibutilide
Procainamide
Sotalol

Antibiotics
Clarithromycin
Erythromycin
Moxifloxacin
Sulfamethoxazole-trimethoprim

Antipsychotics
Haloperidol
Quetiapine
Ziprasidone

Opiates
Methadone

Tricyclic Antidepressants
Amitriptyline
Imipramine

toward nonpharmacological treatments. In addition to a wealth of new surgical and mechanical interventions, the incidence of new arrhythmias has been declining, thanks to rapid treatment of acute coronary syndromes and other precipitating events.

Nonpharmacological Treatment

Depending on the arrhythmia, clinicians can choose among a wide variety of nonpharmacological interventions. When acute arrhythmias threaten a patient's life, the treatment of choice is often direct current cardioversion, using electrical current to reset the heart's conduction system. As made famous by numerous medical dramas, patients are sedated, paddles are placed on the chest, and electrical current is applied to the heart. For patients suffering from severe bradyarrhythmias, pacemakers have become popular treatment options. These small devices, implanted into the pectoral (chest) area, are attached to electrodes embedded into the cardiac tissue. Sophisticated software can sense the patient's heartbeat and take over if the physiologic electrical system can no longer perform its duties. Similar to pacemakers, implantable automatic cardioverter-defibrillators (ICDs)

can be used in patients at risk of developing sudden cardiac death. Like the paddles used in acute treatment of arrhythmias, these devices can sense the onset of ventricular tachycardia or fibrillation and deliver an electrical shock to return the heart to a normal rhythm. Finally, ablation is a surgical procedure used to destroy abnormal conduction pathways that can be sources of arrhythmias. Using a special EKG, the exact location of the abnormal circuit can be discovered and destroyed using radio waves.

Type I Antiarrhythmics

The medications used to treat arrhythmias are divided into four general classes, depending on the electrolyte channels they affect. The type I agents primarily slow the transport of sodium into cardiac cells. Type II agents, the beta blockers, do not directly affect any electrolyte channels but reduce arrhythmic potential by blocking the effect of catecholamines on the SA and AV nodes. Type III agents block the influx of potassium into heart cells, and Type IV agents slow calcium transport.

The type I antiarrhythmic agents are further divided into three subgroups. The type Ia agents include quinidine, procainamide, and disopyramide (Norpace), and all are available generically. In addition to slowing the transport of sodium into cardiac cells, the type Ia agents also prolong the refractory period. As discussed with torsades de pointes, delaying this segment of the depolarization cycle actually increases the risk of developing arrhythmias. In addition to increasing the risk of the very condition they are attempting to treat, low success rates in the treatment of both ventricular and atrial arrhythmias limit the use of these agents significantly. Each agent in this class has unique side effects. Quinidine is notorious for causing severe gastrointestinal complaints, including vomiting, diarrhea, and abdominal cramping. Procainamide has been implicated as a cause of systemic lupus erythematosus, a serious immune disorder that can damage the skin, joints, kidneys, or other organs (see Chapter 14). Disopyramide causes dry mouth, blurry vision, constipation, and urinary retention, as it blocks cholinergic receptors.

PRACTICE POINT

Though procainamide itself is not entirely eliminated by the kidney, it is metabolized to an active compound that can accumulate if the kidneys are not functioning properly. It must be used with caution in patients with renal failure.

The Type Ib agents include generic lidocaine (Xylocaine) and mexiletine (Mexitil) and cause a shortening of the refractory period while slowing sodium influx. These agents are used in the treatment of ventricular arrhythmias. Though it works well, IV lidocaine is limited to the treatment of ventricular arrhythmias in the hospital setting; there is no oral or injectable product suitable for outpatient use. Mexiletine, on the other hand, is available in a tablet formulation but is rarely used due to severe gastrointestinal side effects and poor efficacy.

Type Ic agents slow sodium transport into cardiac cells dramatically and have no impact on the refractory period. These agents, including flecainide and propafenone (Rythmol), are available as oral tablets and can be used to treat both atrial and ventricular arrhythmias. Though the refractory period is not shortened, their potent blockade of sodium transport causes an increased risk of arrhythmias via other mechanisms. Both of the type Ic agents are negative inotropes, meaning they decrease the contractility of the heart. For this reason, this subgroup of antiarrhythmic agents cannot be used in patients with heart failure.

Type II Antiarrhythmics

The type II antiarrhythmic agents are the beta antagonists. In addition to their other therapeutic actions; the beta antagonists can reduce the risk of developing both ventricular and atrial arrhythmias. In the ventricles, these medications block the potentially proarrhythmic (arrhythmia promoting) effects of catecholamines. In atrial arrhythmias, they block the AV node, decreasing the risk of transmitting unwanted contractions to the ventricles. For a full discussion of beta blockers, see Chapter 15.

Type III Antiarrhythmics

Though the use of most antiarrhythmics is limited by either severe side effects or an increased risk of developing arrhythmias, the type III agents are some of the most commonly used treatments. Medications in this subgroup, including amiodarone (Pacerone), dofetilide (Tikosyn), dronedarone (Multaq), ibutilide (Corvert), and sotalol (Betapace), act primarily by slowing the transport of potassium into cardiac cells, though some agents in the class have additional effects.

Amiodarone is available in an injectable dosage form as well as generic oral tablets and is one of the most effective treatments for ventricular and atrial arrhythmias. It has a mixed mechanism of action that borrows from many different classes of antiarrhythmics. The largest drawback with this agent is its numerous side effects. Patients can develop such varying reactions as dizziness, confusion, thyroid problems, eye problems, liver toxicity, bradycardia, or pulmonary fibrosis, a severe and sometimes fatal condition. Clinicians must carefully monitor all patients receiving amiodarone for the many potential side effects. In an effort to discover a safer drug with amiodarone's efficacy, dronedarone was developed. It does lack many of the side effects of amiodarone but may increase mortality in patients with heart failure and is significantly less effective.

CASE?

T. B. has been started on a regimen of amiodarone for her atrial fibrillation. What types of side effects might be expected?

Sotalol's mechanism of action includes both type II and type III properties. This injection or generic oral medication can be used to treat many arrhythmias, but its main use is in atrial fibrillation. Because of its beta blocker effects, patients must be monitored for low blood pressure, bradycardia, and other side effects of that class of medications. Perhaps more concerning, however, is the chance of prolonging the QT interval of the EKG and causing torsades de pointes. The risk is even higher if patients have kidney failure as this can lead to sotalol accumulation.

Dofetilide and ibutilide, oral and IV medications, respectively, are type III antiarrhythmic agents used to convert atrial fibrillation to a normal heart rhythm. Ibutilide and dofetilide are available as generic options. With either agent, clinicians must monitor patients' electrolyte levels closely. If potassium or magnesium levels are low, there is a significant risk for developing torsades de pointes. To avoid this side effect, many experts recommend pretreating all patients with potassium and magnesium supplementation.

Type IV Antiarrhythmics

Calcium channel blockers, discussed at length as antihypertensives in Chapter 15, make up the type IV antiarrhythmic agents. In atrial fibrillation, these agents block the AV node, similar to the beta blockers. They may also play a role in decreasing the risk of developing ventricular arrhythmias caused by increased exertion or catecholamine release. In general, the nondihydropyridines are the agents of choice to treat arrhythmias, as they are more selective for the cardiac tissue. (See Medication Table 16-5.)

SHOCK

At its most basic level, shock is defined as a state of abnormal cellular metabolism. It is a condition where the body cannot provide the materials necessary to keep cells alive and functioning normally. The causes of shock are numerous, spanning a number of body systems and dysfunctions, but all have one issue in common: regardless of its cause, once shock sets in, mortality rates are extremely high and a return to baseline function is very difficult to achieve. In fact, shock is often described as the end stage of all disease states, the ultimate cause of death in nearly every illness.

CASE STUDY

J. S. is a 39-year-old male who has suffered a massive myocardial infarction. He is currently in the intensive care unit because his blood pressure is dropping, his heart rate is elevated, and it appears his cardiac output is not high enough to circulate blood around his body. The cardiologist is concerned that J. S. may be developing shock.

Pathophysiology

When cells are deprived of oxygen or glucose, abnormal routes of metabolism must be used to supply energy. If these states are temporary, very little damage is done and cells can resume their usual function after resolution of the deficiency. Under other circumstances, however, oxygen and glucose may be depleted for extended periods of time. The result is an accumulation of the toxic byproducts of abnormal metabolism. When released into the bloodstream, the toxins cause damage that further impedes the normal delivery of oxygen and glucose to the cells. As neighboring cells are affected and the damage spreads, entire organs begin to shut down and, eventually, the body, as a whole, ceases to function.

Types of Shock

Shock is the root cause of death in many disease states, and the types of shock are numerous. When shock is due to a loss of fluid from the bloodstream, a patient is said to have hypovolemic shock. This condition may arise from a lack of adequate water ingestion, excessive sweating, vomiting,

or diarrhea. A subtype of hypovolemic shock is known as hemorrhagic shock. In these cases, shock sets in due to loss of blood. If the body cannot keep enough volume in its blood vessels, the heart cannot circulate the blood through the vasculature and oxygen cannot be delivered to the tissues.

Severe infections can also cause a patient to develop shock. When the immune system is fighting a foreign invader, the response may be so strong that surrounding tissues become damaged along with the bacteria. To make matters worse, some bacteria can release toxins of their own to damage blood vessels and hasten the onset of septic shock. Yet another immune system–related cause of shock is severe allergic reactions. These patients are said to develop anaphylactic shock, when an outside trigger causes a vigorous immune response that damages the vasculature. In both cases, vascular damage leads to leaky blood vessels and impaired circulation, interfering with oxygen and nutrient delivery.

Other common causes of shock are the result of direct damage to the heart or central nervous system. Cardiogenic shock may be one consequence of severe ischemia after a myocardial infarction. If large areas of the heart are dead, cardiac output can drop to the point where it cannot provide sufficient blood flow to the rest of the body. Traumatic brain injuries lead to a neurogenic shock, where the nervous system can no longer maintain vasoconstriction. When widespread vasodilation occurs, blood pressure can drop so far that tissue perfusion suffers.

Treatment

Regardless of the cause of shock, treatment focuses on restoring blood pressure to appropriate levels. One strategy for raising blood pressure is to administer fluids to the patient. This is typically the first treatment initiated and can lower mortality significantly if started early. Next, clinicians may choose to administer vasopressors, drugs that cause constriction of the blood vessels to raise blood pressure.

CASE?

From what type of shock is J. S. likely suffering?

Fluids

IV 0.9% sodium chloride, also known as normal saline, solution, lactated Ringer's, or 5% dextrose solutions are collectively called the crystalloids. These fluids are usually the agents of choice to restore vascular volume because studies show they are as effective as other treatments but cause fewer side effects and are less costly. In some cases, clinicians turn to fluids called colloids, such as 5% albumin, hetastarch, or dextran. In theory, these solutions, which contain larger molecules than those found in crystalloids, should remain in the vasculature for longer periods of time before diffusing out into the tissues. In practice, however, studies comparing the crystalloids and colloids do not show a significant difference in survival, despite their theoretical advantages and higher cost.

CASE?

What are the theoretical benefits of using colloid fluids to treat J. S.'s shock?

Vasopressors

The most common intravenously administered vasopressors used to treat shock include dopamine, dobutamine, norepinephrine (Levophed), epinephrine (Adrenalin), and phenylephrine, all of which activate the receptors of the autonomic nervous system to cause vasoconstriction, increases in contractility, and increases in stroke volume. The use of vasopressors to increase blood pressure in patients experiencing shock requires close monitoring and careful dose titrations. A balance must be obtained that allows for extra vasoconstriction that supports blood pressure but not excessive constriction that cuts off blood supply entirely. This becomes especially difficult, as extremely high doses of these agents are often required to counteract the symptoms of shock. If patients are stabilized on a vasopressor regimen, care must also be exercised when trying to discontinue these medications. Abrupt withdrawal often results in sudden deterioration of symptoms, so patients are typically weaned off of vasopressors very slowly (see Medication Table 16-6).

ADVANCED CARDIOVASCULAR LIFE SUPPORT MEDICATIONS

When the heart stops, circulation is no longer maintained and cells begin to die throughout the body. If nothing is done to maintain cardiovascular activity, the patient's situation will deteriorate to the point where life cannot continue. Stopping this series of events is known as life support. Basic life support (BLS) consists mainly of cardiopulmonary resuscitation (CPR) techniques and is the mainstay of rescue for patients whose hearts have stopped for whatever reason.[5] CPR is a skill that can be acquired even by people with no other healthcare education; it is widely taught in schools and community settings, as well as in hospitals and healthcare organizations, and it has been shown to be of value when applied in cardiac arrest. The sooner the patient receives CPR, the more likely recovery becomes.

In hospitals and among emergency response personnel, the use of medications and other techniques to augment the BLS activities is termed advanced cardiac life support (ACLS). It involves advanced assessment and monitoring techniques (such as the EKG), placement of airway and IV access devices, and administration of medications. When performed in a hospital setting, it is often called a *code* (or some variation, such as *code blue*) and the personnel responding (physicians, nurses, pharmacists, respiratory therapists) make use of a specialized kit of medications and devices often termed a *crash cart* or *code cart*, that is maintained in readiness to enable a quick response to a potentially fatal patient condition.

Most of the medications kept in the crash cart and used in ACLS have been described in this or other chapters. Administration is generally via the IV route, although if a patient's condition makes placement of an IV line difficult they are sometimes given via the endotracheal route (via a tube placed through the throat and into the tracheal entrance to the lung) or even intraosseously (injected into a bone, usually in the lower leg).

Medications most likely to be used in ACLS include vasopressors (drugs to increase blood pressure), including epinephrine and vasopressin; drugs to control heart rate (adenosine, atropine); and various antiarrhythmics (especially amiodarone, beta antagonists, diltiazem, and lidocaine). Additionally, most code kits or crash carts will include electrolytes such as calcium chloride and magnesium sulfate, along with concentrated (50%) dextrose injection. Because they must be immediately available, these medications are frequently packaged in single-use syringes with specialized needles.

Not every life-threatening emergency originates as a cardiac problem, so crash carts frequently carry medications to treat anaphylaxis (allergic reactions) or medication (particularly narcotic or sedative) overdose, which can also result in fatalities, sometimes by respiratory depression.

Epinephrine, antihistamines, corticosteroids, and inhaled beta-adrenergic agents (such as albuterol) have a place in anaphylactic emergencies. Doses of naloxone (Narcan) and flumazenil can sometimes reverse the effects of narcotics and benzodiazepines, respectively. A list of medications typically kept in an emergency kit or cart can be found in Medication Table 16-7.

Most healthcare organizations have many crash carts ready and placed in various strategic locations so that there is always one close by when an emergency occurs. While maintenance of defibrillators and other equipment and supplies on these carts may vary from one institution to another, maintaining the supply and integrity of the medications is uniformly the responsibility of the pharmacy department. Special packaging, correct (and varied) doses, and even medication placement (so personnel in an emergency situation don't have to be searching for what the patient needs) are vital, and technicians generally stock and restock these supplies, which are checked by the pharmacist before being sealed in a cart certified for use in emergencies.

PRACTICE POINT

Because crash carts and their contents are placed throughout the building and are used with varying (but irregular) frequency, ensuring that all items are in date is an important task. Carts are generally assigned a beyond-use date that corresponds to the earliest expiration date of any medication contained within it. Pharmacy technicians are frequently given a regular (weekly or monthly) assignment of checking the dates on all the carts on the premises and returning any at or near their beyond-use dates to the pharmacy for restocking.

SUMMARY

When the function of the heart is compromised, the consequences are far-reaching and life-threatening. The coronary arteries and the electrical systems of the heart are especially vulnerable to various dysfunctions. The root cause of many of these heart diseases is atherosclerosis. Atherosclerotic plaques can reduce blood flow to the heart, causing damage to the muscle and reducing its ability to function. When oxygen supply is reduced chronically over time, patients develop ischemic heart disease and suffer from chest pain. If the drop in oxygen supply is sudden, patients may experience acute coronary syndromes, an emergent situation that requires immediate attention to restore blood flow and minimize permanent damage to the myocardium. When a significant area of the heart is damaged, however, cardiac output can be reduced or damage can be done to the electrical system of the heart. These circumstances may lead to heart failure and arrhythmias, respectively. In the worst of cases, patients may lose the ability to maintain adequate blood pressure for tissue perfusion, culminating in multiorgan failure and shock. Though numerous treatment strategies exist to help reduce the damage caused by these various heart diseases, prevention remains the best way to ensure a healthy cardiovascular system.

REFERENCES

1. Roth GA, Abate D, Abate KH, et al. Global, regional, and national age-sex-specific mortality for 282 causes of death in 195 countries and territories, 1980–2017: A systematic analysis for the Global Burden of Disease Study 2017. *Lancet.* 2018;392:1736–1788.

2. Duncan MS, Freiberg MS, Greevy RA, et al. Association of smoking cessation with subsequent risk of cardiovascular disease. *JAMA.* 2019;322(7):642–650.

3. American Heart Association. *Heart Disease and Stroke Statistics—2019 At-a-Glance.* Dallas, TX: American Heart Association; 2019.

4. Oladiran O, Nwosu I. Stroke risk stratification in atrial fibrillation: A review of common risk factors. *J Community Hosp Intern Med Perspect.* 2019;9(2):113–120.

5. Panchal AR, Berg KM, Hirsch KG, et al. 2019 American Heart Association focused update on advanced cardiovascular life support: Use of advanced airways, vasopressors, and extracorporeal cardiopulmonary resuscitation during cardiac arrest: An update to the American Heart Association guidelines for cardiopulmonary resuscitation and emergency cardiovascular care. *Circulation.* 2019;140:e881-e894.

6. Lexi-Drugs. Lexicomp. Hudson, OH. http://online.lexi.com. Accessed July 5, 2021.

CHAPTER RESOURCES

Barrett KE, Barman SM, Brooks HL, et al. *Ganong's Review of Medical Physiology*. 26th ed. New York, NY: McGraw-Hill; 2019.

DiPiro JT, Yee GC, Posey M, et al. *Pharmacotherapy: A Pathophysiological Approach*. 11th ed. New York, NY: McGraw-Hill; 2020.

REVIEW QUESTIONS

1. Define ischemic heart disease and angina.

2. Explain the three types of acute coronary syndrome.

3. List the three factors that make up stroke volume.

4. Define heart failure.

5. Why are vasopressors usually tapered off slowly rather than being stopped immediately once a patient stabilizes?

MEDICATION TABLES

MEDICATION TABLE 16-1. Diagnostic Agents[6],[a]

CLASS Generic Name (pronunciation)	Brand Name	Route	Forms	Dose	Notes
Contrast Agents					
IOHEXOL (EYE OH HEX OLE)	OMNIPAQUE	VARIES	SOLUTION	VARIES	
IOPAMIDOL (EYE OH PA MI DOLE)	ISOVUE	VARIES	SOLUTION	VARIES	
Coronary Vasodilators					
Adenosine (a DEN oh seen)	Adenocard	IV	Solution	140 mcg/kg/min	
Regadenoson (re ga DEN oh son)	Lexiscan	IV	Solution	0.4 mg as a single dose	

[a]Pronunciations have been adapted with permission from USP Dictionary of USAN and International Drug Names (USP Dictionary) © 2022.

MEDICATION TABLE 16-2. Treatment of Ischemic Heart Disease[6],[a]

CLASS Generic Name (pronunciation)	Brand Name	Route	Forms	Dose	Notes
Cardioselective Beta Blockers					
Atenolol (a TEN oh lole)	Tenormin	Oral	Tablet	50–100 mg once to twice daily	
Bisoprolol (bis OH proe lol)	Zebeta	Oral	Tablet	5–10 mg once daily	
Metoprolol tartrate (me toe PROE lole)	Lopressor	Oral	Tablet	50–200 mg twice daily	
Metoprolol succinate (me toe PROE lole)	Toprol XL	Oral	Tablet	100–400 mg once daily	
Dihydropyridine Calcium Channel Blockers					
Amlodipine (am LOE di peen)	Norvasc	Oral	Tablet	5–10 mg once daily	Especially useful in patients experiencing angina due to vasospasms
Felodipine (fe LOE di peen)		Oral	Tablet	5–10 mg daily	
Isradipine (iz RA di peen)		Oral	Capsule	5–10 mg twice daily	
Nicardipine (nye KAR de peen)	Cardene	Oral, IV	Capsule, solution	20 mg 3 times daily	
Nifedipine (nye FED i peen)	Procardia XL	Oral	Tablet	30–180 mg once daily	

Continued next page

MEDICATION TABLE 16-2. Treatment of Ischemic Heart Disease[6,a] *(Continued)*

CLASS Generic Name (pronunciation)	Brand Name	Route	Forms	Dose	Notes
Mixed Alpha and Beta Blockers					
Carvedilol (KAR ve dil ol)	Coreg	Oral	Tablet	12.5–50 mg twice daily	
Labetalol (la BET a lole)	Normodyne, Trandate	Oral	Tablet	100–400 mg twice daily	
Nitrates					
Isosorbide dinitrate (eye soe SOR bide dye NYE trate)	Dilatrate SR	Oral	Capsule	40 mg 2–3 times daily	An 8- to 12-hr nitrate-free interval is required to avoid developing a tolerance to these agents
	Isordil	Oral	Tablet	5–40 mg 4 times daily	
Isosorbide mononitrate (eye soe SOR bide mon oh NYE trate)	Generics	Oral	Tablet	5–20 mg twice daily	
		Oral	Tablet	30–240 mg once daily	
Nitroglycerin (nye troe GLI ser in)	Nitro-Time	Oral	Capsule	2.5–26 mg 2–4 times daily	Call 911 immediately if symptoms persist or worsen 5 minutes after 1st dose of nitroglycerin
	Nitro-Stat	Sublingual	Tablet	0.2–0.6 mg q 5 min for 3 doses	
	Nitrolingual	Sublingual	Spray	1–2 sprays q 3–5 min for 3 doses	
	Nitro-Bid	Topical	Ointment	Apply 0.5–2 inches 4 times daily	
	Minitran, Nitro-Dur	Topical	Patch	0.2–0.8 mg/hr patch applied daily	
	Generics	IV	Solution	5 mcg/hr (nonabsorbing set) or 25 mcg/hr (PVC set)	Used in the hospital setting
Nondihydropyridine Calcium Channel Blockers					
Diltiazem (dil TYE a zem)	Cardizem	Oral	Tablet	30–90 mg 4 times daily	Especially useful in patients experiencing angina due to vasospasms
	Cardizem CD, Cartia XT, Tiazac, others	Oral	Capsule	120–480 mg once daily	
	Cardizem LA	Oral	Tablet	120–360 mg once daily	
Verapamil (ver AP a mil)	Calan	Oral	Tablet	80–160 mg 3 times daily	
	Calan SR,	Oral	Tablet	180–480 mg 1–2 times daily	
		Oral	Tablet	180–480 mg at bedtime	

Continued next page

MEDICATION TABLE 16-2. Treatment of Ischemic Heart Disease[6,a] *(Continued)*

CLASS Generic Name (pronunciation)	Brand Name	Route	Forms	Dose	Notes
Nonselective Beta Blockers					
Nadolol (NAY doe lole)	Corgard	Oral	Tablet	40–240 mg once daily	
Propranolol (proe PAN the leen)	Inderal	Oral	Tablet	40–80 mg 2–4 times daily	
	InderalLA, InnoPran XL	Oral	Capsule	80–320 mg once daily	
Timolol (TYE moe lole)	Blocadren	Oral	Tablet	10–40 mg once daily	

[a]Pronunciations have been adapted with permission from USP Dictionary of USAN and International Drug Names (USP Dictionary) © 2022.

MEDICATION TABLE 16-3. Treatment of Acute Coronary Syndromes[6,a]

CLASS Generic Name (pronunciation)	Brand Name	Route	Forms	Dose	Notes
ACE Inhibitors					
Benazepril (ben AY ze pril)	Lotensin	Oral	Tablet	10–40 mg 1–2 times daily	Typically started 12 hr after acute coronary syndrome
Captopril (KAP toe pril)		Oral	Tablet	6.25–50 mg 3 times daily	
Enalapril (e NAL a pril)	Vasotec	Oral	Tablet	5–40 mg 1–2 times daily	
Fosinopril (foe SIN oh pril)		Oral	Tablet	10–40 mg once daily	
Lisinopril (lyse IN oh pril)	Prinivil, Zestril	Oral	Tablet	10–40 mg once daily	
Quinapril (KWIN a pril)	Accupril	Oral	Tablet	5–20 mg 1–2 times daily	
Ramipril (ra MI pril)	Altace	Oral	Capsule	2.5–10 mg 1–2 times daily	
Antiplatelet Agents					
Aspirin (AS pir in)	Ascriptin, Ecotrin, Halfprin, others	Oral	Tablet	162–325 mg × 1 then 75–100 mg daily	Combining antiplatelet agents significantly increases the risk of bleeding
Clopidogrel (kloh PID oh grel)	Plavix	Oral	Tablet	300–600 mg loading dose then 75 mg daily	

Continued next page

MEDICATION TABLE 16-3. Treatment of Acute Coronary Syndromes[6,a] *(Continued)*

CLASS Generic Name (pronunciation)	Brand Name	Route	Forms	Dose	Notes
Antiplatelet Agents					
Prasugrel (PRA soo grel)	Effient	Oral	Tablet	60 mg loading dose, then 10 mg daily	
Ticagrelor (tye KA grel or)	Brilinta	Oral	Tablet	180 mg loading dose, then 90 mg twice daily	
Angiotensin Receptor Blockers (ARBs)					
Candesartan (kan des AR tan)	Atacand	Oral	Tablet	8–32 mg daily	Used as an alternative to ACE inhibitors; typically started 12 hr after acute coronary syndrome
Irbesartan (ir be SAR tan)	Avapro	Oral	Tablet	150–300 mg once daily	
Losartan (loe SAR tan)	Cozaar	Oral	Tablet	50–100 mg 1–2 times daily	
Olmesartan (all mi SAR tan)	Benicar	Oral	Tablet	20–40 mg once daily	
Valsartan (val SAR tan)	Diovan	Oral	Tablet	40–160 mg 1–2 times daily	
Cardioselective Beta Blockers					
Atenolol (a TEN oh lole)	Tenormin	Oral	Tablet	50–100 mg 1–2 times daily	Started as IV therapy in the early phase of treatment, converted to oral therapy and continued indefinitely
Bisoprolol (bis OH proe lol)		Oral	Tablet	2.5–10 mg once daily	
Esmolol (ES moe lol)	Brevibloc	IV	Solution	500 mcg/kg × 1 then 50–150 mcg/kg/min	
Metoprolol tartrate (me toe PROE lole)	Lopressor	IV	Solution	5 mg q 2 min for 3 doses	
	Lopressor	Oral	Tablet	25–100 mg twice daily	
Metoprolol succinate (me toe PROE lole)	Toprol XL	Oral	Tablet	50–200 mg once daily	
Fibrinolytics					
Alteplase (AL te plase)	Activase	IV	Powder	Infusion based on patient weight; 15 mg IV bolus followed by infusion over 60–90 min	Fibrinolytics must be administered with aspirin and heparin
Reteplase (RE ta plase)	Retavase	IV	Powder	10 units followed by 10 units 30 min later	

Continued next page

MEDICATION TABLE 16-3. Treatment of Acute Coronary Syndromes[6,a] *(Continued)*

CLASS Generic Name (pronunciation)	Brand Name	Route	Forms	Dose	Notes
Fibrinolytics					
Tenecteplase (ten EK te plase)	TNKase	IV	Powder	Bolus based on patient weight <60 kg: 30 mg ≥60 to <70 kg: 35 mg ≥70 to <80 kg: 40 mg ≥80 to <90 kg: 45 mg ≥90 kg: 50 mg	
Glycoprotein IIB/IIIA Inhibitors					
Abciximab (ab SIK si mab)	ReoPro	IV	Solution	0.25 mg/kg × 1 then 0.125 mcg/kg/min	Doses of eptifibatide and tirofiban must be reduced in patients with kidney disease
Eptifibatide (ep ti FYE ba tide)	Integrilin	IV	Solution	180 mcg/kg × 1 then 2 mcg/kg/min	
Tirofiban (tye roe FYE ban)	Aggrastat	IV	Solution	UA/NSTEMI: 0.4 mcg/kg/min × 30 min then 0.1 mcg/kg/min STEMI: 25 mcg/kg × 1 then 0.15 mcg/kg/min	
Low Molecular Weight Heparins (LMWHS)					
Dalteparin (dal te PA rin)	Fragmin	SUBQ	Solution	120 International Units/kg q 12 hr	Avoid in patients with heparin-induced thrombocytopenia
Enoxaparin (ee nox a PA rin)	Lovenox	IV, SUBQ	Solution	1 mg/kg q 12 hr	
Mixed Alpha and Beta Blockers					
Carvedilol (KAR ve dil ol)	Coreg	Oral	Tablet	3.125–25 mg twice daily	Continued indefinitely; carvedilol has added benefit in heart failure
	Coreg CR	Oral	Capsule	10–80 mg once daily	
Labetalol (la BET a lole)		IV	Solution	20–80 mg q 10 min	
		Oral	Tablet	200–800 mg twice daily	
Nonselective Beta Blockers					
Nadolol (NAY doe lole)	Corgard	Oral	Tablet	40–120 mg once daily	Continued indefinitely
Propranolol (proe PRAN oh lole)	Inderal	Oral	Tablet	40–120 mg 2–3 times daily	
	Inderal LA, InnoPran XL	Oral	Capsule	80–320 mg once daily	
Timolol (TYE moe lole)		Oral	Tablet	10–40 mg once daily	

Continued next page

MEDICATION TABLE 16-3. Treatment of Acute Coronary Syndromes[6,a] *(Continued)*

CLASS Generic Name (pronunciation)	Brand Name	Route	Forms	Dose	Notes
Statins					
Atorvastatin (a TORE va sta tin)	Lipitor	Oral	Tablet	10–80 mg once daily	Pleiotropic effects may give added benefits in the setting of acute coronary syndrome beyond cholesterol lowering
Lovastatin (LOE va sta tin)	Mevacor	Oral	Tablet	20–80 mg once daily	
Pitavastatin (pit a va STAT in)	Livalo	Oral	Tablet	1–4 mg once daily	
Pravastatin (PRA va stat in)	Pravachol	Oral	Tablet	10–80 mg once daily	
Rosuvastatin (roe SOO va sta tin)	Crestor	Oral	Tablet	5–40 mg once daily	
Simvastatin (sim va STAT in)	Zocor	Oral	Tablet	20–80 mg once daily	
Unfractionated Heparin					
Heparin sodium (HEP a rin) (SOE dee um)		IV, SUBQ	Solution	50- to 100-unit bolus then 12 unit/kg/hr infusion	Dose is adjusted based on aPTT levels (see Chapter 26 for a full discussion)

ACE = angiotensin-converting enzyme; aPTT = activated partial thromboplastin time; IV = intravenous; SUBQ = subcutaneous.
[a]Pronunciations have been adapted with permission from USP Dictionary of USAN and International Drug Names (USP Dictionary) © 2022.

MEDICATION TABLE 16-4. Medications for Heart Failure[6,a]

CLASS Generic Name (pronunciation)	Brand Name	Route	Forms	Dose	Notes
ACE Inhibitors					
Benazepril (ben AY ze pril)	Lotensin	Oral	Tablet	20–40 mg daily; doses may be divided	Titrate slowly while monitoring kidney function and potassium levels
Captopril (KAP toe pril)	Capoten	Oral	Tablet	6.25–50 mg 3 times daily	
Enalapril (e NAL a pril)	Vasotec	Oral	Tablet	2.5–20 mg 1–2 times daily	
Fosinopril (foe SIN oh pril)	Monopril	Oral	Tablet	5–40 mg once daily	
Lisinopril (lyse IN oh pril)	Prinivil, Zestril	Oral	Tablet	2.5–40 mg once daily	

Continued next page

MEDICATION TABLE 16-4. Medications for Heart Failure[6,a] *(Continued)*

CLASS Generic Name (pronunciation)	Brand Name	Route	Forms	Dose	Notes
ACE Inhibitors					
Quinapril (KWIN a pril)	Accupril	Oral	Tablet	10–20 mg twice daily	
Ramipril (ra MI pril)	Altace	Oral	Capsule	1.25–10 mg once daily	
Trandolapril (tran DOLE a pril)	Mavik	Oral	Tablet	1–4 mg once daily	
Angiotensin Receptor Blockers (ARBs)					
Candesartan (kan des AR tan)	Atacand	Oral	Tablet	4–32 mg once daily	Useful in patients who have experienced an ACE inhibitor–induced cough
Irbesartan (ir be SAR tan)	Avapro	Oral	Tablet	150–300 mg once daily	
Losartan (loe SAR tan)	Cozaar	Oral	Tablet	25–100 mg 1–2 times daily	
Olmesartan (all mi SAR tan)	Benicar	Oral	Tablet	20–40 mg once daily	
Valsartan (val SAR tan)	Diovan	Oral	Tablet	40–160 mg twice daily	
Neprilysin Inhibitor/ARB					
Sacubitril/Valsartan (sak UE bi troll/val SAR tan)	Entresto	Oral	Tablet	24/26–97/103 mg twice daily	
Aldosterone Antagonists					
Eplerenone (e PLER en one)	Inspra	Oral	Tablet	25–50 mg once daily	For use in moderate to severe heart failure
Spironolactone (speer on oh LAK tone)	Aldactone	Oral	Tablet	12.5–50 mg once daily	
Cardiac Glycosides					
Digoxin (di JOX in)	Lanoxin	Oral	Tablet	0.125–0.250 mg once daily	Low doses usually sufficient
Cardioselective Beta Blockers					
Bisoprolol (bis OH proe lole)	Zebeta	Oral	Tablet	1.25–10 mg once daily	Should only be initiated in stable patients
Metoprolol succinate (me toe PROE lole)	Toprol XL	Oral	Tablet	12.5–200 mg once daily	

Continued next page

MEDICATION TABLE 16-4. Medications for Heart Failure[6,a] *(Continued)*

CLASS Generic Name (pronunciation)	Brand Name	Route	Forms	Dose	Notes
Loop Diuretics					
Bumetanide (byoo MET a nide)	Bumex	Oral	Tablet	0.5–5 mg 1–2 daily	IV formulations are used to bring acute exacerbations of heart failure under control; patients can be switched to the oral route once stabilized
		IV	Solution	0.5–1 mg 1–2 daily	
Ethacrynic acid (eth a KRIN ik)	Edecrin	Oral	Tablet	50–200 mg 1–2 times daily	
	Sodium Edecrin	IV	Solution	0.5–1 mg/kg × 1 dose	Reserved for patients with hypersensitivity to other loop diuretics
Furosemide (fyoor OH se mide)	Lasix	Oral	Tablet	20–80 mg twice daily	
		IV	Solution	20–200 mg 1–4 times daily	
Torsemide (TORE se mide)	Demadex	Oral	Tablet	5–10 mg once daily	
		IV	Solution	10–200 mg once daily	
Mixed Alpha and Beta Blockers					
Carvedilol (KAR ve dil ol)	Coreg	Oral	Tablet	3.125–50 mg twice daily	Should only be initiated in stable patients
	Coreg CR	Oral	Capsule	10–80 mg once daily	
Positive Inotropes					
Dobutamine (doe BYOO ta meen)		IV	Solution	2.5–20 mcg/kg/min titrated to effect	Use lowest dose for the shortest duration possible; causes increased mortality
Milrinone (MIL ri none)	Primacor	IV	Solution	0.375–0.75 mcg/kg/min	
Vasodilators					
Hydralazine/isosorbide dinitrate (hye DRAL a zeen) (eye soe SOR bide) (dye NYE trate)	Bidil	Oral	Tablet	37.5/20 mg 3 times daily	Monitor patients closely for signs of hypotension and headache
Nitroglycerin (nye troe GLI ser in)		IV	Solution	5–20 mcg/min titrated to effect	
Nitroprusside (nye troe PRUS ide)	Nitropress	IV	Solution	0.3–0.5 mcg/kg/min titrated to effect	

ACE = angiotensin-converting enzyme; IV = intravenous.
[a]Pronunciations have been adapted with permission from USP Dictionary of USAN and International Drug Names (USP Dictionary) © 2022.

MEDICATION TABLE 16-5. Antiarrhythmics[6,a]

CLASS Generic Name (pronunciation)	Brand Name	Route	Forms	Dose	Notes
Type IA					
Disopyramide (dye soe PEER a mide)	Norpace	Oral	Capsule	100 mg 4 times daily	Used in both atrial and ventricular arrhythmias
	Norpace CR	Oral	Capsule	200 mg twice daily	
Procainamide (proe kane A mide)		IV, IM	Solution	IV: 20 mg/min; IM: 0.5–1 g daily in divided doses	
Quinidine gluconate (KWIN i deen)		Oral	Tablet	324–927 mg 2–3 times daily	
Quinidine sulfate (KWIN i deen)		Oral	Tablet	100–600 mg 4–6 times daily	
Type IB					
Lidocaine (LYE doe kane)	Xylocaine	IV	Solution	1–1.5 mg/kg bolus then 0.5–0.75 mg/kg q 5–10 min	Used in ventricular arrhythmias only
Mexiletine (mex IL e teen)	Mexitil	Oral	Capsule	200–300 mg 3 times daily	
Type IC					
Flecainide (FLEK a nide)	Tambocor	Oral	Tablet	50–200 mg twice daily	Used in both atrial and ventricular arrhythmias
Propafenone (proe pa FEEN one)		Oral	Tablet	150–300 mg 3 times daily	
	Rythmol SR	Oral	Capsule	225–425 mg twice daily	
Type II					
Atenolol (a TEN oh lole)	Tenormin	Oral	Tablet	25–100 mg 1–2 times daily	Used to treat ventricular arrhythmias caused by exercise or catecholamines; also useful in blocking the AV node in atrial fibrillation
Bisoprolol (bis OH proe lol)	Zebeta	Oral	Tablet	2.5–10 mg once daily	
Carvedilol (KAR ve dil ol)	Coreg	Oral	Tablet	12.5–50 mg twice daily	
	Coreg CR	Oral	Capsule	20–80 mg once daily	
Labetalol (la BET a lole)	Normodyne, Trandate	Oral	Tablet	200–800 mg twice daily	
Metoprolol tartrate (me toe PROE lole)	Lopressor	Oral	Tablet	100–400 mg twice daily	
Metoprolol succinate (me TOE proe lole)	Toprol XL	Oral	Tablet	50–200 mg once daily	
Nadolol (NAY doe lole)	Corgard	Oral	Tablet	40–120 mg once daily	

Continued next page

MEDICATION TABLE 16-5. Antiarrhythmics[6,a] *(Continued)*

CLASS Generic Name (pronunciation)	Brand Name	Route	Forms	Dose	Notes
Type II					
Propranolol (proe PRAN oh lole)	Inderal	Oral	Tablet	160–480 mg twice daily	
	Inderal LA, InnoPran XL	Oral	Capsule	80–320 mg once daily	
Timolol (TYE moe lole)		Oral	Tablet	10–40 mg once daily	
Type III					
Amiodarone (a MEE oh da rone)	Nexterone, Pacerone	Oral	Tablet	Atrial fibrillation: 10 g load then 200–400 mg once daily; Ventricular arrhythmias: 800–1600 mg 1–2 times daily for 1 mo then 400 mg daily	Amiodarone and sotalol may be used in both atrial and ventricular arrhythmias; dronedarone is used in atrial fibrillation only; Ibutilide and dofetilide are used to convert atrial fibrillation to a normal heartbeat
		IV	Solution	1.2–1.8 g daily until 10 g is administered	
Dofetilide (doe FET il ide)	Tikosyn	Oral	Capsule	500 mcg twice daily	
Dronedarone (droe NE da rone)	Multaq	Oral	Tablet	400 mg twice daily	
Ibutilide (i BYOO ti lide)	Corvert	IV	Solution	1 mg over 10 min	
Sotalol (SOE ta lole)	Betapace	IV	Solution	75–150 mg twice daily	
	Betapace	Oral	Tablet	80–160 mg 2–3 times daily	
Type IV					
Amlodipine (am LOE di peen)	Norvasc	Oral	Tablet	2.5–10 mg once daily	Used to treat ventricular arrhythmias caused by exercise or catecholamines; also useful in blocking the AV node in atrial fibrillation
Diltiazem (dil TYE a zem)	Cardizem SR	Oral	Capsule	180–360 mg twice daily	
	Cardizem CD, Cartia XT, Tiazac, others	Oral	Capsule	120–480 mg once daily	
	Cardizem LA	Oral	Tablet	120–540 mg once daily	
Felodipine (fe LOE di peen)	Plendil	Oral	Tablet	5–20 mg once daily	

Continued next page

MEDICATION TABLE 16-5. Antiarrhythmics[6,a] *(Continued)*

CLASS Generic Name (pronunciation)	Brand Name	Route	Forms	Dose	Notes
Type IV					
Isradipine (iz RA di peen)	(Generics)	Oral	Capsule	5–10 mg twice daily	
Nicardipine (nye KAR de peen)	Cardene SR	Oral	Capsule	60–120 mg twice daily	
Nifedipine (nye FED i peen)	Adalat CC, Procardia XL	Oral	Tablet	30–90 mg once daily	
Verapamil (ver AP a mil)	Calan SR,	Oral	Tablet	180–480 mg 1–2 times daily	
		Oral	Tablet	180–420 mg at bedtime	
	Verelan PM	Oral	Capsule	100–400 mg at bedtime	

AV = atrioventricular; IM = intramuscular; IV = intravenous.
[a]Pronunciations have been adapted with permission from USP Dictionary of USAN and International Drug Names (USP Dictionary) © 2022.

MEDICATION TABLE 16-6. Agents Used in Shock[6,a]

CLASS Generic Name (pronunciation)	Brand Name	Route	Forms	Dose	Notes
Colloids					
5% albumin (al BYOO min)	Albuminar, AlbuRx, Plasbumin, others	IV	Solution	0.5–1 g/kg/dose q 15–30 min	Costly, but theoretically remain in the vasculature for long periods of time
Dextran (DEX tran)	LMD	IV	Solution	500–1000 mL at a rate of 20–40 mL/min	
Hetastarch (HET a starch)	Hextend, Hespan	IV	Solution	500–1000 mL at a rate of 20–40 mL/min	
Crystalloids					
Dextrose (DEX trose)		IV	Solution	500–1000 mL boluses repeated as needed	More affordable than colloids, but theoretically leave the vasculature sooner
Lactated Ringer's (LAK tate id RING ers)		IV	Solution	500–1000 mL boluses repeated as needed	
Sodium chloride (SOE dee um) (klor ide)		IV	Solution	500–1000 mL boluses repeated as needed	

Continued next page

MEDICATION TABLE 16-6. Agents Used in Shock[6,a] *(Continued)*

CLASS Generic Name (pronunciation)	Brand Name	Route	Forms	Dose	Notes
Vasopressors					
Dobutamine (doe BYOO ta meen)		IV	Solution	2.5–20 mcg/kg/min titrated to effect	Must be weaned carefully to avoid a drop in blood pressure
Dopamine (DOE pa meen)		IV	Solution	1–50 mcg/kg/min titrated to effect	
Epinephrine (ep i NEF rin)	Adrenalin	IV	Solution	1–10 mcg/min titrated to effect	
Norepinephrine (nor ep i NEF rin)	Levophed	IV	Solution	0.5–30 mcg/min titrated to effect	
Phenylephrine (fen il EF rin)		IV	Solution	0.1–0.5 mg q 10–15 min	

[a]Pronunciations have been adapted with permission from USP Dictionary of USAN and International Drug Names (USP Dictionary) © 2022.

MEDICATION TABLE 16-7. Typical Crash Cart Medication Contents[6,a]

Drug	Packaging	Strength	Quantity	Uses
Adenosine (a DEN oh seen)	2-mL vial	3 mg/mL	1	Enhances conduction
	4-mL syringe	3 mg/mL	2	Enhances conduction
Amiodarone (a MEE oh da rone)	3-mL vial	50 mg/mL	3	Arrhythmias
Atropine (a TROE peen)	10-mL syringe	0.1 mg/mL	5	Bradycardia, heart block
Calcium chloride (KAL see um) (klor ide)	10-mL syringe	100 mg/mL	1	Circulatory support
Dextrose (DEX trose)	50-mL syringe	50% (0.5 g/mL)	2	Hypoglycemia
Diphenhydramine (dye fen HYE dra meen)	1-mL vial	50 mg/mL	2	Antihistamine (for anaphylaxis)
Dopamine (doe pa MEEN)	250-mg infusion bag	400 mg/250 mL	1	Inotropic vasopressor
Epinephrine (ep i NEF rin)	10-mL syringe	1:10,000 (0.1 mg/mL)	8	Adrenergic stimulant
	30-mL syringe	1:1000 (1 mg/mL)	1	For endotracheal administration
Flumazenil (floo MAZ e nil)	5-mL vial	0.1 mg/mL	2	Benzodiazepine antidote

Continued next page

MEDICATION TABLE 16-7. Typical Crash Cart Medication Contents[6,a] *(Continued)*

Drug	Packaging	Strength	Quantity	Uses
Glucagon (GLOO ka gon)	Powder vial with diluent	1 mg	1	For hypoglycemia
Lidocaine (LYE doe kane)	5-mL syringe	2% (20 mg/mL)	2	Arrhythmias
	250-mg infusion bag	400 mg/mL	1	Arrhythmias
Magnesium sulfate (mag NEE zee um)	2-mL vial	50% (0.5 g/mL)	2	Seizures, arrhythmias
	100-mL infusion bag	10 mg/mL	1	Seizures, arrhythmias
Naloxone (nah LOX own)	1-mL syringe	0.4 mg/mL	4	Narcotic antidote
Norepinephrine (nor ep i NEF rin)	4-mL vial	1 mg/mL	1	Blood pressure
Sodium bicarbonate (SOE dee um) (bye KAR bon ate)	50-mL syringe	1 mEq/mL	2	Treats acidosis
Vasopressin (vas oh PRES in)	1-mL vial	20 units/mL	2	Shock
Verapamil (ver AP a mil)	2-mL vial	2.5 mg/mL	4	Arrhythmias

[a]Pronunciations have been adapted with permission from USP Dictionary of USAN and International Drug Names (USP Dictionary) © 2022.

Chapter 17

Hyperlipidemia

Mate M. Soric, PharmD, BCPS, FCCP

KEY TERMS AND DEFINITIONS

Atherosclerosis—a condition in which arteries have lost their elasticity (hardened) as a result of plaque deposits.

Atherosclerotic plaque—an accumulation of cholesterol and cells that can block the flow of blood through a vessel.

Bile acid sequestrants (BAS)—a class of hyperlipidemia agents that bind to bile acids in the gastrointestinal tract. To produce new bile acid, the liver removes cholesterol from the blood stream, lowering LDL.

Cholesterol—a lipid used in the production of hormones, bile salts, and cell membranes that contributes to atherosclerotic plaque formation when levels are high.

Chylomicrons—a very large lipoprotein that contains 90% triglycerides and 5% cholesterol.

High density lipoprotein (HDL)—the *good* cholesterol that contains 5% triglyceride, 25% cholesterol, and 50% protein.

Hyperlipidemia—elevated levels of one or more lipoproteins in the blood.

Lipids—molecules, including fats, cholesterols, steroids, and others, that are usually insoluble in water.

Lipoprotein—a spherical particle made up of hundreds of lipid and protein molecules.

DOI 10.37573/9781585286638.017

Low density lipoprotein (LDL)—the *bad* cholesterol that contains 6% triglyceride and 65% cholesterol. LDL is highly likely to cause atherosclerosis.

Triglyceride—a lipid that is the storage form of fatty acids, used as an energy source.

Very low density lipoprotein (VLDL)—a lipoprotein that contains 60% triglyceride and 12% cholesterol.

LEARNING OBJECTIVES

After completing this chapter, you should be able to

1. Define hyperlipidemia and recognize its causes, symptoms, and consequences.

2. Identify tests for hyperlipidemias and recognize the conditions under which they are done.

3. Distinguish between total cholesterol, LDL, HDL, VLDL, and triglycerides, know the meaning of each acronym, and recognize target values for each.

4. List nonpharmacologic treatments recommended for each type of hyperlipidemia.

5. List the classes of medications used in the treatment of hyperlipidemia and their basic mechanisms of action.

6. Identify agents and common side effects from each class of medications used to treat hyperlipidemias.

The term lipid is used to describe a wide variety of compounds in the human body. At desired concentrations, these molecules serve many important purposes. One type of lipid, known as a phospholipid, is responsible for making up the cell membranes of nearly every cell in the body, while others, called steroids, are versatile hormones that are integral parts of the reproductive, immune, renal, cardiovascular, and central nervous systems. Some lipids are essential nutrients, such as vitamins A, D, E, and K, that must be obtained from the diet because the body cannot create them on its own. But perhaps the most widely discussed and researched lipid is cholesterol. Like other lipids, cholesterol is vital to the function of the human body; however, more than 50% of American adults have hyperlipidemia or elevated (inappropriately high) levels of lipids in their bloodstreams. When levels rise, whether due to genetics or lifestyle, the chance of developing atherosclerotic plaques increases sharply,

along with the risk for cardiovascular diseases, stroke, and other health problems.

The types, synthesis, and functions of cholesterol are reviewed in this chapter, followed by an examination of the development of atherosclerotic plaques. Next, the techniques used to measure cholesterol levels in the blood and the classification of these results are discussed. Finally, the various treatments, both pharmacological and nonpharmacological, are explored.

CASE STUDY

J. H. is a 48-year-old male who has just had an annual checkup with his primary care physician. His past medical history includes a diagnosis of hypertension. He does not smoke and has no family history of heart disease, though he is overweight. Each year, a blood test has been performed to measure J. H.'s cholesterol. In the past, these levels have been acceptable, but today J. H. learns that his total cholesterol is measured as 285 mg/dL, his HDL is 45 mg/dL, and his triglycerides are 210 mg/dL. His physician has informed him that he has hyperlipidemia. J. H. has now arrived at the pharmacy with a prescription for simvastatin 40 mg at bedtime.

PATHOPHYSIOLOGY OF HYPERLIPIDEMIA

The Role of Cholesterol and Triglycerides in Homeostasis

As described above, there are many different types of lipids present in the body. Cholesterol and triglycerides are the two major lipids involved in the development of atherosclerotic plaques. Normally, cholesterol is an important component of cell membranes throughout the body. This rigid molecule provides a backbone and structure to an otherwise disorganized collection of phospholipids, the major component of the cell membrane. It is also an important ingredient in the formation of a number of hormones and the bile acids, compounds that help the body absorb fat from the gastrointestinal tract. Triglycerides, on the other hand, are the storage form of fatty acids in the bloodstream. They can be used as an energy source when the body's glucose is running low.

CASE?

J. H. is confused about where he got the cholesterol measured in his blood test. Describe the two main sources of cholesterol.

Cholesterol and triglycerides are obtained from two sources, those that the body creates and those that are consumed in the diet. The liver is the main source of production for both these lipids, though cholesterol can also be synthesized by nearly every cell in the body. For this reason, dietary sources are largely unnecessary, as the body can create enough of a supply to function. Whether they are synthesized or consumed, cholesterol and triglycerides must be transported throughout the body on molecules called lipoproteins. These small, spherical molecules travel around the body either delivering cholesterol to cells in need or returning excess cholesterol to the liver to be recycled. Lipoproteins are classified on the basis of their densities and are divided into four major classes: chylomicrons, very low density lipoprotein (VLDL), low density lipoprotein (LDL), and high density lipoprotein (HDL).

The largest of the lipoproteins is the chylomicron. Its main function is to transport triglycerides that are produced from dietary fats, and it is composed primarily of dietary triglycerides. After picking up the triglycerides from the small intestines, chylomicrons travel through the circulatory system to the adipose (fatty) tissue. There, enzymes release the triglycerides from their transporter to be stored in fat cells for later use. After all the triglycerides have reached their destination, the liver will remove the chylomicrons from the circulation until they are needed. After a fast of 8–12 hours, chylomicrons are usually completely absent from the bloodstream. To transport triglycerides being produced by the liver, the body uses VLDL molecules. In a process similar to the one described for the chylomicron, VLDL picks up excess triglycerides in the liver and transports them to the adipose tissue for storage. Unlike the chylomicron, the VLDL molecule can also transport limited amounts of other lipids, with 50% of its composition being triglycerides, 20% being phospholipids, and 20% being cholesterol. After VLDL has delivered its contents to the adipose tissue, half of the remnants are absorbed by the liver, while the other half is used to create LDL molecules.

The major carrier of cholesterol in the bloodstream is the LDL particle. It is made up of 70% cholesterol and 15% phospholipids. Commonly referred to as *bad cholesterol*, LDL particles are the lipoprotein most likely to contribute to atherosclerosis. After sufficient cholesterol has been delivered to the cells of the body, excess LDL particles can begin depositing cholesterol into the smooth muscle of the vascular system. Whether caused by a genetic deficiency or high dietary intake of cholesterol, an elevated LDL level is the first step toward the development of heart disease.

Finally, the smallest of the lipoproteins is the HDL particle. It is made of 5% triglycerides, 30% phospholipids, and 20% cholesterol, with the remainder being protein. These dense particles travel around the body and remove excess cholesterol from cells, returning it to the liver to be eliminated. For this reason, these lipoproteins are typically referred to as *good cholesterol*. Elevated levels of HDL are associated with a decreased risk of developing heart disease.

CASE?

J. H. has heard that there are good and bad types of cholesterol. List the proper name of each lipid particle and explain the differences between them.

Atherosclerosis

Perhaps the most worrisome result of hyperlipidemia is the development of atherosclerosis. The process begins after the circulating LDL particles have delivered a sufficient supply of cholesterol to the cells of the body. Any excess LDL remaining in the bloodstream will begin to deposit into the smooth muscle surrounding the blood vessels, especially in areas of vascular damage. Once beneath the smooth muscle, the LDL particles attract the attention of the immune system. In an effort to remove the particles, white blood cells attempt to digest the cholesterol and are converted into foam cells, causing further irritation in the area. This initial process results in the formation of fatty streaks, which are deposits of cholesterol and foam cells in blood vessel walls. For some patients, the process may end at this stage, with only minimally elevated risks of adverse cardiovascular events. In fact, most people older than 20 years of age have some evidence of fatty streak deposits in their blood vessels. For others, however, the atherosclerosis will progress. As the irritation in the area continues to build and more white blood cells are attracted, the walls of the blood vessel will begin to change. Attempting to wall off the inflamed fatty streak,

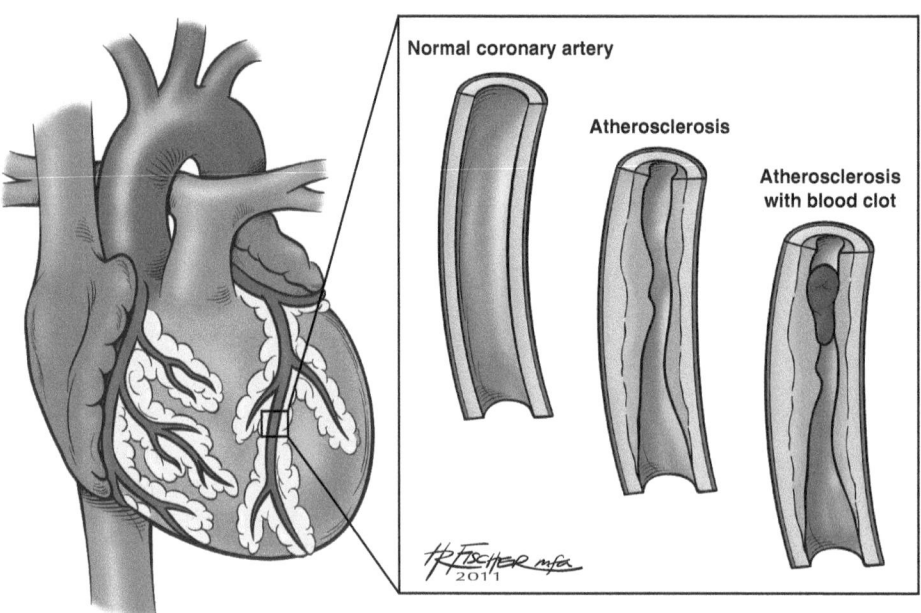

Normal coronary artery

Atherosclerosis

Atherosclerosis with blood clot

FIGURE 17-1. Atherosclerosis is the buildup of a waxy plaque on the inside of blood vessels.

smooth muscle cells, platelets, and collagen begin to bulge into the middle of the blood vessel, forming a true athero-sclerotic plaque (see Figure 17-1).

A number of risk factors for the progression from fatty streak to atherosclerotic plaque have been identified. Some of these risk factors are classified as nonmodifiable, mean-ing they are characteristics that a patient cannot change. A patient's age contributes to the likelihood of plaque forma-tion, with men older than 45 years and women older than 55 years or in premature menopause at highest risk. Addi-tionally, a patient's gender is also an important risk factor, as men are at an increased risk. Finally, a patient's genetics plays a very important role in determining his or her risk for developing atherosclerosis. Clinicians will ask if a patient has any first-degree relatives, meaning a parent or sibling, who suffered an early cardiac death.

Other risk factors, however, are modifiable, mean-ing patients can make decisions that will affect their risk of developing atherosclerosis. These include smoking, body weight, physical activity levels, diet, diabetes, hypertension, and hyperlipidemia. Studies are underway to identify new risk factors, such as the size of LDL particles, number of cho-lesterol receptors, and chronic inflammation markers, which may be important tools to evaluate risk in the future. In addi-tion to these risk factors, cardiovascular risk calculators, such as the ASCVD Risk Score, Framingham, Reynolds, and QRISK calculators, are used to estimate a patient's risk of having an event over a specified number of years.

CASE?

List J. H.'s risk factors for developing atherosclerosis. Which are nonmodifiable? What can J. H. do to change the modifiable ones?

PRACTICE POINT

Cardiovascular risk calculators are available at several online sites. A reliable starting point is the website of the American Heart Association (www.heart.org), where one can enter the search term "risk calculator."

CASE?

J. H. is wondering if following the treatment plan he got from his physician is worth the trouble, because he is currently feeling no symptoms. Describe the risks to J. H. if his new diagnosis goes untreated.

If left untreated, protruding atherosclerotic plaques will eventually decrease blood flow through the narrowing, hardening blood vessel, leading to potentially life-threatening consequences that depend on the location of the plaque. Atherosclerosis of coronary arteries puts patients at risk of developing ischemic heart disease and acute coronary syndromes. If they are present in the arteries supplying the brain with oxygen, patients may develop a stroke. In the rest of the vascular system, blocked arteries may lead to symptoms of atherosclerosis of arteries in the arms or legs that leads to painful cramping and decreased muscle function (termed peripheral vascular disease) or decreased blood flow to vital organs like the kidneys, spleen, or gastrointestinal tract. But perhaps one of the most unnerving characteristics of atherosclerosis is the possibility that patients may not experience any symptoms to warn them of a potentially life-threatening event on the horizon.

DIAGNOSIS OF HYPERLIPIDEMIA

The Lipid Profile

To identify patients with hyperlipidemia, a measurement of the levels of various lipoproteins in the blood must be performed. This blood test is commonly referred to as the lipid panel. In the past, the measurement used to define lipid status was the total cholesterol. This number is determined by adding levels of LDL, HDL, and VLDL into one value. The benefit of this strategy is that patients were not required to fast before obtaining a measurement. The drawbacks, however, were numerous. It is now understood that total cholesterol, alone, does not accurately reflect a patient's risks. Clinicians must look at levels of each lipoprotein individually to assess the patient's status, though the process for obtaining these individual measurements is more complex. Levels of total cholesterol, HDL, and triglycerides can be measured directly in the blood. Next, the triglyceride value must be converted into an estimate of VLDL. Recall that triglycerides are carried by two lipoproteins, chylomicrons and VLDL particles. To get an accurate estimate of VLDL, patients must fast for 8–12 hours before having blood drawn for a lipid panel. This ensures that any triglycerides present in the bloodstream are traveling on VLDL particles and not the temporary chylomicrons. If a patient does not fast, the presence of chylomicrons will affect the measurement of triglycerides and the calculation of LDL, falsely elevating the results. To estimate VLDL levels, the triglycerides of a fasting lipid panel are divided by 5. To obtain a calculated LDL value, the Friedewald formula is used (see Figure 17-2). This entails subtracting

Total Cholesterol = LDL + HDL + VLDL

Since VLDL = Triglycerides/5,

Total Cholesterol = LDL + HDL + Triglycerides/5

To obtain an LDL value,

LDL = Total Cholesterol - (HDL + Triglycerides/5)

FIGURE 17-2. The Friedewald equation for calculating LDL cholesterol values.

the measured HDL and the estimated VLDL levels from the measured total cholesterol.

CASE?

What is J. H.'s calculated LDL level from the values reported to him?

Types of Hyperlipidemia

After the lipid panel has been evaluated, clinicians will attempt to classify patients by type of hyperlipidemia. There are two overarching categories into which patients may fall, either primary or secondary hyperlipidemia. In the case of primary hyperlipidemia, the underlying cause of the disorder is the patient's genetics. At least six different genetic defects have been identified, including deficiencies in the enzyme responsible for cleaving cholesterol from LDL, lacking LDL receptors, excess production of lipoproteins, and abnormal metabolism of lipoproteins. The end result is moderate to extreme elevations in one or more lipoproteins. Treatments can also vary from diet and medication therapy to complete liver transplant.

Much more common than the primary hyperlipidemias, secondary hyperlipidemia is the result of other causes. The most common of these are a diet high in cholesterol and saturated fats and a sedentary lifestyle, leading to being overweight or suffering from obesity. Other secondary causes of hyperlipidemia include certain medications, such as antipsychotics, antivirals, and steroids, and disease states, such as type 2 diabetes, hypothyroidism, and chronic kidney disease.

TREATMENT

For patients with hyperlipidemia, the primary goal is to decrease the risk of developing serious complications due to the development of atherosclerosis. To accomplish this, clinicians will typically begin with lifestyle modifications, such as diet, physical activity, and weight loss. Because lifestyle changes are usually difficult to achieve, pharmacological treatment is added if goal cholesterol levels are not reached with diet and exercise alone. Since LDL is most likely to cause atherosclerosis, the first goal is to bring this value down to acceptable levels. Once this goal is met, HDL and triglycerides can be treated to further minimize the risk of having an adverse cardiovascular event.

Nonpharmacological Treatment

The Therapeutic Lifestyle Changes Diet

The therapeutic lifestyle changes (TLC) diet focuses on reducing dietary saturated fat and cholesterol while promoting a healthy weight loss. The TLC diet recommends that <7% of calories are acquired through saturated fat consumption, as opposed to the typical American diet that receives 11%–17% of calories from these sources. By slowly incorporating healthier options, such as substituting lean meats and skim milk for beef and whole milk, these lifestyle changes are more likely to remain a part of the patient's daily habits. In addition to restricting saturated fats, the TLC diet restricts cholesterol intake to <200 mg/day. As described above, the body can produce enough cholesterol to maintain homeostasis, making dietary cholesterol largely unnecessary. By keeping intake low, LDL cholesterol levels are reduced while HDL levels may increase. As a potential substitute for harmful saturated fats and cholesterol, the TLC diet recommends increasing intake of mono- and polyunsaturated fats, commonly known as the "healthy fats," to 10%–20% of the calories consumed in a day. Found in olives, many seeds, and nuts, the healthy fats can further decrease LDL cholesterol.

CASE?

What type of diet might be best to help J. H. reach his cholesterol goals?

In addition to dietary restrictions, the TLC diet offers a number of options that may be incorporated into the diet to augment LDL reductions. Increasing the amount of soluble fiber in the diet, found in oats, beans, and other plants, to at least 5–10 g daily can reduce LDL by 5%. Consuming 10–15 g daily may cause even larger reductions in LDL. The plant sterols and stanols isolated from soybeans can help reduce the absorption of cholesterol in the gastrointestinal tract. Studies have shown that 2 g daily can reduce cholesterol levels by up to 10%, though higher intake did not result in a greater reduction. Various margarine-like products are available that use plant sterols and stanols to help control LDL levels. It should be noted, however, that these options should be considered as add-on therapy to the dietary options outlined above and not as substitutes for reducing intake of saturated fats and cholesterol.

Other Lifestyle Modifications

In addition to dietary changes, guidelines exist for physical activity and weight loss. Studies have shown that physical activity can cause important changes to lipid metabolism and functioning. Over the long term, exercise causes a reduction in triglycerides, increases HDL, and leads to larger LDL particles that are less likely to contribute to atherosclerosis. To obtain these benefits, it is recommended that at least 30 minutes of moderate physical activity is performed on a near-daily basis. Coupling the dietary and physical activity recommendations will likely lead to another important goal in the treatment of hyperlipidemia: weight loss. Though the emphasis should be placed on the types of food eaten and the amount of physical activity performed, weight loss, itself, can improve a patient's lipid profile. Reductions of as little as 10 pounds can lower LDL and triglycerides while increasing HDL. In general, an initial weight loss goal of 10% of a patient's current weight should be reached over a 6-month period.

The use of alcohol and tobacco has also been examined. Studies have shown that moderate alcohol consumption may actually reduce the risk of heart disease by increasing HDL particles slightly. Moderate intake has been defined as no more than two servings per day for men or no more than one serving per day for women. Patients must be cautioned that consuming more than the recommended amount may actually increase triglyceride levels and contribute to liver damage and cirrhosis. For patients who use tobacco, evidence suggests that not only are HDL levels reduced and LDL levels elevated, but the particles are more prone to cause atherosclerosis. All patients reporting tobacco use should be encouraged to quit, without regard to their lipid status.

CASE?

What are three lifestyle changes that J. H.'s physician might recommend to improve his hyperlipidemia?

Pharmacologic Treatment

HMG-CoA Reductase Inhibitors

Often called the *statins*, the HMG-CoA reductase inhibitors block the function of an important enzyme used in the production of cholesterol. As the body produces less cholesterol, LDL levels begin to drop, possibly by as much as 55%. In addition to dropping LDL cholesterol, triglyceride levels may also fall by up to 30% while HDL levels may rise 15%. Though these favorable effects on the lipid profile are important features of the statin medications, many experts have theorized that there are other benefits of statin use beyond their lipid-lowering effect. The so-called pleiotropic effects of statins range from reducing inflammation to stabilizing atherosclerotic plaques, making them more organized and less likely to rupture. Taken together, their powerful LDL-lowering ability, pleiotropic effects, and benefit on other components of the lipid profile have made the statins the drug of choice for many of the hyperlipidemias.

ALERT!

Statins are usually discontinued for pregnant patients when the risk to the fetus may outweigh possible benefits to the mother. Other agents described later in this chapter, such as the bile acid sequestrants, are considered first line in pregnancy because they are not absorbed into the body, so would be less likely to harm an unborn child.

The agents in this class include atorvastatin (Lipitor), fluvastatin (Lescol), lovastatin, pitavastatin (Livalo, Zypitamag), pravastatin (Pravachol), rosuvastatin (Crestor), and simvastatin (Zocor—see Medication Table 17-1; Medication Tables are located at the end of the chapter). Though many of these medications are available as generics, pitavastatin is brand name only. Clinicians will recommend that they are taken once daily at bedtime to ensure high blood concentrations when the body's cholesterol production is at its peak, during the night (though the some of the newer agents can be taken at any time of day). Depending on which agent and dose is chosen, the effect on LDL levels can vary greatly. See Table 17-1 for a summary of the relative effects of the different doses of the statins.

TABLE 17-1. Potency of Reduction of Low Density Lipoprotein (LDL) for Various Statins[1a]

Statin	Daily Dose		
	Low Intensity (< 30% LDL Reduction)	Moderate Intensity (30%–49% LDL Reduction)	High-Intensity (> 50% LDL Reduction)
Atorvastatin (a TORE va sta tin)		10–20 mg	40–80 mg
Fluvastatin (FLOO va sta tin)	20–40 mg	80 mg	
Lovastatin (LOE va sta tin)	20 mg	40–80 mg	
Pitavastatin (pit A va stat in)		1–4 mg	
Pravastatin (PRA va stat in)	10–20 mg	40–80 mg	
Rosuvastatin (roe SOO va sta tin)		5–10 mg	20–40 mg
Simvastatin (SIM va stat in)	10 mg	20–40 mg	

[a]Pronunciations have been adapted with permission from USP Dictionary of USAN and International Drug Names (USP Dictionary) © 2022.

PRACTICE POINT

Since it is thought that the body synthesizes most cholesterol at night, it is generally recommended that statins be taken at bedtime. Atorvastatin, pitavastatin, and rosuvastatin, however, are longer-acting statins that can be taken any time during the day and retain their effectiveness.

As a class, these medications are fairly well tolerated; however, side effects can occur. One of the most frequently reported side effects is myalgia, or muscle pain, reported in 1%–10% of patients. Patients especially at risk for this adverse event are older adults, patients taking high doses of statins, patients of Asian descent, or those taking other medications that may cause myalgia, such as the fibrates and niacin products also used to treat hyperlipidemia. Clinicians will monitor patients with myalgia closely as it may be a warning sign for a more serious side effect of statin use, called myopathy. This condition is the coupling of muscle pain with an elevation in creatinine kinase levels, an enzyme that is released when muscle tissue is severely damaged. If allowed to progress, myopathy could lead to rhabdomyolysis, a widespread breakdown of muscle fibers that can cause kidney failure and death. All patients who experience unexplained muscle pain should be instructed to call their healthcare providers so that they may be evaluated for these serious side effects. In addition to their effects on muscle tissue, statins may also cause damage to the liver. To avoid this, clinicians will monitor blood levels of liver enzymes. These liver function tests (LFTs) will rise if there is damage to the liver and alert the clinician to stop the offending agent.

ALERT!

Patients should be warned to avoid drinking large amounts of grapefruit juice with statins. This drug–diet interaction can lead to higher levels of statin in the blood and increased risk of side effects.

PRACTICE POINT

Prescribers will choose the appropriate statin dosage based on patient risk factors. Those at highest risk for a myocardial infarction, stroke, or other event tend to receive high-intensity statin therapy (such as atorvastatin 80 mg or rosuvastatin 40 mg daily) to lower LDL by >50%. Patients at lower risk or those who develop side effects to statin therapy tend to receive lower-intensity statin therapy (eg, simvastatin or pravastatin 10 mg daily).

PRACTICE POINT

The pharmacist may counsel patients to watch out for dark brown urine while taking statins. This can be an early warning sign of rhabdomyolysis.

CASE?

What are the common side effects of the medication prescribed to J. H.?

Niacin

Niacin is a B vitamin that, at high doses, can have a favorable effect on each component of the lipid profile. It is thought that niacin's action comes from its ability to inhibit fat breakdown, lowering the amount of fatty acids being delivered to the liver to make lipoproteins. Reductions in LDL tend to be smaller than is seen with the statins, likely dropping by 5%–25%, but the effect on triglyceride and HDL can be dramatic, lowering triglycerides by 20%–40% and increasing HDL up to 35%.

Though niacin has a beneficial effect on each part of the lipid profile, side effects often limit its use. The first, and most bothersome, side effect is known as flushing, a sensation of heat and redness of the face, neck, chest, or body a few hours after a dose of niacin is given. This is the result of vasodilation in the face and neck as niacin levels begin to rise in the body. Though a tolerance to the effect sometimes develops with time, the sensation is unlikely to fully disappear. Gastrointestinal complaints, such as nausea, vomiting, diarrhea, and heartburn, are common, as well. In some patients, symptoms of myopathy can present, similar to those experienced by some statin users. Others may see elevations in blood glucose, making niacin difficult to use in patients with diabetes. Finally, clinicians must closely monitor liver function tests in patients taking niacin products as hepatic injury is a common issue, especially at higher doses.

PRACTICE POINT

The pharmacist or prescriber may recommend taking 325 mg of aspirin 30 minutes before administering a dose of niacin to help reduce the severity of flushing.

Niacin is available in three different formulations, each with a slightly different side effect profile and dosing regimen. The first is an immediate-release tablet or capsule that is available over the counter (Niacor, vitamin B3) started as a once daily dose but increased weekly until the patient is taking it three times a day. The usual target dose is 500 mg three times daily. If lipid profile goals are not met at this dosage, further escalation to doses up to 2 g three times daily may be attempted, though it is unlikely most patients will tolerate these higher doses. The benefit of using immediate-release forms of niacin is that liver damage is unlikely to occur. However, the immediate-release products cause the largest amount of flushing, a consequence that most patients cannot tolerate (see Medication Table 17-1).

Also available over the counter is a sustained-release niacin product (Slo-Niacin). This sustained-release preparation is taken twice daily in doses starting at 500 mg, which can be increased to 1 g if the patient needs and can tolerate the higher dosage. In addition to the benefit of fewer daily doses, sustained-release niacin also reduces the risk of developing flushing. However, these agents should be used with extreme caution and only under the supervision of a healthcare provider because a significant increased risk of liver damage has been discovered.

The final formulation of niacin is an extended-release product (Niaspan). Available only with a prescription, extended-release niacin is absorbed more slowly than an immediate-release product but more rapidly than the sustained-release versions. The result is a lower risk of flushing and little to no risk of liver damage. Dosing typically begins at 500 mg at bedtime and is increased each month by 500 mg to a target of 1–2 g each night. Recently, data from studies suggest that using niacin may not decrease the risk of having heart attacks or strokes in patients with hyperlipidemia so the utility of these agents has been called into question.

ALERT!

Many over-the-counter niacin products are labeled as FLUSH FREE. These supplements are not equivalent to the niacin products outlined above and do not have a role in treating hyperlipidemia.

Fibrates

The fibrates are medications that target primarily triglycerides. Through a series of complex steps, they encourage the breakdown and removal of chylomicrons and VLDL particles from the bloodstream while reducing their production in the liver. They also may have a small role in increasing HDL levels. Reduction in LDL levels, however, is usually modest and the fibrates may even lead to increased LDL in some populations. The newer agents in this class, fenofibrate products (Tricor, Trilipix, and others), are dosed once daily, while the older agent, gemfibrozil (Lopid), is dosed twice daily. For patients with poor kidney function, doses should be reduced to avoid accumulation and the development of side effects. Many different formulations of fenofibrate exist and are available as generic medications. Gemfibrozil is available generically, as well. In general, this class of hyperlipidemia medications is very well tolerated; however, gemfibrozil is associated with slightly higher incidence of upset stomach, myopathy, and liver damage than the fenofibrate products and also carries a higher risk of interacting with statins (see Medication Table 17-1).

PRACTICE POINT

The many different formulations of fenofibrate have slightly different doses and release mechanisms; therefore, they are not interchangeable.

ALERT!

Patients may not gain the full effect of the fibrates until they have completed 6–8 weeks of therapy.

Cholesterol Absorption Inhibitors

The only agent from the class known as the cholesterol absorption inhibitors currently available is ezetimibe (Zetia). This newer class of hyperlipidemia medication, available as a generic and dosed 10 mg once daily, inhibits a cholesterol transporter in the small intestine. The result is a drop in cholesterol absorption by up to 50%, leading to a modest 18% reduction in circulating LDL particles. Because of this relatively small decrease in LDL and no significant effect on other parts of the lipid profile, ezetimibe is usually used as an adjunctive treatment for patients unable to meet their cholesterol goals on other hyperlipidemia treatments. It may also be used in patients who cannot tolerate statins due to adverse events, as it is very well tolerated. Few case reports of muscle-related side effects have been reported with ezetimibe (see Medication Table 17-1).

Omega 3 Fatty Acids

The omega 3 fatty acids are polyunsaturated fats found in oily fish (such as salmon or tuna). When taken at high doses, these substances interfere with the liver's ability to produce VLDL particles, thus reducing serum triglyceride concentrations. Though they are found in certain plants, as well, all available evidence of cardiovascular risk benefit come from fish sources. Available as over-the-counter supplements (various fish oil preparations) and one prescription strength formulation (Lovaza), doses of up to 4 g/day are required to lower triglycerides by up to 50%. As doses approach the 3 g/day threshold, the incidence of adverse effects, including bloating, fishy taste, belching, and indigestion, increases though these agents are generally well tolerated (see Medication Table 17-1).

Bile Acid Sequestrants

Historically, the first agents used to treat hyperlipidemia were the bile acid sequestrants (BAS). When this class of medications is ingested, no drug is absorbed into the bloodstream. Instead, the drug travels through the digestive system binding the bile acids. The bile acids are molecules produced by the liver that are responsible for breaking down and transporting fats from the diet. Bile acid sequestrants can reduce the amount of bile acid by as much as 40%. Sensing this decrease, the body is stimulated to produce new bile acid. Cholesterol is collected from the bloodstream and returned to the liver where it can be reprocessed into new bile acid. The result is a decrease in circulating LDL by up to 25%, with little to no change in the other components of the lipid panel.

The use of bile acid sequestrants has declined in favor of more effective, easier to administer, and more tolerable medications such as the statins. Though they do not get absorbed into the systemic circulation, the gastrointestinal side effects of these agents lead to a > 40% discontinuation rate. Constipation, flatulence, bloating, and abdominal pain

are all likely occurrences as the adsorbed bile acid is eliminated through the feces. In addition to these side effects, administering other medications along with the bile acid sequestrants can lead to significant interactions, as some medications and vitamins become bound to the molecules, and are not absorbed. To avoid this issue, all other medications must be administered at least 1 hour before or 4 hours after a dose of the bile acid sequestrants is administered.

The agents in this class of hyperlipidemia medications are cholestyramine (Questran), colestipol (Colestid), and colesevelam (Welchol). Cholestyramine and colestipol are dosed at 4–5 g and titrated to a maximum dose of 24–30 g/day, respectively. The newer agent colesevelam is dosed at 3.75 g/day. These products are all available in powdered form to be mixed with liquids. Colestipol and colesevelam are also available as oral tablets. Theoretically, the lower dose used with colesevelam reduces the likelihood of the serious gastrointestinal side effects seen with the older bile acid sequestrants (see Medication Table 17-1).

Proprotein Convertase Sutilisin-Kexin Type 9 Inhibitors

The newest class of medication aimed at lowering blood cholesterol levels are the proprotein convertase sutilisin-kexin type 9 (PCSK9) inhibitors. Agents in this class include evolocumab (Repatha) and alirocumab (Praluent), which are available only as brand name injections administered every 2 or 4 weeks. These antibodies bind to an enzyme that would normally promote the degradation of LDL receptors in the liver. In the process, the liver will remove more LDL from the bloodstream. When compared to other medications that treat hyperlipidemia, the PCSK9 inhibitors are very effective at lowering LDL (up to a 76% reduction in many patients), though their higher costs have limited their use. In most cases, these agents are reserved for patients who have elevated LDL levels despite multiple other medications prescribed at their maximum tolerated doses.

CASE?

After 6 months of lifestyle modifications and treatment with simvastatin, J. H. returns to his primary care physician's office and has a lipid panel checked. His LDL is now at goal, but his triglycerides remain slightly elevated. What add-on therapy might the physician prescribe for J. H.? Describe its mechanism of action and potential side effects.

SUMMARY

Cholesterol is an important ingredient in the production of a number of vital substances needed to maintain homeostasis. The body can both produce cholesterol and obtain it through dietary sources. For the typical American, the amount of cholesterol obtained in the diet far exceeds what the body requires, resulting in excess low density lipoprotein (LDL) particles circulating in the bloodstream. When the LDL has delivered sufficient cholesterol to the tissues, leftover particles will begin to deposit into the smooth muscle surrounding the vasculature. This is the first step in the development of atherosclerosis, a hardening and narrowing of the blood vessels. If allowed to continue, the affected blood vessel may become completely blocked or the plaque may rupture, sending fragments and blood clots traveling downstream to smaller vessels that may become blocked, as well. Depending on the affected vessel, the consequences can range from decreased blood flow and organ dysfunction to stroke, myocardial infarction, and death. To reduce the risk of forming deadly plaques, clinicians monitor patients' serum cholesterol levels with a lipid panel. This lab test can give an early warning for patients at risk of developing atherosclerosis. If the levels of cholesterol must be reduced, a combination of lifestyle changes and pharmacological treatment can be initiated to bring the disease under control and reduce the risk of life-threatening consequences.

REFERENCES

1. Grundy SM, Stone NJ, Bailey AL, et al. 2018 AHA/ACC/AACVPR/AAPA/ABC/ACPM/ADA/AGS/APhA/ASPC/NLA/PCNA guideline on the management of blood cholesterol: A report of the American College of Cardiology/American Heart Association Task Force on Clinical Practice Guidelines. *Circulation* 2019;139(25):e1082-e1143.
2. Lexi-Drugs. Lexicomp. Hudson, OH. http://online.lexi.com. Accessed June 22, 2022.

CHAPTER RESOURCES

Barrett KE, Barman SM, Brooks HL, et al. *Ganong's Review of Medical Physiology*. 26th ed. New York, NY: McGraw-Hill; 2019.

DiPiro JT, Yee GC, Posey M, et al. *Pharmacotherapy: A Pathophysiological Approach*. 11th ed. New York, NY: McGraw-Hill; 2020.

The American Heart Association website. Available at http://www.heart.org. Accessed June 22, 2022.

REVIEW QUESTIONS

1. Define the terms lipid, cholesterol, and hyperlipidemia.
2. List the steps involved in the formation of an atherosclerotic plaque.
3. Calculate the LDL of a patient with a total cholesterol level of 170 mg/dL, HDL of 28 mg/dL, and triglycerides of 250 mg/dL.
4. Describe the differences between primary and secondary hyperlipidemias.
5. Describe the mechanism of action of the statins.

MEDICATION TABLE

MEDICATION TABLE 17-1. Hyperlipidemia Pharmacotherapy[2]

CLASS Generic Name (pronunciation)	Brand Name	Route	Forms	Dose	Notes
Bile Acid Sequestrants					
Cholestyramine (koe LESS tir a meen)	Questran, Questran Light, Prevalite	Oral	Powder	4–12 g 1–2 times daily	Significant gastrointestinal side effects limit use; the lower doses needed with colesevelam may reduce this risk
Colesevelam (koh le SEV e lam)	Welchol	Oral	Tablet	3.75 g once daily	
Colestipol (koe LES ti pole)	Colestid	Oral	Powder	5–15 g 1–2 times daily (doses may be divided)	
		Oral	Tablet	2–16 g 1–2 times daily	
Cholesterol Absorbtion Inhibitors					
Ezetimibe (ez ET i mibe)	Zetia	Oral	Tablet	10 mg once daily	No proven cardiovascular risk reduction
Fibrates					
Fenofibrate (fen oh FYE brate)	Antara	Oral	Capsule	30–200 mg once daily	Primarily target is triglycerides
	Lipofen	Oral	Capsule	50–150 mg once daily	
	Tricor	Oral	Tablet	48–145 mg once daily	
	Trilipix	Oral	Capsule	45–135 mg once daily	
Gemfibrozil (jem FI broe zil)	Lopid	Oral	Tablet	600 mg 2 times daily	More likely to interact with statins
Niacin					
Niacin immediate release (NYE a sin)	Niacor	Oral	Tablet	250 mg–2 g 3 times daily	Flushing most common with immediate-release form
Niacin extended release (NYE a sin)	Niaspan	Oral	Tablet	500 mg–2 g at bedtime	
Niacin sustained release (NYE a sin)	Slo Niacin	Oral	Tablet	500 mg–1 g 2 times daily	Liver injury most common with sustained-release form

Continued next page

MEDICATION TABLE 17-1. Hyperlipidemia Pharmacotherapy[2] *(Continued)*

CLASS Generic Name (pronunciation)	Brand Name	Route	Forms	Dose	Notes
Omega 3 Fatty Acids					
Omega 3 fatty acids (oh MAY ga)	Fish oil	Oral	Capsule	3 g once daily	Primarily target triglycerides
	Lovaza	Oral	Capsule	4 g once daily	
Icosapent Ethyl (eye KOE sa pent ETH il)	Vascepa	Oral	Capsule	2 g 2 times daily	
Proprotein Convertase Sutilisin Kexin Type 9 (PCSK9) Inhibitors					
Alirocumab (al i ROK ue mab)	Praluent	SUBQ	Solution	75–150 mg every 2 weeks or 300 mg every 4 weeks	
Evolocumab (e voe LOK ue mab)	Repatha	SUBQ	Solution	140 mg every 2 weeks or 420 mg every 4 weeks	
Statins					
Atorvastatin (a TORE va sta tin)	Lipitor	Oral	Tablet	10–80 mg once daily	Pleiotropic effects may give added benefits; often dosed at bedtime for maximal effect
Lovastatin (LOE va sta tin)	Mevacor	Oral	Tablet	20–80 mg once daily	
Pitavastatin (pit A va stat in)	Livalo	Oral	Tablet	1–4 mg once daily	
Pravastatin (PRA va stat in)	Pravachol	Oral	Tablet	10–80 mg once daily	
Rosuvastatin (roe SOO va sta tin)	Crestor	Oral	Tablet	5–40 mg once daily	
Simvastatin (SIM va stat in)	Zocor	Oral	Tablet	20–80 mg once daily	

Part 6

THE RESPIRATORY SYSTEM

Chapter 18

Overview of the Respiratory System

Celeste Voight, PharmD, BCPS

KEY TERMS AND DEFINITIONS

Alveoli—the terminus (end) of the bronchial tree where primary gas exchange occurs in the lung.

Bronchi—main branches of airways connecting the trachea to the bronchioles in the lung.

Bronchioles—airways connecting the bronchi to the alveoli.

Dry powder inhaler (DPI)—a device used to deliver medication to the lungs using a dry powder without an aerosol propellant.

Hemoglobin—a component of red blood cells that transports oxygen from lungs to cells and tissues throughout the body.

Larynx—a portion of the respiratory tract connecting the pharynx to the trachea. It contains the vocal cords, which vibrate and allow a person to vocalize. The larynx is also referred to as the voice box.

Lungs—the two organs (left and right) located in the chest that take in oxygen from the air by inhalation and distribute it to the bloodstream for use by the body, while removing carbon dioxide waste from the body by exhalation.

Metered dose inhaler (MDI)—a device used to deliver medication to the lungs using an aerosol propellant.

DOI 10.37573/9781585286638.018

Nebulizer—a device used to deliver medication to the lungs using a fine mist that requires a compressor (mechanical device) and nebulizer cup.

Pharynx—the portion of the respiratory tract connecting the larynx and trachea. The pharynx is also referred to as the throat and is part of both the respiratory and gastrointestinal tracts.

Spacer—a tube-like device that connects to the mouthpiece of an MDI allowing more medication to reach the lungs.

Spirometry—a breathing test used to diagnose and monitor lung disease. It measures pulmonary function, with results reported as pulmonary function tests (PFTs).

Thoracic diaphragm—the primary muscle involved in respiration. It sits below the base of the lungs and separates the chest from the abdomen.

Trachea—the portion of the respiratory tract connecting the larynx to the bronchi. The trachea is also referred to as the windpipe.

LEARNING OBJECTIVES

After completing this chapter, you should be able to

1. Identify components of the upper and lower respiratory systems.

2. Recall the basic physiology of the respiratory system.

3. Describe the process of respiratory gas exchange between oxygen and carbon dioxide and explain its importance.

4. Recognize the different pulmonary function tests used to evaluate respiratory function.

5. Describe the proper technique for administration of medications via respiratory routes.

Oxygen is essential to sustain life; it is needed by all cells throughout the body to perform normal metabolic functions. Carbon dioxide is a waste byproduct of cellular metabolism and must be removed from the body. The primary function of the respiratory system is breathing—the inhalation of oxygen and the exhalation of carbon dioxide, with an exchange of gases (oxygen and carbon dioxide) between the air and

blood. Oxygen is transported into the lungs through passageways via inhaled air and, once in the lungs, passively diffuses (moves) into the blood. Once in the blood, it is transported to cells and tissues throughout the body. Carbon dioxide is then released from those cells, where it moves into the blood to be carried to the lungs where it is exhaled. This process is dependent upon the epithelial cells that line the respiratory system; these cells are thin and moist to enable gas exchange between the blood and the air in the lungs.

The respiration process involves the entire respiratory system, including the upper and lower respiratory tracts. These tracts are essentially a network of tubes and passageways that allow air to travel to the lungs. The passageways are lined with the mucus-secreting goblet cells and hair-like cilia that protect the respiratory system from any foreign bodies. The mucus traps foreign bodies, which in turn allows the cilia to sweep the foreign body up out of the respiratory system to be expelled.

RESPIRATORY ANATOMY AND PHYSIOLOGY

Upper Respiratory System

The primary function of the upper respiratory system is to deliver air through passageways to the lungs. The upper respiratory system involves primarily the head and neck region, including the nose, pharynx, and larynx (Figure 18-1).

Air is inhaled through the nose, where it is warmed and moistened within the nasal cavity. The nose also functions as a filter to remove dust particles from the air to protect the lungs from foreign bodies. The nasal cavity empties into the pharynx, the passageway that connects the nose and mouth, commonly referred to as the throat. The pharynx is a component of both the respiratory and digestive systems as it delivers both air to the lungs and food to the stomach. It has three distinct regions: the nasopharynx, oropharynx, and laryngopharynx. The nasopharynx is the uppermost portion (encompassing the upper part of the throat) that is connected to the nasal cavity. The oropharynx is the portion of the pharynx directly below that extends between the soft palate and base of the tongue; it contains the tonsils. The oral cavity empties into the oropharynx. The laryngopharynx lies directly below the oropharynx; it connects to both the larynx (respiratory system) and the esophagus (digestive system), and carries both air and food. The epiglottis is a small piece of cartilage that acts as a tiny "lid" to cover the larynx when

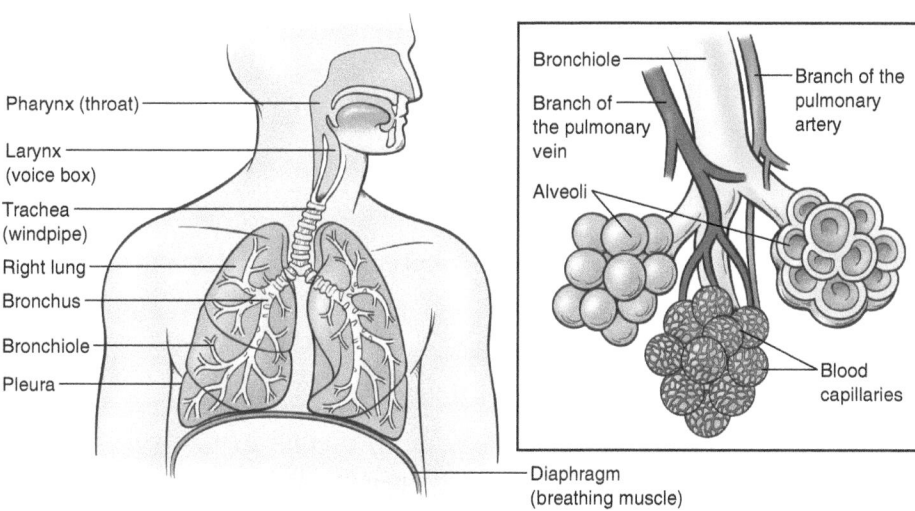

FIGURE 18-1. Anatomy of the respiratory system.

food and drink are being swallowed, directing them to the esophagus. In the absence of solids and liquids, it remains open, allowing air to be delivered to the larynx. The larynx (also called the *voice box*) is located directly below the laryngopharynx and leads into the trachea of the lower respiratory system.

Lower Respiratory System

The lower respiratory system encompasses primarily the chest area of the body and includes the trachea, lungs, and thoracic diaphragm. The primary function of the lower respiratory system is the absorption of oxygen and removal of carbon dioxide from the body. The trachea (commonly referred to as the *windpipe*) is the final passageway leading to the lungs. It is a flexible tube that is approximately 1 inch in diameter that branches into the left and right primary bronchi that enter the left and right lung, respectively. The bronchi are slightly smaller than the trachea, and they continue to branch into smaller and smaller passageways called the secondary bronchi and the bronchioles (see Figure 18-1).

Thoracic Diaphragm

The thoracic diaphragm is the primary muscle involved in respiration. It is a thin, dome-shaped muscle that extends across the body just below the lungs, separating the chest and abdominal cavities; it contracts during inhalation and relaxes during exhalation. As the diaphragm contracts and flattens it allows more room for the lungs to fully expand, causing a negative lung pressure and subsequent suction that further draws air into the lungs. Exhalation occurs due to the

relaxation of the diaphragm combined with elastic recoil of the lungs. This process causes the lungs to decrease back to their original size and increases lung pressure to help draw air out of the lungs.

Bronchial Tree

The trachea branches off into two separate passageways called the primary left and right bronchi at a point called the carina. The carina is the ridge of cartilage between the two bronchi and contains sensitive nerves. When triggered by a foreign body, it produces a strong coughing reflex that helps to expel the material before it can enter the lungs. The primary left bronchus enters the left lung and supplies it with air, while the primary right bronchus enters the right lung and supplies it with air. The primary right bronchus has a slightly larger diameter, when compared to the primary left bronchus, and enters the lung at a slightly more vertical position. The increased diameter and position of the primary right bronchus make it more accessible to foreign bodies, and, thus, more susceptible to infections. The primary left and right bronchi (plural form of bronchus) continue to branch progressively into smaller bronchi (known as the secondary and tertiary bronchi) and finally to the smallest tubes, the terminal bronchioles. The branching of the bronchus is commonly referred to as the bronchial tree, because the structure resembles the branching of a tree. The bronchioles are the smallest passageways within the respiratory system. The terminal bronchioles deliver air to the alveolar ducts, which lead to the alveoli.

The alveoli are the primary site of gas exchange within the lungs. Alveoli are small, sac-like structures located at the end of the bronchial trees, further giving the appearance of a tree. The alveoli resemble a bunch of grapes in appearance. Their structure and shape dramatically increase the available surface area in the lungs, resulting in increased gas exchange to oxygenate the body. The alveoli have very thin walls and are connected to an intricate system of blood vessels that allow oxygen to enter the blood stream and carbon dioxide to leave.

Lungs

The lungs are located inside the thoracic cavity, above the diaphragm and within the protective barrier of the rib cage. Each lung is contained within a separate membranous sac known as a pleural cavity and are separated by the mediastinum. Each pleural cavity is lined with a double layer of a single cell membrane called the pleura. The pleural membranes secrete a small amount of pleural fluid that fills the gap between the two membranes, providing a moist, slippery environment, which allows the two layers to slide against one another during breathing. The pleural space has a slightly decreased air pressure, creating a mild suction that prevents the lungs from collapsing. The lungs are divided into lobes. The right lung has three lobes: upper, middle, and lower; while the left lung only has two lobes: upper and lower.

Respiration

There are two types of respiration: internal and external. Internal respiration occurs within cells when oxygen is utilized to make energy and the waste byproduct, carbon dioxide, is formed. Carbon dioxide is then released from cells into the bloodstream to return to the lungs for removal from the body. External respiration occurs when carbon dioxide is exchanged for oxygen in the lungs. The cycle is continuous; oxygen is distributed throughout the body to be utilized for cellular metabolism and the carbon dioxide is then removed from the body.

MEASURES OF PULMONARY FUNCTION

Pulmonary function tests (PFTs) or lung function tests are used to assess how efficiently the lungs are able to exchange oxygen and carbon dioxide to oxygenate the body. The term "pulmonary function test" refers to several different assessments that attempt to evaluate lung function. PFTs include blood gas measurements, oxygen saturation, and spirometry. The normal values for PFTs vary among patients as they are based on factors such as height, weight, sex, and ethnicity. It is important to establish baseline PFTs (levels taken at

the start of therapy) for each patient. In common respiratory disorders, PFTs are often done at specified intervals to monitor for any changes in their baseline levels indicating a change in lung function. PFTs are used to identify or diagnose a decline in lung function, but they are also used to help classify the type of lung function decline, assess effectiveness of lung treatments, and monitor for adverse lung side effects.[1] PFTs provide information on airflow limitations, lung volumes, and gas exchange.

Arterial blood gas measurements (ABGs) determine how well the body is able to exchange gas based on evaluation of the amount of oxygen and carbon dioxide that is in the blood. Oxygen (PaO_2) and carbon dioxide ($PaCO_2$) are reported as *partial pressures* in mm Hg (the same unit of measurement used for blood pressure). If the lungs are working at a normal capacity, it is expected that the arterial oxygen level would be much higher than the carbon dioxide as the arterial system should be primarily carrying oxygen to the body.

Because the lungs, along with the kidneys, function to regulate the body's acid-base balance (see Chapter 13), changes in blood pH may also indicate respiratory issues. A lower than normal pH (< 7.4), caused by an inability to exhale carbon dioxide efficiently, is termed *respiratory acidosis*.

Oxygen saturation (O_2 sat) is not only a measurement of how much oxygen is in the blood, but also considers the hemoglobin capacity to carry the oxygen. It is expressed as a ratio of the oxygen that is actually bound to hemoglobin versus the amount of oxygen that could be bound to hemoglobin at a specified pressure (to distinguish the difference between respiratory issues and anemia).

Spirometry is a noninvasive examination and only requires the patient to breath in and out through a mouthpiece that is attached to a spirometer. A spirometer is an instrument that measures the amount of air that the patient breathes in and out at specific intervals. The validity of the spirometry results are directly dependent on patient cooperation during the testing process, correct equipment calibration, and experienced test administrators. For spirometry measurements and their definitions, see Table 18-1.

INHALATION AS A ROUTE OF ADMINISTRATION

Inhalation is the preferred method of medication administration for the treatment of most pulmonary conditions. The major benefit of treating pulmonary conditions with an

TABLE 18-1. Spirometry Measurement[a]

Spirometry Value	What Is Measured	Notes
Tidal volume	Volume of air inhaled and exhaled during normal breathing	
Vital capacity	Maximum volume of air exhaled after maximum inhalation	
Residual volume	Amount of residual air in lungs after maximum exhalation	
Total lung capacity (TLC)	Vital capacity plus residual volume	
Forced vital capacity (FVC)	Amount of air exhaled with force after maximum inhalation	
Forced expiratory volume (FEV)	Maximum amount of air exhaled forcefully after maximum inhalation in one breath	This is often measured at second intervals: FEV1, FEV2, FEV3
		FEV1/FVC is calculated and determines the ability to move air through the lungs

[a]Normal values vary depending on factors such as height, weight, gender, age, and ethnicity.

inhaled medication is that the medication is rapidly deposited and absorbed for action directly where it is needed, providing faster symptom relief. The specificity of inhaled medication for the lungs also decreases the likelihood of systemic (body-wide) adverse effects. Inhaled medications must have a particle size small enough to enter the lungs, and the exact particle size of the medication largely determines where in the bronchial tree the medication will be absorbed; the smaller the particle size, the farther down the bronchial tree the medication will reach. There are several types of devices used to administer inhaled medications, including the metered-dose inhaler (MDI), dry powder inhaler (DPI), and nebulizer.

PRACTICE POINT

Patients should be instructed to clean the spacer once a week in warm water, with one drop of liquid dish soap added to the sink, then rinse the mouthpiece only and allow it to air dry in a vertical position.

The MDI and DPI inhalers are effective pulmonary medication delivery devices when used properly. Each inhaler has specific instructions for use to assure that the correct amount of medication reaches the lungs. Improper inhaler technique can result in the medication either being lost in the process or swallowed (and delivered to the gastrointestinal tract instead of the respiratory system). Patients need thorough

instruction on the proper use of inhalers and should be periodically asked to demonstrate to a healthcare professional how they are using their inhalers, to ensure that an improper technique is quickly corrected. Patients using inhalers should be directed to report any symptoms of mouth or throat soreness or hoarseness as this can be a sign of improper technique. Patients should wash their hands prior to using any inhaled delivery device.

To achieve the greatest benefit from MDI inhalers, patients must coordinate inhaler release with their inhaled breath. This can be a particularly difficult task for pediatric and elderly patients; however, most people can benefit from using a spacer. A spacer is a tube-like device that can be attached to the mouthpiece of an MDI to help ensure that the medication is adequately inhaled into the lungs. It includes a new mouthpiece for the patient and can help to ensure inhalation of the medication for absorption into the lungs rather than swallowing it and having it absorbed through the gut. The spacer provides a holding chamber for the medication, allowing the patient additional time to fully inhale the medication. When a spacer is attached, the MDI should still be used exactly as discussed below, including the priming instructions.

The MDIs contain a propellant that helps expel the medication when the canister is depressed. It is important that the patient knows to remove the cap from the inhaler and then shake it prior to each dose. The inhaler should be primed by pressing the canister, wasting one puff prior to the first use of a new inhaler or when the inhaler has not been used recently. (Each inhaler package includes specific instructions for priming.) The inhaler should be held in an upright position while the patient either places the inhaler directly in or 1–2 inches in front of the mouth. The patient should be instructed to exhale completely, then the canister should be pressed at the same time that the patient starts to breathe in slowly and deeply through the mouth. The patient should continue to breathe in slowly for 3–5 seconds and then to hold the breath for 10 seconds or for as long as comfortably possible. This provides the medication time to reach the lungs. The patient should repeat puffs if directed by the physician, but should wait approximately 30 seconds between puffs to ensure optimal absorption of the second puff.

PRACTICE POINT

It is important that the patient understands that the canister should be pressed only once for each puff.

It may be difficult for pediatric or elderly patients using an MDI to get the proper dosage of medication as it requires the patient to coordinate breathing with the release of medication. All patients using an inhaled corticosteroid should be reminded to rinse their mouths after each use to prevent irritation or possible infection. The MDI must be cleaned once a week by removing the canister and rinsing the plastic container with warm water and allowing it to air dry.

ALERT!

Many MDIs and DPIs are packaged in a sealed pouch, and the expiration dating on the package refers to the product in the unopened pouch. Once the seal is broken and the inhaler removed, the medication may be stable for a much shorter time. Most DPIs, for instance, have instructions to discard them 30 days after the pouch is opened; MDIs in pouches are generally said to be good for 12 months. Technicians should call patients' attention to the manufacturers' instructions to reduce the danger of using subpotent expired inhalers.

PRACTICE POINT

Inhalation instructions may vary among MDI brands and should be consulted for the recommended use of that particular product.

The DPIs differ from MDIs because they do not contain a propellant. These inhalers must be activated by either opening the mouthpiece or inserting a power capsule into the unit and then pulling a trigger. Each unit differs and instructions are based on the specific inhaler being used. It is important that the patient does not exhale directly into this inhaler prior to use as this could either waste the medication or decrease the dose delivered. The inhaler should be held level and to the side of the mouth while the patient exhales in preparation to use the inhaler. The DPI requires the patient to inhale quickly and deeply with force as it does not contain a propellant. For maximal benefit, the patient should hold his or her breath for 10 seconds or as long as comfortably possible.

Nebulizers, another type of delivery device, turn liquid medication into a fine mist for inhalation via a mouthpiece or mask. There are several different methods available to reduce the particle size of medications, including compressed air or oxygen, or high frequency vibration to reduce the particle size of medications. They are often used by pediatric and elderly populations as they do not require good coordination for proper medication administration the way MDIs and DPIs do. Each nebulizer unit has specific directions that should be consulted for proper use (Figure 18-2).

The basic directions for using a nebulizer include placing the device on a level surface and plugging it into an electrical outlet. Tubing is then connected to the device at the air outlet connector. The medication must be placed into the nebulizer by either measuring out the correct amount of medication or utilizing a unit dose vial. The mouthpiece and compressor tubing are then connected to the nebulizer and the compressor is turned on. The patient should be instructed to place the mouthpiece between the teeth, sealing the lips, and take deep breaths until the nebulizer sputters, indicating it is out of medication. The machine should be turned off at this point. The nebulizer tubing is washed after each use in warm soapy water, while the mouthpiece, nebulizer, and other parts should be rinsed in warm water. All parts should be allowed to air dry on a clean towel.

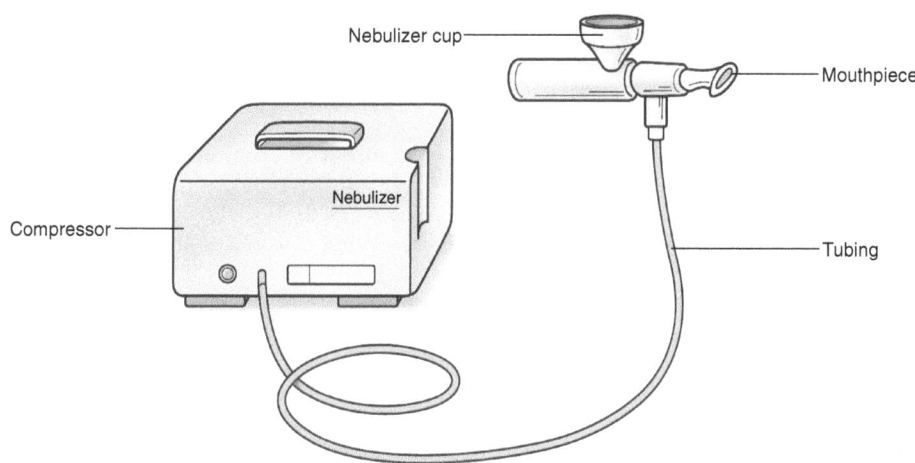

FIGURE 18-2. Nebulizer. A nebulizer changes liquid medicine into fine droplets (in aerosol or mist form) that are inhaled through a mouthpiece or mask. A nebulizer may be used instead of a metered dose inhaler (MDI). It is powered by a compressed air machine and plugs into an electrical outlet. Portable nebulizers, powered by an internal battery or cigarette lighter, are available for individuals requiring treatments away from home.

SUMMARY

The respiratory system provides the essential oxygen and carbon dioxide gas exchange needed to sustain homeostasis and, ultimately, life. A respiratory system that has been damaged or does not function properly has direct adverse effects on quality of life. Once damage has occurred to the respiratory system, it is commonly irreversible, but further progression is preventable in the majority of cases. Progression can be prevented or slowed through close monitoring with the use of pulmonary function tests (PFTs): arterial blood gas measurements (ABGs), oxygen saturation (O_2 sat) measurements, and spirometry. PFTs provide crucial information on progression of the disease and the effects of therapy, including identifying the need for adjustment. Education on the proper administration and storage of inhaled medications is key to successful management of respiratory conditions.

ACKNOWLEDGMENT

The author wishes to acknowledge and thank Christina Bell, PharmD, and Sandra B. Earle, PharmD, BCPS, authors of this chapter in the first edition of this book.

REFERENCES

1. Pulmonary function tests. https://www.nhlbi.nih.gov/health-topics/pulmonary-function-tests. Accessed April 20, 2021.
2. American Thoracic Society. Using your metered dose inhaler. *Am J Respir Crit Care Med*. 2014;190:5–6. https://www.thoracic.org/patients/patient-resources/resources/metered-dose-inhaler-mdi.pdf. Accessed April 20, 2021.

CHAPTER RESOURCES

Herrier RN, Apgar DA, Boyce RW, Foster SL. Asthma and chronic obstructive pulmonary disease (COPD). In: *Patient Assessment in Pharmacy*. New York, NY: McGraw-Hill; 2015; chapter 21. https://accesspharmacy.mhmedical.com/content.aspx?bookid=1074&sectionid=62364556. Accessed April 20, 2021.

Inhalers. https://my.clevelandclinic.org/health/drugs/8694-inhalers. Accessed April 20, 2021.

Home Nebulizer. https://my.clevelandclinic.org/health/drugs/4254-home-nebulizer. Accessed April 20, 2021.

Know How to Use Your Asthma Inhaler. https://www.cdc.gov/asthma/inhaler_video/default.htm. Accessed May 22, 2022.

Teaching Kids About Spirometry. http://kidshealth.org/parent/system/medical/spirometry.html. Accessed April 20, 2021.

Video for DPI Teaching. http://www.mayoclinic.com/health/asthma/MM00406. Accessed April 20, 2021.

REVIEW QUESTIONS

1. Identify the components of the upper and lower respiratory systems and describe the primary function of each.

2. Describe the importance of respiratory gas exchange.

3. Explain the process of respiratory gas exchange between oxygen and carbon dioxide.

4. List the delivery devices available for inhaled medications.

5. What are pulmonary function tests and why are they important?

6. What is a spacer and who could benefit from the use of a spacer?

Chapter 19

Disorders of the Respiratory System

Celeste Voight, PharmD, BCPS

KEY TERMS AND DEFINITIONS

Asthma—chronic lung disease that results from inflammation and bronchoconstriction of the lower airways, characterized by difficulty breathing.

Bronchoconstriction—constriction of the smooth muscle surrounding the airways in the lungs, resulting in a narrowing of the airways, wheezing, and shortness of breath.

Chronic obstructive pulmonary disease (COPD)—chronic lung disease that results in irreversible damage to the lung tissue.

Controller/prevention medication—medications that are taken on a regular schedule to control a disease or prevent its effects, even when symptoms are absent.

Cystic fibrosis (CF)—an inherited condition that causes the production of thickened mucus, resulting in damage primarily to the lungs and pancreas.

Environmental trigger—an environmental factor such as pollen, animal dander, pollution, or tobacco that stimulates a reaction.

Exacerbation—acute worsening of disease symptoms.

Hypersensitivity reaction—an undesirable effect of the body's immune system to an antigen.

Reliever/rescue medications—medications that relax the muscles surrounding the airways within minutes when administered during an episode of bronchoconstriction.

Wheezing—a continuous whistling sound made by constricted airways.

DOI 10.37573/9781585286638.019

LEARNING OBJECTIVES

After completing this chapter, you should be able to

1. Define asthma, chronic obstructive pulmonary disease, and cystic fibrosis.

2. Recall the pathophysiology of asthma, chronic obstructive pulmonary disease, and cystic fibrosis.

3. List nonpharmacologic therapy options for asthma, chronic obstructive pulmonary disease, and cystic fibrosis.

4. List pharmacotherapy options for asthma, chronic obstructive pulmonary disease, and cystic fibrosis.

5. Recognize differences in pharmacotherapy for asthma and chronic obstructive pulmonary disease.

6. State generic and brand names of medications used to treat asthma, chronic obstructive pulmonary disease, and cystic fibrosis.

7. Recognize the doses and common side effects of pharmacologic therapies for disorders of the respiratory system.

Chronic respiratory illness is a growing problem in the United States and the world. The most frequently diagnosed chronic respiratory disease states are asthma, chronic obstructive pulmonary disease (COPD), and cystic fibrosis (CF).[1] Asthma affects roughly 300 million individuals worldwide, with an estimated 25 million of those individuals in the United States.[1,2] Although prevalence rates of asthma increased significantly from 2001 to 2010, the rates remained relatively stable from 2010 to 2017.[1] COPD is currently the fourth leading cause of death worldwide, but as the death rate continues to grow, it is projected to become the third leading cause of death in years to come.[3,4] Due to continued exposure to COPD risk factors and the aging population, the disease burden is likely to increase in the coming years.[4] Cystic fibrosis is a life-threatening condition that affects approximately 70,000 individuals worldwide, with about half of those residing in the United States. In the 1970s, patients were not expected to live past their mid-teens; however, advances in the treatment of CF have extended their life expectancy exponentially.[5,6] These chronic conditions require both nonpharmacologic and pharmacologic approaches to optimize management. Although

these diseases are treated with many of the same drugs, it is important to note that they are used in different ways for each disease. The majority of medications are given via inhalation to limit the systemic side effects of the drugs. It is imperative that patients know how to properly administer inhaled medications–for more information on this see Chapter 18. Patients' quality of life and longevity can be improved by using medications appropriately.[2] This chapter discusses the pathophysiology and management of each condition.

PRACTICE POINT

Many community pharmacies provide health-related literature about respiratory disease and smoking cessation. Pharmacy technicians can contribute to the distribution of this valuable information.

ASTHMA

CASE STUDY

Robert Juner is a 20-year-old college student who runs into the pharmacy wearing jogging clothes and having difficulty breathing. You have not seen him in the pharmacy before. He asks where your asthma medications are with single words. He finds Primatene Mist on the shelf before you can help him, opens the box, and inhales three puffs of medication very quickly. Then he comes to the counter to pay for it. He is breathing a little easier now, but his hands are shaking as he pays for the medication. You hear some whistling sounds in his chest, and he still seems to be in some distress.

Pathophysiology

Asthma is a chronic lung disease that results from persistent inflammation of the lower lung airways. The result of chronic lower lung airway inflammation is bronchoconstriction and decreased airflow, which in turn causes difficulty breathing.

The lung inflammation and airway bronchoconstriction are normally reversible with the use of medications, or occasionally the symptoms will resolve spontaneously (Figure 19-1).[7]

Symptoms of reduced airflow include nighttime and early morning cough, wheezing (a whistling breath sound), shortness of breath, and chest tightness. These symptoms are commonly associated with exercise, but may occur spontaneously or in relation to a known allergen. Although these symptoms are the most common, each symptom does not have to be present for a diagnosis of asthma to be made. For example, a chronic cough may be the only symptom of asthma. The frequency at which these symptoms occur vary significantly, from daily (*persistent asthma*) to periodic (*intermittent asthma*). In addition to variable frequency, severity also differs among patients. Appropriate treatment should be individually tailored to fit each patient's needs based their symptoms, frequency, and severity.[8]

Asthma is a complex condition that is not completely understood, but studies strongly support inherited genetic predisposition in combination with environmental triggers. Common environmental triggers of asthma include airborne allergens (dust mites, animals, molds, and pollen), viral infections (eg, respiratory syncytial virus [RSV] and rhinovirus), environmental pollution, tobacco, and some foods and additives (eg, wheat, eggs, preservatives). For an individual who has a genetic predisposition for asthma, exposure to an environmental trigger may activate what is known as a hypersensitivity reaction. A hypersensitivity reaction can be thought of as an allergic reaction that causes an influx of immune system defensive cells to flood the lungs and their airways. The influx of these defensive cells causes an increase in mucus production, narrowing of the airways, and overall lung airway inflammation, resulting in bronchoconstriction. The typical asthma symptoms of coughing, wheezing, shortness of breath, and chest tightness are a direct result of the inflammation caused by the hypersensitivity reaction. Collectively, the acute worsening of typical asthma symptoms, in combination with difficulty breathing, is referred to as an asthma exacerbation. The typical course for asthma is periods of exacerbation followed by periods of remission, during which asthma symptoms are not evident.[7]

The consequence of untreated chronic inflammation of the lung airways is an increased frequency of asthma exacerbations, possibly causing irreversible lung structural changes (*airway remodeling*). These structural changes can lead to a reduction in the ability of the lung to fully exchange air and completely oxygenate the body, resulting in an increased severity of asthma symptoms. Once airway remodeling is present, the ability to reverse inflammation and bronchoconstriction with medications is reduced (see Figure 19-1). However, with proper asthma therapy and good symptom control these structural changes can be prevented.[2]

Asthma is a condition that most often arises during childhood, with the majority of patients being diagnosed by the age of 5 years.[2] A common theory, the hygiene hypothesis, suggests that susceptible individuals develop asthma and allergies because the allergic immunologic system develops instead of the system to fight infections.[7] Simply

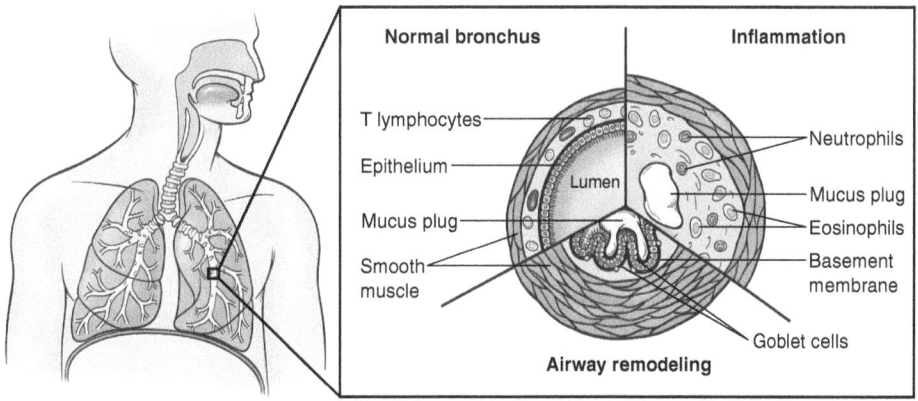

FIGURE 19-1. Asthmatic changes in the bronchus. The upper left section represents an unaffected, normal bronchus. The upper right section shows changes seen in the bronchus in inflammation. (Inflammatory cells infiltrate, producing a cascade of events that fill the lumen with debris.) The bottom section shows airway remodeling (permanent structural changes in the airway that cause a constricted lumen).

put, individuals exposed to more bacteria, common allergens, and less antibiotic therapy have demonstrated a lower risk of asthma.[7] Of those patients with childhood asthma, 30%–40% will have symptoms persist into adulthood.[1] This chapter focuses on the management of adult asthma.

Types of Asthma

1. Acute—severe asthma symptoms that can progress quickly to an emergent, potentially fatal situation. Patients often experience cough, wheezing, and severe shortness of breath and chest tightness. Patients also often have difficulty talking.

2. Chronic—asthma symptoms progress from severe exacerbation to remission, where normal asthma symptoms (cough, wheezing, shortness of breath, and chest tightness) may fluctuate between remission and acute exacerbation. The time between exacerbation and remission is variable and generally depends on asthma control. An exacerbation may be brought on by an environmental trigger such as an allergen, virus, pollution, or tobacco smoke.

3. Cough-variant—a chronic cough is the most bothersome asthma symptom and may be the only asthma symptom experienced. The cough generally occurs during the night in this type of asthma.

4. Drug-induced—an asthma attack that is triggered after ingestion of a drug. Aspirin and nonsteroidal anti-inflammatory drugs (NSAIDs) have both been associated with drug-induced asthma. Beta blockers have also been known to cause drug-induced asthma.

5. Exercise-induced—asthma symptoms are triggered by exercise. Exercise-induced asthma typically occurs after exercise has ended. The exact cause of exercise-induced asthma is not fully understood, but it is thought to be related to hyperventilation that induces constriction of the airway. Exercise-induced asthma will affect most asthma sufferers at some point during their disease course. It is also important to note that for some asthma sufferers, exercise may be the only time that asthma symptoms are experienced, and they have otherwise normal lung function at all other times. Exercise-induced asthma occurs more frequently in regions where the air is cold and dry and seems to be improved in regions where the air is warm and humid. Exercise should not be avoided by patients with exercise-induced asthma but, rather, preventative measures undertaken to ensure adequate exercise capacity.

6. Nocturnal—asthma that occurs during the night while the patient is sleeping. Lung function decreases during the night, falling to its lowest point at approximately 3:00 to 4:00 in the morning. The possible causes of nocturnal asthma include normal nocturnal hormonal functions, exposure to allergens or pollutants, gastroesophageal reflux, obstructive sleep apnea, or sinusitis.

CASE STUDY

From what type of asthma does Robert appear to be suffering?

Asthma Goals

The overall goal of asthma therapy is aimed at increasing asthma control. The Global Initiative for Asthma, *Global Strategy for Asthma Management and Prevention*, states that long-term goals are risk reduction and symptom control.[8] The US Department of Health and Human Services defines asthma control in two separate parts:[2]

1. Reduce impairment

   a. Prevention of chronic asthma symptoms
   b. Fast-acting asthma relief with a short-acting beta$_2$-agonist when needed ≤2 days a week
   c. Maintain (near) normal pulmonary function
   d. Maintain normal activities of daily living (including exercise, other physical activity, and attendance at work or school)
   e. Meet patient and family expectations of and satisfaction with asthma care

2. Reduce risk

   a. Prevent recurrent exacerbations of asthma and minimize the need for emergency department visits or hospitalizations
   b. Prevent progressive loss of lung function; for children, prevent reduced lung growth
   c. Provide optimal pharmacologic therapy with minimal to no adverse effects

Nonpharmacologic Therapy

Nonpharmacologic therapy is an essential component to achieving good asthma control. This may include anything, other than medication therapy, that results in a reduction of asthma symptoms. For example, identifying and avoiding asthma triggers, close management of coexisting disease states, in-depth patient education, and the development of an asthma action plan.

Triggers are factors or conditions that are associated with a worsening in asthma symptoms. See Table 19-1 for examples. The identification of asthma triggers is the first step toward gaining good asthma control. Patient awareness of the environmental triggers that worsen asthma symptoms is crucial in controlling their symptoms. Once they are identified, patients can work to modify exposure to potential triggers in an attempt to reduce or even eliminate particular symptoms and achieve better asthma control. When other health conditions are not well managed, good asthma control is more difficult to achieve. It is important for patients to achieve control of those conditions to optimize their asthma management.

Patient education is an important component of managing any condition but is especially important for managing asthma. The patient should be educated in identifying asthma triggers, recognizing early signs and symptoms of an exacerbation, and how to properly use the inhaler device. Additional information regarding proper inhaler and nebulizer use can be found in Chapter 18. Providing patients with detailed knowledge empowers them to take an active role in their health and managing their condition. Proper education gives each patient the opportunity to achieve greater asthma control through avoidance of triggers, early treatment, and proper inhaler technique.

A written asthma action plan is critical to achieving good asthma control. An asthma action plan is a written set of instructions created by a patient with the healthcare provider. These instructions provide guidance for the patient based on lung function. The plan contains information on daily controller medications, reliever medications, trigger avoidance, and explicit directions on when to seek medical attention for an exacerbation. The action plan should be routinely updated to reflect changes in the patient's medications.[2,7,8]

Pharmacologic Therapy

Asthma pharmacotherapy has two objectives:

1. Quick relief of acute bronchoconstriction and other asthma symptoms

2. Long-term prevention of bronchoconstriction and other asthma symptoms

See Medication Table 19-1. (Medication Tables are located at the end of the chapter).

Reliever/rescue medications are fast-acting medications taken on an as-needed basis for immediate relief of an asthma exacerbation. These medications directly target the bronchoconstriction and provide relief of asthma symptoms within minutes. The reliever medications have a short duration of action (approximately 4–6 hours), which allows them to be safe with multiple uses (up to three times at 20-minute intervals) until adequate relief of asthma symptoms has been obtained. All patients diagnosed with asthma should have a reliever medication available to provide fast relief of bronchoconstriction during acute asthma exacerbations. As-needed reliever medication may provide sufficient asthma control for those patients with intermittent mild asthma or exercise-induced bronchoconstriction when used prior to exercise. Frequency of reliever inhaler use is commonly monitored as a means of evaluating overall asthma control. The need for a quick-relief medication more than twice a week is an indication of poor asthma control and indicates the need for a controller or preventative asthma medication to gain better control.

Controller/prevention medications provide long-term control and prevention of asthma symptoms by decreasing the inflammation that leads to bronchoconstriction and the

TABLE 19-1. Asthma Triggers[7]

Categories	Examples
Allergens	Dust mites, pet dander, airborne pollen (grass, weeds, trees)
Environmental	Wood smoke, occupational exposure, strong odors, cold air
Lifestyle	Stress, exercise, tobacco smoking
Medications	Acetaminophen, aspirin, nonsteroidal anti-inflammatory drugs; nonselective beta-blockers
Infections	Influenza, rhinovirus
Comorbidities	Obesity, obstructive sleep apnea (OSA), allergic rhinitis, gastroesophageal reflux disease (GERD)

other asthma symptoms. This class of medications is used to treat persistent asthma that cannot be controlled with the use of a reliever medication alone. Preventative medications are taken on a routine basis, generally once or twice a day at specified times. They should be taken routinely, whether or not the patient is currently experiencing asthma symptoms, as the goal of these medications is long-term reduction of asthma symptoms. Controller medications should not be used on an as-needed basis due to their delayed onset and longer duration of action. Use of controller medications when immediate relief is desired could result in lack of immediate efficacy or toxic side effects. Standard pharmacologic management of asthma is based on recommendations from the National Asthma Education and Prevention Program and Global Initiative for Asthma, each providing a stepwise approach for asthma therapy management.[2,8]

The goal of asthma pharmacotherapy is to achieve and maintain good asthma control with the least amount of medication possible. The first step is to employ nonpharmacologic measures and only consider pharmacologic therapy if asthma is still not adequately controlled. The first pharmacotherapy given to all patients is a reliever medication, which may be the only medication needed for some patients. If good asthma control is not achieved with the use of a reliever medication alone, the next step is the addition of a controller medication. All steps (step = addition/subtraction of medication or the increase/decrease of medication dose) of therapy are trialed for a sufficient amount of time, and then asthma control is reevaluated before any adjustments in treatment are made. Medication doses are increased and/or the additional medications are added to the therapy regimen until adequate asthma control is achieved. Once a patient has maintained good asthma control for at least three months, decreasing doses and/or removing medications may be considered. This continuous cycle, personalized asthma management, consists of assessing, adjusting, and reviewing the patient's response.[8]

PRACTICE POINT

Patient medication regimens should be reviewed on a routine basis to identify changes in therapy, including the addition of new medications and the discontinuation of any that are no longer used. This process may be referred to as a complete medication review (CMR).

Bronchodilators

Bronchodilators provide rapid relief of bronchoconstriction in the lower lung airways. Many have a quick onset of action and provide rapid relief of asthma symptoms. Bronchodilators have minimal effects on the inflammatory process that is the cause of bronchoconstriction; therefore, their main role in asthma treatment is control of acute symptoms and exacerbations.

Recall (from Chapter 4) that the autonomic nervous system (ANS) regulates many vital body activities, including heart rate, secretions, and breathing. The sympathetic system (SANS) is generally described as the *fight or flight* system as it increases heart rate and dilates the bronchi, while the parasympathetic system (PANS) decreases the heart rate, increases secretions, and constricts the bronchi. A stable internal environment is maintained through the activation and deactivation of these two systems. Sympathetic agonists stimulate receptors in the SANS. Beta agonists are more specific in that they stimulate mainly the beta receptors of the sympathetic system. β_1 (beta$_1$) receptors are located mainly in the heart and kidneys, while β_2 (beta$_2$) receptors are found primarily in the bronchi.

Epinephrine: Quick-Relief Medication

Epinephrine is a hormone that occurs naturally in the body and is released from the adrenal gland in emergency situations. It acts at all types of SANS receptors, including those in the lungs. When administered exogenously (as a medication), epinephrine is a very potent bronchodilator that can be given either as a systemic injection or inhaled directly into the lungs. Epinephrine administration results in profound bronchodilation very quickly, but the duration of action is short, only lasting approximately 60–90 minutes. Epinephrine also has a significant excitatory effect on the heart that limits its usefulness in the treatment of asthma. The excitatory effect of epinephrine on the heart includes symptoms such as fast heart rate and abnormal heartbeat and/or chest pain—all of which are amplified at increased doses.

There are currently two inhaled epinephrine dosage forms available over the counter, a nebulizer solution and a metered-dose inhaler (MDI). The nebulizer products are Asthmanefrin Refill and S2 (Racepinephrine), both containing 2.25% epinephrine. Primatene Mist, the MDI, like the other inhaled bronchodilators, only treats the symptoms, with no effect on the underlying cause of asthma. The use of these products is not recommended for the routine management of asthma. The involvement of a healthcare professional in the diagnosis and management of asthma is important not only to avoid the possibility of drug-induced side effects, but also to ensure good asthma control to avoid long-term irreversible lung structural changes.

ALERT!

It is important to note there are currently two Primatene products available over the counter. In addition to Primatene Mist, there are Primatene tablets. Though the products have the same brand name, the active ingredients are different. Primatene asthma tablets contain ephedrine and guaifenesin, while Primatene Mist contains epinephrine.

CASE?

When Robert comes to the counter to pay for the Primatene Mist, how might a pharmacy technician be able to help him?

Beta$_2$ agonists

The main action of beta$_2$ agonists is relaxation of the smooth muscles of the lung airways, resulting in dilation of the airways and relief of bronchoconstriction. Beta$_2$ agonists have no effect on the inflammatory process that leads to bronchoconstriction and therefore provides only symptomatic asthma relief, with little direct effect on the heart. They can be separated into two groups based on duration of action: short-acting beta$_2$ agonists (SABAs) and long-acting beta$_2$ agonists (LABAs).

SABAs used in the treatment of asthma include albuterol (Ventolin, Proventil, and ProAir) and levalbuterol (Xopenex). These may be used as reliever medications during acute asthma attacks. SABAs can produce rapid relief of acute asthma symptoms during an acute exacerbation. The National Asthma Education and Prevention Program *2020 Focused Updates to the Asthma Management Guidelines* report has updated recommendations regarding the use of SABAs.[2] The report states that SABAs administered as needed remain the preferred management for intermittent asthma. However, the updated guidelines now recommend the use of combination low-dose inhaled corticosteroid (ICS)-formoterol as needed over SABAs in select individuals with persistent asthma. These changes in recommendations

better align with the current Global Initiative for Asthma guideline.[8] For adults and adolescents 12 years and older, the 2022 GINA guidelines recommend as needed low-dose ICS-formoterol therapy as the preferred reliever. However, the 2020 NAEPP report only recommends low-dose ICS-formoterol as reliever therapy for patients on Step 3 or 4. As discussed earlier, bronchodilators (SABAs) do not have any effect on the underlying cause of asthma and provide only rapid symptomatic asthma relief. Consequently, regular use of SABAs is associated with increased airway inflammation, while over-use shows an increased risk of asthma exacerbations. The use of SABAs in mild intermittent asthma must be monitored closely to assure adequate asthma control. Asthma is considered to be under good control if reliever therapies are used on two or fewer days per week. Exercise-induced bronchospasm may be prevented with the use of SABAs prior to exercise. SABAs are available in two inhalation preparations: inhaler and nebulizer solution. Inhalation reduces the incidence of side effects and is associated with a faster onset of action.

The duration of action of SABAs also varies, with the inhalation preparation having a shorter duration of action. The typical SABA inhaler dose is one to two puffs every 4–6 hours (depending on medication) as needed or three times at 20-minute intervals. SABAs are generally well tolerated, with side effects most notable at high doses. Side effects include angina (chest pain), atrial fibrillation (rapid heartbeat), arrhythmia (problems with heartbeat), cough, and tremor. SABAs should be used cautiously in patients with a history of cardiac problems.

CASE?

What treatment for Robert's asthma is suggested by the guidelines described?

Long-acting beta$_2$ agonists (LABAs) are similar to SABAs in that they also provide symptomatic relief of bronchoconstriction. LABAs vary in their onset of action, but can provide bronchodilation for a much longer time than SABAs. The duration of action is at least 12 hours, which limits administration to once or twice daily. The majority of LABAs have a slower onset of action when compared with a SABA, so they must not be used as a reliever medication. Formoterol, a LABA, has a similar onset of action to those of SABAs. Formoterol, in combination with an ICS, is the only LABA that may be used as a reliever therapy for acute asthma symptoms. The role of LABAs in asthma therapy is prevention of chronic bronchoconstriction, as they do not treat the underlying disease process causing the bronchoconstriction. Currently, LABAs (except formoterol) are only indicated for use as part of combination therapy with ICSs for persistent asthma patients unable to achieve adequate asthma control with an ICS alone.

LABA monotherapy is not recommended due to a lack of data suggesting an improvement in asthma control, and a small but significant increase in risk of asthma-related death. LABAs should be taken routinely on a daily basis, regardless of asthma symptoms and should be continued even when the patient is not experiencing any asthma symptoms. When LABAs are taken routinely in combination with an ICS, they can help to prevent irreversible airway changes that can occur with uncontrolled asthma. Due to their longer duration of action, LABAs are conveniently taken once or twice daily. These are generally well-tolerated medications, with the most common side effects reported being headache, hypertension, dizziness, and chest pain.

Muscarinic antagonists

The primary action of muscarinic antagonists is blocking the effects of acetylcholine at the muscarinic receptors, blocking the action of acetylcholine at these receptors preventing bronchoconstriction and reducing mucus secretion. These agents can be separated into two groups based on duration of action: short-acting muscarinic antagonist (SAMA) and long-acting muscarinic antagonist (LAMA). The use of muscarinic antagonists for asthma management is limited, as they are predominantly used for COPD. A SAMA/SABA (e.g. ipratropium/albuterol) combination may be used for the treatment of an acute asthma exacerbation, either via a nebulizer or MDI. One LAMA, tiotropium, is approved as maintenance therapy for moderate to severe asthma for those 12 years and older. It is more commonly prescribed in the following situations: 1) in addition to an ICS and LABA or 2) in addition to an ICS for patients intolerant of LABA therapy. For additional information on muscarinic antagonist therapy, see the COPD section.

CASE?

Might long-acting beta$_2$ agonists (LABAs) be dangerous for Robert?

Theophylline

Theophylline provides mild to moderate bronchodilation and, as a result, relief of asthma symptoms. Theophylline also possesses a mild anti-inflammatory effect, which reduces some of the inflammation that is causing the bronchodilation and asthma symptoms. Although theophylline therapy can address both the cause and symptoms of asthma, it is not a potent bronchodilator or anti-inflammatory agent. In addition to limited efficacy in asthma, side effects are common and can be life threatening. Therefore, sustained-release theophylline is not recommended for routine use in the management of asthma.

Theophylline use for the treatment of asthma is limited because of the availability of better medications. Theophylline has a very small range between where it is therapeutic (helpful) and toxic (harmful). Thus, theophylline blood concentrations must be monitored very closely via blood draws to assure good therapeutic outcome without serious toxic side effects. It is also highly reactive with other medications and has a serious side effect profile that increases with increased doses. The most common side effects associated with theophylline are tachycardia, nausea, vomiting, headache, dizziness, jitteriness, and insomnia. Persistent vomiting is a sign of theophylline toxicity (poisoning). The theophylline dose should never be doubled, even if the previous dose was missed, due to dose-related increased side effects and drug interactions, as well as the possibility of death.

Theophylline is available as a liquid, sustained-released capsules, and extended-release tablets.[9] The dose is individualized for each patient based on weight and then adjusted based on blood theophylline concentrations. This is intended to assure that each patient receives just enough theophylline to achieve good asthma control, but not so much that dose-related side effects would be likely. Oral extended- or sustained-release theophylline is typically dosed once daily.

Glucocorticoid Therapy: Prevention Medication

As discussed in Chapter 9, hormonal steroids are produced naturally by the adrenal glands. While mineralocorticoids function to regulate the retention of salt and water, and the adrenal androgens regulate the reproductive system, glucocorticoids act on metabolism and the immune system. The effects of glucocorticoid steroids on the immune system make them a useful option for the treatment of asthma, and they will be the focus of this discussion.

Glucocorticoid steroids act on glucocorticoid receptors to elicit a specific function, which is based on the location of the target receptor. Glucocorticoid receptors are found throughout the body, making glucocorticoid steroids capable of causing systemic (body-wide) effects on the immune system and metabolism, including both desirable and undesirable effects. The challenge with using glucocorticoid therapy for treatment of asthma has been specifically targeting the respiratory system while minimizing effects on the rest of the body. The development of inhaled glucocorticoid therapy has helped enhance the desired anti-inflammatory effects of the steroid while reducing the undesired side effects by localizing therapy to the lungs through inhalation.

It should be noted that, while glucocorticoid is the technical name for this class of hormonal steroids that have an effect on the immune system, they are also commonly referred to as corticosteroids. The terms glucocorticoids and corticosteroids are used interchangeably when discussing this class of hormonal steroids. Glucocorticoid hormonal steroid therapy that is administered through inhalation is often referred to as inhaled corticosteroids (ICSs).

ICSs relieve inflammation through a reduction in the body's normal immune response. Thus, they directly treat the underlying cause of bronchoconstriction and asthma symptoms, chronic inflammation. In asthma, the immune system is activated by an environmental trigger that induces a hypersensitivity reaction, which stimulates defensive cells to flood into the lungs and cause inflammation and bronchoconstriction. ICSs are able to block the immune system response to the environmental trigger so that defensive cells are never stimulated into action.

ICSs do not have a direct effect on bronchoconstriction and should not be used as a reliever medication, unless in combination with formoterol. ICSs primarily function as controller therapy that, when taken daily, significantly reduce the risk of asthma exacerbations and hospitalizations. When ICSs are used regularly these medications typically result in an overall decrease in bronchoconstriction, a direct result of controlling the underlying inflammation, and this can reduce reliever inhaler usage. It is important that all asthmatic patients have a reliever inhaler (SABA or ICS-formoterol combination) for rapid asthma relief, even if they are on daily controller therapy with an ICS.

ICSs are the most effective class of medications for achieving and sustaining good long-term asthma control and are the first-line medication therapy for any type of persistent asthma. ICS-formoterol as needed may be used for the management of mild intermittent symptoms.[2] ICSs are typically administered as one to two puffs once to twice daily, but the exact dosing regimen is dependent on the particular medication. The dose of ICSs is highly variable because it depends on patient-specific factors and asthma severity. The exact dose must be determined through medication trials and individual patient response. Due to the side effects associated with corticosteroid therapy, the lowest effective dose should be used, to minimize the likelihood of systemic side effects associated with ICSs. Doses can be divided among three broad ranges: low, medium, or high daily dose. Leukotriene modifiers are considered alternative controller therapy or add-on therapy

to ICS therapy.[1,2] Alternative therapies are reserved for when patients are unable to tolerate ICS therapy at all or unable to tolerate dose increases necessary to achieve good asthma control. Leukotriene modifier therapy has been proven less effective than ICS for the treatment of asthma, especially in the reduction of exacerbations. Consequently, leukotriene modifiers are not recommended as first-line agents for the management of asthma, but may be used for the prevention of exercise-induced bronchoconstriction.

Leukotriene modifiers available include montelukast (Singulair), zafirlukast (Accolate), and zileuton (Zyflo). NAEPP 2020 and GINA 2022 consider oral leukotriene-modifying agents as alternative first-line controller therapy for adults and adolescents 12 years and older. Montelukast is approved for use in patients 12 months to adult and may be preferred for younger patients based on once daily dosing and variety of available preparations. The different oral preparations available include tablet, chewable tablet, and granule packet. The typical once daily dose for montelukast is 4–5 mg for children and 10 mg for patients aged 15 years or older. Montelukast has been associated with behavioral and mood changes, although the most common side effects for leukotriene modifiers are less severe, and include abdominal pain, cough, dizziness, and nasal congestion. Liver enzymes must be closely monitored as zafirlukast has been associated with liver impairment.

Mast Cell Stabilizer: Prevention Medication

Cromolyn sodium primarily functions as an asthma preventative agent aimed at increasing long-term asthma control. It targets the underlying inflammation that is caused when mast cells are stimulated by an environmental trigger. These mast cells release histamine and stimulate other cells to flood the airways, resulting in an increase in mucus production and bronchoconstriction. This medication has no direct effect on the symptoms of asthma, so is not generally used as a reliever medication for an acute exacerbation. Cromolyn sodium is not recommended for routine use due to the availability of more effective therapies, but may be considered an alternative to ICS therapy for control of mild persistent asthma, prevention of exercise-induced bronchoconstriction, and allergy-induced asthma when administered prior to a known exposure. Overall, cromolyn sodium has limited use in chronic asthma management due to its minimal efficacy compared to ICSs.

Cromolyn sodium is available as a nebulizer solution. It takes approximately 4–6 weeks of treatment to achieve the full effect, although some improvement is often seen in 1–2 weeks. Cromolyn sodium is dosed four times a day until the maximum effectiveness is reached, indicated by increased asthma control, at which time the dosing can be tapered to the lowest effective dose. It is very well tolerated, with the most common complaints being transient coughing and mild wheezing.

CASE?

If Robert continues to have asthma symptoms, but ICSs are not indicated or tolerable, what other treatment might his healthcare provider prescribe?

Immunomodulator Therapy: Prevention Medication

Immunomodulator medications are sometimes referred to as monoclonal antibodies. They are a class of medications that have been designed using a combination of human and mouse protein to target a specific immune system cell, with the intention of either activating or deactivating the cell. By targeting specific cells within the inflammatory pathway, inflammation is directly prevented along with indirectly preventing the symptoms associated with inflammation. This therapy can result in a reduction of unwanted side effects because the medication has an effect only on the particular cell that induces the asthma symptoms. Targets for these drugs include immunoglobulin E (IgE) for allergic asthma and interleukin (IL)5/5R and IL4R for eosinophilic asthma. In recent years there has been an increase in the types of available immunomodulators for the management of asthma. Current immunomodulators available for the treatment of asthma include omalizumab (Xolair; anti-IgE), dupilumab (Dupixent; anti-IL4R), mepolizumab (Nucala;

ALERT!

Omalizumab administration can result in a severe allergic reaction known as an anaphylaxis. This reaction is triggered when the immune system recognizes the mouse protein portion of omalizumab as foreign and rallies to fight off the foreign substance that has entered the body. The result is a severe life-threatening reaction that must be treated immediately. To minimize the risk, patients initially receive therapy while being observed by a clinician for up to 2 hours following injection. Select patients may be approved for self-administration based on a risk assessment.

---

anti-IL5), reslizumab (Cinqair; anti-IL5), benralizumab (Fasenra; anti-IL5R), and tezepelumab (Tezspire; anti-TSLP). In many cases, these medications are effective only in specific types of asthma. For example, omalizumab targets the immune system cell, IgE, that is released when activated by an allergen; therefore it is only useful for patients with allergic asthma. Immunomodulator therapy is currently recommended for difficult-to-treat patients with an allergic or eosinophilic asthma diagnosis uncontrolled on high-dose ICS/LABA therapy. The addition of immunomodulator therapy may allow a dose reduction of ICS therapy.

These immunomodulator therapies are not available orally due to inactivation of the drug in the gastrointestinal tract. Consequently, they must be administered subcutaneously (SUBQ) or intravenously (IV) at regular intervals. The

---

PRACTICE POINT

Omalizumab vials must be reconstituted with sterile water prior to administration. Using a 3-mL syringe and 18-gauge needle, a total of 1.4 mL of sterile water is added to the vial. After the addition of the sterile water, the medication vial must be kept upright and gently swirled for 1 minute to ensure that the entire product is evenly wet. The medication must be gently swirled for 5–10 seconds every 5 minutes until the medication is completely dissolved. The reconstitution process takes approximately 20 minutes but no more than 40 minutes. If the medication has not dissolved within 40 minutes, it should be discarded. The reconstituted medication should be inverted for 15 seconds prior to withdrawal. Using a 3-mL syringe and 18-gauge needle, all medication should be removed from the inverted vial. After all medication has been removed, the needle plunger should be pulled back to the end of the barrel to ensure that all medication is removed from the vial. The needle should be changed to a 25-gauge for subcutaneous injection. All air, large bubbles, and excess solution should be discarded from the syringe at this time, preserving the 1.2-mL (150 mg) dose. A thin layer of small bubbles may be present.

doses of these medications may vary from weight-based (mg/kg) to fixed dosing based on immune cell levels. The most common side effects of these medications include injection site reactions (pain and bruising) and headache.

Combination Therapy: Prevention Medication

Combination therapy can consist of two or more medications within a single inhaler. As discussed earlier, the most effective medications for achieving long-term asthma control are ICSs, and as such, they are the first-line medication for intermittent and persistent uncontrolled asthma. When ICS medications fail to adequately control asthma symptoms, the next option is to consider either an increase in the ICS dose or the addition of another medication. An increased dose of the ICS may not be a viable option due to the increased side effects associated with higher doses. The addition of another asthma medication from a different class may significantly improve management of asthma symptoms as the two medications are both targeting the condition but at different points in the pathway. The addition of two medications from different classes can result in a greater reduction of asthma symptoms as both medications work together compared to either medication alone. The most common asthma medications to be used in combination are ICSs and LABAs. The ICS targets the inflammation and the LABA relieves the bronchoconstriction that is caused by the inflammation. This medication should be taken once or twice a day regardless of asthma symptoms. The side effects associated with combination therapy are consistent with the side effects experienced for each individual medication as discussed above.

CASE?

Why might Robert eventually need more than one kind of inhaler or medication for his asthma? What is the difference between a reliever inhaler and a controller medication?

CHRONIC OBSTRUCTIVE PULMONARY DISEASE

Pathophysiology

COPD is similar to asthma in that it is also a chronic lung disease associated with chronic inflammation of the lung airways and decreased lung airflow. The main difference between asthma and COPD is that the decreased airflow in asthma

CASE STUDY

Joe Button is a 56-year-old man who is a regular patient in your pharmacy. He is classified as GOLD Grade 2/Group C and was started on salmeterol (Serevent Diskus) one puff twice daily about 4 weeks ago in addition to his tiotropium (Spiriva Respimat) two puffs once daily. Joe states that he experiences shortness of breath when going up or down a flight of stairs. He smoked two packs of cigarettes per day for 35 years but quit smoking about 2 years ago. He comes into the pharmacy to have his monthly tiotropium refilled but does not ask to have his salmeterol refilled.

is reversible, whereas in COPD it is only partially reversible and progresses over time. The immune system defensive cells that trigger the inflammation also differ between asthma and COPD. Asthma is typically diagnosed early in life whereas COPD is diagnosed in mid- to late life.

The lung inflammation and damage associated with COPD is due primarily to toxic gas exposure. Toxic gas exposure causes a significant amount of inflammation in the lung airways extending into the lung vasculature. This inflammation, over time, leads to destruction of the lung tissue. As the body attempts to repair the damaged lung tissue, the tissue becomes scarred, making it incapable of fully exchanging air, and the end result is reduced lung function. The most common cause of COPD is smoking tobacco, but occupational pollutant exposure and environmental pollution can also be sources of toxic gas exposure. There also appears to be a genetic predisposition to COPD as not all patients who are exposed to toxic gas develop COPD, although the exact mechanism isn't clearly understood at this time. The risk of COPD is additive, meaning that the risk increases with prolonged exposure times and multiple toxin exposures.

The inflammatory process in COPD differs from asthma, with different cells activating the inflammatory process. The inflammation pathway in COPD activates hypersecretion (excess secretion) of mucus. The cilia cells are also damaged from the toxic gas exposure; consequently, they are unable to protect the lungs from foreign particles as they do when they are functioning normally. The increased mucus production combined with the decreased ability of the cilia to protect the lungs lead to a persistent cough and increased sputum production that are the characteristic symptoms of COPD. The most frequent symptoms associated with COPD include shortness of breath, cough, and increased mucus and sputum production.

The inflammatory damage and resultant decreased lung function associated with COPD are mainly irreversible, and lung function will continue to worsen over time. There are currently no treatment options available to repair and restore damaged lung tissue. The major challenge with COPD is that many patients have already suffered significant irreversible lung tissue damage before a diagnosis of COPD has been established. Typically, COPD is diagnosed later in life and often after many years of repeated toxic gas exposure. Although the lung damage is not able to be fully reversed, further damage can be prevented and the progression of COPD possibly slowed with removal of toxic gas exposure, including smoking cessation.

The disease process of COPD is classified using two different systems. First, the degree of airflow limitation is divided into four grades based on lung function determined by spirometry, discussed in Chapter 18. The four grades are Gold 1, 2, 3, and 4, with the higher numbers correlating with more limited airflow (Table 19-2). Second, the degree of symptom burden is divided among four different groups

TABLE 19-2. COPD Grades[10]

Grade	Spirometry Results (FEV$_1$ % of predicted)
GOLD 1	≥80%
GOLD 2	50%–79%
GOLD 3	30%–49%
GOLD 4	<30%

TABLE 19-3. COPD Groups[10]

Group	Symptom and Exacerbation Assessment
A	1. Lower symptom burden 2. Lower exacerbation risk
B	1. Higher symptom burden 2. Lower exacerbation risk
C	1. Lower symptom burden 2. Higher exacerbation risk
D	1. Higher symptom burden 2. Higher exacerbation risk

based on the severity of symptoms and risk of exacerbations. The four groups are A, B, C, and D (Table 19-3). The initial and follow-up treatment recommendations are based on the appropriate COPD group.

The goals of COPD therapy include the following:[10]

1. Relieve symptoms

2. Improve exercise tolerance

3. Improve health status

4. Prevent disease progression

5. Prevent and treat exacerbations

6. Reduce mortality

Nonpharmacologic Therapy

Smoking cessation therapy reduces the risk of developing COPD and slows the progression of COPD. Smoking cessation should be strongly encouraged as this can slow the decline in lung function and may also improve the typical COPD symptoms of persistent cough and increased sputum production. Although smoking cessation clearly improves overall COPD outcomes, it is difficult for many patients to achieve sustained smoking cessation and it often takes numerous attempts until the patient is successful. By the time of COPD diagnosis, many patients have smoked most of their lives, increasing the difficulty of smoking cessation. (For additional information about smoking cessation therapies, refer to Chapter 7.)

Pulmonary rehabilitation programs can decrease COPD symptoms, enabling patients to resume general activities of daily living (showering, dressing, and walking), resulting in marked improvement in their quality of life. These programs are centered on patient education and involve healthcare providers from several different specialties, including dietary, physical therapy, occupational therapy, and respiratory. Pulmonary rehabilitation programs involve close patient follow up with the healthcare team as they work toward improving their overall health status through guided exercise programs, special breathing techniques, and nutritional education.

Chronic oxygen therapy is recommended to increase the survival of COPD patients suffering from severe hypoxemia (low oxygen level) at rest, and as a quality-of-life improvement mechanism. A reduction in mortality (death) has been proven with continuous oxygen therapy for at least 15 hours per day compared to those not receiving oxygen therapy. It is important that all patients receiving oxygen therapy are instructed on the dangers associated with smoking and concurrent oxygen use.

Pharmacologic Therapy

There are no medications currently available that have been shown to decrease the progressive lung function decline associated with COPD. Instead, the goal of COPD pharmacotherapy is to reduce symptoms and exacerbations in an effort to improve overall health and thereby improve quality of life.; The Global Initiative for Chronic Obstructive Lung Disease provides guidelines for management based on the severity of disease, with medication therapy added in a step-wise approach based on patient response to therapy.[10] This step-wise approach to therapy is similar to that for asthma. Proper inhaler technique may be difficult for some patients with COPD, considering many are elderly and this may have an impact on medication choice. See Medication Table 19-2.

Bronchodilator Therapy

Bronchodilator therapy is the primary treatment for COPD patients. As discussed earlier in the section on pharmacotherapy for asthma, bronchodilator therapy relieves bronchoconstriction by relaxation of the smooth muscles of the lung airways and provides symptomatic COPD relief. The three bronchodilator therapies that may be utilized in COPD are anticholinergics, beta$_2$ agonists, and theophylline. No bronchodilator has been proven to be better than the others in the treatment of COPD.[11] The choice of specific bronchodilator therapy is made based on airflow limitation, symptom burden, exacerbation risk, individual patient response to treatment, and patient-specific factors. Bronchodilator medications are available in short-acting and long-acting preparations and may be administered on an as-needed basis for immediate relief of symptoms or prescribed as routine therapy to prevent and reduce symptoms. Short-acting bronchodilators are preferred for as-needed therapy and are not recommended for use on a routine basis. Long-acting bronchodilators are recommended for use on a routine basis for the prevention and reduction of symptoms. Again, the exact medication regimen should be based on COPD severity and patient-specific factors.

Anticholinergics

The parasympathetic part of the autonomic nervous system (PANS) has many actions, including bronchoconstriction and increased secretions. Agents that interfere with acetylcholine,

the primary neurotransmitter of the PANS, are referred to as anticholinergics, and they oppose PANS actions. Because of these effects (opposing bronchoconstriction and secretions), anticholinergics, especially of the antimuscarinic category (see Chapter 4) are indicated in the treatment of COPD symptoms. Anticholinergic medication is available in short-acting (SAMA—short-acting antimuscarinic) and long-acting (LAMA) preparations. Anticholinergic medications are generally well tolerated, with the most common side effects reported associated with upper respiratory tract infections, palpitations, dry mouth, metallic taste, and throat irritation.

Ipratropium is available as an inhaler and nebulizer solution in two preparations: ipratropium alone and as a combination with the beta$_2$ agonist albuterol. Ipratropium is a short-acting bronchodilator with a duration of about 4–6 hours and an onset of effect of approximately 15–20 minutes. Ipratropium may be used for symptomatic relief on an as-needed basis, but SABAs may be preferred due to a faster onset (approximately 5 minutes). The combination of ipratropium and albuterol has been shown to increase bronchodilation more than either medication given alone.[11] Ipratropium inhalation therapy is typically dosed as one to two inhalations four times a day, with a maximum of 12 inhalations in 24 hours. Nebulizer therapy may be given as one vial three to four times a day, with doses 6–8 hours apart.

There are several different LAMAs available, including tiotropium, umeclidinium, aclidinium, and glycopyrronium bromide. These medications are available in various formulations; either as singular agents or in combination with a LABA and/or ICS. LAMAs have been proven to reduce COPD exacerbations and improve patient response to pulmonary rehabilitation.[11] LAMAs have a greater impact on reducing exacerbations compared to LABAs. Combination therapy with a LABA and a LAMA is a common regimen due to the reduction in exacerbations compared to either given alone. Such combinations are administered once or twice daily due to their long duration of action. Due to the prolonged duration of action and delayed onset of effect compared to SAMAs, these medications are not used as needed for immediate relief of COPD symptoms. LAMAs are indicated for daily administration to prevent and reduce symptoms.

Beta$_2$ agonists

The effects of beta$_2$ agonists are the same as were discussed previously in the section on asthma pharmacotherapy. SABAs are an appropriate treatment for as-needed relief of acute exacerbations due to the fast onset of their bronchodilator effects (approximately 5 minutes). They can be used on a routine basis, but the short duration of action of SABAs and frequent dosing inhibits their usefulness as a daily therapy to decrease symptoms. As discussed earlier, the combination of ipratropium and albuterol has been found to result in better bronchodilation. The inhalation preparation of SABA is preferred over oral and parenteral forms—although all preparations have equivalent efficacy, the specificity of inhalation preparation to the lungs results in decreased side effects.

The available LABA preparations include salmeterol, formoterol, arformoterol, olodaterol, indacaterol, and vilanterol. These medications are available in various formulations, either as singular agents or in combination with a LAMA and/or ICS. The onset of action for LABAs is approximately 15–20 minutes, except for formoterol, which has an onset of 5 minutes. LABAs are appropriate for the prevention and reduction of COPD symptoms and are conveniently administered once or twice daily due to their long duration of action.

CASE?

How would the medications prescribed for Joe be expected to improve his COPD?

Theophylline

Theophylline has shown modest bronchodilator effects for stable COPD patients.[10] The effect on exacerbation rates is not well known at this time due to limited data. Theophylline therapy is associated with a wide variety of side effects and possible toxicity, including arrhythmias (irregular heartbeat) and seizures. Due to the limited effectiveness and side effects associated with therapy, theophylline is not routinely recommended for the management of COPD.

Phosphodiesterase-4 Enzyme Inhibitor

Roflumilast belongs to a class of drugs, the phosphodiesterase-4 enzyme inhibitors, which regulate inflammatory mediators in a variety of conditions. Roflumilast is the only one in this group used to treat COPD (as of this writing), and can reduce the risk of exacerbations in a small population of patients with COPD. It is reserved for patients with severe to very severe COPD, who have chronic bronchitis with a history of exacerbations requiring oral glucocorticoid therapy (discussed in the next section). It increases lung tissue levels of cyclic adenosine monophosphate (cAMP), a chemical that acts as a messenger in many cellular processes and reduces the numbers of some cells in the lung fluids. It is administered as an oral tablet on a routine (preventive) basis and is not useful as an as-needed bronchodilator for sudden

breathing problems. The most common adverse reactions are diarrhea, decreased appetite, nausea, weight loss, headache, and insomnia. The adverse effects generally lessen over time. Though rarely, roflumilast can cause neuropsychiatric events and should be used with caution in patients experiencing depression or suicidal thoughts.

Glucocorticoid Therapy

The routine use of inhaled corticosteroids (ICS) is not recommended for the management of COPD, except under certain circumstances. ICS monotherapy has not been shown to have long-term effects on the decline of lung function or mortality of patients with COPD. However, in combination with long-acting bronchodilators, they are more effective at improving lung function and reducing exacerbations compared to either medication alone. Patients with COPD who have an extensive exacerbation history may exhibit a greater benefit from ICS compared to patients who do not have frequent or severe exacerbations. A reduction in acute exacerbations can lead to an improved overall health status.[10]

Treatment with oral glucocorticoids is reserved for the management of acute exacerbations. As discussed in the section on asthma, glucocorticoids act on specific receptors throughout the body to reduce inflammation. There is an extensive list of long-term side effects of glucocorticoids, including bone weakening, easy bruising, increased risk of infections, and increased blood sugar. When used short term for the treatment of an exacerbation, systemic glucocorticoids have been shown to lessen the rate of treatment failure and rate of relapse, and to improve lung function and breathlessness. Prednisone is commonly used, and the recommended dose is 40 mg once daily for 5 days. Ultimately, when used for acute exacerbation, systemic glucocorticoids shorten recovery time and improve lung function in patients with COPD.

Preventive Immunization Therapy

Common and normally mild respiratory infections, such as the flu or pneumonia, can have serious and sometimes deadly consequences in patients with COPD. These patients already have reduced lung function and any infection that further reduces it could have deadly consequences. Preventive measures should be undertaken to ensure that the risk of infection is as low as possible. Patients with COPD should be advised to get the inactivated influenza vaccine (flu shot) every year. The pneumococcal vaccination (pneumonia vaccine) is normally one dose, but a second dose of the vaccination may be given 5 years after the first vaccination in some patient populations.[11]

CASE?

Should the pharmacy technician inquire about the lack of refill of the salmeterol? Why might Joe not have his salmeterol prescription refilled?

CYSTIC FIBROSIS

CASE STUDY

Peter Jacobs is the father of a 10-year-old boy with cystic fibrosis. He has come into the pharmacy to get some cough syrup for his son's terrible hacking cough.

Pathophysiology

Cystic fibrosis (CF) is an inherited chronic disease caused by a gene mutation. This gene mutation causes an alteration in the normal secretion and absorption of chloride and sodium in the mucus-secreting exocrine glands. The result of the altered sodium and chloride levels is a change in the consistency of the normal mucus secretion. The mucus secretions are abnormally thickened and sticky, making them difficult to clear, allowing the mucus to cover and clog several organ systems. The most notable effects of the thickened mucus are on the lungs and pancreas.

Pulmonary disease is considered the hallmark of CF; all patients with CF have concurrent pulmonary disease. The lungs normally have a thin layer of mucus that protects the lungs from foreign particles, but in CF this layer is thick and sticky. The thick mucus not only clogs the lungs, making it difficult to fully exchange oxygen, it also traps bacteria and foreign particles in the lungs, leading to chronic respiratory infections and continual inflammation. The result of the mucus on the lungs is damage and progressive decrease in lung function followed by respiratory failure.

Pancreatic enzyme deficiency is also a common difficulty in patients with CF. The thick mucus plugs the pancreatic ducts and blocks the release of pancreatic enzymes into the intestine. The pancreatic enzymes are needed for the digestion of fat and protein and the absorption of vitamins A, D, E, and K (fat-soluble vitamins). Without these pancreatic enzymes, malnutrition will occur. The signs and symptoms of decreased pancreatic enzymes are abdominal distension; foul-smelling, loose bowel movement; flatulence; and malnourishment. CF patients must replace the pancreatic enzymes to ensure proper nutrition and normal growth.

CF can also adversely affect other organs and organ systems in the body, causing problems with the intestines, liver, reproduction, and anemia to name a few. The effects on these systems are patient specific, whereas the issues with the lungs and pancreas are more global CF issues although the extent differs by patient. CF is a serious chronic disease that must include continual lifelong management to prevent and quickly control serious life-threatening exacerbations of the disease. The life expectancy of CF patients has steadily increased with the development of better management techniques and increased education on the importance of these techniques to reduce symptoms and improve quality of life and life expectancy.

Goals

The goals of CF therapy include:[5]

1. Ensuring adequate nutrition for optimal growth and development through pancreatic enzyme replacement

2. Preventing lung damage and lung function decline by decreasing inflammation and aggressive infection prevention strategies, including airway clearance techniques and pharmacotherapy

3. Maintaining normal activities and quality of life

Nonpharmacologic Therapy

Nutritional Therapy

Patients with CF require increased caloric intake to maintain normal growth and development due to reduced nutrient absorption and increased calorie expenditures from difficulty breathing.[5] The increased caloric intake recommendation may be anywhere between 110% and 200% of persons who do not have CF. All patients with CF should receive close nutritional guidance from a dietitian experienced with CF as dietary needs vary at different stages of life. For patients who are consistently underweight, nutritional supplements or enteral tube feedings may be required to maintain adequate nutrition. Adequate nutrition is essential to fight infections and maintain normal growth and development. A daily CF-specific multivitamin containing optimized doses of fat-soluble vitamins (A, D, E, and K) can ensure an adequate supply of vital nutrients.

Pancreatic enzyme replacement therapy (PERT) ensures proper absorption and utilization of protein, carbohydrates, and fats by the body. Pancreatic enzyme capsules contain microbeads that are covered with a protective coating. This protective coating ensures that the microbeads will reach the small intestine where they are needed for effective absorption. Consequently, the capsules must be swallowed whole or they may be opened and the microbeads swallowed, but they must not be chewed. The pancreatic enzymes must be given right before a meal or snack. The enzymes should not be mixed with hot foods as the heat will inactivate the enzymes. Pancreatic enzyme products differ in their enzyme ratios, and it is generally recommended that patients do not change products, as dosages may vary between products. Generic products are not recommended. The dose of pancreatic enzymes is highly individualized and tailored to

individual patient needs. Pancreatic enzymes are generally well tolerated and are available in several formulations. All except Viokase have a protective coating but have differing amounts of lipase (for fat absorption), protease (protein absorption), and amylase (carbohydrate absorption). Examples of various pancreatic enzyme products are listed in Medication Table 19-3.

Mechanical Clearance Techniques

Mechanical clearance techniques loosen lung mucus, allowing it to be expelled from the lungs. Removing the mucus from the lungs helps increase lung function and decreases the likelihood of infection by preventing bacteria from getting trapped within the lungs. The techniques are normally performed twice a day but may be performed up to 6 times a day during an exacerbation. The cough is an important way that a patient with CF clears the lungs; therefore, cough suppressants should never be recommended for a patient with CF.

Postural drainage and percussion is an external vibration technique used to loosen mucus to enhance its removal from the lungs. This technique involves the patient's chest, sides, and back being rapidly vibrated manually with rapidly alternating cupped hands. This method requires the help of another person. The vibrations loosen the mucus, allowing it to be expelled through a forced cough. A similar technique involves the use of an inflatable vest that provides external mechanical vibration to the chest and back to help free the mucus for removal through a cough. The advantage of the inflatable mechanical vest is that therapy can be performed by the patient without the aid of another individual. A flutter valve device is a handheld device that causes an internal airway vibration when air is blown through it. The internal vibration, similar to the external vibrations, helps to free and mobilize the mucus, allowing it to be coughed up and expelled.

Pharmacologic Therapy

The goal of pharmacologic therapy is to preserve lung function through aggressive prevention techniques, with mucus removal as well as anti-inflammatory and anti-infective medications while maintaining normal growth and development.[5] Exacerbations must be treated quickly and aggressively to prevent life-threatening complications. Inhalation with the use of a metered dose inhaler or a nebulizer is the preferred route of administration as the medications are delivered directly to the lungs.

A primary part of treatment for patients with CF is airway clearance therapy, and it should be started within the first few months of life. The typical medications included in airway clearance therapy are albuterol (inhaled bronchodilator), hypertonic saline (short-acting inhaled mucolytic), mannitol (short-acting inhaled mucolytic), acetylcysteine (short-acting inhaled mucolytic), and dornase alfa (inhaled mucolytic). If the patient is using a bronchodilator regularly, the bronchodilator should be inhaled first, followed by the short-acting mucolytic therapy, and lastly dornase alfa. Inhaled antibiotics and other inhaled medications such as asthma inhalers should be administered after airway clearance therapy.

Mucolytic Therapy

Mucolytic medications help to dissolve and thin the mucus to enhance the mucus removal techniques discussed earlier. Mucolytic products are administered via inhalation to ensure the mucolytic medication reaches the lungs. Dornase alfa is targeted to break up the accumulated deoxyribonucleic acid (DNA), resulting in thinned mucus and improved airflow to the lungs. The dose of dornase alfa is 2.5 mg one or two times a day to thin mucus secretions and help increase mucus clearance from the lungs. Side effects may include a sore throat and hoarse voice.

Hypertonic saline is a 7% sodium chloride solution. When administered by a nebulizer, this concentrated salt solution "pulls" more water into the lung fluid, resulting in

thinner, less viscous bronchial secretions. It is typically given two to four times a day. Side effects of this medication may include cough, chest tightness, sore throat, and sneezing. If a patient is unable to tolerate the 7% solution, a 3 or 3.5% inhaled solution may be used.

Anti-Inflammatory Therapy

The use of anti-inflammatory medication can result in a reduction of lung inflammation and has been found to decrease the rate of decline in lung function over time. Ibuprofen anti-inflammatory treatment involves high doses of ibuprofen that require close monitoring, including obtaining regular blood ibuprofen levels. The effects of ibuprofen therapy are seen with long-term use and as a result a patient may not notice any change in overall health status. There are few patients in the United States currently on this therapy possibly due to the required routine blood draws. The most common side effect of ibuprofen therapy is stomach upset, with possible gastrointestinal bleeding. Azithromycin has been found to have anti-inflammatory effects. It is commonly given in lower anti-infective doses (three times weekly) to reduce inflammation in the patient with CF and not for its antibiotic effects.

Anti-Infective Therapy

With time, patients with CF develop chronic lung infection that is due to the thick mucus trapping pathogens in the lungs and causing infection. The chronic lung infection proliferates and causes an acute exacerbation of symptoms.

The goal of anti-infective therapy is to improve lung function and prevent respiratory failure. Antibiotics used in patients with CF are available in a variety of formulations—oral, intravenous, and inhaled—depending on the indication. Choosing the appropriate antibiotic regimen is based on sputum cultures and the antibiotic sensitivity of pathogens. Commonly, patients with CF require higher doses and longer durations of antibiotic therapy than patients without CF to adequately recover from an infection. Unfortunately, the pathogens are not entirely cleared from the airways of patients with CF, which commonly leads to resistance. The development of resistant pathogens limits the antibiotic options available to treat infections and ultimately contributes to the decline in lung function. Antibiotics used for anti-infective therapy of cystic fibrosis are discussed in detail in Chapter 27.

Cystic Fibrosis Transmembrane Conductance Regulator Therapy

Cystic fibrosis transmembrane conductance regulator (CFTR) modulators are a new class of medications that focus on the central defect of CF, gene mutations. These medications work to keep channels open longer, causing fluid to move into the airways, thinning secretions for easier clearance. There are over 2,000 different mutations requiring different medications for different mutations. Some of the medications are effective for multiple types of mutations. Specific tests must be performed prior to patients receiving CFTR modulator therapy to identify which gene mutations they have. Currently, there are four agents available for the treatment of CF, including elexacaftor/tezacaftor/ivacaftor (Trikafta), ivacaftor (Kalydeco), lumacaftor/ivacaftor (Orkambi), and tezacaftor/ivacaftor (Symdeko). These medications should be taken with a food high in fat and pancreatic enzymes if pancreatic insufficient. Side effects may include liver dysfunction, stomach pains, diarrhea, headache, and rash. Representative pharmacologic agents used in the treatment of cystic fibrosis are included in Medication Table 19-4.

SUMMARY

Asthma, chronic obstructive pulmonary disease (COPD), and cystic fibrosis (CF) are all chronic lung diseases that can severely affect a patient's life and life expectancy. Beta agonists, anticholinergics, and glucocorticoids, as well as other medication classes, are commonly used to treat these diseases. Many of these drugs are administered via inhalation with a spacer or nebulizer. Ensuring that the patient has received adequate education on the proper use and cleaning techniques of this equipment is important to assure maximum patient health benefit. Patients should be encouraged to stop smoking and keep their immunizations up to date. Proper use of both nonpharmacologic and pharmacologic interventions can significantly improve their health status and quality of life. Pharmacists and pharmacy technicians can play an important role by ensuring that patients understand and use their medications properly.

ACKNOWLEDGMENT

The author wishes to acknowledge and thank Christina Bell, PharmD, and Sandra B. Earle, PharmD, BCPS, authors of this chapter in the first edition of this book.

REFERENCES

1. American Lung Association. Asthma Trends and Burden. American Lung Association Epidemiology & Statistics Unit, Research and Health Education Division. Aug 2019. http://www.lung.org. Accessed April 24, 2021.

2. US Department of Health and Human Services. *2020 Focused Updates to the Asthma Management Guidelines: A Report from the National Asthma Education and Prevention Program Coordinating Committee Expert Panel Working Group*. Washington, DC: US Department of Health and Human Services; 2020.

3. Lozano R, Naghavi M, Foreman K, et al. Global and regional mortality from 235 causes of death for 20 age groups in 1990 and 2010: A systematic analysis for the Global Burden of Disease Study 2010. *Lancet* 2012;380(9859): 2095-2128.

4. Mathers CD, Loncar D. Projections of global mortality and burden of disease from 2002 to 2030. *PLS Med* 2006;3(11):e442.

5. American Lung Association. Learn About Cystic Fibrosis. April 2018. https://www.lung.org/lung-health-diseases /lung-disease-lookup/cystic-fibrosis. Accessed July 27, 2021.

6. Cystic Fibrosis Foundation. Cystic Fibrosis Foundation Patient Registry. 2020 Annual Data Report to the Center Directors. Bethesda, MD: Cystic Fibrosis Foundation; 2021.

7. Blake KV, Lang JE. Asthma. In: DiPiro JT, Yee GC, Posey L, et al., eds. *Pharmacotherapy: A Pathophysiologic Approach*. 11th ed. New York, NY: McGraw-Hill Medical; 2020.

8. Global Initiative for Asthma. *Global Strategy for Asthma Management and Prevention Updated 2022*. https:// ginasthma.org/wp-content/uploads/2022/05/GINA

-Main-Report-2022-FINAL-22-05-03-WMS.pdf. Accessed July 6, 2022.

9. Lexi-Drugs. Lexicomp Online. Wolters Kluwer; 2021. https://online.lexi.com. Accessed April 30, 2021.

10. Bourdet SV, Williams DM. Chronic obstructive pulmonary disease. In: DiPiro JT, Yee GC, Posey L, et al., eds. *Pharmacotherapy: A Pathophysiologic Approach*. 11th ed. New York, NY: McGraw-Hill Medical; 2020.

11. Global Initiative for Chronic Obstructive Lung Disease. *Global Strategy for the Diagnosis, Management, and Prevention of Chronic Obstructive Pulmonary Disease 2020 Report*. Bethesda, MD: Global Initiative for Chronic Obstructive Lung Disease; 2020.

CHAPTER RESOURCES

Blake KV, Lang JE. Asthma. In: DiPiro JT, Yee GC, Posey L, et al., eds. *Pharmacotherapy: A Pathophysiologic Approach*. 11th ed. New York, NY: McGraw-Hill Medical; 2020.

Fletcher C, Petro R. The natural history of chronic airflow obstruction. *BMJ* 1977;1(6077):1645-1648.

Walters JA, Tan DJ, White CJ, et al. Systemic corticosteroids for acute exacerbations of chronic obstructive pulmonary disease. *Cochrane Database Syst Rev*. 2014;(9):CD001288.

Leuppi JD, Schuetz P, Blingisser R, et al. Short-term vs conventional glucocorticoid therapy in acute exacerbations of chronic obstructive pulmonary disease: The REDUCE randomized clinical trial. *JAMA* 2013;309(21):2223-2231.

Wright CC, Vera YY. Cystic Fibrosis. In: DiPiro JT, Yee GC, Posey L, et al., eds. *Pharmacotherapy: A Pathophysiologic Approach*. 11th ed. New York, NY: McGraw-Hill Medical; 2020.

Mogayzel PJ, Naureckas ET, Robinson KA, et al. Pulmonary Clinical Practice Guidelines Committee. Cystic fibrosis pulmonary guidelines: Chronic medications for maintenance of lung health. *Am J Respir Crit Care Med*. 2013 Apr;187(7):680-689. https://www.atsjournals.org/doi/10.1164/rccm.201207-1160oe?url_ver=Z39.88-2003&rfr_id=ori:rid:crossref.org&rfr_dat=cr_pub%20%200pubmed. Accessed April 30, 2021.

REVIEW QUESTIONS

1. Define asthma and list the characteristics of the different types of asthma that have been identified.

2. What is meant by the acronym COPD? What are the characteristics of this disease?

3. What organ systems are affected by cystic fibrosis?

4. What types of medication therapy are used for both asthma and COPD? Which medications are used for one disease but not the other?

5. How is the autonomic nervous system involved in respiratory system disorders?

MEDICATION TABLES

MEDICATION TABLE 19-1. Asthma Pharmacotherapy[9]

Generic Name	Brand Name	Dosage Forms	Typical Dose	Clinical Use	Side Effects	Notes
Bronchodilators						
Epinephrine (e pi NEF rin)	Primatene Mist, Asthmanefrin Refill, S2 (Racepinephrine)	MDI 0.125 mg/puff; nebulizer solution 2.25%	MDI 1–2 puffs q 4 hr PRN; nebulizer 1 vial q 3 hr PRN	Not recommended for routine management of asthma	Tachycardia, hypertension, nervousness, sleeplessness	OTC inhaler, OTC nebulizer solution; use with caution
Albuterol (al BYOO ter ole)	Ventolin/Proventil/ ProAir HFA, generics	DPI/MDI 90 mcg/puff; nebulizer 0.63 mg/3 mL, 1.25 mg/3 mL, 2.5 mg/3 mL	MDI or DPI 2–4 puffs q 4–6 hr PRN; nebulizer solution 2.5 mg q 4–6 hr PRN	Quick relief of mild asthma symptoms; reliever therapy; prevention of exercise-induced bronchospasm	Dose related: nervousness, chest pain, increased serum glucose, cough, tremor	SABA
Levalbuterol (lev al BYOO ter ol)	Xopenex	MDI 45 mcg/puff; nebulizer 0.31 mg/3 mL, 0.63 mg/3 mL, 1.25 mg/3 mL, 1.25 mg/0.5 mL	MDI 1–4 puffs q 4–6 hr PRN; nebulizer 0.63–1.25 mg q 6–8 hr PRN;			
Salmeterol (sal ME te role)	Serevent Diskus	DPI 50 mcg/puff	1 puff q 12 hr	Symptom prevention; controller therapy	Headache, hypertension, dizziness, chest pain	LABA; not appropriate for monotherapy; must always be prescribed with ICS or other control medication
Theophylline (the OFF i lin)	Elixophyllin, Theo-24	Elixir/oral solution 80 mg/15 mL; Theo-24 100 mg, 200 mg, 300 mg, 400 mg; 24 hour-ER tablet 400 mg, 600 mg; 12 hour-ER tablet 300 mg, 450 mg	Individualize dose based on theophylline blood levels	Symptom prevention; controller therapy; not routinely recommended	Tachycardia, nausea/vomiting, headache, dizziness, insomnia	Oral; never increase or double a missed dose; increased side effects and drug interactions

Continued next page

MEDICATION TABLE 19-1. Asthma Pharmacotherapy[9] (Continued)

Generic Name	Brand Name	Dosage Forms	Typical Dose	Clinical Use	Side Effects	Notes
Inhaled Corticosteroids						
Beclomethasone (be kloe METH a sone)	QVAR RediHaler	MDI 40 mcg/puff, 80 mcg/puff	80–640 mcg/day	Symptom prevention; controller therapy for persistent asthma	Oral thrush, hoarse voice, dysphonia	2 weeks needed to see full effect; rinse mouth after each use
Budesonide (byoo DES oh nide)	Pulmicort Flexhaler Pulmicort suspension for inhalation	DPI 90 mcg/puff, 180 mcg/puff; suspension 0.25 mg/2 mL, 0.5 mg/2 mL, 1 mg/2 mL	DPI 180–1,440 mcg/day; suspension 0.5–2 mg/day			
Fluticasone (floo TIK a sone)	Flovent HFA/Diskus, Arnuity Ellipta, ArmonAir Digihaler	DPI Diskus 50 mcg/ blister, 100 mcg/blister, 250 mcg/blister; MDI 44 mcg/puff, 110 mcg/ puff, 220 mcg/puff; DPI (furoate) 50 mcg/ puff, 100 mcg/puff, 200 mcg/puff; DPI (propionate) 55 mcg/ puff, 113 mcg/puff, 232 mcg/puff	DPI 200–2,000 mcg/day; MDI 176–1,760 mcg/day; DPI (furoate) 100–200 mcg/day; DPI (propionate) 110–464 mcg/day			
Mometasone (moe MET a sone)	Asmanex Twisthaler, Asmanex HFA	DPI 110–220 mcg/puff; MDI 50–200 mcg/puff	DPI 110–880 mcg/day; MDI 400–800 mcg/day			
Ciclesonide (sye KLES oh nide)	Alvesco	MDI 80 mcg/puff, 160 mcg/puff	160–640 mcg/day			
Combinations						
Fluticasone/salmeterol (floo TIK a sone) (sal ME te role)	Advair Diskus/HFA, AirDuo RespiClick/ Digihaler, Wixela Inhub	Diskus and Inhub DPI 100/50 mcg/ puff, 250/50 mcg/ puff, 500/50 mcg/puff; HFA MDI 45/21 mcg/ puff, 115/21 mcg/ puff, 230/21 mcg/puff; RespiClick/Digihaler MDI 55/14 mcg/puff, 113/14 mcg/puff, 232/14 mcg/puff	1–2 puffs twice daily	Symptom prevention; controller therapy for persistent asthma	Oral thrush, hoarse voice, dysphonia, headache, hypertension, dizziness, chest pain	ICS/LABA; 2 weeks needed to see full effect; use MDI with spacer; dry powder inhalers (DPI) and breath-actuated inhalers CANNOT be used with a spacer; rinse mouth after each use

Continued next page

MEDICATION TABLE 19-1. Asthma Pharmacotherapy[9] (Continued)

Generic Name	Brand Name	Dosage Forms	Typical Dose	Clinical Use	Side Effects	Notes
Fluticasone/vilanterol (floo TIK a sone) (VYE lan ter ol)	Breo Ellipta	DPI 100/25 mcg/puff, 200/25 mcg/puff	1 puff once daily	Symptom prevention; controller therapy for persistent asthma		ICS/LABA; 2 weeks needed to see full effect; rinse mouth after each use
Budesonide/formoterol (byoo DES oh nide) (for MOH te rol)	Symbicort	MDI 80/4.5 mcg/puff, 160/4.5 mcg/puff	2 puffs twice daily	Symptom prevention; controller therapy for persistent asthma		ICS/LABA; 2 weeks needed to see full effect; use with spacer; rinse mouth after each use
Mometasone/ fomoterol (moe MET a sone) (for MOH te rol)	Dulera	MDI 50/5 mcg/puff, 100/5 mcg/puff, 200/5 mcg/puff	2 puffs twice daily	Symptom prevention; controller therapy for persistent asthma		ICS/LABA; 2 weeks needed to see full effect; use with spacer; rinse mouth after each use
Fluticasone/ umeclidinium/ vilanterol (floo TIK a sone) (ue me kli DIN ee um) (VYE lan ter ol)	Trelegy Ellipta	DPI 100/62.5/25 mcg/ puff, 200/62.5/25 mcg/ puff	1 puff once daily	Symptom prevention; maintenance therapy	Oral thrush, hoarse voice, dysphonia, URI, dry mouth, metallic taste, throat irritation, cough, headache, hypertension, dizziness, chest pain,	ICS/LAMA/LABA; 2 weeks needed to see full effect; rinse mouth after each use; not for rapid symptom relief
Leukotriene Modifiers						
Montelukast (mon te LOO kast)	Singulair	Chewable tablet 4 mg, 5 mg; granule packet 4 mg; tablet 10 mg	4–10 mg/day	Symptom prevention; prevention of exercise-induced bronchospasm; allergic rhinitis	Headache, dizziness, heartburn, stomach pain, tiredness, mood/ behavior changes	Doses above 10 mg will not increase effect in adults; give at bedtime; not for rapid symptom relief
Zafirlukast (za FIR loo kast)	Accolate	Tablet 10 mg, 20 mg	20–40 mg/day	Symptom prevention; allergic rhinitis	Nausea, loss of appetite, pain in the right upper part of the abdomen, excessive tiredness, lack of energy	Take on empty stomach; check liver function; many drug interactions; not for rapid symptom relief

Continued next page

MEDICATION TABLE 19-1. Asthma Pharmacotherapy[9] (Continued)

Generic Name	Brand Name	Dosage Forms	Typical Dose	Clinical Use	Side Effects	Notes
Zileuton (zye LOO ton)	Zyflo	Tablet 600 mg (IR or ER)	IR 600 mg 4 times daily; ER 1,200 mg twice daily	Symptom prevention	Headache, heartburn, diarrhea, muscle pain, nose and throat irritation, pain or fullness in the face	Do not chew or crush; adults only; check liver function; many drug interactions; not for rapid symptom relief
Immunomodulators						
Omalizumab (oh mah lye ZOO mab)	Xolair	SUBQ prefilled syringe 75 mg/0.5 mL, 150 mg/1 mL; reconstituted 150 mg	150–375 mg SUBQ q 2–4 weeks	Prevention of symptoms for moderate to severe allergic asthma; add-on therapy	Bruising at site, redness, pain, stinging, delayed anaphylaxis	Not effective for rapid symptom relief; allow pre-filled syringe to warm to room temperature for 15 to 30 minutes; leave in carton to protect from light; monitor for 2 hours post-dose for anaphylaxis
Benralizumab (ben ra LIZ ue mab)	Fasenra, Fasenra Pen	SUBQ prefilled syringe/auto-injector 30 mg/mL	30 mg SUBQ q 4 weeks × 3 doses followed by 30 mg q 8 weeks	Prevention of symptoms for severe eosinophilic asthma; add-on therapy	Headache, sore throat	Not effective for rapid symptom relief; warm at room temperature for 30 min prior to administration
Dupilumab (doo PIL ue mab)	Dupixent	SUBQ prefilled syringe 100 mg/0.67 mL, 200 mg/1.14 mL, 300 mg/2 mL; pen injector 200 mg/1.14 mL, 300 mg/2 mL	400-600 mg SUBQ × 1 dose followed by 200-300 mg SUBQ every other week; child/ adolescent dosing based on age and weight	Prevention of symptoms for severe eosinophilic asthma or corticosteroid-dependent asthma; add-on therapy	Bruising at site, redness, pain, itchiness, headache, inflammation of the eyes	Not effective for rapid symptom relief; warm at room temperature for 30 min (100 and 200 mg syringe or pen) or 45 min (300 mg syringe or pen) prior to administration

Continued next page

MEDICATION TABLE 19-1. Asthma Pharmacotherapy[9] (Continued)

Generic Name	Brand Name	Dosage Forms	Typical Dose	Clinical Use	Side Effects	Notes
Mepolizumab (me poe LIZ ue mab)	Nucala	SUBQ auto-injector, prefilled syringe, reconstituted 100 mg/mL; 40 mg/0.4 mL prefilled syringe	40–100 mg SUBQ q 4 weeks	Prevention of symptoms for severe eosinophilic asthma; add-on therapy	Bruising at site, redness, pain, itchiness, headache, fatigue	Not effective for rapid symptom relief; prefilled syringe/ auto-injector warm at room temperature for 30 min prior to administration; do not shake reconstituted solution
Reslizumab (res LIZ ue mab)	Cinqair	IV solution 100 mg/10 mL	3 mg/kg IV q 4 weeks	Prevention of symptoms for severe eosinophilic asthma; add-on therapy	Throat irritation	Not effective for rapid symptom relief; allow diluted solution to reach room temperature
Tezepelumab	Tezspire	210 mg/1.91 mL prefilled syringe	210 mg SUBQ q 4 weeks	Prevention of symptoms for severe asthma; add-on therapy	Bruising at site, pain, throat irritation	Not effective for rapid symptom relief; warm prefilled syringe at room temperature for 60 min prior to administration

DPI = dry powder inhaler; ER = extended release; ICS = inhaled corticosteroid; IR = immediate release; IV = intravenous; LABA = long-acting beta₂ agonist; MDI = metered-dose inhaler; OTC = over the counter; PRN = as needed; SABA = short-acting beta₂ agonist; SUBQ = subcutaneous.

MEDICATION TABLE 19-2. Chronic Obstructive Pulmonary Disease Pharmacotherapy[9]

Generic Name	Brand Name	Dosage Forms	Typical Dose	Clinical Use	Side Effects	Notes
Bronchodilators						
Albuterol (al BYOO ter ole)	ProAir Digihaler/ HFA/RespiClick, Proventil HFA, Ventolin HFA	DPI/MDI 90 mcg/puff; nebulizer 0.63 mg/3 mL, 1.25 mg/3 mL, 2.5 mg/3 mL	MDI/DPI 2 puffs q 4–6 hr PRN; nebulizer solution 2.5 mg q 4–6 hr PRN	Quick relief ofsymptoms	Dose-related: ner- vousness, chest pain, increased serum glu- cose, cough, tremor	SABA; quick onset; use spacer with MDI
Ipratropium (i pra TROE pee um)	Atrovent HFA	MDI 17 mcg/puff; nebulizer solution 0.02%	MDI 2 puffs q 4–6 hr prn OR 4 times a day scheduled; nebulizer 1 vial q 4–6 hr prn OR 6–8 hr scheduled	Quick relief of symptoms	URI, bronchitis, dry mouth, nausea, metallic taste, throat irritation	SAMA; quick onset; use spacer with MDI
Ipratropium/albuterol (i pra TROE pee um (al BYOO ter ole)	Combivent Respimat, generics	Respimat 20/100 mcg/ spray; nebulizer solution 0.5/2.5 mg/3 mL	MDI 1 puff 4 q 4–6 hr prn OR 4 times a day scheduled; nebulizer 1 vial q 4–6 hr prn OR 6 hr scheduled	Quick relief or maintenance therapy depending on COPD severity	URI, palpitations, dry mouth, metallic taste, throat irritation	SAMA/SABA
Tiotropium (ty oh TRO pee um)	Spiriva HandiHaler, Spiriva Respimat	Capsule 18 mcg; aerosol solution 1.25 mcg/puff, 2.5 mcg/puff	1 capsule inhaled once daily; 2 puffs once daily	Symptom prevention; maintenance therapy	URI, dry mouth, metallic taste, throat irritation, cough	LAMA; capsule is not to be taken orally
Umeclidinium (ue me kli DIN ee um)	Incruse Ellipta	DPI 62.5 mcg/puff	1 puff once daily	Symptom prevention; maintenance therapy	URI, dry mouth, metallic taste, throat irritation, cough	LAMA; administer at the same time every day
Aclidinum (a kli DIN ee um)	Tudorza Pressair	DPI 400 mcg/puff	1 puff twice daily	Symptom prevention; maintenance therapy	URI, dry mouth, metallic taste, throat irritation, headache, cough	LAMA; administer at the same time every day
Glycopyrrolate (glye koe PYE roe late)	Seebri Neohaler, Lonhala Magnair Starter and Refill Kit	Capsule 15.6 mcg; inhalation solution 25 mcg/mL	1 capsule inhaled twice daily; 1 vial of solution inhaled twice daily	Symptom prevention; maintenance therapy	URI, metallic taste, throat irritation, cough	LAMA; capsule is not to be taken orally
Revefenacin	Yupelri	175 mcg/3 mL inhalation solution	Nebulizer 1 vial daily	Symptom prevention; maintenance therapy	URI, headache, throat irritation	LAMA; administer at the same time every day

Continued next page

MEDICATION TABLE 19-2. Chronic Obstructive Pulmonary Disease Pharmacotherapy[9] *(Continued)*

Generic Name	Brand Name	Dosage Forms	Typical Dose	Clinical Use	Side Effects	Notes
Salmeterol (sal ME te role)	Serevent Diskus	DPI 50 mcg/puff	1 puff twice daily (12 hours apart)	Symptom prevention; maintenance therapy	Headache, chest pain, hypertension, URI, dizziness, throat irritation, dry mouth	LABA; not for rapid symptom relief
Arformoterol (ar for MOE ter ol)	Brovana	Nebulizer solution 15 mcg/2 mL	15 mcg twice daily	Symptom prevention; maintenance therapy	Chest pain, back pain, URI, diarrhea	LABA; not for rapid symptom relief
Formoterol (for MOH te rol)	Perforomist	Nebulizer solution 20 mcg/2 mL	20 mcg twice daily	Symptom prevention; maintenance therapy	Insomnia, dizziness, chest pain, nausea, dry mouth, URI, throat irritation	LABA; quickest onset of LABAs; not for rapid symptom relief
Olodaterol (oh loe DA ter ol)	Striverdi Respimat	Aerosol inhaler 2.5 mcg/puff	2 puffs once daily	Symptom prevention; maintenance therapy	URI, back pain, UTI, bronchitis	LABA; not for rapid symptom relief
Theophylline (the OFF i lin)	Elixophyllin, Theo-24	Elixir/oral solution 80 mg/15 mL; Theo-24 100 mg, 200 mg, 300 mg, 400 mg; 24 hour-ER tablet 400 mg, 600 mg; 12 hour-ER tablet 300 mg, 450 mg	Individualize dose based on theophylline blood levels	Symptom prevention; maintenance therapy; not routinely recommended	Tachycardia, nausea/vomiting, headache, dizziness, insomnia	Oral; never increase or double a missed dose; increased side effects and drug interactions
Roflumilast (roe FLUE mi last)	Daliresp	Tablet 250 mcg, 500 mcg	250 mcg once daily × 4 weeks followed by 500 mcg once daily	Symptom prevention; maintenance therapy; add-on therapy	Diarrhea, headache, weight loss, decreased appetite, nausea, suicidal behaviors (rare)	PDE-4 inhibitor; oral; dose titration for tolerability
Combinations						
Umeclidinium/vilanterol (ue me kli DIN ee um) (VYE lan ter ol)	Anoro Ellipta	DPI 62.5/25 mcg/puff	1 puff once daily	Symptom prevention; maintenance therapy	URI, dry mouth, metallic taste, throat irritation, cough	LAMA/LABA; not for rapid symptom relief
Glycopyrrolate/formoterol (glye koe PYE roe late) (for MOH te rol)	Bevespi Aerosphere	Aerosol inhalation 9/4.8 mcg/puff	2 puffs twice daily	Symptom prevention; maintenance therapy	URI, metallic taste, throat irritation, cough, headache, hypertension, dizziness, chest pain	LAMA/LABA; not for rapid symptom relief; MDI may be used with a spacer

Continued next page

MEDICATION TABLE 19-2. Chronic Obstructive Pulmonary Disease Pharmacotherapy[9] (Continued)

Generic Name	Brand Name	Dosage Forms	Typical Dose	Clinical Use	Side Effects	Notes
Aclidinum/formoterol (a klii DIN ee um) (for MOH te rol)	Duaklir Pressair	DPI 400/12 mcg/puff	1 puff twice daily	Symptom prevention; maintenance therapy	URI, dry mouth, metallic taste, throat irritation, cough, headache, hypertension, dizziness, chest pain	LAMA/LABA; not for rapid symptom relief
Tiotropium/olodaterol (ty oh TRO pee um) (oh loe DA ter ol)	Stiolto Respimat	Aerosol inhaler 2.5/2.5 mcg/puff	2 puffs once daily	Symptom prevention; maintenance therapy	URI, dry mouth, metallic taste, throat irritation, cough, back pain	LAMA/LABA; not for rapid symptom relief
Fluticasone/ umeclidinium/vilanterol (floo TIK a sone) (ue me kli DIN ee um) (VYE lan ter ol)	Trelegy Ellipta	DPI 100/62.5/25 mcg/ puff, 200/62.5/25 mcg/puff	1 puff once daily	Symptom prevention; maintenance therapy	Oral thrush, hoarse voice, dysphonia, URI, dry mouth, metallic taste, throat irritation, cough, headache, hypertension, dizziness, chest pain,	ICS/LAMA/LABA; 2 weeks needed to see full effect; rinse mouth after each use; not for rapid symptom relief
Budesonide/ glycopyrrolate/formoterol	Breztri Aerosphere	Aerosol inhalation 160/9/4.8 mcg/puff	2 puffs twice daily	Symptom prevention; maintenance therapy	Oral thrush, URI, metallic taste, throat irritation, cough, head-ache, hypertension, dizziness, chest pain	ICS/LAMA/LABA; 2 weeks needed to see full effect; may use MDI with spacer; rinse mouth after use; not for rapid symptom relief

DPI = dry powder inhaler; ICS = inhaled corticosteroid; LABA = long-acting beta₂ agonist; LAMA = long-acting muscarinic antagonist; MDI = metered-dose inhaler; PRN = as needed; SABA = short-acting beta₂ agonist; SAMA = short-acting muscarinic antagonist; URI = upper respiratory tract infection; UTI = urinary tract infection.

MEDICATION TABLE 19-3. Representative Pancreatic Enzyme Preparations [9]

Generic Name	Brand Name	Dosage Form(s)	Representative Strengths (USP units lipase/protease/amylase
Pancrelipase (pan kre LYE pase)	Creon (5 strengths available)	Capsule, delayed-release particles	Creon Strengths: 3,000/9,500/15,000 6,000/19,000/30,000 12,000/38,000/60,000 24,000/76,000/120,000 36,000/114,000/180,000
	Pancreaze (6 strengths available)		Pancreaze strengths: 2,600/8,800/15,200 4,200/14,200/24,600 10,500/35,500/61,500 16,800/56,800/98,400 21,000/54,700/83,900 37,000/97,300/149,900
	Pertzye (4 strengths available)		Pertzye strengths: 4,000/14,375/15,125 8,000/28,750/30,250 16,000/57,500/60,500 24,000/86,250/90,750
	Zenpep (7 strengths available)		Zenpep strengths: 3,000/10,000/14,000 5,000/17,000/24,000 10,000/32,000/42,000 15,000/47,000/63,000 20,000/63,000/84,000 25,000/79,000/105,000 40,000/126,000/168,000
	Viokace (2 strengths)	Tablet	Viokace strengths: 10,440/39,150/39,150 20,880/78,300/78,300

MEDICATION TABLE 19-4. Representative Cystic Fibrosis Pharmacotherapy[9]

Generic Name	Brand Name	Dosage Form(s)	Strength
Mucolytic			
"Hypertonic" sodium chloride (SOW dee um KLOR ide)	HyperSal	Nebulization solution	3%, 3.5%, 7%
Dornase alfa (DOOR nase AL fa)	Pulmozyme	Inhalation solution	1 mg/mL
Mannitol	Aridol Inhalation Kit, Bronchitol	Dry powder inhaler	40 mg capsules for inhalation
Acetylcysteine	Mucomyst	Inhalation solution	10%, 20%
Cystic Fibrosis Transmembrane Conductance Regulator (CFTR) Modulators			
Ivacaftor (eye va KAF tor)	Kalydeco	Packet, oral	25 mg, 50 mg, 75 mg
		Tablet, oral	150 mg
Lumacaftor and ivacaftor (loo ma KAF tor, eye va KAF tor)	Orkambi	Packet, oral	Lumacaftor 100 mg/ivacaftor 125 mg Lumacaftor 150 mg/ivacaftor 188 mg
		Tablet, oral	Lumacaftor 100 mg/ivacaftor 125 mg Lumacaftor 200 mg/ivacaftor 125 mg
Tezacaftor and ivacaftor (tez a KAF tor, eye va KAF tor)	Symdeko	Tablet therapy pack, oral	Tezacaftor 50 mg/ivacaftor 75 mg and ivacaftor 75 mg Tezacaftor 100 mg/ivacaftor 150 mg and ivacaftor 150 mg
Elexacaftor, tezacaftor, and ivacaftor (e lex a KAF tor, tez a KAF tor, eye va KAF tor)	Trikafta	Tablet therapy pack, oral	Elexacaftor 50 mg/tezacaftor 25 mg/ivacaftor 37.5 mg and ivacaftor 75 mg Elexacaftor 100 mg/tezacaftor 50 mg/ivacaftor 75 mg and ivacaftor 150 mg

THE GASTROINTESTINAL SYSTEM

Chapter 20

Acid-Related Diseases of the Upper Gastrointestinal Tract

Patrick J. Gallegos, PharmD, BCPS

KEY TERMS AND DEFINITIONS

Dyspepsia—(literally "bad digestion") persistent or recurrent discomfort (indigestion) in the upper abdomen characterized by a range of symptoms, including bloating, belching, nausea, stomach fullness (inability to finish a normal meal), and heartburn. Dyspepsia may be related to certain foods, beverages, or medications and is a common symptom of acid-related diseases such as peptic ulcer disease.

Erosions—single or multiple superficial lesions (areas of tissue damage), which may occur in the esophagus, stomach, or duodenum and affect primarily the mucosal lining of the gastrointestinal (GI) tract.

Esophagitis—injury to the lining of the esophagus (esophageal mucosa) related to abnormal gastric acid exposure. Esophagitis ranges from mild to severe and symptoms do not correlate directly with the degree of severity.

Gastritis—inflammation of the lining of the stomach (gastric mucosa) without ulceration. Gastritis may be acute (eg, related to medications such as nonsteroidal anti-inflammatory drugs, alcohol) or chronic (eg, related to *Helicobacter pylori* infection).

Gastroesophageal reflux disease (GERD)—an acid-related disorder caused primarily by malfunctioning of the lower esophageal sphincter (valve) and altered esophageal motility leading to a backward flow

DOI 10.37573/9781585286638.020

(reflux) of stomach contents into the esophagus. Although gastroesophageal reflux is a normal process, it is a disease when symptoms such as heartburn or esophageal injury occur.

Heartburn—heartburn is the most common typical symptom of gastroesophageal reflux disease and is characterized by a burning discomfort arising from behind the breast bone and moving up toward the neck and throat. Heartburn may also be associated with certain foods, medications, and other acid-related diseases such as peptic ulcer disease.

Hiatal hernia—passage of the upper portion of the stomach from below the diaphragm into the chest secondary to weakening of the diaphragm muscles and abdominal pressure. Some patients are asymptomatic while others have symptoms related to gastroesophageal reflux disease.

Peptic ulcer disease (PUD)—peptic ulcers occur in the stomach (gastric ulcer) and duodenum (duodenal ulcer) and are considered a chronic disease. Ulcers are typically singular, confined, and in contrast to erosions, extend deeper into the submucosa and the muscle layer.

Stress-related mucosal bleeding (SRMB)—bleeding that is associated with stress-related damage to the lining of the GI tract ("stress ulcer").

Stress-related mucosal damage (SRMD) or stress ulcer—the terms stress-related mucosal damage or stress ulcer are used to describe acute, superficial, scattered damage to the lining of the stomach of critically ill patients. Unlike chronic peptic ulcers, stress ulcers are painless, but both can lead to life-threatening bleeding.

Upper endoscopy—upper endoscopy, sometimes referred to as esophagogastroduodenoscopy (EGD), is a procedure performed by a physician and involves placing a tube with a light (called an endoscope) through the mouth into the esophagus, stomach, and duodenum. It has a small camera that allows the operator to view the upper gastrointestinal tract, which is magnified on an outside viewing monitor. The endoscope can be fitted with surgical instruments to allow the operator to perform procedures or obtain tissue samples for biopsy.

Upper gastrointestinal (UGI) bleeding—bleeding that occurs within the upper gastrointestinal tract, which may be related to medications, diseases, or other causes.

Upper gastrointestinal (UGI) radiography—a noninvasive radiologic procedure, which consists of the patient drinking a solution of barium sulfate. The barium coats the upper gastrointestinal tract and when exposed to x-rays, abnormalities (eg, ulcers, erosions, strictures) of the esophagus, stomach, or small intestine become visible.

Upper gastrointestinal (UGI) tract—the gastrointestinal tract is responsible for digestion, absorption, and elimination of food. It is divided into "upper" and "lower" sections beginning with the mouth and ending with the anus. The main structures of the upper gastrointestinal tract include the mouth, pharynx, esophagus, stomach (gastrum), and duodenum (first part of the small intestine). The lower GI tract (subject of Chapter 22) includes the remainder of the small intestine, along with the large intestine, rectum, and anus.

pH—a scale used to express a solution's acidity or alkalinity. The scale ranges from 0 to 14, with lower values being more acidic and higher values being more basic. Seven is neutral.

Prodrug—a medication that is inactive until it is ingested and metabolized by the body into a pharmacologically active medication.

LEARNING OBJECTIVES

After completing this chapter, you should be able to

1. Define the following:
   - Upper gastrointestinal tract.
   - Acidic pH.
   - Basic pH.
   - Dyspepsia.
   - Gastritis.
   - Gastric erosions.
   - Peptic ulcer disease.
   - Gastroesophageal reflux disease.
   - Heartburn.
   - Esophagitis.
   - Hiatal hernia.
   - Stress-related mucosal damage or stress ulcer.

2. Describe the anatomy and normal physiology of the upper gastrointestinal tract and discuss the role of gastric acid in acid-related diseases.

3. Identify the causes and risk factors for dyspepsia, peptic ulcer disease, gastroesophageal reflux disease, and upper gastrointestinal bleeding.

4. List the most common signs, symptoms, and complications of dyspepsia, peptic ulcer disease, gastroesophageal reflux disease, and upper gastrointestinal bleeding.

5. Describe the nonpharmacologic treatment of dyspepsia, peptic ulcer disease, and gastroesophageal reflux disease.

6. Explain the pharmacotherapeutic effects of antacids, H_2-receptor antagonists, proton pump inhibitors, sucralfate, bismuth salts, and misoprostol, and list their most common side effects and drug interactions.

7. State the brand and generic names of the most widely used antacids, H_2-receptor antagonists, proton pump inhibitors, sucralfate, bismuth salts, and misoprostol, along with their routes of administration, available dosage forms, and common dosages.

8. Recognize common drug regimens for the treatment of dyspepsia, peptic ulcer disease, gastroesophageal reflux disease, and upper gastrointestinal bleeding.

Diseases of the upper gastrointestinal (UGI) tract include a wide range of disorders, the majority of which involve stomach (gastric) acid. Acid plays an important role in the development of symptoms and the damage that is caused to the lining (mucosa) of the UGI tract. The most common acid-related diseases include dyspepsia (indigestion), peptic ulcer disease (PUD), gastroesophageal reflux disease (GERD), and stress-related mucosal damage (SRMD) or stress ulcers.[1] A serious complication of PUD, GERD, and SRMD is upper gastrointestinal (UGI) bleeding, which may be life threatening. Stress-related mucosal bleeding (SRMB) is usually asymptomatic and is associated with a high mortality.

Acid-related diseases of the UGI tract in the United States are associated with decreased quality of life, time away from work, mortality, and a large financial burden on the healthcare system.[1] Billions of dollars are spent annually on the diagnosis of acid-related diseases, hospitalizations, and medications used to treat these diseases. In some cases, patients can self-treat with oral over-the-counter (OTC)

medications, while others require more complicated drug regimens and/or parenteral drug therapy.

ANATOMY AND PHYSIOLOGY OF THE UPPER GASTROINTESTINAL TRACT

The UGI tract begins with the mouth and ends in the small intestine at the junction of the duodenum (first part of the small intestine) and jejunum (second part of the small intestine). The esophagus is a muscular tube, which lies behind the heart and connects the oropharynx to the stomach (Figure 20-1). It is lined with a thick layer of mucosa, which protects it from abrasive and irritating foods, beverages, and medications. The lower esophageal sphincter (LES) is a valve that guards against stomach contents refluxing back into the esophagus. When the sphincter relaxes, it permits food to empty into the stomach. Spontaneous motility (peristalsis) of the esophagus moves swallowed substances toward the stomach. Alterations in the esophageal mucosa, weakening of the LES, and decreased esophageal motility can contribute to GERD.

The esophagus delivers substances such as food, beverages, and medications to the stomach. The stomach is a very acidic environment, which aids in the digestion or breakdown of ingested substances and delivers these substances to the small intestine. Figure 20-1 shows the relationship of the stomach to the esophagus and the duodenum. This figure also

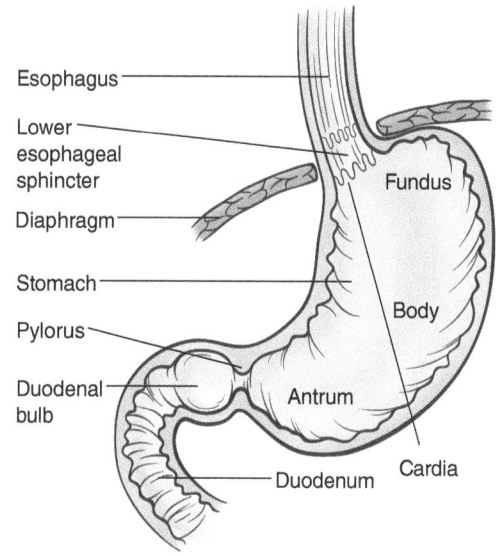

FIGURE 20-1. Diagram of the upper gastrointestinal tract.

demonstrates the four regions of the stomach (cardia, fundus, body, and antrum). The stomach contains many specialized cells important to digestion, as well as to protection of the stomach lining. Parietal cells in the stomach secrete hydrochloric acid, which aids in digestion; G cells secrete gastrin, which regulates acid secretion; chief cells secrete pepsinogen, which is converted to pepsin and helps digest protein; and mast cells secrete histamine, which is one of the three major stimulants of gastric acid (along with gastrin and acetylcholine). Epithelial cells in the stomach lining secrete mucus and bicarbonate, which work together with prostaglandins to maintain blood flow to this protective mucosal layer. The protective stomach lining has a neutral pH of 7.0, which helps repel stomach acid and is the primary reason why the stomach lining is not damaged by hydrochloric acid (which in the fasting state has an acidic pH of approximately 2.0). Medications, including nonsteroidal anti-inflammatory drugs (NSAIDs), alcohol, and bacteria such as *Helicobacter pylori* (*H. pylori*) can damage the protective mucosal barrier, allowing stomach acid to enter and resulting in ulcers and erosions.[2]

The small intestine consists of three sections: the duodenum, jejunum, and ileum. The duodenum extends from the pylorus to the jejunum where the UGI tract ends, and the lower GI tract begins. The pylorus (Figure 20-1) regulates the passage of partially digested foods and other substances into the duodenum and acts like a sphincter, which guards the opening between the stomach antrum and the duodenum. Peptic ulcers occur most frequently in the duodenal bulb (first part of the duodenum) as acidic gastric contents enter the duodenum from the stomach.

PHARMACOLOGIC AGENTS USED TO TREAT ACID-RELATED DISEASES OF THE UPPER GASTROINTESTINAL TRACT

Medications used to treat acid-related UGI tract diseases are divided into two groups: drugs that decrease stomach acidity and drugs that do not alter stomach acid.[1-3] (Medication Table 20-1; Medication Tables are located at the end of the chapter). Antacids, the histamine$_2$-receptor antagonists (H$_2$RAs), and the proton pump inhibitors (PPIs) all decrease stomach acidity and thus increase stomach pH. Sucralfate, bismuth salts, misoprostol, and alginic acid all provide benefits without altering stomach acid. This section focuses on how these medications work, their effectiveness, use in special populations, the most important side effects,

and major drug interactions. The therapeutic uses of each drug group are discussed in the sections on the treatment of the specific UGI diseases.

Antacids

Antacids are oral dosage formulations of inorganic salts used to relieve infrequent mild to moderate UGI symptoms, such as indigestion, sour stomach, and heartburn.[1-3] They are available OTC as tablets and liquid suspensions of a single salt (calcium, magnesium, aluminum, and sodium) or as a combination of several salts (eg, magnesium and aluminum). Antacid salts undergo a chemical reaction with acid in the stomach, which results in neutral salts and other neutralization products. By neutralizing some of the acid in the stomach, antacids can lead to a reduction in symptoms associated with acid-related UGI disorders. This requires neutralizing enough acid to raise the pH of the gastric environment to 4.0–5.0. All antacid neutralization reactions utilize similar chemical reactions, but depending on the initial salt, different neutralization products may result. Calcium carbonate is the most potent antacid, followed by sodium bicarbonate, and then the magnesium and aluminum salts, but differences in antacid potency can be adjusted for by increasing or decreasing the antacid dose. Antacids relieve symptoms quickly (within minutes), but the effect is short-lived and lasts only about 30 minutes when taken on an empty stomach.[1-3]

PRACTICE POINT

The duration of antacid effect may be prolonged by administering the antacid within 1 hour of a meal, thus increasing the duration of action for up to 3 hours. Symptom relief often depends on the antacid dose, with a larger dose resulting in greater neutralization of acid, higher pH, and greater relief of UGI symptoms. Some patients may require relatively large and frequent dosages to achieve symptomatic relief.

Specific antacid salts are associated with different adverse effects, which often guide the selection of an antacid. For instance, aluminum-containing antacids are associated with constipation, especially when taken in higher daily dosages. In contrast to aluminum salts, magnesium-containing antacids are associated with a dose-related diarrhea. At low doses, diarrhea may not occur, but as the daily dose is increased, diarrhea may become troublesome. Some antacids combine magnesium and aluminum salts to counter their different adverse effects, but diarrhea usually remains the predominant effect.

Prolonged use of calcium can result in high levels of calcium in the blood (hypercalcemia).[1] Although calcium salts are often associated with constipation, most individuals who take calcium-containing antacids do not experience constipation or diarrhea. If calcium salts are taken in combination with sodium bicarbonate, milk-alkali syndrome may result. Milk-alkali syndrome is a disorder in which high calcium blood concentrations increase the pH of the blood above its normal level, causing alkalosis. This pH change can reduce kidney function.

Sodium can cause the body to retain fluid. For this reason, antacids containing sodium should not be selected for patients with fluid-affected disorders such as hypertension, heart failure, ascites, and chronic kidney disease. They also may disrupt the natural electrolyte balance if used for prolonged periods. On a practical level, the carbon dioxide that is produced in the neutralization reaction between sodium bicarbonate and stomach acid can cause belching, bloating, flatulence (excess gas in the stomach or intestine), and distension (stretching or enlarging of the abdomen).

All antacids have the potential to interfere with the body's uptake of medications that depend on an acidic environment in the stomach for either dissolution or absorption.[1] Drugs for which this is a particular concern include the antifungal medications ketoconazole and itraconazole (Sporanox®), iron, the antituberculosis medication isoniazid, and the anticonvulsant medication phenytoin (Dilantin®). By increasing stomach pH (decreasing acidity), antacids can also hasten the dissolution of enteric-coated medications such as aspirin. Finally, aluminum, calcium, and magnesium ions produced during acid neutralization can bind to certain medications, such as tetracycline (eg, doxycycline) and fluoroquinolone antibiotics (eg, ciprofloxacin), to decrease their absorption and ultimately their effectiveness.

> ### PRACTICE POINT
>
> *It is possible to avoid most of the major drug interactions associated with antacids by dosing other medications 2 hours before or 4 hours after taking the antacid.*

Alginic Acid and Simethicone

Alginic acid or simethicone are sometimes combined with antacids, but neither has any effect on stomach acid. Alginic acid forms a foam layer that floats on top of the stomach contents and is thought to provide added protection to the esophagus when the acidic stomach contents reflux into the esophagus. Simethicone is a defoaming agent that is often added to antacid preparations as an antiflatulent to help break up gas bubbles in the GI tract and aid in the elimination of intestinal gas.

H₂-receptor Antagonists

The H$_2$RAs block histamine at the H$_2$-receptor on the parietal cells in the stomach, thus inhibiting acid secretion. There are currently three H$_2$RAs available in the United States, cimetidine (Tagamet®), famotidine (Pepcid®), and nizatidine, available by prescription, as well as cimetidine and famotidine OTC products (Medication Table 20-1). The oral H$_2$RAs are slower to act (30–45 minutes) than antacids but provide symptom relief over a longer period (about 6–8 hours). Famotidine is also available as a combination product with antacids, thus providing a quick onset of action as well as a longer duration of effect. Cimetidine and nizatidine are available as oral solutions that are stable almost indefinitely at room temperature and may be used until the expiration date assigned by the manufacturer. Famotidine is available as an oral suspension that is only stable for 30 days at room temperature (77°F) once reconstituted. Only cimetidine and famotidine are available for injection.

> ### PRACTICE POINT
>
> *The famotidine and nizatidine liquid formulations contain sugar, whereas cimetidine formulations are flavored with sugar alcohols or artificial sweeteners. Formulations without added sugar may be more appropriate for patients with diabetes or other conditions requiring control of carbohydrate intake.*

Famotidine is the most potent of these medications and cimetidine is the least potent. However, when the H$_2$RAs are taken in recommended dosages to treat a specific indication, they provide similar relief of symptoms and rates of ulcer or esophageal healing. Because H$_2$RA action is not tied to meals, they can be used to treat nocturnal (nighttime) or fasting symptoms.

Cimetidine and famotidine are eliminated from the body through metabolism in the liver and excretion by the kidney. Nizatidine is primarily eliminated by the kidneys. Dosage reductions for all three H_2RAs are recommended in patients with reduced kidney function. In general, no adjustment is needed in patients with liver dysfunction.

The oral H_2RAs are safe and well tolerated. Some of the more common adverse effects include diarrhea, constipation, mild dizziness, headache, drowsiness, lethargy, confusion, and rashes. A reversible fall in blood platelet numbers (thrombocytopenia) may occur with all H_2RAs, but the incidence is low. The injectable formulations are generally safe as well. Cimetidine has been associated with antiandrogen effects, including enlargement of breast tissue (gynecomastia) and erectile dysfunction (impotence). Both effects are reversible with discontinuation of cimetidine. The risk of adverse effects is increased in the elderly, patients with reduced kidney function, and those taking high H_2RA doses.

The H_2RAs share the potential to alter the dissolution and absorption of drugs that are dependent on an acidic gastric environment. The list of affected medications is like that of the antacids (eg, the antifungals ketoconazole and itraconazole). Cimetidine inhibits the liver metabolism of many medications and can lead to clinically important drug interactions. This is the case for medications that have a narrow therapeutic window, such as warfarin and phenytoin. The concurrent use of agents that interact with cimetidine generally leads to the recommendation of another H_2RA. Famotidine and nizatidine do not interact in a way that disrupts the metabolism of other drugs, so they are free from these drug interactions.[1-3]

One of the effects seen with the H_2RAs is tachyphylaxis.[4] Tachyphylaxis is a decreased response (or developing tolerance) to a drug after repeated doses in a relatively short period of time. Increasing the dose of the drug will not increase or restore response. This is a particular problem with intravenous (IV) dosage forms of H_2RAs, and it has been observed with oral H_2RAs as well. It may occur in a few days to several weeks or months.

Proton Pump Inhibitors

The PPIs are used for more frequent symptoms and more severe forms of acid-related diseases, as they are potent inhibitors of gastric acid secretion.[1] They act by binding to H^+/K^+ ATPase, or the so-called proton pump, of the parietal cells in the stomach. This is involved in the last step in the secretion of gastric acid. PPIs achieve a sustained increase in stomach pH (reduced acidity) even after meals when acid secretion would otherwise tend to increase greatly. The PPIs are prodrugs that require an acidic environment in the parietal cells of the stomach where they are converted to their active form. Thus, the PPI must be either enteric-coated in the form of enteric-coated granules or tablets or mixed with sodium bicarbonate (Medication Table 20-1). This provides protection for the drug from stomach acid until it is absorbed into the vascular system and gets to the parietal cell, where it is activated. The PPIs work best when taken before a meal so that the proton pumps are actively secreting acid.

PRACTICE POINT

To achieve the best effect, it is recommended that patients take a PPI 30–60 minutes prior to eating. One common dosing recommendation is to take the medication in the morning 30 minutes before the first meal of the day. If a second dose is needed, it is best taken 30 minutes before the evening meal.

The PPIs currently available in the United States include omeprazole (Prilosec®), omeprazole/sodium bicarbonate (Zegerid®), lansoprazole (Prevacid®), rabeprazole (Aciphex®), pantoprazole (Protonix®), esomeprazole (Nexium®), and dexlansoprazole (Dexilant®)[1-3] All are available by prescription in a variety of dosage forms (Table 20-1). Omeprazole (Prilosec OTC®), generic omeprazole, omeprazole/sodium bicarbonate (Zegerid OTC®), and lansoprazole (Prevacid 24 HR®) are available OTC. Only pantoprazole and esomeprazole are currently available for injection.

The acid-inhibiting effects of the PPIs usually last for about 20–24 hours, which exceeds their time in the body. All PPIs are similar when taken in recommended doses to relieve symptoms and heal peptic ulcers and esophagitis. Standard PPI dosages are superior to the H_2RAs in relieving acid-related symptoms as well as ulcer and esophageal healing. Dosage reductions are recommended in patients with severe liver impairment but not required in patients with kidney failure.

The PPIs are well tolerated, and adverse effects associated with their short-term use are similar to those observed with the H_2RAs. However, there are various safety warnings from the U.S. Food and Drug Administration (FDA) concerning the association of potential side effects with long-term use of PPIs. These side effects are increased risk of fractures, low magnesium (hypomagnesemia), pneumonia, *Clostridium difficile*-associated diarrhea, vitamin B_{12} deficiency, dementia, kidney failure, and systemic lupus erythematosus.[5-11] It is important to note that the majority of published studies in this area are "observational," meaning that they do not prove a cause and effect relationship between PPIs and these outcomes; instead they show an association with these issues to the extent that the FDA has provided safety warnings.

TABLE 20-1. Proton Pump Inhibitor Alternative Dosage Formulations and Administration[1,2a]

Proton Pump Inhibitor	Administration Options
Omeprazole (oh ME pray zol)	Capsule opened and granules mixed in juice or sprinkled on soft food (applesauce) and given orally or by NG tube; oral suspension containing sodium bicarbonate in package for NG tube; extemporaneously compounded suspension in sodium bicarbonate can be compounded and administered by NG tube
Lansoprazole (lan SOE pra zole)	Capsule opened and granules sprinkled on soft food (applesauce); capsule granules mixed in juice and given orally or by NG tube; extemporaneously compounded suspension in sodium bicarbonate can be prepared and administered by NG tube; oral suspension in package for oral use (not NG); orally disintegrating tablet for oral or NG tube use
Pantoprazole (pan TOE pra zole)	Extemporaneously compounded suspension in sodium bicarbonate can be prepared and administered by NG tube; IV administration
Esomeprazole (es oh ME pray zol)	Capsule opened and granules sprinkled on soft food (applesauce); capsule granules mixed in water and given by NG tube; capsule granules mixed in juice and given orally or by NG tube; IV administration
Dexlansoprazole (dex lan SOE pra zole)	Capsule opened and granules sprinkled on soft food (applesauce)

IV = intravenous; NG = nasogastric.
[a]Pronunciations have been adapted with permission from USP Dictionary of USAN and International Drug Names (USP Dictionary) © 2022.

The PPIs, like the H$_2$RAs, have been associated with a decreased dissolution and absorption of medications that depend on an acidic environment. All the PPIs are metabolized by the liver, but omeprazole and esomeprazole have the greatest potential to interact with medications metabolized by the liver, such as warfarin and phenytoin. However, drug interactions with omeprazole and esomeprazole are much less common than those observed with cimetidine. The concurrent use of omeprazole or esomeprazole with clopidogrel may decrease the antiplatelet effects of clopidogrel via a CYP-450 2C19 drug interaction. This is a category D drug interaction,[12] which means practitioners should likely consider modifying therapy to avoid the drug interaction. Data suggests that pantoprazole, rabeprazole, or lansoprazole may not interact with clopidogrel to the same extent (category C).[13] Clinical studies and platelet function data have inconsistently demonstrated clinically significant outcomes (eg, negative cardiac-related outcomes and mortality).[14-17] Therefore, the current recommendation is to avoid the drug interaction with clopidogrel and omeprazole or esomeprazole and to use an alternative PPI (eg, pantoprazole).

Sucralfate

Sucralfate (Carafate®) is an aluminum salt of a complex sugar known as a disaccharide (Medication Table 20-1). It is available only by prescription. Sucralfate heals peptic ulcers by forming a protective barrier that coats the lining of the stomach, thus permitting the ulcer to heal by protecting it from damage due to acid, pepsin, and bile salts. It may also stimulate prostaglandins in the stomach lining, which could lead to further protective effects. In contrast to the antacids, H$_2$RAs, and PPIs, sucralfate does not neutralize or decrease gastric acid secretion.

Constipation is the most common adverse effect seen with sucralfate and is related to the aluminum content of the drug. Aluminum also binds dietary phosphate and could lead to low serum phosphate levels. Sucralfate may be associated with the development of a bezoar (a mass of undigested material in the stomach). Because of the aluminum content, sucralfate should be avoided in patients with kidney failure. Sucralfate potentially interacts with many medications by binding to them in the esophagus and stomach, thereby decreasing their availability. Medications that can be affected include warfarin, fluoroquinolone antibiotics (eg, ciprofloxacin, levofloxacin), phenytoin, levothyroxine, and ketoconazole.

Bismuth Salts

Bismuth salts are used for a wide range of GI complaints, although they do not neutralize or inhibit gastric acid secretion. The mechanisms by which they exert beneficial effects are not completely understood, but bismuth may have a topical (local) effect on the stomach lining, promoting protective responses. It is likely that bismuth also has some antimicrobial activity, particularly with regard to *H. Pylori*. The two bismuth salts with GI indications in the United States are bismuth subsalicylate (Pepto Bismol)—see Medication Table 20-1—and bismuth subcitrate (as a combination product for treatment of *H. pylori*).

> ## ALERT!
>
> Bismuth subsalicylate should be avoided in children recovering from or suffering with influenza. The risk of Reye's syndrome, a potentially fatal condition, increases with exposure to salicylates.

> ## ALERT!
>
> The risk of bleeding and toxicity increases when the patient is taking bismuth subsalicylate concurrently with other salicylate medications. Bismuth subsalicylate should be avoided in patients with kidney failure as salicylates can accumulate and result in salicylate toxicity. Patients who are allergic to salicylates, such as aspirin, are likely to be allergic to bismuth subsalicylate.

> ### PRACTICE POINT
>
> *Tablet and liquid formulations containing bismuth cause a blackening of the stool, but the tongue may also blacken with liquid formulations. Normal coloration returns after stopping the bismuth product. Black-colored stools (melena) may also be a sign of UGI bleeding.*

Misoprostol

Misoprostol (Cytotec) acts to reduce the risk of ulcers or ulcer-related bleeding in patients taking aspirin or other NSAIDs. It is a man-made analog of a naturally occurring prostaglandin. In the body, misoprostol contributes to numerous effects that are protective to the stomach. It increases the production of mucus and bicarbonate, increases

blood flow to the stomach lining, and decreases the rate of turnover of mucosal cells. Misoprostol also inhibits the secretion of stomach acid, but the effect is less than that seen with the H_2RAs.

> ## ALERT!
>
> Misoprostol carries a warning that indicates that it can cause abortion, premature birth, or birth defects and therefore is contraindicated in pregnant women.

Misoprostol also has abortive properties and should not be used in women of childbearing age without adequate birth control. Women must have a negative serum pregnancy test and must be capable of effectively using contraception before receiving a prescription for misoprostol.

> ### PRACTICE POINT
>
> *For women of childbearing potential, initiation of the misoprostol should only occur on the second or third day of the menstrual period.*

Misoprostol's major adverse effect is dose-dependent diarrhea (diarrhea increases as the dose increases) that occurs in about one-third of patients. Abdominal cramping is also troublesome. Less common adverse effects include nausea, flatulence, and headache.

TREATMENT OF ACID-RELATED DISEASES OF THE UPPER GASTROINTESTINAL TRACT

This section briefly discusses the etiology, pathophysiology, risk factors, clinical presentation, and complications of dyspepsia, PUD, GERD, and UGI bleeding. Emphasis is placed on nonpharmacologic (nondrug) and pharmacologic treatment.

Dyspepsia

Dyspepsia is a very common complaint among patients, although patients with dyspepsia do not often seek medical attention. In many cases, occasional dyspepsia is brought on by ingesting spicy foods, acidic foods, or beverages (eg, tomato or orange juice), or eating too much or too fast. Avoidance of troublesome foods and beverages and improved eating habits usually lead to improvement or elimination of symptoms. Medications such as the NSAIDs (eg, aspirin, naproxen, ibuprofen, piroxicam) are the most important cause of drug-induced dyspepsia, but symptoms do not necessarily correlate with damage to the stomach lining (eg, erosions or ulcers). Other medications that may produce dyspepsia include theophylline, potassium supplements, and digoxin. In most cases, taking the medication with food, decreasing the dose, or stopping the drug reduces or eliminates symptoms.

In contrast, some patients complain of relapsing and long-lasting dyspeptic symptoms, which may or may not be associated with a known underlying cause. Occasionally, chronic dyspeptic symptoms occur in otherwise healthy individuals for whom diagnostic tests do not reveal a cause (eg, peptic ulcer) for their symptoms.[18] Thus, *nonulcer dyspepsia* is used to describe this condition. However, in a subset of patients with chronic dyspepsia, diagnostic tests confirm the presence of PUD, GERD, or gastric malignancy.[19]

Because it is not always possible to determine the cause of dyspepsia, treatment is aimed at relieving the dyspeptic symptoms with an antacid, H_2RA, or PPI. Food-induced symptoms can be avoided by eliminating troublesome foods and beverages or can be treated with an antacid or an OTC H_2RA. Reducing the dose or discontinuing treatment usually relieves drug-induced dyspepsia, but antacids, H_2RAs, or a PPI may be necessary if the drug dose cannot be reduced, or the drug cannot be discontinued. Dyspepsia, which is neither food- nor drug induced, is initially managed by physicians with a 1-month trial of either an H_2RA or PPI. Treatment of PUD- or GERD-related dyspepsia is aimed at treating the underlying disease. A small number of patients, for whom the etiology cannot be determined, do not respond well to drug treatment.

Peptic Ulcer Disease

PUD is a chronic acid-related disease characterized by a distinct, confined, lesion (ulcer) found most often in the lining of the stomach (gastric ulcer) or the first part of the small intestine (duodenal ulcer) of ambulatory patients. Although peptic ulcers usually occur as a single lesion, multiple ulcers may be present. Stress ulcers (stress-related mucosa damage) in contrast, are multiple acute ulcers that occur primarily in critically ill hospitalized patients. About 10% of the U.S. population develops chronic PUD in their lifetime, with a similar prevalence in men and women. The natural course of PUD is characterized by ulcer recurrence and is influenced by *H. pylori* infection and NSAID use.

CASE STUDY

Eugene Gonzalez is a 48-year-old man who is seen by his doctor for complaints of burning stomach pain. Several weeks ago, he noticed the gradual onset of a localized burning pain in the upper stomach (epigastric region) that occurred daily, especially between meals and sometimes at night. Mr. Gonzalez indicates that taking antacids relieves the pain but that it often returns within 30 minutes. He denies any NSAID use and has a negative history for PUD.

CASE STUDY

Julia Rosenberg is a 66-year-old woman with a long history of PUD related to various NSAIDs she has taken to relieve symptoms of arthritis. She currently takes ibuprofen 400 mg twice daily, aspirin 81 mg daily, and atenolol 50 mg daily. Two months ago, she was hospitalized for a bleeding gastric ulcer. The ibuprofen was stopped temporarily, and a PPI was prescribed to heal the ulcer. Last week an EGD was performed, and ulcer healing was confirmed. Her physician tells her to reinstitute the ibuprofen 400 mg twice daily.

Etiology, Pathophysiology, Risk Factors

Most peptic ulcers in the stomach and duodenum are caused by *H. pylori* bacteria or NSAIDs and occur in the presence of normal gastric acid secretion. Zollinger-Ellison syndrome (ZES), a rare form of PUD, is caused by increased gastric acid secretion resulting in multiple, severe ulcers. Certain viral infections, chemotherapy, or radiation exposure may cause peptic ulcers, but these ulcers are uncommon.

Helicobacter pylori-Related Ulcers

H. pylori is a spiral-shaped, gram-negative bacterium that, when acquired, resides in the lining of the stomach or the duodenum. It attaches to the gastroduodenal lining and secretes toxic substances that cause chronic gastritis and peptic ulcers. Although 30% to 40% of the U.S. population is infected with the organism, only 20% of infected individuals develop ulcer symptoms.[20] A small number (1%) of individuals with long-standing *H. pylori*-related gastritis will develop gastric cancer.[20] The prevalence of *H. pylori* varies worldwide, but it is linked to poor socioeconomic conditions. Most individuals acquire *H. pylori* during childhood and likely co-infect other individuals living in the same household.

Nonsteroidal Anti-inflammatory Drug-Induced Ulcers

NSAIDs, including aspirin (acetylsalicylic acid; ASA), are available by prescription and OTC and rank among the most widely used class of medications in the United States, especially in individuals older than 65 years.[19] There is overwhelming evidence linking NSAIDs with stomach erosions, stomach ulcers, and ulcer-related complications, as hospitalizations and mortality are increased in chronic NSAID users.[19] NSAIDs act directly on the stomach lining to cause erosions, but ulcers (which are deeper than erosions) are related to the ability of the NSAID to systemically inhibit naturally occurring protective prostaglandins in the stomach lining (see the section on Anatomy and Physiology).

Prostaglandins in the body are produced by two pathways: cyclooxygenase-1 (COX-1) and cyclooxygenase-2 (COX-2). The COX-1 pathway promotes gastroduodenal protection while the COX-2 pathway mediates inflammation and pain. Thus, depletion of COX-1 by NSAIDs and ASA promotes the formation of ulcers and bleeding. Currently available NSAIDs inhibit both COX-1 and COX-2 to varying degrees and have both a beneficial anti-inflammatory action and a potentially toxic effect on the stomach lining. Rofecoxib (Vioxx) and valdecoxib (Bextra), previously available selective COX-2 inhibitors, were withdrawn from the U.S. market because of risk for cardiovascular events (eg, myocardial infarction and thrombotic stroke). Celecoxib (Celebrex) remains available but has a similar risk profile to nonselective COX inhibitors.

CASE?

Which of the peptic ulcer patients in the cases included here is more likely to be infected with H. pylori?

The risk of developing an NSAID-induced ulcer increases in individuals with a previous ulcer or ulcer complication, those older than 60 years of age, taking multiple or high dosages of NSAIDs, taking an NSAID plus ASA (even low cardioprotective ASA dosages such as 81 mg/day), and those taking concomitant corticosteroids, anticoagulants, or antiplatelet drugs.[19]

Clinical Presentation, Complications, and Diagnosis

Patients with PUD present with mild to severe epigastric pain (pain located in the upper abdomen) or an acute life-threatening UGI complication. The pain is often described as burning but may be a feeling of abdominal discomfort or fullness. Some individuals complain of dyspeptic symptoms, including bloating or belching, while others may have nocturnal pain that awakens them from sleep. In some patients, ulcer pain is precipitated by food while in others pain is relieved by food. The absence of epigastric pain does not necessarily imply that an ulcer is not present. Changes in the character of the pain or signs and symptoms such as nausea, vomiting, and weight loss may suggest ulcer-related complications such as UGI bleeding, perforation, or pyloric obstruction, which is related to the formation of scar tissue. Ulcer pain typically resolves with treatment, but recurrence of pain may suggest that the ulcer is not healed or that it recurred.

The diagnosis of PUD is usually based on the history and physical examination, visualization of the ulcer either by upper endoscopy or upper gastrointestinal (UGI) radiography, and tests to confirm *H. pylori* infection. Gastric acid secretory studies and fasting serum gastrin tests are reserved for patients with severe or complicated disease. Routine laboratory tests may not be very helpful, except in patients suspected of having ulcer-related complications. Patients with PUD have a high probability of *H. pylori* infection and should be tested so that appropriate treatment can be instituted.

H. pylori infection may be diagnosed by either endoscopic or nonendoscopic methods. Endoscopy not only permits direct visualization of the ulcer, but also enables tissue samples (biopsies) to be obtained and tested for the presence of *H. pylori*. The nonendoscopic tests, however, are less invasive and are inexpensive. The most widely available and most often used nonendoscopic tests include a blood test (serology) that detects antibodies to *H. pylori* and a breath test that uses radiolabeled urea (urea breath test, UBT) to detect active infection. Serology (blood testing) is most convenient as it can be performed in the physician's office, but its diagnostic accuracy is less than that of the UBT. A stool antigen test is also available, but it is not widely used in the United States. Please note, both the *H. pylori* breath test and the stool antigen test can have false negatives in patients taking a PPI, bismuth, or antibiotics.

Goals of Therapy

The goals for treating PUD are to accelerate ulcer healing, prevent ulcer recurrence, and reduce ulcer-related complications with cost-effective and safe medications. Failure to cure the *H. pylori* infection may cause recurrent ulcers and the continuing risk of ulcer complications. Patients at risk of NSAID-induced ulcers should receive prophylactic cotherapy to reduce the risk of ulcer recurrence.

Nonpharmacologic (Nondrug) Therapy

There is no specific "ulcer diet" for patients with PUD. However, patients who are unable to tolerate certain spicy foods, citrus, caffeine, or alcohol-containing beverages should avoid these items. Patients should be encouraged to reduce stressful situations and stop cigarette smoking. Endoscopic or radiologic procedures may be required for diagnosis, and surgery may be necessary for ulcer-related complications such as UGI bleeding.

Pharmacotherapy

Helicobacter pylori-Related Ulcers

Successful eradication of *H. pylori* and ulcer healing require combining an antisecretory drug (eg, PPI) with multiple antibiotics with or without a bismuth salt. The effectiveness of clarithromycin triple therapy is limited in areas where *H. pylori* resistance exceeds 15%.[2] Typically, three- and four-drug regimens are recommended, but only those regimens that have been adequately studied should be used for eradication and ulcer healing.[20]

CASE?

In-office serologic (blood) testing for *H. pylori* was positive and UGI radiology confirmed a small duodenal ulcer. Mr. Gonzalez's physician prescribed a three-drug regimen to eradicate the infection and heal the ulcer. Why does he have to take three drugs to treat his peptic ulcer?

PRACTICE POINT

A PPI-based, three-drug regimen is usually the first-line treatment for H. pylori-*positive patients with an active ulcer, a documented history of a prior ulcer, or a history of ulcer-related complications.*

The recommended treatment for *H. pylori* infection (Table 20-2) in the United States consists of either bismuth

quadruple therapy or concomitant (non-bismuth quadruple) therapy. It is recommended not to substitute for the primary antibiotics with either of these regimens. Bismuth-containing quadruple therapy (10 or 14 days) is a first-choice treatment as it results in satisfactory eradication rates, but nonadherence to the complicated drug regimen can make this challenging for patients if not previously used. This regimen consists of metronidazole, tetracycline, a PPI or H_2RA, and bismuth subsalicylate. All medications except the PPI should be taken four times a day with meals and at bedtime.

The concomitant (non-bismuth quadruple) therapy (10 or 14 days) is another first-line treatment with good efficacy. This regimen consists of clarithromycin, amoxicillin, metronidazole, and a PPI. All medications should be taken twice daily. The PPI should be taken 30–60 minutes before a meal along with the three antibiotics, but it should not be continued beyond 2 weeks after stopping the antibiotics unless it is used to treat another disease (eg, GERD). A single daily PPI dose may be less effective than twice daily when used as part of a four-drug *H. pylori* treatment regimen.

A three-drug regimen containing a PPI, clarithromycin, and either amoxicillin or metronidazole for 7, 10, or 14 days has a higher incidence of resistance in the United Sates. This combination should only be used in areas where clarithromycin resistance is < 15%. Sequential treatment consisting of 5 days of a PPI plus amoxicillin, followed by 5 additional days of a PPI plus clarithromycin plus metronidazole has been shown to be more effective than the combination of a PPI plus both amoxicillin and clarithromycin for 7 days.[20]

Third-choice treatment options are used when other regimens are unsuccessful and typically include antibiotics from other classes, such as a fluoroquinolone (eg, levofloxacin), LOAD (levofloxacin, omeprazole or other PPI, nitazoxanide, [brand name Alinia®], and doxycycline) therapy, or hybrid therapy (Table 20-2).

PRACTICE POINT

Substitution of one PPI for another in the regimens described is acceptable and does not improve or worsen H. pylori *eradication. An H_2RA should not be substituted for a PPI in a three-drug regimen, as the H_2RA may not be as effective as the PPI. However, an H_2RA may be used as part of the bismuth-based, four-drug regimen. Comparable eradication rates occur when bismuth subcitrate is used in place of bismuth subsalicylate.*

TABLE 20-2. Drug Regimens Used to Treat *Helicobacter pylori*-Related Peptic Ulcers[2,20,21a]

Regimen/Medications	Frequency	Duration
Clarithromycin-Based Three-Drug Regimen		
Clarithromycin 500 mg (kla RITH roe mye sin)	Twice daily	14 days
Amoxicillin 1 g (a mox i SIL in) or Metronidazole 500 mg (me troe NI da zole)	Twice daily 2 or 3 times daily	14 days
PPI	Twice daily	14 days
Levofloxacin-Based Three-Drug Regimen		
Levofloxacin 500 mg (lee voe FLOKS a sin)	Once daily	14 days
Amoxicillin 1 g (a mox i SIL in)	Twice daily	14 days
PPI	Twice daily	14 days
Levofloxacin-Based Sequential Therapy		
Amoxicillin 1 g (a mox i SIL in)	Twice daily	Days 1–10
Levofloxacin 500 mg (lee voe FLOKS a sin)	Once daily	Days 6–10
Metronidazole 500 mg (me troe NI da zole)	Twice daily	Days 6–10
Load		
Levofloxacin 250 mg (lee voe FLOKS a sin)	Once daily	7–10 days
PPI (eg, omeprazole [oh MEP ra zole])	Once daily	7–10 days
Nitazoxanide (nye ta ZOX a nide) 500 mg	Twice daily	7–10 days
Doxycycline 100 mg (doks i SYE kleen)	Once daily	7–10 days
Rifabutin-Based Three-Drug Regimen		
Rifabutin 50 mg (rif a BYOO tin)	3 times daily	14 days
Amoxicillin 1 gram (a mox i SIL in)	3 times daily	14 days
PPI (omeprazole 40 mg)	3 times daily	14 days
High-Dose Dual Therapy		
Amoxicillin 1 g 3 times daily or 750 mg 4 times daily (a mox i SIL in)	3-4 times daily	14 days
PPI	3-4 times daily	14 days
Clarithromycin-Based Sequential Therapy		
Amoxicillin 1 g (a mox i SIL in)	Twice daily	Days 1–5
Clarithromycin 500 mg (kla RITH roe mye sin)	Twice daily	Days 6–10
Metronidazole 500 mg (me troe NI da zole)	Twice daily	Days 6–10
PPI	Twice daily	Days 1–10
Clarithromycin-Based Hybrid Therapy		
Amoxicillin 1 g (a mox i SIL in)	Twice daily	Days 1–14
Clarithromycin 250-500 mg plus	Twice daily	Days 7–14
Metronidazole 250-500 mg (me troe NI da zole)	Twice daily	Days 7–14
PPI	Once or twice daily	14 days

Continued next page

TABLE 20-2. Drug Regimens Used to Treat *Helicobacter pylori*-Related Peptic Ulcers[2,20,21a] *(Continued)*

Regimen/Medications	Frequency	Duration
Bismuth-Based Four-Drug Regimen[b]		
Tetracycline 500 mg (tet ra SYE kleen)	Four times daily	10–14 days
Metronidazole 250-500 mg (me troe NI da zole)	Four times daily	10–14 days
Bismuth subsalicylate 525 mg (BIZ muth) (sub sa LIS i late)	Four times daily	10–14 days
PPI or H₂RA	Once or twice daily	10–14 days
Non-Bismuth-Based Four-Drug Regimen		
Clarithromycin 250-mg (kla RITH roe mye sin)	Twice daily	1–10 days
Amoxicillin 1 g (a mox i SIL in)	Twice daily	1–10 days
Metronidazole 250-500 mg (me troe NI da zole)	Twice daily	1–10 days
PPI	Once or twice daily	1–10 days

H₂RA = histamine₂-receptor antagonist; PPI = proton pump inhibitor.
[a]Pronunciations have been adapted with permission from USP Dictionary of USAN and International Drug Names (USP Dictionary) © 2022.
[b]Commercially available, prepackaged products include Helidac®, which contains bismuth subsalicylate, metronidazole, and tetracycline, and Pylera®, which contains bismuth subcitrate, metronidazole, and tetracycline.

The antibiotics that have been most studied as part of an initial *H. pylori* regimen are clarithromycin, amoxicillin, metronidazole, tinidazole, nitazoxanide, rifabutin, doxycycline, and tetracycline.[2,20] Substitution of clarithromycin for tetracycline is acceptable, but adverse effects are increased. Other antibiotic substitutions may be less effective. Specifically, ampicillin should not be substituted for amoxicillin, doxycycline should not be substituted for tetracycline, and azithromycin or erythromycin should not be substituted for clarithromycin.

ALERT!

Amoxicillin should not be prescribed for penicillin-allergic patients, and metronidazole should be avoided if ethanol (as part of alcoholic beverages or even as a component of some liquid medications) is consumed because metronidazole reacts with ethanol to cause numerous adverse effects (this is called a disulfiram-like reaction).

Adverse effects vary with different drug regimens. Metronidazole increases the frequency of adverse effects when the dose is greater than 1 g/day. Taste disturbances (metallic taste) may occur with metronidazole and clarithromycin. Antibiotic-associated diarrhea may also occur.

Nonsteroidal Anti-inflammatory Drug-Induced Ulcers

Drugs used to treat acid-related diseases are also used to heal an active ulcer caused by NSAIDs and to reduce the risk of (prevent) an NSAID-induced ulcer and ulcer-related UGI complications (eg, bleeding). When the patient has an active ulcer, the NSAID should be discontinued. Consider switching to acetaminophen, tramadol, or a short-acting narcotic. Most ulcers heal with a standard dosage regimen of an H₂RA, PPI, or sucralfate (Medication Table 20-1) if the NSAID is stopped. Treatment with a PPI is preferred because it provides a more rapid rate of symptom relief and ulcer healing (4 weeks) than an H₂RA or sucralfate (6–8 weeks).[1,2] The PPIs are interchangeable for this indication as long as they are used in their recommended oral dosages (Medication Table 20-1).

If NSAID therapy must be continued despite ulceration, consideration should be given to using a potentially less ulcerogenic NSAID or reducing the NSAID daily dose. Ulcer healing can occur if the NSAID is continued, but it will take longer (12 weeks) and requires the use of a potent acid suppressant.[1,2] Thus, the PPIs are also the drugs of choice when the NSAID cannot be discontinued.[1,19] If *H. pylori* is present, the patient should be treated with an eradication regimen that contains a PPI.[1,2]

Various management strategies have been used to reduce the risk of NSAID-induced ulcers and UGI bleeding in high-risk patients. The use of enteric-coated preparations such as aspirin reduces the irritating effects on the stomach but does not stop ulcers from forming. Taking an NSAID with food or milk may reduce NSAID-related dyspepsia but does not prevent ulcers. Antacids and sucralfate should not be used for preventive purposes, as there is insufficient evidence to support their use for this indication. Taking an H_2RA along with the NSAID (cotherapy) works to reduce NSAID dyspepsia, but it is not effective in reducing the risk of stomach ulcers when given in standard prescription dosages (eg, famotidine 40 mg/day).[2] It is possible that higher H_2RA dosages (eg, famotidine 40 mg twice daily) may reduce the risk of NSAID-induced stomach ulcers, but it most likely does not reduce the risk of UGI bleeding. Misoprostol (Medication Table 20-1) cotherapy reduces the risk of NSAID-induced stomach ulcers and ulcer-related complications such as UGI bleeding. However, multiple daily dosing, abdominal cramping, dose-related diarrhea, and abortive effects limit adherence as well as its effectiveness.

The PPIs are as effective as misoprostol for reducing the risk of NSAID ulcers and have the added advantage of fewer troublesome adverse effects. The PPIs are superior to the H_2RAs when used for this indication. All PPIs, when used in recommended oral dosages, reduce the risk of NSAID-induced stomach ulcers and ulcer-related UGI complications. All the PPIs have a similar efficacy and safety profile and are interchangeable.

Selective COX-2 inhibitors such as rofecoxib and valdecoxib are associated with a lower risk of GI toxicity, but they are no longer available in the United States because of their association with serious cardiovascular thrombotic effects. Celecoxib is a currently available COX-2 inhibitor; however, it bears the same FDA labeling in regard to GI and cardiovascular risks as all other available NSAIDs. Data shows that celecoxib has a lower relative risk of GI and cardiovascular events compared to nonselective NSAIDS and therefore may be used more in practice. Gastroprotective benefits are reduced in patients using aspirin with celecoxib. Thus, it is recommended to use PPI cotherapy with celecoxib if low-dose aspirin is being used. Finally, increased cardiovascular risk and the acute side effects possible with NSAIDs (eg, fluid retention, hypertension, renal toxicity) require that the lowest effective dose of celecoxib be used as it is at least as beneficial as a nonselective NSAID plus a PPI.

Gastroesophageal Reflux Disease

GERD is a common acid-related disease caused by the reflux (backward movement) of acid and other stomach contents into the esophagus, which results in symptoms such as heartburn and may cause damage to the esophageal lining. The prevalence of GERD (including symptoms of heartburn and esophageal damage) in the Western world is about 10%–20%.[1] Patients with GERD may have a decreased quality of life and are at risk for serious complications, which includes esophageal cancer.[1]

Etiology, Pathophysiology, Risk Factors

The most common cause of gastroesophageal reflux is temporary relaxation of the LES (Figure 20-1). The LES remains contracted (at high pressure) unless food or liquid is being swallowed. When relaxation of the LES occurs, gastric contents, including acid, bile, and other stomach enzymes, enter the esophagus. This is a very common occurrence (even in healthy individuals), and although these acidic contents encounter the esophageal lining, most individuals do not develop symptoms or esophageal damage. This is because waves of esophageal contractions and relaxations force contents back into the stomach, while swallowing saliva (containing bicarbonate) acts to reduce the acidity of the stomach contents.[1] In patients who develop GERD, transient relaxations of the LES become more common and the contact time of the acid and esophageal lining is increased, which leads to mucosal damage and symptoms. Other risk factors include diet and lifestyle, medications, and medical conditions, which either reduce LES pressure or the ability of the LES to function properly. Obesity, bending over, and wearing tight-fitting clothing increases intra-abdominal pressure and places more strain on the LES. Some foods (eg, high-fat meals, chocolate, and mint) can reduce the LES pressure, while acidic foods and beverages (eg, tomatoes, citrus) can irritate the esophageal lining. Medications, including the calcium channel blockers, benzodiazepines, narcotic analgesics, beta-adrenergic agonists, and nitrates, decrease LES pressure. The most common medical conditions associated with GERD are hiatal hernia and gastroparesis, a partial paralysis of the stomach, which can occur in patients with diabetes.

Clinical Presentation, Complications, and Diagnosis

The most common typical symptoms of GERD are heartburn and acid regurgitation, a sour taste in the back of the throat caused by refluxed stomach acid. Other symptoms include belching, hiccups, nausea, vomiting, and feeling full earlier during a meal (early satiety). More worrisome (alarm) symptoms include difficult or painful swallowing, unexpected weight loss, vomiting, and blood in vomit or stool.[3]

CASE?

What are the most serious consequences that could result from Mrs. Dryden's GERD?

Complications associated with GERD include erosive esophagitis, stricture formation (narrowing of the esophagus, which can cause difficulty in swallowing), Barrett's esophagus, and adenocarcinoma (a type of cancer) of the esophagus. Erosive esophagitis results from damage of the lining (mucosa) of the esophagus caused by exposure to stomach acid or other irritating substances and varies in severity, from mild inflammation and redness to ulceration and bleeding. Barrett's esophagus, a precancerous condition, occurs in about 10% of patients who undergo endoscopy for GERD and results from continuous acid exposure and esophageal injury in patients with long-standing GERD. Barrett's esophagus is associated with an increased risk of adenocarcinoma of the esophagus.[22]

Some patients have symptoms of GERD that do not appear to involve the esophagus. These manifestations include noncardiac chest pain, nonallergic or nonseasonal asthma, chronic hoarseness or laryngitis, and even dental erosions. These may be the only symptoms the patient describes to the doctor. Specialized testing and evaluation are necessary to determine if GERD is the cause of these symptoms.

There are numerous methods available to establish a diagnosis of GERD and determine if complicated disease is present. Upper endoscopy allows the physician to visualize and determine the extent of the damage to the esophageal lining, identify hiatal hernia or strictures, and screen for Barrett's esophagus or cancer. Upper GI radiography or barium esophagram (also sometimes called a barium swallow test) permits identification of erosions, ulcerations, strictures, and hiatal hernia. Continuous 24-hour intra-esophageal pH monitoring enables the physician to determine when and at what times the pH in the esophagus is low; this demonstrates the reflux of acid into the esophagus. The most common test to evaluate GERD is an empiric trial (test) of a PPI.[23] Patients who respond to a short trial of PPI once or twice daily receive a tentative diagnosis of GERD and are managed without costly workups. However, a positive response does not differentiate between GERD and other acid-related diseases such as PUD.

PRACTICE POINT

Patients should keep a diary to record their GERD symptoms and attempt to relate them to lifestyle or diet. This diary should be brought to their healthcare provider for discussion and review to determine the best course of action in eliminating the patient's symptoms.

Goals of Therapy

The goals for treating GERD are to relieve symptoms, promote esophageal healing, prevent symptomatic relapse and complications, and provide cost-effective and safe drug therapy. Remember that GERD is a chronic disease with the potential for serious complications like those of diabetes or hypertension and may require long-term maintenance therapy.

Nonpharmacologic (Nondrug) Therapy

The first step in managing GERD is to discuss lifestyle and dietary changes, which may benefit the patient's symptoms.[3] Lifestyle recommendations include the elevation of the head of the bed by 6–8 inches using wooden blocks under the headboard, not eating within 3 hours of bedtime, weight loss, smoking cessation, and avoidance of alcohol. Specific dietary recommendations include avoiding those foods known to worsen GERD symptoms (eg, foods with high fat content, spicy foods, caffeinated beverages, and citrus- or tomato-containing foods). While these modifications may have some benefit in reducing GERD symptoms, they are not likely to completely cure most patients. Nonetheless, patients should be made aware of these recommendations. Some OTC and prescription medications can cause or worsen GERD symptoms and should be avoided or changed to medications without such effects when possible.

CASE?

Why do you think Mrs. Dryden's doctor changed her medication for GERD from famotidine to omeprazole?

Pharmacotherapy

Mild Disease

Most patients with mild or infrequent heartburn can be managed with OTC medications, sometimes with advice from a pharmacist. Patients must first be evaluated to determine if they are a candidate for self-treatment. Exclusions for self-treatment include evidence of alarm symptoms, and non-esophageal or severe symptoms as described in the Clinical Presentation, Complications, and Diagnosis section under the Gastroesophageal Reflux Disease heading.[3] Those who present with these symptoms should be referred to their physician for further evaluation. Antacids and H$_2$RAs remain the OTC drugs of choice for managing mild and infrequent symptoms. Antacids (Medication Table 20-1) provide the fastest relief of symptoms and can be dosed every 1–2 hours as long as the maximum dosage is not exceeded and adverse effects are not problematic. For patients who do not respond adequately to antacids or who require substantial doses to control symptoms, an OTC H$_2$RA or PPI may be considered.

The OTC H$_2$RAs are indicated for patients with infrequent mild to moderate heartburn. They have a longer duration of action than antacids but can take up to an hour for the onset of symptom relief. They can be taken before meals or at bedtime before most heartburn occurs. The OTC H$_2$RAs may be taken at either one half or full prescription dose (Medication Table 20-1). They are all similar in potency

when used in recommended dosages. Patients should not use more than two doses a day or continue treatment for more than 2 weeks at a time.

Another option is the OTC PPIs omeprazole and lansoprazole, but they should be reserved for patients with frequent heartburn (2 or more days per week). Although the onset of symptom relief (2–3 hours) is slower than with the H$_2$RAs, they provide superior relief of symptoms throughout the day and night when compared to the H$_2$RAs. Patients should be instructed to take OTC PPIs 30 minutes prior to breakfast on an empty stomach to maximize its acid-inhibiting action.

PRACTICE POINT

OTC omeprazole and OTC lansoprazole should be reserved for patients with frequent heartburn and should be taken daily for 2 weeks. A second course of therapy should be separated by at least 4 months unless directed by a physician as the need for more frequent use might indicate more severe disease.[3]

ALERT!

Patients who continue to require OTC medications beyond 2 weeks, do not achieve adequate relief of symptoms, or develop symptoms suggesting more complicated disease should be referred to a primary care provider for further evaluation.

Moderate to Severe Disease

Patients with moderate to severe GERD symptoms will most likely require a PPI, and 75%–85% of patients will obtain acceptable relief with this option.[1] Studies have also suggested that patients may not gain any greater heartburn relief by increasing to maximum doses. Healing of esophageal erosions is possible after 8–12 weeks of continuous H$_2$RA therapy, but it requires the highest doses and only approximately 50% of patients will achieve complete healing.[1] One of the factors that may be responsible for these findings is that tolerance (the body becomes less responsive to the drug's effects) develops with continued therapy.

CASE?

Over the next few months after starting famotidine, Mrs. Dryden described partial relief of her symptoms but was still having some heartburn after meals. What might be the next type of therapy her doctor would prescribe? Would it be a replacement for the famotidine or an addition to it?

The PPIs are the drugs of choice for most patients because of their ability to reduce stomach acid for a prolonged period. Numerous studies have demonstrated that the PPIs are superior to the H$_2$RAs in relief of symptoms and healing of erosive esophagitis.[22] The majority of patients will have an acceptable response to once daily dosing; however, those with severe or nocturnal symptoms and those presenting with severe esophagitis may require twice daily dosing. There is little data to suggest that one PPI is better than another when used in equivalent doses, but newer options may be more beneficial in healing patients with very severe disease when dosed once a day.[1]

Some patients may have nocturnal (nighttime) symptoms despite once or twice daily PPI therapy and may require the addition of an H$_2$RA at bedtime. There is no conclusive evidence for this practice as tolerance to the H$_2$RA may develop with continued use.[4,23] One way to avoid potential tolerance is for the patient to take the H$_2$RA only at bedtime if nighttime symptoms are anticipated (eg, after eating foods known to cause late-night symptoms or eating within 3 hours of bedtime).

CASE?

How long should Mrs. Dryden plan on continuing medication treatment for her GERD?

Long-term Maintenance Therapy

GERD is a chronic disease and in many cases patients will require long-term or even lifelong therapy. Depending on the severity of the disease, up to 80% of patients will have a recurrence of symptoms or esophagitis within 6 months of discontinuing therapy.[1] This may place patients at an increased risk of developing complications. For this reason, long-term maintenance therapy is often recommended. Patients with moderate to severe symptoms or esophagitis

who have received 8–12 weeks of a PPI and are symptom-free, should be continued on PPI maintenance therapy to reduce the risk of symptomatic recurrence. Patients with mild disease who are well controlled on a PPI may be "stepped down" to an H$_2$RA to determine if they can be maintained on a less potent agent. However, most studies indicate that only about 50% of these patients remain asymptomatic on an H$_2$RA, while the others must be restarted on a PPI.[1] Thus, patients should remain on the least potent medication that prevents symptom recurrence.

Upper Gastrointestinal Bleeding: A Very Serious Complication

CASE STUDY

Jose Vasquez is a 69-year-old man who comes to the emergency department complaining of black tarry stools during his last bowel movement. He is quite pale and during his initial examination is found to have a low blood pressure and elevated heart rate. After further questioning, he states that he has taken large amounts of ibuprofen over the last few months for his back pain.

UGI bleeding occurs in approximately 300,000 patients per year in the United States. These patients are at high risk of dying from this serious condition (approximately 10%) and despite advances in medical and drug therapy, this death rate has not changed for more than 40 years. Patients at highest risk for mortality (death) include older patients (>60 years of age) and patients who already have additional serious chronic diseases, such as cardiac, liver, or kidney disease. Although most patients with UGI bleeding will survive, patients who rebleed after therapy to stop the bleeding or who develop initial bleeding while they are in the hospital have a high mortality rate (approximately 40%–50%).[1]

Etiology, Pathophysiology, Risk Factors

PUD and SRMD (stress-related mucosal damage, or stress ulcer) are the most common reasons for UGI bleeding. Other causes include variceal bleeding (bleeding within the esophagus associated with liver disease), erosive esophagitis, Mallory Weiss tears (tearing of the tissue between the stomach and esophagus, which is usually associated with coughing or vomiting), and cancer. The most common causes of PUD bleeding are NSAID-induced ulcers and *H. pylori*-related ulcers.[1]

Patients admitted into the intensive care units (ICUs) of hospitals are at an especially high risk of bleeding from SRMD, which is associated with critical illness. Bleeding from these lesions can begin very quickly (within 24 hours of admission). Although stomach acid is central to the development of SRMD, numerous other factors are involved. Normally, prostaglandins within the stomach lining provide a protective barrier against stomach acid (see the section on Anatomy and Physiology). Stress associated with critical illness depletes the protective prostaglandins, resulting in an imbalance between the protective factors in the stomach lining and stomach acid, which causes the SRMD. Risk factors associated with SRMD and bleeding include pulmonary failure, which requires mechanical ventilation, and disruption in blood clotting (referred to as coagulopathy). Severe sepsis syndrome (the body's overactive response to infection) is sometimes considered a risk factor as well. Other risk factors include organ failure, transplants, burns, head injuries, and use of blood thinners or corticosteroids.[1]

Peptic Ulcer Bleeding

Clinical Presentation, Complications, and Clinical Course

Patients with bleeding peptic ulcers usually present with coffee ground emesis (coagulated blood in vomit), hematochezia (red or maroon blood in stools—typically from a massive GI bleed), or melena (dark tarry stools).[21] Patients with these signs or symptoms represent a medical emergency that must be dealt with immediately as these patients can quickly go into hypovolemic shock (cardiovascular instability caused by a substantial loss in blood volume). The patient needs to be rapidly stabilized with volume resuscitation by giving large amounts of intravenous (IV) fluids (e.g. normal saline) and may potentially require blood products.[24]

The patient will usually have a nasogastric tube inserted and be placed on suction to determine if the GI tract is the source of the bleed, to remove gastric contents (lavage), and to determine if the patient is continuing to bleed. Most patients will have an endoscopy performed within 24 hours of admission to the hospital to determine the site and significance of the bleeding.[24] This will allow the physician to test for H. pylori infection and perform interventions to attempt to stop the bleeding. Most identified peptic ulcers have a low risk of rebleeding with appropriate therapy. However, some ulcers are so deep that a blood vessel is visible, or the ulcer continues to bleed. These ulcers are associated with a high risk of rebleeding and mortality. Patients with UGI bleeding require close monitoring and medications aimed at reducing stomach acid to allow for more rapid ulcer healing.

Goals of Therapy

The primary goals of therapy when managing PUD bleeding is to quickly stabilize the patient with IV fluids and possibly blood products and to restore hemostasis (stop bleeding and restore blood volume) through endoscopic and pharmacologic intervention. For patients with serious GI bleeding, this usually means giving an agent that increases stomach pH to >6 for a prolonged period.[1] Finally, attempts will be made to prevent further complications, such as rebleeding or the development of new ulcers. This is accomplished through long-term pharmacotherapy directed at reducing stomach acid to allow for complete ulcer healing (see the discussion earlier of NSAID-induced ulcers). For patients with H. pylori infection, treatment is aimed at eradicating the infection (see the section on H. pylori-related ulcers).

CASE?

What are the goals of therapy if Mr. Vasquez's UGI bleed was related to a peptic ulcer?

Pharmacotherapy

Drug therapy directed toward reducing stomach acid is the preferred way to improve hemostasis and prevent rebleeding in patients with peptic ulcer bleeding. Although once a mainstay in managing patients with UGI bleeding, the H_2RAs have fallen out of favor because of their inability to maintain a stomach pH of >6 (near neutral) over a 24-hour period and because tolerance to their effects may develop. The PPIs are the drugs of choice for prevention of PUD rebleeding after successful endoscopy as they reduce rates of rebleeding, the need for surgery, and additional endoscopic procedures.

CASE?

The ICU physician has ordered IV pantoprazole for Mr. Vasquez, even though he is taking other medications by mouth. When can the hospital pharmacy expect the IV to be discontinued and changed to an oral PPI?

The most appropriate PPI dose and method of administration remains uncertain. Patients at low risk of bleeding are usually managed with an oral PPI and discharged from the hospital after endoscopic intervention. Patients at high risk of rebleeding are usually started on IV PPI therapy consisting of a rapid IV loading dose (80 mg of pantoprazole or esomeprazole) and a continuous IV infusion (8 mg/hr of esomeprazole or pantoprazole). The IV infusion should be continued for up to 72 hours (as the patient is at highest risk of rebleeding during this time), after which the patient should be converted to oral PPI therapy, which is continued for at least 8–12 weeks.[21]

Stress-Related Mucosal Bleeding

Clinical Presentation, Complications, and Clinical Course

Patients with SRMB may present with small amounts of blood in the stomach contents when a nasogastric tube is being used for feedings or medication administration, or small amounts of blood may be identified in stool samples that are tested for its presence. Others may present with large amounts of blood or coffee ground–like material in the patient's vomit, in nasogastric aspirates, or with bloody diarrhea.[1] This type of bleeding, along with a drop in blood pressure, increase in heart rate, or drop in laboratory blood volume measurements, is considered life-threatening bleeding and must be evaluated immediately.

The stomach ulcerations associated with SRMD differ from chronic peptic ulcers in that they are numerous, do not extend as deeply into the stomach lining, develop very early in the critically ill hospitalized patient, and progress to a very serious condition, which can lead to increased hospital lengths of stay or even death. One major drawback in managing SRMB is that, due to their extensive distribution throughout the stomach, they usually cannot be managed with endoscopic therapy and must be treated with medications.[1] Thus, the most important consideration in SRMB is prevention of the bleeding.

Goals of Therapy

The primary goal of therapy associated with SRMD is prevention of bleeding. Patients must be assessed for risk and started on optimal prophylactic therapy when warranted. Patients with one of the three primary indications (intubation, blood clotting disruption, or sepsis) or who have two or more of the other risk factors discussed should have SRMB prophylaxis started immediately, unless contraindicated.

Pharmacotherapy

Numerous options exist for the prevention of SRMB, with the majority directed at reducing stomach acid. The use of liquid antacids is superior to placebo, but their administration is cumbersome because of the need for frequent administration (eg, every 1–2 hours) and the need to provide continuous stomach acid pH monitoring. Liquid antacids are

also associated with a number of adverse events (eg, electrolyte abnormalities, constipation, and diarrhea).[2]

Sucralfate is another option with proven benefit, but up to four doses per day are needed, and the fact that it does not increase stomach pH may limit its usefulness. Sucralfate only acts as a barrier between the acidic environment and the stomach lining. It also inhibits the absorption of other medications, may clog nasogastric tubes, cause constipation, and may cause aluminum toxicity in renal failure.[2]

The H$_2$RAs have been widely used for SRMB prophylaxis. Benefits include the fact they can be given IV as a continuous or intermittent infusion and have demonstrated superiority in reducing SRMB when compared to antacids and placebo. All the H$_2$RAs require a dosage reduction in renal dysfunction (a common finding in critically ill patients).[1] The H$_2$RAs also have the potential to cause pneumonia in hospitalized patients since acid is protective against microbes within the stomach. When stomach pH is increased, these pathogens might survive, and if stomach contents are aspirated into the lungs this could lead to the development of pneumonia.[1] The PPIs are the preferred option for prevention of SRMB because of their profound effect on stomach acid. Although there is very little evidence to indicate that PPIs are superior to H$_2$RAs, more potent acid suppression appears to provide improved efficacy, but the potential for pneumonia remains.[1]

> ### PRACTICE POINT
>
> *Some IV preparations may be given by slow IV push while others require that they be diluted in an appropriate volume of fluid for IV administration. Always refer to the package insert for appropriate administration options and corresponding labeling.*

As noted earlier, there are a number of PPI administration options available (Table 20-1), which allow for use in different circumstances encountered in the critical care setting (eg, patients who cannot take anything by mouth, have nasogastric tubes, or have difficulty swallowing). Adverse events associated with PPI prophylaxis are rare, but there may be an increased risk of hospital-acquired pneumonia and increased GI infections due to bacterial overgrowth.[1,2]

Regardless of which SRMB prophylaxis regimen is selected, the patient must be continually monitored for signs and symptoms of bleeding (presence of blood in nasogastric aspirate, vomit, or stool). Finally, it is important to ensure that medications used to prevent SRMB are discontinued when the patient is no longer at risk or has been transferred from the critical care setting, as many are continued and eventually the patient is discharged on these medications without an appropriate indication.

SUMMARY

Acid-related diseases of the upper gastrointestinal (UGI) tract involve stomach acid and include dyspepsia, peptic ulcer disease (PUD), gastroesophageal reflux disease (GERD), and stress-related mucosal damage (SRMD). The proper selection and use of antacids, H_2RAs, proton pump inhibitors (PPIs), sucralfate, bismuth salts, and misoprostol, will relieve symptoms, heal or prevent ulcers and esophagitis, as well as treat or prevent PUD and SRMB, thus improving quality of life, decreasing mortality, and decreasing the medical and financial burden to our society.

ACKNOWLEDGMENT

The author wishes to acknowledge Randolph V. Fugit, PharmD, BCPS, Stuart D. Rockafellow, PharmD, and Rosemary R. Berardi, PharmD, FCCP, FASHP, FAPhA, authors of this chapter in the first edition of this text.

REFERENCES

1. Law EJ, Fong JJ. Upper gastrointestinal disorders. In: Zeind C, Carvalho MG, eds. *Applied Therapeutics: The Clinical Use of Drugs*. 11th ed. Philadelphia, PA: Lippincott Williams and Wilkins; 2018:480-517.

2. Love BL, Mohorn PL. Peptic ulcer disease and related disorders. In: DiPiro JT, Yee GC, Posey L, et al., eds. *Pharmacotherapy: A Pathophysiologic Approach*. 11th ed. New York, NY: McGraw-Hill; 2020.

3. Whetsel T, Garofoli G. Heartburn and dyspepsia. In: *Handbook of Nonprescription Drugs*. 20th ed. Washington, DC: American Pharmaceutical Association; 2020, Chapter 13.

4. McRorie JW, Kirby JA, Miner PB. Histamine2-receptor antagonists: Rapid development of tachyphylaxis with repeat dosing. *World J Gastrointest Pharmacol Ther*. 20145(2):57-62.

5. Turner T. Proton pump inhibitor (PPI) lawsuits. Drugwatch. https://www.drugwatch.com/proton-pump-inhibitors/lawsuits/. Updated January 7, 2020. Accessed January 28, 2020.

6. Schoenfeld AJ, Grady D. Adverse effects associated with proton pump inhibitors. *JAMA Intern Med*. 2016;176(2):172-174.

7. Johnson DA, Oldfield EC. Reported side effects and complications of long-term proton pump inhibitor use: Dissecting the evidence. *Clin Gastroenterol Hepatol*. 2013;11(5):458-464.

8. Gray SL, LaCroix AZ, Larson J, et al. Proton pump inhibitor use, hip fracture, and change in bone mineral density in postmenopausal women: Results from the Women's Health Initiative. *Arch Intern Med*. 2010;170(9):765-771.

9. Cheungpasitporn W, Thongprayoon C, Kittanamongkolchai W, et al. Proton pump inhibitors linked to hypomagnesemia: A systematic review and meta-analysis of observational studies. *Ren Fail*. 2015;37(7):1237-1241.

10. Gomm W, von Holt K, Thomé F, et al. Association of proton pump inhibitors with risk of dementia: A pharmacoepidemiological claims data analysis. *JAMA Neurol*. 2016;73(4):410-416.

11. Aggarwal N. Drug-induced subacute cutaneous lupus erythematosus associated with proton pump inhibitors. *Drugs—Real World Outcomes*. 2016;3(2):145-154.

12. Omeprazole and clopidgrel. Interactions. Lexicomp. Wolters Kluwer Health, Inc. Riverwood, IL. http://online.lexi.com. Accessed January 28, 2020.

13. Pantoprozole and clopidgrel. Interactions. Lexicomp. Wolters Kluwer Health, Inc. Riverwood, IL. http://online.lexi.com. Accessed January 28, 2020.

14. Kwok CS, Jeevanantham V, Dawn B, Loke YK. No consistent evidence of differential cardiovascular risk amongst proton-pump inhibitors when used with clopidogrel: Meta-analysis. *Int J Cardiol*. 2013;167(3):965-974.

15. Niu Q, Wang Z, Zhang Y, et al. Combination use of clopidogrel and proton pump inhibitors increases major adverse cardiovascular events in patients with coronary artery disease: A meta-analysis. *J Cardiovasc Pharmacol Therap*. 2017;22(2):142-152. doi: 10.1177/1074248416663647.

16. Melloni C, Washam JB, Jones WS, et al. Conflicting results between randomized trials and observational studies on the impact of proton pump inhibitors on cardiovascular events when coadministered with dual antiplatelet therapy: Systematic review. *Circ Cardiovasc Qual Outcomes*. 2015;8:47-55.

17. Bundhun PK, Teeluck AR, Bhurtu A, Huang WQ. Is the concomitant use of clopidogrel and proton pump inhibitors still associated with increased adverse cardiovascular outcomes following coronary angioplasty? A systematic review and meta-analysis of recently published studies (2012-2016). *BMC Cardiovasc Disord*. 2017;17:3.

18. Talley NJ, Holtmann G. Approach to the patient with dyspepsia and related functional gastrointestinal complaints. In: Yamada T, Alpers DH, Kalloo KN, et al., eds. *Principles*

of Clinical Gastroenterology. 1st ed. Hoboken, NJ: Wiley-Blackwell; 2008:38-61.

19. Soll AH, Graham DY. Approach to the patient with dyspepsia and peptic ulcer disease. In: Yamada T, Alpers DH, Kalloo KN, et al., eds. *Principles of Clinical Gastroenterology*. 1st ed. Hoboken, NJ: Wiley-Blackwell; 2008:99-121.

20. Chey WD, Grigorios IL, Howden CW et al. ACG clinical guideline: Treatment of *Helicobacter pylori* infection. *Am J Gastroenterol*. 2017;112:212-238.

21. Elta GH, Takami M. Approach to the patient with gross gastrointestinal bleeding. In: Yamada T, Alpers DH, Kalloo KN, et al., eds. *Principles of Clinical Gastroenterology*. 1st ed. Hoboken, NJ: Wiley-Blackwell; 2008:122-151.

22. Richter JE. Approach to the patient with gastroesophageal reflux disease. In: Yamada T, Alpers DH, Kalloo KN, et al., eds. *Principles of Clinical Gastroenterology*. 1st ed. Hoboken, NJ: Wiley-Blackwell; 2008:83-98.

23. American Gastroenterological Association Institute. American Gastroenterological Association medical position statement on the management of gastroesophageal reflux disease. *Gastroenterology*. 2005;135:1383-1391.

24. Barkun A, Almadi M, Kuipers EJ, et al. Management of nonvariceal upper gastrointestinal bleeding: Guideline recommendations from the International Consensus Group. *Ann Intern Med*. 2019;171(11):805-822.

REVIEW QUESTIONS

1. Why does Mr. Gonzalez have to take three drugs to treat his peptic ulcer?

2. Would Ms. Rosenberg be a candidate for prophylactic cotherapy once the ulcer is healed? If so, what is the preferred agent?

3. What are the most serious consequences of long-standing GERD?

4. Why might Mrs. Dryden's doctor have changed her medication for GERD from ranitidine to omeprazole?

5. What are the goals of therapy if Mr. Vasquez's UGI bleed is related to a peptic ulcer?

MEDICATION TABLE

MEDICATION TABLE 20-1. Selected Oral Medications Used to Treat Acid-Related Upper Gastrointestinal Disorders in Adults[1-3a]

Class/Agents	Brand Name	Generic	Rx	Usual Adult Dosage Range (Rx)	OTC	Usual Adult Dosage Range (OTC)	Notes
Antacids (selected)							
Calcium-containing (KAL see um)	Tums Regular Strength	X			X	2–4 tablets as needed; up to 15 tablets/day	Each tablet contains 500 mg calcium carbonate; chew tablets
	Tums EX 750	X			X	2–4 tablets as needed; up to 10 tablets/day	Each tablet contains 750 mg calcium carbonate; chew tablets
	Maalox Quick Dissolve Regular Strength	X			X	2–3 tablets as needed; up to 12 tablets/day	Each tablet contains 600 mg calcium carbonate; chew tablets
	Mylanta Ultimate Strength	X			X	2–4 tablets between meals and at bedtime as needed; up to 10 tablets/day	Each tablet contains 700 mg calcium carbonate and 300 mg magnesium hydroxide; chew tablets
Magnesium-containing (mag NEE zhum)	Philips Milk of Magnesia Original	X			X	1–3 tsp q 4 hr as needed; up to 4 times/day	Each 5 mL contains magnesium hydroxide 400 mg
Magnesium- and aluminum-containing (mag NEE zhum) (a LOO mi num)	Mylanta Maximum Strength Liquid	X			X	2–4 tsp before meals and at bedtime as needed; up to 12 tsp/day	Each 5 mL contains aluminum hydroxide 400 mg, magnesium hydroxide 400 mg, and simethicone 40 mg
	Maalox Regular Strength Liquid	X			X	2–4 tsp 4 times a day as needed; up to 16 tsp/day	Each 5 mL contains aluminum hydroxide 200 mg, magnesium hydroxide 200 mg, and simethicone 20 mg
	Gaviscon Extra Strength Liquid	X			X	2–4 tsp 4 times a day as needed; up to 16 tsp/day	Each 5 mL contains aluminum hydroxide 254 mg, magnesium carbonate 237 mg, and alginic acid as an inactive ingredient
Magnesium- and calcium-containing (mag NEE zhum) (KAL see um)	Mylanta Supreme Liquid	X			X	2–4 tsp 4 times a day as needed; up to 18 tsp/day	Each 5 mL contains magnesium hydroxide 135 mg, and calcium carbonate 400 mg

Continued next page

MEDICATION TABLE 20-1. Selected Oral Medications Used to Treat Acid-Related Upper Gastrointestinal Disorders in Adults[1-3a] (Continued)

Class/Agents	Brand Name	Generic	Rx	Usual Adult Dosage Range (Rx)	OTC	Usual Adult Dosage Range (OTC)	Notes
Aluminum-containing (a LOO mi num)	Alternagel	X			X	1-2 tsp 4 times a day as needed; up to 18 tsp/day	Each 5 mL contains aluminum hydroxide 600 mg
Sodium-containing (SOE dee um)	Alka Seltzer Heartburn Relief	X			X	2 tablets in 4 ounces of water q 4 hr as needed; up to 8 tablets/day	Each tablet contains 1,940 mg sodium bicarbonate and 1,000 of citric acid
	Alka Seltzer Original	X			X	2 tablets in 4 ounces of water q 4 hr as needed; up to 8 tablets/day	Each tablet contains 1,916 mg sodium bicarbonate, 1,000 mg citric acid, and 325 mg aspirin
Histamine-2 Receptor Antagonists							
Cimetidine (sye MET i deen)	Tagamet	X	X	400 mg 4 times daily or 800 mg twice daily			
	Tagamet HB	X			X	200–400 mg daily	
Famotidine (fa MOE ti deen)	Pepcid	X	X	20–80 mg daily	X	10–20 mg daily (maximum 40 mg/day)	
	Pepcid AC	X			X	10–20 mg daily	
	Pepcid AC Maximum Strength				X	20–40 mg daily	
	Pepcid Complete	X			X	10–20 mg daily	Contains famotidine 10 mg, calcium carbonate 800 mg, and magnesium hydroxide 165 mg
Nizatidine (ni ZA ti deen)		X	X	150–300 mg daily			
Proton Pump Inhibitors							
Omeprazole (oh ME pray zol)	Prilosec	X	X	20-80 mg daily			Take 30 min before morning meal; if twice daily, take second dose 30 min before dinner
	Prilosec OTC	X			X	20 mg daily	Take 30 min before morning meal; take daily for 14 days

Continued next page

MEDICATION TABLE 20-1. Selected Oral Medications Used to Treat Acid-Related Upper Gastrointestinal Disorders in Adults[1-3a] *(Continued)*

Class/Agents	Brand Name	Generic	Rx	Usual Adult Dosage Range (Rx)	OTC	Usual Adult Dosage Range (OTC)	Notes
Omeprazole/sodium bicarbonate (oh ME pray zol) (SOE dee um bye KAR bon ate)	Zegerid	X	X	20–80 mg daily			Take 30 min before morning meal; if twice daily, take second dose 30 min before dinner; each capsule contains 20 or 40 mg omeprazole with 1,100 mg sodium bicarbonate (equivalent to 304 mg of sodium); because 20- and 40-mg dosages contain the same amount of bicarbonate, two 20-mg capsules should not be substituted for the 40-mg capsule
Pantoprazole (pan TOE pra zole)	Protonix	X	X	40–80 mg daily			Take 30 min before morning meal; if twice daily, take second dose 30 min before dinner
Lansoprazole (dex lan SOE pra zole)	Prevacid	X	X	15–60 mg daily			Take 30 min before morning meal; if twice daily, take second dose 30 min before dinner
	Prevacid 24 HR	X			X	15 mg daily	Take 30 min before morning meal; take daily for 14 days
Rabeprazole (ra BE pray zole)	Aciphex	X	X	20–40 mg daily			Take 30 min before morning meal; if twice daily, take second dose 30 min before dinner
Esomeprazole (es oh ME pray zol)	Nexium	X	X	20–80 mg daily	X	20 mg daily	Take 30 min before morning meal; if twice daily, take second dose 30 min before dinner
Dexlansoprazole (dex lan SOE pra zole)	Dexilant		X	30–60 mg daily			Take 30 min before morning meal; if twice daily, take second dose 30 min before dinner
Other							
Sucralfate (soo KRAL fate)	Carafate	X	X	1–4 g daily			Take potentially interacting oral medications 1 hr before the next dose of sucralfate

Continued next page

MEDICATION TABLE 20-1. Selected Oral Medications Used to Treat Acid-Related Upper Gastrointestinal Disorders in Adults[1-3a] (Continued)

Class/Agents	Brand Name	Generic	Rx	Usual Adult Dosage Range (Rx)	OTC	Usual Adult Dosage Range (OTC)	Notes
Misoprostol (mye soe PROST ole)	Cytotec	X	X	400–800 mcg daily			Contraindicated in pregnant women; serum pregnancy test required in women of childbearing age; diarrhea is dose dependent
Bismuth subsalicylate (biz muth) (sub sa LIS i late)	Pepto Bismol Original Liquid	X			X	2 tbsp q 30 min to 1 hr as needed; up to 16 tbsp/day	Each 15 mL contains bismuth subsalicylate 262 mg; caution in patients with salicylate allergy; bismuth salts darken stool; liquid products may darken tongue

OTC = over the counter; Rx = prescription.
[a]Pronunciations have been adapted with permission from USP Dictionary of USAN and International Drug Names (USP Dictionary) © 2022.

Chapter 21

Nausea, Vomiting, and Upper Gastrointestinal Tract Motility Disorders

Tibb F. Jacobs, PharmD, BCPS | Jamie M. Terrell, PharmD

KEY TERMS AND DEFINITIONS

Antiemetic—a preparation or medication that relieves nausea and vomiting.

Chemoreceptor trigger zone (CTZ)—the neural center for emesis, located in the brain.

Emesis—the medical term for vomiting.

Gastroparesis—condition that delays or stops stomach emptying, resulting in nausea, vomiting, bloating, discomfort, and weight loss. Usually the result of nerve damage, but may also be related to other medical conditions.

Motion sickness—the uncomfortable dizziness, nausea, and vomiting that people experience when their sense of balance and equilibrium is disturbed by constant motion.

Nausea—the feeling of needing to vomit.

Vestibular—related to the structures of the ear, which are linked to the maintenance of balance and perception of spatial positioning.

Vomiting—the forcible ejection of the contents of the stomach through the mouth (also called emesis).

DOI 10.37573/9781585286638.021

LEARNING OBJECTIVES

After completing this chapter, you should be able to

1. Define the following:
   - Antiemetic
   - Chemoreceptor trigger zone
   - Emesis
   - Gastroparesis
   - Motion sickness
   - Nausea
   - Vestibular
   - Vomiting

2. Identify the causes and risk factors for developing nausea/vomiting and gastroparesis.

3. List the most common signs and symptoms of nausea/vomiting and gastroparesis.

4. Describe nonpharmacologic therapies for nausea and vomiting.

5. Explain the pharmacotherapeutic effects of antacids, histamine$_2$-receptor antagonists, anticholinergics, antihistamines, dopamine antagonists, cannabinoids, corticosteroids, benzodiazepines, serotonin antagonists, and neurokinin$_1$-receptor antagonists and list their most common side effects and major drug interactions.

6. State the brand and generic names of the most widely used antiemetic and promotility medications, along with their routes of administration, dosage forms, and available doses.

7. Recognize common regimens for the treatment of nausea, vomiting, and gastroparesis.

Nausea and vomiting (N/V) usually present in a fairly straightforward manner. Nausea is defined as the feeling of needing to vomit, while vomiting is defined as the ejection of gastric contents. While the definitions of N/V are simple, the conditions have a variety of causes. Nausea and vomiting can be self-limiting or they can signal a more complex medical problem. This chapter will focus on the treatment of N/V, including both nonpharmacological and pharmacological therapies.

NAUSEA, VOMITING, AND GASTROPARESIS

Pathophysiology

The process of emesis can be divided into three stages: nausea, retching, and vomiting. Nausea is the feeling of needing to vomit. It can be accompanied by pallor (paleness), tachycardia (increased heart rate), sweating, and salivation. Retching is the labored movement of the chest and abdominal muscles that occurs before vomiting. Vomiting is the forceful ejection of the gastric contents through the mouth. Regurgitation is a more passive process, where the stomach contents move up the gastrointestinal (GI) tract into the mouth.[1]

Nausea and vomiting (N/V) are triggered by impulses sent from the vomiting center in the medulla of the brain. The vomiting center can be stimulated by impulses sent from the cerebral cortex, vestibular system (considered later in this chapter), the chemoreceptor trigger zone (CTZ), or from the GI tract or pharynx. Neuroreceptor transmitters are located in the vomiting center. They include cholinergic, histaminic, dopaminergic, opiate, serotonin, neurokinin, and benzodiazepine receptors. Stimulation of these receptors can lead to emesis. Therefore, medications that block these receptors are helpful in the treatment of N/V.

CASE STUDY

Mr. Bill Jones, a regular customer, comes into the pharmacy and says that he has been experiencing some N/V since early this morning. He called his doctor's office and was told to try to manage his symptoms with over-the-counter (OTC) products. If the N/V do not resolve by tomorrow, the doctor would like to see him.

Causes of Nausea and Vomiting

There can be many different causes of N/V. GI diseases, as well as other types of disorders (including cardiovascular, infectious, neurologic, or metabolic diseases), can cause N/V. Certain medications (particularly medications associated with the treatment of cancer), as well as conditions

TABLE 21-1. Causes of Nausea and Vomiting[1,2]

Gastrointestinal	Neurologic	Therapy-Induced
Obstruction disorders	Vestibular disorders	Chemotherapy
Constipation	Migraines	Antibiotic
Gastroparesis	Increased intracranial pressure	Radiation therapy
Nonulcer dyspepsia	Depression	Opiates
Irritable bowel syndrome	Psychiatric illness	Oral contraceptives
Pancreatitis	Anticipatory	Digoxin
Peptic ulcer disease	Bulimia and anorexia nervosa	Operative procedures
Gastroenteritis		Oral hypoglycemics
Cardiac		**Endocrine/Metabolic**
Acute myocardial infarction		Pregnancy
Congestive heart failure		Renal disease
		Diabetes

such as pregnancy, postoperative states, motion sickness, and motility disorders, can also cause N/V. See Table 21-1 for a more complete list of causes of N/V.

Clinical Presentation

Patients may present with mild or more severe symptoms. Simple N/V are usually mild and self-limiting and only require symptom management. Complex N/V can be more severe and not easily relieved with antiemetic medications. Complex N/V tend to be caused by more difficult-to-manage disease states (for example, chemotherapy or diabetic gastroparesis). These patients may become dehydrated and develop electrolyte imbalances and weight loss.

TREATMENT

The desired treatment outcome for all patients is the relief of N/V and prevention of any more serious adverse effects, such as dehydration, malnourishment, and electrolyte imbalances. Treatment can consist of nonpharmacological therapy and/or pharmacological therapy.

Nonpharmacological Therapy

Nonpharmacological therapy can include dietary measures, acupuncture, or acupressure, as well as relaxation and self-hypnosis techniques. Dietary approaches to N/V are frequently recommended for pregnant patients. These include eating frequent, small meals, avoiding spicy or fatty foods, eating crackers before arising in the morning, taking small sips of carbonated beverages or fruit juices when nauseated, and eating high-protein snacks. Acupressure and acupuncture are based on the theory that bodily functions are controlled by certain points on the body, and the P6 (neiguan or pericardium) point is used by acupuncturists to treat N/V. This is the same point stimulated by acupressure wristbands, which have been used with nausea and vomiting of pregnancy (NVP), postoperative nausea and vomiting (PONV), and motion sickness.[1,2]

Nonpharmacological therapy can be used with or without pharmacological treatment to avoid or reduce unwanted adverse effects from the medications used in the treatment of N/V. Patients who are pregnant may not wish to use medications due to concerns about possible teratogenic effects (related to or causing malformation of the embryo or fetus).

CASE?

What are some nonpharmacological methods that can be recommended for Mr. Jones's N/V?

Pharmacologic Therapy

A variety of prescription and OTC medications are used to treat N/V, and many classes of medications can be used as antiemetics. The causes, frequency, and severity of the patient's N/V help to determine which medication and route of administration is most appropriate for an individual. (See Medication Table 21-1; Medication Tables are located at the end of the chapter).

Antacids

Antacids work locally in the stomach to neutralize gastric acid. They are available without a prescription, so they are often used as a first-line therapy for acute or occasional N/V. They are especially effective for N/V associated with heartburn. Magnesium hydroxide, aluminum hydroxide, and calcium carbonate are the most common antacid ingredients. Side effects associated with infrequent use of these preparations are mild and tend to be limited to diarrhea with magnesium products and constipation with aluminum or calcium products.

Histamine$_2$-receptor antagonists

Like antacids, histamine$_2$ (H$_2$)-receptor antagonists also act locally in the stomach to reduce the amount of acid secreted from gastric parietal cells. These products (ranitidine, famotidine, cimetidine, nizatidine) are all also available without a prescription. They are effective for N/V associated with heartburn or gastroesophageal reflux disease (GERD). These products are typically safe for occasional use. As noted in Chapter 20, however, cimetidine has quite a few drug interactions and would not be a good first choice for a patient already taking multiple medications.

In April 2020, the U.S. Food and Drug Administration (FDA) asked all manufacturers of ranitidine to remove products containing it from public shelves. In its investigation leading to the removal, the FDA found the contaminant N-nitrosodimethylamine (NDMA) in certain lots and discovered it may accumulate when stored improperly. Currently, ranitidine is not available in prescription or over-the-counter formulations in the United States. Following that action, voluntary recalls of certain lots of nizatidine have occurred as well. As of this writing, there is no evidence of trace NDMA in famotidine or cimetidine.[3,4]

Anticholinergics

Scopolamine is a commonly used anticholinergic for motion sickness. It blocks muscarinic receptors (see Chapter 4) found in the vomiting center and vestibular system and prevents N/V associated with motion sickness. It is available as a transdermal patch that can be applied and left on for up to 72 hours. This makes it an effective treatment for patients who cannot take oral medications or patients who need

constant therapy (for example, patients traveling on cruise ships). Adverse effects seen with anticholinergic medications include dry mouth, drowsiness, blurred vision, and urinary retention.

Antihistamines

Medications that block histamine (H$_1$) receptors in the vestibular center are called antihistamines. These medications act similarly to anticholinergic medications and are effective for the treatment and prevention of motion sickness and vertigo (the sensation of rotation of oneself or one's surroundings while actually still). There are quite a few antihistamines and many are available OTC, which makes it easy for patients to self-treat. Dimenhydrinate, diphenhydramine, and meclizine are available without a prescription, while hydroxyzine requires a prescription. Adverse effects for this class of medications are very similar to those of the anticholinergic medications and include dry mouth, drowsiness, blurred vision, and urinary retention.

CASE?

What classes of medications are available OTC that Mr. Jones could try to help relieve his N/V?

PRACTICE POINT

Meclizine is available both OTC and Rx. It tends to cause less drowsiness than dimenhydrinate or diphenhydramine for most patients. The OTC products include Bonine and Travel-Ease.

Dopamine Antagonists

Phenothiazines are often used in the treatment of N/V. They block the dopaminergic receptors in the CTZ, causing a decrease in N/V. Available products include promethazine, prochlorperazine, and chlorpromazine (a medication discussed in Chapter 7 as an antipsychotic). They are available as oral tablets and liquids, rectal suppositories, and injections. This makes them convenient to use in a variety of patients and situations. They are available as generic products and are relatively inexpensive. Phenothiazines can be used for motion sickness, vertigo, gastritis, NVP, PONV, and chemotherapy-induced nausea and vomiting (CINV). Side effects seen with this class of medications include sedation, orthostatic hypotension, and extrapyramidal symptoms. (Extrapyramidal symptom effects are involuntary movement disorders that can be permanent.)

ALERT!

LOOK-ALIKE/SOUND-ALIKE—Hydroxyzine (an antihistamine) can be easily confused with hydralazine, which is used for the treatment of high blood pressure.

PRACTICE POINT

Promethazine gel can be compounded for application to the skin as a transdermal preparation.[5] This dosage form can be used when patients are unable to take oral medications and do not wish to use a suppository.

CASE?

Mr. Jones returns to the pharmacy the next day. His doctor has given him a prescription for promethazine. The prescription says "promethazine 25 mg one every 4–6 hours as needed." What is wrong with this prescription?

Benzamides

Metoclopramide and trimethobenzamide are considered benzamides. They block the dopamine receptors in the CTZ and act in the GI tract, where they promote gastric motility. Metoclopramide is available in solid and liquid oral dosage forms, as well as an injection. It has been used for the treatment of gastroparesis (discussed extensively later in this chapter) since it stimulates the movement of food through the gut. It is also useful in the treatment of PONV and CINV. Metoclopramide has a black-box warning for having the possibility to cause tardive dyskinesia, which is an often-irreversible movement disorder, and should not be used for more than 12 weeks. Side effects include drowsiness, fatigue, dystonic reactions, and diarrhea.[6] Trimethobenzamide is available as a capsule and an injection. It can be used

for simple N/V and PONV. Its side effects are also drowsiness and fatigue.

ALERT!

All patients receiving metoclopramide must be provided a medication guide with their prescriptions.

Butyrophenones

Butyrophenones include haloperidol (also used as an antipsychotic and discussed in Chapter 7) and droperidol. They block dopamine in the CTZ to decrease N/V. They are not used very frequently in the treatment of N/V. Droperidol has a black box warning stating that it can cause life-threatening arrhythmias in certain patients. Besides arrhythmias, these medications can cause sedation, agitation, restlessness, and extrapyramidal symptoms as well.

Cannabinoid

Dronabinol is a drug used to prevent and treat refractory CINV. It is available as oral formulations, and its exact mechanism of action is unknown. Some of the common adverse effects seen when using cannabinoids are drowsiness, euphoria, hypotension, ataxia, impaired vision, and dizziness.

PRACTICE POINT

The cannabinoids used to treat N/V are synthetic products but are chemically related to the principal active ingredient in marijuana. They are, thus, controlled substances and must be handled according to the regulations of the Drug Enforcement Agency and the State Board of Pharmacy.

Corticosteroids

Corticosteroids (discussed extensively in Chapter 9) can be used alone or in combination with other products to treat N/V, and are especially useful for CINV or radiation-induced N/V. The most commonly used corticosteroid for these indications is dexamethasone. It can be given orally or intravenously, and adverse effects (diabetes, cataracts, reduction in bone mineral density) typically seen with long-term use are not usually encountered with short-term treatment of

N/V. Some adverse effects that may be seen with short-term use are GI upset, insomnia, increased energy, and hyperglycemia (increased blood sugar). Corticosteroids are thought to reduce or prevent N/V by releasing serotonin, decreasing the permeability of the blood–brain-barrier, and reducing inflammation.[1]

Benzodiazepines

Lorazepam, discussed in Chapter 7, is often used to prevent and treat CINV. It is thought to be effective by preventing messages from the cerebral cortex and limbic system from reaching the vomiting center in the brainstem. Common side effects seen when using lorazepam are sedation and amnesia, although patients receiving it should also be monitored for respiratory depression.

Serotonin Antagonists

Chemotherapeutic and anesthetic agents cause the release of serotonin from cells in the intestinal mucosa, which can trigger N/V by stimulating the visceral vagal nerve fibers and the CTZ, where there is an abundance of serotonin receptors known as 5-hydroxytryptamine$_3$ (5-HT$_3$) receptors. Selective 5-hydroxytryptamine (5-HT, serotonin) antagonists are used in the prevention and treatment of CINV and PONV, and they work by blocking the 5-HT$_3$ receptors. The 5-HT$_3$ receptor antagonists include dolasetron, granisetron, ondansetron, and palonosetron, and they are available in both oral and injectable dosage forms. These agents are generally very well tolerated; however, some adverse effects that may be seen include headache, GI upset, asthenia, dizziness, and somnolence. It is important to note that these agents can also cause asymptomatic electrocardiograph changes, which reflect alterations in cardiac rhythms, and proper precautionary measures should be taken.

CASE?

Mr. Jones comes back to your pharmacy several months later. He has been diagnosed with colon cancer and will have a course of chemotherapy. His doctor told him this type of chemotherapy would make him very nauseated. The doctor gave Mr. Jones a prescription for ondansetron. Mr. Jones puts the prescription on hold but doesn't want to fill it until he sees how the chemo makes him feel. Should Mr. Jones have his prescription for ondansetron filled before he takes the first dose of chemo or wait until later? Why?

PRACTICE POINT

Some oral serotonin antagonists (especially ondansetron) are sometimes prescribed for severe or refractory NVP as an off-label use.

Neurokinin$_1$-Receptor Antagonists

Neurokinin$_1$ (NK$_1$) receptors are involved in CINV due to their presence in the GI tract and CTZ. Aprepitant was the first NK$_1$-receptor antagonist and is effective in the prevention of acute and delayed CINV. It is available as an oral capsule, suspension, and as an intravenous (IV) preparation and is used in combination with a 5-HT$_3$ antagonist and a corticosteroid. Rolapitant is another NK$_1$-receptor antagonist available in the United States as an oral tablet and is also used in combination with serotonin antagonists. Possible adverse effects seen with neurokinin$_1$-receptor antagonist use include fatigue, neutropenia (reduced white blood count), and hiccups.

PRACTICE POINT

While both the oral and IV forms of aprepitant have the same brand name (Emend), the IV form has a different generic name, fosaprepitant dimeglumine. Fosaprepitant dimeglumine is converted in the body to aprepitant.

ALERT!

Pharmacy technicians preparing fosaprepitant dimeglumine for IV infusion must take special care to read the included directions for mixing, as it is incompatible with many common solutions and requires gentle handling (no shaking).

Over-the-Counter Therapy

OTC therapies can be used as a first-line therapy by patients seeking reprieve from their N/V symptoms. They may also be very useful for patients who cannot be seen by a physician immediately but want to try a pharmacologic agent for their ailments. While OTC medications are often the first choice for many patients with these symptoms, some patients should not be treated with them and must be referred to their primary care provider or an emergency department for further evaluation. These patients include those with severe right upper quadrant pain (just below the ribs); N/V with fever or diarrhea; severe abdominal pain in the middle or right lower quadrant; patients with a diagnosis of glaucoma, benign prostatic hypertrophy, chronic bronchitis, emphysema, or asthma; patients who are pregnant or breastfeeding; or patients with blood in their vomitus.[2]

There are many different agents available OTC for N/V symptoms. Antacids, anticholinergics, and antihistamines are drug classes used for N/V and all have products that are available OTC. Please see earlier sections for further discussion of these drug classes.

Bismuth Products

Bismuth subsalicylate is available without a prescription and is used to treat N/V associated with overindulgence in food and drink. It is also used to treat indigestion, heartburn, and gas complaints and may cause fecal discoloration (grayish black). It is available as a liquid, chewable tablet, or caplet. Products with bismuth subsalicylate are recommended only for adults.

Phosphorated Carbohydrate Solution

Phosphorated carbohydrate solution is available OTC and contains fructose, dextrose, and phosphoric acid. The solution is used in patients with nausea associated with intestinal influenza and also for food or drink indiscretions. This solution acts to relieve N/V by decreasing smooth muscle contraction in the GI tract and also by delaying gastric emptying. Due to the high sugar content of this preparation, patients should be counseled to avoid this product if

ALERT!

Administering acetylsalicylic acid or salicylates to children or teenagers who have a viral illness like the flu or chickenpox can cause a rare but serious illness called Reye's syndrome. Because viral illness is so hard to identify, especially in its early stages, children (especially children with fever) should never be given salicylate-containing medications. Salicylates include products such as Pepto-Bismol and Kaopectate, as well as aspirin.

they have diabetes. Also, if the patient's symptoms do not improve after the maximum stated dose or time, the patient should be referred for further evaluation.[2]

Complementary Therapies

Pyridoxine (vitamin B_6) is available without a prescription and is often used in NVP. It is water soluble and has been used successfully since the 1940s. The exact mechanism of action is unknown. While side effects are rare, as the dose of pyridoxine increases, so does the risk of peripheral sensory neuropathic disturbances. Inhibited prolactin secretion has also been noted at extremely high doses.

Pyridoxine has also been used in combination with doxylamine. While the two drugs were originally in a combination product together, due to the possibility of teratogenicity, the combined drug was pulled from shelves in 1983. It is important to understand that no evidence of teratogenicity has been found. Both products are available OTC and are recommended by many obstetricians for their pregnant patients with NVP.

Ginger (*Zingiber officinale*), which does not cause central nervous system depression like other OTC medications, has been used to relieve NVP, PONV, and motion sickness. It is thought that ginger works directly at the digestive tract to reduce nausea. Two other natural products are also commonly used in the United States. Chamomile (*Matricaria recutita*) and peppermint oil (*Mentha piperita*) are both thought to have antispasmodic properties. Both are labeled GRAS (Generally Recognized as Safe by the FDA) in the United States.[7,8]

CHEMOTHERAPY-INDUCED NAUSEA AND VOMITING

CINV can be divided into three categories: acute, delayed, and anticipatory. Acute CINV occurs within 24 hours after receiving chemotherapy, while delayed CINV occurs more than 24 hours after the therapy. Anticipatory N/V happens before the chemotherapy dose in some patients who have experienced acute or delayed N/V previously. Risk factors for an increased chance of CINV include previous experience of CINV, female gender, low chronic alcohol ingestion, younger age, history of motion sickness, or nausea and vomiting during pregnancy.[1] Chemotherapeutic agents are classified according to their emetogenicity (tendency to induce vomiting). Knowing which agent is to be used and which category (lowest, low, moderate, high, or highest) it is in is the most important factor considered by clinicians when choosing an agent to prevent CINV.[1,2]

POSTOPERATIVE NAUSEA AND VOMITING

While not all patients experience N/V following surgical procedures, it can be very uncomfortable for those who do. It can also require that the patient be admitted to the hospital or prolong a hospital stay. Those patients who may experience PONV can be identified through risk factors that have already been established. History of PONV or motion sickness, female gender, nonsmoker, use of volatile anesthetics (halothane, enflurane, isoflurane, sevoflurane, and desflurane), use of opioids for pain control, and duration and type of surgery may all increase the risk of PONV to the patient. Clinicians try to decrease or eliminate as many risk factors as possible for their patients.

Several different drugs have been identified to help prevent PONV. Droperidol or a serotonin antagonist is effective in many high-risk patients. Other drugs that may be used include dexamethasone (given prior to undergoing anesthesia), anticholinergics, or antihistamines. Combinations of drugs may also be needed to achieve the best result.[1]

NAUSEA AND VOMITING OF PREGNANCY

Any woman of childbearing age who presents with N/V should be evaluated for pregnancy because pregnancy is the most common endocrinologic cause of N/V.[7] A majority of pregnant women will experience nausea and/or vomiting at some point during the pregnancy, most notably during the first trimester. When choosing a therapeutic agent for this population, teratogenic potential should be of primary concern. Nonpharmacologic alternatives, such as behavioral, dietary, and physical modifications, should be considered before pharmacologic therapy is initiated. Drugs that have been used and are considered to be safe during pregnancy include pyridoxine, doxylamine, promethazine, metoclopramide, and trimethobenzamide. Risks versus benefits must be weighed in all situations.

MOTION SICKNESS AND VESTIBULAR DISTURBANCES

Disorders of the vestibular system in the inner ear can be the cause of N/V in some patients. Infection, injury, neoplasm, and motion can all cause vestibular disturbances, which in turn, can result in dizziness, vertigo, and N/V. Some patients may experience motion sickness while riding in cars, trains, or boats. In patients who know that they are susceptible to this ill feeling, precautionary measures should be taken to minimize or avoid the exposure if possible, ensure adequate ventilation, and try to take part in distracting activities. It is recommended that patients take medication to control the N/V before it occurs to allow for adequate absorption of the oral therapy. Anticholinergics and antihistamines are usually the drugs of choice. However, if vomiting has already ensued and absorption of the oral medication is unpredictable, a scopolamine patch may be the best therapy.

MOTILITY DISORDERS

Gastroparesis, or delayed gastric emptying, can present in some patients as nausea, vomiting, bloating, constipation, or diarrhea. It is commonly seen in poorly controlled diabetic patients who have autonomic neuropathy. Under normal circumstances, the muscles in the stomach force food through the digestive tract. However, in patients with gastroparesis, those muscles do not function appropriately and food is not pushed through the stomach into the intestines properly.

Fortunately for sufferers of gastroparesis, there are drugs, termed promotility agents, available to help this condition by speeding the clearance of food and acid from the esophagus and stomach. Metoclopramide is effective for this disorder, but it also has side effects that may be intolerable to some patients (see the earlier discussion of dopamine antagonists) and it should not be used long term. Erythromycin, an antibiotic, has actions on receptors in the stomach to increase motility. Patients may develop a tolerance to this medication and would then need to be switched to a different agent. Also, erythromycin has several drug interactions, which must all be considered when the drug is prescribed or dispensed. The lower GI tract is also subject to motility disorders. These are covered in Chapter 22.

SUMMARY

There are many classes of medication that can be used to treat nausea and vomiting (N/V). It is important to first determine the cause of a patient's N/V before treatment is recommended or prescribed. Patients who are pregnant may wish to try nonpharmacological measures first. Patients who are experiencing simple N/V from gastritis or another self-limiting illness will probably benefit from nonpharmacological or over-the-counter (OTC) products initially. Patients who are traveling and have problems with motion sickness have both OTC products, such as diphenhydramine and meclizine, and prescription options, such as scopolamine patches, available. There are also many options for patients with more severe causes of N/V, such as chemotherapy-induced nausea and vomiting (CINV) or postoperative nausea and vomiting (PONV). These patients will need a prescription product. The medication selected should be chosen based on patient-specific characteristics. It is often necessary to try several options before finding one that works best for each patient.

REFERENCES

1. Wilhem S, Lepari M. Nausea and vomiting. In: Chisholm-Burns MA, Wells BG, Schwinghammer TL, et al., eds. *Pharmacotherapy: Principles and Practice*. New York, NY: McGraw-Hill; 2019:329-338.

2. Welch AC. In: Krinsky DL, Ferreri SP, Hemstreet B, et al., eds. *Handbook of Nonprescription Drugs: An Interactive Approach to Self-Care*. 19th ed. Washington, DC: American Pharmacists Association; 2017:335-354.

3. Questions and answers: NDMA impurities in ranitidine (commonly known as Zantac). Food and Drug Administration Website. https://www.fda.gov/drugs/drug-safety-and-availability/questions-and-answers-ndma-impurities-ranitidine-commonly-known-zantac. Accessed January 27, 2020.

4. FDA requests removal of all ranitidine products (Zantac) from the market [news release]. Washington, DC: U.S. Food and Drug Administration; April 1, 2020. https://www.fda.gov/news-events/press-announcements/fda-requests-removal-all-ranitidine-products-zantac-market. Accessed April 15, 2021.

5. Loyd VA Jr. Promethazine HCl 50 mg/mL in PLO gel. *Int J Pharm Compound*. 2001;5(1):51.

6. Lexicomp®. Hudson, OH: Wolters Kluwer Clinical Drug Information; 2021. http://online.lexi.com. Accessed April 15, 2021.

7. Murphy PA. Alternative therapies for nausea and vomiting of pregnancy. *Obstet Gynecol*. 1998;91:149-155.

8. Niebyl JR, Goodwin TM. Overview of nausea and vomiting in pregnancy with an emphasis on vitamins and ginger. *Am J Obstet Gynecol*. 2002:S253-S255.

REVIEW QUESTIONS

1. Discuss nonpharmacological therapies for nausea and vomiting and which patients can most benefit from this type of therapy.

2. List and discuss treatment options for patients who suffer from nausea associated with motion sickness.

3. What is the best way to manage motion sickness and vestibular disturbances?

4. What is PONV, who is at risk of experiencing it, and how can it be managed?

5. Discuss the development and treatment of gastroparesis.

MEDICATION TABLE

MEDICATION TABLE 21-1. Pharmacologic Treatment of Nausea and Vomiting[6,a]

CLASS Generic Name (pronunciation)	Brand Name	Route	Forms	Dose	Rx/OTC
Antacids (also see Chapter 20 Medication Tables)					
Magnesium hydroxide (mag NEE zhum) (hye DROX ide)	Various products	Oral	Liquid	5–15 mL up to 4 times/day as needed	OTC
Aluminum hydroxide (a LOO mi num) (hye DROX ide)	Various products	Oral	Liquid	10 mL 5–6 times daily after meals and at bedtime as needed	OTC
Calcium carbonate (KAL see um) (KAR bon ate)	Various products	Oral	Tablet, liquid	1–4 tablets as symptoms occur; 10–15 mL q 2–4 hr as needed	OTC
H$_2$-Receptor Antagonists (also see Chapter 20 Medication Tables)					
Cimetidine (sye MET i deen)	Tagamet HB	Oral	Tablet, liquid	200 mg up to twice daily as needed	OTC
Famotidine (fa MOE ti deen)	Pepcid AC	Oral	Tablet, liquid	10–20 mg up to twice daily as needed taken 10–60 min before meals	OTC
Nizatidine (ni ZA ti deen)	Axid AR	Oral	Tablet, solution	150 mg up to twice daily as needed	OTC
Proton Pump Inhibitors (also see Chapter 20 Medication Tables)					
Dexlansoprazole (dex lan SOE pra zole)	Dexilant	Oral	Tablet	30 mg once daily	Rx
Esomeprazole (es oh ME pray zol)	Nexium	Oral	Tablet	20 mg once daily as needed	OTC
Lansoprazole (lan SOE pra zole)	Prevacid	Oral	Tablet	15 or 30 mg once daily as needed	OTC
Omeprazole (oh ME pray zol)	Prilosec	Oral	Tablet	20 mg once daily as needed	OTC
Pantoprazole (pan TOE pra zole)	Protonix	Oral	Tablet	20–40 mg once daily as needed	Rx
Rabeprazole (ra BE pray zole)	AcipHex	Oral	Tablet	20 mg once daily as needed	Rx
Anticholinergics					
Scopolamine (skoe POL a meen)	Transderm Scop	Transdermal	Patch	1 mg q 72 hr as needed	Rx
Antihistamines					
Dimenhydrinate (dye men HYE dri nate)	Dramamine	Oral, IV, IM	Tablet, injection	Oral: 50–100 mg q 4–6 hr as needed; IM, IV: 50 mg q 4 hrs	OTC

Continued next page

MEDICATION TABLE 21-1. Pharmacologic Treatment of Nausea and Vomiting[6,a] *(Continued)*

CLASS Generic Name (pronunciation)	Brand Name	Route	Forms	Dose	Rx/OTC
Diphenhydramine (dye fen HYE dra meen)	Benadryl	Oral, IV, IM	Tablet, capsule, liquid, injection	Oral: 25 mg q 4–6 hr or 50 mg q 6–8 hr as needed; IM, IV: 10–50 mg q 6 hr as needed	OTC
Hydroxyzine (hye DROX i zeen)	Vistaril	Oral	Tablet, liquid	25–50 mg q 6 hr as needed	Rx
Meclizine (MEK li zeen)	Bonine, Antivert, Dramamine Less Drowsy	Oral	Tablet	25–50 mg 1 hr before travel or 25–100 mg daily in divided doses	OTC
Phenothiazines					
Chlorpromazine (klor PROE ma zeen)	Thorazine	Oral, IV, IM	Tablet, injection	Oral: 10–25 mg q 4–8 hr as needed; IM, IV: 10–25 mg q 3–4 hr as needed	Rx
Prochlorperazine (proe klor PER a zeen)	Compazine, Compro	Oral, rectal, IV, IM	Tablet, suppository, injection	Oral: 5–10 mg 3–4 times daily as needed; rectal: 25 mg twice daily as needed; IM: 5–10 mg q 3–4 hr as needed; IV: 2.5–10 mg q 3–4 hr as needed	Rx
Promethazine (proe METH a zeen)	Phenergan	Oral, rectal, trans-dermal, IV, IM	Tablet, liquid, suppository, injection	12.5–25 mg q 4–6 hr as needed	Rx
Butyrophenones					
Droperidol (droe PER i dole)	Inapsine	IV, IM	Injection	0.625–1.5 mg after surgery	Rx
Haloperidol (ha loe PER i dole)	Haldol	Oral, IM, IV	Tablet, injection	0.5–1 mg q 6 hrs as needed for CINV; 0.5–2 mg as a single dose at end of surgery for PONV	Rx
Benzamides					
Metoclopramide (met oh KLOE pra mide)	Reglan	Oral, IM, IV	Tablet, liquid, injection	N/V: IV or oral; IV, 10 or 20 mg as a single dose; oral, 10 mg as a single dose and may repeat after 4–6 hr if needed CINV: oral 10 mg before chemotherapy or 10 mg q 6 hr as needed; can also be used 10–20 mg four times/day on post-chemotherapy days 2–4 and can be given in combination with dexamethasone; delayed CINV: 0.5 mg/kg or 20 mg q 6 hr as needed, 2–4 days	Rx

Continued next page

MEDICATION TABLE 21-1. Pharmacologic Treatment of Nausea and Vomiting[6,a] *(Continued)*

CLASS Generic Name (pronunciation)	Brand Name	Route	Forms	Dose	Rx/OTC
Trimethobenzamide (trye meth oh BEN za mide)	Tigan	Oral, IM	Capsule, injection	Oral: 300 mg 3–4 times daily; IM: 200 mg 3–4 times daily	Rx
Corticosteroids					
Dexamethasone (dex a METH a sone)	Decadron	Oral, IM, IV	Tablet, injection	Can be given with NK_1-receptor antagonist and serotonin-receptor antagonist with or without olanzapine; 10 mg prior to chemotherapy; 12 or 20 mg oral or IV, depending on specific NK_1 antagonist used; on post-chemotherapy days, can be given 8 mg once or twice daily on days 2–4, depending on which agents dexamethasone was administered with	Rx
Cannabinoids					
Dronabinol (droe NAB i nol)	Marinol, Syndros	Oral	Capsule	Capsule: 5 mg/m^2 before chemotherapy, then q 2–4 hr as needed for a total of 4–6 doses/day; increase dose in increments of 2.1 mg/m^2 based on response (max 12.6 mg/m^2 dose); solution: 4.2 mg/m^2 then q 2–4 hr as needed for a total of 4–6 doses/day; increase dose in increments of 2.1 mg/m^2 based on response (max 15 mg/m^2 dose)	Rx-CIII
Benzodiazepines					
Lorazepam (lor A ze pam)	Ativan	Oral, IV	Tablet, injection	0.5–2 mg q 4–6 hr as needed	Rx-CIV
Serotonin Antagonists					
Dolasetron (dol A se tron)	Anzemet	Oral, IV	Tablet, injection	100 mg orally within 2 hr before chemotherapy; may be used with dexamethasone, an NK_1-receptor antagonist, and olanzapine	Rx

Continued next page

MEDICATION TABLE 21-1. Pharmacologic Treatment of Nausea and Vomiting[6,a] *(Continued)*

CLASS Generic Name (pronunciation)	Brand Name	Route	Forms	Dose	Rx/OTC
Granisetron (gra NI se tron)	Sancuso, Sustol	IV, oral, transdermal	Injection, tablet, oral liquid, transdermal patch	IV: 10 mg within 30 min before chemotherapy; PO: 1 mg twice daily or 2 mg daily 1 hr before chemotherapy; SUBQ: 10 mg 30 min prior to chemotherapy in combination with dexamethasone or an NK_1-receptor antagonist; transdermal: apply 24–48 hr before chemotherapy; remove no sooner than 24 hr after chemotherapy; may be worn up to 7 days	Rx
Ondansetron (on DAN se tron)	Zofran	IV, oral	Injection, tablet, liquid	Postop N/V: 4 mg IV or 8 mg PO Chemo: 8 mg or 0.15 mg/kg IV or 8 mg BID × 2 doses; schedule and dosing varies depending on chemo regimen.	Rx
Palonosetron (pal oh NOE se tron)	Aloxi	IV	Injection	0.25 mg IV 30 min prior to chemo	Rx
Neurokinin$_1$ Antagonist					
Aprepitant (ap RE pi tant)	Emend	Oral	Capsule	130 mg IV 30 min prior to chemotherapy in combination with a serotonin antagonist and dexamethasone OR 125 mg capsule or 3 mg/kg suspension (max 125 mg/dose) 1 hr prior to chemotherapy, followed by 80 mg once daily for 2 days, in combination with serotonin antagonist and dexamethasone	Rx
Fosaprepitant dimeglumine (fos ap RE pi tant di ME gloo meen)	Emend	IV	Injection	150 mg 30 min prior to chemotherapy, given in combination with serotonin antagonist and dexamethasone	Rx
Rolapitant (roe LA pi tant)	Varubi	Oral	Tablet	180 mg 2 hr prior to chemotherapy in combination with dexamethasone, with or without serotonin antagonist	Rx

Continued next page

MEDICATION TABLE 21-1. Pharmacologic Treatment of Nausea and Vomiting[6,a] *(Continued)*

CLASS Generic Name (pronunciation)	Brand Name	Route	Forms	Dose	Rx/OTC
Miscellaneous Agents					
Bismuth subsalicylate (biz muth) (sub sa LIS i late)	Pepto-Bismol, various additional products containing bismuth	Oral	Caplet, liquid, suspension	524 mg q 30–60 min or 1,050 mg q 60 min for up to 2 days (maximum 4,200 mg/24 hr)	OTC
Phosphorated carbohydrate solution	Emetrol	Oral	Liquid	15–30 mL; repeat dose q 15 min until distress subsides; not to be administered over more than 1 hr (5 doses)	OTC
Pyridoxine (peer i DOX een)	Aminoxin, Pyri-500	IM, IV, oral	Capsule, injection solution, liquid, tablet, sustained-release tablet	10–25 mg PO daily 3–4 times daily, alone or in combination with doxylamine	OTC
Erythromycin (er ith roe MYE sin)	Erythrocin, EryPEd, E.E.S., Ery-Tab, others	Oral, IV	Capsule, granules for suspension, injection, powder for suspension, tablet	250–500 mg 3 times daily before meals; 3 mg/kg every 8 hr	Rx

IM = intramuscular; IV = intravenous; OTC = over the counter; PO = orally; Rx = prescription; SUBQ = subcutaneous.

*C-IV = schedule IV controlled substance.

*According to the FDA, schedule IV describes drugs, substances, or chemicals that are defined as drugs with a low potential for abuse and low risk of dependence.

aPronunciations have been adapted with permission from USP Dictionary of USAN and International Drug Names (USP Dictionary) © 2022.

Chapter 22

Lower Gastrointestinal Tract

Shelby P. Brooks, PharmD, BCPS |
Jeffery D. Evans, PharmD

KEY TERMS AND DEFINITIONS

Appendicitis—inflammation of the vermiform appendix usually occurring because of an obstruction of the appendix.

Colitis—inflammation in the colon (another name for the large intestine). Different diseases may cause this inflammation, which can lead to significant disease, including cancer.

Colonoscopy—examination with a flexible, lighted, tubular instrument using fiber optics to permit visualization of the colon. Patients undergoing a colonoscopy are expected to use bowel preparations the day before the scope to ensure the entire colon has been thoroughly cleansed, and there are no feces remaining in the lower gastrointestinal tract. This aids in a clearer visual inspection of the colon.

Duodenal ulcer—chronic inflammation of the duodenal area of the gastrointestinal tract most commonly linked to the *Helicobacter pylori* bacteria or from nonsteroidal anti-inflammatory medications (ibuprofen, naproxen) or aspirin. Duodenal ulcers are the most common form of peptic ulcer.

Gastroenteritis—inflammation of the gastrointestinal tract, involving both the stomach and the small intestine, which results in acute diarrhea. The inflammation is caused most often by an infection from certain viruses or less often by bacteria, their toxins, parasites, or an adverse reaction to food contamination or medication.

DOI 10.37573/9781585286638.022

Lower gastrointestinal tract—the portion of the digestive system that includes the cecum, appendix, large intestine, and anus. Water is actively absorbed in this portion of the system to help form the stool.

Prodrug—a medication that is given in an inactive form and is converted in the body to an active form. Prodrugs may be used to reduce side effects of the active medication or to permit administration via an alternate route.

LEARNING OBJECTIVES

After completing this chapter, you should be able to

1. Define the following:
   - Lower gastrointestinal tract.
   - Duodenal ulcer.
   - Appendicitis.
   - Gastroenteritis.
   - Colonoscopy.

2. Review the anatomy and normal physiology of the lower gastrointestinal tract.

3. Identify the causes, risk factors, and clinical presentation for diarrhea, constipation, hemorrhoids, inflammatory bowel disease, irritable bowel syndrome, flatulence, and parasitic infections.

4. Review the treatment goals for diarrhea, constipation, hemorrhoids, inflammatory bowel disease, irritable bowel syndrome, flatulence, and parasitic infections.

5. List the nonpharmacologic, pharmacologic, and alternative treatments for diarrhea, constipation, hemorrhoids, inflammatory bowel disease, irritable bowel syndrome, flatulence, and parasitic infections.

6. Discuss the therapeutic effects, drug properties, dosages, and routes of administration for each class of medications listed above, and list their most common side effects and drug interactions.

The lower gastrointestinal (GI) tract is the site of important functions of the body, including many of importance to the absorption and action of medications. Several diseases have an impact on this region of the body. This chapter provides a summary of the major disorders affecting the lower GI system and the medications that are used most frequently to treat them.

CASE STUDY

Paul Hernandez is a 55-year-old male who comes into the pharmacy every month to fill his prescriptions. This afternoon he seems unusually distant and pale in the face. He states, "You might want to stay away from me. I think I have a stomach virus." When asked about his illness, Mr. Hernandez replies, "I can't keep a thing down, no water or food. I've been having diarrhea since last night, and it has kept me up all night. I'm extremely tired and weak, and my mouth is dry as a bone." The pharmacist asks Mr. Hernandez a series of questions and finds out that Mr. Hernandez has a slight fever, severe abdominal cramping, and thought he saw blood in one of his bowel movements. He is not taking any antibiotics currently, just his usual blood pressure and high cholesterol medication. He has not traveled outside of the country in the last 6 months, but he states that he and Mrs. Hernandez ate at the local buffet yesterday for lunch.

ANATOMY AND PHYSIOLOGY OF THE LOWER GASTROINTESTINAL TRACT

The lower GI tract begins with the end of the small intestine, or small bowel, and ends with the anus (external GI tract opening—Figure 22-1).

The large intestine is the portion of the lower GI tract extending from the ileocecal junction to the anus. It consists of the cecum, colon, rectum, and anal canal (see Figure 22-1). Normally, 18 to 24 hours are required for material to pass through the large intestine. Attached to the cecum is a small tube called the vermiform appendix. If this tube becomes obstructed (blocked), secretions from the appendix cannot pass the obstruction and accumulate, causing enlargement,

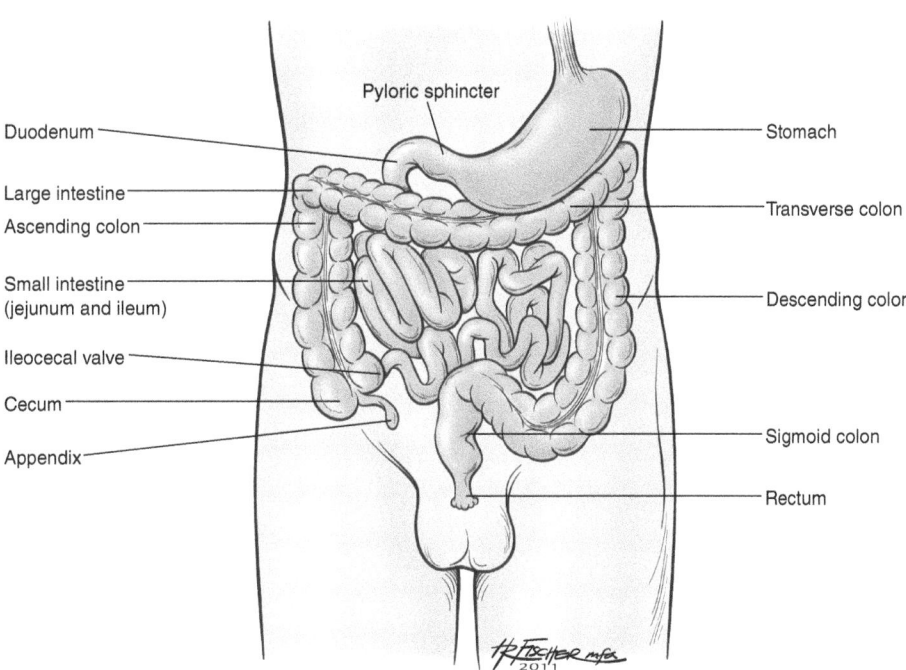

FIGURE 22-1. Anatomy of the lower gastrointestinal tract.

pain, and inflammation. This condition is known as appendicitis. Bacteria in the area can cause infection of the appendix. Symptoms include sudden abdominal pain, particularly in the right lower portion of the abdomen; a slight fever; loss of appetite; constipation or diarrhea; nausea; and vomiting. If the appendix bursts, the infection can spread throughout the abdomen or even the whole body, with life-threatening results.

The colon, which is responsible for converting chyme to feces and containing feces until it is eliminated by defecation, consists of four parts: the ascending colon, transverse colon, descending colon, and sigmoid colon. The ascending colon extends superior to (above) the cecum and ends at the right colic flexure near the right inferior (lower) margin of the liver. The transverse colon extends from the right colic flexure to the left colic flexure, and the descending colon extends from the left colic flexure to the superior opening of the true pelvis where it becomes the sigmoid colon. Peristaltic waves are responsible for moving chyme along the ascending colon. About three or four times each day, large parts of the transverse and descending colon undergo several strong contractions, called mass movements. Mass movements are very common after meals, especially breakfast, because the presence of food in the stomach or duodenum initiates them. The sigmoid colon forms an S-shaped

tube that extends into the pelvis and ends at the rectum. The rectum is a straight, muscular tube that begins at the termination of the sigmoid colon and ends at the anal canal. The last 2 to 3 cm of the digestive tract is the anal canal. It begins at the inferior (lower) end of the rectum and ends at the anus with the external sphincter.

Drugs administered orally pass through various parts of the GI tract and are absorbed. Any leftover drug residue exits the body through the anus. The total time it takes for a drug to move through the GI tract is from about 10 hours to 5 days. Some medications are administered in an inactive form, termed a prodrug, intended to reduce the incidence of side effects caused by taking a medication in its active form or to permit a drug to be administered via a route that would not be possible with its active version. The duodenum is the site where many prodrugs are hydrolyzed during absorption, being converted to their active forms. Drugs with a very low pH (acidic drugs) will dissolve best in the ileum, and drugs in an oral sustained-release dosage form will be more likely absorbed in the colon. Rectal suppository dosage forms have variable drug absorption. A portion of the drug dose may be absorbed via the lower hemorrhoidal veins, from which the drug enters directly into the systemic circulation (absorption within the body); other drugs may be metabolized (broken down) before systemic absorption, so will exert only a local effect.

DIARRHEA

Diarrhea is a symptom characterized by increased stool (feces) frequency, decreased consistency or liquidity (watery), and increased weight as compared to an individual's normal bowel pattern. The normal frequency and consistency vary between individuals. More than three bowel movements per day is considered abnormal.

CASE?

What type of diarrhea is Mr. Hernandez experiencing? What might be the cause of his diarrhea?

Diarrhea can be acute, persistent, or chronic. Acute diarrhea is abrupt-onset diarrhea in a healthy individual most often related to an infectious agent, and lasts anywhere from 1 to 14 days. Persistent diarrhea is diarrhea lasting from 14 days to 4 weeks. Chronic diarrhea is a decrease in fecal consistency lasting more than 4 weeks. Persistent and chronic diarrhea illnesses are often secondary to other chronic medical conditions, which are outside the scope of this chapter.

Acute diarrhea can be caused by viruses, bacteria, protozoa, or from traveling to some countries, where poor sanitation and hygiene are prevalent. Ingestion of contaminated water or food can lead to infectious diarrhea. Noroviruses are the predominant cause of acute diarrhea, and most norovirus infections often occur after consuming contaminated water or food.[1] Viruses in this group cause the "stomach flu," or gastroenteritis. Typically these viruses are spread person to person by the fecal-oral route. They are self-limiting, usually lasting 1 to 3 days and affecting infants and children less than 5 years of age most often.

Patients may present with vomiting, nausea, headache, muscle ache, fever, or watery diarrhea. This type of viral diarrhea is often referred to as "the stomach bug." The rotavirus accounts for about 12% of all acute diarrhea cases and up to 50% of infant viral diarrhea.[2] Cases peak in the winter season and in children between 4 and 23 months of age. The rotavirus is also spread by the fecal-oral route and the effects typically last 5 to 8 days. Most of the cases exhibit watery diarrhea accompanied by vomiting. Nearly all children in both industrialized and developing countries have been infected with rotavirus by the time they are 3 to 5 years of age.[2] Risk factors for the contraction of virus causing diarrhea (gastroenteritis) include daycare attendance, recent antibiotic use, having a compromised immune system (the body's ability to fight infection is weak), or spending time in institutional settings, schools, and nursing homes. These infections can also occur in other group settings, such as banquet halls, cruise ships, dormitories, and campgrounds.

CASE?

What signs and symptoms suggest bacterial causes for the illness Mr. Hernandez describes?

Bacterial diarrhea or bacterial gastroenteritis affects 15% to 20% of people in the United States annually and can be caused by numerous types of bacteria, including, most prominently, *Escherichia coli, Salmonella*, and *Campylobacter*.[2] Typically, bacterial diarrhea is spread by eating contaminated food or water and improperly cooked or refrigerated poultry and dairy products. Bacterial diarrhea can present within 8 to 12 hours of eating contaminated food. Outbreaks of food-borne bacterial infections have been traced to poor sanitary conditions in meat-processing plants, grocery stores, and restaurants. Symptoms include nausea, abdominal cramping and bloating, occasional vomiting, and watery diarrhea. Depending on the bacteria causing the gastroenteritis, bloody diarrhea may result.

Another bacterial diarrhea is caused by *Clostridioides difficile*. These bacteria, also known as *C. diff*, not only cause diarrhea but can also result in more serious intestinal conditions such as colitis. The prime risk factor for contracting *C. diff* infection includes prolonged use of antibiotics, with elderly patients having a greater risk. People can become infected if they touch items or surfaces that are contaminated with infected feces, then touch their mouths or mucous membranes. Healthcare workers can spread the bacteria to other patients or contaminate surfaces through hand contact. To prevent spread, healthcare workers must wash their hands with soap and water to eliminate the spores that cause the growth of *C. diff*; hand sanitizers will not eliminate the spores. Patients typically present with watery diarrhea (at least three bowel movements per day for 2 or more days), fever, loss of appetite, nausea, and abdominal pain/tenderness. *C. diff* can be hard to treat and requires prescription antibiotics (oral vancomycin or fidaxomicin). Other diarrheal diseases can be treated with over-the-counter (OTC) products.

Protozoal infections account for about 10% to 15% of diarrhea cases. These types of infections occur most frequently in travelers entering or returning from endemic areas—relatively secluded places with contaminated water supplies harboring protozoa (single-celled, nonbacterial organisms). Protozoal contamination is uncommon in developed countries, such as the United States, Canada, Australia, New Zealand, Japan, and countries in northern and western Europe.[3] *Cryptosporidium parvum* and *Cyclospora* are the most common protozoal parasites among children, while *Giardia lamblia* is more common among traveling adults. Protozoal infections result in sudden-onset diarrhea 3 to 7 days after arrival in a foreign location and are generally accompanied by profuse watery or pale, greasy stool, nausea and vomiting, and occasional fecal evidence of inflammation (mucus). Preventative measures for travelers include awareness of parasites or bacteria known to the area and carrying small containers of hand-sanitizing solutions or gels when handwashing is not possible. Some oversights include brushing teeth with contaminated water, ingesting ice cubes, or eating cold salads or meats. Depending on the type of protozoan causing the diarrhea, symptoms may last up to 3 weeks but are self-limiting (will resolve on their own) and will end with adequate treatment unless the patient is severely immunocompromised.

CASE?

What signs and symptoms suggest dehydration in Mr. Hernandez? What is an appropriate treatment for his dehydration?

Goals for treating patients with diarrhea are to (1) prevent dehydration or correct fluid and electrolyte imbalance, (2) relieve symptoms, (3) identify and treat the cause, and (4) prevent complications. Most acute cases of diarrhea can be treated with nonpharmacological therapy or OTC medications, as most cases of diarrhea are self-limiting. Replacement of fluid loss and electrolytes is the standard for efficacious and cost-effective management of acute diarrhea. Clear liquids at room temperature, such as broth, carbonated beverages (without caffeine), and rehydrating fluids such as Pedialyte or Gatorade, are good options for replacing fluid loss. Pedialyte and Gatorade contain a mix of water and electrolytes (sodium, chloride, glucose, potassium, and citrate), which are all needed to adequately hydrate a person and allow bodily processes to continue.

For children with body weight less than 10 kg, 60 to 120 mL of oral rehydration is needed for each diarrheal stool or vomiting episode.[2] For patients who cannot be managed on oral rehydration therapy, intravenous (IV) rehydration (with solutions of sodium chloride, dextrose, and/or other electrolytes such as potassium or magnesium) may be necessary.

Antidiarrheal Agents

Loperamide

Among hundreds of OTC products promoted as antidiarrheal agents, only loperamide and bismuth subsalicylate have sufficient evidence of efficacy and safety to bear U.S. Food and Drug Administration (FDA)-approved labeling for this condition. Loperamide is available in OTC and prescription (Rx) strength as brand and generic. It is available in tablets, capsules, and a liquid formulation. Some brands are listed in Medication Table 22-1 (Medication Tables are located at the end of the chapter). Loperamide works by slowing intestinal motility (reducing small and large intestine movement), thereby reducing the daily fecal volume and diminishing the loss of fluid and electrolytes. Loperamide's effect lasts for approximately 11 hours. Peak levels are reached in 2.5 hours with the liquid formulation and in 5 hours with the tablets and capsules. Improvement in diarrhea is usually seen within 48 hours. Most common side effects include increased blood glucose, abdominal pain, dry mouth, dizziness, and fatigue. Drug interactions have been noted with an antiretroviral medication (saquinavir), an antifungal medication (itraconazole), and a medication for high triglycerides (gemfibrozil). All of these drugs are known to increase the concentration of loperamide in the bloodstream.

ALERT!

Loperamide should not be used in diarrhea associated with antibiotic use, if there is blood present in the stool, or the diarrhea is caused by *C. diff* infection. If constipation occurs, loperamide should be discontinued.

CASE?

What OTC therapy might Mr. Hernandez try to treat his bacterial diarrhea?

CASE?

What dose of bismuth subsalicylate would be appropriate for Mr. Hernandez?

Bismuth Subsalicylate

Bismuth subsalicylate (BSS) is effective in the treatment of acute diarrhea, including travelers' diarrhea, by significantly reducing the number of diarrheal stools. It is also effective in treating upset stomach, indigestion, heartburn, and nausea. BSS is available as an OTC tablet or suspension with multiple brand names. BSS is also available as a combination product in prescriptions used to treat peptic ulcers. The exact mechanism is not known, but it seems to exert its antidiarrheal action by stimulating absorption of fluid and electrolytes across the intestinal wall (antisecretory action) and by reducing intestinal inflammation and hypermotility (excess intestinal movement) by the subsalicylate portion. In addition, the bismuth component may exert direct antimicrobial effects against bacterial and viral pathogens. Bismuth

is poorly absorbed in the GI tract. The subsalicylate in a dose of BSS is comparable to a 200-mg dose of aspirin with a similar effect in the body. An antidiarrheal effect should occur within 48 hours of use. The most common adverse events include a temporary and harmless darkening of the tongue and/or black stool, ringing in the ears (tinnitus), and fecal impaction.

Diphenoxylate HCl/Atropine Sulfate

Diphenoxylate HCl/atropine sulfate is better known as Lomotil®. It is a prescription antidiarrheal medication available as a Schedule V controlled drug. It is indicated as adjunct treatment (in addition to other therapies) of diarrhea.

Diphenoxylate is an opioid (opium derivative similar to those discussed in Chapter 5) that acts both locally, at the gut level, and centrally, in the central nervous system (CNS), to slow intestinal contractions and peristalsis, prolonging the gut transit time. This allows moisture to be drawn out of the intestines thereby stopping the formation of loose and liquid stools. Atropine is an anticholinergic combined with diphenoxylate to prevent abuse or overdose. Diphenoxylate begins working in 45 to 60 minutes, with effects lasting up to 3 to 4 hours. Improvement is usually observed within 48 hours.

Common side effects include abdominal discomfort, nausea and vomiting, dizziness, sedation, somnolence (sleepiness), euphoria, and malaise. Serious side effects include possible anaphylaxis in sensitive patients, pancreatitis, and toxic megacolon. Toxic megacolon refers to a rapid widening of the large intestine leading to bloating, abdominal pain, fever, and possibly shock if left untreated. Diphenoxylate is contraindicated for patients with myasthenia gravis or patients taking potassium chloride supplements.

Diphenoxylate should not be used in combination with monoamine oxidase inhibitors (MAOIs). The combination of the two can significantly raise a patient's blood pressure. Because diphenoxylate is an opioid, combining it with barbiturates, tranquilizers, or alcohol can significantly increase the depressive effects of each medication. Use in women of childbearing potential is only indicated when, in the opinion of the prescriber, the potential benefits outweigh the potential risk to the fetus. Use in breastfeeding mothers should be cautioned as Lomotil can be found in breast milk. In addition, the atropine component can decrease the production of milk in the breastfeeding mother. Patients with bacterial diarrhea should be cautioned when using this medication, as it may prolong or aggravate the diarrhea further.

ALERT!

The use of Lomotil® is contraindicated in children younger than 2 years of age. If used in children, the liquid formulation is recommended when the child is less than 13 years of age. The maximum dose for adults and children is 20 mg/day. For children experiencing severe dehydration or electrolyte imbalance, Lomotil® should be withheld until the child is adequately hydrated because of the risk of intoxication from diphenoxylate when patients are severely dehydrated.

PRACTICE POINT

When measuring the liquid formulation for children, the plastic dropper provided should always be used to prevent accidental overdose.

Opium

Opium is an effective and fast-acting nonspecific antidiarrheal agent that exerts its action by both enhancing the tone and preventing contraction of the intestinal muscles, thus inhibiting the propulsive contractions of the GI tract. Its principal active ingredient is morphine and it is available as opium 10% tincture (10 mg morphine/mL). It is indicated for the treatment of diarrhea and used for unlabeled indications, which include the relief of pain, neonatal abstinence

syndrome, and the management of short bowel syndrome. Common side effects include constipation, nausea, and vomiting; pruritus (itching) and urticaria (skin rash similar to hives) have also been observed related to the morphine in opium. Opium can be addictive, and a person can become tolerant of the medication and eventually require higher doses to achieve the same beneficial effect. Because morphine is a CNS depressant, other medications such as pain medications, anxiety medications, and antidepressant medications can worsen the depressant effects of opium.

Opium tincture may be used in children, but it is imperative that it is diluted appropriately. To administer to children, a 25-fold dilution must be used for a final concentration of 0.4 mg/mL of morphine. Opium should be used with caution in the elderly, in debilitated individuals, and in patients with liver or lung problems or bleeding disorders.

PRACTICE POINT

Opium tincture is a Drug Enforcement Administration (DEA) Schedule II controlled preparation, available to patients only by nonrefillable prescription.

ALERT!

In diarrhea caused by poisoning, the toxin must be eliminated from the GI tract before opium can be given.

Complementary and Alternative Therapy: Lactobacillus acidophilus

Probiotics are dietary supplements of live microorganisms. According to the currently adopted definition by the World Health Organization, probiotics are "Live microorganisms, which when administered in adequate amounts, confer a health benefit on the host."[2] Probiotics include several *Lactobacillus* species and *Bifidobacterium lactis*, which both have strain-specific benefits in controlling some aspect of a person's health. The most common species useful in the treatment or prevention of acute, uncomplicated diarrhea is *Lactobacillus acidophilus*. Lactobacilli are bacteria that normally live in the human small intestine and vagina. Probiotic formulations are available commercially in food products such as yogurt, nutrition bars, beverages, and many others that are becoming more popular. *Lactobacillus acidophilus* is also available as a capsule, tablet, granules for suspension, powder for suspension, and a concentrate solution. Some probiotics include other helpful bacteria to treat ailments in addition to diarrhea. Because *Lactobacillus* is naturally occurring bacteria in the lower GI tract, it is useful in the restoration and stabilization of the normal intestinal flora (harmless microorganisms that inhabit the intestinal tract and are essential for its normal functioning). *Lactobacillus* also interferes with the ability of pathogenic bacteria to adhere (attach) to intestinal mucosal cells and establish an infection. Patients who are sensitive to milk or have lactose intolerance should refrain from using *Lactobacillus* probiotics. Burping, intestinal gas (or flatulence), constipation, hiccups, and vomiting have been reported during treatment; however, it is unknown whether this symptom was due to *Lactobacillus* therapy or to concomitant antibiotic therapy. *Lactobacillus* is commonly used in both hospital and retail settings where patients are taking broad spectrum antibiotics as a way to restore the normal gut flora and prevent antibiotic-associated diarrhea.

Probiotics such as *Lactobacillus acidophilus* have been shown safe and effective for use in children. Product dosing will vary, but the typical daily dose for both adults and children is 3 to 4 times a day. Unless directed by a healthcare provider, use should be limited to 2 days of therapy.

PRACTICE POINT

The microorganisms in probiotic preparations are encapsulated for stability and are viable for a year from the shipping date. Lactobacillus granules must be stored in the refrigerator at 2°C to 8°C for optimum benefit.

CASE STUDY

Mr. Jones is a 58-year-old truck driver who recently lost his wife. He has come to the pharmacy to inquire about a remedy for the awful stomach cramping he has had in the past week. When asked if he has noticed any changes in his stool, he mentions that he "has not had a bowel movement for as long as he can remember." Mr. Jones tells the pharmacist that his diet consists of fast-food lunches and dinners with truck-stop snacks along the way. He doesn't drink as much water as he once did, and now he relies on coffee and sodas to stay alert. He is tired all the time but attributes this to his recent 25-pound weight gain. Mr. Jones is taking two blood pressure medicines, amlodipine and lisinopril, and amitriptyline to help with his sad feelings and difficulty sleeping. He has picked up a value pack of ibuprofen and three boxes of Tums Extra Strength saying, "My knees are killing me from driving all the time and my stomach just can't get right."

CONSTIPATION

The importance of regularity of defecation is often greatly overstated. Many people have the misleading notion that a daily bowel movement is critical for good health, but what is "normal" differs from person to person. Some will defecate once or twice daily, while other healthy adults may defecate only once every 2 days. A defecation rate of fewer than three per week is defined as constipation. Symptoms often include straining, lumpy or pellet-like hard stools, and a sensation of incomplete defecation or evacuation of stool.[4] There are many causes of constipation, and most are poorly understood. Some causes include insufficient nutrition, impaired colon motility, psychiatric factors, or anatomical (structural) abnormalities. Structural abnormalities and to some degree psychiatric factors are beyond the scope of this chapter; however, some common psychiatric causes that could be recognized by pharmacy technicians include depression, sexual abuse, high levels of stress, and/or unusual attitudes toward food and bowel function. Insufficient nutrition can be a direct result of inadequate fiber or fluid intake. A diet low in calories, carbohydrates (e.g., Atkins diet), or fiber may lead to diet-related constipation. Some fiber-based foods (e.g., breakfast cereals, nutrition bars) could contribute to constipation because of the processed sugar they contain. Impaired colon motility can result from a slow transit time (GI tract moving slowly), irritable bowel syndrome (which will be discussed in detail later in the chapter), nerve damage (which stimulates gut motility), drugs, or other neurological causes (spinal cord injury, Parkinson disease, multiple sclerosis, etc.).[4] Representative medications known to cause constipation can be found in Medication Table 22-2.

Some patients are more likely to develop constipation than others. Infants and children, as well as adults over the age of 55 are more at risk. Functional fecal retention (slow GI movement) and fecal withholding (unwillingness to defecate) are two of the more common causes of pediatric constipation. The urge to defecate is a stimulus received from the brain. When this is ignored or suppressed, rectal muscles can lose tonicity and become less effective in eliminating stool. The leading contributors to constipation in adults are poor diet, lack of exercise, medication use, and poor bowel habits. Polypharmacy (use of multiple medications by a patient) and sedentary lifestyle are the primary factors leading to chronic constipation in older adults. Other populations at risk for constipation include pregnant women (especially in the last trimester), terminal care patients, those with limited mobility or sedentary lifestyles, and travelers.

Some patients who present with constipation complaints require medical attention. Those who report bloody stools, fever associated with constipation, sudden weight loss, or severe nausea and vomiting should be referred to a physician for follow-up and OTC medications should not be recommended. In managing constipation, the goal is to first relieve constipation and reestablish normal bowel function, then focus on establishing dietary and exercise habits that will prevent recurrences. If there are medications causing constipation, the medication may be stopped or changed, after the patient consults with their healthcare provider, to a product less likely to cause this side effect.

Bulk-forming laxatives and stool softeners are good initial therapy in addition to increasing fiber and fluid in the diet. If no contraindications to fiber exist (anatomic abnormalities, some diseases), daily fiber intake should be increased and patients advised to drink approximately 2 L of fluid per day and increase aerobic exercise (walking, running, and swimming) to help stimulate GI motility. The American Dietetic Association recommends 14 g of dietary fiber per 1,000 kcal or 25 g for adult women and 38 g for adult men.[5]

Bulk-Forming Agents

Bulk-forming laxatives are derived from natural plant sources, synthetic cellulose derivatives, or analogs. The most common plant source is psyllium, branded as Metamucil® and many generics. A synthetic cellulose derivative, methylcellulose, is often used and another agent is calcium polycarbophil, the calcium salt of a synthetic polyacrylic resin. (See Medication Table 22-1 for products and dosage forms.) Bulk-forming laxatives are often recommended as first line because they closely mimic the body's physiologic mechanism in promoting evacuation. They dissolve or swell in the intestinal fluid, forming emollient gels that facilitate passage of the intestinal contents and stimulate gut movement. The actions of these agents are localized in the gut and they do not undergo systemic absorption. This enables treatment while avoiding systemic drug interactions, but these agents should be taken at least 2 hours before or 2 hours after taking an oral prescription medicine to prevent a delay in absorption of some medications.

Psyllium is approved for the relief of occasional constipation and for restoring regular bowel function. It is also useful when recommended by a physician for the treatment of constipation associated with GI disorders and in patients with irritable bowel syndrome, diverticular disease, and hemorrhoid treatment, which will be discussed later in the chapter. Psyllium also appears to be useful in the reduction of cholesterol levels as an adjunct to a dietary program. It is available in a granule, seed husk, whole seed, wafer, capsule, and powder for oral suspension. Psyllium products are indicated for children older than 6 years of age and adults.

PRACTICE POINT

Psyllium and other bulk-forming laxatives must be taken with at least 240 mL (8 ounces, a full glass) of water or other liquid either before or after meals. Without adequate fluid, the product can swell and block the throat or esophagus, which could lead to choking. Patients who have difficulty swallowing should not take these products.

Psyllium produces an effect in 12 to 72 hours. If constipation persists for longer than a week and psyllium has not produced an effect, patients should be advised to see a doctor. Psyllium should not be used for acute relief of constipation for longer than 7 days. If other adverse events such as chest pain, vomiting, or difficulty in swallowing or breathing occur after taking this product, patients should seek immediate medical attention. Two side effects that occur most often with bulk-forming laxatives are abdominal distention and flatulence.

Methylcellulose is approved for the same indications as psyllium, with a bowel movement expected within 12 to 72 hours. The side effects and drug interactions are the same as for psyllium. These products are available in a powder for oral suspension, tablets, and chewable tablets.

Polycarbophil laxatives produce a defecation response by increasing bulk volume and water content of the stool, which produces a bowel movement in 12 to 72 hours. Polycarbophils are approved for the same indications as psyllium. Additional uses, although not FDA approved, include bacterial vaginosis (bacterial infection of the vaginal tract), and diarrhea. Polycarbophil has been shown to lower the vaginal pH, which creates an unfavorable environment for bacterial growth. Polycarbophil is used in chronic watery diarrhea, due to its ability to absorb substantial amounts

of water. The products are available as tablets that can be swallowed or chewed. Flatulence occurs less with calcium polycarbophil as compared to psyllium.

ALERT!

Prescription medications should be taken at least 1 hour before or 2 hours after polycarbophils (especially antibiotics containing any form of tetracycline).

ALERT!

Polycarbophil products contain approximately 150 mg of calcium per tablet. Patients susceptible to hypercalcemia (those who are elderly, have a malignancy, HIV/AIDS, or renal disease) should be cautioned.

PRACTICE POINT

Bulk-forming agents are the recommended constipation remedies for patients who are pregnant or postpartum, need additional fiber added to their diet, and diabetic patients. The powder, wafer, and granule dosage form of psyllium should be kept at room temperature away from moisture or humidity.

Surfactants

Surfactants, more commonly known as stool softeners, include docusate sodium (Colace®) and docusate calcium. Stool softeners are not considered laxatives. They work by actively drawing water into the stool, thus softening the stool and achieving ease in bowel movement. Their action takes place in the small and large intestines, with an onset of 24 to 72 hours. Most patients will achieve a bowel movement within 48 hours; however, for some patients it may take as long as 3 to 5 days. Surfactants should not be taken for more than 7 days. A 240-mg dose of docusate calcium and a 100-mg dose of docusate sodium contain the same quantity of dioctyl sulfosuccinic acid, the active ingredient. Occasionally docusate calcium is selected over docusate sodium by the physician based on its lack of sodium. This is a concern in patients who are sodium restricted (examples may include patients with hypertension or renal insufficiency). However, it should be noted that if no additional sodium is added during the manufacturing process, a 100-mg dose of docusate sodium contains only 10 mg of sodium.

Docusate sodium is available as a tablet, soft-gel capsule, syrup, rectal enema, and liquid formulation. It is approved for use in adults and children over the age of 2 years. The tablets and capsules are indicated for relief of occasional constipation (irregularity), while the syrup and liquid formulation are indicated for constipation due to hard stools, in cardiac and other conditions in which maximum ease of stool passage is desirable to avoid difficult or painful defecation, and when peristaltic stimulants (laxatives) are contraindicated. Docusate calcium is available as a soft gel capsule and as a regular capsule indicated for adults and children over the age of 12 years. It is approved for the treatment of occasional constipation and for the prevention of dry, hard stools. It is useful as a prophylactic agent to prevent straining during defecation in patients following anal or rectal surgery and in patients who have recently suffered with a heart attack. Docusate products are commonly used for preventing constipation. In terminally ill patients who are primarily confined to a bed or those taking scheduled doses of opiates for pain relief, docusate products are recommended as first line for prevention. Although docusate products appear to be safe for use in pregnancy since there is minimal absorption from the GI tract, there is not enough evidence to recommend their use in pregnant patients.

> ## ALERT!
>
> Dulcolax Stool Softener is a brand name for docusate sodium and Dulcolax is a brand name for bisacodyl, which is a stimulant laxative. Another product, Dulcolax Soft Chews, has still a different active ingredient. Similarly, Kaopectate Liqui-gels (stool softener docusate calcium) can be easily confused with Kaopectate Antidiarrheal (bismuth subsalicylate). Patients choosing OTC remedies may be confused by these similarities in product names.

Docusate should not be taken if constipation is accompanied by significant abdominal pain, nausea, vomiting, or sudden changes in bowel habits that persist for more than 2 weeks. Some uncommon reactions that have occurred with the use of docusate include development of a rash, bitter taste in the mouth, nausea, and diarrhea. Additional side effects from docusate calcium include perianal irritation, bloating, flatulence, and cramps.

> ## ALERT!
>
> Docusate should not be taken along with mineral oil, as this may increase mineral oil absorption and result in systemic toxicity.

> ### PRACTICE POINT
>
> *For administration purposes, the docusate syrup formulations should be mixed with 6 to 8 oz of milk or fruit juice prior to administration to improve taste.*

Hyperosmotic Laxatives

Hyperosmotic laxatives can be classified as saline or nonsaline. Nonsaline hyperosmotic agents include glycerin, polyethylene glycol (PEG) 3350 (MiraLax®), lactulose, and sorbitol. Bowel cleansing preparations, most often used for GI scopes or surgeries include PEG solutions such as Golytely® and Colyte™. This group of agents works by promoting local irritation and by drawing water into the feces, stimulating evacuation.

Glycerin is available as a suppository and rectal enema for the short-term treatment of constipation and to evacuate the colon prior to rectal and bowel examinations for adults and children older than 2 years of age. It usually produces a bowel movement within 15 minutes to 1 hour. Use of liquid glycerin as an enema is not recommended in adults and older children as this may cause considerable rectal irritation. The rectal suppositories must be retained for about 15 minutes for glycerin to have its full effect. They may cause rectal discomfort or a burning sensation. Contraindications for using the suppository include nausea, vomiting, recent abdominal surgery, fecal impaction, intestinal obstruction, or undiagnosed abdominal pain. Some side effects include perianal (around the anus) irritation, sweating, excessive bowel activity, abdominal cramps, bloating, and flatulence. There are no appreciable drug interactions.

PRACTICE POINT

Glycerin suppositories should be stored in a cool place, away from any excessive heat.

Polyethylene glycol (PEG) 3350 (MiraLax®) consists of very large, poorly absorbable ethylene glycol molecules that act as osmotic agents, causing water to be retained with the stool, resulting in a softer stool and more frequent bowel movements. It appears to have no effect on active absorption or secretion of glucose or electrolytes; therefore, it does not contribute to a loss of much-needed nutrients. It is approved for the treatment of constipation and has been used for chronic constipation and preparation of the bowel for a colonoscopy. PEG 3350 is available as an OTC and prescription product. The dosage form available is an oral powder to be mixed in 8 oz of water, juice, soda, coffee, or tea prior to administration. A bowel movement is typically produced in 2 to 4 days, with dosing options available to adults and children 18 months of age and older. In contrast to other products useful in the treatment of constipation, PEG 3350 can be used for up to 14 days, which is 7 days longer than the recommendations for other products. Some common side effects include bloating, abdominal discomfort, cramping, and flatulence. For patients suffering with known or suspected bowel obstruction, this medication is contraindicated. There are no documented drug-drug interactions with PEG 3350.

ALERT!

Patients who have renal disease should be cautioned to consult their prescriber before using PEG 3350 products. There are currently no sufficient data to confirm the safety of this laxative in pregnancy.

Sorbitol is available OTC for the treatment of constipation. It is available alone as a 70% oral solution and as a component of combination laxative products. (It is also available as a prescription but indicated for urinary bladder irrigation.) Sorbitol functions as an osmotic laxative but is not among the most commonly used agents. It has the tendency to cause hyperglycemia and electrolyte disturbances, so it is not considered first line as a laxative. GI upset such as abdominal pain, nausea, or vomiting has also been associated with sorbitol. However, in infants younger than 1 year of age, fluids, particularly juices containing sorbitol, such as prune, pear, and apple juices, are recommended as first-line treatment in constipation within the context of a healthy diet. An increased risk for colonic necrosis (local cell death) has been shown when sorbitol is used in conjunction with sodium polystyrene sulfonate (medication used for the reduction of potassium in the body).

Lactulose is a synthetic disaccharide used for the treatment of constipation in adults and infants and is available as an oral or rectal solution and as crystals for reconstitution. In patients with a history of chronic constipation, lactulose therapy increases the number of bowel movements per day and the number of days on which bowel movements occur. Lactulose is poorly absorbed from the GI tract, and no enzyme capable of hydrolysis of this synthetic disaccharide is present in human GI tissue. As a result, oral doses of lactulose reach the colon virtually unchanged. In the colon, lactulose is broken down primarily to lactic acid, and small amounts of formic and acetic acids by the action of colonic bacteria, which results in an increase in osmotic pressure and slight acidification of the colonic contents. This in turn causes an increase in stool water content and softens the stool. Since transit time through the colon may be slow, 24 to 48 hours may be required to produce the desired bowel movement. Side effects that can occur with lactulose include gaseous distention with flatulence or belching and abdominal discomfort such as cramping. Excessive dosage can lead to diarrhea with potential complications such as loss of fluids, hypokalemia (low potassium levels), and hypernatremia

ALERT!

When lactulose crystals are dissolved in water, the resulting solution may be colorless to a slightly pale yellow. Under recommended storage conditions, a normal darkening of color characteristic of sugar solutions may occur and does not affect therapeutic action. Prolonged exposure to temperatures greater than 30°C (86°F) or to direct light, however, may cause extreme darkening and clouding to the point where the products should not be used.

(high sodium levels). Patients requiring a galactose-free diet should not take lactulose, and patients with diabetes should be cautioned about its use as well. Conflicting reports have shown that some antibiotics and antacids have the ability to decrease the effects of lactulose, most probably because of the change in pH in the colon. Patients should be cautioned about the concomitant use of these products with lactulose and space them out by 1 or 2 hours.

ALERT!

Patients with diabetes should use caution when taking lactulose as it has 3 g of carbohydrates per 15 mL.

PRACTICE POINT

A 10-g packet of lactulose crystals should be dissolved in half a glass of water before administration. Lactulose syrup can be mixed with fruit juice, water, or milk to increase palatability. Lactulose solution should be kept at room temperature, but not frozen (it becomes too thick to pour). Lactulose should be dispensed in a tightly closed, light-resistant container with a child-resistant closure.

In terminally ill patients, prevention of constipation is extremely important. Glycerin suppositories or docusate sodium are recommended; lactulose is an alternative to docusate, although it can lead to bloating and possible postural hypotension (due to fluid shift to the bowel).

Bowel cleansing preparations such as Golytely® are considered hyperosmotic laxatives, but they are only used for procedural or surgery situations that require a complete emptying of bowel contents. These hyperosmotic laxatives (bowel cleansing preparations) all contain a combination of polyethylene glycol (PEG) 3350, sodium bicarbonate, potassium chloride, and sodium chloride. The ingredients are important to supply the body with needed electrolytes to prevent dehydration related to bowel evacuation. Bowel cleansing preparations are supplied as a powder to be mixed with water; sometimes flavor packs are included. Once

mixed as directed, the final volume is 4 L (about 1 gallon). Typical dosing is 240 mL (1 cup) every 10 minutes until all 4 L are consumed or until the rectal effluent is clear. Bowel cleansing preparations are contraindicated in patients with GI obstruction, gastric retention, bowel perforation, or other serious inflammatory bowel condition. Safety and efficacy have not been determined in children; therefore, bowel cleansing preparations are only recommended for adults. The first bowel movement should occur within 1 hour of beginning the preparation. The most common side effects include nausea, abdominal fullness, and bloating.

ALERT!

Oral medications given within 1 hour of the start of drinking the material may be flushed from the body before adequate absorption so required doses should be administered at least 2 hours before starting the bowel cleansing preparation. The patient should fast 3 to 4 hours prior to ingestion of the solution. No foods, except clear liquids, are permitted after the solution is started.

PRACTICE POINT

While Golytely is not recommended for children, there are some pediatric forms of bowel cleansing preparations that can be used. These include GaviLyte-N, and MoviPrep that are administered orally at a rate of 25 mL/kg/hour until rectal effluent is clear. Similar side effects can occur in children as with adults using bowel cleansing preparations.

PRACTICE POINT

Rapid drinking of each portion is preferred to drinking small amounts continuously. The solution should be refrigerated once it is reconstituted and used within 48 hours. Refrigeration also helps to increase the palatability of the drug.

Saline Laxatives

Saline laxatives are a group of hyperosmotic laxatives, which include magnesium citrate, magnesium hydroxide, and the sodium phosphates. Products in this group encourage bowel movements by drawing water into the bowel from surrounding body tissues. This provides a soft stool mass and increased bowel action. Most commonly, these products are used for bowel cleansing prior to surgery, similar to the PEG/electrolyte preparations discussed earlier. Their onset of action is between 30 minutes and 3 hours for oral doses and 2 to 5 minutes for rectal doses. Typically, the rectal formulations are safe for use in adults and children over the age of 2, and the oral formulations should not be used in children younger than 5 years of age. Saline laxatives also can interact with many medications, such as oral anticoagulants (warfarin or aspirin), medications that affect the heart rhythm (digoxin), and some antinausea medications (chlorpromazine).

Magnesium citrate is available as oral solution 1.75 g/30 mL. The typical dose is 150 to 300 mL once, which can be repeated if needed. The citrate form is more easily digested and better absorbed than other forms of magnesium. It is best taken on an empty stomach. In addition to renal insufficiency, patients with heart block or on a low sodium (salt) diet should not use magnesium citrate. Some important side effects include diarrhea, dizziness, abdominal pain, nausea, and vomiting. Severe dehydration can result if the patient is not consuming enough fluids while taking this medication.

PRACTICE POINT

Much like hyperosmotic bowel preparations, refrigeration and rapid drinking is preferred to increase the palatability of magnesium citrate.

Magnesium hydroxide (Phillips'® Milk of Magnesia) is used for the treatment of constipation and as an antacid. It is available as a chewable tablet, oral liquid suspension, and an oral concentrate suspension. It can be given to adults and children older than 2 years of age. Magnesium hydroxide should not be used when abdominal pain, nausea, or vomiting are present, and it should not be taken for longer than 1 week. Multiple drug interactions exist with the use of magnesium hydroxide. Some drugs to use with caution include amphetamines (attention deficit hyperactivity disorder [ADHD] medications) or quinidine, as it can cause a

decrease in their absorption. The effects of anticholinergics, iron preparations, folic acid, penicillin antibiotics, digoxin, some antifungals, and phenytoin could all be reduced and these medications should be spaced from doses of magnesium hydroxide, preferably with magnesium hydroxide given 2 to 4 hours after the prescription medication. Use of magnesium hydroxide with fluoroquinolone antibiotics such as levofloxacin and ciprofloxacin (even spaced 2 to 4 hours apart) can cause crystals in the urine and eventually lead to toxicity of the kidney.

ALERT!

Magnesium-containing laxatives should not be used long term or for repeated correction of constipation. Up to 20% of an orally administered dose may be absorbed, leading to toxicity in patients with compromised renal function. Magnesium toxicity can lead to severe cardiovascular changes such as decreased blood pressure and slow heart rate, especially in newborns or older adults.

ALERT!

A healthcare provider should be consulted and specific weight-based dosing should be followed if magnesium hydroxide is being considered for use in a child under the age of 2 years.

PRACTICE POINT

Magnesium hydroxide doses should always be followed with a full glass (240 mL) of liquid. It should be shaken well before using (suspension).

Sodium phosphate bowel evacuants such as sodium phosphate dibasic anhydrous (OsmoPrep®) were once available as OTC products, but the manufacturers voluntarily removed their OTC status after reports of patients suffering from acute phosphate nephropathy, a type of kidney injury, when using them for bowel cleansing prior to colonoscopy or other procedures. Now they are prescription-only products.

Sodium phosphate preparations are indicated for cleansing of the colon as a preparation for colonoscopy in adults 18 years of age or older. They work by inducing diarrhea, which effectively cleanses the entire colon. Each administration has an effect for approximately 1 to 3 hours. The primary mode of action is thought to be through the osmotic effect of sodium, causing large amounts of water to be drawn into the colon, promoting evacuation. The more common side effects include abdominal bloating and pain, nausea, and vomiting. Patients should be advised to hydrate adequately before, during, and after taking sodium phosphate preparations.

ALERT!

Medication guides are required when sodium phosphate bowel preps are dispensed.

PRACTICE POINT

Sodium phosphate bowel cleansing kits have complex directions, which must be followed precisely. It is a good idea to have patients review the instructions before leaving the pharmacy to be sure they understand how these are to be taken.

Mineral Oil (Lubricant Agent)

Mineral oil is used in many different products for its laxative effects and as an emulsifier for oral and topical preparations. This section focuses on mineral oil as an emollient laxative. Mineral oil is indicated in adults for the relief of constipation when straining must be avoided, such as before and after surgery for hemorrhoids or other painful anorectal disorders (conditions affecting the anus and rectum) and in patients with hypertension, coronary occlusion, and hernia. It acts only as a nonirritating intestinal lubricant. Mineral oil can also be administered rectally for bowel cleansing. In children 2 years of age and older, it is indicated primarily for chronic constipation.

Mineral oil works by slowing down colonic absorption of fecal water and therefore softening the stool. It coats fecal material to prevent or reduce colonic absorption of fecal water and lubricate hard stools, easing their passage without irritating the mucosa. If given orally, mineral oil will exert its

effect within 6 to 8 hours; if given rectally, the effect occurs in 5 to 15 minutes. The nonemulsified plain mineral oil given orally and mineral oil given rectally have minimal absorption; however, the emulsified mineral has 30% to 60% absorption. Mineral oil use can decrease the absorption of fat-soluble vitamins (vitamins A, D, E, and K) from the GI tract. Mineral oil can also cause anal pruritus (itching), diarrhea, nausea and vomiting, bloating, flatulence, and abdominal cramps. Mineral oil should not be given if docusate products are also being used; docusate can increase the absorption of mineral oil, thereby increasing its systemic effect. Mineral oil should not be used by patients with appendicitis (inflammation of the appendix), history of a colostomy (removal of the colon) or ileostomy (removal of the ileum), diverticulitis, or fecal impaction. It should not be given to bedridden patients or patients with difficulty swallowing. It should not be used in pregnant patients.

ALERT!

Oral mineral oil is only indicated for adults and children older than 6 years of age. Only the rectal administration of mineral oil is recommended in children 2 to 6 years of age.

PRACTICE POINT

Mineral oil should not be taken with meals; it should be administered on an empty stomach. The bottle of mineral oil should be kept tightly closed and protected from sunlight.

Castor oil is indicated for the preparation of the small and large bowel for procedures and for isolated bouts of constipation. It is approved for use in adults and children over the age of 2 years; however, it can be used in infants with much smaller dosing. The exact mechanism of action for castor oil is unknown. It is believed that within the small intestine, pancreatic enzymes break castor oil down to glycerol and ricinoleic acid. Ricinoleic acid reduces the net absorption of fluid and electrolytes and stimulates intestinal peristalsis. A bowel movement occurs within 2 to 6 hours. If constipation is accompanied by abdominal pain, intestinal obstruction, nausea and vomiting, and symptoms of appendicitis, castor oil should not be used. Prolonged use of castor oil may result in loss of electrolytes, fluid, and nutrients in addition to habituation (habit forming) and laxative abuse. Nausea, vomiting, diarrhea, cramps, and abdominal pain have been reported with castor oil.

ALERT!

The use of castor oil should be avoided in pregnancy and lactating mothers. It has the ability to possibly induce labor and can be excreted in breast milk. It should also be avoided in the elderly as long-term therapy except if being used for constipation associated with opiate analgesic use.

PRACTICE POINT

A full glass (8 oz) of water should be ingested 1 hour after taking castor oil. This is necessary to flush the colon thoroughly and prevent cramping.

CASE?

If Mr. Jones decided to try Senokot for the treatment of his constipation, when should he expect a bowel movement, and what is the appropriate dose for him to take?

Stimulant Laxatives

Anthraquinone Laxatives

Anthraquinone laxatives include aloe, cascara sagrada, casanthranol, senna, aloin, danthron, rhubarb, and frangula. The two drugs here discussed are cascara sagrada and senna (includes the sennosides), which are the most commonly used. Cascara is available as a dietary supplement as a tablet, capsule, fluid extract (liquid), and a tea for use in adults and children over the age of 2 years. It is an all-natural laxative designed for the relief of occasional constipation. The plant-derived compounds present in cascara are laxative prodrugs, which pass unabsorbed through the GI tract until they reach the colon. There they exert their action by increasing motility

and affecting secretion and absorption. A bowel movement typically occurs in 6 to 8 hours. Abdominal pain, excessive bowel activity, diarrhea, nausea, and perianal irritation are the primary adverse effects with anthraquinone laxatives. Symptoms of appendicitis, bowel obstruction, and fecal impaction are contraindications for the use of this medication. This medication should not be used for more than 1 week.

ALERT!

Patients taking cascara for more than 1 to 2 weeks may experience a decrease in serum potassium level. A reduction in potassium could predispose patients to heart irregularities and affect concomitant medications. The risk of digoxin toxicity is much greater if serum potassium decreases.

PRACTICE POINT

Discoloration of acidic urine to yellow-brown or black may occur. Pink-red, red-violet, or red-brown discoloration of alkaline urine may occur with cascara.

Sennosides (senna) can be found alone or in combination with other products in OTC formulations. Some common dosage forms include tablets, chocolate tablets (Ex-Lax®), granules, oral liquid, oral drops, and even a tea. They are approved for the relief of occasional constipation in adults and children over the age of 2 years. All senna products should be taken with a full glass of water or juice. All anthraquinones are passed unchanged to the colon where they are converted to their active product (very similar to cascara). Senna is converted to its active anthraquinones known as sennosides, which are then metabolized to an active byproduct. They appear to act by preventing water and electrolyte absorption from the large intestine, resulting in increased intestinal volume and pressure that stimulates colonic motility. Defecation is typically seen within 6 to 12 hours, but effects may not occur for 24 hours. Some absolute contraindications to using this medication include acute inflammatory conditions such as Crohn's disease (CD) and appendicitis (which will be discussed later), bowel obstruction, severe nausea and vomiting, or undiagnosed abdominal pain.

> ## ALERT!
>
> Pregnant patients and lactating mothers should not use cascara products. Although not recommended for pregnant patients, senna products can be used in lactating mothers. Sennosides are not excreted in breast milk.

Two important side effects that can occur as a result of using senna products include a condition called melanosis coli. Melanosis coli is a harmless darkened pigmentation of the colonic mucosa resulting from chronic use of anthraquinone derivatives. Once the medication is stopped, melanosis coli will improve in 4 to 12 months.[6] The same urine discoloration that is caused from cascara preparations can also occur with senna. Acidic urine will change from yellow to brown or black, while alkaline urine will change to a pink-red, red-violet, or red-brown color. Other more common side effects while taking this medication may include diarrhea, nausea, vomiting, perianal irritation, fainting, bloating, flatulence, and cramps. There are no drug interactions known with sennosides.

> ## ALERT!
>
> While some senna products are labeled for use in children 2 to 6 years of age, others are not recommended for children under 12 years. If there is any doubt, the pediatrician should be consulted.

Bisacodyl

Bisacodyl is one of the more commonly used stimulants. Bisacodyl products are available OTC as enteric-coated tablets, tablets, and rectal suppositories. They are also available in some bowel preparation kits. Bisacodyl is indicated for the relief of occasional constipation and irregularity in adults and children over the age of 12 years. Bisacodyl works in the large intestine, where it stimulates the bowel muscles to contract, and thereby push the bowel's contents along. It produces strong but brief peristaltic movements. It also helps ease elimination by accumulating water to soften the

bowel's contents. The effect is both to help soften the stool and make it pass through more quickly. Rectal suppositories will stimulate a bowel movement in 15 minutes to 1 hour. Defecation is usually seen in 6 to 12 hours with the tablets. Absolute contraindications to using this medication include appendicitis, intestinal obstruction, and gastroenteritis. Patients should be cautioned about taking bisacodyl products if they are experiencing severe abdominal pain, nausea, vomiting, rectal bleeding or failure to have bowel movements after administration, inflammatory bowel disease (CD or appendicitis), or ulcerated hemorrhoid. The more common side effects include abdominal cramping, which may be worse in severely constipated patients. The use of bisacodyl products beyond 7 days is not recommended.

> ## ALERT!
>
> Multiple laxatives have the same brand name followed by a qualifier (such as Stool Softener) although they may have completely different active ingredients. Additionally, some products are combined to include a stimulant laxative and a stool softener. It is important to be proficient with reading drug labels on OTC products and becoming familiar with the active ingredients in those products to assist consumers in making appropriate choices and avoiding contraindications.

> ### PRACTICE POINT
>
> *Bisacodyl products should not be taken within 1 hour of any antacids or other stomach medications that may increase the pH of the stomach. It has the possibility of preventing bisacodyl from working effectively.*

> ### PRACTICE POINT
>
> *Bisacodyl products have been shown to be safe in pregnancy and lactating mothers.*

Stimulant laxatives have the tendency to cause drug abuse and dependence. Chronic use (overuse for long periods of time) of laxatives may result in fluid and electrolyte imbalances, fatty stool, softening of the bones, diarrhea, and liver disease. This condition is also known as laxative abuse syndrome (LAS) and is difficult to diagnose. It is often seen in women with depression, personality disorders, or anorexia nervosa.

HEMORRHOIDS

Hemorrhoids are abnormally large, bulging, symptomatic bundles of the blood vessels (arteries and veins) supplying blood to the anal and rectal region (anorectal region) of the lower GI tract. Hemorrhoids can be considered external or internal. External hemorrhoids are dilated veins at the outer side of the external sphincter (outer opening of the anus). Internal hemorrhoids are dilated veins beneath the mucous membrane within the sphincter. There is limited information on the causes of hemorrhoids; however, a few things have been associated with their development: pregnancy, prolonged standing or sitting, lack of dietary fiber, constipation, diarrhea, and heavy lifting with straining. The diagnosis is initially based on symptoms, then confirmed with a sigmoidoscopy, which is a visual scope looking at the sigmoid region of the lower GI tract. Hemorrhoids can cause symptoms such as bleeding, pain, itching, discomfort, irritation, burning, inflammation, and swelling. Hemorrhoidal bleeding is bright red and can appear as scanty blood on the toilet paper or blood squirting into the toilet bowl.

The goals of hemorrhoid treatment are to alleviate and maintain remission and to prevent complications. The mainstay of therapy is an adequate intake of fiber and water and improving diet to avoid aggravating symptoms. Patients should avoid lifting heavy objects and discontinue intake of irritating substances such as caffeine or spicy foods. Patients should avoid sitting on the toilet for longer than 10 minutes to reduce straining and decrease pressure on the hemorrhoidal vessels. OTC nonsteroidal anti-inflammatory drugs (ibuprofen, naproxen) and aspirin should be avoided; both may cause excessive bleeding. Pharmacological OTC and prescription treatments are available to treat hemorrhoids. They consist of a range of psyllium or methylcellulose products to increase fiber, corticosteroids, which act as antipruritic and anti-inflammatory agents, analgesics, anesthetics, and vasoconstrictors. Antipruritic agents are used to relieve or prevent itching. In addition to previously discussed oral products, including stool softeners and psyllium, the most prescribed medications for hemorrhoids are topical preparations such as hydrocortisone, pramoxine, phenylephrine, and lidocaine.

Hydrocortisone Preparations

Hydrocortisone products for hemorrhoids may contain hydrocortisone alone (as hydrocortisone acetate) or include pramoxine or lidocaine. All three are available as rectal creams. Additionally, hydrocortisone/lidocaine is available as a rectal gel and as a topical pad; hydrocortisone/pramoxine is available as a rectal foam aerosol and rectal lotion; and hydrocortisone acetate is available as a rectal suppository and rectal foam aerosol. Topical hydrocortisone works by constricting the blood vessels, reducing itching and inflammation. Hydrocortisone is the only OTC corticosteroid and is available at a maximum concentration of 1%. The prescription hydrocortisone products can be found in concentrations as high as 2.5%. The rectal foam aerosol is available at a concentration of 10%. Lidocaine and pramoxine are both local anesthetics, which work by inhibiting the conduction of nerve impulses from sensory nerves, thereby causing a loss of sensation and reducing itching, burning, and pain in 30 to 60 seconds. Absorption is variable as with all rectal products, and sometimes the relief will not occur for much longer. Typically, intact skin will not respond as well as damaged or abraded skin, but hydrocortisone products should not be used on weeping or exudative (fluid that leaks out of blood vessels into nearby tissues) lesions. The dosing for these products ranges from one to three times a day for 1 to 2 weeks depending on symptom severity. Some of the more common side effects include stinging, tenderness, sloughing (skin peeling), and redness. Patients with traumatized or extremely irritated skin should consult a physician before using the product. Mixing other rectal medications along with any of the hydrocortisone preparations is not recommended. There are no appreciable drug interactions with the use of topical hydrocortisone preparations. If the hemorrhoids worsen, or if symptoms persist unaltered for greater than 7 days or clear up and occur again within only a few days, patients should discontinue use of these product(s) and consult a doctor.

ALERT!

Hydrocortisone products should be avoided in children younger than 2 years of age unless recommended or prescribed by a physician.

PRACTICE POINT

After applying the preparation, patients should be told to wash their hands immediately and to avoid contact with the eyes.

Phenylephrine Preparations

Phenylephrine products for hemorrhoids are branded as Preparation H and may contain hydrocortisone, aloe vera, or lidocaine for additional relief. OTC phenylephrine products are available as a suppository or an ointment with a maximum concentration of 0.25%. Phenylephrine is an alpha-adrenergic agonist, which produces local vasoconstriction that helps reduce hemorrhoids. These products are usually dosed four times a day and since they are topical preparations, systemic absorption is minimal, which reduces side effects. Phenylephrine products can be used in adults and children 12 years of age or older. If symptoms do not improve within 7 days or rectal bleeding occurs, a physician should be consulted.

Although systemic side effects are rare, patients with cardiovascular disease, especially ischemic heart disease, should use caution with extensive use of these topical preparations. There is limited information about the use of topical phenylephrine in pregnancy, but systemic (IV) phenylephrine does cross the placenta. Currently, it is recommended to avoid topical preparations of phenylephrine for pregnant and lactating patients.

INFLAMMATORY BOWEL DISEASE

CASE STUDY

Kelsey Fratner is a 24-year-old Caucasian woman who comes into the pharmacy regularly. She asks to speak to the pharmacist and mentions that she has been having an "upset stomach" and frequent diarrhea for more than 2 months. She has been using loperamide daily and does not feel it has been working; she wants to know what other OTC products she might consider. She reports that she has had frequent mouth ulcers over the last couple of months, but they generally heal and are not that painful. She also states that she has had blood mixed in with her diarrhea.

Inflammatory bowel disease (IBD) occurs in more than 1 million patients in the United States. Just like joints in the body may become swollen and painful (arthritis), the intestines can become inflamed and swollen. Also, like arthritis, there is more than one cause for IBD. The two most common causes of IBD are Crohn's disease (CD) and ulcerative colitis (UC).

CD is an autoimmune disorder, meaning the body's defenses against bacterial and viral infections have turned against the body and have started to attack body tissues (other autoimmune diseases discussed in this book include type 1 diabetes in Chapter 10 and rheumatoid arthritis in Chapter 13). CD may appear at almost any age but is most often diagnosed when patients are in their 30s or over the age of 50 years. This condition may affect the entire length of the GI tract. Although the majority of patients have symptoms in their colon, fewer than one out of five patients have the disease restricted to that portion of the GI tract. Affected locations appear like a road made of cobblestones where there are areas of ulcers surrounded by areas of thickness from where other ulcers have healed and left scar tissue behind. Among the patches of cobblestone areas, there may be portions of the GI tract where no disease is present. This type of disease is called *discontinuous* as it only has an effect on portions of the GI tract at one time. CD can also be *continuous* in which the entirety of the GI tract is affected. Patients with CD have a wide range of GI symptoms, including frequent diarrhea (sometimes more than 10 times a day), with some bleeding when defecating (passing feces), diffuse (widespread) abdominal pain, and ulcers of the mouth that may spread down the esophagus. Symptoms that may occur outside of the GI tract include skin ulcers and joint pain. Both types of symptoms are relieved by the same medications; however, currently there are no medications or therapies that cure CD. Due to the autoimmune nature of the disease, patients may have symptoms relapse and remit (come and go).

Another form of IBD is UC. The majority of patients with UC are diagnosed with the disease earlier in life than patients with CD and are female. People who have family members that have UC are at a higher risk of being diagnosed with UC than the general population. The cause of UC is less well defined than that of CD, and while there is evidence that it is related to genetics, there could also be nongenetic contributing factors. Though the cause of the inflammation may be different, the end result of both diseases is similar. Patients with UC frequently present with diarrhea accompanied by blood and mucus. Patients may also complain of diffuse abdominal pain.

UC is similar to CD in that the patient will develop ulcers in parts of their GI tract. However, unlike CD, the ulcers only appear in the colon and usually in the rectum. The ulcers in UC are continuous through the affected areas of the colon, which is different than what is seen in CD. There are pharmacologic treatments for UC, but these only reduce the symptoms of the disease and do not address its underlying causes. The only curative procedure is to remove the patient's colon; however, this is generally done only in patients with significant disease that does not respond to other treatments. The treatments for IBD depend on which of the major types of the disease the patient has. However, many of the treatments are the same in duration and dose, with the end goal of forcing the disease into remission.

CASE?

Which type of IBD correlates with the symptoms that Kelsey is having?

Anti-inflammatory Medications

Anti-inflammatory agents have a direct impact on the symptoms of IBD; however, they do not impact the root causes of the disease. Since there is an inflammation reaction occurring that leads to swelling and ulcerations, these agents help reduce the reaction and allow the tissue to heal.

Generally, when anti-inflammatory agents are discussed, the most common agents like ibuprofen, naproxen, and celecoxib are mentioned. However, these are not generally used in the treatment of IBD due to an increased risk in ulcer formation with these particular agents. Sulfasalazine, mesalamine, balsalazide, and olsalazine are used for the treatment of both CD and UC. Though similar in action, these agents do have different dosage regimens and side effects.

Sulfasalazine (Azulfidine®)

Sulfasalazine is an older anti-inflammatory agent. It is unique in that it contains a sulfonamide moiety (part of its chemical structure contains a sulfur molecule in the same configuration as sulfa antibiotics) that can lead to patients developing allergies to the medication. Additionally though, this sulfa moiety acts like an antibiotic that may help in treating the ulcers that develop from IBD. Sulfasalazine is activated by the bacteria in the gut to its active form, mesalamine, an anti-inflammatory and sulfapyridine. Sulfasalazine is usually started at a dose of 1 to 2 g divided in two doses daily and gradually increased to as much as 4 g divided into two doses for UC and up to 6 g daily for CD. It is expected that the full potential of the medication will not be achieved until at least 4 weeks of therapy. Even though the medication is working, the body may still need additional time to heal the inflamed areas.

Sulfasalazine has side effects that impact the skin and GI system. One of the most common side effects is a rash that may develop after the start of the drug or after a dose increase. If the rash is significant, the patient can be started on a desensitization protocol (which allows the body to slowly adjust to the medication, thus not causing a rash). In rare cases, sulfasalazine has been linked to Stevens-Johnson syndrome (a very serious and deadly skin rash).

ALERT!

Screening for two allergies should be performed before sulfasalazine is dispensed. The first is sulfonamide allergy, which may be inferred if the patient is allergic to sulfa antibiotics. The second is aspirin, as mesalamine, a metabolite of sulfasalazine, is similar in structure to aspirin. If the patient has an allergy to aspirin or has any disease state (such as asthma or severe allergies) the patient should not use the medication.

Indigestion, loss of appetite, nausea, and vomiting have all been associated with sulfasalazine in up to one out of three patients taking the medication. If the patient has significant adverse effects to the medication, one of the other anti-inflammatory agents should be used.

Mesalamine (Asacol® and Others)

Mesalamine is one of the active metabolites of sulfasalazine. The benefit of mesalamine over sulfasalazine is that there is no sulfonamide produced by mesalamine, thus fewer patients are hypersensitive (allergic) to the medication. Mesalamine, also known as 5-ASA (it looks like aspirin to the body), works by inhibiting the inflammation in the GI tract by blocking prostaglandin (a chemical in the body that can cause inflammation) synthesis.

Mesalamine also will take a few days to a few weeks to work before the patient starts seeing a benefit from the medication. It is dosed as two 400-mg tablets twice daily for mild to moderate, active UC and two 800-mg tablets twice daily for more significant active disease. Once the patient has responded to therapy with the agent, the dose is usually a total of 1,600 mg daily. For patients with CD, the dose is higher. The target dose for CD is two 400-mg tablets 3 times a day. This dose was found to be as effective as a 4-g daily dose in clinical trials.

Mesalamine can lead to several side effects. The most common side effects include diarrhea (which is already caused by IBD so it may worsen initially), flatulence, nausea, and upper abdominal pain (which may be related to IBD). In addition to these GI side effects, mesalamine has been linked to headache and can cause nasopharyngitis (sore throat).

> ### PRACTICE POINT
>
> *Some prescriptions written for mesalamine will have its abbreviation of 5-ASA on them in place of mesalamine.*

> ### PRACTICE POINT
>
> *Mesalamine has multiple different formulations (ie, immediate release, extended release, delayed release, etc.). These formulations are not interchangeable and correlate to where the medication will be released in the GI tract.*

Balsalazide

Balsalazide is a prodrug for mesalamine. The benefit is that it is not active in the upper part of the GI tract but is metabolized to its active form once it reaches the lower GI tract where it can have an effect. As mesalamine, it works in the lower GI tract by reducing prostaglandin synthesis, thereby reducing inflammation. Balsalazide is used in the treatment of active UC and in patients whose UC is in remission. For active disease, the patient should take 2.25 g (three 750 mg tablets) three times daily for 6 weeks to induce remission. After this high-dose start, the dose is reduced to 1.5 g twice daily or 3 g twice daily. The patient should expect to see an effect from the medication within 10 to 14 days of starting the higher dose.

Balsalazide has fewer side effects, especially GI and skin related, than either mesalamine or sulfasalazine. This is most likely because it does not start to work until it is in the lower intestines. It can cause rash (very infrequently) and some GI tract issues, such as abdominal pain, diarrhea, nausea, and vomiting (occurring about one-half as much as the other agents). There is still concern that the patient must be screened to see if they have an allergy to aspirin as mesalamine is very similar to aspirin and other salicylates.

Olsalazine

Olsalazine is another prodrug for mesalamine. It is actually two mesalamine molecules attached together that are then separated in the lower GI tract. Once separated from each other, the two molecules have the same mechanism of action as mesalamine. The usual dose for olsalazine is 1 g/day in two divided doses. Like balsalazide, olsalazine has fewer side effects than sulfasalazine most likely because it is not activated until it reaches the lower GI tract. The primary side effect of therapy with olsalazine is diarrhea. Again, the disease also causes diarrhea so it is difficult to determine if it is the disease causing the diarrhea or olsalazine. Some patients will require a dose reduction to tolerate therapy with olsalazine.

> ### PRACTICE POINT
>
> *Though they have fewer side effects, both olsalazine and balsalazide cost more than mesalamine or sulfasalazine. Thus, if a patient has difficulty paying for medication, the pharmacist might recommend one of the older medications to the physician.*

Corticosteroids

Corticosteroids have been covered elsewhere (Chapter 9), thus a full review of them will not be done here. However, corticosteroids play an important role in the management of IBD when the nonsteroidal medications have failed. Corticosteroids reduce inflammation by preventing the arachidonic acid pathway, which will reduce several key inflammatory agents such as prostaglandins and chemokines (chemicals in the body that help cause inflammation). Corticosteroids are also immunosuppressants.

Oral steroid therapy with either prednisone or methylprednisolone is not indicated for the long-term management of IBD. Due to the significant side effects associated with long-term steroid use, such as weight gain, osteoporosis (bone loss over time), and hyperglycemia (high blood sugar), the limited effectiveness in chronic use discourages their use. However, corticosteroids are very effective for the short-term treatment of an acute episode of IBD.

Immunomodulators

Due to the immunogenic (related to the body's own immune system) causes of CD and the possible link to UC, medications that can have an impact on the immune system and thus reduce its targeting of the body's tissues may be prescribed. The following medications are primarily used to treat only IBD that is diagnosed as CD; however, some prescribers may use the agents for UC, though effectiveness is very limited.

PRACTICE POINT

The immunomodulators are now considered first-line therapy, with the biologics or biologics plus thiopurine agents (azathioprine and mercaptopurine) carrying a more substantial recommendation than the thiopurine agents alone.

Azathioprine and Mercaptopurine

Azathioprine is rapidly metabolized inside the body to 6-mercaptopurine so these will be considered together. 6-Mercaptopurine is thought to suppress the immune system by inhibiting the body's synthesis of new proteins, including antibodies, which contribute to inflammation. With fewer antibodies circulating in the bloodstream, inflammation should diminish. These agents have been used primarily in host versus graft disease (which happens after organs are transplanted) and other autoimmune disorders but have been studied in both CD and UC. Azathioprine and mercaptopurine are dosed based on the weight of the patient. (See Medication Table 22-1.) Patients should not expect to see any positive effects until 3 months after starting the medication.

Because of their mechanism of action, these drugs can have significant effects not only on the immune system but also on other body functions. Thrombocytopenia (low platelet counts) and leukopenia (low levels of white blood cells) have been noted with patients taking these agents. Nausea, vomiting, and diarrhea may occur within the first few months of therapy. Studies recommend giving the drugs in smaller doses throughout the day to minimize the threat of these side effects. Finally, pancreatitis (inflammation of the pancreas, which can be deadly) has occurred in about 6% of patients taking azathioprine in some clinical trials and patients should be alert to changes in their abdominal pain (location or intensity).

ALERT!

Azathioprine should not be used with mercaptopurine since azathioprine is metabolized to it.

Monoclonal Antibodies

Because IBD, like rheumatoid arthritis, is an autoimmune disorder, the monoclonal antibodies (infliximab, adalimumab, and certolizumab) discussed in Chapter 13 are also useful in the treatment of IBD. Infliximab, ustekinumab, adalimumab, and vedolizumab are used to treat both CD and UC, whereas certolizumab (alternative therapy option) is used for CD only.

PRACTICE POINT

The dosing of monoclonal antibodies changes over the therapy period. Initially (usually the first week), patients receive higher doses than in subsequent periods. While standard doses of adalimumab, certolizumab, ustekinumab, and vedolizumab are prescribed for most patients, infliximab dosing is based on patient weight.

Natalizumab (Tysabri)

Natalizumab is another monoclonal antibody. It targets receptors on the leukocytes (white blood cells) that make them less likely to hurt normal tissue. Natalizumab was discussed in Chapter 6 in its role in therapy of multiple sclerosis. It is dosed once a month in patients with moderate to severe CD (as an alternative treatment agent) but is not used to treat UC. The 300-mg dose is infused through an IV line over about 1 hour once every month. Only patients who respond (indicated by disease remission) should continue to receive this medication.

Progressive multifocal leukoencephalopathy (PML) is a viral disease that has been linked to the use of natalizumab. The disease is severe and may cause death. This is the reason why the medication is only available through the TOUCH (Tysabri Outreach: Unified Commitment to Health) program. The program requires frequent visits with the prescribing physician to monitor for complications of PML. Additional side effects include rash, nausea, arthralgias, headache (around one-third of patients), urinary and respiratory tract infections, and fatigue. The majority of these side effects occur less commonly in patients with CD as compared to patients with multiple sclerosis.

IRRITABLE BOWEL SYNDROME

Irritable bowel syndrome (IBS) is a collection of symptoms that, when found together, are considered IBS (IBS should not be confused with IBD described above). The hallmark of IBS is chronic or recurrent abdominal pain or discomfort that occurs along with a change in bowel habits. Patients may have symptoms that include unusual frequency of bowel movements (either less than three per week or more than three per day), abnormal stool consistency (hard and lumpy or soft and watery), straining during defecation, urgency of defecation, a feeling of not completely defecating after finishing, passing mucus, or bloating. Additionally, these patients may either present as constipated, having diarrhea with frequent bowel movements, or a mix of the two. These symptoms are all GI related; however, IBS patients also report other pain disorders and generalized issues throughout their bodies. Patients who are diagnosed with IBS are also likely to have GERD (gastroesophageal reflux disease), fibromyalgia, and chronic fatigue syndrome.

A clear cause for the disease is not known, but there are theories that it is related to stress and an overactive pain response. During stressful situations in life, the body changes hormone levels to prepare the body for whatever is going to happen. Some scientists believe that these changes cause patients with IBS to start developing symptoms as their GI systems are being affected by the change of hormone levels. The involvement of overactive pain receptors, known as hyperalgesia, relates IBS to fibromyalgia and pain disorders. Scientists think that the overactive pain response best explains IBS symptoms because IBS patients are more responsive to both internal and external stimuli, demonstrating a lower threshold for pain. Additionally, when stressed, a natural response is to be more sensitive to stimuli; thus, both theories may be tied together.

Because there is no known cause for IBS, therapies for it deal mostly with treatment of anxiety or depression. The first-line treatment for IBS, though, is diet. A diet that is high in fiber is recommended to regulate patients. Additionally, patients are asked to identify food triggers that can worsen the disease. If patients are unable to reduce or control their symptoms through diet, pharmacologic agents are then recommended. For these patients a determination, if possible, of whether they have constipation- or diarrhea-dominant IBS must occur. If the patient has constipation more frequently, laxatives and other agents to increase the number of bowel movements are recommended. The opposite is true for patients with diarrhea. The recommended therapies are the medications for constipation and diarrhea covered earlier in this chapter. Additionally, some patients begin therapy and see benefit from selective serotonin reuptake inhibitors (SSRIs) or tricyclic antidepressants (TCAs); these are used at the same doses used to treat depression. These agents are covered in Chapter 7. There are three other classes of medication that have shown to be effective in relieving the symptoms of IBS: serotonergic agents, antispasmodics, and guanylate cyclase activators.

Serotonergic Agents

There are two agents in this class of drugs: tegaserod and alosetron. Both agents affect serotonin receptors; however, one is an agonist and one is a receptor antagonist. They are used to treat different types of the disease, one for constipation dominant and the other for diarrhea dominant. They both are in restricted access programs due to side effects.

Alosetron (Lotronex)

Alosetron is a serotonin ($5\text{-}HT_3$) receptor antagonist that helps slow down the gut and reduce the frequency of diarrhea. It is very selective and potent at the receptor site; thus, unlike other serotonin antagonists, there is not much concern of it having effects at other receptor sites. By blocking the actions of $5\text{-}HT_3$ in the GI tract, it decreases gut motility. Alosetron originally was approved only for IBS with diarrhea; however, it was used for treating patients with diarrhea only, which led to the occurrence of significant (and deadly) side effects. These side effects lead to the removal of the product from the U.S. market, but public demand resulted in the product being re-released but as part of a limited access program. The dosing for alosetron starts at the lowest possible dose and is increased later to minimize side effects. The use

of alosetron has been approved for females only as it was not found to be effective in men. Significant side effects related to the use of alosetron, including toxic megacolon (rapid expansion of the diameter of the colon that can lead to death), obstruction, and ischemic colitis were reported. Other than these GI-related side effects, the medication is well tolerated.

PRACTICE POINT

The Prescribing Program for Lotronex (PPL) requires a physician to undergo training to monitor the medication and its effects. The FDA requires a medication guide each time the drug is dispensed. Additional Information on the program may be found at http://www.lotronexppl.com/.

Tegaserod (Zelnorm)

Tegaserod is a serotonin receptor agonist, which appears to accelerate the motility of the GI tract. It is also thought to have some effect on 5-HT1. Tegaserod increases the secretion of intestinal fluids and increases the peristaltic reflex,

---

PRACTICE POINT

The safety and efficacy of tegaserod have not been established in males. This agent is contraindicated for women 65 and over.

ALERT!

Cardiovascular risk factors that must be considered before tegaserod is prescribed and used include active smoking, high blood pressure or history of being treated with medicines that lower blood pressure, high cholesterol or medicine to lower blood cholesterol levels, history of diabetes, age 55 years or over, or obesity.[7] A medication guide must accompany every tegaserod prescription dispensed.

which will help expel the contents of the intestines. Tegaserod is used for short periods of time only for constipation-dominant IBS in adult women under 65 years of age who do not have a history of ischemic cardiovascular disease and who have no more than one risk factor for cardiovascular disease.[7] Patients taking tegaserod have complained of GI side effects such as flatulence, abdominal pain, and headaches. Most significantly, however, tegaserod has been linked to an increased risk of major cardiovascular events (stroke and heart attack).

Antispasmodics

Dicyclomine and Hyoscyamine

Dicyclomine and hyoscyamine are the most commonly used antispasmodics for the management of symptoms associated with IBS. These agents work by relaxing intestinal smooth muscles, which reduces GI motility. Each medication may be dosed multiple times a day, but is not intended for long-term use. Hyoscyamine is available in multiple dosage forms, including immediate- and extended-release tablets, intramuscular injection, intravenous, or subcutaneous injection. Dicyclomine is available only as an oral capsule or solution. Please refer to the medication table at the end of the chapter for dosing specifics, as there are many. Common side effects of these agents include drowsiness or blurred vision, diarrhea, increased sensitivity to hot environments, and dry mouth.

Dicyclomine is approved for use in adults and children older than 2 years of age. If an antispasmodic is needed for a child, hyoscyamine is the better agent to use, especially with infants and children younger than 2 years of age. Both dicyclomine and hyoscyamine cross the placenta, therefore use in pregnant women is not recommended due to the potential fetal adverse effects. These agents are also present in breast milk and can suppress lactation, so they are not recommended for use in breast feeding mothers.

Guanylate Cyclase Activators

Linaclotide and Plecanatide

Linaclotide (Linzess) and plecanatide (Trulance) are agonists of guanylate cyclase-C on the luminal surface of the intestinal epithelium. This causes a chain reaction that ultimately increases the secretion of chloride and bicarbonate into the intestines, which increases intestinal fluid concentrations and GI transit time. Linaclotide and plecanatide are only used for chronic idiopathic constipation and IBS syndrome

with constipation in adult patients, and are recommended as first-line agents.

PRACTICE POINT

Linaclotide is a capsule, which can be taken whole, or its contents sprinkled into applesauce or mixed with 30 mL of room-temperature water for sipping or tube feeding. Plecanatide is a tablet that can be swallowed whole or crushed and administered with applesauce or water. When opened or crushed for mixing, the medications should be administered immediately.[8]

These medications are well tolerated, with the most common side effect being diarrhea within the first month of use. This usually subsides the longer the patient is on the medication, but if it does not decrease after the first month of use, then a physician should be consulted.

ALERT!

The use of linaclotide and plecanatide should be avoided in children younger than 6 years of age and is contraindicated for those under 2 years. In younger patients, these medications can cause severe dehydration leading to death.[8]

FLATULENCE

Flatulence, or gassiness, occurs when there is an accumulation of gas in the intestines. Frequently patients will also complain of pain or bloating that goes along with flatulence. There are several causes of flatulence. A common cause that is correctable with behavior changes is aerophagia (swallowing air). People who frequently chew gum, drink carbonated drinks, or smoke are more prone to swallowing air, which can end up in the intestines and lead to flatulence. Other causes of flatulence are mechanical obstructions (such as cancers or adhesions of the inner part of the intestine to itself); poor absorption of certain nutrients that are then metabolized by bacteria to gaseous products; movement disorders of the bowels where slowdown of the gut may occur, leading to gas accumulation; and bacterial overgrowth that occurs with other disease states.

Treatment for flatulence varies by cause. Obstructions, for example, sometimes require surgery, whereas aerophagia can be regulated through behavior modifications. There are a limited number of medications that are approved for use to reduce flatulence. Their mechanisms of actions vary from trying to assist the patient in passing the gas earlier (thus preventing painful accumulation) to absorbing the gas into a solid to prevent it from being expelled as a gas.

Simethicone

Simethicone works to reduce the surface tension of gas bubbles in the intestines. This allows the bubbles to come together and form larger, more movable gas bubbles. Thus, simethicone will not reduce the quantity of gas, but it may help the patient mobilize intestinal gas. Simethicone is available in OTC products and in some prescription products. The dosing of simethicone depends on the age of the patient and is described in Medication Table 22-1. The side effects of simethicone are mild, with diarrhea and nausea being the most common. These side effects generally will not limit the use of the medication if the patient is still in pain or feels bloated.

PRACTICE POINT

The effectiveness of simethicone has long been questioned; however, since it has few side effects and no adverse effects it is still recommended.

Charcoal, Activated

Charcoal is one of nature's great purifiers. It actively binds a host of chemicals to it, and prevents those molecules from reentering the system around it. This is the mechanism of action for charcoal in intestinal gas, as it binds the gas and then enables the patient to expel the bound gas through defecation. In addition to its uses for intestinal gas, it is also used in acute poisonings with several different agents. Charcoal is available as an OTC product and can be used for adults to treat intestinal gas. The normal dose for adults is 520 mg given after meals or when the patient first feels discomfort from gas or bloating. The patient should not consume more than 4 g charcoal/day.

Side effects from charcoal ingestion are generally mild and cosmetic. All patients taking charcoal will notice black,

dark stools after usage as the charcoal passes from their systems. In patients where there are concerns about GI bleeding this may be an issue as it will be hard to distinguish the dark stool of melena (blood in the feces) from that caused by charcoal. Care must also be advised when giving charcoal to patients with swallowing difficulties as aspiration of the medication into the lungs is possible and is harmful.

ALERT!

Charcoal interacts with numerous drugs because it binds medications as well as gas, thus the doses of charcoal and medications must be separated by at least 2 hours.

Alpha-Galactosidase-A

Alpha-galactosidase-A is considered to be a dietary supplement and is widely used to reduce the incidence of intestinal gas caused by eating beans. Beans contain a complex carbohydrate that is metabolized by gas-producing bacteria in the lower GI tract. Alpha-galactosidase-A is an enzyme that converts the complex carbohydrates into glucose and other simple carbohydrates, which can be absorbed by the body and made unavailable to the bacteria, thus reducing gas production.

ALERT!

Beano should be put only on cool foods. If placed on hot foods, the enzyme will be deactivated.

PRACTICE POINT

Alpha-galactosidase-A is only effective in gas that results from beans, not just everyday gas.

PARASITE INFECTIONS

As mentioned earlier in the chapter, parasitic infections are a common occurrence, especially in underdeveloped countries or parts of countries where sanitation is poor.

This section will focus on helminths (worms) that live in the intestines. Common worms that live inside the human intestines include *Ascaris lumbricoides*, *trichuris trichiura* (whipworm), *Enterobius vermicularis* (pinworm), *Taenia solium* and *Taenia sanguinata* (tapeworm), and *Necator americanus* and *Ancylosoma duodenale* (hookworm). The various worms, though different, have similar life cycles where the adult worm lives and feeds in the intestines of a human. Once the worm matures, eggs are laid in the intestines that are then excreted with the feces. The eggs then need to mature outside of the body, and at some point, they may be ingested by a human again. This is considered to be a fecal-oral route of transmission. The human does not need to eat feces to be exposed, because when feces dry out, it is common for the eggs to disperse in the wind or be carried away by water or other animals. Once the eggs are inside the human body, they hatch and the cycle begins again.

Most patients with worm infections do not notice them. However, certain populations, especially children, may have lifelong complications from worm infections early in life, as the worms compete for the same nutrients that the child needs for growth and development. So even though a child is eating normally, there may be signs of malnutrition, growth retardation, and failure to thrive syndrome related to a worm infection.

Treatments that help eliminate worms from the body usually work in one of two ways. They either attack the adult worm, or they inhibit the ability of the eggs to form and grow, terminating the life cycle. These mechanisms support the pulse therapy (short "bursts" of medications) that is common with antiparasite treatment. There are several treatments available for each of the types of parasites. One of the choices, metronidazole is covered in Chapter 27.

Mebendazole

Mebendazole is an antiparasite (worm) agent that is taken by mouth and can impede the growth of and eventually kill several different types of intestinal parasites. Mebendazole interferes with the parasite's cellular transport of glucose, eventually starving it of needed energy. This causes the parasite's death. It is believed that mebendazole also has an effect on the eggs of the parasite and the larvae of the parasites that are living in tissues and not in the intestinal lumen.

The dosage of mebendazole depends on the species of the parasite (see Medication Table 22-1) and is not dependent on the age of the patient, though the medication is not recommended for patients younger than 2 years of age. Each of the dosing regimens may be repeated in 3 weeks if complete resolution of the infection has not occurred. The medication is not effective for hydatid disease, and thus should not be used to treat this infection. Side effects of mebendazole are generally mild due to the short-term nature of the therapy. However, the most common are skin rash, headache, or diarrhea/constipation. Rarely has the medication been believed to cause hepatitis.

Albendazole

Albendazole is similar to mebendazole as it is effective against different types of worms and works at multiple stages of the life cycle of the worm, primarily by blocking glucose transport inside of the worm. This leads to an energy starvation of the worm, eventually paralyzing it, and allowing the patient to pass it with the stool. Albendazole is also effective in certain species of worms in the larval and egg phases.

Dosing for albendazole also depends on the worm infection the patient has. This cycle is repeated three times to ensure that all of the larvae are destroyed. Doses are adjusted for patients who weigh less than 60 kg (132 pounds). Since the medication targets processes that are different in the worm and are not shared with humans, the side effects of this medication are generally mild. However, headache, nausea and vomiting, and abdominal pain are common side effects of the medication. Additionally, although rare, Stevens-Johnson syndrome and agranulocytosis have occurred with the medication, and hepatoxicity and acute renal failure have occurred in patients taking the medication.

SUMMARY

The lower gastrointestinal (GI) tract is a complex system of different organs that are affected by several different diseases. As shown in this chapter, the diseases that affect the lower GI system cause significant issues in patients who have them. However, there are treatments that are safe and effective in the management of these diseases. The knowledgable pharmacy technician, in collaboration with a pharmacist, can have a significant impact on the lives of these patients.

REFERENCES

1. Walker PC. Diarrhea. In: Krinsky D, Hume A, Ferreri S et al., eds. *Handbook of Nonprescription Drugs*. 20th ed. Washington, DC: American Pharmacists Association; 2020:307-331.

2. Centers for Disease Control. http://www.cdc.gov. Accessed August 8, 2022.

3. World Health Organization. http://www.who.int/. Accessed November 2021.

4. World Gastroenterology Organization. WGO Practice Guidelines on Constipation; 2010. http://www.worldgastroenterology.org/guidelines. Accessed November 2021.

5. Slavin JL. Position of the American Dietetic Association: Health implications of dietary fiber. *J AM Diet Assoc.* 2008;108:1716-1731.

6. Tabbers MM, Dilorenzo C, Berger MY, et al. Evaluation and treatment of functional constipation in infants and children: Evidence-based recommendations from ESP-GHAN and NASPGHAN. *J Pediatr Gastroenterol Nutr.* 2014;58(2):265-281.

7. Alfasignma USA, Inc. Zelnorm (tegaserod) tablets [prescribing information]. https://www.myzelnorm.com/. Accessed July 12, 2022.

8. Lexicomp. Lexi-Drugs [database]. Hudson, OH: Wolters Kluwer. http://online.lexi.com.

REVIEW QUESTIONS

1. What are the goals of treatment for diarrhea and which drug classes are available without a prescription?

2. What are some of the common causes of constipation?

3. What are the major differences between the treatments of Crohn's disease and ulcerative colitis?

4. Explain the differences between the different anti-inflammatory agents used to treat IBD.

5. Discuss why the two serotonergic agents used to treat irritable bowel syndrome have been pulled off of the market. Consider both effectiveness and safety.

MEDICATION TABLES

MEDICATION TABLE 22-1. Representative Medications for Disorders of the Lower Gastrointestinal Tract[8]

Generic Name	Brand Name	Rx/OTC	Dosage Forms	Adult Dosages	Pediatric Dosages
Medications for the Treatment of Diarrhea					
Loperamide (loe PER a mide)	Imodium A-D, Diamode	OTC	Tablets and capsules: 2 mg	4 mg once, 2 mg after each unformed stool (max 16 mg)	8–12 years (<30 kg): 2 mg 3 times/day (max 6 mg) 5–8 years (20–30 kg): 2 mg 2 times/day (max 4 mg) 2–5 years (13–20 kg): 1 mg 3 times/day (max 3 mg)
			Liquid: 1 mg/5 mL, 1 mg/7.5 mL	4 mg once, 2 mg after each unformed stool (max 16 mg)	Not intended for children <6 years of age
Bismuth subsalicylate (BIZ muth) (sub sa LIS i late)	Bismatrol, Pepto-Bismol	OTC	Tablet, chewable tablet: 262 mg	2 tablets, repeat every 30 min to 1 hr (max 16 tablets)	9–11 years: 1 tablet 6–8 years: tablet 3–5 years: tablet; not intended for children <3 years of age (max 8 doses)
			Liquid, children's: 87 mg/5 mL, 130 mg/15 mL, 262 mg/15 mL Liquid, extra strength: 524 mg/15 mL	30 mL of 262 mg/15 mL or 15 mL of 524 mg/15 mL, repeat every 30 min to 1 hr (max 16 tablets)	9–11 years: 15 mL 6–8 years: 10 mL 3–5 years: 5 mL of 87 mg/5 mL; not intended for children <3 years of age (max 8 doses)
Diphenoxylate/ atropine sulfate (dye fen OX i late) (A troe peen)	Lomotil	Rx (Schedule V controlled substance)	Tablet: 2.5 mg/0.025 mg Liquid: 2.5 mg/0.025 mg/5 mL; liquid should be used in children <13 years of age	5 mg 4 times/day PRN	9–12 years (23–55 kg): 1.5–3 mL 4 times/day 6–8 years (17–32 kg): 2.5–5 mL 4 times/day 5 years (16–23 kg): 2.5–4.5 mL 4 times/day 4 years (14–20 kg): 2–4 mL 4 times/day 3 years (12–16 kg): 2–3 mL 4 times/day 2 years (11–14 kg): 1.5–3 mL 4 times/day; not intended for children <2 years
Opium (OH pee um)		Rx (Schedule II)	Tincture: 10%	0.6 mL 4 times/day	If used for children, must be diluted 25-fold

Continued next page

MEDICATION TABLE 22-1. Representative Medications for Disorders of the Lower Gastrointestinal Tract[8] (Continued)

Generic Name	Brand Name	Rx/OTC	Dosage Forms	Adult Dosages	Pediatric Dosages
Medications for the Treatment of Constipation					
Bulk-forming Agents					
Psyllium (SIL i yum)	Metamucil, Konsyl, others	OTC	Capsules: 0.52 g	2–6 capsules with 8 oz liquid 3 times/day PRN	Not intended for children <12 years
			Powder: 3.4–3.5 g	1 rounded tsp with 8 oz liquid 1–3 times/day PRN	6–12 years: ½ rounded tsp with 8 oz liquid 1–3 times/day PRN
			Granules: 4.03 g	1–2 rounded tsp with 8 oz liquid 1–2 times/day PRN	7–11 years: 1 rounded tsp with 8 oz liquid 1–2 times/day PRN
			Wafers: 3.4 g	2 wafers with 8 oz liquid 3 times/day PRN	6–12 years: 1 wafer with 8 oz liquid 3 times/day PRN
Methylcellulose (meth ill SEL yoo lose)	Citrucel, Maltsupex	OTC	Tablets: 500 mg	2 tablets with 8 oz liquid PRN (max 12)	6–12 years: 1 tablet with 8 oz liquid PRN (max 6)
			Powder: 2 g	11.5 g with 8 oz liquid 3 times/day PRN	6–12 years: 5.75 g with 8 oz liquid daily
Polycarbophil (pol i KAR boe fil)	Equalactin, Fiber-Lax, Fiber	OTC	Tablets, chewable tablets: 500 mg	2 tablets with 8 oz liquid 1–4 times/day PRN	6–12 years: 1 tablet with 8 oz liquid 1–3 times/day PRN
Surfactants					
Docusate sodium (DOK yoo sate) (SOE dee um)	Colace, Dulcolax Stool Softener, and many others	OTC	Tablets: 100 mg	100–300 mg daily	6–12 years: 100 mg daily
			Capsules: 50–250 mg	100–300 mg daily	6–12 years: 50–150 mg daily
			Syrup: 4 mg/mL (available as 20 mg/5 mL and 60 mg/15 mL)	60–180 mg daily	6–12 years: 40–120 mg daily; 3–6 years: 20–60 mg daily; <3 years: 10–40 mg daily
			Syrup: 3.33 mg/mL (available as 50 mg/15 mL and 100 mg/30 mL)	50–100 mg daily	6–12 years: 50 mg daily; 3–5 years: 33 mg daily
			Liquid: 10 mg/mL	50–200 mg daily	6–12 years: 40–120 mg daily; 3–6 years: 20–60 mg daily

Continued next page

MEDICATION TABLE 22-1. Representative Medications for Disorders of the Lower Gastrointestinal Tract[8] (Continued)

Generic Name	Brand Name	Rx/OTC	Dosage Forms	Adult Dosages	Pediatric Dosages
Hyperosmotic Laxatives					
Glycerin (GLI ser in)	Fleet Glycerin Suppositories, Pedia-Lax, others available	OTC	Suppository	1 suppository daily	Do not use in children <2 years of age
	Fleet Liquid Glycerin		Rectal liquid	Not indicated for adults	2–6 years: 1 unit as directed by physician
Polyethylene glycol (PEG) 3350 (pol ee ETH i leen) (GLYE col)	Gavilax, MiraLAX, others	OTC	Powder for oral solution: 17 g packets 225 g, 510 g, and 527 g bottle	17 g (approx. 1 heaping tbsp) in 8 oz of water daily	18 months to 11 years: 0.25–1.42 g/kg/day; in children >20 kg, use adult dose
Polyethylene glycol/electrolyte solutions: (PEG ES) polyethylene glycol (PEG) 3350, sodium bicarbonate, potassium chloride, and sodium chloride (pol ee ETH i leen) (GLYE col)	Golytely, Nulytely, Gavilyte, MoviPrep	Rx	Packets, disposable jugs	4 L of oral solution prior to GI exam; patients should drink 240 mL every 10 min until 4 L are consumed or until the rectal effluent is clear	Not recommended
Sorbitol (SOR bi tal)		Rx	70% solution	2–3 tbsp PO daily as a single dose (1 part 70% solution: 2.3 parts water) 120 mL rectally daily	2–12 years: 30–60 mL (1 part 70% solution: 2.3 parts water) rectally daily
Lactulose (LAK tyoo lose)	Constulose, Enulose, Generlac, Kristalose	Rx	Oral solution: 10 g/15 mL	15–45 mL 3–4 times/day (max 40 g or 60 mL)	Children: 40–90 mL/day in divided doses Infants: 2.5–10 mL/day in divided doses

Continued next page

MEDICATION TABLE 22-1. Representative Medications for Disorders of the Lower Gastrointestinal Tract[8] (*Continued*)

Generic Name	Brand Name	Rx/OTC	Dosage Forms	Adult Dosages	Pediatric Dosages
Hyperosmotic Saline Laxatives					
Magnesium citrate (mag NEE zhum) (SYE trate)	Citroma	OTC	Oral solution: 1.75 g/30 mL	150–300 mL once	6–12 years: 0.5 mL/kg (max 200 mL every 4–6 hr for bowel procedure)
Magnesium hydroxide (mag NEE zhum) (hye DROX ide)	Milk of Magnesia	OTC	Chewable tablet: 311 mg	6–8 tablets before bedtime with 8 oz of water	6–11 years: 3–4 tablets at bedtime with 8 oz of water 2–6 years: 1–2 tablets at bedtime with 8 oz of water
			Liquid suspension: 400 mg/5 mL	30–60 mL daily in 2 divided doses	6–12 years: 15–30 mL daily in 2 divided doses 2–6 years: 5–15 mL daily in 2 divided doses <2 years: 0.5 mL/kg in 2 divided doses 4 times/day PRN
			Liquid suspension: 800 mg/5 mL	15–30 mL daily in 2 divided doses	6–12 years: 7.5–15 mL daily in 2 divided doses 2–6 years: 2.5–7.5 mL daily in 2 divided doses
			Liquid suspension: 1,200 mg/5 mL	10–20 mL daily in 2 divided doses	Not recommended in children <12 years
Sodium phosphate (SOE dee um) (FOS fate)	OsmoPrep®	Rx	Oral tablet	As directed (32–40 tablets starting the evening prior to the procedure)	Not recommended in children <18 years
		Rx	Oral liquid	45 mL the evening prior to the procedure	Not recommended in children <18 years
Mineral oil	Fleet Oil	OTC	Rectal enema (118 mL)	1 bottle daily	2–12 years: ½ bottle daily
	GoodSense Mineral Oil	OTC	Oral solution	15–45 mL daily	6–12 years: 5–15 mL daily
Castor oil	GoodSense Castor Oil	OTC	Oral liquid	15–60 mL daily	2–12 years: 5–15 mL daily

Continued next page

MEDICATION TABLE 22-1. Representative Medications for Disorders of the Lower Gastrointestinal Tract[8] (Continued)

Generic Name	Brand Name	Rx/OTC	Dosage Forms	Adult Dosages	Pediatric Dosages
Stimulant Laxatives					
Senna (SEN a)	Ex-Lax, Senokot, Perdiem Overnight Relief, others	OTC	Tablets: 8.6–25 mg sennosides	2 tablets 1–2 times/day with water	6–12 years: 1 tablet 1–2 times/day with water
		OTC	Granules: 15 mg/5 mL	1 tsp daily (max 2 tsp 2 times/day)	6–12 years: ½ tsp (max 1 tsp 2 times/day) 2–6 years: ¼ tsp (max ½ tsp 2 times/day)
		OTC	Granules: 20 mg/5 mL	As a tea: ¼–½ cup daily	
		OTC	Oral syrup: 8.8 mg/5 mL	2–3 tsp daily (max 3 tsp 2 times/day)	6–12 years: 1–1½ tsp daily (max 1½ tsp 2 times/day) 2–6 years: ½–¾ tsp daily (max ¾ tsp 2 times/day)
		OTC	Oral concentrate (Fletcher's Castoria)	Not intended for adults	6–15 years: 10–15 mL daily
		OTC	Oral drops: 8.8 mg/mL	Not intended for adults	2–5 years: 5–10 mL daily 6–12 years: 1–1.5 mL daily (max 1.5 mL 2 times/day) 2–6 years: 0.5–0.75 mL daily (max 0.75 mL 2 times/day)
Bisacodyl (bis AK oh dill)	Dulcolax, Ex-Lax Ultra, others	OTC	Tablets, enteric-coated: 5 mg	1–3 tablets daily	6–12 years: 1 tablet daily
		OTC	Rectal suppository: 10 mg	1 suppository daily	½ suppository daily
Medications for Hemorrhoids					
Hydrocortisone (hye droe KOR ti sone)	Preparation H, others	OTC	Cream/suppository	Cream: apply sparingly up to twice daily Suppository: insert 1 suppository rectally 2 times/day	None
Phenylephrine (fen il EF rin)	Preparation H	OTC	Gel/ointment/ suppository	Gel/ointment: apply up to 4 times daily Suppository: insert 1 suppository rectally 2 times/day	None

Continued next page

MEDICATION TABLE 22-1. Representative Medications for Disorders of the Lower Gastrointestinal Tract[8] *(Continued)*

Generic Name	Brand Name	Rx/OTC	Dosage Forms	Adult Dosages	Pediatric Dosages
Medications for Inflammatory Bowel Disease					
Anti-inflammatory Medications					
Sulfasalazine (sul fa SAL a zeen)	Azulfidine	Rx	Tablets: 500 mg Enteric-coated tablets: 500 mg	Starting dose: 1–2 g in 2 divided doses Maintenance dose: 3–4 g in 2 divided doses	Starting dose: 40–60 mg/kg/day divided into 4 or fewer doses/day Maintenance dose: 30 mg/kg/day divided into 4 or fewer doses/day; do not exceed 2 g
Mesalamine (me SAL a meen)	Apriso, Asacol, Canasa, Lialda, Pentasa, Rowasa	Rx	Rectal enema: 4 g/60 mL Extended-release tablets: 0.375 g, 800 mg Extended-release capsule: 250 mg, 500 mg Enteric-coated tablets: 400 mg Rectal suppository 1 g	Enema: 4 g once daily HS; Rectal suppository: 1 g daily Oral: 800–1.6 g TID or 2.4–4.8 g daily, depending on patient status and dosage form	Oral, 5 years and up: dose based on weight; not indicated for children <5 Rectal: not labeled for pediatric use.
Balsalazide (bal SAL a zide)	Colazal	Rx	Capsule: 750 mg	Initial dose: 2,250 mg 3 times/day Maintenance dose: 1,500 mg 2 times/day	5 years and above: 2,250 mg 3 times/day initially; no maintenance dose for pediatrics
Olsalazine (ole SAL a zeen)	Dipentum	Rx	Capsule: 250 mg	1.5 g in 2 or 3 doses daily	Dosing not established
Immunomodulators					
Adalimumab (a dal AYE mu mab)	Humira	Rx	SUBQ solution: 20 mg/0.4 mL, 40 mg/0.8 mL	160 mg the first week, 80 mg the second week, then 40 mg every other week	No recommend dose for IBD
Azathioprine (ay za THYE oh preen)	Azasan, Imuran	Rx	Tablet: 50 mg, 75 mg, 100 mg	1.4–2.5 mg/kg/day; however, clear dose is unknown	Dosing not established
Certolizumab pegol (ser toe LIZ oo mab)	Cimzia	Rx	SUBQ solution: 200 mg/mL	400 mg every other week over 6 weeks, then 400 mg every 4 weeks	Dosing not established

Continued next page

MEDICATION TABLE 22-1. Representative Medications for Disorders of the Lower Gastrointestinal Tract[8] (Continued)

Generic Name	Brand Name	Rx/OTC	Dosage Forms	Adult Dosages	Pediatric Dosages
Infliximab (in FLIX i mab)	Remicade	Rx	IV powder for solution: 100 mg	5 mg/kg every 2 weeks × 3 doses, then 5 mg/kg every 8 weeks	For children 6 years and older: 5 mg/kg every 2 weeks × 3 doses, then 5 mg/kg every 8 weeks; no dose established for children younger than 6 years
Mercaptopurine (6-MP) (mer kap toe PURE een)	Purixan	Rx	Oral tablet	1.5–2.5 mg/kg daily	1–1.5 mg/kg/day
Natalizumab (na ta LIZ you mab)	Tysabri	Rx (limited access program)	IV solution: 20 mg/mL	300 mg every month IV	Dosing not established
Irritable Bowel Syndrome					
Alosetron (al OH se tron)	Lotronex	Rx	Tablet: 0.5 mg, 1 mg	Females only: 0.5 mg 2 times/day × 4 weeks, then 1 mg 2 times/day	Not recommended
Tegaserod (te GAS a rod)	Zelnorm	Rx	Tablet: 6 mg	Females <55 years only: 6 mg 2 times/day up to 12 weeks	Not recommended
Flatulence					
Alpha-galactosidase-A (AL fa gal lak TOE si days)	Beano, Gas-X	OTC	Tablets and suspension	Use after meals containing beans	Use after meals containing beans
Charcoal, activated	Various brands available	OTC	Capsules: 250 mg, 260 mg	520 mg after meals or with discomfort; NTE 4,160 mg	Not recommended in children
Simethicone (sye METH i kone)	Mylicon, Gas-X, Phazyme, others	OTC	Chewable tablets: 80 mg, 125 mg Capsule: 125 mg, 166 mg, 180 mg Suspension: 20 mg/0.3 mL, 40 mg/0.6 mL	40–360 mg PO 4 times/day and nightly; NTE 500 mg	<2 years: 20 mg 4 times/day and nightly; NTE 240 mg 2–12 years: 40 mg 4 times/day and nightly; NTE 240 mg

Continued next page

MEDICATION TABLE 22-1. Representative Medications for Disorders of the Lower Gastrointestinal Tract[8] (Continued)

Generic Name	Brand Name	Rx/OTC	Dosage Forms	Adult Dosages	Pediatric Dosages
Parasite Infections					
Albendazole (al BEN da zole)	Generics	Rx	Tablet: 200 mg	Ancylostomiasis, necatoriasis, ascarisis: 400 mg × 1 dose Echinococcosis, patients >60 kg: 400 mg 2 times/day × 28 days, then 14 days off × 3 cycles Echinococcosis, patients <60 kg: 15 mg/kg/day in 2 doses; NTE 800 mg	Ancylostomiasis, necatoriasis, ascarisis: 400 mg × 1 dose Echinococcosis, patients >60 kg: 400 mg 2 times/day × 28 days, then 14 days off × 3 cycles Echinococcosis, patients <60 kg: 15 mg/kg/day in 2 doses; NTE 800 mg
Mebendazole (me BEN da zole)	Emverm	Rx	Chewable tablets: 100 mg	Ancylostomiasis, necatoriasis, ascariasis, trichuriasis: 100 mg 2 times/day × 3 days Enterobiasis: 100 mg × 1 dose	For patients >2 years, the adult dose is used; no dose is recommended for patients <2 years

GI = gastrointestinal; IBD = inflammatory bowel disease; IV = intravenous; NTE = not to exceed; OTC = over the counter; PO = by mouth; PRN = as needed; Rx = prescribed; SUBQ = subcutaneous.

MEDICATION TABLE 22-2. Medication Classes That Cause Constipation (Examples of Drugs within Those Classes—Not All Inclusive)

Opioids (morphine, naloxone, codeine, hydrocodone, oxycodone, propoxyphene/APAP, tramadol, fentanyl)
Anticholinergics (diphenhydramine or other antihistamines, atropine agents, neuroleptics, antiparkinsonian drugs, overactive bladder medications such as tolterodine, trospium, and tiotropium)
Antidepressants (monoamine oxidase (MAO) inhibitors: selegiline, amitriptyline)
Antipsychotics (aripiprazole, clozapine, quetiapine, haloperidol)
Antacids (aluminum, calcium carbonate)
Antihypertensives (calcium channel blockers, diuretics, clonidine, hydralazine)
Calcium-channel blockers (diltiazem, verapamil, amlodipine, nicardipine)
Diuretics (furosemide, hydrochlorothiazide)
Ganglionic blockers (mecamylamine)
Iron supplements (slow Fe, iron sulfate)
Nonsteroidal anti-inflammatory drugs (naproxen, ibuprofen, meloxicam)
Resins (cholestyramine, polystyrene)

Chapter 23

Hepatic and Pancreatic Disorders

Brian A. Hemstreet, PharmD, FCCP, BCPS

KEY TERMS AND DEFINITIONS

Ascites—an abnormal accumulation of fluid in the abdominal cavity. This is a common complication of cirrhosis.

Cirrhosis—a chronic liver disease that is a result of longstanding or repeated damage to the liver. Scar tissue replaces normal tissue, resulting in many complications related to loss of normal liver function. Cirrhosis is often referred to as *end-stage liver disease*.

Hepatic encephalopathy (HE)—a dysfunction of the brain and nervous system that occurs in patients with cirrhosis. This disorder is thought to be due to the presence of waste products in the bloodstream, such as ammonia, that are normally detoxified by the liver.

Hepatitis—inflammation of the liver that may be caused by a variety of diseases, toxins, and drugs. Hepatitis may by acute or chronic and patients may exhibit symptoms, such as abdominal pain, jaundice, or nausea. Hepatitis may also be severe enough to require hospitalization.

Jaundice—yellow discoloration of the skin, whites of the eyes, and mucous membranes that occurs in patients with hepatitis or cirrhosis. This is due to accumulation of a substance called bilirubin that is normally detoxified by the liver.

Malabsorption—the inability to absorb nutrients from the gastrointestinal tract. This is often seen in patients with chronic pancreatitis, who lose the ability to digest orally ingested food (maldigestion) due to a lack of pancreatic enzymes.

DOI 10.37573/9781585286638.023

Nonalcoholic fatty liver disease (NAFLD)—chronic liver disease related to fatty infiltration of the liver, often found in patients with obesity, type 2 diabetes, and metabolic syndrome.

Pancreatitis—inflammation of the pancreas due to toxins, drugs, trauma, structural abnormalities, or other causes. Pancreatitis can be acute or chronic.

Pancreatic exocrine insufficiency—the inability of the pancreas to supply adequate enzymes for normal digestion of food. This results in maldigestion and symptoms such as steatorrhea.

Portal hypertension—increased pressure in the portal vein, due to a backup of blood flow as a result of the presence of fibrosis due to cirrhosis.

Pseudocyst—a large fluid collection that forms in or around the pancreas as a result of inflammation due to pancreatitis.

Varices—enlarged veins located in the lower part of the esophagus or the stomach that are close to the surface. These form as a result of portal hypertension. The veins become so large that they may burst, leading to life-threatening bleeding.

LEARNING OBJECTIVES

After completing this chapter, you should be able to

1. Define the following:
   - Hepatitis.
   - Cirrhosis.
   - Ascites.
   - Encephalopathy.
   - Jaundice.
   - Esophageal varices.
   - Portal hypertension.
   - Pancreatitis.
   - Pancreatic exocrine insufficiency.
   - Malabsorption.
   - Pseudocyst.

2. Recall common causes and complications of chronic liver disease.

3. Review the role and mechanism of common drug treatments for cirrhosis.

4. Review adverse effects and drug interactions for medications used in the treatment of chronic liver disease.

5. Identify key patient counseling points for medications used to treat complications of chronic liver disease.

6. Describe the anatomy and normal physiology of the liver and pancreas.

7. Recognize common medications used in the management of acute pancreatitis.

8. Review adverse effects, drug interactions, and key patient counseling points for medications used in the treatment of chronic pancreatitis.

Hepatic disorders are those that directly affect the liver. Given that the liver is a vital organ that is involved in many important functions in the human body, diseases of the liver can result in very serious consequences for patients. There are many different causes of both acute and chronic liver disease. These include infections, such as those due to hepatitis B virus or hepatitis C virus, exposure to drugs and alternative medications or other toxins, inherited or genetic disorders, autoimmune disorders (where the body's immune system attacks its own organs), and metabolic disorders, among others. Approximately 1 million deaths per year are attributed to complications of cirrhosis.[1] This makes the prevention and treatment of liver disease and its complications a significant area of healthcare focus and utilization.

Traditionally, the most common causes of chronic liver disease in the United States are chronic alcohol abuse and hepatitis C virus infection.[1,2] However the increasing prevalence of obesity and type 2 diabetes in the United States has led to nonalcoholic fatty liver disease (NAFLD) now being recognized as the most common cause of chronic liver disease in the United States.[3] While some drug treatments may target the acute processes involved in liver disease, such as those caused by viruses or autoimmune conditions, much of the drug management revolves around management of chronic liver disease and its associated complications. Therefore, this chapter focuses on common medications used in the chronic management of advanced nonviral-associated liver diseases and its complications.

CASE STUDY

Jessica Worthy is a 47-year-old woman who is 5 feet 6 inches tall and weighs 128 lb. She has a history of alcohol abuse and reports drinking 8–10 beers daily during the past 20 years. She is seen today at the clinic with complaints of abdominal swelling, swollen ankles, mild shortness of breath, and a 10-lb weight gain over the past 3 weeks. She has noticed that the whites of her eyes and her skin are turning yellow. She currently takes no medications and reports no allergies to medications or foods. After review of her physical exam, laboratory tests, and radiology results, her healthcare provider tells her that she has developed cirrhosis due to chronic alcohol abuse.

ANATOMY AND PHYSIOLOGY OF THE LIVER

The liver is a large organ that consists of two major sections, called lobes, and is located in the right upper portion of the abdominal cavity (Figure 23-1). It performs many important functions, including metabolism of drugs and nutrients; detoxification of metabolic waste products and toxins; synthesis of proteins, cholesterol, and bile; excretion of waste products; and participation in host immunity. The blood flow coming into the liver is unique in that it comes mostly from a large blood vessel called the portal vein.

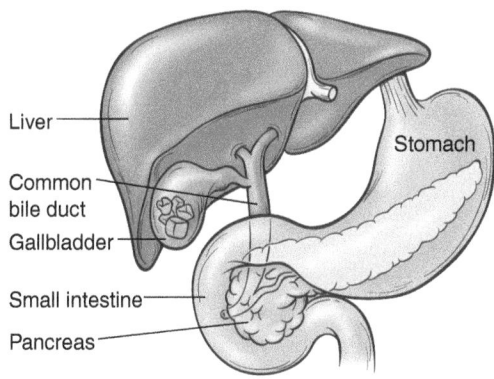

FIGURE 23-1. Position of liver and pancreas.

A small portion of blood flow comes also from the hepatic artery, which carries oxygen-rich blood to the liver. The portal vein drains blood from the stomach and intestines and delivers it to the liver. Therefore, any nutrient or drug that is orally ingested passes through the portal vein and goes to the liver first before making its way to the systemic circulation. This is often referred to as the "first pass effect." Based on this blood flow the liver is able to act as a filter to help metabolize or detoxify any potentially harmful substances that are orally absorbed before they reach the bloodstream.

Once blood enters the liver it passes slowly through small cavities called sinusoids. As the blood passes through the sinusoids it is exposed to the various types of cells located in the liver. The largest number of cells are called hepatocytes. These cells perform most of the detoxification and metabolic processes within the liver. The hepatocytes also produce important proteins, such as albumin and various proteins involved in the normal blood clotting process. Specialized cells, called Kupffer cells, help to remove any bacteria that may have entered the liver through the portal vein. Once filtered, the blood then leaves the liver and enters the systemic circulation through the hepatic veins.

The liver also produces a substance called bile, which helps to remove fat-soluble substances, including some drugs, from the body. Bile contains molecules known as bile acids, which also aid in fat absorption in the small intestine. Bile leaves the liver and travels through a series of tube-like structures called bile ducts. All the bile ducts that collect and drain bile from the liver are referred to collectively as the biliary system. The biliary system drains into series of larger ducts that exit the liver and eventually empty into the small intestine. Most substances that are secreted into the bile are eliminated in the feces after entering the small intestine. Bile also includes some important waste products such as bilirubin, which, if not excreted properly, accumulates in the body and leads to jaundice, a yellowish discoloration of the skin and eyes. For most patients additional symptoms from jaundice are rare, but in severe cases they may experience intense itching or dark-colored urine.

CASE?

Do Ms. Worthy's abdominal swelling, ankle swelling, and shortness of breath indicate that she has most likely developed a major complication of cirrhosis? Which complication would match these symptoms?

CHRONIC COMPLICATIONS OF HEPATIC DISORDERS

Cirrhosis

As the liver sustains repeated injury and inflammation over a long time, a process referred to as fibrosis takes place. Fibrosis leads to the replacement of normal liver cells with scar tissue. The function of the remaining normal liver cells is often able to compensate for the initial fibrosis. Once the fibrosis gets severe enough, the structure of the liver cells and blood vessels is altered, and the liver starts to lose the ability to perform its normal functions. This advanced stage is referred to as cirrhosis, also sometimes called end-stage liver disease. The development of cirrhosis is a slow process and patients may not be aware that they have it until complications are present or abnormalities are identified on laboratory examination of liver function tests. Patients with cirrhosis may develop complications such as jaundice, an enlarged spleen, ascites, hepatic encephalopathy (HE), edema, and an increased risk for liver cancer.[4-6] When these complications are present patients are then referred to as having decompensated cirrhosis.[7]

Laboratory abnormalities seen in patients with cirrhosis often include increased or normal AST/ALT (liver function tests), low serum albumin, increased serum bilirubin and prothrombin time (or INR), anemia, and low platelets. Once cirrhosis develops, the damage to the liver is generally considered to be irreversible. Patients may ultimately require a liver transplant as a consequence of cirrhosis.

Variceal Bleeding

Blood entering the liver through the portal vein can usually flow through the sinusoids without much resistance. Once patients develop cirrhosis, the structural changes and presence of scar tissue in the liver cause increased resistance to blood flow within the liver. This limits the ability of blood to flow easily into the liver from the portal vein and leads to a backup of blood flow and increased pressure in the portal vein. This process ultimately results in increased pressure within the portal vein, referred to as portal hypertension. This increased pressure in the portal vein causes a backup of blood flow in the blood vessels in the surrounding area that empty into the portal vein leading to collateral vessel formation. These blood vessels, located mostly in the esophagus or stomach, significantly enlarge and protrude close to the surface. These enlarged vessels are referred to as varices. Approximately 50% of patients with cirrhosis have gastroesophageal varices, and the percentage of patients with varices increases as the liver disease becomes more severe.[5-7]

Once varices are present, they can continue to increase in size and may protrude into the center of the esophagus. The most serious (and sometimes even fatal) complication that can occur is bleeding secondary to rupture of the varices. Following an acute bleeding episode, patients are at high risk for rebleeding, with this risk being highest within the first 5 days after the bleeding episode.[5] Certain drug and nondrug therapies may be used to prevent a first episode of bleeding in patients with varices (referred to as primary prevention) or to prevent future bleeding in patients who have already experienced a variceal bleeding episode (called secondary prevention).

Ascites

By definition, ascites is the presence of fluid in the peritoneal cavity. It is one of the most common complications of cirrhosis and occurs in up to 50% of patients within 10 years of their diagnosis.[6] The development of ascites is related to both portal hypertension and dilation of the blood vessels that supply the liver and the gastrointestinal (GI) system. This dilation of blood vessels is due to the increased local production of substances such as nitric oxide, which cause the blood vessels to relax and increase blood flow. The shift in blood flow causes the blood volume in the rest of the arterial system to decrease. The body senses this and institutes processes that lead to sodium and water retention to try and maintain arterial blood volume. Since blood flow through the liver is already compromised in cirrhosis, excessive sodium and water retention causes fluid to leak out of the surface of the liver into the peritoneal cavity. The rate of death due to ascites is approximately 44% within 5 years.[6]

Patients with ascites may have several liters of fluid present in their peritoneal cavity. This causes patients to develop serious abdominal swelling, which can limit mobility and cause shortness of breath if the fluid presses on the diaphragm and does not allow the lungs to expand normally. Patients often complain of abdominal discomfort and may gain several pounds of weight because of the large amount of fluid that is retained. Patients may also develop hernias due to the increased pressure in the abdominal cavity. The fluid may also become infected with bacteria, leading to the development of spontaneous bacterial peritonitis. Samples of the ascitic fluid may be taken by inserting a needle through the abdominal wall into the peritoneal cavity. This is called paracentesis. Patients who don't respond to drug treatment for ascites may need paracentesis on a regular basis to remove large amounts of fluid (more than 5 liters) to relieve their symptoms. Alternatively, patients may require placement of a stent, called a TIPS (transjugular intrahepatic portosystemic shunt), to reduce pressure in the portal vein with the hopes of reducing the rate of ascitic fluid production.[4] The ultimate cure for ascites is liver transplantation.

Hepatic Encephalopathy

Hepatic encephalopathy (HE) is a metabolic disorder that is another common complication of cirrhosis. Patients with HE experience alterations in mental status, consciousness or alertness, behavior, and muscle function. The primary reason patients develop HE is thought to be the accumulation of various substances in the bloodstream that are normally detoxified by the liver. The major substance involved in the development of HE is ammonia. Ammonia is produced by various tissues in the body but is mostly produced in the colon as a byproduct of bacterial protein metabolism. Ammonia enters the bloodstream via the portal vein. The hepatocytes metabolize the ammonia to urea, which is then mostly excreted through the kidney. Some urea does diffuse back into the intestines from the bloodstream, where bacteria convert it back into ammonia. In patients with liver disease, less ammonia is converted into urea, and the excess may enter the central nervous system, leading to significant dysfunction. Other substances may also contribute to the development of HE but to a lesser extent than ammonia. Several additional factors may precipitate HE, and ammonia may sensitize the brain to the effects of these factors. Precipitating factors include excess protein intake, infection, GI bleeding, electrolyte disturbances, acidosis, and drugs that have sedative or central nervous system depressant effects, such as narcotics.[8]

Patients with HE require a lot of focused care. They may appear sleepy or confused and may be unable to cooperate with their caregivers. They may also be unable to perform routine tasks that require fine motor function and be confined to a bed in severe cases. Patients with HE may also have disturbances in their sleep patterns and may exhibit bizarre or aggressive behavior. If untreated, patients may fall into a coma. Fortunately, HE may be reversible with the removal of precipitating factors, restriction of protein intake, and initiation of drug treatment.

Spontaneous Bacterial Peritonitis

Infections are another common complication of cirrhosis. Spontaneous bacterial peritonitis (SBP) is an often-fatal complication, and occurs when bacteria cause infection of the ascitic fluid within the peritoneal cavity.[6,7] Infection is thought to occur by a process known as bacterial translocation, in which bacteria migrate from the intestinal tract into the bloodstream and ultimately end up in the ascitic fluid. This is secondary to the reduced immune system function that develops in patients with cirrhosis, possible bacterial overgrowth in the intestines, and reduced GI motility. Once bacteria enter the ascitic fluid, the dysfunction of the immune system caused by chronic liver disease results in a lack of clearance of the bacteria. The most common bacteria that cause SBP are organisms that normally reside in the intestinal tract, such as *Escherichia coli*, *Klebsiella*, or *Proteus*. Gram positive organisms, such as *Staphylococcus* or *Streptococci*, may also be present. Risk factors for the development of SBP include a low ascitic fluid protein, increased serum bilirubin, and the presence of variceal bleeding.[7,8]

Patients who develop SBP may have signs or symptoms that include fever, abdominal pain or tenderness, altered mental status, vomiting, or diarrhea. Laboratory values may indicate an elevated white blood cell count in the ascitic fluid or presence of an elevated blood urea nitrogen (BUN) or lowered bicarbonate concentration (acidosis). The diagnosis is ultimately made by performing a paracentesis. The presence of inflammation secondary to SBP may also lead to decreased perfusion of the kidney. Kidney dysfunction is a major concern and is a leading cause of mortality in patients with SBP.[7] Once patients have SBP they often require lifelong antibiotic treatment to prevent further SBP episodes.

CASE?

Ms. Worthy's healthcare provider has referred her to a liver specialist for management of her cirrhosis. The specialist performs an endoscopy and finds several large esophageal varices. What is the major complication associated with untreated esophageal varices?

PHARMACOLOGIC AGENTS USED IN THE MANAGEMENT OF HEPATIC DISORDERS

A wide variety of medications are used to treat and prevent the complications of chronic liver disease and cirrhosis. Most medications that have favorable effects are used for other non-liver associated conditions, while some are specifically used to treat or prevent certain complications of cirrhosis.

Beta Blockers for Prevention of Variceal Bleeding

Beta-adrenergic antagonists (often referred to as "beta blockers") are traditionally used for patients with cardiovascular conditions such as high blood pressure, heart failure, heart attack, or rapid heart rate (as discussed in Chapters 15 and 16). However, in patients with cirrhosis, beta blockers are used for the prevention of variceal bleeding. Beta blockers work by inhibiting the actions of epinephrine and norepinephrine at the beta-receptor. Stimulation of beta$_1$ (β_1) receptors causes increases in heart rate and blood pressure, while stimulation of beta$_2$ (β_2) receptors causes relaxation of the smooth muscles in the airways and in the blood vessels in the GI system. The stimulation of the beta$_2$ receptor causes the blood vessels in the GI system to dilate, therefore increasing blood flow to the portal vein.

Beta blockers are thought to prevent variceal bleeding by reducing heart rate and cardiac output (β_1 effects), therefore reducing the amount of blood that is pumped to the GI system and portal vein. This results in reductions in portal vein pressure. They also prevent the dilation of the blood vessels in the GI system (β_2 effects), causing these blood vessels to constrict and further reduce blood flow to the portal vein. To have these favorable effects, the use of agents that block both β_1 and β_2 receptors, also referred to as "nonselective" beta blockers, is required. The most commonly used nonselective beta blockers are propranolol, carvedilol, and nadolol. Beta blockers that only target the β_1 receptor, such as atenolol or metoprolol, are less effective and therefore are not recommended for the prevention of variceal bleeding. Patients who are candidates for the use of beta blockers for primary prevention are those with advanced cirrhosis and "high-risk varices," which are either small varices that have certain characteristics, called red wale marks (seen during endoscopy), or any patient with medium or large varices. Any patient who experiences an episode of variceal bleeding should receive a nonselective beta blocker for secondary prevention of a future episode.

Beta blockers can significantly reduce the rate of variceal bleeding. Propranolol is typically started at a low dose of 20 mg orally twice daily or 10 mg orally 3 times daily. A typical starting dose for nadolol is 40 mg once daily. The goal is to reduce the heart rate by at least 25% from baseline to a goal of 55–60 beats/minute. Once patients reach the maximum effective dose, they may be switched to long-acting formulations that are given once daily to improve adherence.

Unfortunately, beta blockers may be associated with many side effects, including fatigue, low blood pressure and heart rate, shortness of breath, lightheadedness, nausea, insomnia, and sexual dysfunction. Increases in blood sugar or potassium levels may also occur. Patients with asthma, those with diabetes who experience frequent hypoglycemia, those with peripheral vascular disease or preexisting low heart rate should not receive beta blockers. For patients who cannot tolerate beta blockers, the preferred method of prevention is endoscopic variceal ligation. This procedure involves placing rubber bands around the varices during endoscopy, which cause the varices to become necrotic and die.

CASE?

Which medication(s) might be prescribed as initial therapy to help remove fluid and reduce Ms. Worthy's abdominal and ankle swelling?

Diuretics for Management of Ascites and Edema

Diuretics are medications that work by increasing fluid and sodium loss through the kidney. The main role of diuretics in patients with cirrhosis is the treatment of ascites and edema (leg and ankle swelling). The main goals of diuretic therapy are to reduce patient symptoms and remove an adequate amount of fluid and sodium. Prior to starting diuretics, patients should restrict their intake of sodium to less than 2,000 mg/day. This will help to prevent further formation of ascites and edema; however, these restrictions are very difficult to follow for most patients.

The most common diuretic regimen used in the treatment of ascites is the combination of furosemide and spironolactone.[6,7] Furosemide is a potent loop diuretic that causes rapid excretion of water and sodium from the kidney. Furosemide is typically started at an oral dose of 40 mg once daily in the morning.[6] It is also available as an intravenous (IV) preparation that can be used in hospitalized patients with severe ascites and edema, or in patients who cannot swallow. IV doses range from 20–80 mg and may be repeated several times throughout the day. Spironolactone is a potassium-sparing diuretic that works synergistically with furosemide. While its diuretic effects are much weaker than furosemide, spironolactone also has favorable effects on blocking the effects of aldosterone, the main hormone that leads to excessive sodium and water retention in patients with cirrhosis. It also helps to offset the loss of potassium that occurs with furosemide. A typical starting dose of spironolactone is 100 mg once daily in the morning, given in combination with 40 mg furosemide.[6]

Once diuretic therapy is started urine output should be monitored to ensure effectiveness. Most patients will also be weighed daily to mark fluid loss. The use of furosemide may cause excessive loss of sodium and potassium, so these laboratory values are usually monitored closely. Furosemide may also cause increases in ammonia production in the kidney, which may precipitate HE. Spironolactone use may be associated with elevated blood concentrations of potassium. In addition, male patients may experience painful breast swelling, called gynecomastia, because spironolactone may cause reduced effects of testosterone in the body. If the patient experiences gynecomastia an alternate potassium-sparing diuretic, such as amiloride, may be substituted, although this drug may be less effective and is more costly.

PRACTICE POINT

One way to gauge the effectiveness of diuretics in patients with ascites is to have patients monitor their weight. Patients should initially weigh themselves daily to monitor for adequate weight reduction due to fluid loss, especially if they have edema.

For patients who are acutely symptomatic from massive ascites or those who are unresponsive to diuretic therapy, removal of fluid by performing periodic paracentesis may be needed. Paracentesis, while faster at removing fluid than diuretics, is only a symptomatic intervention and does not address the underlying process that leads to formation of ascites. Removal of large quantities of fluid (>5 L) via paracentesis may cause shifting of fluid from the bloodstream back into the peritoneal cavity. This may reduce blood flow to the kidney, leading to kidney failure. IV albumin may be administered in this setting to help prevent kidney failure. Ultimately, patients may need a liver transplant or placement of a TIPS shunt to alleviate ascites.

Lactulose for Treatment and Prevention of Hepatic Encephalopathy

As discussed earlier, the major substance thought to contribute to the development of HE is ammonia. Thus, therapies that are effective at managing HE are those that reduce

blood concentrations of ammonia. One such drug is the non-absorbable sugar lactulose. Lactulose is available as a solution that contains 10 g lactulose/15 mL (tablespoon) or as 10-g or 20-g powder packets that can be dissolved in water. When ingested orally lactulose is not absorbed—it remains in the intestine and is broken down by bacteria in the colon to acetic acid and lactic acid. This makes the environment of the colon more acidic. Ammonia (the chemical designation is NH_3) in the acidified colon is converted to a charged form called ammonium ion (NH_4^+) that cannot pass back through the intestine into the bloodstream. Additionally, lactulose acts as a laxative and causes increased frequency of bowel movements. This leads to excretion of ammonia in the stool, which ultimately reduces blood ammonia concentrations and improves the symptoms of HE. A typical starting dose of lactulose is 20–30 g (30–45 mL) every 1–2 hours until one-two soft bowel movements occur. Once this happens the dose is reduced to maintain two to three bowel movements a day. A typical maintenance dose is 10–20 g (15–30 mL) orally two or three times a day.

PRACTICE POINT

For hospitalized patients who cannot swallow, 300 mL of lactulose may be mixed with 700 mL of water and administered as a retention enema (retained in the colon for at least 1 hour).

Lactulose therapy is commonly used for both acute and chronic management of HE. Since lactulose is a laxative, the main adverse effect seen in practice is diarrhea. Doses may be reduced in patients who experience more than two to three bowel movements daily. Patients may have difficulty with adherence to lactulose therapy because of the need to have frequent bowel movements. Diarrhea may lead to dehydration in severe cases, as well as loss of potassium through the GI tract. Lactulose may also cause abdominal cramping and distension, as well as flatulence. Lactulose tastes very sweet, which may not be appealing to some patients.

CASE?

Ms. Worthy was hospitalized last night for altered mental status. The medical team in the hospital started her on oral lactulose for treatment of HE. What major adverse effect is expected with the use of lactulose?

Antibiotics for Prevention and Treatment of Spontaneous Bacterial Peritonitis and Hepatic Encephalopathy

Antibiotics have various roles in the management of the complications of chronic liver disease, including both prevention and treatment of SBP and HE. These drugs are discussed extensively in Chapter 27 but will be introduced here in context. For patients who have not had a prior episode of SBP, antibiotics may be prescribed on a chronic basis to select patients to prevent a first episode (primary prevention). Antibiotics also reduce the rate of development of SBP and improve rates of survival in the setting of acute variceal bleeding.

The most common antibiotics used for SBP prevention in patients with acute variceal bleeding are third-generation cephalosporins, such as ceftriaxone 1 g IV every 24 hours.[6,7] Alternatively, systemic antibiotic therapy with ciprofloxacin or levofloxacin may be considered. There is concern, however, for an increase in potential adverse effects with these agents.

Patients who develop an acute episode of SBP are typically hospitalized and require systemic IV antibiotic treatment as initial therapy for a total of 5 days. This is usually a third-generation cephalosporin, such as ceftriaxone, often in combination with IV albumin. Albumin where indicated based on lab values, is thought to prevent the development of kidney failure in patients with SBP.[6,7] More broad-spectrum antibiotics, such as piperacillin/tazobactam or meropenem, may be required if the patient has a previous history of SBP or develops the infection during hospitalization. Ciprofloxacin and levofloxacin may be options in patients with serious penicillin allergies; however, the potential for serious adverse effects needs to be considered. Aminoglycoside antibiotics, such as gentamicin or tobramycin, should be avoided, as they can cause serious injury to the kidney. The antibiotics should also be dose-adjusted properly for the patient's kidney function.

Once patients recover from an acute episode of SBP they typically receive lifelong oral antibiotic therapy to prevent further episodes (secondary prevention), unless there is a significant improvement in their liver disease over time. The antibiotic used should preferably be one that is poorly absorbed and thus targets the bacteria in the GI tract, although systemically absorbed antibiotics are also routinely used and are effective. The choice of antibiotic may be made based on several factors, including cost, presence of allergies, frequency of administration, and potential for drug interactions and adverse effects. Recent guidelines recommend norfloxacin or ciprofloxacin daily as preferred agents. Trimethoprim/sulfamethoxazole, one double-strength tablet given once daily for 5–7 days per week, is often prescribed as a starting regimen. The use of antibiotics for treatment or prevention of SBP may be associated with adverse effects. These are discussed in Chapter 27.

The other main use for antibiotics in patients with cirrhosis is the treatment and prevention of HE. Antibiotics are considered therapeutic alternatives to lactulose.[7,8] This is based on the fact that a large proportion of ammonia is produced by the bacteria that normally live in the colon. By reducing the number of bacteria, the amount of ammonia that is produced and absorbed into the systemic circulation is significantly reduced, thus improving symptoms of HE. Antibiotics may also be combined with lactulose in patients who do not completely respond to appropriate doses of lactulose. Similar to prevention of SBP, antibiotics that are poorly absorbed can be used for the treatment of HE. The most widely studied antibiotic for HE is neomycin 3–6 g daily orally in divided doses. When taken orally, less than 1% of an oral dose of neomycin is absorbed. Nevertheless, there is concern for kidney dysfunction with long-term use and thus, its use has largely fallen out of favor.

ALERT!

Over time, the small portion of neomycin that is absorbed may accumulate and cause kidney damage or hearing loss.

Rifaximin has become the most common antibiotic used for HE. When taken orally, only about 0.5% (about 1/200th of the dose) is absorbed; thus, its effects are localized to the GI tract. Unlike neomycin, rifaximin is not associated with kidney or hearing dysfunction. Overall, it may be better tolerated than lactulose. Rifaximin's main role is for the prevention of recurrent episodes of HE, often in combination with lactulose. The recommended rifaximin dose is 550 mg orally twice daily.

CASE?

Ms. Worthy's HE was caused by spontaneous bacterial peritonitis. Which drug regimen would be appropriate as initial treatment for this infection?

Octreotide for Acute Variceal Bleeding

As mentioned, acute variceal bleeding is associated with significant morbidity and mortality in patients with cirrhosis. When patients develop acute variceal bleeding, the treatment is typically a combination of direct therapies administered via endoscopy, such as endoscopic variceal ligation or sclerotherapy (injection of an irritating substance into the bleeding varices that causes local inflammation and coagulation). In addition, drugs that cause constriction of the vessels in the intestinal system may also help to reduce blood flow into the portal vein. This may reduce acute bleeding. Octreotide is a drug that constricts the intestinal blood vessels in this setting. It is thought to act by reducing the release of substances that cause dilation of GI blood vessels and is administered as an initial IV bolus dose of 50 mcg, followed by a continuous infusion of 50 mcg/hour IV for a total of 2–5 days. Potential adverse effects of octreotide include nausea, headache, dizziness, low calcium, and increased or decreased blood glucose.

PRACTICE POINT

Octreotide is available in two formulations, a solution for IV or subcutaneous injection and a suspension that is administered intramuscularly. The solution is used for the IV infusion that patients with acute variceal bleeding receive. Octreotide multidose vials may be reconstituted with either normal saline or 5% dextrose. A typical preparation for infusion would be 1,000 mcg of octreotide injected into either a 100-mL or 250-mL bag of normal saline or 5% dextrose. This would yield concentrations of 10 mcg/mL or 4 mcg/mL, respectively.

Albumin

Albumin is one of the primary circulating proteins in the bloodstream and is a major product of the liver. One of albumin's main functions is to help maintain the appropriate amount of fluid in the bloodstream by virtue of its osmotic effects. In advanced liver disease, the ability of the liver to produce albumin is significantly reduced. As the blood concentration of albumin becomes lower, fluid that is normally retained in the bloodstream leaks into the tissues, causing edema. Additional fluid may leak into the peritoneal cavity, worsening ascites. Likewise, blood flow to vital organs, such as the kidney, may be reduced as blood volume decreases. Therefore, administration of IV albumin has a role in patients with cirrhosis who are at high risk for kidney dysfunction, such as those with SBP and those patients who are undergoing large-volume paracentesis. In these settings IV infusions of albumin are thought to help maintain blood volume and possibly bind inflammatory substances.

In SBP an IV dose of 25% albumin 1.5 g/kg given on day 1, followed by 1 g/kg on day 3 given in conjunction with IV antibiotics has been shown to reduce the incidence of kidney impairment.[6] In patients who undergo paracentesis, fluid may shift from the bloodstream back into the peritoneal cavity. This may reduce perfusion (blood flow) to the kidney and cause kidney failure. This typically does not happen unless more than 5 L is removed at any one time. Albumin infusions can help maintain blood volume and prevent this shift of fluid following paracentesis. Recommendations are to use 6–8 g albumin/liter of fluid removed in patients who have 5 or more liters removed at one time.[6,7] Albumin is well tolerated, with allergic reactions occurring very rarely.

PRACTICE POINT

The major obstacle to use of albumin is that it is very costly. A treatment course used for SBP or for large-volume paracentesis may cost several hundred dollars. This makes the use of albumin restricted at many institutions.

INTRODUCTION TO PANCREATIC DISORDERS

The pancreas is an accessory organ to the GI system that is involved in many important endocrine and exocrine (digestive) processes. The pancreas works in conjunction with the liver to facilitate nutrient digestion and absorption, regulate blood glucose concentrations, and produce many other important hormones involved in normal GI and metabolic processes. Dysfunction of the pancreas can lead to serious metabolic consequences and may adversely affect nutritional status if chronic dysfunction develops. While many disorders may affect the pancreas, this chapter focuses on pancreatitis, particularly the medications used in the management of acute and chronic pancreatitis.

CASE STUDY

Donald Bradley is a 58-year-old man who is 5 feet 10 inches tall and weighs 190 lb. He has a history of alcohol abuse and reports drinking one pint of vodka daily for the past 22 years. He is admitted to the hospital with complaints of severe abdominal pain, nausea, and vomiting. He currently takes no medications and reports no drug allergies. Laboratory tests reveal an elevated lipase and white blood cell count. He is diagnosed with acute pancreatitis.

ANATOMY AND PHYSIOLOGY OF THE PANCREAS

The pancreas is located just underneath the liver, in close proximity to the duodenum (first part of the small intestine—see Figure 23-1). It is a long and narrow organ that has a larger section, referred to as the head, which then tapers into the section known as the tail. The pancreas contains several different cell types. The endocrine cells secrete important hormones such as insulin and glucagon, which regulate blood glucose, as well as other hormones, such as somatostatin. These substances can enter the bloodstream directly from the pancreas and exert their effects on other organs or cells in the body. The exocrine cells store and secrete pancreatic enzymes, which are important in the digestion of food. The major groups of pancreatic enzymes that are involved in food digestion are amylases, which digest sugars and carbohydrates; proteases, which digest proteins; and lipases, which digest fats.

Pancreatic enzymes are stored in inactive forms within the pancreas and are released during food intake. The pancreatic enzymes are secreted through a series of ducts that drain the pancreas. These ducts are lined with cells that produce bicarbonate, which is secreted along with the pancreatic enzymes. The bicarbonate helps to protect the enzymes from the acidic contents that enter the small intestine from the stomach. The pancreatic enzymes are released into the common bile duct, which also receives and drains secretions from the liver. The common bile duct empties the liver and

pancreatic secretions into the small intestine at the time food is present. Thus, as food leaves the stomach it is exposed to the pancreatic enzymes and the secretions of the liver. The digestion of fat by the pancreatic enzymes also helps facilitate the absorption of the major fat-soluble vitamins A, D, E, and K in the small intestine.[9]

CASE?

What are the primary causes of acute pancreatitis in the United States? Which one most likely caused Mr. Bradley's condition?

PATHOPHYSIOLOGY OF ACUTE AND CHRONIC PANCREATITIS

The pancreas may be susceptible to injury from a wide variety of causes. Injury to the pancreas may be short term and reversible, as in the case of acute pancreatitis. Acute pancreatitis is an inflammatory process within the pancreas that is thought to be triggered by an initial event that causes the premature release of pancreatic enzymes within the pancreas. This local release of pancreatic enzymes causes damage and inflammation within the pancreas. This inflammation can then extend into the areas surrounding the pancreas. In severe cases inflammation can cause serious systemic complications. The most common causes of acute pancreatitis are gallstones, chronic alcohol use, and extremely elevated triglycerides.[9,10] Several different medications are also associated with the development of acute pancreatitis. Drugs that have a definite association with the development of acute pancreatitis include azathioprine, estrogens, valproic acid, and enalapril, among others.[10] Up to 20% of cases have no identifiable cause and are referred to as idiopathic.

Patients with acute pancreatitis almost always require hospitalization. Cases may range from mild to severe, with severe cases typically managed in an intensive care unit. Patients often exhibit abdominal pain, nausea, vomiting, and fever. Patients may have an elevated white blood cell count, low serum calcium, and elevated liver function tests and blood glucose. Blood tests often reveal an abnormally elevated lipase, which is very indicative of pancreatic inflammation. Most patients have localized pancreatic inflammation, but some may progress to necrosis (cell death) of the pancreatic tissue. Of these, many will develop a secondary infection.[9,10] Other local complications may include the development of an abscess or pseudocyst, a large fluid collection that forms in or around the pancreas. This fluid often requires surgical drainage and may become infected with bacteria.

In severe cases of pancreatitis patients may develop organ failure, respiratory distress, and shock. Some of these complications can be fatal. In most cases acute pancreatitis is reversible and once the cause is removed the pancreatitis should resolve, although any complications may need further management.

Chronic pancreatitis develops when there is progressive inflammation and damage to the pancreas over time that results in irreversible endocrine and exocrine function. Chronic alcohol use is the most common cause of chronic pancreatitis. Genetic disorders, structural abnormalities, and autoimmune processes are other potential causes of chronic pancreatitis.[11] Repeated episodes of acute pancreatitis can also contribute to the development of chronic pancreatitis. Over time chronic pancreatitis is associated with the development of fibrosis, obstruction, and tissue atrophy within the pancreas.

When patients progress to chronic pancreatitis, they typically develop chronic abdominal pain. This often leads to the need for chronic pain medications. Patients may develop intermittent acute flares of pancreatitis with associated pain on top of their chronic disease. Patients may also exhibit intermittent nausea and vomiting. Irreversible endocrine dysfunction leads to the loss of insulin secretion. Therefore, patients with chronic pancreatitis often develop diabetes. Finally, exocrine dysfunction leads to a lack of production and secretion of pancreatic enzymes. This is referred to as pancreatic exocrine insufficiency (PEI).[12] Patients lose the ability to digest food properly due to the lack of pancreatic enzyme secretion. The inability to digest fat in the GI tract leads to the development of frequent fatty, greasy, foul-smelling bowel movements, referred to as steatorrhea. This lack of fat digestion and absorption also leads to the inability to absorb fat-soluble vitamins. Therefore, patients are at risk for vitamin A, D, E, and K deficiency. Collectively, these irreversible abnormalities in pancreatic function result in patients becoming extremely malnourished. Overall, chronic pancreatitis is a slowly progressive and often fatal process.

CASE?

Which medication(s) would you expect the healthcare provider to prescribe for treatment of Mr. Bradley's pain due to his acute pancreatitis?

PHARMACOLOGIC AGENTS USED IN THE MANAGEMENT OF PANCREATIC DISORDERS

Nonpharmacologic

The management of patients with acute pancreatitis mostly involves removal of the cause and treatment of symptoms. Most patients require hospitalization. Oral intake may be withheld to prevent stimulation of the pancreas. Oxygen and IV fluid administration may be required if the patient has difficulty breathing or appears dehydrated.[9,10] For patients with gallstone-induced pancreatitis, performance of an endoscopy with a procedure to remove the gallstone from the biliary tract is sometimes required. In some instances, the gallstone will pass out of the biliary tract by itself. Formation of abscesses or pseudocysts may require surgical drainage and antibiotic therapy.

Nutritional Support

The development of acute pancreatitis is associated with high energy consumption. Resuming oral nutritional intake within 24–48 hours of onset is recommended.[9,10] Oral intake is preferred; however, enteral nutrition products administered through a feeding tube (also called tube feeding) is an alternate method of providing nutrition if the patient cannot tolerate oral intake. Several different brands of enteral feedings are available; many are discussed in Chapter 24. The choice of these products is tailored based on individual patient needs. The use of orally administered nutrition prevents the GI tract tissue from atrophying and helps maintain the function of the GI tract. This helps to prevent bacteria from entering the bloodstream through the GI tract. The use of IV total parenteral nutrition is associated with many more complications such as infections, and electrolyte and blood glucose abnormalities, and therefore its use is generally reserved for patients who will have prolonged periods of time that they cannot receive oral nutrition.

Pharmacologic Treatments

Since abdominal pain is often the most common symptom patients have, the use of IV analgesics is often required. Intravenous acetaminophen may be added to supplement pain control.[10] Narcotics, discussed extensively in Chapter 5, are the most commonly used medications in this setting. Examples include morphine, hydromorphone, and fentanyl. The use of patient-controlled analgesia for administration may be preferred, as patients often require frequent doses. Potential adverse effects include sedation, nausea, itching, constipation, and respiratory depression. Patients with acute pancreatitis often have nausea and vomiting, so antiemetic drugs are usually required. Examples include promethazine, prochlorperazine, or ondansetron. IV or rectal (suppository) administration is often required. For patients who are in the intensive care unit, the administration of acid-suppressive drugs, such as histamine-receptor antagonists or proton pump inhibitors, is required to prevent GI bleeding. Patients who develop pancreatic necrosis with infection may need broad-spectrum IV antibiotics such as imipenem, meropenem, or doripenem.

Since many cases of acute pancreatitis are associated with chronic alcohol use, hospitalization and cessation of alcohol use is required. During this time patients are at risk for alcohol withdrawal. Many hospitals have protocols that are used to screen for and manage alcohol withdrawal. This involves frequent monitoring of the patient's mental status and vital signs. Haloperidol may need to be administered for treatment of delirium or mental status changes. Patients may develop alcohol withdrawal seizures. Benzodiazepine drugs such as alprazolam, diazepam, or chlordiazepoxide are frequently administered to relieve most symptoms of alcohol withdrawal. Patients are also given IV multivitamins, folic acid, and thiamine to prevent complications related to deficiencies in vitamins. If the offending cause of the acute episode is removed, the patient should ultimately recover and be able to go home.

CHRONIC PANCREATITIS

Pain Management

Once patients develop chronic pancreatitis, drug treatment is used primarily to relieve symptoms, promote nutrient absorption, and treat diabetes. Chronic abdominal pain is the most common symptom that patients experience. Patients initially may experience intermittent episodes of intense abdominal pain. These episodes eventually increase in frequency and ultimately progress to continuous pain. Analgesics are commonly used for the management of pain in patients with chronic pancreatitis. The initial use of nonnarcotic medications, such as acetaminophen or nonsteroidal anti-inflammatory drugs (NSAIDs), is usually preferred. Unfortunately, most patients will not get adequate relief with these drugs.

Narcotics are often required to manage chronic pain. Patients should receive scheduled medications around

> **ALERT!**
>
> Patients who continue to drink alcohol may experience liver toxicity if they use acetaminophen and may also be at higher risk for GI bleeding if NSAIDs are used.

the clock, with additional doses of short-acting drugs for episodes of breakthrough pain. Morphine or oxycodone are commonly used and are available in both long-acting preparations that may require less frequent dosing and short-acting versions that can be used for breakthrough pain. Fentanyl is available as a patch that is administered once every 3 days (72 hours), but there is no corresponding oral preparation. Methadone is another oral option for long-term management. Less potent narcotics, such as tramadol, may also be tried. The use of long-term narcotics may be associated with dependence, constipation, nausea, and delayed gastric emptying. Patients may develop tolerance to narcotics, which may require increases in dosing over time. Patients may ultimately require nerve blocks to manage pain. The use of pancreatic enzymes may help to reduce pain as well as improve maldigestion and nutritional status.

Pancreatic Enzymes

One of the major complications of chronic pancreatitis is malnutrition. This is directly related to the loss of pancreatic enzyme secretion, or PEI. Lack of pancreatic enzyme activity in the GI tract leads to the inability to digest nutrients, a process known as maldigestion. Maldigestion leads to undigested food and nutrients being present within the GI tract in forms that cannot be absorbed. This is referred to as malabsorption. Normally, digestion of carbohydrates and starches starts upon ingestion, as amylase enzymes present in the saliva begin to break down these molecules. Other enzymes present in the intestinal tract break the molecules into smaller pieces that are readily absorbed in the small intestine. Protein digestion begins in the stomach following exposure to pepsin and gastric acid. Enzymes present in the intestinal wall further break the proteins into smaller molecules to be absorbed. The amylase and protease enzymes that are normally secreted by the pancreas contribute to this digestive process, but as pancreatic function declines, loss of pancreatic amylase and protease does not substantially impair the absorption of carbohydrates and proteins as these other digestive processes can compensate.

Unlike carbohydrates and proteins, up to 90% of fat absorption is facilitated by pancreatic lipases, and loss of pancreatic function significantly affects fat digestion. When pancreatic lipase falls too low, as happens in patients with chronic pancreatitis, fat cannot be digested and absorbed. This leads to loss of fat in the stool and the development of steatorrhea, as well as impaired absorption of fat-soluble vitamins. Another major contributor to maldigestion is the loss of pancreatic bicarbonate secretion. Pancreatic enzymes are normally secreted into the duodenum and require a local pH of least 5 in the GI tract to function properly. At a pH of below 5 pancreatic enzymes are inactivated and destroyed by the acid environment. Bicarbonate secretion from the pancreas normally helps neutralize the acidic contents of the stomach and allows the pancreatic enzymes to function appropriately. Since patients with chronic pancreatitis not only have a lack of enzymes but also a loss of bicarbonate secretion from the pancreas, the digestive and absorptive processes are shifted to further down in the small intestine, leading to faster passage of nutrients through the GI tract and further malabsorption.

To help correct maldigestion and malabsorption, pancreatic enzymes can be orally administered with ingested nutrients. This goal of pancreatic enzyme replacement is to simulate the normal digestive process as closely as possible by delivering the enzymes to the duodenum in close proximity to ingested nutrients.[12] This ultimately allows the patient to properly digest and absorb nutrients. Oral pancreatic enzyme replacement products are derived from pig pancreatic enzymes (also called pancrelipase) and, much like human enzymes, contain lipases, amylase, and protease. They are available as capsules containing enteric-coated mini-microspheres or micro-tablets, or as immediate-release tablets. Pancreatic enzyme products are discussed in depth in Chapter 19, as they relate to cystic fibrosis.

When initiating pancreatic enzyme replacement therapy for patients with chronic pancreatitis, approximately 40,000–50,000 units of lipase activity should be provided per standard adult meal.[12] In children, 500–2,500 units/kg of lipase activity per meal can be used. One-half the standard dose is often used for snacks. Therefore, capsules containing the appropriate amount of lipase activity should be used for each dose. Patients often require more than one capsule per meal. For instance, an adult patient requiring 40,000 units per meal could use two 20,000-unit capsules.

Once pancreatic enzyme therapy is initiated, the patient is monitored for reductions in steatorrhea and improvement in weight gain. Steatorrhea may be significantly reduced or even go away completely in some patients. The patient's enzyme dose can be adjusted based on the improvement in steatorrhea and the amount of weight gained. Pancreatic enzyme products are generally well tolerated. Patients

may experience diarrhea or constipation from the enzymes. At very high doses blood concentrations of uric acid may be elevated. Doses above the recommended maximum daily dose of 10,000 units/kg/day or 2,500 units/kg per meal have been associated with inflammation and scarring of the inside of the intestinal tract, a condition known as fibrosing colonopathy. This adverse effect is rare if doses are kept below this amount. If the patient is on an appropriate dose of enzymes and is not responding by gaining weight or having fewer symptoms related to steatorrhea, this may be potentially due to the pH in the duodenum being too low for the enteric-coated enzyme products to be released. In this case, the addition of an acid-suppressive drug, such as a proton pump inhibitor or histamine$_2$-receptor antagonist (as described in Chapter 20), may be added to the patient's regimen.[12]

One last effect that may be achieved by the use of pancreatic enzymes is pain relief. Pain in patients with chronic pancreatitis is thought to be partially due to continuous stimulation of the pancreas by a substance called cholecystokinin. A protein that causes release of cholecystokinin is secreted in the small intestine. This protein is normally destroyed by proteases that are released by the pancreas, so patients who lack proteases, such as those with chronic pancreatitis, are unable to slow the release of cholecystokinin. To restore the process of slowing cholecystokinin release, pancreatic enzymes must be delivered to the duodenum in their active, uncoated form. This necessitates the use of non-enteric-coated products. Thus, non-enteric-coated products may be used for patients with severe pain who have not responded to other medications. If non-enteric-coated products are used, administration of an acid-suppressive drug is required to help minimize destruction of the enzymes by gastric acid. It may not be practical to use non-enteric-coated enzymes, as enteric-coated products generally require administration of fewer capsules and generally result in better symptom improvement and weight gain.

Fat-Soluble Vitamins

Since a major component of chronic pancreatitis involves maldigestion and malabsorption of fat, patients are at risk for fat-soluble vitamin deficiency. Vitamin preparations that deliver adequate amounts of vitamins A, D, E, and K are required. This may be accomplished though the administration of tablet, capsule, or liquid formulations that are designed specifically to provide higher amounts of these vitamins (Medication Table 23-1; Medication Tables are located at the end of the chapter). These products also often contain other substances, such as B vitamins, folic acid, selenium, and coenzyme Q10. Liquid or chewable formulations may be preferred for children and patients who have difficulty swallowing. Some products are formulated to include different forms of some of the fat-soluble vitamins or may be formulated in a dose form that may enhance absorption. Since products differ in content in formulation, substitution of one for another may not be possible.

SUMMARY

Chronic liver disease and subsequent development of cirrhosis is most commonly caused by chronic alcohol abuse or viral hepatitis infection. Complications of cirrhosis can include variceal bleeding, SBP, ascites, and HE. Various drugs may be effective at treating and preventing the complications of cirrhosis but do not correct the underlying liver disease itself. Since patients may be on several medications to treat or prevent their complications, it is important that they know the appropriate ways to use the medications, as well as potential side effects that they may encounter. Likewise, certain medications have roles for use only in the hospital setting. Unfortunately, cirrhosis is largely irreversible.

Like cirrhosis, most cases of acute and chronic pancreatitis are due to chronic alcohol abuse. Drug management of acute pancreatitis is mostly supportive and involves removal of the underlying cause and treatment of symptoms such as pain and nausea. Once patients develop chronic pancreatitis, they lose both endocrine and exocrine function and develop chronic pain. The use of pain medications, such as narcotics, is almost always necessary to treat the chronic pain. Pancreatic enzymes are used orally to treat PEI by providing replacement enzymes to help food digestion. In some instances, the use of pancreatic enzymes may also help to improve pain. Patients may also require supplementation with fat-soluble vitamins. Unfortunately, chronic pancreatitis is irreversible, and patients will require long-term drug therapy.

REFERENCES

1. Asrani SK, Devarbhavi H, Eaton J, Kamath PS. Burden of liver diseases in the world. *J Hepatol*. 2019;70:151-171.
2. Mellinger JL, Shedden K, Winder GS, et al. The high burden of alcoholic cirrhosis in privately insured persons in the United States. *Hepatology*. 2018;68:872-882.
3. Ando Y, Jou JH. Nonalcoholic fatty liver disease and recent guideline updates. *Clin Liver Dis*. 2021;17(1):23-28.
4. Crabb DW, Im GY, Szabo G, et al. Diagnosis and treatment of alcohol-related liver diseases: 2019 practice guidance from the American Association for the Study of Liver Diseases. *Hepatology*. 2020;71(1):306-333. Doi: 10.1002/hep.30866.
5. Garcia-Tsao G, Abraldes JG, Berzigotti A, Bosch J. Portal hypertensive bleeding in cirrhosis: Risk stratification, diagnosis, and management—2016 practice guidance by the American Association for the Study of Liver Diseases. *Hepatology* 2017;65(1):310-335.
6. Biggins SW, Angeli P, Garcia-Tsao G, Ginès P, Ling SC, Nadim MK, Wong F, Kim WR. Diagnosis, evaluation, and management of ascites, spontaneous bacterial peritonitis and hepatorenal syndrome: 2021 practice guidance by the American Association for the Study of Liver Diseases. *Hepatology*. 2021;74:1014-1048. https://doi.org/10.1002/hep.31884
7. Angeli P, Bernardi M, Villanueva C, et al. EASL clinical practice guidelines for the management of patients with decompensated cirrhosis. *J Hepatol*. 2018;69(2):406-460.
8. Vistrup H, Amodio P, Bajaj J, et al. Hepatic encephalopathy in chronic liver disease: 2014 practice guideline by the American Association for the Study of Liver Diseases and the European Association for the Study of the Liver. *Hepatology*. 2014;60(2):715-735.
9. Crockett SD, Wani S, Gardner TB, et al. American Gastroenterological Association Institute guideline on initial management of acute pancreatitis. *Gastroenterol*. 2018;154:1096-1101.
10. Waller A, Long B, Koyfman A, Gottlieb M. Acute pancreatitis: Updates for emergency clinicians. *J Emerg Med*. 2018;55(6):769-779.
11. Barry K. Chronic pancreatitis: Diagnosis and treatment. *Am Fam Physician*. 2018;97(6):385-393.
12. Dominguez JE, Diagnosis and treatment of pancreatic exocrine insufficiency. *Curr Opin Gastroenterol*. 2018;34:349-354.
13. *AHFS Drug Information2021 Updates*. Bethesda, MD: American Society of Health-System Pharmacists; 2021.

CHAPTER RESOURCE

American Association of the Study of Liver Disease Practice Guidelines, https://www.aasld.org/publications/practice-guidelines.

REVIEW QUESTIONS

1. Which medication(s) would be preferred as initial therapy to help remove excess fluid in patients with ascites?

2. For a patient with hepatic encephalopathy caused by spontaneous bacterial peritonitis, which drug regimen would be prescribed as initial treatment for this infection? Why would these drugs be chosen?

3. Mr. Bradley requires administration of pancreatic enzymes to treat his malnutrition and malabsorption. What are the three major groups of enzymes found in pancreatic enzyme replacement products? What does each do?

4. How should Mr. Bradley be instructed to take his pancreatic enzyme replacement product?

5. Why do encapsulated pancreatic enzyme products require enteric coatings?

MEDICATION TABLE

MEDICATION TABLE 23-1. Representative Medications Used in the Management of Hepatic and Pancreatic Disorders[13a]

Class Generic Name	Brand Name	Generic	Rx	Usual Adult Dosage	Notes
Beta Blockers					
Carvedilol (kar-VE-dil-ol)	Coreg	X	X	3.125–25 mg twice daily	Non-selective agent with alpha receptor blocking properties
Propranolol (proe PRAN oh lole)	Inderal, Inderal LA, INNOPRAN XL	X	X	20–240 mg orally in divided doses	Nonselective agent; start with immediate release and then switch to long acting to improve adherence
Nadolol (NAY doe lole)	Corgard	X	X	20–320 mg orally in divided doses	Nonselective agent
Diuretics					
Furosemide (fyoor OH se mide)	Lasix	X	X	40–600 mg orally or IV in 2–3 divided doses	May cause low potassium and magnesium levels and dehydration
Spironolactone (spire on oh LAK tone)	Aldactone, Carospir	X	X	100–400 mg orally once daily	Potassium-sparing agent; may cause gynecomastia in male patients
Antibiotics (selected)					
Metronidazole (me troe NI da zole)	Flagyl	X	X	1,000–1,500 mg orally in 3-4 divided doses	Significant interaction with alcohol; may cause nausea and metallic taste; use 500-mg tablets
Rifaximin (ri FAX i men)	Xifaxan		X	1,100 mg orally in 2 divided doses	Poorly absorbed; much more expensive than other options; 200-mg or 550-mg tablets
Ceftriaxone (sef try AX one)	NA	X	X	1–2 g IV once daily	Dosed once daily; no adjustment for kidney disease; caution with severe penicillin allergy
Cefotaxime (sef oh TAKS eem)	NA	X	X	2–8 g IV in 2–3 divided doses	Need to adjust dose for severe kidney disease; caution with severe penicillin allergy
Other agents					
Octreotide (ok TREE oh tide)	Sandostatin	X	X	50 mcg/hr	Requires continuous IV infusion for 3–5 days; may cause hyperglycemia or hypoglycemia, constipation, and dizziness
25% Albumin (al BYOO min)	Various	X	X	1–1.5 g/kg or 6–8 g/L of fluid removed	Very expensive; indicated for SBP and large-volume paracentesis
Lactulose (LAK tyoo lose)	Enulose, Kristalose, Constulose	X	X	20–60 g 3–4 times daily	10 g/15 mL solution or 10-g or 20-g powder packet; may also be compounded as a retention enema (300 mL mixed with 700 mL water or saline)

Continued next page

MEDICATION TABLE 23-1. Representative Medications Used in the Management of Hepatic and Pancreatic Disorders[13a] *(Continued)*

Class Generic Name	Brand Name	Generic	Rx	Usual Adult Dosage	Notes
Pancreatic enzyme replacement products (selected)					
Pancrelipase (pan cre LI pase)	Creon		X	3,000 units per 120 ml formula (infants up to 12 months) Max of 2,500 units/kg/meal or 10,000 units/kg/day for ages great than 12 months	Capsules with enteric-coated spheres; 3,000, 6,000, 12,000, 24,000, 36,000 lipase units per capsule
	Pancreaze		X	2,600 units per 120 ml formula (infants up to 12 months) Max of 2,500 units/kg/meal or 10,000 units/kg/day for ages great than 12 months	Capsules containing enteric-coated microtablets; 2,600, 4,200, 10,500, 16,800, 21,000, 37,000 lipase unit strengths
	Zenpep		X	3,000 units per 120 ml formula (infants up to 12 months) Max of 2,500 units/kg/meal or 10,000 units/kg/day for ages great than 12 months	Capsules with enteric-coated beads; 3,000, 5,000, 10,000, 15,000, 20,000, 25,000, and 40,000 lipase unit strengths
	Pertzye		X	4,000 units per 120 ml formula (infants up to 12 months) Max of 2,500 units/kg/meal or 10,000 units/kg/day for ages great than 12 months	Capsules with bicarbonate-buffered enteric-coated microspheres; 4,000, 8,000, 16,000, 24,000 lipase units per capsule
	Viokace	X	X	500–2,500 units/kg per meal	Immediate-release tablet with 10,440 or 20,880 lipase units per tablet
Fat-soluble vitamins					
Multivitamin	DEKAs Essential	X		0.5 mL daily or 1 capsule daily	Liquid, capsules
	genADEKs			1–2 mL daily or 1–2 tablets daily	Liquid or softgel capsules
	MVW Complete		X	1–2 capsules or tablets daily, or 0.5–1 mL daily	Softgels, chewable tablets (bubblegum, grape, or orange), pediatric drops

IV = intravenous; NA = none available; SBP = spontaneous bacterial peritonitis.
[a]Pronunciations have been adapted with permission from USP Dictionary of USAN and International Drug Names (USP Dictionary) © 2022.

Chapter 24

Nutritional Pharmacology

*Steve W. Plogsted, PharmD, BCNSP, CNSC, FASPEN |
Mary Ann Stuhan, PharmD, RPh |
Julie Cunningham, MPH, RDN, LDN, CDCES, IBCLC*

KEY TERMS AND DEFINITIONS

Carbohydrates—nutrients made up of hydrogen and oxygen (in the same proportions as in water), along with carbon. They include sugar, starch, and fiber. The primary function of carbohydrates is to provide the most efficient fuel (energy) for the cells. Carbohydrates provide approximately 3.4–4 kcal/g.

Lipids—a group of substances composed of carbon, hydrogen, and oxygen, which includes fats, phospholipids, and cholesterol. Fats are considered nutrients. Composed of carbon, hydrogen, and oxygen, fats of all types are the most calorie-dense of the energy nutrients, supplying 9 kcal/g.

Malnutrition—a condition in which the body is not being provided the proper amounts of nutrients to sustain health. While this term is usually used for undernutrition (insufficient nutrients), it can also be applied to overnutrition, especially when excessive amounts of fat or calories are consumed.

Minerals—inorganic elements that are included in a variety of substances used for body processes. They come from the earth, soil, and water and are absorbed by plants. Humans obtain minerals from the plants and animals they eat.

DOI 10.37573/9781585286638.024

Nutrients—specific substances found in food that perform one or more physiological or biochemical functions in the body that are necessary to sustain health. There are six classifications of nutrients: carbohydrate, protein, lipids, vitamins, minerals, and water.

Nutrition—the provision of nutrients to the body to sustain its processes. Enteral nutrition is delivery of nutrients via the gastrointestinal tract. Parenteral nutrition is delivery of nutrients using the intravenous route of administration.

Proteins—the essential building blocks of the body, they are substances composed of combined chains of amino acids. Dietary proteins are digested so that the body can recombine the amino acids to form human proteins. Nutritionally, they provide 4 kcal/g.

Recommended Dietary Allowance (RDA)—the average daily dietary intake level that is sufficient to meet the nutrient requirement of most healthy individuals.

Vitamins—essential nutrients that are necessary for a variety of biological processes, including growth, digestion, and nerve function. They are needed in small amounts and must be obtained from external sources, as the body does not produce them.

LEARNING OBJECTIVES

After completing this chapter, you should be able to

1. Identify the vitamins and minerals necessary to the human body, their functions, and key food sources.

2. List the three energy nutrients and the calories they contribute to the dietary intake.

3. List some reasons why nutritional and vitamin supplementation may be necessary.

4. List the benefits and risks of vitamin supplementation.

5. Identify the components of nutrition support formulations.

6. Review the preparation and administration of nutrition support.

7. Discuss obesity and list approved medication therapies for this condition.

Good nutrition is vital to good health for all people and essential for the healthy growth and development of children and adolescents. Major causes of disease and death in the United States are related to poor diet. According to the Surgeon General of the United States, what we eat influences long-term health more than anything other than smoking and taking in excessive amounts of alcohol. Specific diseases and conditions linked to poor food choices include cardiovascular disease, hypertension, dyslipidemia, type 2 diabetes, obesity, osteoporosis, constipation, diverticular disease, iron deficiency anemia, oral disease, malnutrition, and some cancers.

People do not always take in all the nutrients they need, but fortunately healthy people have reserves that will get them through short bouts of poor food choices. In the United States, malnutrition from low vitamin and mineral intake does not pose a significant threat, but overweight and obesity are major nutrition problems. An energy imbalance (more calories taken in than used) due to poor food choices and limited physical inactivity are the primary factors contributing to the steady increase in obesity seen in the United States since the 1970s. Health risks related to overweight and obesity include several chronic diseases, such as diabetes, hypertension, and heart disease. More than 70% of U.S. adults are overweight and about 40% are obese.[1] The U.S. Departments of Agriculture and Health and Human Services have published dietary guidelines for Americans. These are federal government recommendations to promote health, reduce the risk of chronic diseases, and reduce the prevalence of overweight and obesity through improved nutrition and physical activity.

The general recommendations described in the Dietary Guidelines for Americans are:[2]

1. Follow a healthy eating pattern at every life stage to meet nutrient needs, help achieve a healthy body weight, and reduce the risk of chronic disease.

2. Customize and enjoy nutrient-dense food and beverage choices to reflect personal preferences, cultural traditions, and budgetary considerations.

3. Focus on meeting food group needs with nutrient-dense foods and beverages, and stay within calorie limits. The core elements that make up a healthy dietary pattern include:
   - Vegetables of all types—dark green; red and orange; beans, peas, and lentils; starchy; and other vegetables
   - Fruits, especially whole fruit
   - Grains, at least half of which are whole grain

- Dairy, including fat-free or low-fat milk, yogurt, and cheese, and/or lactose-free versions and fortified soy beverages and yogurt as alternatives
- Protein foods, including lean meats, poultry, and eggs; seafood; beans, peas, and lentils; and nuts, seeds, and soy products
- Oils, including vegetable oils and oils in food, such as seafood and nuts

4. Limit foods and beverages higher in added sugars, saturated fat, and sodium, and limit alcoholic beverages.

Specifically, "An underlying premise of the Dietary Guidelines is that nutritional needs should be met primarily from foods and beverages—specifically, nutrient-dense foods and beverages. Nutrient-dense foods provide vitamins, minerals, and other health-promoting components and have no or little added sugars, saturated fat, and sodium. A healthy dietary pattern consists of nutrient-dense forms of foods and beverages across all food groups, in recommended amounts, and within calorie limits."[2] The Guidelines also remind us that, "because foods provide an array of nutrients and other components that have benefits for health, nutritional needs should be met primarily through foods. Thus, the Dietary Guidelines translates the Academies' nutrient requirements into food and beverage recommendations. The Dietary Guidelines recognizes, though, that in some cases, fortified foods and dietary supplements are useful when it is not possible otherwise to meet needs for one or more nutrients (e.g., during specific life stages such as pregnancy)."[2] The amount of each nutrient sufficient to meet the daily needs of healthy individuals is known as the Recommended Dietary Allowance (RDA), although other, similar values include the newer Dietary Reference Intake (DRI).

CASE?

What foods are likely to be prohibited in Mrs. Broskie's weight loss plan?

CASE STUDY

The Broskies have just moved to a new home they built on farmland that has been in their family for three generations. Mr. and Mrs. Broskie are both 39 years old. He is a paramedic and works for the local fire department. Mrs. Broskie has a degree in elementary education. They have two sons, 15-year-old Hugh and 7-year-old Henry, and a daughter, 6-month-old Helen (who is still nursing). Mrs. Broskie has gained a lot of weight in the past few years, and she is considering going on a low-carb diet that limits many foods but lets her continue to have fried eggs and bacon for breakfast and eat her favorite foods, meat and cheese.

ENERGY NUTRIENTS

Carbohydrates, fat, and protein are the only nutrients that provide energy. Alcohol also provides calories, but it is not a nutrient. The measurement unit for energy is the calorie—the energy needed to increase the temperature of 1 mL of water by 1°C. That is such a small value that we consider the energy value of food in kilocalories (usually called Calories with a capital C, as listed on food nutrition labels). A kilocalorie is equal to 1000 calories, and is the energy necessary to raise the temperature of 1,000 mL of water by 1°C.

Carbohydrates

Carbohydrates include sugar, starch, and fiber. Carbohydrates are made up of carbon, hydrogen, and oxygen. *Carbo* means carbon and *hydrate* means water. Dietary carbohydrates are estimated to provide 4 kilocalories (kcal or Calories, with a capital C) per gram ("/g") and intravenous (IV) dextrose infusions are calculated at 3.4 kcal/g. The primary function of carbohydrate is to provide the most efficient fuel (energy) for the cells. A small amount of carbohydrate energy can be stored in the body in the form of glycogen. The energy is used for body movement but also for every process that takes place and by every cellular function. Complex carbohydrates (starch) are broken down to simple ones (sugars, usually glucose) in the body by digestive enzymes so they can circulate in the blood and reach every cell.

Simple carbohydrates consist of monosaccharides and disaccharides. These are commonly known as sugar and include not only table sugar (sucrose, a disaccharide), but also the sugars found in milk (lactose) and fruit and vegetable sources (fructose). Blood sugar is a monosaccharide called glucose (also known as dextrose). Glucose can be eaten in food or beverage, but it is also made by the body. Simple sugars are also bound together to form the polysaccharides. Food sources for simple carbohydrates include table sugar, honey, syrups, sweets, candy, soda, and other sweetened beverages.

Complex carbohydrates include starch, which is composed of long chains of simple sugars (polysaccharides), and fiber, which is made up of monosaccharides. Fiber cannot be digested by humans but plays an important role in maintaining digestive health. Good food sources for starch include breads and cereals from wheat, rice, oats, and barley, and starchy vegetables like corn, peas, legumes (kidney beans, navy beans, black beans, etc.), and potatoes. Good food sources for fiber are whole grains, seeds, nuts, vegetables, and fruits. There is no RDA for carbohydrates, but the recommendation is that, for healthy individuals, 45% to 65% of total calories should come from carbohydrates and that not more than 10% of total calories should come from added sugars.[2]

PRACTICE POINT

A 12-ounce can of sugar-sweetened (nondiet) soda contains 33 g of sugar.

CASE?

What macronutrients will be replacing the carbohydrates Mrs. Broskie has eliminated from her diet?

Lipids

Lipids are a group of substances that includes fats, phospholipids, and cholesterol, as well as other types of substances not relevant to nutrition. Lipids, like carbohydrates, are composed of carbon, hydrogen, and oxygen. The fats are considered nutrients; cholesterol and phospholipids are not. Humans make both cholesterol and phospholipids, so they do not need to acquire them from food. Fats of all types are the most calorie-dense of the energy nutrients, supplying 9 kcal (Calories)/g.

Saturated Fats

Saturated fats are those that are solid at room temperature (except for coconut and palm oils). Chemically, the saturated fats contain long chains of fatty acids whose carbon bonds are fully taken up and no hydrogen can be introduced.

Unsaturated Fats

Unsaturated fats are liquid at room temperature and are divided into polyunsaturated (more than one double bond with carbons that can take up hydrogen) and monounsaturated fats (only one double bond).

Trans Fats

Trans fats are found in nature, but the majority of dietary trans fats are found in foods that have been chemically modified. The production of trans fat requires adding hydrogen to polyunsaturated fats (liquid oils) under pressure. This makes the oils into a soft solid (stick margarine is one example). Trans fats were widely found in processed foods until recently when, due to their propensity to contribute to cardiovascular disease, the processed food manufacturers were forced to state the amount of trans fat on the nutrition facts label. Since then, trans fats have been removed from or included in significantly lower amounts in many foods.

Triglycerides

Triglycerides are the common form of fat found in food and in the body, either stored as body fat or circulating in the blood. Chemically, they have a glycerol base (a three-carbon "skeleton") on which three fatty acids, usually a combination of saturated and unsaturated fatty acids, are attached.

Phospholipids

Phospholipids are widely dispersed in foods as well as made by the human body. They are not essential nutrients although they are a component of cell membranes and supply fatty acids for cellular metabolism, blood clotting, and cellular regeneration. The structure of a phospholipid is similar to a triglyceride, but one of the fatty acids has been replaced with one of several phosphorus-containing compounds.

Cholesterol

Cholesterol is made by animals and humans (but not plants). It is a component of cell membranes, hormones (including sex hormones, cortisol, and others), and bile. It is not a nutrient because the body can manufacture it. It cannot be utilized to produce energy because it has a different structure than fatty acids.

Lipids are necessary structural components of many body parts, as well as necessary body substances such as hormones. Each body cell contains fat as a part of the cell membrane. There is a layer of fat under the skin that helps regulate body temperature by keeping heat in during exposure to cold. The same layer of fat cushions a person against minor bruises. Fats provide a source of stored energy because they can be converted to glucose when necessary.

Fat in foods plays a role in the pleasure acquired from eating, as fat carries flavor, odor, and mouth feel. Fat is also the last foodstuff to empty from the stomach. Since it stays in the gut longer, it creates a feeling of fullness that signals a person to stop eating and indicates that one is satisfied with the meal.

Lipids are not soluble in water and do not mix with water or blood. In the blood, lipids must have a protein wrap to be transported through the bloodstream. They are then called lipoproteins. In food, lipids gravitate to the top of any mixture containing water. To mix lipids and water, one must use an emulsifier that suspends small particles of lipid throughout the solution. Within the digestive system, bile acts as an emulsifier. It suspends small particles of fat throughout the digestive contents and allows the fat particles to be absorbed. Without bile, fat particles would clump together and most fat would not be absorbed.

Two of the polyunsaturated fatty acids are essential nutrients. These are alpha-linolenic acid (an omega-3 fatty acid) and linoleic acid (an omega-6 fatty acid). Alpha-linolenic acid is used by the body to make eicosapentaenoic acid (EPA) and docosahexaenoic acid (DHA). Linolenic acid is used by the body to make arachidonic acid (AA). EPA, DHA, and AA are then used to make prostaglandins that promote a response to inflammation, control blood pressure, cause uterine contractions, and more. Essential fatty acids are necessary for growth. Infants with too low an intake of essential fatty acids can have multiple physical problems.

Although there is no RDA for fats, studies suggest an amount labeled *Adequate Intake* (AI) for the essential fatty acids. The AI for alpha-linolenic acid is 1.6 g/day for men and 1.1 g/day for women. The AI for linoleic acid is 17 g/day for men and 12 g/day for women. The recommendation for cholesterol is to limit intake to 300 mg or less per day regardless of gender or caloric intake.[3]

Protein

Protein provides 4 kcal/g. Compared to carbohydrates and fats, proteins are unique. Like carbohydrates and fats, they are composed of carbon, hydrogen, and oxygen; however, protein adds nitrogen, which is an element that all cells need to make key biological compounds and structural components. Proteins are formed from groups of amino acids. (*Amino* means nitrogen containing.) There are 20 basic amino acids that the body uses to build structure, and of those nine are essential, meaning they must be obtained from food sources. The nine essential amino acids are tryptophan, threonine, valine, histidine, isoleucine, leucine, lysine, methionine, and phenylalanine. Proteins containing all nine of the essential amino acids are known as *complete* or *high quality*. Animal products (meat, fish, milk, eggs, cheese, yogurt, and some fortified food products) are complete proteins. Incomplete *(low quality)* proteins are those lacking one or more essential amino acids. Incomplete proteins are found in plant products (vegetables, grains, legumes, seeds, and nuts).

Proteins are the building blocks of the body (the brick and mortar of the structure) and the substance in enzymes, hormones, and antibodies. Proteins are the transport vehicles for nutrients, oxygen, waste, and more throughout the body. It is the basis for bones, skin, muscles, connective tissue, and more.

Vegetarians exclude some or all forms of animal protein. Vegetarians are classified by the protein sources they choose to eat. Those who avoid meat, fish, and poultry but will eat eggs and dairy are lacto-ovo vegetarians. They will get all their essential amino acids. Vegans take in no animal products (including foods produced by an animal, such as milk or eggs). A vegan must be careful to consume grains with legumes or legumes as well as seeds or nuts to obtain all of the essential amino acids required by the body. Just as an omnivore (person who eats both plant and animal products) must eat a balanced diet to get all of the nutrients, so must a vegan balance intake to take in the proper amount of nutrients. Both omnivores and vegans can have very healthy diets, and both can choose unwisely and have diets that are not health enhancing.

The RDA for protein is 0.8 g/kg of body weight. This translates to 360 mg per pound of body weight. A 156-pound (70-kg) person would need 56 g of protein per day. Because the protein recommendation is based on body weight, it cannot be included in the Nutrition Facts Panel on food labels. The energy nutrients are summarized in Table 24-1.

CASE?

What vitamins may Mrs. Broskie be losing by eliminating carbohydrate-rich foods from her meals?

TABLE 24-1. Energy Nutrients

Nutrient	Energy Factor	Type	Dietary Sources	Notes
Carbohydrates	4 kcal/g (3.4 kcal/g for IV dextrose)	Simple	Table sugar, honey, syrups, sweets, candy, soda, and other sweetened beverages	
		Complex		
		Starch	Breads and cereals from wheat, rice, oats, and barley; starchy vegetables like corn, peas, legumes (kidney beans, navy beans, black beans, etc.), and potatoes	
		Fiber	Whole grains, seeds, nuts, vegetables, and fruits	
Fat	9 kcal/g	Saturated fat	Animal sources (milk, butter, cheese, beef fat, pork fat, lard) and tropical oils (coconut and palm oil)	Except for the tropical oils, saturated fats are solid at room temperature
		Unsaturated fat	Monounsaturated fats: olive oil, canola oil, peanut oil Polyunsaturated fats: sunflower oil, safflower oil, soybean oil, corn oil	Liquid at room temperature
		Trans fat	Processed foods	These are not necessary to the diet and should be avoided
		Triglycerides	Processed foods	
		Phospholipids	Eggs, liver, peanuts, wheat germ, dairy products	Lecithin is a common phospholipid often added to processed foods as a stabilizer; there is no health benefit to supplementing the diet with lecithin powder
Protein	4 kcal/g		Meat, fish, milk, eggs, cheese, yogurt, legumes, seeds, nuts	The legumes (beans) have more protein than other plant foods; a combination of grains and legumes can be used as a meat substitute

Vitamins

Vitamins are essential nutrients needed in small amounts that are necessary to achieve a healthy, productive life. Vitamins are necessary for a variety of biological processes, including growth, digestion, and nerve function. There are 13 vitamins that the body absolutely needs from external sources: vitamins A, C, D, E, K, and the B vitamins (thiamine, riboflavin, niacin, pantothenic acid, biotin, vitamin B6, vitamin B12, and folate). Although most people get all the vitamins they need from the foods they eat, some cannot obtain optimal nutritional intake for a variety of reasons (such as intestinal malabsorption syndromes) and must rely on supplemental vitamins to achieve a good nutritional intake.

Fat-Soluble Vitamins

Fat-soluble vitamins include vitamins A, D, E, and K. They are absorbed into the body with the help of bile acids, which are made in the liver, and in the presence of dietary fat. People who have impaired digestive systems or who have too low an intake of fat may have deficiencies of these vitamins and require supplementation. Vitamins A and D work together in calcium metabolism and bone health, so they are often administered together in combination products. The fat-soluble vitamins, with their characteristics, uses, food sources, and drug interactions are listed in Medication Table 24-1 (Medication Tables are located at the end of the chapter).

ALERT!

The body stores fat-soluble vitamins for use as needed, but if people take in too much of these nutrients, they can accumulate and cause toxicity in the long term.

Water-Soluble Vitamins and Nutrients: B Vitamins, Vitamin C, and Choline

Although water-soluble vitamins are easily absorbed by the body, they are not stored in significant amounts the way the fat-soluble vitamins are. The kidneys can usually remove the excess water-soluble vitamins from dietary or supplemental sources. The B vitamins have a wide and varied range of functions in the human body, but their primary function is to facilitate the process of converting blood sugar into energy.

B-vitamin deficiencies are uncommon in the United States, but when they occur, they usually involve several B vitamins, since many of them come from the same food groups. Alcohol interferes with the absorption of these vitamins, and some of the physical and mental problems that alcoholics experience may be attributed to a deficiency of B vitamins. Elderly people are also at risk for deficiencies because of inadequate diets and the possible interference with B-vitamin absorption by medications. Deficiencies can occur in severely malnourished people or in those receiving long-term dialysis or IV feeding. The water-soluble vitamins, with their characteristics, uses, and food sources are listed in Medication Table 24-1.

PRACTICE POINT

Because the B vitamins are water soluble and eliminated in the urine, toxic reactions from oral administration of most B vitamins are extremely rare (exceptions are niacin and vitamin B6.)

CASE?

When the Broskies moved to the country and started using well water, Helen's pediatrician wrote a prescription for a vitamin supplement drop to replace the over-the-counter product recommended when she was born. What is in this new supplement that Helen didn't need when she lived in the city?

Minerals

Minerals are inorganic elements that come from the earth, soil, and water and are absorbed by plants. Humans obtain minerals from the plants and the animal products they eat. Minerals are not destroyed by food processing or food storage methods. Minerals are categorized according to the amounts present in the normal human body. Major minerals (macrominerals) are present in amounts greater than 5 g. Trace minerals (minor minerals, trace elements) are present in quantities less than 5 g. The mineral nutrients, with their characteristics, uses, and food sources are listed in Table 24-2.

TABLE 24-2. Minerals[3]

Mineral	Functions	Food Sources	Adult Dietary Reference Intake (DRI) (male/female aged 31-50 years)	Deficiency	Toxicity	Notes
Major Minerals						
Calcium	Maintain and grow healthy bones and teeth, nerve conduction, muscle contraction, blood clotting, production of energy, immunity to disease	Dairy products, seafood, green leafy vegetables, meat, eggs	1,000 mg/day (TUI 2,500 mg/day)	Muscle weakness, bone pain, osteoporosis	Calcification of soft tissue (frequently the kidneys)	Most abundant mineral in the body
Phosphorus	Maintain strong bones, all cell functions, cell membranes	Dairy products, fish, meats, poultry, soda	700 mg/day (TUI 4,000 mg/day)	Inability to utilize calcium	Electrolyte imbalances	
Magnesium	Part of every major biologic process, use of glucose in the body, synthesis of nucleic acids and protein, cellular energy	Green leafy vegetables, fish, nuts	420 mg/day male 320 mg/day female (TUI 350 mg/day)	Electrolyte imbalances, heart failure, neuromuscular symptoms	Flushing, sweating, CNS depression, cardiac abnormalities	Toxicity can occur with excess supplementation or from magnesium in laxatives and antacids; magnesium is used in pregnant women suffering from eclampsia
Sodium	Maintaining body's fluid and electrolyte balance, muscle contraction	Table salt, processed foods, canned foods, cured meats, fast food	1,500 mg/day	Fatigue, nausea/vomiting, muscle weakness, mental status changes (confusion, hallucination, coma)	Edema, high blood pressure	It is generally recommended that sodium intake be limited to 2,000 mg per day but no TUI has been determined
Chloride	Maintaining body's fluid and electrolyte balances, part of hydrochloric acid in the stomach	Table salt, processed foods, meat, dairy, eggs	2,300 mg/day (TUI 3,600 mg/day)	Dehydration or fluid loss may be noted, but many patients will have no symptoms	Vomiting	
Potassium	Part of many major biologic processes, muscle contraction, nerve impulses, synthesis of nucleic acids and protein, energy production	Fresh vegetables, fresh fruits	3,400 mg/day male 2,600 mg/day female	Irregular heartbeat, glucose intolerance	Vomiting, weakness, cardiac arrhythmia	TUI not determined
Trace Minerals						
Chromium	Insulin utilization and glucose tolerance	Whole grains, meats, brewer's yeast	35 mcg/day male 25 mcg/day female	Glucose intolerance	Kidney impairment	TUI not determined

Continued next page

TABLE 24-2. Minerals[3] (Continued)

Mineral	Functions	Food Sources	Adult Dietary Reference Intake (DRI) (male/female aged 31-50 years)	Deficiency	Toxicity	Notes
Trace Minerals						
Copper	Part of iron absorption and incorporation into hemoglobin, necessary for melanin formation and maintaining myelin sheaths	Seafood, nuts, whole grains	900 mcg/day (TUI 10 mg/day)	Anemia also causes neutropenia	Liver damage, psychoses	
Fluoride	Binding calcium in bones and teeth	Fluoridated water	4 mg/day male 3 mg/day female (TUI 10 mg/day)	Dental decay	Changes in teeth and bone, CNS abnormalities, heart failure	Fluoride supplements and multivitamins with fluoride are used to provide adequate amounts of this nutrient for children who drink primarily well water or in areas where water is not fluoridated
Iodine	Part of thyroid hormones that help regulate energy metabolism, growth, and development	Seafood, iodized salt, plants grown in iodine-rich soil	150 mcg/day (TUI 1,100 mcg/day)	Goiter, cretinism (mental retardation and poor physical growth in infants)	Zinc hyper- or hypothyroidism, GI irritation	
Iron	Hemoglobin synthesis and function; production of collagen, elastin, neurotransmitters; melanin formation	Meats, fish, poultry, eggs, dried fruit	8 mg/day male 18 mg/day female (TUI 45 mg/day)	Iron deficiency anemia, fatigue, weakness	GI impairment, organ damage	Absorbed better in the presence of vitamin C; poorly absorbed in the presence of calcium
Manganese	Part of several enzymes, bone development	Whole grains, leafy green vegetables, nuts	2.3 mg/day male 1.8 mg/day female (TUI 11 mg)	Enzyme malfunction	CNS abnormalities	
Molybdenum	Part of several enzymes	Liver, cereals, nuts, legumes	45 mcg/day (TUI 2,000 mcg/day)	Enzyme malfunction	Liver damage	
Selenium	Antioxidant, thyroid hormone regulator	Seafood, meat, whole grains, eggs	55 mcg/day (TUI 400 mcg/day)	Heart disease	Brittle nails, hair loss, rash, fatigue, garlic breath odor	
Zinc	Immunity and healing, good eyesight, involved with numerous enzymes	Whole grains, brewer's yeast, fish, meats, enriched cereals	11 mg/day male 8 mg/day female (TUI 40 mg/day)	Impaired growth and maturation, diminished immune response, loss of appetite	Low HDL, decreased taste and smell, hair loss	Zinc supplements have been used to treat colds and promote wound healing but are not FDA approved for these indications

CNS = central nervous system; FDA = U.S. Food and Drug Administration; GI = gastrointestinal; HDL = high density lipoprotein; TUI = Tolerable Upper Intake Level.

Supplements

Supplements are only useful when they fill a specific identified nutrient gap that cannot be or is not otherwise being met by the individual's intake of food. Nutrient supplements cannot replace a healthy diet. Individuals who are already consuming the recommended amount of a nutrient in food will not gain any health benefit if they also take the nutrient as a supplement. It is important to note that supplements and fortified foods may cause intakes to exceed the safe levels of nutrients. Nutrients taken in as supplements are actually drugs and no longer considered nutrition.

PRACTICE POINT

Dietary studies have shown that the following nutrients are most likely to be deficient in the American diet for adults: calcium, choline, potassium, fiber, magnesium, and vitamins A (as carotenoids), C, D, and E. Iron also is under-consumed by many adolescent girls and women aged 19 to 50 years.

Individual vitamins and minerals are sometimes prescribed by physicians to treat specific patient problems or issues. Alcoholics, for example, often receive thiamin to relieve deficiencies; folic acid supplements are recommended to all women of childbearing age to prevent birth defects; and some patients with anemia may need iron. Pediatricians may prescribe fluoride-enhanced vitamins for children who drink primarily well water or live in areas where the water is not fluoridated. Some ophthalmologists recommend a multivitamin high in antioxidant vitamins and zinc to prevent age-related eye issues. Those who are on restricted diets or otherwise unable to fulfill their nutritional needs through normal food sources may also be candidates for supplementation. Sometimes medication therapies deplete vitamins and minerals, making supplements necessary or advisable in combination with those medications. Examples of these are listed in the drug/nutrient interactions column in Medication Table 24-1.

CASE?

Mr. Broskie has an artificial heart valve and takes warfarin to prevent a blood clot. What vitamin in some supplements might interfere with his therapy?

Many patients choose to take a nonprescription vitamin supplement for a variety of reasons, some better than others. These include those who take a multivitamin product for insurance against nonspecific vitamin deficiencies or hoping to prevent disease. Others select specific vitamins to supplement, based on claims in popular literature or Internet sources. The National Institutes of Health's position is that people who might benefit from multiple vitamin and mineral supplementation include postmenopausal women (calcium with vitamin D), women of childbearing age (folic acid), people over the age of 50 (vitamin B12), pregnant women (iron), and breastfed infants (vitamin D), as well as those with poor dietary nutrient intake, patients on restricted (eg, vegan) or low-calorie diets, and those with medical conditions that interfere with the absorption or use of nutrients.[4] The American Academy of Pediatrics recommends a supplement of 400 IU of vitamin D daily for all partially and exclusively breastfed infants, as well as infants who consume less than 1 L of fortified infant formula per day.[5]

Since many multiple vitamin supplements contain the full recommended dietary allowance of several ingredients, it is possible that people who take them regularly could exceed the recommended maximum levels for those nutrients. Additionally, some vitamin supplements can interfere with medication therapy. (Examples of these are listed in the drug/nutrient interactions column in Medication Table 24-1.) Many patients, thinking that vitamins are natural and, therefore, harmless, are not aware of this issue and should be directed to seek the advice of the physician or pharmacist before choosing a supplement.

PRACTICE POINT

Patient profiles should list not only prescription preparations the patients are taking, but also over-the-counter products, including vitamins, dietary supplements, and herbals as well. As many people do not consider these to be medications, they will not mention that they take these products, so they should be specifically asked about them at the same time they are asked about their medications, and they should be advised to mention supplements to their physicians.

CASE?

Hugh Broskie is on the track team at his high school and wants to be sure he is getting enough vitamins. Mrs. Broskie has a leftover supply of her prenatal vitamins and thinks Hugh should use those up before spending a lot of money on the stress-formula tablets his teammates are taking. Should they talk to the pharmacist about this? What issues do you think are involved?

There are so many supplements and combinations available, both brand and generic, on pharmacy shelves, in grocery and convenience stores, and on the Internet that listing all would be impractical. A representative sampling is included in Table 24-3. The Academy of Nutrition and Dietetics and the National Institutes of Health recommend that consumers take care in choosing over-the-counter (OTC) vitamin supplements. Many available supplements have ingredients that could interact with patients' conditions or other therapies. More is not necessarily better; often supplements can be harmful when taken in high amounts, for a long time, or in combination with certain other substances. Consumers should evaluate whether the product is worth the cost.

Many supplements are quite expensive and may not offer the expected effect. This is especially true of water-soluble vitamins (B vitamins and vitamin C) that the body does not store and excretes the excess. The medical team should be made aware of any and all supplements being taken as some can cause inaccurate medical test results or alter the effect of medications.

CASE STUDY

Henry Broskie is 7 years old and weighs 21 kg (46 lb). He was normal at birth, but at 2 years of age he started to experience problems with swallowing food so a gastrostomy tube (GT) was placed and he was started on PediaSure feedings. When he was 4, he had bowel surgery and received parenteral nutrition until tube feedings could be restarted. The PediaSure was restarted slowly and while the volume was advancing, he showed signs of formula intolerance (intestinal pain and diarrhea). The formula was changed to Peptamen Junior, which he seemed to tolerate.

TABLE 24-3. Representative Multiple Vitamin Supplements[8]

Category	Brand Name	Nutrients	Target/Purpose
Daily multivitamin	Flintstones, One A Day	All or most of the recognized vitamins, generally at levels close to the Recommended Dietary Allowances (RDAs)	Formulations for children, adults, men, women, pregnant women, and seniors typically provide different amounts of the same vitamins and minerals based on the reported specific needs of these groups
Multivitamins with minerals	Centrum, Theragran-M	All or most of the recognized vitamins and minerals, generally at levels close to the RDAs	
Multivitamins with fluoride	Poly-Vi-Flor, Floriva, Tri-Vi-Flor	Similar to daily multivitamins, with 0.25-1 mg fluoride per dose	Supplement for children living in areas where drinking water is not fluoridated (prescription only)
Stress-formula vitamins	StressTabs, BioStress, Super B-complex	Water-soluble vitamins (B and C) in doses 2-10 times the RDA, sometimes with minerals, fish oil, or other additives	Marketed to people with stressful or active lives; could cause overdoses
Renal formula vitamins	Nephro-Vite RX, Nephroplex	B and C vitamins at RDA levels with additional B6, folate, and biotin	Patients with chronic kidney disease
Prenatal vitamins	Foltabs, CitraNatal Rx	Multiple vitamins with higher doses of folate and calcium and often zinc, copper, and/or iodine	Pregnant women; high folate products are RX only

NUTRITION SUPPORT

Nutrition is the provision of nutrients to the body and is necessary to sustain life. While it is recommended that people get their nutrition from consuming a healthy diet of nutrient-rich foods, sometimes illness and disease make this an unrealistic or impossible goal. When a person cannot eat at all or is unable to consume an adequate quantity of food due to an adverse physical condition, additional nutrition must be supplied in a different way. Nutrition support is the provision of oral, enteral, or parenteral nutrients to treat or prevent malnutrition in patients who are unable to fulfill their nutritional needs by consuming food for reasons including, but not limited to, illness, decreased appetite, difficulty swallowing, or surgery that interferes with eating. Nutrition support can enhance the rate of recovery from certain conditions and enable sustained life in others. Nutrition support includes, among other means, the provision of total enteral or parenteral nutrition support and therapeutic nutrients to maintain or restore optimal nutrition status and health. The amount, type, and route of nutrition support are tailored specifically to each patient, with the goal being to improve patient outcomes, minimize infections, and allow patients to live their lives as normally as possible.

Enteral Nutrition

Enteral nutrition (EN) provides nutrition via tube feedings or by mouth into the digestive tract. In most healthcare settings, however, the terms enteral nutrition and tube feeding are used synonymously. EN can be administered through different types of tubes. Feeding tubes can be placed in many ways, for example, through the nose into the stomach (nasogastric, NG) or intestines (nasoenteral), or may be placed via incision into the stomach (gastrostomy, GT or PEG) or intestine (jejunostomy). EN or tube feeding is a mixture of the energy nutrients (carbohydrate, fat, and protein), vitamins, and minerals in liquid form. Usually a commercial liquid nutrient product is used.

ALERT!

Tube feedings can also be homemade, but that is not recommended for sanitary reasons, as well as the potential for tube clogging of homemade feedings.

Supplemental nutrition refers to the use of liquid nutrient mixtures in addition to a person's diet. The person may be able to eat but not enough to provide adequate nutrition. This could be due to poor appetite (anorexia), extreme weakness due to illness, or an increased need for calories and nutrients beyond what a normal diet can provide. When increasing the nutritional intake is necessary, the first step should always be to add additional foods at or between meals if tolerated. Supplemental nutrition is generally given by mouth rather than via tube. Many people can tolerate liquids better than solids and for many the liquid nutrition can be milk, milkshakes, or instant breakfast drinks. Sometimes it is necessary to use commercial liquid nutrient products. When clinicians select an EN product, they consider the osmolarity of the product. Osmolarity is defined as the number of particles in solution. Different parts of the gastrointestinal tract have different tolerances to the osmolar load that is associated with the various enteral products. For example, a product that is intended strictly for gastric feeding may not be tolerated when administered directly into the jejunum.

In addition to supplemental products primarily administered by mouth to patients who are eating but unable to consume enough to satisfy their nutritional needs, there are four types of commercial nutrient products: modular, intact or polymeric, elemental (predigested), and disease-specific formulas.

CASE?

Use Table 24-3 to compare nutrition formulations. Why might Peptamen Junior be working better for Henry than PediaSure?

Modular formulas consist of one nutrient and are used for people who only need supplementation of one or two of the energy nutrients. They are supplied in liquid form or as a powder to be added to foods, beverages, or other types of oral supplements. Polycose, for instance, has only carbohydrates, while ProMod is considered a protein product with added carbohydrate. Pro-Phree, by contrast, contains no protein, supplying all of its calories from carbohydrate and fat. Examples of lipid products are Microlipid and medium chain triglyceride (MCT) oil.

Intact (polymeric) formulas are used when the person has a functioning gastrointestinal tract, but nutritional intake is limited to a specific volume. These liquid nutrient products must contain all of the nutrients the person needs. They may be used orally or as a tube feeding. These products vary widely. Some products are in the form of pudding, some are lactose free or contain fiber, and some are strictly for use as tube feedings and are not flavored for oral use. The common goal of all of them is to provide a source of complete nutrition.

Elemental (predigested) feedings are formulated for persons with impaired gastrointestinal function or with metabolic disorders. These are intended as tube feedings and are seldom used for oral feedings because of taste issues. Elemental formulas vary, but most have had one or more energy nutrient treated with enzymes to compensate for insufficient amounts of digestive enzymes in the gut. In some products, some portions of an energy nutrient may be absent. Lactose (milk sugar) is frequently kept out of an elemental product. Protein may be pretreated partially or totally to allow absorption of amino acids. Fats that are used may be either those that are easier to absorb or partially digested.

ALERT!

Because of their ingredients and osmolarity considerations, tube feeding products are not uniformly interchangeable, in spite of having similar names. Technicians involved in dispensing these products must be conscious of the differences and be sure to select the correct one ordered for the patient.

Disease-specific formulas are most often used for diseases of the liver, respiratory system, and kidneys. Examples of disease-specific products are Hepatic Aid (liver), Pulmocare (respiratory), and Nepro (kidney). Representative formulations of each type mentioned are listed in Table 24-4, with their caloric density, energy nutrient composition, and osmolarity for comparison.

Adverse effects of EN can occur because of incorrect ordering, administration, or monitoring. The liquid nutrient solution should be selected by a clinician and quantified based on the person's individual nutrition needs. One size fits all is not appropriate. Dietitians should carefully monitor each patient's nutrition and electrolyte status.

Parenteral Nutrition

Parenteral nutrition (PN) supplies nutrients to the body when the stomach and intestines are not working or no longer present, or the patient is unable to meet nutritional demands enterally. PN consists of a sterile nutrient liquid that is administered intravenously, directly into the bloodstream. Consisting of protein and energy nutrients, vitamins, and minerals and adequate fluid, PN has also historically been referred to as total parenteral nutrition (TPN) or total nutrient admixture (TNA).

CASE?

A case of Peptamen Junior costs the Broskies more than $150, and Henry's medical bills are really stretching their budget. There is currently a deal on Peptamen 1.5 for about 10% less. Should Mrs. Broskie get that for Henry this month instead? Why or why not?

PRACTICE POINT

When parenteral nutrition was first developed it was called hyperalimentation, but this term is no longer used.

An IV nutrition solution can be administered through a peripheral vein or a central vein. The back of the hand or in the forearm area is the location where an IV catheter is placed for peripheral administration. It is easy to insert and requires minimal skill; the catheter doesn't travel too far from the insertion site. This type of insertion is used mainly for short-term access. Since the veins are small and the rate of blood flow past the catheter is relatively slow, they are prone to failing when high dextrose concentrations are infused. The veins also do not tolerate high concentrations of electrolytes. Dextrose concentrations greater than 10% are often not tolerated peripherally, and veins can become irritated or damaged when concentrations are too high. In these cases, a central catheter must be used for PN administration. There are several types, but they share one important feature. The tip of the catheter usually rests directly above the right atrium in the superior vena cava. This is a large vein that enjoys a high blood flow rate, which produces a dilution effect on the concentrated solutions. When a physician orders a PN, there is usually a place on the order form where peripheral or central access is indicated.

TABLE 24-4. Representative Enteral Nutrition Products[13]

Product	Type	Caloric Density (kcal/mL)	Osmolarity (mOsm/mL)	Protein (% of Total)	Carbohydrate (% of Total)	Fat (% of Total)
Polycose	Modular	3.8 kcal/g used	1.6/g used	0	100	0
Pro-Phree	Modular	5.1 kcal/g used	205	0	50.8	49.2
MCT oil	Modular	7.7 kcal/mL	NA	0	0	100
Tolerex	Elemental	1	550	8.2	90.5	1.3
Vivonex TEN	Elemental	1	630	15	82	3
Jevity	Standard	1.06	300	17	54	29
Nutren	Standard	1	300	16	51	33
Jevity 1.2, Fibersource HN	Standard	1.2	450	19	53	29
Nutren 2, TwoCal HN	Standard	2	746	16	39	45
Peptamen, Vital HN	Semi-elemental	1	270	16	51	33
Peptamen 1.5, Vital 1.5	Semi-elemental	1.5	550	18	49	33
Nutren Pulmonary, Pulmocare	Pulmonary	1.5	330	18	27	55
Nutrihep, Hepatic Aid II	Hepatic	1.5	790	11	77	12
Abbott, Nepro	Renal	1.8	960	17	35	48
Glucerna 1.0	Diabetic	1	355	17	34	49
Glucerna 1.5	Diabetic	1.5	875	22	33	48
Oxepa	Immune	1.5	535	17	28	55
Kindercal TF	Pediatric	1.06	290	11	51	38
PediaSure	Pediatric	1	278	12	44	44
Peptamen Junior	Pediatric	1.06	255	12	54	34
Carnation Instant Breakfast	Supplement	1	480	14	51	35
Boost	Supplement	1	625	17	67	16

MCT = medium chain triglyceride; NA = not available.

CASE?

Henry's bowel is diseased, and he must have surgery to remove a large portion of it. He will no longer be able to absorb nutrients from enteral feedings. What can be done to keep him alive and growing?

PN must meet each patient's individual nutritional, electrolyte, and fluid needs. The main components are the energy nutrients: carbohydrate, protein, and fat. These are also known as macronutrients. Additionally, PN usually includes electrolytes (minerals such as sodium, potassium, and chloride) and vitamins, as well as trace elements. These are known as micronutrients. Finally, sterile water is usually added to the nutrition admixture to adjust the volume and ensure that the patient's fluid requirements are being met.

PRACTICE POINT

Most adults require an intake of fluid of 25–35 mL per day for every kg (2.2 lb) of body weight. This means that a 150-lb patient would be expected to require 1,700–2,400 mL of fluid daily.

The process of ordering and compounding PN solutions is complex and involves numerous steps before the final product can be dispensed and administered to the patient. Someone knowledgeable about nutrition and authorized to do so must first initiate the order, based on the patient's size, medical condition, and nutritional needs (including the results of lab work). PN orders are usually written by a physician, dietitian, or pharmacist, and in some settings, a nutrition support team involves all three disciplines in the process. Once the order has been transmitted to the pharmacy, an overall evaluation of the order is performed to ensure that the formulation ordered is practical and can be compounded safely.

Non-nutrients commonly added to PN admixtures include heparin, insulin, and histamine$_2$ antagonists. Heparin is frequently added to the PN to keep clots from forming in the vein used for administration. Insulin is sometimes included to ensure patients metabolize the dextrose being infused. Histamine$_2$-receptor antagonists such as famotidine (discussed in Chapter 20) can prevent stress ulcers in patients whose stomachs may still be producing digestive acids (which are not being utilized when the patient is being fed intravenously).

Since the IV route has already been established for the patient on PN, physicians may want to have as many medications as possible added to the PN for convenience. The issue with this is that the stability of the medications may not have been adequately studied under these conditions, and interactions between them and the components of the PN solution have not been evaluated. For instance, the pH (acidity) of the PN solution may be very different from a regular IV fluid and this could affect stability.

Some common additives in the PN have limited stability, especially when mixed with one another, and that must be considered when compounding. The multivitamins that are a routine component of the PN can lose their potency over time. For this reason, the vitamins should be one of the last items added. These vitamins are also sensitive to light and many pharmacies place a brown plastic wrap over the finished product to minimize the light exposure. Some institutions wrap the IV tubing for light protection once the PN is hung on the patient. Insulin is a medication that is commonly added to PN solutions. Insulin can react or adhere to the plastic from the bag or tubing, decreasing its potency or effectiveness. If it is to be added to the PN bag, this should also be one of the last steps. This is a more stable additive less likely to cause incompatibilities than those previously mentioned.

Another issue that merits consideration when compounding is the order of mixing of the ingredients. Most electrolytes are compatible with each other. Calcium and phosphorus, however, are only conditionally compatible. In fact, if you were to mix calcium and phosphorus in a plain dextrose bag, it is likely that they would precipitate almost immediately. Fortunately, in a PN solution, calcium and phosphorus are protected, to some extent, from interacting with each other by the presence of the protein component. This protection is limited by how much calcium and phosphorus are added, how much protein is in the mixture, the pH of the mixture, and the temperature of the final product. Colder solutions, a lower pH, and sufficient amount of protein make the solution more stable.

ALERT!

Precipitates are not acceptable in PN solutions, as particles should not be administered intravenously.

PRACTICE POINT

When compounding PN, add the phosphorus to the PN before adding calcium to dilute it to a lower concentration. Reactive electrolytes such as phosphorus are usually added near the end of the compounding process to maximize the total volume of solution to which they are added (thereby minimizing their concentrations). In general, it is inadvisable to have a ratio of more than 10 mEq/L of calcium in solutions with 30 mM or more of phosphates.

Some PN formulations include carbohydrate (dextrose), protein (amino acids), and fat (intravenous lipid emulsion) in the same bag, often called a *three-in-one or all-in-one (AIO)*, while others *(two-in-one)* require the fat component to be administered separately from the carbohydrate/protein admixture that carries the electrolytes and vitamins. The obvious advantage of the three-in-one admixture is the requirement for a single bag at a single rate to deliver all of the patient's nutrient needs. The disadvantage is that addition of the lipid component makes the admixture milky and precipitation may not be visually detected.

Standardized commercial PN products are available. These products are designed to meet the nutrition requirements of general population groups (specific for age, stress, or disease) and come in a range of protein (amino acid) and carbohydrate (dextrose) concentration combinations. (See Table 24-5.) These standardized commercial PN products require fewer additions or compound adjustments before they are administered. The standard products are complex but preferred over pharmacy-compounded products for a multitude of reasons that include sterility, stability, and nutritional balance. Challenges occur when the person's formula must be individualized.

Adverse events are often related to the ordering process consisting of creating the correct order and communicating the order. For these reasons, many institutions require special forms or utilize an automated compounding device tied to their institution's computer system when ordering PN. Labels should provide information that matches the order in a manner that allows the person administering the PN to verify its accuracy.

PN support is administered using a variety of protocols. The most common method is through continuous infusion over a 24-hour period. This is especially helpful when initiating PN, advancing calorie content (especially dextrose calories), or administering it in a metabolically unstable patient. Glucose is the component of the PN solution that causes the greatest amount of intolerance if the administration rate is not regulated correctly. Infusing glucose at a high rate can produce hyperglycemia in the patient receiving it, and this can cause a variety of metabolic complications. Once the patient is at goal nutrition or is stable, it is possible to infuse the PN over a shorter period. This is known as cycling the PN and offers several benefits. First, the patient is free of all the tubing and pumps for several hours each day and can move freely about the environment. This is especially advantageous in long-term outpatient settings. It is difficult to attempt to lead a relatively normal life when receiving PN 24 hours a day. People who work or attend school usually prefer not to be hooked to the PN solution while out of the house. Another benefit is that it gives the liver a rest from metabolizing the components. Long-term infusion of PN can often damage the liver, and cycling allows the liver a period of recovery that may minimize potential damage. The component most related to liver damage is the intravenous fat emulsion, especially the omega-6 fatty acid content. Lipid emulsions contain varying amounts of omega-6 fatty acid, depending on the brand used. Minimizing the amount of lipids or

TABLE 24-5. Representative Parenteral Nutrition Products[7]

Product	Amino Acid %	Dextrose %	Fat	Electrolytes	Notes
Aminosyn II	10, 15	–	–	–	Sulfite free; 15% used in bulk compounding
Aminosyn PF	7, 10	–	–	–	Infants/children; sulfite free
Premasol	6, 10	–	–	–	Infants/children; sulfite free
Travasol	10	–	–	–	
Prosol	20	–	–		Used in bulk compounding
Clinisol	15	–	–	–	Used in bulk compounding
FreAmine III	10	–	–	–	Contains phosphate
Freamine HBC	6.9	–	–	–	Can be used via peripheral vein or central vein with appropriate dextrose; used for patients in metabolic stress
Plenamine	15	–	–	–	Designed for bulk compounding
Procalamine	3	3	–	–	Contains 3% glycerol; can be used via peripheral catheter
Trophamine	6, 10	–	–	–	Infants/children; sulfite free
Clinimix	4.25, 5, 6, 8	5, 10, 15, 20, 14	–	–	Sulfite free, comes in a variety of combinations; comes in a 2-chambered bag, unclamp before dispensing
Clinimix E	2.75, 4.25, 5, 8	5, 10, 15, 20, 14	–	Varies	Sulfite free, comes in a variety of combinations; comes in a 2-chambered bag, unclamp before dispensing
Kabiven	3.3	9.8	3.9%	Yes	3-chambered bag, unclamp before dispensing; lipid is soy based
Peri-Kabiven	2.4	6.8	3.5%	Yes	3-chambered bag, unclamp before dispensing; can be used via peripheral catheter; lipid is soy based
Hepatamine	8	–	–	–	Hepatic formula
NephrAmine	5.4	–	–	–	Renal formula
Intravenous Lipids[7,8]					
Intralipid	20, 30	–	2 kcal/mL, 3 kcal/mL	–	100% soy oil; 30% used in compounding
Nutrilipid	20	–	2 kcal/mL	–	
SMOFlipid	20	–	2 kcal/mL	–	30% soy, 30% medium chain triglyceride, 25% olive, 10% fish oils
Omegaven	10	–	1.1 kcal/mL	–	100% fish oil
Clinolipid	20	–	2 kcal/mL	–	20% soy, 80% olive oil

the omega-6 component can lessen the chance of developing liver disease. Reducing the number of days the lipid is administered may also prevent or slow the progression of liver damage associated with lipid infusion. For some patients, it may be possible to administer lipids only one to three times per week. The periods without lipids allow the liver to clear the fats so they don't build up in the liver and cause damage. For those patients who do not depend on PN for 100% of their nutrition, the PN can also be given fewer than 7 days per week.[14]

OBESITY

Overweight and obesity refer to body weights above those generally considered healthy. Because total weight includes total body composition (bone, muscle, water, fat), a healthy weight varies with height, gender, and age. Weights that fall into the ranges of overweight and obesity have been shown to increase the likelihood of certain diseases and other health problems.[3] While in the past, weight status was based on charts of population averages for gender and height, it is now defined on the basis of body mass index (BMI), a measure of total body weight relative to height. A BMI of 18.5–24.9 is termed *normal* weight, while a BMI of 25–29.9 is considered overweight, a BMI of above 30 indicates obesity, and a BMI above 40 defines severe obesity. [9]

CASE?

Mrs. Broskie has been spending a lot of time in the hospital with Henry and relying on the vending machines there for snacks. Her weight is increasing and she wants to try an OTC product to help her lose weight. What might the pharmacist recommend?

PRACTICE POINT

An individual who is 5'9" tall and weighs 125–168 lb would have a BMI in the healthy range but would be considered obese with a weight above 203 lb. The Centers for Disease Control and Prevention provide online BMI calculators for adults at https://www.cdc.gov/healthyweight/assessing/bmi/adult_bmi/english_bmi_calculator/bmi_calculator.html and for children and teens at https://www.cdc.gov/healthyweight/bmi/calculator.html.

Weight loss can contribute to improved health. Modest weight loss (5% to 10% of total weight) can decrease risk factors for weight-related health problems and reduce blood pressure, blood sugar, and cholesterol.[6] Most dietitians and other medical professionals recommend gradual weight loss programs emphasizing reduced calorie intake and increased exercise, but some patients request or require pharmaceutical assistance to accomplish their weight goals. Medications approved for use in weight loss programs work either by decreasing nutrient absorption or suppressing appetite. Prescription weight loss medications are generally individualized based on patient goals and health issues.

Because calories are absorbed through the gastrointestinal tract, reducing energy-nutrient absorption can cause weight loss. While various products have been marketed as *blockers* of carbohydrate absorption, the only weight loss medication approved by the U.S. Food and Drug Administration (FDA) to decrease calorie absorption is a lipase inhibitor, orlistat, which reduces the ability of the gastrointestinal tract to process dietary fats. Orlistat prevents absorption of about 30% of dietary fat, which then passes through the bowel for evacuation. Because excess unabsorbed fat can cause uncomfortable side effects, including fecal incontinence, urgency, and intestinal gas, patients who reduce their fat consumption find the drug more tolerable, thus losing even more weight from additional caloric restriction. It is recommended that patients begin a reduced-fat diet 3 or more days before beginning to take orlistat. Doses are taken only with meals containing fat and skipped when meals are skipped or are without fat. Because orlistat interferes with fat absorption, it can also reduce absorption of fat-soluble vitamins (A, D, E, and K), so it is recommended that patients also take a multivitamin, timed at least 2 hours before or after the orlistat dose.

Orlistat is available as an OTC product, Alli, which is packaged with extensive instructions and access to an online diet plan. Patients purchasing Alli should be reminded to read all of the accompanying literature. A higher-strength capsule, Xenical, is available only by prescription, but it is the same drug with the same actions. Alli is approved for use in weight-loss plans of up to 6 months, but Xenical also carries an indication for maintenance of weight loss.

CASE?

Mrs. Broskie purchased Alli at the pharmacy but was too busy to read the directions. She complains that she has an upset stomach, especially when she eats her favorite fried eggs and bacon breakfast in the hospital cafeteria. Should she stop taking Alli? What do you think the pharmacist might advise?

Appetite suppressants, called anorexiants, can assist patients in following a calorie-restricted diet. Anorexiants currently approved by the FDA are benzphetamine, diethylpropion, phentermine (also available as a combination product, with topiramate), and phendimetrazine. They work by stimulating the sympathetic (adrenergic) nervous system, increasing norepinephrine release and/or transmission in the central nervous system. (Refer to Chapters 4 and 5.) These drugs, related to amphetamines, are effective in suppression of appetite and are recommended only for short-term use as part of a weight-reduction plan based on caloric restriction. All are considered to have abuse potential, and extended use (longer than a few weeks) is contraindicated. While results are not dramatic, these drugs have been shown to cause increased weight loss in some patients. Common side effects of drugs in this category include cardiovascular issues (palpitations, increased heart rate, and blood pressure), central nervous system effects (stimulation, insomnia, restlessness), and gastrointestinal effects (nausea, constipation, stomach pain), along with mouth dryness and changes in urinary frequency and libido. Patients with diabetes may experience changes in their patterns of blood sugar and insulin needs that do not necessarily parallel their weight loss. Anorexiants are not currently recommended for patients with cardiovascular disease, severe chronic kidney disease or liver impairment, psychosis, or glaucoma.[10]

A combination product containing naltrexone, an opioid antagonist, and bupropion, also used in substance use disorders, has been shown to be effective for weight management in some patients, and is classified as an anorexiant combination. Its use is contraindicated in patients with uncontrolled hypertension, severe kidney or liver disease, glaucoma, seizure disorders, and most patients diagnosed with substance use disorders. It is also not recommended for patients with binge eating disorders, or for adolescents and young adults suffering from depression.[10]

ALERT!

The combination product naltrexone and bupropion (Contrave) used for weight management carries a boxed warning for suicidal thoughts or actions and a medication guide must be dispensed along with all prescriptions for it.

PRACTICE POINT

Currently all approved anorexiants except naltrexone/bupropion are considered by the Drug Enforcement Administration (DEA) as controlled substances in schedule III or IV, with prescribing restrictions and limited refills.

Glucagon-like peptide 1 (GLP-1), a substance normally produced in the body, has many actions related to glucose metabolism and insulin release (see Chapter 10). A group of agents known as GLP-1 receptor agonists that mimic the actions of naturally produced GLP-1 is used in the treatment of type 2 diabetes. GLP-1-receptor agonists are known to reduce appetite and/or increase feelings of fullness, so a logical extension is use in weight management. Although five different GLP-1-receptor agonists are available for diabetes therapy, only one of these, liraglutide, has FDA approval for use in weight management. The product with this approval, Saxenda, has the same generic name as one approved for diabetes, but only Saxenda is labeled for this indication (and *not* for diabetes mellitus). Unlike other pharmacotherapy for weight management, liraglutide must be administered not by mouth but by subcutaneous injection every day. It is a recommended weight management treatment for patients who suffer from or are at risk for type 2 diabetes, but should not be used for this purpose by patients who are already being treated with a GLP-1-receptor agonist.

PRACTICE POINT

In the pharmacy, liraglutide must be refrigerated (at 2°C–8°C), and discarded if freezing occurs. After initial use, patients may choose to keep it in the refrigerator or at room temperature (below 86°F). Each pen syringe must be discarded 30 days after first use regardless of storage conditions.[11]

FDA-approved medications for use in weight loss are listed in Medication Table 24-2.

Numerous other therapies, some prescription and some OTC, have been and continue to be used to promote weight management. Some physicians favor off-label prescribing (for indications not approved by the FDA) of other drugs, including antidepressant agents, for weight loss. If enough

> **ALERT!**
>
> Liraglutide is currently classified as a hazardous drug, although the prefilled syringes may be excluded from some handling requirements. Gloves should be worn while receiving, unpacking, and placing the product in storage.[12]

> **ALERT!**
>
> Liraglutide has a black box warning for risk of thyroid tumors. Patients must receive the required medication guide when the product is dispensed.

data can be collected, some of these may, like bupropion, eventually be approved for use in weight management.

Finally, a wide variety of complementary and alternative therapies are available OTC and used by some patients hoping for assistance in weight management. These include bitter orange, guarana extract, and various diet teas, which appear to act in ways similar to the FDA-approved appetite suppressants, although recommended safe doses have not been documented (and they could be dangerous if added to prescription anorexiant therapy). Other "natural" supplements popularized on the Internet and in lay publications for weight loss include calcium pyruvate, chromium picolinate, chitosan, *Garcinia*, and *Hoodia*. These have not been studied scientifically, and most are unclear on even their mechanism of action, let alone a recommended safe dose, and should be avoided until further information is available. Products containing the herb *Ephedra* have been promoted for weight loss and may still be obtained from international sources, but the FDA has banned their legal sale in the United States.

SUMMARY

Adequate and proper nutrition is vital to the life and health of all human beings. Energy and nonenergy nutrients must be supplied in proper amounts to maintain body function and, while the best way to accomplish this is by consumption of a balanced diet, some patients require nonfood supplementation. Overweight and obesity are conditions that can contribute to health problems, and medication therapy can be useful in weight management.

ACKNOWLEDGMENT

The authors wish to acknowledge and thank Carol Battles, PhD, RD, LD, CHES, coauthor of this chapter in the first edition of this book.

REFERENCES

1. Centers for Disease Control and Prevention, National Center for Health Statistics. Obesity and overweight. https://www.cdc.gov/nchs/fastats/obesity-overweight.htm. Accessed March 9, 2021.

2. Dietary Guidelines for Americans. *Dietary Guidelines for Americans, 2020–2025* and online materials. https://www.dietaryguidelines.gov/resources/2020-2025-dietary-guidelines-online-materials. Accessed March 9, 2021.

3. National Institutes of Health, Office of Dietary Supplements. Nutrient recommendations: Dietary Reference Intakes (DRI). https://ods.od.nih.gov/HealthInformation/Dietary_Reference_Intakes.aspx. Accessed March 9, 2021.

4. National Institutes of Health, Office of Dietary Supplements. Multivitamin/mineral supplements: Fact sheet for health professionals. https://ods.od.nih.gov/factsheets/MVMS-HealthProfessional/. Accessed October 28, 2021.

5. Wagner CL, Greer FR. Prevention of rickets and vitamin D deficiency in infants, children, and adolescents. *Pediatrics*. 2008;122(5):1142-1152. doi: 10.1542/peds.2008-1862.

6. Centers for Disease Control and Prevention. Healthy weight, nutrition, and physical activity: Losing weight. https://www.cdc.gov/healthyweight/losing_weight/index.html. Accessed March 9, 2021.

7. Facts and Comparisons eAnswers [database]. Hudson, OH: Wolters Kluwer.

8. Lexicomp Online [database]. Hudson, OH: Wolters Kluwer Clinical Drug Information; 2021.

9. Fryar CD, Carroll MD, Afful J. Prevalence of overweight, obesity, and severe obesity among adults aged 20 and over: United States, 1960–1962 through 2017–2018. NCHS Health E-Stats. 2020. https://www.cdc.gov/nchs/data/hestat/obesity-adult-17-18/obesity-adult.htm. Accessed March 9, 2021.

10. Sheehan A, Chen JT, Yanovski JA. Obesity. In: DiPiro JT, Yee GC, Posey L, et al., eds. *Pharmacotherapy: A Pathophysiologic Approach. 11th ed.* New York, NY: McGraw-Hill; 2020.

11. Novo Nordisk. Saxenda prescribing information. https://www.novo-pi.com/saxenda.pdf. Accessed April 6, 2022.

12. Connor TH, MacKenzie BA, DeBord DG, et al. NIOSH list of antineoplastic and other hazardous drugs in healthcare settings, 2016. Cincinnati, OH: National Institute of Occupational Safety and Health; 2016. https://www.cdc.gov/niosh/docs/2016-161/pdfs/2016-161.pdf?id=10.26616/NIOSHPUB2016161. Accessed March 10, 2021.

13. https://www.nutritioncare.org/Guidelines_and_Clinical_Resources/EN_Formula_Guide/EN_Adult_Formulas/. Accessed July 6, 2022.

14. Cober P, Gura K, Mirtallo J, Ayers P, Boullata J, Anderson C, Plogsted S. ASPEN Parenteral Nutrition Safety Committee. ASAPEN Lipid Injectable Emulsion Safety Recommendations Part 2: Neonate and Pediatric Considerations. Nutr Clin Pract 2021; 36:1106-1125.

CHAPTER RESOURCES

Dietary Guidelines for Americans. https://www.dietaryguidelines.gov/. Accessed April 6, 2022.

National Institutes of Health, Office of Dietary Supplements. Dietary supplement fact sheets. https://ods.od.nih.gov/. Accessed April 6, 2022.

REVIEW QUESTIONS

1. Name the energy nutrients and give the energy yield and common dietary sources of each.

2. List the fat-soluble vitamins and explain why it is dangerous for patients to over-supplement with them.

3. What are the components of enteral nutrition products? How can they be administered?

4. What are the components of PN? How is it administered?

5. How does orlistat work to promote weight loss?

MEDICATION TABLES

MEDICATION TABLE 24-1. Vitamins and Essential Nutrients[2,3,7,8a]

Type	Vitamin	Chemical Name(s)	Functions	Food Sources	Adult Recommended Dietary Allowance or Daily Adequate Intake ages 31–50 (male/female)	Tolerable Upper Intake (TUI)	Deficiency May Result In	Toxicity	Drug/Nutrient Interactions[5]	Brand Name
Fat Soluble	A	Retinol (REH tin ol), Beta carotene (bay tuh KAYR oh teen)	Vision, protein synthesis, skin, reproduction, growth	Fortified milk, egg yolks, and cheese; dark leafy green vegetables and broccoli; dark orange fruits and vegetables	Male/female 900/700 mcg	3,000 mcg/day	Skin disorders, diarrhea, eye damage, night blindness, total blindness, dry skin, poor growth, poor immune response	Liver damage, bone fractures, dry skin, intestinal disturbances	Statins and oral contraceptives can increase levels; cholestyramine, orlistat, and neomycin decrease absorption	Aquasol-A
	D	Calcitriol (kal si TRYE ole), cholecalciferol (kol eh kal SIF er ol), ergocalciferol (ER goh kal SIF er ol), paricalcitol (payr ih KAL si tol)	Bone growth/maintenance through calcium and phosphorus absorption	Fish liver oils, fatty fish, liver; sunshine on skin; fortified milk and cereals	Male/female 15 mcg (600 IU)	100 mcg (4,000 IU)	Osteomalacia, rickets in children	Kidney damage, mineral deposits in soft tissue	Anticonvulsants, cimetidine, heparin, isoniazid, and neomycin may interfere with absorption and/or activity	Rocaltrol, Drisdol, Zemplar
	E	Alpha-tocopherol (AL fa toh KOF er ol)	Antioxidant	Wheat germ, nuts, seeds, vegetable oils, egg yolks, dark leafy green vegetables	Male/female 15 mg	1,000 mg alpha-tocopherol	None established	Bleeding due to interference with vitamin K	May increase effects of oral anticoagulants	E-400, Nutr-E-Sol, Vita E

Continued next page

MEDICATION TABLE 24-1. Vitamins and Essential Nutrients[2,3,7,8a] *(Continued)*

Type	Vitamin	Chemical Name(s)	Functions	Food Sources	Adult Recommended Dietary Allowance or Daily Adequate Intake ages 31–50 (male/female)	Tolerable Upper Intake (TUI)	Deficiency May Result In	Toxicity	Drug/Nutrient Interactions[5]	Brand Name
Fat Soluble	K	Phytona-dione (fye toe na DYE one)	Blood clotting, prevention of bleeding, bone health, fracture healing	Liver, cabbage, dark leafy vegetables, broccoli, citrus fruits	Male/female 120/90 mcg	TUI not determined	Easy bruising/bleeding	Rare	May interact with aspirin, antibiotics, anticoagulant/antiplatelet drugs, doxorubicin, laxatives, weight-loss medications, antiseizure medications, and warfarin; individuals should consult a physician before beginning a vitamin K regimen	Mephyton
Water Soluble	B1	Thiamin, Thiamine (THYE a min)	Coenzyme in energy metabolism, nerve function	Pork, enriched breads/cereals, black beans, nuts	Male/female 1.2/1.1	TUI not determined	Beriberi (weak; poor muscle coordination, digestion, nerve function, cardiovascular function, and digestion)		Deficiencies have been associated in patients on phenytoin and some diuretics; people who consume a lot of carbohydrates or high-calorie diets need more thiamin	
Water Soluble	B2	Riboflavin (RYE boh FLAY vin)	Coenzyme in energy metabolism	Milk, milk products, whole grains, enriched breads/cereals	Male/female 1.3/1.1 mg	TUI not determined	Skin, mucous membranes deficient, cracks on lips and corners of mouth	None known	Chlorpromazine, doxorubicin, and possibly oral contraceptive medications reduce the conversion of riboflavin to its active form	B-2-400

Continued next page

MEDICATION TABLE 24-1. Vitamins and Essential Nutrients[2,3,7,8a] (Continued)

Type	Vitamin	Chemical Name(s)	Functions	Food Sources	Adult Recommended Dietary Allowance or Daily Adequate Intake ages 31–50 (male/female)	Tolerable Upper Intake (TUI)	Deficiency May Result In	Toxicity	Drug/Nutrient Interactions[5]	Brand Name
Water Soluble	B3	Niacin (NYE a sin)	Coenzyme in energy metabolism, protein and fat metabolism; vasodilator	Protein-rich foods: meats, fish, poultry, dairy, eggs, enriched breads/cereals	Male/female 16/14 mg	35 mg/day	Pellagra (diarrhea, dementia, dermatitis, death)	Red skin flush, upset digestion	May interfere with diabetes medications and increase toxicity of statins and carbamazepine	
	B5	Pantothenic acid (pan TOE then ik)	Coenzyme in energy metabolism, fat, and protein metabolism, production of essential body compounds	Whole grains, legumes, nuts, seeds, animal protein	Male/female 5 mg	TUI not determined	None known			Panto-250
	B7 (also known as vitamin H or coenzyme R)	Biotin (BYE oh tin)	Coenzyme in carbohydrate metabolism, production of proteins and fats	Eggs, milk, liver, mushrooms, bananas, tomatoes, whole grains, nuts, brewer's yeast; also produced by bacteria in the intestines	Male/female 30 mcg	TUI not determined	Rare: skin rash, hair loss, damage to nerves			Meribin

Continued next page

MEDICATION TABLE 24-1. Vitamins and Essential Nutrients[2,3,7,8a] *(Continued)*

Type	Vitamin	Chemical Name(s)	Functions	Food Sources	Adult Recommended Dietary Allowance or Daily Adequate Intake ages 31–50 (male/female)	Tolerable Upper Intake (TUI)	Deficiency May Result In	Toxicity	Drug/Nutrient Interactions[5]	Brand Name
Water Soluble	B6	Pyridoxine (peer i DOX een)	Coenzyme in amino acid metabolism, especially for nervous system, red and white blood cell production, and heart disease	Meats, fish, poultry, whole grains, nuts and seeds, dried fortified cereals, soybeans, avocados, baked potatoes with skins, watermelon, plantains, bananas, peanuts, and brewer's yeast	Male/female 1.3 mg/day	100 mg/day	Associated with heart disease, skin problems and nervous system disorders, mouth sores, small-cell type anemia, insulin sensitivity; increased risk for kidney stones	Nerve damage to the limbs, which may cause numbness, trouble walking, and pain; very high doses can cause symptoms of instability and numbness in the feet and hands, which may be permanent in some cases; of specific concern are possible adverse effects on nerve development in the offspring of pregnant women who take large doses, such as for morning sickness	The following drugs interfere with vitamin B6 status: isoniazid, hydralazine, phenelzine, cycloserine, estrogens, theophylline, corticosteroids, erythromycin, gentamicin, neomycin, sulfonamides, alcohol, and caffeine	Pyri-500

Continued next page

MEDICATION TABLE 24-1. Vitamins and Essential Nutrients[2,3,7,8a] (Continued)

Type	Vitamin	Chemical Name(s)	Functions	Food Sources	Adult Recommended Dietary Allowance or Daily Adequate Intake ages 31–50 (male/female)	Tolerable Upper Intake (TUI)	Deficiency May Result In	Toxicity	Drug/Nutrient Interactions[5]	Brand Name
Water Soluble	B9 (this name is seldom used)	Folic acid, folate (FOE lik) (FOE late)	Important for the formation of RNA and DNA as well as new cell formation, protein metabolism, and growth; it is used in the manufacturing of neurotransmitters (chemical messengers in the brain), in protecting the heart via its influence on homocysteine	Liver, legumes, avocado, bananas, orange juice, cold cereal, asparagus, green leafy vegetables, and yeast; folic acid is now added to commercial breads and cereals	Male/female 400 mcg/day (600 mcg/day in pregnancy, 500 mcg/day in lactation)	1,000 mcg/day	Megaloblastic anemia, depression, poor growth, nerve growth and impairments in concentration, memory, and hearing	High levels may, especially in older adults, hide signs of B12 deficiency, a condition that can cause nerve damage	May interfere with anticonvulsants and methotrexate; absorption and activity can be decreased by including oral contraceptives, aspirin, indomethacin, famotidine, some antibiotics (tetracycline, isoniazid, cycloserine, erythromycin, sulfonamides), and cholestyramine; may reduce blood levels of levodopa and some anticonvulsants	FA-8

Continued next page

MEDICATION TABLE 24-1. Vitamins and Essential Nutrients[2,3,7,8a] *(Continued)*

Type	Vitamin	Chemical Name(s)	Functions	Food Sources	Adult Recommended Dietary Allowance or Daily Adequate Intake ages 31–50 (male/female)	Tolerable Upper Intake (TUI)	Deficiency May Result In	Toxicity	Drug/Nutrient Interactions[5]	Brand Name
Water Soluble	B12	Cyanocobalamin (sye an oh koe BAL a min), hydroxycobalamin (hye drox ee koe BAL a min)	Production of red blood cells, manufacturing genetic material (DNA and RNA), and healthy functioning of the nervous system; B12 works closely with folate	Animal products only (not in vegetables), including meats, dairy products, eggs, and fish (clams and oily fish are very high in B12); B12 is added to commercial dried cereals	Male/female 2.4 mcg/day	TUI not determined	Low levels of folate during pregnancy increase risk of birth defects in newborns	B12 requires an intrinsic factor that is produced in the stomach for absorption; without the intrinsic factor dietary B12 is useless	Folic acid supplementation may mask B12 deficiencies; vitamin C and iron supplements may interfere with its bioavailability; blood levels may be reduced by zidovudine, antacids, metformin, oral contraceptives, and some antibiotics	Nascobal
	C	Ascorbic acid (a SKOR bik)	Acts as an antioxidant (reduces harm from damaging chemical processes in the body) and as such plays a role in the immune system;	Citrus fruits and juices, strawberries, papayas, hot chili peppers, bell peppers, broccoli, potatoes, dark leafy greens, kale, red cabbage, and brussels sprouts	Male/female 90/75 mg/day	2,000 mg/day	Scurvy is the primary deficiency disease; it affects most body tissues, particularly bones, teeth, and blood vessels; symptoms include bleeding gums, wounds that won't heal, rough skin, and wasting away of the muscles; deficiencies may contribute to periodontal disease and gallstones;	High doses may cause nausea and diarrhea, may increase risk of kidney stones; ascorbic acid increases iron absorption so people with blood disorders, such as hemochromatosis, thalassemia, or sideroblastic anemia, should avoid high doses;	Increases absorption of iron; may interfere with absorption of copper and chromium and reduce efficacy of some chemotherapy	Acerola-C, Fruit C

Continued next page

MEDICATION TABLE 24-1. Vitamins and Essential Nutrients[2,3,7,8a] *(Continued)*

Type	Vitamin	Chemical Name(s)	Functions	Food Sources	Adult Recommended Dietary Allowance or Daily Adequate Intake ages 31–50 (male/female)	Tolerable Upper Intake (TUI)	Deficiency May Result In	Toxicity	Drug/Nutrient Interactions[5]	Brand Name
			essential for the production of collagen, the basic protein in bones, cartilage, tendons, and ligaments				uncommon in the U.S., usually occurring in the elderly, alcoholics, cancer patients, and some people on severely limited diets low in fresh fruits and vegetables	large doses may also thin blood and interfere with anticoagulant medications, blood tests used in diabetes, and stool tests		
Water Soluble	Choline (KOE leen) No letter assigned; while choline is an essential water-soluble nutrient, it is not a vitamin	Essential for fetal brain development and for learning and memory; it aids with the movement of fat into cells and decreases fat content in the liver, choline is a precursor of acetyl-choline, a neurotransmitter, and it plays a role in phospholipid and homocysteine synthesis	Liver, peanuts, eggs, and milk	Male/female 550/425 mg/day	3,500 mg/day	Fishy body odor, vomiting, sweating, low blood pressure, and gastrointestinal problems	Liver damage		

[a] Pronunciations have been adapted with permission from USP Dictionary of USAN and International Drug Names (USP Dictionary) © 2022.

MEDICATION TABLE 24-2. Agents Used for Weight Loss[7,8]

Category	Generic Name	Brand Name	Dosage Form	Usual Dose	Length of Therapy	Regulatory Status
Lipase inhibitor	Orlistat (OR li stat)	Alli	Capsule	60 mg 1-3 times daily	Up to 6 months	OTC
		Xenical	Capsule	Up to 120 mg 3 times daily	Up to 2 yr	Rx
Anorexiant	Benzphetamine (benz FET a meen)	Various generics	Tablet	25-50 mg 1-3 times daily	2-4 wk	aRx (C-III)
	Diethylpropion (dye eth il PROE pee on)	Various generics	Tablet, IR	25 mg 3-4 times daily	2-4 wk	Rx (C-IV)
			Tablet, CR	75 mg daily	2-4 wk	Rx (C-IV)
	Phendimetrazine (fen dye ME tra zeen)	Various generics	Capsule, ER	105 mg every morning before breakfast	Up to 12 weeks	Rx (C-III)
			Tablet, IR	17.5-35 mg 2-3 times daily one hour before meals		
	Phentermine (FEN ter meen)	Adipex-P and generics	Tablet	15-37.5 mg total per day in 1 or 2 doses	2-4 wk	Rx (C-IV)
			Capsule			
		Lomaira	Tablet	8 mg 3 times daily		
Glucagon-like Peptide-1 antagonist	Liraglutide (lir a GLOO tide)	Saxenda	Solution (pen injector)	0.6-3 mg SUBQ once daily	Indefinite	Rx
Combination products	Naltrexone and Bupropion (nal TREKS one, byoo PROE pee on)	Contrave	Tablet, ER (naltrexone 8 mg and bupropion 90 mg)	2 tablets twice daily	Indefinite; discontinue after 12 weeks if 5% weight loss not achieved	Rx
	Phentermine and topiramate (FEN ter meen, toe PYRE a mate)	Qsymia	Capsule, ER (phentermine/topiramate 3.75 mg/23 mg, 7.5 mg/46 mg, 11.25 mg/69 mg, 15 mg/92 mg)	1 capsule of prescribed strength once daily	Indefinite; gradually discontinue after 12 weeks if 5% weight loss not achieved on maximum dose	Rx (C-IV)

CR = controlled release; ER = extended release; IR = immediate release; OTC = over the counter; SUBQ = subcutaneous.

Part 8

THE HEMATOLOGIC SYSTEM

535

Chapter 25

Overview of the Hematologic System

Mate M. Soric, PharmD, BCPS, FCCP

KEY TERMS AND DEFINITIONS

Albumin—the most common protein found in plasma.

Antigen—a substance that provokes the immune system.

Basophils—the least common white blood cell; plays a role in allergic reactions.

Blasts—cells formed from stem cells during the differentiation process that will, in turn, produce mature blood cells.

Clotting cascade—the complex series of reactions that must take place before fibrin can be produced.

Clotting factors—the proteins that make up the clotting cascade, identified by roman numerals.

Coagulation—the process of forming a blood clot.

Complete blood count (CBC)—a laboratory test that evaluates the number of cells and level of hemoglobin in the blood.

Differentiation—the process of stem and precursor cells developing into mature cells.

Eosinophils—white blood cells that play a role in allergic reactions and parasitic infections.

Erythrocytes—mature red blood cells.

DOI 10.37573/9781585286638.025

Erythropoiesis—the process of producing red blood cells.

Erythropoietin (EPO)—hematopoietic growth factor that controls the production of red blood cells.

Ferritin—the storage form of iron in the blood.

Granulocytes—certain white blood cells, including neutrophils, basophils, and eosinophils.

Hematopoiesis—the development of blood cells.

Hematopoietic stem cell—a cell in the bone marrow that is capable of differentiating into many different blood cell types.

Hemoglobin—a protein in red blood cells consisting of heme, globin, and iron that is responsible for carrying oxygen.

Hemostasis—the process of stopping blood loss.

Leukocytes—white blood cells.

Leukocytosis—an increase in the number of white blood cells.

Leukopenia—a decrease in the number of white blood cells.

Lymphocytes—white blood cells, categorized as T or B lymphocytes that attack viruses and tumor cells, and produce antibodies.

Myeloid stem cell—a cell that can differentiate into a number of blood cells depending on the growth factor that acts on it.

Neutrophils—white blood cells that serve as the first response to infection.

Plasma—the liquid component of blood.

Plasma cells—mature B lymphocytes that produce antibodies.

Plasmin—an enzyme that dissolves blood clots.

Platelets—blood cells responsible for forming clots to stop bleeding.

Polymorphonuclear cells (PMNs)—neutrophils.

Red blood cells (RBCs)—a blood cell containing hemoglobin that carries oxygen throughout the body.

Reticulocytes—immature red blood cells.

Thrombocytes—platelets.

White blood cells (WBCs)—a group of six blood cells that contribute to allergic reactions, fight infections, and attack tumor cells.

LEARNING OBJECTIVES

After completing this chapter, you should be able to

1. Describe the developmental process of red blood cells, white blood cells, and platelets.

2. List nutritional requirements for the proper development of red blood cells.

3. Explain the structure and function of red blood cells, white blood cells, and platelets.

4. Describe the processes the body uses to achieve hemostasis: vasoconstriction, platelet plug formation, and the clotting cascade.

5. List the utility of the most common laboratory tests of the blood.

The blood being pumped throughout the circulatory system is the foundation for virtually every system in the body. Blood vessels act as the equivalent of a vast highway, and blood, in its travels over this highway, transports oxygen, nutrients, and hormones to the tiniest of capillaries while carrying away carbon dioxide, cellular debris, and harmful chemicals. The volume of blood in the body depends on a number of factors, including age, gender, and body type. Blood consists of fluid or plasma, formed elements or cells, and cell fragments called platelets. The cells are suspended within the plasma and move along the blood vessel highway to the various body systems like cars on the interstate. The formed elements of blood consist of red blood cells (RBCs) or erythrocytes, white blood cells (WBCs) or leukocytes, and platelets (thrombocytes).

Plasma or whole blood contains varying amounts of each of the formed elements. The volume percentage of RBCs in whole blood is called the packed cell volume (PCV) or hematocrit. A normal range of hematocrit is between 37% and 49% dependent on gender and age. WBCs make up less than 1% of blood volume, and plasma constitutes the remainder of the blood volume. When the percentages of these elements are outside of the normal range, changes can occur within the body that can lead to health concerns. For example, a decreased number of RBCs can lead to a disease such as anemia (discussed later in the chapter), and too few WBCs can compromise the immune system. In this chapter, the development of the blood elements is explained, and the role each plays in the maintenance of the overall health of the human body is explored.

HEMATOPOIESIS: THE DEVELOPMENT OF BLOOD CELLS

Hematopoiesis, the development of blood cells, begins deep in the bone marrow in the hollow center of bones. Though there are many different blood cells with numerous functions, they all originate from the same hematopoietic stem cells located in the bone marrow. Hematopoietic stem cells have the potential to mature into many different cell types, including RBCs, WBCs, and platelets. The process of maturing into a particular type of cell is known as differentiation. The final cell type formed by differentiation depends on the signals stem cells receive. Figure 25-1 summarizes the complex developmental process of blood cells.

Development of Red Blood Cells

The hematopoietic stem cell is the starting point for RBC production. The first step in the development of RBCs is the differentiation of myeloid stem cells into blasts or precursor cells, after being exposed to the hormone erythropoietin, or EPO. Precursor cells then mature into reticulocytes, immature RBCs that will enter the bloodstream via capillaries in the bone marrow to continue their maturation. After 24–48 hours in the circulation, reticulocytes become mature RBCs.

PRACTICE POINT

A reticulocyte count is a laboratory test that can be used to examine how well the body is producing RBCs.

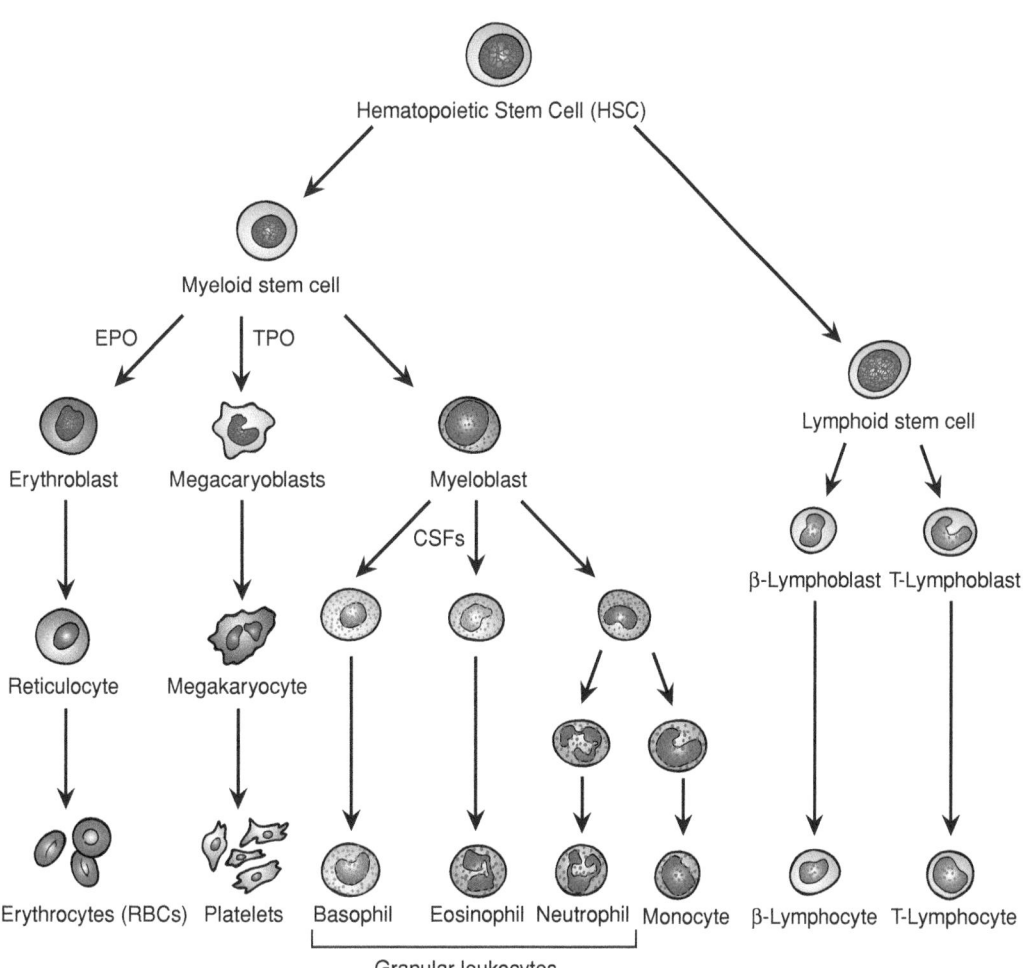

FIGURE 25-1. The development of blood cells. CSF = colony stimulating factor; EPO = erythropoietin; TPO = thrombopoietin.

Development of Platelets

When a myeloid stem cell is exposed to thrombopoietin, or TPO, the result is the formation of megakaryocytes, giant cells that are about 10 to 15 times the size of a typical RBC and made of up to 5,000 interconnected platelets. Under the influence of TPO, this large cell will begin to crumble, releasing platelets (or thrombocytes) into the bloodstream.

Development of White Blood Cells

There are actually six different cell types grouped together as WBCs: monocytes, neutrophils, basophils, eosinophils, B (β-) lymphocytes, and T lymphocytes. These cells are responsible for defending the body from outside attacks. The development of WBCs closely mirrors that of the RBCs, with a few important differences.

Granulocytes and Monocytes

Once again, the hematopoietic stem cells, which have differentiated into myeloid stem cells, serve as the starting point for the development of granulocytes (neutrophils, basophils, and eosinophils) and monocytes. In this case, however, they respond to colony stimulating factors (CSFs). Once produced, monocytes enter the bloodstream and travel to various tissues to differentiate into mature macrophages. The mature granulocytes, on the other hand, remain in the bloodstream to fend off invaders.

Lymphocytes

In contrast to RBCs, monocytes, and granulocytes, the lymphocytes begin their development as hematopoietic stem cells that differentiate into lymphoid stem cells. These stem cells mature directly into T and B lymphoblasts (immature cells). The T lymphoblasts travel through the bloodstream to an organ called the thymus, located behind the sternum. Here they mature to T lymphocytes. Mature T cells travel from the thymus to the spleen and peripheral lymph nodes, where they play a central role in fighting viral infections. T lymphocytes that do not survive to maturity are cleared from the thymus by macrophages.

PRACTICE POINT

The majority of mature T cells are produced before puberty. As a person ages, the thymus atrophies and its capacity for developing T cells decreases.

The B lymphoblasts remain in the bone marrow to develop into mature B lymphocytes. When an antigen (immune system stimulant, such as a microorganism fragment or byproduct) binds to the B cell receptor, the B cell is activated. Some activated B cells will enlarge and convert to plasma cells that secrete antibodies to help fight infections, while others will become memory B cells that lie in wait for future infections carrying the same antigen.

STRUCTURE AND FUNCTION OF THE COMPONENTS OF BLOOD

Red Blood Cells

In each drop of blood, the normal range is 240–270 million RBCs. Mature RBCs have a characteristic biconcave shape (Figure 25-2) and a flexibility that allows them to safely travel through the turbulent circulatory system. They are relatively small, with a diameter of 7–8 μm (micrometer, or millionth of a meter), so about 10 RBCs can fit inside a single speck of dust. They are packed with hemoglobin to transport oxygen.

Hemoglobin is made of a protein called globin and four heme units. At the center of each heme is an iron ion that not only gives the RBC its distinctive red color but is also responsible for the ability to carry oxygen. Each RBC contains roughly 280 million hemoglobin molecules, making up about a third of the cell's weight. If iron supplies cannot meet the demand of RBC production, small, pale RBCs will be formed that will not carry oxygen efficiently and may

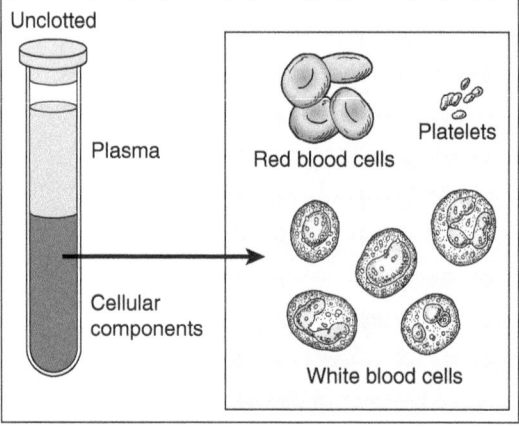

FIGURE 25-2. Cellular components of the blood. Each has a characteristic form. Note the biconcave shape of the RBCs and the platelets, which are cellular fragments.

TABLE 25-1. Recommended Daily Allowances of Iron[1]

Age	Males (mg/day)	Females (mg/day)	Pregnancy (mg/day)	Lactation (mg/day)
7–12 months	11	11	N/A	N/A
1–3 yr	7	7	N/A	N/A
4–8 yr	10	10	N/A	N/A
9–13 yr	8	8	N/A	N/A
14–18 yr	11	15	27	10
19–50 yr	8	18	27	9
51+ yr	8	8	N/A	N/A

cause symptoms of an iron deficiency anemia. The recommended daily allowance (RDA) of iron varies by age, gender, and pregnancy status and is shown in Table 25-1.

PRACTICE POINT

Iron can be found in many foods such as meats, beans, eggs, and whole grains or can be replaced using iron supplements.

Like iron, vitamin B_{12} and folate are two other important nutrients that play roles in the development of RBCs. If intake falls below the RDA of 2–3 mcg/day of vitamin B_{12} or 400 mcg/day of folate, cell division is delayed, resulting in a decreased production of RBCs. The RBCs that are produced tend to be larger than normal and are called macrocytes, causing a macrocytic anemia.

ALERT!

Iron supplements come in many different varieties. Each of the different iron salts contains a different amount of elemental iron; therefore, dosing is different for each type of iron supplement and the correct one must be chosen.

As RBCs enter areas of high oxygen concentration, such as the lungs, each iron ion located in the hemoglobin molecules can temporarily bond to a single molecule of oxygen. The RBC then leaves the lung and travels via the bloodstream to the farthest reaches of the circulatory system:

PRACTICE POINT

Vitamin B_{12}-rich foods include meats, dairy products, and fortified cereals. Folate can be found in spinach, beans, and rice, among other foods.

the capillaries. Here, the oxygen concentration is low and the bonds holding the oxygen molecules to the hemoglobin are broken, allowing the free oxygen to diffuse into the tissue where it is needed most. On the return trip, the hemoglobin plays a role in bringing carbon dioxide away from the tissues and delivering it to the lungs for exhalation. While most carbon dioxide is simply dissolved in the plasma, 13% is transported on hemoglobin molecules.

The average RBC will circulate for 120 days, traveling from the heart to the lungs to capillaries and back. A considerable amount of damage takes place as the cells race around the body in blood vessels and are crammed through tiny capillaries. RBCs at the end of the life cycle are cleared out by macrophages in the spleen and liver, but the important pieces that make up hemoglobin are conserved. The iron is stored in the blood as ferritin and is transferred to the bone marrow on transferrin molecules so that it can be recycled into new hemoglobin for newly formed RBCs.

To keep up with the rapid breakdown of RBCs, the bone marrow must produce 2 million RBCs per second. This process, called erythropoiesis, is regulated by the oxygen concentration in tissues throughout the body. When oxygen concentration drops for any number of reasons in a condition called hypoxia, the body sends signals to the kidneys to produce additional EPO. The hematopoietic growth factor then travels to the bone marrow to increase the production of RBCs, which will eventually lead to an increase in oxygen concentration. The same cycle is repeated in reverse when oxygen levels are high. Signals are sent to the kidneys to decrease EPO production, which will, in turn, decrease the number of RBCs produced in the bone marrow and decrease oxygen supply in the tissues. This type of regulation is known as a feedback loop and is commonly found in a number of body systems.

PRACTICE POINT

EPO can be made synthetically and used as a treatment for several anemias. Synthetic erythropoietins are discussed at length in Chapter 26.

White Blood Cells

As mentioned in the previous section, there are six different WBCs found in the blood. Collectively, the neutrophils, basophils, and eosinophils are known as granulocytes because of the granules containing various substances found in each cell that fight infection, signal other WBCs, or cause allergic reactions. Slightly larger than RBCs, granulocytes are about 8–12 μm in diameter. At about 60% to 70%, the neutrophils are the most common of the WBCs and are also called polymorphonuclear cells (PMNs) due to their strangely shaped nuclei (see Figure 25-1). Neutrophils are often the first responders to outside invaders and leave the bloodstream to attack pathogens head on. Eosinophils, the WBCs usually linked with allergic reactions and fighting parasites, are much less common than neutrophils, accounting for only 2% to 4% of all WBCs. Basophils, however, are even rarer, making up only 0.5% to 1% of the WBCs.

Lymphocytes come in a variety of sizes ranging from 6–14 μm in diameter. They are the second most common WBC at 20% to 25%. The T lymphocytes are responsible for fending off viral infections and destroying human cells that have become cancerous. By using special receptors found on the outside surface of cells, T lymphocytes can differentiate *self* from *nonself* and launch attacks on anything that is seen as a foreign body.

PRACTICE POINT

Unfortunately, the process by which T lymphocytes discern self from nonself also results in attacks on organs that may be transplanted from other people or species.

B lymphocytes, on the other hand, act as the memory bank of the immune system, creating antibodies that circulate in blood vessels and attach themselves to invading organisms. Some B lymphocytes mature into memory cells that can survive many years in the bloodstream, ready to unload countless antibodies when a known pathogen returns.

PRACTICE POINT

Memory B cells are also responsible for conferring long-term immunity when a vaccine is administered.

Monocytes and their counterparts in the tissues, the macrophages, make up 3% to 8% of all WBCs. They are roughly twice the size of RBCs at 12–20 μm in diameter, but they can grow many times that size in the face of an immune response. Though neutrophils are usually the first WBCs to respond to sites of infection, the macrophages tend to do most of the defending. The function of the macrophage is phagocytosis, or the swallowing of pathogens and cellular debris. Once it has ingested a pathogen, the macrophage will attempt to destroy or contain it while it sends out signaling chemicals, called cytokines, to call additional WBCs to the area.

Even though RBCs outnumber WBCs by a ratio of at least 500:1, 75% of the bone marrow is dedicated to the production of WBCs. These numbers show that the turnover rate for WBCs is high, particularly when an immune response is ongoing. For instance, a macrophage, which has a typical life span of 1–3 months in normal tissue, may only survive a few hours when it is battling an infection at full capacity. Similar to the effect of EPO on RBCs, the production of WBCs is increased by CSFs and cytokines released from cells at the site of infection and is decreased when the infection resolves.

Plasma

The cells discussed above make up approximately 45% of the blood volume. Though they perform the bulk of the hematological processes, they could not function without the remaining 55%, made up of plasma. The largest component of plasma is water (more than 91%), which acts as the conduit through which all blood cells flow. Suspended in this water are numerous proteins, such as albumin, antibodies, and fibrinogen, along with dissolved nutrients, electrolytes, gases, and waste products. Also located in the plasma are the numerous enzymes that make up the clotting cascade, a complex system of checks and balances that lead to the production and breakdown of blood clots.

HEMOSTASIS

When significant damage occurs to a blood vessel, the body works quickly to minimize the loss of blood. This process, known as hemostasis, is made up of three important steps: a narrowing of the damaged blood vessel known as vasoconstriction, the formation of a platelet plug, and the formation of a blood clot through the clotting cascade. While the response must be quick and definitive, the body must also be careful to avoid an overreactive hemostatic response that could lead to thrombogenesis, the formation of an unwanted blood clot. When a thrombus is formed, the risk for heart attack, stroke, and other cardiovascular events is drastically increased. As in most body systems, there is a delicate balance between coagulation and anticoagulation to form clots in appropriate areas and dissolve those that are not needed.

Vasoconstriction

After an initial injury, damaged cells send a signal to the surrounding smooth muscle to contract immediately. This is an effort to decrease the size of the blood vessel and limit the amount of blood flowing through it. If the injury is significant, the vasoconstriction may even result in the complete closure of the blood vessel. While this is an effective short-term measure to decrease blood loss, it is usually temporary, buying time for platelets to congregate in the area and to initiate the clotting cascade.

Platelet Plug Formation

As discussed earlier, platelets are released from megakaryocytes in the bone marrow in response to TPO. These smallest of blood cells are only 2–4 µm in diameter and are essentially only fragments of the much larger megakaryocyte precursor cell. Once they enter the circulation, platelets live for an average of 5–9 days.

Circulating platelets are attracted to damaged areas of vessel walls. Once attached, the platelet is activated and releases signaling chemicals that cause additional vasoconstriction and attract other platelets to the area. As more platelets arrive, the normally disc-shaped cells spread out and become sticky. This change makes it easier for platelets to interact with one another and form the platelet plug to fill any gaps in the vessel wall.

The Clotting Cascade

The platelet plug, though an important step in hemostasis, usually cannot stop a bleed alone. It is a loose mass of platelets that can be dislodged from the area of injury unless strengthened by fibrin threads, which are the end products of the clotting cascade (see Figure 25-3). Made up of a series of reactions, the clotting cascade involves the sequential activation of clotting factors.

The cascade is divided into three parts: the intrinsic, extrinsic, and common pathways. As described above, when tissue damage is present, the body needs to respond quickly to repair the damaged site. The extrinsic pathway is designed to be a fast track to the development of a clot. In cases of severe damage, the extrinsic pathway can form a clot in seconds. For this pathway to be used, damaged tissue must supply the starting ingredient, a protein called tissue factor (TF). Even without obvious tissue damage, however, it is still possible for a clot to form. When no TF is released, the intrinsic pathway must be used to form a clot. This longer pathway requires multiple steps and could take several minutes to form a clot. The delay is a natural protection against unwanted clot formation, allowing time for the body's anticoagulants to take effect, if necessary. The intrinsic and extrinsic pathways converge to form the common pathway. Here, the final steps in the conversion of fibrinogen (one of the soluble proteins found in the plasma) to active fibrin threads occur. Once formed, the fibrin threads interact with the platelet plug, interweaving between platelets and entangled RBCs and lending strength to the new clot. At this point, blood loss is contained and the body can begin to heal the damaged area, replacing the injured vessel wall with new cells.

The ability of the clotting cascade to function normally depends heavily on the body having enough vitamin K. This important nutrient is found in most green, leafy vegetables and is essential to the production of clotting factors II, VII, IX, and X. If the body's stores are low, the production of these factors will decrease and clot formation will be more difficult to achieve, increasing the risk of bleeding. Conversely, some medications, such as warfarin, will intentionally interfere with vitamin K to anticoagulate a patient. These and other anticoagulants (commonly known as *blood thinners*) are discussed in Chapter 26.

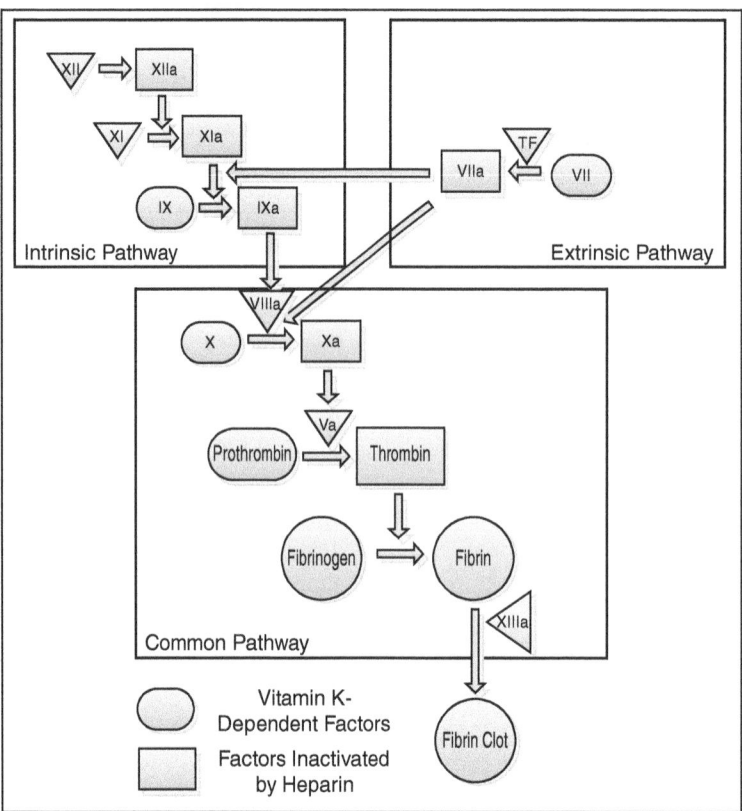

FIGURE 25-3. The clotting cascade. TF = tissue factor.

Regulation of Hemostasis

When clots are formed at inappropriate locations or appropriate clots are no longer needed, the fibrinolytic cascade works to undo the effects of the clotting cascade. Incorporated into each formed clot is an inactive enzyme called plasminogen. The inactive enzyme can be converted to plasmin, which acts to dissolve fibrin threads and inhibit many clot-forming substances. Circulating in the blood are the body's own natural anticoagulants, such as heparin and others, working to block the clotting cascade at various points, as well. After these substances were discovered, many were developed into powerful medications, which are discussed in Chapter 26. In this, as in many other body systems, it is the interplay between these two opposing systems that allows the hemostatic system to function properly.

COMMON BLOOD TESTS

A number of blood tests are available to healthcare providers to assess the status of the hematological and hemostatic systems. The most widely used is the complete blood count (CBC). In each CBC, the WBC count, platelet count, hemoglobin level, and hematocrit are measured. The WBC count is a useful tool to identify infections, check the health of the immune system, or screen for cancers of the bone marrow. Typical WBC counts range between 5,000 and 10,000 cells per microliter (µL, or 0.1 mL) of blood. When the number of WBCs is higher than expected, the patient is said to have a leukocytosis, while those that have low counts have a leukopenia. If a CBC is ordered with differential, the lab will also include counts of each individual type of WBC for comparison. See Table 25-2 for more details. Platelet counts can show the ability of the body to form clots. Normal platelet counts are between 150,000 and 450,000 cells per microliter of blood. These levels can be affected by certain platelet disorders, cancers, and medications. The hemoglobin and hematocrit levels are two of the most important laboratory tests to screen for anemias. Hemoglobin is usually between 13.1 and 17.3 g/dL in adults. Though the hemoglobin level is very useful in determining the presence of an anemia, it does little to describe the cause. Additional lab tests, such as the mean corpuscular volume (MCV), ferritin, total iron binding capacity (TIBC), vitamin B_{12} and folate levels, need to be ordered. These tests are discussed in greater detail in

TABLE 25-2. Components of a Complete Blood Count with Differential[2]

Blood Test	Reference Range[a]	Common Causes of High Values	Common Causes of Low Values
RBC count	3.5–6.0 million/µL	• Certain cancers	• Anemias
WBC count	4,500–11,000/µL	• Infections • Steroids	• Chemotherapy or radiation
Platelet count	150,000–450,000/µL	• Certain cancers	• Heparin-induced thrombocytopenia • Certain immune diseases
Hemoglobin	12.0–17.5 g/dL	• Living at high altitudes • Smoking	• Anemias • Bleeding
Hematocrit	35%–49%	• Dehydration (falsely high) • Smoking	• Anemias • Bleeding
Neutrophils	50%–70% of WBCs	• Bacterial infection • Severe burns	• Chemotherapy or radiation • Certain medications
Lymphocytes	20%–40% of WBCs	• Viral infection • Certain cancers	• AIDS • Steroids
Monocytes	2%–6% of WBCs	• Chronic inflammation • Infections	• Certain cancers • Steroids
Eosinophils	1%–4% of WBCs	• Allergic reaction • Parasitic infection	• Often low without significant issues • Stress
Basophils	0%–1% of WBCs	• Allergic reaction • Chronic inflammation	• Often low without significant issues • Stress

RBC = red blood cell; WBC = white blood cell.
[a]Reference ranges may vary depending on individual laboratory techniques used.

Chapter 26. Finally, when a patient's hemostatic system is in need of closer examination, tests such as the international normalized ratio (INR) and activated partial thromboplastin time (aPTT) describe the ability of the body to form clots and helps keep the doses of powerful anticoagulants in the proper range. These tests are discussed in Chapter 26, as well.

SUMMARY

Blood is made up of a number of cells, proteins, and other substances that work together to transport substances, defend the body from invaders, and stop blood loss after an injury occurs. All blood cells begin as hematopoietic stem cells found in bone marrow. The stem cells differentiate into red blood cells (RBCs), white blood cells (WBCs), and platelets when influenced by hematopoietic growth factors, such as erythropoietin (EPO).

The RBCs are responsible for the transport of oxygen from the lungs to tissues all over the body. When hemoglobin

in the RBCs is exposed to an oxygen-rich environment, the iron ions can bind to oxygen molecules. The blood is then pumped to distant capillaries where the oxygen supply is low. As the concentration drops, the oxygen molecules break free of the hemoglobin and diffuse into the tissue.

Neutrophils, eosinophils, basophils, monocytes, and lymphocytes are collectively known as the WBCs. The WBCs are responsible for defending the body from infection. When a pathogen enters the body, neutrophils are the first cells to respond. They attack the invader and try to engulf it while sending out signals to attract other WBCs. Monocytes and their counterparts in the tissues, the macrophages, arrive next and also swallow pathogens. Lymphocytes are broken down into two groups. The T lymphocyte helps the body fight viral infections and kills off tumor cells. B lymphocytes, once activated, produce antibodies against antigens. The eosinophils and basophils, the least common WBCs, are responsible for allergic reactions in the body.

The hemostatic system stops the loss of blood from damaged blood vessels. The initial reaction to injury at a blood vessel is vasoconstriction. This tightening of smooth muscles decreases the amount of blood flowing through the area of injury, buying time for the rest of the system to go into effect. Platelets are blood cells that form plugs to stop blood loss. When exposed to an area of blood vessel damage, platelets are activated, becoming sticky and larger in size. Activated platelets also send signals to other platelets to converge. As more platelets arrive, they form a loose mass called a platelet plug. On its own, the platelet plug cannot adequately stop blood loss. It needs to be strengthened by the addition of fibrin threads. Fibrin threads are formed when soluble fibrinogen is converted into fibrin at the end of the clotting cascade. For blood clots to form rapidly when tissue damage is present, the extrinsic pathway of the clotting cascade shortens the usually complex series of steps necessary to form clots. The intrinsic pathway, however, allows clots to form even in the absence of tissue damage. To minimize the inappropriate clotting of blood, this pathway requires many steps to occur in sequence for clot formation. Other natural checks and balances are in place in the body to keep blood clots where they are needed, such as the fibrinolytic cascade, a system of many enzymes and anticoagulants that regulate the process of thrombogenesis.

Healthcare providers have a number of tests at their disposal to evaluate the condition of the hematologic system. The most commonly used blood test is the complete blood count (CBC). WBC counts, platelet counts, hemoglobin, and hematocrit levels are typically reported in a CBC. A high WBC count, a condition called leukocytosis, is usually present in patients with an infection, cancer, or on certain medications. Platelet counts can show how well a person can form blood clots, and the hemoglobin and hematocrit levels are usually used to detect the presence of an anemia.

REFERENCES

1. National Institutes of Health, Office of Dietary Supplements. Nutrient recommendations: Dietary Reference Intakes (DRIs). https://ods.od.nih.gov/Health_Information/Dietary_Reference_Intakes.aspx. Accessed April 5, 2022.
2. Nicoll D, Mark Lu C, McPhee SJ. *Guide to Diagnostic Tests*. 7th ed. New York, NY: McGraw-Hill; 2017.

CHAPTER RESOURCES

Barrett KE, Barman SM, Brooks HL, et al. *Ganong's Review of Medical Physiology*. 26th ed. New York, NY: McGraw-Hill; 2019.

DiPiro JT, Yee GC, Posey M, et al., eds. *Pharmacotherapy: A Pathophysiological Approach*. 11th ed. New York: NY: McGraw-Hill; 2020.

REVIEW QUESTIONS

1. Describe the developmental processes that lead to the body's production of blood cells.
2. Name the WBCs and the function of each type.
3. Describe the effects of a vitamin B_{12} or folate deficiency on RBC shape, production, and hemoglobin levels.
4. Describe the three components of the hemostatic system.
5. List the most common laboratory blood tests and why each is used.

Chapter 26

Disorders of the Hematologic System

Marcia E. Honisko, PharmD, RPh, BCOP |
Megan A. Kaun, PharmD, RPh, BCACP

KEY TERMS AND DEFINITIONS

Anemia—a condition in which red blood cell mass and hemoglobin are below normal, leading to clinical symptoms, including pallor, fatigue, difficulty breathing, and rapid heartbeat.

Deep vein thrombosis (DVT)—formation of a blood clot in the deep vessels carrying blood back to the heart. DVT occurs most commonly in the veins of the legs but can also occur in the arms and other locations in the body.

Embolus—a piece of a blood clot that has broken off and traveled via the bloodstream to a distant location in the body.

Endothelial damage—damage to the inner lining of the blood vessel wall (promotes clot formation).

Erythropoiesis—the production of red blood cells from the bone marrow.

Hematocrit—a calculation of the percentage of blood volume that is occupied by red blood cells.

Hemoglobin—a protein in red blood cells consisting of heme, globin, and iron that transports oxygen to tissues.

Hemolysis—the destruction of red blood cells.

Hypercoagulability—a state in which the body forms blood clots more readily than considered normal.

International normalized ratio (INR)—a blood test used to measure the degree of anticoagulation in a patient taking warfarin.

DOI 10.37573/9781585286638.026

Intrinsic factor—a small protein secreted by glands in the stomach that is required for absorption of vitamin B_{12}.

Macrocytic—a term used to describe large red blood cells.

Megaloblastic—a term used to describe anemia in which red blood cells are large.

Microcytic—a term used to describe small red blood cells.

Normocytic—a term used to describe normal-sized red blood cells.

Pernicious anemia—anemia resulting from a deficiency in intrinsic factor and absorption of vitamin B_{12}.

Pulmonary embolism (PE)—all or part of a blood clot that has become dislodged from its point of origin and traveled to the lung causing a blockage.

Stasis—a condition in which blood flow is significantly slowed or halted within certain areas of the blood vessels.

LEARNING OBJECTIVES

After completing this chapter, you should be able to

1. List the different types of anemia.

2. Describe the presentation and laboratory abnormalities associated with the different types of anemia.

3. State the therapies used to treat each type of anemia.

4. List medications that can cause neutropenia and thrombocytopenia, and state drugs that are useful for neutropenia.

5. Explain the factors that cause clot formation and list the most common sites of clot formation.

6. Describe acute and chronic treatment of clots.

7. Explain the therapeutic effects, most common side effects, and adverse reactions of anticoagulant medications.

8. State brand and generic names of anticoagulant medications, along with routes of administration, dosage forms, and available doses.

Red blood cells (RBCs), or erythrocytes, circulate through the blood and function to carry oxygen to tissues. The lifespan of RBCs is about 120 days, at which time they are removed from the system by macrophages. To ensure the RBC mass stays constant, erythropoiesis takes place with the help of erythropoietin. Anemia occurs when there is not sufficient

RBC mass and is determined by several different measurements. These laboratory values or calculations include hemoglobin, hematocrit, the number of RBCs, indices of RBC size and color, and other factors depending on the type of anemia (see Table 26-1).

Anemia can be classified based on the cause (excessive blood loss, destruction of blood cells, hemolysis, or ineffective production of RBCs) or based on the RBC size: microcytic (small), normocytic (normal), or macrocytic (large). Within each type, there are specific causes of the anemia; that is, anemia is a component of an underlying disease or problem. Anemic patients may present with varying clinical effects. In general, patients may experience fatigue, pallor (paleness to the skin), dizziness, faintness, difficulty breathing, rapid heart rate, headache, and lack of concentration. Other manifestations may occur, specific to the type of anemia, and will be described with each type of anemia.

CASE

Mr. Felow, a 67-year-old male, was brought to the hospital by his wife, who was concerned about her husband's significant unsteadiness, tiredness, and pale coloring noticeable over the past couple of days. Workup was initiated to explain these symptoms. Blood work was obtained and included a hemoglobin level of 7.1 g/dL. The physician explained to the patient and his wife that the patient has iron deficiency anemia.

CASE?

Mr. Felow was told he needed to have a colonoscopy as part of the workup for his newly diagnosed anemia. What is the reasoning for this procedure?

MICROCYTIC ANEMIA

The classic origin of microcytic anemia is iron deficiency. Deficiency of iron may result from a number of different causes, including lack of sufficient iron in the diet, inadequate absorption of iron, and blood loss. Absorption may be altered due to surgery or the absence of acid in the stomach, which could occur in patients taking medications like proton pump inhibitors. Gastrointestinal (GI) bleeding is a main

TABLE 26-1. Normal Laboratory Values Utilized in Evaluating Anemia[1,a]

Laboratory Value	Normal Range	
	Male	Female
Hemoglobin (g/dL)	14–18	12–16
Hematocrit (%)	42–52	37–47
RBCs (millions/mm³)	4.3–5.9	3.5–5.5
Mean corpuscular volume (MCV)	76–96	76–96
Mean corpuscular hemoglobin (MCH)	27–32	27–32
Serum iron (mcg/dL)	50–160	40–150
Ferritin (ng/mL)	20–300	20–200
Iron saturation (%)	20–50	20–50
Total iron binding capacity (TIBC; mcg/dL)	255–450	255–450
Vitamin B_{12} (pg/mL)	200–800	200–800
Folic acid (ng/mL)	≥3	≥3
Reticulocyte count (%)	0.5–1.5	0.5–1.5
Haptoglobin (mg/dL)	38–208	38–208
Lactate dehydrogenase (LDH; international units/L)	100–225	100–225
Bilirubin Total (mg/dL) Direct (mg/dL)	0.1–1 0–0.4	0.1–1 0–0.4

aValue ranges may vary slightly.

cause of blood loss, although menstruation, other types of hemorrhaging, and blood donation may also be contributors.

Regardless of the cause, hemoglobin is below normal in iron deficiency anemia, and other laboratory values help describe this type of anemia. Mean corpuscular volume (MCV) is the measure of the average volume of RBCs and relates to RBC size. MCV is low in iron deficiency anemia. Serum iron, ferritin, iron saturation, and total iron binding capacity (TIBC) are also used to evaluate the anemia. Serum iron is low, as is ferritin, which is considered the storage form of iron. TIBC is the capacity of iron to be bound by transferrin, a transport protein of iron. TIBC is high in patients with iron deficiency anemia because with the lack of iron, there is plenty of availability for iron to be bound to transferrin.

Patients with low iron levels, as defined by typical laboratory assessment, present with classic symptomatology of tiredness, weakness, and pallor. Tongue soreness, thin/brittle nails, and koilonychia (concave surface to nails) may also be present. Patients may also experience cravings for dirt, clay, or ice chips; this phenomenon of craving substances not fit to eat is referred to as pica.

Therapy to correct the objective and subjective signs of this anemia involves treatment of an underlying cause and the use of exogenous (produced by a manufacturer other than the body) iron. If, for example, a GI bleed or other type of hemorrhage is the contributing factor, it should be treated appropriately. Replenishing iron may be accomplished through the use of oral iron products. Ferrous sulfate

CASE?

What other abnormal laboratory values may have been noted on Mr. Felow's initial blood work besides the below-normal hemoglobin?

CASE?

List the symptoms Mr. Felow is experiencing that are consistent with iron deficiency anemia.

is most often used and is inexpensive, though other salt forms, such as ferrous gluconate and ferrous fumarate, are available (see Medication Table 26-1; Medication Tables are located at the end of the chapter). Approximately 200 mg of elemental iron per day is needed to treat iron deficiency.

PRACTICE POINT

Iron salts, by definition, have components other than elemental iron. Ferrous sulfate, for instance, has only about 65 mg of elemental iron in a 325-mg tablet. Based on that value, ferrous sulfate 300–325 mg administered three times daily yields a dose of 200 mg of elemental iron per day.

Iron is best absorbed when taken on an empty stomach and in an acidic environment. Many patients, however, are not able to tolerate this administration technique due to nausea and GI irritation and, therefore, the dose is titrated (gradually increased to the desired dose) or is taken with a light meal or snack. Other adverse effects of oral iron include constipation, dark stools, heartburn, and abdominal cramping. To ensure iron absorption, milk and antacids should not be ingested at the same time iron is taken. Vitamin C (ascorbic acid) may increase the absorption if taken with iron in the form of vitamin C supplements or orange juice. There are iron-containing products that also contain vitamin C and other vitamins in the dosage form (see Medication Table 26-2).

PRACTICE POINT

Oral iron products are available as prescription or over the counter. Some products are combined with other agents, such as ascorbic acid, vitamin B$_{12}$, or folic acid. Review the latest product information for up-to-date specifics on ingredients, dosing, and availability.

Another consideration for the optimal absorption of iron is the understanding that iron is mainly absorbed in the duodenum. Enteric-coated products are formulated with a barrier to control the location of absorption and are thought to reduce GI upset. Iron products that are enteric coated, however, may reach the small intestine, where absorption is not the most favorable, and these products are not the

best option. Similarly, sustained-release iron formulations do not allow for duodenal absorption. Oral iron therapy usually continues for a 3- to 6-month period, though it is usually individualized to patient need and response.

ALERT!

Accidental overdose of iron can be fatal in children. Care should be taken to keep iron-containing products out of the reach of children.

PRACTICE POINT

Iron may interfere with the absorption of other medications, including fluoroquinolone antibiotics, tetracycline antibiotics, bisphosphonates for osteoporosis, and thyroid supplements. A few hours should separate the ingestion of these medications before or after iron ingestion.

Patients who are not able to tolerate oral iron, have absorption problems, or are losing iron rapidly, may require intravenous (IV) iron for correction of their deficits. A few IV iron products are available: iron dextran (INFeD), iron sucrose (Venofer), sodium ferric gluconate (Ferrlecit), ferumoxytol (Feraheme), ferric derisomaltose (Monoferric), and ferric carboxymaltose (Injectafer) (see Medication Table 26-3). Iron dextran may be administered in daily doses or as a total dose infusion over several hours based on the hemoglobin level and deficit. The calculation used for iron dextran dosing is based on the hemoglobin deficit and the patient's ideal body weight.

CASE?

After being discharged from the hospital, Mr. Felow arrives at the pharmacy with a prescription for iron. What information should the pharmacist give to the patient about how to take the ferrous sulfate he is now going to purchase and what to expect? Along with the iron, his wife would like to purchase a bottle of magnesium hydroxide in case Mr. Felow experiences constipation with the iron. What other information should be provided to the patient?

Besides allergic reactions, iron dextran may also cause pain at the IV site, fever, and muscle or joint pain. Iron sucrose, sodium ferric gluconate, ferumoxytol, and ferric carboxymaltose have less potential to cause allergic reactions and do not require a test dose, but they cannot be administered as a single total dose infusion. Instead, these IV iron forms are administered in smaller, repeated doses. For example, ferumoxytol is administered to patients with iron deficiency in chronic kidney disease as a single 510-mg dose followed by a second 510-mg dose 3–8 days later; similarly, ferric carboxymaltose is administered as two 750-mg doses one week apart. Iron sucrose may be administered in several daily doses or an alternative schedule with a maximum amount of 1,000 mg in a 14-day period. Ferric derisomaltose is the newest approved product; the dose is dependent on the patient's weight and is administered over at least 20 minutes. It does also require observation after infusion for potential hypersensitivity reaction.

ALERT!

Due to the possibility of allergic reactions, the first dose of iron dextran is preceded by a test dose followed by a period of observation for signs and symptoms of low blood pressure, swelling, hives, itching, or difficulty breathing.

MACROCYTIC ANEMIA

Macrocytic anemia falls at the other end of the spectrum of RBC size and results from deficiency of vitamin B_{12} and/or folic acid; it is also referred to as megaloblastic (large cell) anemia. In macrocytic anemia, vitamin B_{12} and folic acid levels are below normal on laboratory data, and MCV is above normal. Causes of vitamin B_{12} deficiency may be dietary deficiency or deficiency of intrinsic factor, which is secreted by the parietal cells in the stomach and is essential for the absorption of vitamin B_{12}. Lack of vitamin B_{12} due to deficiency of intrinsic factor is referred to as pernicious anemia and is determined by the Schilling test, which uses intramuscular and radio-labeled vitamin B_{12} to evaluate the renal elimination of B_{12}. Radio-labeled vitamin B_{12} has been tagged with a radioactive substance to be more readily identified and measured for testing purposes. If less than 5% of the administered vitamin B_{12} is detected in the urine, pernicious anemia is diagnosed. Due to shortages of the radio-labeled product, this test may be difficult to perform. Causes of folic

acid deficiency include a deficient diet, impaired absorption such as after gastric bypass surgery, alcoholism, pregnancy, or medication. Examples of drugs involved in folic acid deficiency are phenytoin (Dilantin), trimethoprim (Primsol), methotrexate (Rheumatrex), carbamazepine (Tegretol), or sulfasalazine (Azulfidine).

CASE?

After several weeks, Mr. Felow has been having a lot of difficulty tolerating the ferrous sulfate tablets. He has been experiencing significant nausea and stomach cramping interfering with eating and meeting his dietary needs. As a result, his physician decides to order IV iron dextran. What symptoms should he watch for while receiving the iron?

Presentation of macrocytic anemia involves weakness and pallor. Other signs may include a sore, beefy, red tongue and central nervous system symptoms, including paresthesias (abnormal burning or tingling sensations) and numbness. Replacing vitamin B_{12} and folic acid is the treatment for macrocytic anemia. Vitamin B_{12} (cyanocobalamin) is administered intramuscularly as a daily injection for 7 days, then once a week for 4 weeks, and then monthly as a maintenance dose. A similar response may be seen with the use of oral cobalamin products, although high doses are required to ensure adequate absorption, as is patient adherence with daily dosing. Folic acid may be taken orally as a 1-mg dose once daily for approximately 2–3 weeks. Macrocytic anemia should not be treated using folic acid alone without vitamin B_{12} because although the MCV and anemia would normalize, the neurological symptoms would not be addressed or improved.

NORMOCYTIC ANEMIA

Anemia may also be classified as normocytic, in which the RBCs are of normal size and the MCV is within normal values. Patients with long-standing disease states often also experience anemia that is normocytic in nature. Examples of chronic diseases associated with anemia are congestive heart failure, malignancy (cancer), systemic lupus, rheumatoid arthritis, endocarditis (inflammation of the inner layer of the heart), osteomyelitis (infection and inflammation of the bone or bone marrow), and chronic lung infections. This anemia is also referred to as anemia of inflammation. In addition to low hemoglobin and a normal MCV, laboratory data may show a low TIBC, decreased iron, and a normal to high ferritin level. Correction of this anemia is to treat the underlying chronic disease state.

Chronic kidney disease is another example of disease that can lead to normocytic/normochromic anemia. In this situation, erythropoietin is not effectively produced by the kidney, and RBCs have an abbreviated lifespan; however, other causes for the anemia should be evaluated and ruled out to ensure appropriate therapy. Erythropoietin-stimulating agents (ESAs) may be utilized for patients with chronic kidney disease, dialysis dependent or not, to maintain hemoglobin in the range of 10–12 g/dL. The available ESAs, epoetin alfa (Procrit, Epogen), epoetin alfa-epbx (Retacrit, a biosimilar agent), and darbepoetin alfa (Aranesp), are administered either subcutaneously or intravenously. Dosing of epoetin alfa is 50–100 units per kilogram of body weight (units/kg) 3 times a week, while the usual darbepoetin alfa dosing is 0.45 microgram per kilogram of body weight (mcg/kg) once weekly or 0.75 mcg/kg every other week for patients not on dialysis. Sufficient iron is needed to ensure an appropriate response to the ESAs and may be supplemented orally or intravenously.

ESAs may also be considered for anemia resulting from cancer therapy. Some chemotherapeutic agents are myelosuppressive, meaning they tend to cause a reduction of blood cells, including RBCs, white blood cells, and platelets formed in the bone marrow. ESAs may be part of the cancer therapy to treat anemia and low hemoglobin for patients receiving myelosuppressive therapy. They are not recommended when the anticipated outcome of the therapy is cure as some studies have shown risk of progression of the cancer and shortened survival with the use of ESAs in certain types of cancer. The main goal of this therapy, therefore, is to improve quality of life and to reduce the need for blood transfusions in patients with a significantly low hemoglobin level or symptoms from the anemia.[2] There are guidelines, however, for ESA initiation, dose adjustments, and duration of therapy in this indication. The dose is adjusted based on response and hemoglobin levels. High blood pressure and thromboembolic events are side effects that have been related to ESA usage. In fact, uncontrolled high blood pressure is a contraindication for epoetin alfa and darbepoetin alfa (see Medication Table 26-4).

PRACTICE POINT

A medication guide for ESA therapy must be provided to each patient prior to administering or dispensing epoetin alfa and darbepoetin alfa.

ALERT!

Using the lowest dose of ESAs sufficient to reduce the need for RBC transfusions decreases the incidence of serious cardiovascular events.

HEMOLYTIC ANEMIA

Classified based on its cause, hemolytic anemia occurs when RBCs are destroyed prematurely. Hemolytic anemia may be caused by a variety of factors, including an autoimmune process; infections such as malaria; drugs or chemicals such as sulfonamides, nitrates, nitrofurantoin, salicylates, lead, or copper; and radiation. Specific laboratory work that reveals hemolytic anemia includes an elevated reticulocyte count, a low level of haptoglobin (the protein that binds to free hemoglobin), elevated lactate dehydrogenase (LDH), and bilirubin. For autoimmune hemolytic anemia, further testing involves a Coombs' test, which helps determine if patients have warm or cold antibodies on RBCs. Splenomegaly (enlarged spleen), hepatomegaly (enlarged liver), weakness, and lymphadenopathy (enlarged lymph nodes) may be present with warm hemolytic anemia and involves immune globulin (IgG) antibodies. Treatment strategies may include corticosteroids, folic acid, removal of the spleen, blood transfusions, and IV IgG. Cold autoimmune hemolytic anemia involves IgM antibodies and may be associated with malignancy. Transfusions with warm blood and avoiding cold exposure are therapies for this type of anemia.

DRUG-INDUCED NEUTROPENIA

Neutropenia is a condition involving a white blood cell (WBC) count below normal and is defined as having an absolute neutrophil count (ANC) below 1,500/µL. The ANC is calculated by multiplying the WBC count by the percent of mature (segmented) neutrophils and immature WBCs (bands) from the differential report on the complete blood count laboratory data. Causes of neutropenia include infection, congenital factors, primary immune neutropenia, and drug-related causes. Drug-induced neutropenia may further be divided into chemotherapy-involved and nonchemotherapy-involved drugs.

As discussed previously, cytotoxic or myelosuppressive chemotherapeutic agents have the ability to reduce blood counts, including WBCs. Examples of these agents include methotrexate, cyclophosphamide (Cytoxan), and doxorubicin (Adriamycin, Doxil), among several others or combinations of drugs. Patients receiving these medications are at risk for developing febrile neutropenia (reduced WBC count with fever), severe infections, and morbidity and fatality related to the infections. Granulocyte colony-stimulating factors (G-CSFs) are available to prevent or treat chemotherapy-induced neutropenia to reduce the related infections and potential time spent in the hospital (see Medication Table 26-5). Some chemotherapy regimens put patients at high risk for neutropenia, and certain patient factors, such as older age and comorbidities (coexisting medical conditions), also increase the risk of developing neutropenia. Filgrastim (Neupogen) is a G-CSF used to prevent and treat neutropenia. It is dosed as a 5 mcg/kg daily subcutaneous (SUBQ) injection. Pegfilgrastim (Neulasta) is a G-CSF with a longer action than filgrastim; therefore, this drug is used only for prevention of the neutropenia at a dose of 6 mg subcutaneously. Both medications should be administered starting 24–72 hours after the chemotherapy is given, and the pegfilgrastim should not be administered within 2 weeks of the next cycle of chemotherapy. Both drugs also have biosimilar agents approved for use. The most common side effect of filgrastim and pegfilgrastim is bone pain. Other less common adverse effects include rupture of the spleen and allergic reactions with manifestations of rash, wheezing, and low blood pressure.

PRACTICE POINT

Pegfilgrastim may be administered as a conventional subcutaneous injection or with an on-body injector, a device that injects the drug over 45 minutes 27 hours after being placed on the patient.

PRACTICE POINT

The side effect of bone pain may be treated with non-narcotic analgesics, such as nonsteroidal anti-inflammatory drugs or acetaminophen.

In addition to cancer chemotherapy, other medications may also cause neutropenia, or agranulocytosis, though less commonly. The drugs either produce an immune-mediated process in which the drug or drug metabolite binds to the neutrophil membrane and forms antibodies or has a direct toxic effect on the cells. A list of drugs from varying classes of medications with probability of causing neutropenia has been formulated based on case reports and population studies. Some of the more common offenders include clozapine (Clozaril), antithyroid drugs, sulfasalazine, and ticlopidine. The low WBC count may be delayed 3–6 months after the drug treatment begins but could occur within days to weeks if the cause is immune-mediated. Patients may be asymptomatic or may present with a sore throat or fever. Treatment involves discontinuing the suspected drug although identifying the specific drug may be difficult, especially if patients are taking multiple medications. The neutropenia usually resolves within 1–3 weeks of stopping the drug. Treatment may also include treating the infection or using a G-CSF though high-grade evidence for their use is not available. Table 26-2 lists some medications that have been implicated as causes of neutropenia.

TABLE 26-2. Drugs with High Risk for Inducing Neutropenia[3]

Drug Class	Medications
Antithyroid	Methimazole Propylthiouracil
Anti-inflammatory	NSAIDs Sulfasalazine
Psychotropic	Clozapine Phenothiazines Tricyclic antidepressants
Cardiovascular	Antiarrhythmics: flecainide, procainamide Ticlopidine Angiotensin-converting enzyme inhibitors Propranolol Dipyridamole Digoxin
Dermatologic	Dapsone Isotretinoin
Antibacterial	Macrolides Trimethoprim/sulfamethoxazole Chloramphenicol Sulfonamides Vancomycin Cephalosporins Penicillin G
Antimalarial	Chloroquine Quinine

Continued next page

TABLE 26-2. Drugs with High Risk for Inducing Neutropenia *(Continued)*

Drug Class	Medications
Antifungal	Amphotericin B Flucytosine
Anticonvulsants	Carbamazepine Phenytoin Valproic acid
Diuretics	Thiazides Furosemide Spironolactone
Sulfonylureas	Chlorpropamide

PRACTICE POINT

Clozapine is only available through a restricted REMS (Risk Evaluation and Mitigation Strategy) program. Prescribers and dispensing pharmacies must be certified, and patients must be educated regarding the risk of neutropenia and be enrolled in the program.

DRUG-INDUCED THROMBOCYTOPENIA

Medications may also cause a reduction in the platelet count, or thrombocytopenia, caused by drug-dependent antibodies that allow destruction of platelets. Several medications have caused thrombocytopenia. The drugs with the most frequent reports of reduction of platelets include heparin, abciximab (ReoPro), quinine, quinidine, sulfonamides, vancomycin, gold salts, beta-lactam antibiotics, and valproic acid (Depakote, Depakene) products.

Heparin is the most common drug that is implicated as a cause of thrombocytopenia. Low molecular weight heparin (LMWH) products also may cause thrombocytopenia, but the incidence is lower compared to heparin. There are two types of heparin-induced thrombocytopenia: heparin-induced thrombocytopenia type I (HIT-I) (sometimes referred to as heparin-associated thrombocytopenia [HAT]) and heparin-induced thrombocytopenia type II (HIT-II). HIT-I involves a direct effect on platelets and a lesser reduction of platelets, while HIT-II involves an immune-mediated effect with antibodies directed against heparin complexes and a significant reduction of platelets. A test for heparin antibodies may be used to determine if a patient has HIT-II, although it is not very sensitive, giving false negative results. The serotonin release assay is also a test used to verify HIT-II and carries high sensitivity and specificity, which are statistical measures of how good a test is at identifying true positives and negatives over false positives and negatives. In HIT-II, the platelet count begins to fall within 5–10 days of the heparin initiation, and the formation of clots is a risk. Consequently, it may sometimes be referred to as HITT for heparin-induced thrombocytopenia and thrombosis.

Treatment of drug-induced thrombocytopenia includes stopping the causative drug. Because of the risk of thrombosis in HIT-II, other types of anticoagulants should be utilized. These drugs include the direct thrombin inhibitor argatroban, the factor Xa inhibitor fondaparinux (Arixtra), and the direct oral anticoagulant drugs (DOACs). Details of these drugs are described later in the chapter. Once the platelet count has recovered to greater than 150,000/μL and the patient has been on a stable dose of a direct thrombin inhibitor, warfarin may be initiated as oral therapy as an option if the DOACs and fondaparinux are not used and continued.

ALERT!

A history of heparin hypersensitivity should be noted in the patient's record and profile if the patient has experienced HIT-II.

COAGULATION DISORDERS

CASE STUDY

Mr. Parton is in the hospital after having right knee replacement surgery. Two days after his surgery he developed redness and swelling in his right lower leg. He was subsequently diagnosed with a deep vein thrombosis (DVT).

Inappropriate Formation of Blood Clots

Blood clots (also known as thrombi) are formed by the body to stop blood loss when an injury occurs. Without them, even a minor cut could result in excessive bleeding and eventually death. Blood clots are constantly being formed and broken down in a process called hemostasis. When working properly, hemostasis ensures that clots are formed in the right number and size to stop bleeding but that they are not too many or too large to stop blood from flowing freely in the body.

Hemostasis

Hemostasis is a complex process that receives input from many sources. The coagulation cascade, discussed in Chapter 25, is the primary regulatory mechanism for this process. The cascade receives input from internal and external sources that initiate the clotting process. Once this process has begun it feeds back on itself. This feedback prevents the process from continuing indefinitely such that all the blood in the body clots and stops flowing.

CASE?

What factors did Mr. Parton have that may have contributed to his blood clot?

The input that initiates the cascade can be classified into one of three categories, called Virchow's triad of coagulability.[4] Rudolf Virchow, a renowned scientist and physician in Berlin in the 1800s, is credited with describing three factors that contribute to the development of venous thrombosis. These three categories include stasis, hypercoagulability,

and endothelial damage. Table 26-3 illustrates examples of each group. When one or more of these factors occur, a clot could be formed that can cause damage to the body. Some factors provide stronger input than others.

Clinical Manifestations

The area in which a clot is formed determines the clinical manifestations (ie, signs and symptoms) of that clot. The formation of a thrombus in any location will block blood flow to that area and cause damage and even death of the surrounding tissue. The three most common sites for clot formation are the heart, the brain, and the legs. A blood clot in the heart results in a myocardial infarction, also known as a heart attack (described in detail in Chapter 16). A blood clot in the brain results in a cerebrovascular accident (stroke) and a blood clot in the leg results in a deep vein thrombosis (DVT). Once a clot is formed, it is possible for part of that clot to break off and travel through the blood. Once the blood vessels narrow, the clot becomes stuck in that area and blood flow to the new location is compromised. This is called an embolus. The most common site of embolus is the lungs; this is known as a pulmonary embolus.

Deep Vein Thrombosis and Pulmonary Embolism

A DVT presents with a wide range of symptoms, from no symptoms at all to redness, pain, and swelling in the area of the clot. Many patients have DVTs with no long-lasting effects while others may have serious consequences. The two most serious complications are post-thrombotic syndrome, extensive serious tissue damage resulting from prolonged lack of blood flow to the area, and death secondary to pulmonary embolism (PE). Untreated DVT can be associated with fatal PE.

TABLE 26-3. Virchow's Triad of Coagulability[4]

Stasis	Hypercoagulability	Endothelial Damage
• Immobilization (such as bed rest after surgery) • Narrowed blood vessels • Atrial fibrillation • Long-distance plane or car travel	• Cancer • Genetic defects in the clotting cascade • Medications • Estrogen products (estrogen, estradiol, conjugated estrogens) • Tamoxifen, raloxifene • Nicotine/nicotine products	• Injury/trauma • Surgery • Cholesterol plaque rupture (which can result in a heart attack)

CASE?

Mr. Parton was given heparin in the hospital and then started on rivaroxaban (Xarelto). He was told he must take rivaroxaban for the next 3 months. Why was it important for him to receive immediate treatment for his DVT?

A pulmonary embolus is formed when a DVT (usually from the leg) breaks off, travels through the veins, and ultimately becomes lodged in the lungs. Symptoms of a pulmonary embolus include sudden-onset shortness of breath, chest pain, or sudden death.

Treatment of Deep Vein Thrombosis and Pulmonary Embolism

If left untreated, a blood clot would eventually be dissolved by the body (if the patient survived); however, treatment must be provided for clots to prevent them from getting bigger, breaking off, or forming new clots. The treatment of all clots is divided into one of two categories: drugs that break up clots (thrombolytics) and drugs that prevent clot growth (embolization) or formation (anticoagulants). Antiplatelet medications also prevent clot formation. Thrombolytics are used only in severe cases of DVT and PE and are discussed in detail along with antiplatelet agents in Chapter 17 so this chapter focuses primarily on anticoagulant medications.

Patients who develop a clot will receive anticoagulant medications for as little as 3 months and some will require therapy for the rest of their lives. The circumstances in which the clot is formed and whether this is a first episode or a recurrence are the primary determining factors for duration of therapy.

Anticoagulants

Patients often refer to anticoagulants as "blood thinners." This can be misleading because they do not in fact thin the blood; instead, they change the ability of the blood to form clots. This makes the blood flow more freely when the skin is cut, making the blood appear thinner. All anticoagulant medications stop the clotting cascade at some point in the pathway. Anticoagulants affect all blood in the body, not just the blood in the area of the clot. For this reason, bleeding (inside and outside of the body) and bruising are the most common risks associated with any anticoagulant. Bleeding is most commonly seen from the mucous membranes (nose and mouth); from the GI tract, manifesting as bright red or very dark tarry stools; and from the genitourinary tract, manifesting in red- or pink-tinged urine. Bruising can occur anywhere on the body.

It should be noted that all anticoagulant medications have different doses depending on the reason for administration. If the patient already has a clot, a high dose of anticoagulant (known as the treatment dose) is prescribed and if the patient is at high risk for a clot, but does not have one yet, a lower dose (called the prophylaxis dose) is used to prevent a clot from forming. Anticoagulant medications are divided into classes based on the area of the clotting cascade each type affects. These are listed in Medication Table 26-6. Figure 26-1 shows the clotting cascade that was discussed in Chapter 25 showing the step that each medication inhibits.

Heparin

Heparin (also called unfractionated heparin or UFH) is a protein normally produced in the body. The heparin that is used in therapy is usually derived from porcine (pig) sources but is chemically similar to human heparin. Physiologically, heparin controls the coagulation cascade by accelerating the activity of antithrombin, a blood factor that "ties up" several different clotting factors (mainly IIa and Xa) and preventing them from contributing to the formation of a thrombus (see Figure 26-1).

ALERT!

Regular vials of heparin sodium have been confused with vials of heparin sodium lock flush, resulting in severe over- or under-dosing of the patient. The concentration of heparin sodium vials ranges from 1,000 units/mL up to 40,000 units/mL and heparin lock flush vials range from 10 units/mL to 100 units/mL. The ISMP (Institute for Safe Medication Practices) considers heparin a high-risk medication because of the potential for fatal dosing errors. Double check all doses before dispensing.

UFH has a wide variety of indications, including the prevention and treatment of DVT/PE, heart attack, stroke, and the prevention of clot formation during surgery, dialysis, and blood transfusions, just to name a few. Also, very low doses of heparin are used to ensure that a clot does not form in an IV line—this is called a heparin lock flush or Hep-Lock.

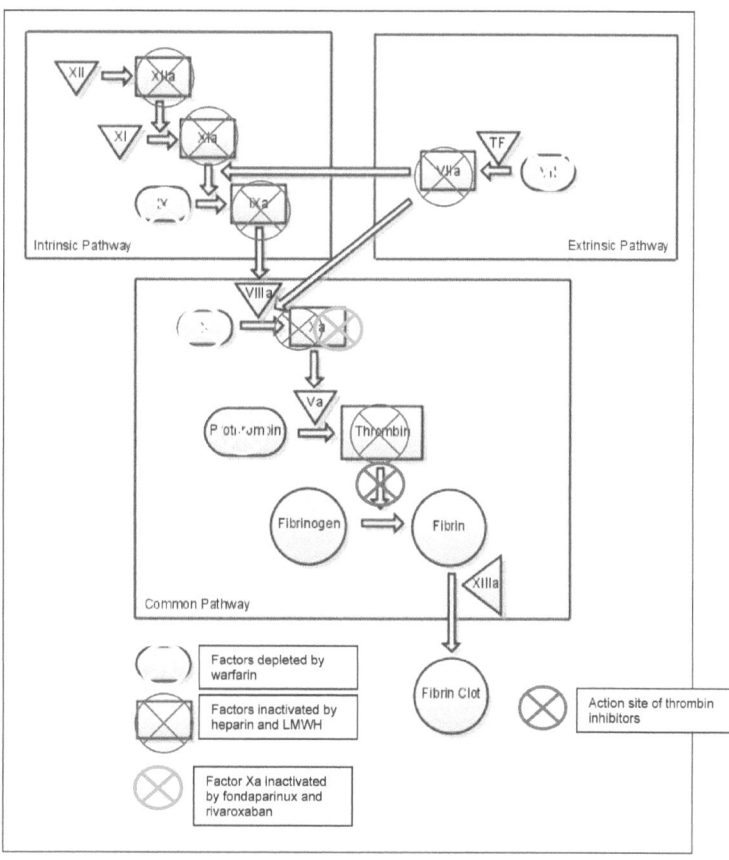

FIGURE 26-1. The clotting cascade shows the factors that each medication inhibits.

Heparin may be administered by continuous IV infusion, intermittent IV injection, or intermittent SUBQ injection. The dose and route of administration depend on the reason for giving heparin. The healthcare team can confirm heparin is working by measuring one of two lab tests; the activated partial thromboplastin time (aPTT) or the anti-Xa assay (the X represents the Roman numeral 10 and the *a* stands for active—this may also be called the heparin assay). Both of these blood tests show an increase when heparin is in the body. If the number is too high, there is too much heparin and the patient is at risk for bleeding; if it is too low, there is not enough heparin and the patient is not receiving the desired effect. Most commonly, IV infusions are dosed using an institution-specific dosing protocol. This is a sheet with dosing instructions for the nurse based on the patient's weight, aPTT or anti-Xa test results, and reason for taking heparin. It usually includes a bolus dose (used to kick-start the inhibition of the clotting cascade), an initial infusion rate based on the patient's weight, and directions for dose adjustment based on aPTT/anti-Xa results. Intermittent IV

and SUBQ dosing is based on weight, and the aPTT/anti-Xa is not always tested when these methods are used. IV infusions are most commonly used to provide a treatment dose and intermittent dosing is most commonly used for prophylaxis dosing.

CASE?

Which was most likely used on Mr. Parton in the hospital: IV continuous infusion, IV intermittent, or SUBQ heparin?

If too much heparin is given to the patient, the aPTT/anti-Xa will rise too high and the patient will be at risk for bleeding. If this occurs, a drug called protamine can be administered to reverse the effects of heparin. Heparin is safe to be used in adults, infants and children, and pregnant or lactating women.

PRACTICE POINT

Protamine sulfate is a drug that is approved by the U.S. Food and Drug Administration (FDA) only for the reversal of heparin overdose. It is available as a 10-mg/mL solution for slow IV injection (over 10 minutes). Each milligram of protamine neutralizes approximately 100 heparin units, so the usual dose of 50 mg should neutralize a 5,000-unit dose of heparin.

Low Molecular Weight Heparin

Low molecular weight heparins (LMWHs) are derived from natural heparin and have a very similar action. They are primarily indicated for the prevention and treatment of DVT, PE, and the treatment of heart attacks. Two LMWHs are available in the United States: enoxaparin (Lovenox) and dalteparin (Fragmin). There are several important differences between unfractionated heparin and LMWHs. First, LMWHs stay active in the body longer so doses are given less often. Second, blood tests are not often used in the dosing of these medications. Doses of LMWHs are determined by the patient's body weight and may require adjustment in patients with poor kidney function. Also, LWMHs are dosed subcutaneously only, are not administered intravenously, and are safe to use in adults and pregnant women.

PRACTICE POINT

LMWHs are supplied in prefilled syringes and may be used by the patient at home. Counseling by a pharmacist will be needed to ensure that the patient knows how to use a prefilled syringe and to self-inject properly.

ALERT!

LMWHs can be reversed with the administration of protamine, although this is currently an unlabeled use, and the reversal is less complete than occurs with protamine reversal of heparin.

Vitamin K Antagonist

Warfarin (still commonly known as Coumadin, although this is no longer an available brand name) is a widely used oral anticoagulant available generically in the United States. It acts by antagonizing the action of vitamin K, a nutrient essential to the formation of clotting factors II (prothrombin), VII, IX, and X, reducing the effectiveness of these factors in the body. Because of its mechanism, it may be a few days before the body responds to the drug (while current levels of clotting factors are eventually depleted), and it also takes time for its effects to end (while new clotting factors are being synthesized). Warfarin is a drug that has what is called a "narrow therapeutic window." This means that the dosing must be adjusted precisely at all times. Too little and the patient is at risk for having clots; too much and the patient is at risk for bleeding. Because of this, patients must remember to take each dose at the same time every day. Frequent blood testing is required to make sure the dose is appropriate for the patient and to adjust it if necessary. The test, called the international normalized ratio (INR), may also be abbreviated PT/INR (for prothrombin time/INR). The INR evaluates how long it takes the sample blood to clot compared to "normal" blood (blood that is not under the influence of anticoagulant medications). Normal blood has an INR of approximately 1 (there are no units of measure associated with an INR). When warfarin is administered the INR increases, thus indicating that it takes longer for the blood to form a clot. A specific INR goal range will be determined for

PRACTICE POINT

The management of warfarin therapy can be complex. It is common for a patient to be managed through an anticoagulation clinic in addition to the oversight of the primary physician. Anticoagulation clinics may be run by pharmacists, nurses, or other healthcare professionals. The purpose of these clinics is to make sure that anticoagulation is being managed properly. INR levels are drawn in these clinics, and the practitioner will decide what action to take regarding the warfarin dose. Technicians may be employed in these settings to assist in the INR measurements and administrative tasks associated with the clinic.

each patient based on the reason they are taking the warfarin. For example, a patient who is taking warfarin to treat a DVT will most commonly have an INR goal of between 2 and 3. Patients will typically have an INR drawn at least once per month while on warfarin and may have it drawn as frequently as every few days. Doses are adjusted based on the INR results: too low and more warfarin is given; too high and less is given. Patients frequently may come into the pharmacy with new prescriptions for warfarin as their provider attempts to find the right dose for that patient. It may take days to weeks to get the INR in the correct range.

ALERT!

It is common for patients beginning warfarin therapy to remain on LMWH or another anticoagulant until the INR reaches the correct range and even for a few days after to guarantee the full effect of the dose is seen. This may appear as a "duplicate therapy" warning in some patient profile software, and it will be up to the pharmacist to follow up or dismiss it.

Warfarin interacts with many other drugs so careful review of the profile by the pharmacist is required for any patient using warfarin. INR levels may change when patients change their eating habits (far more or less) of foods containing medium to high levels of vitamin K (such as green leafy vegetables). Patients need pharmacist counseling regarding these issues.

PRACTICE POINT

A medication guide must be provided to patients whenever warfarin is dispensed.

For patient safety, warfarin tablets are color coded. Tablet size ranges from 1–10 mg, and each strength is always the same color regardless of the manufacturer. For example, warfarin 1 mg (all manufacturers) and Jantoven 1 mg tablets are always pink. This helps the patient identify when a pill is the wrong strength, and it helps providers determine what strength the patient is on at home when the patient does not remember the dose.

When the INR is too high (indicating a relative overdose of warfarin), the practitioner may decide to let it come down

on its own or, in order to prevent or stop a bleeding episode, that more intervention is necessary. If bleeding is severe the patient may need a blood product called fresh frozen plasma to stop it. In less severe cases of bleeding or when warfarin must be reversed to *prevent* a bleeding episode, vitamin K (phytonadione, Mephyton) may be used. Vitamin K may be administered orally, IV, or subcutaneously.

PRACTICE POINT

Severe allergic reactions have been associated with IV administration of vitamin K. For safety, all IV doses of vitamin K should be in an IV bag, not sent to the nursing unit in a vial to be given IV push. Dispensing in this way dilutes the dose and allows administration to be stopped before the entire dose is given if a reaction is noticed, minimizing the consequences.

The heparins and warfarin reduce the ability of the blood to coagulate (form clots) by interfering with a number of different processes in the coagulation cascade. Recent advances in anticoagulation therapy have produced more focused treatments that act on fewer and more specific processes in the cascade, which may lead to fewer side effects and more precise control.

Factor Xa Inhibitors

The use of oral factor Xa (FXa) inhibitors has been increasing steadily in the United States over the last 10 years (X is the Roman numeral 10, and *a* is for active). FXa inhibitors available in the United States include Fondaparinux (Arixtra) for SUBQ injection, as well as rivaroxaban (Xarelto), apixaban (Eliquis), and edoxaban (Savaysa) oral tablets. Fondaparinux is similar to LMWH in indications and administration (SUBQ only). The oral FXa inhibitors have a variety of indications, including atrial fibrillation and treatment and prevention of DVT and PE. The factor Xa inhibitors are synthetic molecules, manufactured rather than derived from human or animal sources. Fondaparinux dose is decided based on patient weight and reason for using the drug. Doses are reduced or the drug is stopped in patients with low kidney function. Oral FXa inhibitors are dosed once or twice daily, require no monitoring tests and have relatively few drug-drug or drug-food interactions. Caution is used in patients with low kidney or hepatic function. In the event of an overdose or bleeding event, FXa inhibitors can be difficult to reverse. Andexanet alpha (Andexxa) is indicated for the reversal of apixaban and rivaroxaban and may be used off-label to reverse edoxaban. This intravenous medication is expensive, typically >$10,000 per dose, and frequently has use restricted to very specific situations.

PRACTICE POINT

The oral forms of FXa inhibitors and direct thrombin inhibitors include rivaroxaban, apixaban, edoxaban, and dabigatran. These medications are known collectively as direct oral anticoagulants, or DOACs.

PRACTICE POINT

The need to switch between different anticoagulant medications is common, especially going from injectable to oral. Careful timing is required to ensure that the effect of the first anticoagulant wears off just as the new anticoagulant starts working. This requires in-depth understanding of the pharmacokinetic properties of the medications. This is commonly referred to as an anticoagulant transition.

Direct Thrombin Inhibitors

Three direct thrombin inhibitors are available in the U.S. market, including Argatroban (no alternate name), bivalirudin (Angiomax), and dabigatran (Pradaxa). Bivalirudin is available for IV administration and is used short term during certain cardiac procedures. Argatroban is a continuous IV infusion and is used to provide anticoagulation to a patient who has had HIT-II (as mentioned earlier in the chapter). It requires constant monitoring and careful dose adjustment. No reversal agent is available for argatroban. These agents are not commonly used for anticoagulation unless other options are contraindicated or otherwise not available for use.

The newest direct thrombin inhibitor, dabigatran (Pradaxa), is available orally. Similar to the oral FXa inhibitors, dabigatran requires little or no monitoring and has very few drug-drug and drug-food interactions that impact how

it works. GI side effects such as nausea, vomiting, and GI bleeding have been the primary side effects associated with dabigatran and can result in patients discontinuing therapy. Because of the potential for loss of potency upon exposure to moisture, dabigatran capsules should be stored and dispensed only in the original manufacturer's bottle or blister packaging. A bleeding episode or overdose associated with dabigatran can be treated with intravenous idarucizumab (Praxbind). This is a monoclonal antibody that binds to dabigatran and its metabolites, rendering it ineffective.

PRACTICE POINT

Pharmacies should not repackage dabigatran in standard vials, and patients should not remove the capsules from their packaging to place them in pill boxes or organizers. Once the original manufacturer's bottle is opened, its contents of dabigatran capsules are stable for up to 4 months assuming tight reclosure and proper storage.[5] The FDA requires a medication guide with each dabigatran prescription.

Prevention

Active blood clot prevention is indicated for any patient at high risk for clots. This includes patients with one or more risk factors contained in Virchow's triad. Appropriate prevention measures include low-dose (prophylaxis-dose) anticoagulants, certain antiplatelet medications (as discussed in Chapter 16), and nondrug therapy. There are ways other than medication that patients can help prevent blood clots. Some of these methods include ambulation (getting up and moving around), external pneumatic compression cuffs (EPC cuffs), and support/TED (thromboembolic disease) stockings. Any or all of these therapies may be recommended or prescribed for a patient at high risk for developing a clot. EPC cuffs are generally only used in the hospital setting, but many pharmacies fit and sell TED stockings.

CASE?

Did Mr. Parton have risk factors that warranted active blood clot prevention?

SUMMARY

Anemia is characterized by a reduction in red blood cells (RBCs) or hemoglobin, thereby reducing the oxygen-carrying capacity of the blood. Different laboratory values are utilized to describe anemia, and clinical symptoms can result from it. Anemia may be classified in different ways based on the specific cause or on the cell structure. The main type of microcytic anemia is iron deficiency anemia, which is treated through the administration of oral or intravenous (IV) iron. Macrocytic anemia involves vitamin B_{12} or folic acid deficiency, and their replacement is the appropriate therapy for correction. Anemia of chronic disease is a type of normocytic anemia. Treatment of the underlying disorder will improve the anemia and for kidney disease, erythropoietin-stimulating agents (ESAs) may be used due to the impaired release of erythropoietin from the kidneys. ESAs may also be used, within certain guidelines, to improve quality of life and reduce the need for blood transfusion support in patients receiving myelosuppressive chemotherapy. Other types of anemia include hemolytic anemia, sickle cell anemia, thalassemia, and sideroblastic anemia.

Neutropenia may be caused by chemotherapeutic medications and nonchemotherapeutic medications through direct toxic effects, as well as through antibody formation and immune-mediated processes. Due to the risk of febrile neutropenia, interruptions in chemotherapy regimens, and hospitalizations, the G-CSFs, filgrastim and pegfilgrastim, are used for the treatment and prevention of chemotherapy-induced neutropenia. The most common nonchemotherapy drugs implicated in neutropenia are clozapine, methimazole (Tapazole), sulfasalazine, and trimethoprim/sulfamethoxazole (Bactrim). The suspected drug should be stopped, and G-CSFs may be considered.

Drug-induced thrombocytopenia may involve a number of different medications, with the most common one being heparin. There are two types of heparin-induced thrombocytopenia: HIT-I and HIT-II. HIT-II is an immune-mediated process that puts patients at risk of developing thromboses. Direct thrombin inhibitors, the factor Xa inhibitor fondaparinux, or newer oral agents may be used to prevent thrombosis once the heparin is discontinued. Other medications thought to cause thrombocytopenia should also be discontinued, and the platelet count should soon recover.

Blood clots are formed by a number of internal and external factors coming together to inappropriately activate the clotting cascade. Blood clots can manifest in several ways, including heart attacks, strokes, deep vein thrombosis (DVT),

and pulmonary embolism (PE). These clots can have serious consequences, including severe tissue damage and even death. Treating clots usually involves giving an anticoagulant to prevent the clot from getting any bigger or breaking off while the body dissolves it over a period of weeks to months. Available anticoagulants include heparin, low molecular weight heparin (LMWH), direct thrombin inhibitors, factor Xa inhibitors, and warfarin. The most common side effect of all anticoagulants is bruising and bleeding. Some anticoagulants have antidotes or reversal agents and others do not. Active prevention in high-risk patients is very important, and this includes drug therapy and nondrug therapy.

REFERENCES

1. Bakerman S. *Bakerman's ABC's of Interpretive Laboratory Data*. 4th ed. Scottsdale, AZ: Interpretive Laboratory Data; 2002.

2. Bohlius J, Bohlke K, Castelli R, et al. Management of cancer-associated anemia with erthyropoiesis-stimulating agents: ASCO/ASH clinical practice guideline update. *J Clin Oncol*. 2019;37:1336-1351.

3. Coates TD. Drug-induced neutropenia and agranulocytosis. Uptodate.com. Available at http://www.uptodate.com/contents/drug-induced-neutropenia-and-agranulocytosis. Accessed 11 April 2022.

4. Witt DM, Clark NP, Vazquez SR. Venous thromboembolism. In: DiPiro JT, Yee GC, Posey L, Haines ST, Nolin TD, Ellingrod V. eds. *Pharmacotherapy: A Pathophysiologic Approach*, 11e. McGraw Hill; 2020. Accessed April 29, 2022.

5. Taking and storing Pradaxa capsules. Boehringer Ingelheim. https://www.pradaxa.com/staying-on-track. Accessed July 5, 2021.

6. Lexicomp Online, Lexi-Drugs [Database]. Hudson, OH: Wolters Kluwer; 2021. http://online.lexi.com. Accessed 11 April 2022.

REVIEW QUESTIONS

1. What is anemia and what clinical effects could be experienced in patients with anemia?

2. How is anemia classified?

3. List five risk factors for clot development.

4. Which oral anticoagulant medication has special storage requirements to keep in the original bottle?

5. How are anticoagulants different from thrombolytics?

MEDICATION TABLES

MEDICATION TABLE 26-1. Oral Iron Products[6,a]

Iron Salt (pronunciation)	Percent Elemental Iron	Dosage Forms	Notes
Ferrous sulfate (FER us) (SUL fate)	20	Tablets: 325 mg Elixir: 220 mg/5 mL Syrup: 300 mg/5 mL Solution: 75 mg/1 mL	Liquid iron may stain teeth
Ferrous fumarate (FER us) (FYOO ma rate)	33	Tablets: 324 mg, 325 mg	
Ferrous gluconate (FER us) (GLOO koe nate)	12	Tablets: 324 mg	

[a] Pronunciations have been adapted with permission from USP Dictionary of USAN and International Drug Names (USP Dictionary) © 2022.

MEDICATION TABLE 26-2. Representative Polysaccharide-Iron Complex and Oral Iron Combination Products[6]

Example Products		Other Ingredients in Addition to Iron
EZFE 200 Ferrex 150 Ferric x-150	Myferon 150 Nu-Iron Poly-Iron 150	
IFerex 150 Forte Myferon 150 Forte Poly-Iron 150 Forte		Vitamin B_{12} and folic acid

Note: Other products are available by prescription or over the counter and may include other ingredients, such as vitamin C (ascorbic acid).

MEDICATION TABLE 26-3. Intravenous Iron Products[6,a]

IV Iron (pronunciation)	Brand Name	Elemental Iron Concentration	Test Dose Required?
Iron dextran (EYE urn) (DEX tran)	INFeD	50 mg/mL	Yes
Iron sucrose (EYE urn) (SOO krose)	Venofer	20 mg/mL	No
Sodium ferric gluconate (SOE dee um) (FER ik) (GLOO koe nate)	Ferrlecit	12.5 mg/mL	No
Ferumoxytol (FER ue) (MOX i tol)	Feraheme	30 mg/mL	No
Ferric carboxymaltose	Injectafer	750 mg/15 mL	No
Ferric derisomaltose	Monoferric	100 mg/mL	No

[a] Pronunciations have been adapted with permission from USP Dictionary of USAN and International Drug Names (USP Dictionary) © 2022.

MEDICATION TABLE 26-4. Erythropoietin-Stimulating Agents (ESAs)[6,a]

ESA (pronunciation)	Brand Name	Route	Dosage Form	Notes
Epoetin alfa (e POE e tin) (AL fa) Epoetin alfa-epbx	Procrit, Epogen Retacrit (biosimilar)	SUBQ or IV	Injection, solution: 2,000 units/mL, 3,000 units/mL, 4,000 units/mL, 10,000 units/mL, 20,000 units/mL, 40,000 units/mL	IV administration preferred for hemodialysis patients; injections contain albumin; do not shake; protect from light; refrigerate product
Darbepoetin alfa (DAR be POE e tin) (AL fa)	Aranesp	SUBQ or IV	Injection, solution: 25 mcg, 40 mcg, 60 mcg, 100 mcg, 150 mcg, 200 mcg, 300 mcg, 500 mcg	Available as single-dose vials or autoinjectors; do not shake; protect from light; refrigerate product

IV = intravenous; SUBQ = subcutaneous.
[a] Pronunciations have been adapted with permission from USP Dictionary of USAN and International Drug Names (USP Dictionary) © 2022.

MEDICATION TABLE 26-5. Granulocyte Colony-Stimulating Factors (G-CSF)[6,a]

G-CSF (pronunciation)	Brand Name	Route	Dosage Forms	Dose	Notes
Filgrastim (fil GRA stim) Tbo-filgrastim *Biosimilars:* Filgrastim-aafi Filgrastim-sndz	Neupogen Granix Nivestym Zarxio	SUBQ or IV	Injection, solution: 300 mcg/mL, 480 mcg/1.6 mL	5 mcg/kg daily until WBC recovery; not to be administered within 24 hr before to 24 hr after chemotherapy administration	Available as single-dose vials or prefilled syringes; refrigerate product; do not shake; protect from light
Pegfilgrastim (peg fil GRA stim) Pegfilgrastim on-body injector *Biosimilars:* Pegfilgrastim-jmdb Pegfilgrastim-apgf Pegfilgrastim-cbqv Pegfilgrastim-bmez	Neulasta Neulasta Onpro Fulphila Nyvepria Udenyca Ziextenzo	SUBQ	Injection, solution: 6 mg/0.6 mL	6 mg once per chemotherapy cycle (but not within 14 days before or 24 hr after chemotherapy dose) Do not used fixed 6 mg dose in infants, children, or adolescents <45 kg	Refrigerate product; do not shake; protect from light

IV = intravenous; SUBQ = subcutaneous; WBC = white blood cell.
[a] Pronunciations have been adapted with permission from USP Dictionary of USAN and International Drug Names (USP Dictionary) © 2022.

MEDICATION TABLE 26-6. Anticoagulants[6]

CLASS Generic Name (pronunciation)	Brand Name	Route	Forms	Dose	Notes
Vitamin K Antagonists					
Warfarin (WAR far in)	Jantoven	Oral	Tablet	1–10 mg, adjust to INR	Many drug interactions; patient should only use one manufacturer; tablet color indicates dose (brand and generic the same)
Heparin					
Heparin (HEP a rin)	Hep-Lock U/P, Hep-Lock, HepFlush-10	IV, SUBQ	Solution	Dosed in units/kg; concentrations range from 1–20,000 units/mL	Many uses; dose depends on indication; check doses carefully; heparin sodium 10,000 units/mL may be confused with Hep-Lock 10 units/mL
Low Molecular Weight Heparins					
Enoxaparin (ee nox a PA rin)	Lovenox	SUBQ	Solution	Usually weight based; 1 mg/kg q 12 hr or 1.5 mg/kg once daily	Many uses; dose depends on indication and whether it is for prophylaxis or treatment of condition; supplied as prefilled syringes
Dalteparin (dal TE pa rin)	Fragmin	SUBQ	Solution	2,500–5,000 units once daily	Supplied as prefilled syringes or multidose vial
Factor Xa Inhibitors					
Fondaparinux (fon da PARE i nux)	Arixtra	SUBQ	Solution	2.5–7.5 mg once daily	Supplied as prefilled syringes; dose depends on indication and weight of patient
Rivaroxaban (riv a ROX a ban)	Xarelto	Oral	Tablet	10–20 mg once daily	Indicated for atrial fibrillation, DVT treatment and prophylaxis and coronary artery disease; doses >15 mg give with food, may be crushed
Apixaban (a PIX a ban)	Eliquis	Oral	Tablet	2.5–10 mg twice daily	Indicated for atrial fibrillation, DVT treatment, and postsurgical prophylaxis; give with or without food, may be crushed
Edoxaban (e DOX a ban)	Savaysa	Oral	Tablet	30–60 mg once daily	Indicated for atrial fibrillation and treatment of DVT/PE; administer without regard to food, may be crushed; efficacy reduced in patients with CrCl >95 ml/min

Continued next page

MEDICATION TABLE 26-6. Anticoagulants[6] (Continued)

CLASS Generic Name (pronunciation)	Brand Name	Route	Forms	Dose	Notes
Direct Thrombin Inhibitors					
Argatroban (ar GA troh ban)	Argatroban	IV infusion	Solution	Weight based; usually started at 2 mcg/kg/min and not exceeding 10 mcg/kg/min	Very specific dosage protocol; dose is based on aPTT and is quite variable; rate of administration is dependent on dose
Bivalirudin (bye VAL i roo din) (bivalrudin is also a hirudin)	Angiomax	IV bolus, IV infusion	Powder	Weight-based dosing Bolus dose: 0.1–0.75 mg/kg Infusion: 0.2–1.75 mg/kg/hr	Needs to be reconstituted with sterile water, gently swirl to dissolve. Must dilute further with D5W or NS prior to use to a concentration of 5 mg/ml; usually given IV bolus followed by IV infusion; dose based on aPPT and is quite variable; infusion usually given at rate of 2.5 mg/hr
Dabigatran (da bi GAT ran)	Pradaxa	Oral	Capsule	150 mg twice daily	Must be dispensed and stored in original manufacturer's bottle or blister pack
Reversal Agents					
Vitamin K (phytonadione) (fye toe na DYE own)	Mephyton	Oral	Tablet	2.5–10 mg dependent on INR	Dose is based on INR and amount of bleeding; many routes of administration, although oral is preferred; injectable formulation may be given orally undiluted; use NS or D5W for dilution of IV form
	generics	SUBQ	Solution		
Protamine sulfate (PROE ta meen) (SUL fate)		IV bolus	Solution	Most common dose: 1–1.5 mg/100 units of heparin given previously	Dosed based on heparin dose received, route it was given, and timeframe since heparin was received by patient; given slowly over 10 min; does not need to be diluted
Andexanet alpha	Andexxa	IV bolus plus infusion	Solution	400–800 mg bolus followed by 4–8 mg/min infusion	Indicated for reversal of rivaroxaban or apixaban; used off-label for reversal of edoxaban and betrixaban; use of an in-line filter is required
Idarucizumab (Eye da roo ciz u mab)	Praxbind	IV bolus	Solution	5 grams administered as 2 × 2.5 g doses not more than 15 minutes apart	Indicated for reversal of dabigatran

a PTT = activated partial thromboplastin time; D5W = 5% dextrose in water; DVT = deep vein thrombosis; INR = international normalized ratio; IV = intravenous; NS = normal saline; PE = pulmonary embolism; SUBQ = subcutaneous.

Part 9

INFECTIOUS DISEASES

Chapter 27

Bacterial Infections

Rachael Craft, PharmD, BCIDP

KEY TERMS AND DEFINITIONS

Antibiotic—a substance that kills or inhibits the growth of bacteria.

Bacteria—unicellular (single-celled) microorganisms. The singular of this term is bacterium.

Bactericidal—able to kill bacteria.

Bacteriostatic—suppressing the growth of bacteria.

Broad-spectrum—a term describing an agent that has activity against a wide variety of microorganisms.

Infection—invasion by pathogenic microorganisms, which multiply in a host.

Microorganism—a life form of microscopic size (not visible to the unaided eye).

Normal flora—microorganisms inhabiting the human body that under normal circumstances do not cause illness or disease.

Nosocomial—acquired in or associated with a healthcare facility.

Pathogen—organism that causes illness or disease.

Prophylaxis—prevention of illness or disease. (adjective = Prophylactic).

Resistance—the ability of microorganisms to withstand the effects of antibiotics.

DOI 10.37573/9781585286638.027

LEARNING OBJECTIVES

After completing this chapter, you should be able to

1. Define:
   - Infection
   - Bacteria
   - Normal flora
   - Pathogen
   - Resistance

2. Outline the concept of normal flora bacteria and the mechanism behind the development of pathogenicity.

3. Describe host defense mechanisms.

4. Recognize the types of bacteria and bacterial infections.

5. Explain the therapeutic effects of antibiotics and the most common indications for each class.

6. Identify factors relevant to antibiotic selection.

7. Outline the management of patients with bacterial infections, including monitoring for efficacy and safety.

Bacteria are single-celled microscopic organisms that live in soil, water, and humans. Bacteria are found everywhere on earth and in all types of environments. There are approximately five nonillion (5×10^{30}) bacteria on earth.[1]

In humans, bacteria reside on the skin and in the digestive tract, genitourinary tract, airways, and mouth. When these bacteria stay in a particular part of the body and do not cause harm or infection, they are referred to as normal flora or colonizing bacteria. Normal flora protects the body against disease-causing organisms. Normal flora also performs tasks that are useful to the human host. Skin flora prevents pathogenic organisms from colonizing the surface of the skin by utilizing nutrients for themselves and/or being hostile to pathogenic organisms. The flora that resides in the gastrointestinal (GI) tract are often referred to as *gut flora*. These organisms are responsible for many functions, such as preventing the overgrowth of pathogenic organisms, carbohydrate metabolism, production of certain vitamins (biotin, vitamin K), and various other functions. It is important to understand that not all bacteria are infectious when they reside in their normal environment and that they perform many important functions.

CASE STUDY

G. F. is a 16-year-old male who presents to the emergency room (ER) with shortness of breath and increased sputum production. G. F. states he has not felt well for the past couple of days but today has trouble breathing. Upon examination in the ER, breath sounds are positive for wheezing with crackles, temperature 102.1°F, oxygen saturation 89%, and white blood cell (WBC) count = 15.7 (normal WBC count = 4–10). Blood and sputum cultures are obtained and sent to the laboratory for analysis.

Bacteria that cause illness or disease are known as pathogens; they are referred to as pathogenic. Bacteria become pathogenic when they produce toxins and/or gain access to a body location where they are not tolerated as *normal flora*. Toxin production or invasion by pathogenic organisms are considered infection. Many host factors may influence the likelihood of infection. Host defense mechanisms can be classified as natural barriers, nonspecific immune responses, and specific immune responses.

Natural barriers to infection include the skin, mucous membranes, respiratory tract, and GI tract. The skin usually provides protection unless its barrier is physically disrupted (eg, injury, abrasion, incision, burns, or intravenous catheter). Mucous membrane barriers include secretions that are produced by the body (eg, cervical mucus, tears, or saliva). Many of these secretions contain immunoglobulins, which are proteins that are used by the immune system to identify and neutralize foreign substances, such as IgA and IgG that prevent organisms from attaching to host cells. The respiratory tract barrier consists of cilia (short hair-like structures that extend from a cell and move in locomotion). The lining of the respiratory tract serves as a filter mechanism as it transports invading organisms away from the lung. In addition, coughing serves as a barrier to remove these organisms. GI barriers include the acidic content of the GI tract and antibacterial activity of pancreatic enzymes, bile, and secretions released by the intestine. As mentioned earlier, the normal flora of the GI tract can serve as a barrier because they inhibit pathogenic organisms by competing for environmental resources.

Once a pathogenic organism is recognized, the body's natural defenses are initiated. Nonspecific immune responses are usually produced first. This response involves fever and the increased production of neutrophils, WBCs capable of ingesting microorganisms or particles (discussed in Chapter 25). The inflammation that occurs during an infection directs the immune system response to the site of injury or infection by increasing blood flow to that site and increasing vascular permeability. This allows the WBCs to penetrate tissues and access the site to begin inhibiting the spread of the infectious organism.

Specific immune responses occur after infection. The body produces antibodies and immunoglobulins that adhere to specific targets on the infecting organisms. The antibodies help cells ingest antigens, inactivate toxic substances that are produced by bacteria, and attack bacteria directly. In addition, the specific immune response activates systems responsible for clearing pathogens from a host.

When there are breakdowns or deficiencies in the body's defense system, the host is vulnerable to many types of infections. Defects in natural barriers include impaired cough, loss of gastric acidity, loss of cutaneous (skin tissue) integrity, and loss of normal flora. Defects in immune barriers, which include disease states that limit or inhibit the production or replication of the body's immune cells, are referred to as immunosuppression or immunodeficiency. Diseases, such as HIV infection, lupus, leukemia, and megaloblastic anemia, and decreases in numbers of WBCs lead to immunosuppression. Additionally, certain medications can contribute to deficiencies in the host's immune response. These medication classes include some cancer chemotherapies, some biologics, and corticosteroids.

SIGNS AND SYMPTOMS OF BACTERIAL INFECTIONS

Signs and symptoms in the infected host are based on the location and the type of infection. Infection can be confirmed by fever, other signs and symptoms, and predisposing factors. Fever is defined as a controlled elevation of body temperature above the normal range of 36°C to 37.8°C (98.2°F to 99.5°F). The increase in body temperature is a defense mechanism. Some organisms are susceptible to moderate temperature elevations and, in addition, the elevation of temperature activates many of the body's other defense mechanisms. Recall from Chapter 25 that certain WBCs are responsible for providing defense against invading pathogens. Most infections cause an elevation of the body's WBC count, known as leukocytosis.

Identification of the pathogen assists with confirming the presence of infection. Infected body materials are often sampled for this purpose. Such sampling is known as culturing. It is most effective if cultures are obtained prior to antibiotic therapy.

CASE?

What signs and symptoms of infection does G. F. have?

Several types of cultures can be obtained from the infected host. These include blood, sputum, tissue, wound, urine, stool, cerebral spinal fluid, and samples from other body fluids. The interpretation of the culture is important in determining whether the organisms identified (if any) are pathogenic, contaminant, or normal flora from the site of collection. Another test used to assist in obtaining useful information regarding the type of organism present is known as a Gram stain. Gram staining rapidly classifies bacteria into broad groups based on their shape and color and may provide useful information to assist in the initial selection of antibiotic therapy before culture results are completed.

For certain types of infections, such as pneumonia, other methods can be used to diagnose or confirm the presence of infection. This includes chest x-rays to review the patient's lungs for images that may reveal infiltration in the lobes of the lung. Computed tomography (CT) scans along with magnetic resonance imaging (MRI) can allow the clinician a better view of infectious processes in many parts of the body.

TABLE 27-1. Signs and Symptoms of Bacterial Infections

Type of Infection	Location	Signs and Symptoms
Meningitis	Central nervous system	Fever, stiffness of neck and back, altered mental status, headache
Brain and meningeal abscess	Central nervous system	Fever, altered mental status
Encephalitis	Central nervous system	Fever, altered mental status
Sinusitis (sinus infection)	Respiratory (upper)	Fever, nasal discharge, facial pain
Otitis media (ear infection)	Respiratory (upper)	Fever, irritability, discharge
Pneumonia	Respiratory (lower)	Fever, chills, shortness of breath, productive cough
Bronchitis	Respiratory (lower)	Persistent cough, malaise
Enteritis	Gastrointestinal tract	Fever, diarrhea, dehydration
Peritonitis	Intra-abdominal	Fever, nausea, vomiting, abdominal guarding
Bacteremia	Blood	Fever, chills, malaise
Cellulitis	Skin/soft tissue	Edema, erythema, fever
Gonorrhea	GU tract	Dysuria, urethritis, discharge
Urinary tract infection (UTI)	GU tract	Dysuria, urgency, frequency

There are many different types of infections that occur in humans. Bacterial infections can form in every system of the human body. Table 27-1 classifies various types of infections, location, and some of the most common signs and symptoms.

CASE?

What organisms are the most likely cause of G. F.'s infection?

CLASSIFICATION OF BACTERIA

There are several types of bacteria that are responsible for causing infections. The classification of bacteria includes the association of bacteria into an organized form of naming referred to as taxonomy. This includes the genus and species names of the bacteria. For example, with the bacterium known as *Staphylococcus aureus*, *Staphylococcus* is the genus or family name and *aureus* is the specific species. In addition, bacteria are classified by their shapes, known as morphology. There are three basic morphologies of bacteria: round (coccus), rod-shaped (bacillus), or spiral-shaped (spirillum). Bacteria are also classified by their color after a stain is applied. This staining process is referred to as a Gram stain. As mentioned previously, Gram staining is an empirical method of differentiating between the main groups of bacteria: Gram positive, Gram negative, and acid fast. Gram-positive bacteria have a thick cell wall that stains purple. Gram-negative bacteria have a thin cell wall that stains pink. Acid-fast bacteria resist Gram staining because the cell walls contain a high concentration of lipids. Finally, bacteria can be classified based on oxygen requirements. Those bacteria that require oxygen to live and grow are referred to as aerobic and those not needing oxygen are referred to as anaerobic.

The two most common groups of Gram-positive cocci (round) are staphylococci and streptococci. These are the genus names and there are several species within each group. When viewed microscopically, staphylococci appear in clumps (clusters) like a bunch of grapes and streptococci form chains. The most common pathogen in the *Staphylococcus* group is *Staphylococcus aureus*. Further tests can differentiate *Staphylococcus aureus* from other staphylococci. All species of staphylococci are normal flora and colonize on the skin and mucous membranes of humans.

Streptococci are classified according to their ability to break down blood in fresh blood agar plates. Some streptococci have no effect on blood and are termed *nonhemolytic* streptococci. The most important of the nonhemolytic streptococci are the enterococci, such as *Enterococcus faecalis* and *Enterococcus faecium,* both of which are normal flora in the GI tract. Other streptococci cause partial breakdown of blood and are called alpha-hemolytic streptococci, which are often referred to as viridans (green) streptococci. The viridans streptococci are a large and heterogeneous group of bacteria and include organisms that play a role in tooth decay and those that can cause endocarditis (infection of the tissue surrounding the heart) and brain abscesses. The most common pathogen of the alpha-hemolytic streptococci family is *Streptococcus pneumoniae* (the cause of pneumococcal pneumonia and meningitis). The beta-hemolytic streptococci cause the complete breakdown of blood in fresh blood agar plates. Clinically, the most important of the beta-hemolytic streptococci is *Streptococcus pyogenes,* the infecting organism for strep throat.

The Gram-positive bacilli (rods) can be divided according to their ability to produce spores. Spores of Gram-positive rods are highly resistant structures that may add considerably to their pathogenic capacity. Gram-positive rods that are spore forming are grouped in the genus *Bacillus.* Important members of this genus include *Bacillus anthracis* (the cause of anthrax) and *Bacillus cereus* (a cause of food poisoning). Gram-positive rods that are anaerobic spore formers are grouped in the class clostridia. These include *Clostridium perfringens,* a principal cause of gangrene, *Clostridium tetani* (the cause of tetanus), *Clostridium botulinum* (the cause of the fatal food poisoning botulism), and *Clostridioides difficile* (*C. diff*), a growing cause of infectious diarrhea following antibiotic therapy.

The non-spore-forming Gram-positive rods include coryneform bacteria and lactobacilli. Some lactobacilli are important members of the normal vaginal flora of women of child-bearing age. A common pathogen of this group includes *Listeria monocytogenes,* which is one of the most virulent foodborne pathogens. Table 27-2 organizes the Gram-positive bacteria by shape, oxygen use (ie, aerobic or anaerobic), and enzyme-producing groups.

The Gram-negative bacteria have an outer thin cell wall and stain pink on a Gram stain. The Gram-negative cocci include the genera *Moraxella* and *Neisseria.*[2] The most pathogenic *Neisseria* organisms include *Neisseria meningitidis* (the cause of bacterial meningitis) and *Neisseria gonorrhoeae* (the cause of gonorrhea). These organisms are most often seen in pairs and are commonly referred to as diplococci.

Gram-negative bacilli include the order enterobacterales. This group is differentiated into types based on whether they can grow in the presence (aerobic) or absence (anaerobic) of oxygen and are frequently found in the GI tract of humans and animals. Some pathogens in this group include *Yersinia pestis* (the cause of plague), *Salmonella typhi* (the cause of typhoid), *Shigella dysenteriae* (the cause of bacillary dysentery), *Pseudomonas aeruginosa* (the cause of many types of infections associated with high mortality rates), and *Salmonella enteritidis* (the cause of food poisoning). Additional members of this class include *Escherichia coli* and members of the genus *Klebsiella.* The *Vibrio* and *Campylobacters* are Gram-negative rods that appear curved or spiral in shape. These bacteria are commonly found in natural waters, both

TABLE 27-2. Classification of Common Gram-Positive Microorganisms

Aerobic Gram Positive
Cocci
Streptococci: *Streptococcus pneumoniae, Streptococcus viridans*
Enterococci: *Enterococcus faecalis, Enterococcus faecium*
Staphylococci: *Staphylococcus aureus, Staphylococcus epidermidis*
Bacilli (rods)
Corynebacterium
Listeria
Anaerobic Gram Positive
Cocci
Peptococcus
Peptostreptococcus
Bacilli (rods)
Clostridia: *Clostridium perfringens, Clostridium tetani, Clostridioides difficile*
Propionibacterium

freshwater and marine. *Vibrio cholerae* (the cause of the waterborne infection cholera), *Campylobacters* (the cause of bacterial enteritis), and *Helicobacter pylori* (the cause of stomach ulcers) are common pathogens in this group.

Some Gram-negative bacilli appear so short that they often resemble cocci under the microscope. These are sometimes referred to as cocco-bacilli. This group includes members of the genera *Haemophilus* and *Acinetobacter*, the latter being a cause of hospital-acquired (nosocomial) infections. Other Gram-negative bacteria are very fastidious (specific) in their nutritional requirements, including members of the genus *Legionella*, which cause atypical pneumonias and Legionnaires' disease. Anaerobic Gram-negative bacilli include the genus *Bacteroides*, which causes infections of the peritoneal (abdominal) cavity and GI tract, and *Fusobacteria*, which causes periodontal (gum) infections. Table 27-3 organizes the Gram-negative bacteria by shape, oxygen use, and enzyme-producing groups.

The next group of bacteria includes the acid-fast bacteria, which possess a waxy cell wall, and they rarely stain using the basic Gram stain technique. These bacteria are identified using a different technique of staining that requires acid and alcohol. The most pathogenic organisms in this group include *Mycobacterium tuberculosis*, which causes tuberculosis, and *Mycobacterium leprae*, which causes leprosy.

A final group of bacteria is referred to as atypical. They are smaller in size than normal bacteria. The most common pathogenic forms are those in the *Mycoplasma*, *Chlamydia*, and *Rickettsia* groups. *Mycoplasma* lack cell walls and are highly pleomorphic, meaning they can change shape. The most common pathogen is *Mycoplasma pneumoniae*, which can cause both upper and lower respiratory infections, including tracheobronchitis and atypical pneumonia. Members of the genus *Chlamydia* have cell walls and are coccoid in shape. The most common pathogen in this group is *Chlamydia trachomatis*, a cause of female reproductive problems, pelvic inflammatory disease (PID), and neonatal respiratory and eye infections. The rickettsiae appear as pleomorphic (form-changing) bacillary or coccobacillary (short rod or oval) forms. The most common pathogens in this group include *Rickettsia rickettsii*, the cause of Rocky Mountain spotted fever (transmitted by ticks), and *Rickettsia prowazekii*, the cause of epidemic typhus fever (transmitted by infected human body lice).

BACTERIAL RESISTANCE

When antibiotics first came into use in the 1930s, they were effective against most bacterial infections. Over time, many antibiotics have lost effectiveness against common bacterial infections due to the increase of antibiotic resistance. Bacteria may be naturally resistant to different classes of antibiotics or may acquire resistance from other bacteria through the exchange of resistant genes. Bacteria

TABLE 27-3. Classification of Common Gram-Negative Microorganisms

Aerobic Gram Negative
Cocci
Neisseria: *Neisseria meningitidis, Neisseria gonorrhoeae*
Moraxella catarrhalis
Bacilli (rods)
Enterobacterales: *Escherichia coli, Klebsiella, Enterobacter, Citrobacter, Proteus, Serratia, Salmonella, Shigella*
Pseudomonas
Legionella
Helicobacter pylori
Cocco-bacilli
Haemophilus
Anaerobic Gram Negative
Cocci
Veillonella
Bacilli (rods)
Bacteroides: *Bacteroides fragilis*
Fusobacterium
Prevotella

can be resistant to antibiotics in many ways. There are four main mechanisms by which bacteria exhibit resistance to antibiotics:

1. Inactivation or modification of the antibiotic—Bacteria produce enzymes that deactivate the antibiotic (eg, bacteria produce an enzyme called beta-lactamase that inactivates penicillins).

2. Alteration of the target site for the antibiotic—For example, penicillin binds to penicillin-binding protein (PBP) on some bacteria, but certain bacteria have altered this protein and the antibiotic cannot bind to the organism.

3. Alteration of metabolic pathways—For example, sulfonamide antibiotics work by disrupting the synthesis of folic acid by altering para-aminobenzoic acid (PABA). Some sulfonamide-resistant bacteria are able to utilize preformed folic acid and are not dependent on PABA for folic acid synthesis.

4. Reduction of drug transport across the cell wall—This occurs by genetic alterations in certain bacteria that decrease the permeability of the cell wall to the drug or increases active efflux (pumping out) of the antibiotic across the surface of the cell.

SUSCEPTIBILITY

Susceptibility refers to the sensitivity of a microorganism to a given antibiotic. Susceptibility testing is often used to determine the likelihood that a particular antibiotic regimen will be effective in eliminating or inhibiting the infection. Susceptibility testing is performed by growing the bacterial isolate in the presence of varying concentrations of several antimicrobials and then examining the amount of growth to determine which concentrations of antimicrobials inhibit the growth of the bacteria. Results are reported as susceptible (likely to inhibit the pathogenic microorganism), intermediate (may be effective at a higher-than-normal concentration), and resistant (not effective at inhibiting the growth of the organism). The organism is categorized as susceptible, intermediate, or resistant by determining the minimum inhibitory concentration (MIC) of the antibiotic. The MIC is the lowest concentration of an antibiotic that inhibits the growth of the bacteria. This information is then used to determine the best option for treating the infection. While broad-spectrum antibiotics are often ordered as initial therapy (to begin treatment of an apparent infection before all tests are complete), prolonged or inappropriate use of such

agents can lead to antibiotic resistance, and more specific therapy is generally prescribed once the susceptibility of the infecting organisms has been determined.

PRACTICE POINT

Once the organism is identified and antibiotic sensitivities are known, antibiotic therapy should be changed, if necessary, to the narrowest-spectrum agent that will treat the infection. This way we can prevent antibiotic resistance and unnecessary side effects caused by broad-spectrum antibiotics. This is why antibiotic orders are sometimes revised after a few days of treatment.

ANTIBIOTIC MEDICATIONS

Antibiotics are the drugs of choice for the treatment of bacterial infections. The goal of antibiotic therapy is to kill invading bacteria without harming the host. Antibiotic effectiveness depends on the mechanism of action of the antibiotic, distribution of the drug to the site of infection, immune status of the host, and resistance patterns of the organism.

The first class of antibiotics discussed here are those that are categorized in the beta-lactam group (because they have a beta-lactam ring in their chemical structure). Beta-lactam antibiotics work by inhibiting cell wall synthesis of bacteria. The first antibiotic class in this group to be discovered was penicillin. It was discovered by Alexander Fleming in 1928 and developed as a treatment for human infections in the late 1930s.[3] Over the years, as a result of research prompted by bacterial resistance, the beta-lactam class has grown into several groups with various spectra of activity (ie, activity against specific types of microorganisms).

Penicillins are bactericidal. They kill bacteria by activating enzymes that destroy the bacterial cell wall.[3] Some organisms produce beta-lactamase, an enzyme that inactivates penicillins. This effect can be blocked by adding a beta-lactamase inhibitor (clavulanic acid, sulbactam, or tazobactam) to the penicillin. Penicillins are primarily used for Gram-positive organisms and some Gram-negative cocci. A minority of Gram-negative bacilli are also susceptible to large parenteral (intravenous, or IV) doses of penicillin.

All classes of penicillins have the same adverse effects and reaction, which include anaphylaxis, drug-fever, serum sickness, rash, nephritis, hemolytic anemia, and leucopenia. Side effects patients may experience when taking these medications include diarrhea, colitis, nausea, and vomiting. Most of the penicillins are renally excreted and dose modifications are necessary for patients with impaired kidney function. The lists that follow detail the characteristics of the major groups of penicillin antibiotics. Pronunciations, brand names, and dosage forms for these agents are detailed in Medication Table 27-1 (Medication Tables are located at the end of the chapter).

Natural Penicillins

Penicillin G (IV) Penicillin VK (Oral) Penicillin benzathine/procaine (IM)

- Spectrum of activity
  - Gram-positive organisms (e.g., streptococci)
  - Gram-negative organisms (*Neisseria meningitides*)

- Avoid use for staphylococci infections

- Advantages: good oral absorption; inexpensive; IM formulation utilized for syphilis, as well as some respiratory tract infections and antibacterial prophylaxis in patients with rheumatic heart disease

- Disadvantages: frequent dosing (q 4 hr to q 6 hr) for oral and IV dosage forms; increasing resistance

Aminopenicillins

Ampicillin (IV, Oral) Amoxicillin (Oral) Ampicillin/Sulbactam (IV) Amoxicillin/Clavulanate (PO)

- Semisynthetic (chemically altered) derivatives of natural penicillins

- Are not susceptible to acid hydrolysis in the digestive tract (unlike natural penicillins)

- Spectrum of activity
  - Gram-positive organisms (enterococci, streptococci, *Listeria*)
  - Gram-negative organisms (better activity compared with natural penicillins)

- Ampicillin/sulbactam and amoxicillin/clavulanate include beta-lactamase inhibitors, which increases the spectrum of activity, including coverage against anaerobic bacteria

- Advantages: broader spectrum than natural penicillins; good tissue distribution

- Disadvantages: superinfections (an infection following a previously treated infection, typically caused by an overgrowth of bacteria that were not affected by antibiotic therapy treating the initial infection); GI intolerance more commonly seen with oral formulations that contain a beta-lactamase inhibitor.

Antistaphylococcal (Penicillinase-Resistant) Penicillins

Nafcillin (IV) Oxacillin (IV) Dicloxacillin (PO)

- Have activity against organisms (*Staphylococcus*) that produce beta-lactamase (penicillinase), which inactivates natural penicillins (no need for added beta-lactamase inhibitor)

- Spectrum of activity
  - Gram-positive organisms, staphylococci (main target)

- No Gram-negative activity

- Advantages: preferred agents for methicillin-susceptible *Staphylococcus aureus* (MSSA); no dosing adjustment needed for renal function impairment

- Disadvantages: frequent dosing (q 4 hr); no activity against methicillin-resistant *Staphylococcus aureus* (MRSA) or Gram-negative organisms

Extended-Spectrum Penicillins

Piperacillin/Tazobactam (IV)

- Activity against organisms that produce beta-lactamase, which inactivates penicillin (penicillinase)

- Spectrum of activity
  - Gram-positive organisms (streptococci, enterococci, staphylococci)
  - Gram-negative organisms; adds coverage to more resistant bacteria, including *Pseudomonas*
  - Anaerobic activity, including *Bacteroides fragilis*

- Advantages: broad spectrum of coverage, including *Pseudomonas*; good tissue distribution

- Disadvantages: formulations contain large amounts of sodium, may contribute to renal impairment

The next group of beta-lactam antibiotics is the cephalosporins, which are bactericidal, with both Gram-positive and Gram-negative activity. Like the penicillins, they inhibit cell wall synthesis. Cephalosporins penetrate well into most body fluids, especially in the presence of inflammation. Hypersensitivity reactions are the most common adverse effect of cephalosporins (urticaria and anaphylaxis are rare). Since the cephalosporins have a beta-lactam ring in the chemical structure like penicillins, some patients who have had an allergic reaction to penicillin may also react to a cephalosporin. Cross-reactivity rates between cephalosporins and penicillins is uncommon and is around 2% to 5%.[4] Cephalosporins can be given cautiously to patients with a history of delayed hypersensitivity to penicillin if necessary, but a different class of antibiotics is usually chosen if possible.

Many patients complain of pain with IM injections. Thrombophlebitis (inflammation of the vein) after IV use is possible. Most of the cephalosporins are renally excreted and dose modifications are required for patients with impaired kidney function. All cephalosporins can produce leukopenia and thrombocytopenia and prolonged use can contribute to the development of *Clostridioides difficile* (pseudomembranous) colitis. The cephalosporins are classified in *generations*, numbered first through fifth. Later generations generally have an expanded spectrum against aerobic Gram-negative bacilli. The lists that follow detail the characteristics of each generation; additional details are summarized in Medication Table 27-2.

First-Generation Cephalosporins

Cefazolin (IV) Cefadroxil (Oral) Cephalexin (Oral)

- Spectrum of activity
  - Gram-positive organisms (staphylococci, streptococci)
  - Gram-negative organisms (*E. coli, Proteus, Klebsiella*)

- Commonly used for surgical prophylaxis

- Advantages: inexpensive, good Gram-positive coverage, especially methicillin-susceptible *Staphylococcus aureus* (MSSA)

- Disadvantages: little Gram-negative coverage, no *Enterococcus* coverage

> ## ALERT!
> LOOK-ALIKE/SOUND-ALIKE—Both generic names and brand names of many cephalosporins begin with "cef" or "ceph" and are easily confused.

Second-Generation Cephalosporins

Cefaclor (Oral) Cefuroxime (IV, IM, Oral) Cefprozil (Oral) Cefotetan (IV) Cefoxitin (IV)

- Often used for polymicrobial infections (multiple microorganisms) involving Gram-negative bacilli and Gram-positive cocci

- Cefotetan and cefoxitin are referred to as the cephamycins; they have anaerobic activity and are, therefore, mainly used prophylactically for intra-abdominal procedures

- Advantages: better Gram-negative coverage than the first generations

- Disadvantages: Increasing resistance; no *Enterococcus* coverage

> ## ALERT!
> LOOK-ALIKE/SOUND-ALIKE—Keflex, a brand name of cephalexin, has been confused with Keppra, an anticonvulsant.

Third-Generation Cephalosporins

Cefdinir (Oral) Cefditoren (Oral) Cefixime (Oral) Cefotaxime (IV, IM) Cefpodoxime (Oral) Ceftazidime (IV, IM) Ceftibuten (Oral) Ceftriaxone (IV, IM)

- Spectrum of activity
  - Gram-positive organisms (streptococci)
  - Gram-negative organisms (adds coverage of *Neisseria meningitides* and *H. influenzae*)
    - Ceftazidime is the only third-generation cephalosporin with *Pseudomonas* activity

- Ceftriaxone and cefotaxime are used empirically (initiation of antibiotic therapy based on the most common organisms that cause the type of infection) for acute meningitis due to suspected *Streptococcus pneumoniae, H. influenzae,* or *Neisseria meningitides*

- Advantages: many therapeutic uses; used to treat nosocomial infections

- Disadvantages: relatively poor activity against Gram-positive cocci, especially methicillin-sensitive *Staphylococcus aureus* (MSSA), and no *Enterococcus* coverage

Fourth-Generation Cephalosporin

Cefepime (IV, IM)

- Spectrum of activity
  - Gram-positive organisms; maintains activity against staphylococci and streptococci
  - Gram-negative organisms; adds *Pseudomonas* activity and beta-lactamase–producing enterobacteriaceae, such as *Enterobacter*

- Advantages: broad spectrum of activity

- Disadvantage: available in IV formulations only, no *Enterococcus* activity

Fifth-Generation Cephalosporin

Ceftaroline (IV)

- Spectrum of activity
  - Gram-positive organism; activity against MRSA
  - Gram-negative organism; similar to third-generation cephalosporins (eg, Ceftriaxone)
- Advantages: approved for community-acquired pneumonia as well as skin and soft tissue infections
- Disadvantage: available in IV formulations only, no *Enterococcus* activity

Cephalosporins with Beta-lactamase Inhibitors

Ceftazidime/Avibactam (IV)
Ceftolozane/Tazobactam (IV)

Ceftazidime and Ceftolozane act like other beta-lactams by inhibiting cell wall synthesis. Avibactam and tazobactam have little antibacterial effect but instead inactivate certain enzymes, allowing for a broader spectrum of coverage. Ceftazidime/avibactam and Ceftolozane/tazobactam are utilized for complicated urinary tract infections (UTIs) and, with the addition of metronidazole, complicated intra-abdominal infections.

Ceftazidime/avibactam has activity against both carbapenem-resistant organisms and *Pseudomonas aeruginosa*. Ceftolozane/tazobactam also has activity against resistant Gram-negative bacteria and is used most commonly for resistant *Pseudomonas aeruginosa*.

- Advantages: Good tissue distribution, activity against resistant Gram-negative bacteria
- Disadvantages: Expensive; dosage may need to be adjusted for patients with impaired renal function

Cefiderocol (IV)

The newest of the cephalosporins, approved for community-acquired UTIs, as well as hospital-acquired/ventilator-associated pneumonia (HAP/VAP). Known to have good Gram-negative activity against more carbapenem-resistant organisms, along with *Pseudomonas* and *Acinetobacter*.

- Advantages: Activity against resistant Gram-negative bacteria

- Disadvantages: There is an increase in all cause mortality in patients with carbapenem-resistant Gram negative bacterial infections

Other Beta-Lactam Antibiotics

Penicillins and cephalosporins are not the only antibiotics with a beta-lactam ring incorporated into their chemical structures. Carbapenems and monobactams also have this ring and work by inhibiting bacterial wall synthesis. They differ in spectrum of action, effectiveness, and side effect profiles and are included in the beta-lactam summary in Medication Table 27-2.

Carbapenems

Imipenem-Cilastin (IV) Meropenem (IV)
Ertapenem (IV, IM) Doripenem (IV)

The carbapenems are bactericidal drugs that have an extremely broad spectrum of activity. All the carbapenems can cause GI disorders, rash, phlebitis, and headache. In rare cases they may cause hypotension (decreases in blood pressure). Imipenem-cilastin can also increase seizure risk. Carbapenem doses must be adjusted in patients with impaired kidney function. There is a possible cross-reaction with penicillins and these drugs should therefore be avoided in severe allergies.

- Spectrum of activity
  - Gram-positive organisms; broad coverage including enterococci, except ertapenem
  - Gram-negative organisms; broad coverage including *Pseudomonas*, except ertapenem
  - Anaerobic activity
- Advantages: broad spectrum of activity
- Disadvantages: more serious adverse reactions than penicillins and cephalosporins

Meropenem/Vaborbactam (IV)

The first carbapenem with a beta-lactamase inhibitor approved by the U.S. Food and Drug Administration (FDA). Vaborbactam inhibits the degradation of meropenem from bacterial enzymes, allowing for activity against carbapenem-resistant enterobacteriaceae (CRE). Meropenem-vaborbactam is approved for UTI, including pyelonephritis. Known for its broad Gram-negative coverage.

Imipenem-Cilastin-Relebactam (IV)

This is the newest carbapenem with a beta-lactamase inhibitor. The purpose of relebactam is to restore the activity of resistant organisms to imipenem-cilastin. This includes carbapenem-resistant *Klebsiella* and *Pseudomonas*. Imipenem-cilastin-relebactam is approved for complicated UTIs and intra-abdominal infections.

Monobactams

Aztreonam (IV, IM, Inhalation)

The monobactams are cell wall–inhibiting bactericidals. They can cause similar side effects to carbapenems and must be dose-adjusted in patients with impaired kidney function. The only agent in this group currently available in the United States is aztreonam and this antibiotic only has Gram-negative activity, including *Pseudomonas*.

- Advantages: excellent safety profile; can be used safely in penicillin-allergic patients

- Disadvantages: no Gram-positive or anaerobic coverage, increasing resistance in *Pseudomonas* sp.

Non-Beta-Lactam Antibiotics

Fluoroquinolones

Levofloxacin (IV, Oral) Ciprofloxacin (IV, Oral, Otic, Ophthalmic) Moxifloxacin (IV, Oral) Ofloxacin (Oral, Otic, Ophthalmic) Delafloxacin (IV, Oral)

The fluoroquinolones (often called *quinolones* for short) are bactericidal and act by inhibiting the activity of enzymes essential for bacterial DNA replication. Fluoroquinolone doses must be adjusted for patients with impaired kidney function. They can cause nausea, vomiting, and diarrhea, as well as altered mental status and confusion when not properly adjusted for renal function. They can cause cardiac dysfunction in patients with cardiac conduction problems or when used in combination with other medications that have cardiac effects, which can predispose patients to ventricular tachyarrhythmia. Another downside to these antibiotics is the concern for tendon rupture. Characteristics of the fluoroquinolones are listed below; additional details are summarized in Medication Table 27-3.

- Spectrum of activity
  - Gram-positive organisms; Moxifloxacin and Levofloxacin overall have good activity against streptococci infections
  - Gram-negative organisms; Levofloxacin and Ciprofloxacin have *Pseudomonas* activity
  - Adds atypical coverage (*Mycoplasma* spp., *Chlamydophilia* spp., *Mycobacterium*)
  - Anaerobic activity with Moxifloxacin (only one in its class)
  - Delafloxacin has activity against *Pseudomonas* and MRSA (only one in its class)

- Advantages: convenient dosing (q 12 hr, q 24 hr), good tissue distribution

- Disadvantages: should not be administered to children younger than 16 years (cartilage dysfunction); some serious side effects

Aminoglycosides

Amikacin (IV, IM) Gentamicin (IV, IM, Ophthalmic) Neomycin (Oral) Paromomycin (Oral) Plazomicin (IV) Streptomycin (IV, IM) Tobramycin (IV, IM, Inhalation, Ophthalmic)

The aminoglycosides are bactericidal and work by inhibiting bacterial protein synthesis. Aminoglycosides are poorly absorbed orally and are administered by inhalation, intravenously, topically, and in the eye and ear. Oral dosage forms are indicated only for intestinal infections and for the treatment and prevention of hepatic encephalopathy (see Chapter 23).

The aminoglycosides have a narrow *therapeutic range*, meaning that, while a minimum concentration is necessary for bactericidal action, at higher concentrations they can cause serious adverse effects. These adverse events include nephrotoxicity (kidney damage), which in most cases is reversible, and ototoxicity (hearing loss/impairment), which is often irreversible. To prevent these adverse events from occurring, clinicians must base the dose of these medications on several pharmacokinetic parameters, including patient weight, site of infection, and renal function. Pharmacokinetic equations (of the type introduced in Chapter 2) are used to determine the proper dose and dosing interval to achieve therapeutic drug levels, to ensure eradication of the infecting organism without causing harm to the patient. *Peak levels* are determined within 30–60 minutes after a dose has been administered and are presumed to be the highest blood concentration of antibiotic that is achieved. *Trough levels* are determined shortly before the next scheduled dose is given and are presumed to be the lowest level to which antibiotic concentrations fall in a specific treatment regimen. Characteristics of the aminoglycosides are listed below; additional details are summarized in Medication Table 27-3.

- Spectrum of activity
  - Gram-positive; only in combination with cell wall inhibitors (eg, beta-lactams) for synergy
  - Gram-negative; can be used alone or, for serious infections, in combination with other antibiotics
- Advantages: excellent Gram-negative coverage; provides synergistic activity for Gram-positive infections
- Disadvantages: nephrotoxicity, ototoxicity, cost of monitoring when used systemically

Macrolides

Azithromycin (IV, Oral) Clarithromycin (Oral) Erythromycin (IV, Oral, Ophthalmic, Topical) Fidaxomicin (Oral)

Unlike the groups discussed above, the macrolide antibiotics are primarily bacteriostatic. They kill bacterial cells by inhibiting protein synthesis and, thus, suppress bacterial replication.

Erythromycin, the prototype macrolide, has peristalsis activity, therefore causing GI disturbances, including nausea, vomiting, abdominal cramps, and diarrhea. These side effects are less common with clarithromycin and azithromycin, which were developed later. Erythromycin may cause dose-related tinnitus (ringing of the ears), dizziness, and reversible hearing loss. Erythromycin has numerous drug interactions because it inhibits hepatic metabolism through the cytochrome P-450 system, so it can increase drug levels of other medications that are metabolized through the same pathway. This interaction can lead to toxic drug levels that predispose patients to adverse drug reactions and side effects. The macrolides can cause cardiac dysfunction in patients with cardiac conduction problems or when used in combination with other medications that have certain cardiac effects. This may then predispose a patient to ventricular tachyarrhythmia. Erythromycin and clarithromycin can further elevate the PT/INR (prothrombin time/international normalized ratio) when taken with warfarin. Azithromycin has the lowest tendency of the macrolides to cause drug interactions. Characteristics of the macrolides are listed below; additional details are summarized in Medication Table 27-3.

- Spectrum of activity
  - Gram-positive organisms (streptococci)
  - Gram-negative organisms (limited activity)
  - Atypical bacteria: *Mycoplasma pneumoniae*, *Chlamydia trachomatis*, *Chlamydophila pneumoniae*, *Legionella sp.*, *Corynebacterium diphtheriae*, *Campylobacter*, *Treponema pallidum*, *Propionibacterium acnes*, and *Borrelia burgdorferi*
  - Clarithromycin is used for *Helicobacter pylori*

- Fidaxomicin's only place in therapy is for *Clostridioides difficile* colitis

- Advantages: good for community-acquired infections, convenient dosing (azithromycin), dosage not adjusted for renal impairment (exception clarithromycin)

- Disadvantages: high side effect profile; many drug interactions with other medications that have cardiac effects (QT prolongation) and predisposes to ventricular tachyarrhythmia; increased resistance

Tetracyclines

Doxycycline (IV, Oral) Minocycline (IV, Oral) Tetracycline (Oral) Tigecycline (IV) Omadacycline (IV, Oral) Eravacycline (IV)

The tetracyclines are bacteriostatic antibiotics that slow bacterial growth by inhibiting bacterial protein synthesis. Because tetracycline absorption is decreased by metallic cations such as aluminum, calcium, magnesium, and iron, preparations containing these ions should not be taken with this class of antibiotics. All tetracyclines can cause nausea, vomiting, and diarrhea. They can also exacerbate gastroesophageal reflux disease (GERD, discussed in Chapter 20). Tetracyclines can cause photosensitivity (increased incidence of sunburns when exposed to the sun). They can cause staining of teeth, hypoplasia (defects) of dental enamel, and abnormal bone growth in children.

Tigecycline, a derivative of tetracycline designed to overcome bacterial resistance, exhibits activity against community-acquired pneumonia, complicated intra-abdominal infections, and complicated skin and skin structure infections caused by susceptible organisms. This includes MRSA and vancomycin-sensitive *Enterococcus faecalis*. It is only administered intravenously.

Eravacycline is a fluorocycline that is structurally similar to tigecycline, with slight modifications. It is a newer drug in this class, typically used for complicated intra-abdominal infections. It is typically reserved for use against drug-resistant bacteria. It has activity against vancomycin-resistant *Enterococcus* (VRE), MRSA, anaerobes, and resistant enterobacterales. It is only administered intravenously.

Omadacycline, a semisynthetic tetracycline derivative, is also a newer drug in this class, with activity against community-acquired pneumonia and complicated skin and skin structure infections by susceptible organisms, including MRSA, *Enterococcus faecalis*, and *Enterobacter*. In addition to the intravenous form, it is available as an oral tablet. Patients

taking omadacycline by mouth should follow the same precautions mentioned for the older tetracyclines.

PRACTICE POINT

While it penetrates tissues very well, tigecycline cannot be used to treat bloodstream infections because it does not reach high enough concentrations there. It is also very expensive; thus, it is reserved for infections that cannot be treated effectively by other antibiotics.

ALERT!

Because of their interactions with bone and dental enamel, tetracyclines should be avoided after the first trimester of pregnancy and in mothers who are breastfeeding, as well as in children below the age of 8.

Characteristics of the tetracyclines are listed below; additional details are summarized in Medication Table 27-3.

- Spectrum of activity
  - Gram-positive (community-acquired MRSA coverage)
  - Gram-negative (*Neisseria gonorrhea* and *Helicobacter pylori*)
  - Atypical (rickettsia, spirochetes [*Treponema pallidum*, *Borrelia burgdorferi*], *Vibrio* sp., *Brucella* sp., *Bacillus anthracis*, *Mycoplasma*, and *Chlamydia*)

- Advantages: activity against community-acquired MRSA; inexpensive, not adjusted for impaired renal function

- Disadvantages: high side effect profile; increasing resistance

---

PRACTICE POINT

Patients taking tetracyclines and related agents should avoid direct sunlight as well as tanning beds and use a sunblock of SPF 15 or higher on areas exposed to the sun (including the lips).

Glycopeptides

Vancomycin (IV, Oral) Telavancin (IV) Dalbavancin (IV) Oritavancin (IV)

Glycopeptides are bactericidal antibiotics that inhibit cell wall synthesis. Vancomycin can be associated with ototoxicity and nephrotoxicity if drug concentrations in the body become too high. As with the aminoglycosides, several pharmacokinetic parameters must be considered by doctors and pharmacists deciding on dose and frequency of administration. Patients at the highest risk for drug accumulation are the elderly and those with impaired kidney function. The oral formulation of vancomycin is not systemically absorbed and is only effective for treating *Clostridioides difficile* colitis (a local effect in the GI tract). Vancomycin intended for use in treating systemic infections must be infused intravenously over at least 60 minutes. Telavancin is a synthetic derivative of vancomycin indicated only for skin and skin structure infections by certain Gram-positive cocci. It is administered only by IV infusion, over at least 60 minutes. Dalbavancin and oritavancin, like telavancin, are semisynthetic derivatives.

> ### PRACTICE POINT
>
> *IV vancomycin doses should be limited to concentrations of 5 mg/mL, unless patients are fluid-restricted, and infused at rates not to exceed 10 mg/min.*

> ### PRACTICE POINT
>
> *The FDA requires distribution of a medication guide to patients receiving telavancin.*

> ### ALERT!
>
> Glycopeptides can cause a dangerous reaction termed "red man syndrome" that is characterized by redness, flushing, and itching. This is not an allergic reaction; it occurs when IV infusion of the drug is too rapid. Glycopeptides can still be used but the infusion needs to be slowed down.

Oritavancin can be given as a single dose, whereas dalbavancin can be given in either one to two doses. Both are indicated for skin and skin structure infections for Gram-positive organisms. Oritavancin is administered only by IV, over at least 3 hours, whereas dalbavancin can be administered over 30 minutes.

- Spectrum of activity
  - Only covers Gram-positive bacteria
  - Gram-positive cocci (staphylococci including MRSA, streptococci, enterococci) and Gram-positive bacilli
  - Oral vancomycin only used for *Clostridioides difficile*

- Advantages: very effective against penicillin and cephalosporin-resistant strains of Gram-positive organisms; vancomycin is the drug of choice for MRSA; dalbavancin and oritavancin only require one or two doses

- Disadvantages: Vancomycin and telavancin can accumulate in patients with impaired kidney function leading to increased drug concentrations and incidence of toxicity

> ### ALERT!
>
> Vancomycin injection is very irritating and is never administered via the IM route.

Sulfonamides

Co-trimoxazole (IV, Oral) Sulfacetamide (Topical, Ophthalmic) Sulfadiazine (Topical, Oral)

The sulfonamides, sometimes called *sulfa drugs* or *sulfas*, were the earliest antibiotics marketed for human therapy.[3] First used in 1932, they represented a dramatic change in the way infections were treated. Although the penicillins and newer antibiotics, along with the widespread emergence of bacterial resistance to them, have reduced the importance of this class, several are still in use today.

Sulfonamides are bacteriostatic; they inhibit bacterial replication by interfering with folic acid synthesis in bacteria unable to utilize preformed folate for cellular processes. Since the introduction of sulfonamides, many bacterial strains have acquired the ability to skip the metabolic step blocked by sulfonamides and incorporate absorbed folate into their metabolism, so they have become resistant to these antibiotics.

Sulfonamides were named because their chemical structure includes an altered version of the folic acid precursor PABA (the one used by bacteria to make folic acid) that has a sulfate molecule attached.[3] A similar structure is also found in other medications, including thiazide diuretics and some diabetes medications.

Co-trimoxazole, a combination of the sulfonamide antibiotic sulfamethoxazole and another agent, trimethoprim (which also interferes with bacterial folic acid production), is the most commonly used sulfa anti-infective. It is active against a wide variety of Gram-positive and Gram-negative organisms and is prescribed for the treatment of bacterial infections of the ears (otitis media), GI tract (travelers' diarrhea), respiratory system, and urinary tract. Co-trimoxazole has also been found to be an effective prophylaxis and treatment for pneumonia caused by the organism *Pneumocystis jiroveci*, a fungal infection (PJP) that affects immunosuppressed patients, especially HIV-infected individuals. It appears to be effective against toxoplasmosis, a protozoal parasite, as well. Important to note if giving the IV formulation of sulfamethoxazole/trimethoprim, the weight-based dosing is determined using the trimethoprim component.

Other sulfa antibiotics include sulfadiazine (used orally for bacterial infections and topically as silver sulfadiazine, for burns), sulfacetamide (used only for ophthalmic infections), sulfasalazine (used in the management of ulcerative colitis—see Chapter 22), and sulfisoxazole (available in combination with erythromycin for the treatment of ear infections). Facts to remember about sulfonamide antibiotics are listed below; additional information is included in Medication Table 27-3.

- Spectrum of activity
  - Co-trimoxazole, wide range of activity
  - Susceptible enterobacterales
  - *Pneumocystis jiroveci* pneumonia
  - *Toxoplasma gondii*
  - *Listeria monocytogenes*
  - Community-acquired MRSA
  - *Stenotrophomonas maltophilia*

- Advantages: inexpensive; useful for less common bacterial infections
- Disadvantages: allergic/hypersensitivity reactions; increasing resistance; drug interactions (eg, warfarin); monitor for hyperkalemia

Miscellaneous Antibiotics

A number of antibiotics are not classified in groups and are discussed here as miscellaneous. They are listed below with their most prominent characteristics (see also Medication Table 27-3).

Chloramphenicol (IV)

Like many of the other antibiotics, chloramphenicol exerts its antimicrobial action by inhibiting protein synthesis. It is bacteriostatic for a wide variety of microorganisms but is considered bactericidal for *H. influenzae*, *Neisseria meningitidis*, and *S. pneumoniae*.[3] Chloramphenicol is an older antibiotic and resistant strains of some pathogens are common.

Unfortunately, chloramphenicol's protein synthesis inhibition is not limited to microorganisms.[3] Some human cells, particularly those of the blood-forming system, are also affected by its action, and it has been known to cause serious, even fatal, blood disorders. For this reason, use of chloramphenicol is limited to serious infections by pathogens with documented sensitivity to the drug and only when less dangerous drugs cannot be used (because of resistance or patient factors such as allergy).

- Broad spectrum of activity against a wide variety of organisms
- Used infrequently in the treatment of typhoid fever, meningitis, Rocky Mountain spotted fever, and anthrax when other drugs cannot be used
- Advantages: broad spectrum, good penetration of spinal fluid for central nervous system infections such as meningitis
- Disadvantages: resistant organisms; life-threatening adverse reactions; allergic/hypersensitivity reactions

Clindamycin (IV, Oral, Vaginal, Topical)

Clindamycin is classified as lincosamide, which is bacteriostatic by inhibiting protein synthesis of bacteria.

- Spectrum of activity
  - Activity against anaerobic organisms (above the diaphragm)
  - Community acquired MRSA infections

- Advantages: option for patients with severe penicillin allergies; renal function dose adjustments are not necessary
- Disadvantages: high rate of *Clostridioides difficile* colitis with use

Daptomycin (IV)

Daptomycin is classified as a lipopeptide that is bactericidal by disrupting multiple aspects of bacterial cell membrane function and inhibition of protein, DNA, and RNA synthesis, which results in bacterial cell death.

- Spectrum of activity
  - Gram-positive cocci (staphylococci, including MRSA, streptococci, enterococci, including vancomycin-resistant *Enterococcus* [VRE]) and Gram-positive bacilli
- Advantages: excellent activity for resistant Gram-positive organisms
- Disadvantages: expensive; cannot be used for pneumonia due to inactivation by lung surfactant; weekly monitoring of creatinine kinase levels

ALERT!
LOOK-ALIKE/SOUND-ALIKE—Daptomycin has been confused with dactinomycin, a cancer chemotherapy.

Linezolid (IV, Oral)

Linezolid is classified as an oxazolidinone that is bacteriostatic by inhibiting bacterial replication. However, it does display some bactericidal activity against certain bacteria.

- Spectrum of activity
  - Gram-positive cocci (staphylococci, including MRSA, streptococci, enterococci, including vancomycin-resistant *Enterococcus* [VRE]) and Gram-positive bacilli
- Advantages: available in IV and oral formulations; excellent tissue penetration; dose not adjusted for renal function
- Disadvantages: thrombocytopenia and neuropathies with prolonged use; monoamine oxidase inhibitor drug interactions

Metronidazole (IV, Oral, Topical, Vaginal)

Metronidazole demonstrates bacteriostatic action by disrupting bacterial DNA structure, resulting in inhibition of protein synthesis.

- Spectrum of activity
  - Excellent activity against anaerobic bacterial (below the diaphragm) and protozoal infections

- Advantages: available in IV, oral, and topical formulations; does not require renal function dose adjustments

- Disadvantages: patients have to avoid alcohol while taking medication due to disulfiram-like reaction (severe nausea and vomiting); drug interactions (eg, warfarin)

Rifaximin

Rifaximin works by inhibiting bacterial RNA synthesis. It is used for travelers' diarrhea and as an alternative for treatment of *Clostridioides difficile*-associated diarrhea.

- Activity against *Escherichia coli, Acinetobacter, Bacteroides, Enterobacter cloacae*, and various other organisms that reside in the GI tract

- Advantages: low resistance rates; available in oral formulation

- Disadvantages: superinfections; not for use in children younger than 12 years

Quinupristin/Dalfopristin (IV)

Quinupristin/dalfopristin is classified as a streptogramin, an antibiotic that is bacteriostatic by inhibiting bacterial protein synthesis.

- Activity against vancomycin-resistant *Enterococcus faecium* bacteremia; treatment of complicated skin and skin structure infections caused by methicillin-susceptible *Staphylococcus aureus* or *Streptococcus pyogenes*

- Advantages: good activity against resistant Gram-positive organisms

- Disadvantages: may cause arthralgias and/or myalgias with use and can cause hyperbilirubinemia

Colistimethate (IV, IM, Inhaled)

Colistimethate has bacteriostatic activity by acting as a cationic detergent, which damages the bacterial cytoplasmic membrane, causing leaking of intracellular substances and cell death.

- Has activity against resistant strains of Gram-negative bacilli (*Pseudomonas aeruginosa, Enterobacter aerogenes, Escherichia coli*, and *Klebsiella pneumoniae*)

- Advantages: active against resistant organisms; may be used as inhalation therapy to treat lung infections

- Disadvantages: must be dose adjusted in patients with impaired kidney function

Nitrofurantoin (Oral)

Nitrofurantoin is a bactericidal antibiotic with a unique mechanism of action. It is chemically changed by bacteria to a product that inactivates or alters bacterial ribosomal proteins and other macromolecules, inhibiting energy metabolism and DNA synthesis.

- Only indicated for urinary tract infections

- Spectrum of activity
  - Common urinary organisms (eg, *E. coli, Klebsiella, Proteus, Enterococcus*) if susceptible

- Advantages: inexpensive

- Disadvantages: should not be used in patients with impaired renal function; avoid for pyelonephritis

Fosfomycin (Oral)

- Only indicated for urinary tract infections

- Spectrum of activity
  - Common urinary organisms (eg, *E. coli*, *Klebsiella*, *Proteus*, *Enterococcus*) if susceptible

- Advantages: one-time dose

- Disadvantages: avoid for pyelonephritis

Antimycobacterials/Antituberculosis Antibiotics

These agents are used in the treatment of tuberculosis and other infections caused by the organisms from the genus *Mycobacterium*. Because the mycobacteria are slow-growing organisms, tuberculosis infection may be active or latent (not causing signs and symptoms of active infection) in the host. At any time, the latent infection can develop into an active disease. The treatment of these infections is complex due to the multidrug-resistant strains of *Mycobacterium*. Many of the antibiotics used to treat these infections have severe side effects and patient compliance or adherence to treatment regimens is often poor. This has led to bacterial resistance and the need for multiple medication combinations to overcome resistance patterns. A single drug may be given for 4–6 months upon discovery of a latent infection without symptoms, but treatment of active disease usually involves a regimen of two to four drugs, chosen based on the tested sensitivity of the infecting organism.[2] Treatment with these drug combinations can range from 18 weeks up to 18 months.

Rifampin (IV, Oral)

Rifampin is a bactericidal antibiotic that inhibits bacterial RNA synthesis by preventing attachment of an enzyme to DNA, thus blocking initiation of RNA transcription.

- Activity against tuberculosis in combination with other agents; also has activity against *Haemophilus influenzae*, *Legionella* pneumonia; used in combination with other anti-infectives in the treatment of staphylococcal and *M. leprae* infections

- Disadvantages/considerations: may permanently discolor soft contact lenses; causes red–orange discoloration of urine, feces, saliva, sweat, and tears. There is an increase in bacterial resistance; multiple drug interactions; hepatic dysfunction

ALERT!

LOOK-ALIKE/SOUND-ALIKE—Rifampin looks and sounds like rifaximin, an antibiotic that is not indicated for the treatment of tuberculosis.

Ethambutol (Oral)

Ethambutol is a bacteriostatic antibiotic that interferes with cellular metabolism, resulting in the impairment of bacteria replication and cell death.

- Used in combination with other antibiotics to treat tuberculosis; has activity against *Mycobacterium avium complex* (MAC) and *Mycobacterium tuberculosis*

- Disadvantages: many side effects, including optic neuritis with decreased visual acuity, dermatitis, pruritus, headache, fever, and mental confusion

Cycloserine (Oral)

Cycloserine may be bactericidal or bacteriostatic, depending on its concentration at the site of infection and the susceptibility of the organism. It interferes with bacterial cell wall synthesis.

- Used in combination with other antibiotics to treat tuberculosis; has activity against strains of *E. coli* and *Enterobacter* for the treatment of urinary tract infections

- Disadvantages: many side effects, including drowsiness, somnolence, headache, dizziness, anxiety, nervousness, vertigo, and confusion; dose must be adjusted in patients with altered kidney function

Isoniazid (IM, Oral)

Isoniazid is a bactericidal antibiotic with activity against many types of mycobacteria, primarily those that are actively dividing. Its exact mechanism of action is not known, but it may be related to the inhibition of mycolic acid synthesis and disruption of the cell wall.

- Used in monotherapy or in combination with other antibiotics to treat tuberculosis, as well as in the treatment of both latent and active tuberculosis; has activity against *Mycobacterium bovis*, *M. tuberculosis*, and *M. kansasii*

- Disadvantages: many side effects; U.S. Black Box Warning: severe and sometimes fatal hepatitis may occur, usually within the first 3 months of treatment, although may develop even after many months of treatment; peripheral neuropathies (tingling, numbness in toes/fingers); vitamin B_6 depletion

Pyrazinamide (Oral)

Pyrazinamide may be bacteriostatic or bactericidal, depending on its concentration and the susceptibility of the organism. The exact mechanism of action is unknown but is partially related to the conversion of medication to pyrazinoic acid, which lowers the pH of the environment, leading to the suppression of bacterial growth.

- Used in combination with other antibiotics to treat tuberculosis; has activity only against *Mycobacterium tuberculosis*

- Disadvantages: many side effects; liver toxicity; dosage must be reduced in patients with renal dysfunction, myalgia, nausea, and vomiting

Other antimycobacterial drugs include aminosalicylic acid, capreomycin, ethionamide, rifabutin, and rifapentine. These are used infrequently in cases of resistant disease or patients who do not respond to other therapies. Their pronunciations, brand names, routes of administration, and dosage forms are included in Medication Table 27-3 along with those of the antituberculosis drugs described above. Table 27-4 summarizes types of infection, likely organisms, and first- and second-line antibiotic choices.

TABLE 27-4. Empiric Treatment of Common Infections

Site of Infection	Likely Organism	First-Line Agent	Second-Line Agent
Skin infection	*Staphylococcus* sp., *Streptococcus* sp.	Antistaphylococcal penicillins (PCNs), 1st-generation cephalosporin	Vancomycin (if methicillin-resistant *Staphylococcus aureus* [MRSA] is suspected or severe allergy to PCN)
Urinary tract	*Escherichia coli*, *Proteus, Klebsiella, Enterococcus*	Nitrofurantoin, fosfomycin, sulfamethoxazole/trimethoprim	Fluoroquinolone (levofloxacin and ciprofloxacin) Beta-lactam (amoxicillin/clavulanate, ampicillin/sulbactam, cefdinir cefaclor, cefpodoxime, cephalexin)
Respiratory	Atypical, *Streptococcus pneumoniae*, *Haemophilus influenzae* (community acquired), MRSA, *Pseudomonas* (hospital-acquired)	**Community**: azithromycin, fluoroquinolone (levofloxacin, moxifloxacin), amoxicillin, doxycycline, amoxicillin/clavulanate, 3rd-generation cephalosporin (ceftriaxone, cefpodoxime, cefotaxime), ceftaroline **Hospital**: Vancomycin, linezolid, piperacillin/tazobactam, cefepime, ceftazidime, meropenem, imipenem, fluoroquinolone (levofloxacin, ciprofloxacin), aminoglycosides	
Intra-abdominal	Anaerobes, *E. coli*	**Community**: 2nd-generation cephalosporin, ertapenem, moxifloxacin, tigecycline, piperacillin-tazobactam; combination options are cefazolin, cefuroxime, ceftriaxone, cefepime, levofloxacin with metronidazole **Hospital**: Meropenem, piperacillin-tazobactam. Combination options are levofloxacin or cefepime with metronidazole	

ANTIBIOTIC SELECTION

Several factors must be considered for antibiotic selection. First, the clinician must determine the goal of therapy. In some cases, this will be to prevent an infection following surgery or another procedure. This is known as surgical prophylaxis. Not all surgeries or procedures require the patient to receive antibiotic therapy. Treatment with antibiotics is recommended for patients with valvular heart disorders or artificial joints, as well as those who are immunosuppressed, or otherwise at high risk for infection. Procedures carrying a higher risk of bacterial infections are those performed in the mouth, GI tract, and genitourinary tract. If prophylactic antibiotic therapy is indicated, antibiotic selection is based on the normal flora that resides in the location of the procedure. For example, a patient at risk for endocarditis (infection of the heart valves or lining of the heart) who is scheduled for a dental procedure would receive amoxicillin 2,000 mg orally 30–60 minutes prior to the procedure. Amoxicillin has activity against those organisms that inhabit the oral cavity. The goal of using amoxicillin in this patient is to prevent the bacteria that enter the bloodstream (from the dental procedure) from causing an infection in the heart. As stated earlier, not all patients need antibiotic prophylaxis; it is routinely used for those with risk factors for infectious processes. There are several guidelines available for prophylactic antibiotic dosing for various procedures.

In other cases, the goal of therapy will be to treat an infection that has already developed. Regardless of the goal, antibiotic selection is determined by the most likely organism to cause an infection based on the location of the infectious process or type of surgery performed. Empiric therapy refers to the selection of an antibiotic based on the organisms most commonly encountered at the site of the infection prior to obtaining culture results. Finally, definitive treatment refers to antibiotic selection that has activity toward a known pathogen based on the results of culture and sensitivity testing. In addition, the following factors must be considered for antibiotic selection.

- Allergies or history of adverse drug reactions to certain antibiotics (cross-sensitivity of antibiotic class)
- Patient's age (FDA approval for specified ages or known toxicity within certain age groups)
- Genetic or metabolic abnormalities (drug accumulation/toxicity)
- Renal (kidney) function (dose adjustment if renally excreted)
- Hepatic (liver) function (dose adjustment if hepatically metabolized)
- Site of infection (drug distribution/tissue penetration)
- Pregnancy/lactation (safe use in pregnancy or lactation)
- Concomitant drug therapy (drug interactions)
- Concomitant disease states (drug/disease interaction)
- Antibiogram (hospital-specific susceptibility and resistance patterns)
- Resistance patterns

COMBINATION THERAPY

Combination therapy refers to the use of more than one antibiotic to treat an infection. The concept behind combination therapy is to achieve one of the following: broaden antimicrobial coverage for a suspected organism or multiple organisms, improve efficacy though synergistic activity, and help overcome bacterial resistance. Many infections, such as pneumonia and hospital-acquired (nosocomial) infections, are treated with combination therapy for the reasons listed earlier. In addition, when patients are started on empiric therapy and the organism is yet to be identified, they may be placed on multiple antibiotics until the cultures and sensitivities are reported. At that time, the clinician may narrow down the antibiotic regimen based on the results and patient response.

CASE?

Why do you think G. F. was started on both ceftriaxone and azithromycin?

PATIENT MONITORING

Patient monitoring begins once antibiotic therapy is initiated. This includes monitoring the patient for safety, efficacy, response, and completion of therapy. Safety monitoring includes watching for both allergic reactions and adverse drug events associated with the selected antibiotic(s). As with all medications, the patient's allergies must be reviewed prior to any medication being dispensed. Antibiotic allergies range from nausea to anaphylaxis. If a patient is allergic to penicillin, there is a small chance of cross allergy to other antibiotics in the beta-lactam class. For mild reactions to penicillins, such as nausea or a mild rash, most clinicians will confidently dispense an antibiotic in a different beta-lactam group, such as a cephalosporin. If the patient reports an incident of anaphylactic reaction to penicillin, an antibiotic from a different class altogether (ie, fluoroquinolone) should be used to ensure patient safety. Allergies are often a class effect and antibiotics from a different class should be used for severe allergies to avoid additional reactions.

In addition to allergies, patients should be monitored for adverse drug reactions. It is important for clinicians to be familiar with the common side effects of different antibiotic classes to be able to properly monitor the patient. Adverse reactions to antibiotics include the side effects one may experience while taking the medication. They can also be the result of a drug interaction that increases the chance of a known adverse reaction or unwanted effect due to altered drug absorption, distribution, and elimination.

It is important for clinicians to monitor patients for response to antibiotic therapy, ensuring efficacy of the antibiotic(s) selected to treat the infection. As mentioned earlier, cultures are obtained to help identify the pathogenic organism(s). These cultures are monitored for growth, identification, and sensitivity of the organism to specific antibiotics. Commonly, cultures may remain negative and no organism(s) grow in the culture obtained. If this is the case, the patient's laboratory and physical condition will be monitored to determine the efficacy of the selected therapy. In cases where cultures do grow, the clinician will review the identified organism(s) and compare it to the antibiotic regimen the patient is receiving to ensure proper antimicrobial coverage. If sensitivities are reported, the clinician may modify the regimen to an antibiotic that is more effective against the specific pathogen. Whenever possible, therapy is adjusted to provide coverage for only those organisms isolated or suspected. This is an important factor in reducing the possible development of resistant organisms.

Patient-specific values, such as the WBC count and temperature, are monitored closely to determine if the patient is responding to antibiotic therapy. A baseline WBC count is obtained and monitored closely thereafter. If the WBC count trends downward, it is a good indication the patient is responding to antibiotic therapy and improving. If the patient's WBC count increases or continues to increase despite antibiotic therapy, it may be a sign of treatment failure. A patient's temperature is also monitored for response to therapy. Like the WBC count, if the temperature was elevated at baseline and the patient becomes afebrile and maintains an afebrile state, it is a good indication that the patient is responding to therapy.

Alternatively, if the temperature remains elevated or spikes, it may be a sign of treatment failure.

Finally, other diagnostic tests may be reordered to evaluate for continued or worsening infection. A repeat chest x-ray can be obtained for patients who are worsening on therapy to determine if the initial infection has not responded or if there may be a new infection that may warrant a change in therapy. Clinicians must also determine duration of therapy for antibiotic use based on the type and severity of infection being treated. There are several guidelines available for various infections that serve as treatment suggestions for both selection of antibiotic therapy and duration of treatment. Although these guidelines provide recommendations for duration of therapy, it is important to also evaluate the clinical response of the patient and adjust the duration based on response. In some cases, a longer duration of therapy may be warranted.

Duration of treatment is not only important to prevent treatment failure but also to help prevent antibiotic resistance. Often patients start to feel better and do not finish their course of antibiotics. This may lead to bacterial resistance as the pathogenic organism(s) may not be completely eradicated.

PRACTICE POINT

Antibiotic treatment often continues after the symptoms of an infection have disappeared. It is important that patients complete the full prescribed course of an antibiotic treatment, even if they feel cured, to prevent recurrence of the infection and the development of resistant strains.

CASE?

After 48 hours of IV antibiotics, G. F.'s breathing has improved and his WBC count has become lower. Does this mean it is time to discontinue therapy and send him home?

Prevention of infection is the best and most effective medicine. Handwashing is the most important and effective way to limit the spread of infectious organism(s). In hospital settings, many measures are in place to limit the number of hospital-acquired infections. These include the proper use of hand sanitizer, surveillance of employee handwashing, limiting contact with patients with highly contagious organisms (known as isolation), and monitoring of patients' IV and urinary catheters, which can increase the risk of patients getting a hospital-acquired infection.

SUMMARY

Bacteria live among us and reside in our bodies as normal flora that helps us fight off other invading organisms and assist with many important functions in various organ systems. Our bodies have various natural defenses that assist normal flora in providing protection against invading organisms. When these natural defenses fail or breakdown, normal flora can become pathogenic and cause infection. Once an infection occurs, the body's immune system starts the process of attacking the pathogen and inhibiting the replication of the pathogen. Every system in the body is susceptible to infection. In most cases, patients are febrile and have elevated WBCs that are consistent with infection. The location of the infection determines the type of disease or illness that occurs. The patient usually exhibits signs and symptoms that are specific to the type of infection. The signs and symptoms of the infection can guide the clinician regarding the most likely organism causing the infection. Depending on the type of infection and patient history, empiric antibiotic therapy is initiated. If bacterial resistance is suspected, broader coverage may be initiated. Risk factors for bacterial resistance include recent prior antibiotic use, and history of prior resistant organisms. Samples from the patient are usually cultured in hopes of identifying the offending organism and also to determine the susceptibility of that organism to various antibiotics. When the cultures reveal the infecting organism(s), the initial empiric therapy can be changed, if necessary, to agents chosen to treat the specific infection.

There are several antibiotic classes that cover specific organisms and each has specific indications for use. Once antibiotic therapy is initiated, patients are monitored for safety and for efficacy. Safety includes monitoring for allergic reactions and adverse reactions or side effects. Efficacy refers to signs of improvement and eradication of the organism(s). Monitoring cultures and sensitivities allows the clinician to modify empiric therapy to target the specific organism(s) identified and use the most effective agent based on sensitivities. A patient's vital signs and laboratory values allow the clinician to determine if a patient is improving.

Over the years, bacteria have "learned" many methods to become resistant to antibiotics. Every year new antibiotics are developed to combat resistant organisms but not at the rate of bacterial resistance that is occurring. One way to slow the development of resistance is with the proper use of antibiotic regimens, with clinicians choosing an agent with the narrowest spectrum that includes the infecting organism and treating the infection for the optimal length of time.

ACKNOWLEDGMENT

The author wishes to acknowledge the work of John Flanigan, PharmD, BCNSP, James Adams, PharmD, BCPS, and Catherine W. Davis, PharmD, BCPS on this chapter in the first edition of this text.

REFERENCES

1. Whitman WB, Coleman DC, Wiebe WJ. *Proc Natl Acad Sci USA*. 1998;95:6578-6583.

2. DiPiro JT, Talbert RL, Yee GC, et al., eds. *Pharmacotherapy: A Pathophysiologic Approach*. 11th ed. New York, NY: McGraw-Hill; 2020.

3. Brunton LL, Hillal-Dandan R, Knollmann BC, eds. *Goodman & Gilman's The Pharmacological Basis of Therapeutics*. 13th ed. New York, NY: McGraw-Hill; 2017.

4. Macy E, Blumenthal KG. Are cephalosporins safe for use in penicillin allergy without prior allergy evaluation? *J Allergy Clin Immunol Pract*. 2018;6:82-89.

CHAPTER RESOURCE

AHFS Drug Information 2019. Bethesda, MD: American Society of Health-System Pharmacists; 2019.

REVIEW QUESTIONS

1. What are some ways that bacteria become resistant to antibiotics?

2. What factors should be considered when selecting an antibiotic to treat an infection?

3. Describe the difference between using antibiotics for surgical prophylaxis and empiric treatment of an infection.

4. Why is it important for patients to finish their full prescribed course of antibiotics even if it extends for several days after they feel completely better?

5. Why are beta-lactamase inhibitors added to penicillins but not to fluoroquinolones?

MEDICATION TABLES

MEDICATION TABLE 27-1. The Penicillins [a]

Agent (pronunciation)	Brand Name	Dosage Form	Route
Natural			
Penicillin G benzathine (pen i SILL in) (BENZ a theen)	Bicillin L-A	Suspension	Intramuscular (IM)
Penicillin G potassium (pen i SILL in) (poe TAS ee um)	Pfizerpen-G	Solution	Injection
Penicillin G procaine (pen i SILL in) (PROE kane)	—	Suspension	IM
Penicillin V potassium (pen i SILL in) (poe TAS ee um)	—	Tablet, solution	Oral
Aminopenicillins			
Amoxicillin (a mox i SIL in)	—	Tablet, capsule, suspension	Oral
	Moxatag	Extended-release tablet	Oral
Amoxicillin/clavulanate (a mox i SIL in) (KLAV yoo la nate)	Augmentin	Tablet, suspension	Oral
Ampicillin (am pi SILL in)	—	Capsule, suspension	Oral
	—	Solution	Injection
Ampicillin/sulbactam (am pi SILL in) (sul BAK tam)	Unasyn	Solution	Injection
Penicillinase-Resistant (antistaphylococcal)			
Dicloxacillin (dye klox a SILL in)	—	Capsule	Oral
Nafcillin (naf SILL in)	Nallpen	Solution	Injection
Oxacillin (ox a SILL in)	Bactocill	Solution	Injection
Extended Spectrum			
Piperacillin/tazobactam (pi PER a sil in) (ta zoe BAK tam)	Zosyn	Solution	Injection

[a] Pronunciations have been adapted with permission from USP Dictionary of USAN and International Drug Names (USP Dictionary) © 2022.

MEDICATION TABLE 27-2. Cephalosporins and Beta-Lactam Antibiotics[a]

Agent (pronunciation)	Brand Name	Dosage Form	Route
First Generation			
Cefazolin (sef A zoe lin)	Kefzol	Premixed solution, powder for reconstitution	Intravenous (IV), intramuscular (IM)
Cefadroxil (sef a DROX il)	Duricef	Capsule, tablet (as hemihydrate and monohydrate); suspension	Oral
Cephalexin (sef a LEX in)	Keflex	Capsule, suspension, tablet	Oral
Second Generation			
Cefaclor (SEF a klor)	—	Capsule, powder for suspension, extended-release tablet	Oral
Cefuroxime (se fyoor OX eem)	Zinacef	Premixed solution; powder for reconstitution	IV
	Ceftin	Suspension, tablet	Oral
Cefprozil (sef PROE zil)	—	Suspension, tablet	Oral
Cefotetan (SEF oh tee tan)	Cefotan	Powder for reconstitution	IV, IM
Cefoxitin (se FOX i tin)	Mefoxin	Premixed solution, powder for reconstitution	IV, IM
Third Generation			
Cefdinir (SEF di ner)	Omnicef	Capsule, suspension	Oral
Cefditoren (sef DIT or in)	Spectracef	Tablet	Oral
Cefixime (sef IX eem)	Suprax	Suspension, capsule, tablet	Oral
Cefotaxime (sef oh TAKS eem)	Claforan	Premixed solution, powder for reconstitution	IV, IM
Cefpodoxime proxetil (sef pode OX eem)	—	Suspension, tablet	Oral
Ceftazidime (SEF tay zi deem)	Fortaz, Tazicef	Premixed solution, powder for reconstitution	IV, IM
Ceftibuten (sef TYE byoo ten)	Cedax	Capsule, suspension	Oral
Ceftriaxone (sef trye AX one)	Rocephin	Premixed solution, powder for reconstitution	IV, IM
Fourth Generation			
Cefepime (SEF e peem)	Maxipime	Premixed solution, powder for reconstitution	IV, IM

Continued next page

MEDICATION TABLE 27-2. Cephalosporins and Beta-Lactam Antibiotics [a] *(Continued)*

Agent (pronunciation)	Brand Name	Dosage Form	Route
Fifth Generation			
Ceftaroline fosamil (sef TAR oh line) (FOS a mil)	Teflaro	Powder for reconstitution	IV
Cepahlosporin/Beta-Lactamase Combination			
Ceftazidime/Avibactam (SEF tay zi deem) (a vi BAK tam)	Avycaz	Powder for reconstitution	IV
Ceftolozane/Tazobactam (sef TOL oh zane) (taz oh BAK tam)	Zerbaxa	Powder for reconstitution	IV
Siderophere Cephalosporin			
Cefiderocol (SEF I DER oh kol)	Fetroja	Powder for reconstitution	IV
Carbapenems			
Doripenem (dor i PEN em)	Doribax	Powder for reconstitution	IV
Ertapenem (er ta PEN em)	Invanz	Powder for reconstitution	IV, IM
Imipenem/cilastatin (i mi PEN em) (sye la STAT in)	Primaxin	Powder for reconstitution	IV
Meropenem (mer oh PEN em)	Merrem	Powder for reconstitution	IV
Carbapenem/Beta-Lactamase Combination			
Meropenem/Vaborbactam (mer oh PEN em) (va bor BAK tam)	Vabomere	Powder for reconstitution	IV
Imipenem/cilastin/relebactam (i mi PEN em) (sye la STAT in) (REL e BAK tam)	Recarbrio	Powder for reconstitution	IV
Monobactam			
Aztreonam (AS tree oh nam)	Azactam	Premixed solution, powder for reconstitution	IV, IM
	Cayston	Powder for reconstitution (nebulizer solution)	Inhalation

[a] Pronunciations have been adapted with permission from USP Dictionary of USAN and International Drug Names (USP Dictionary) © 2022.

MEDICATION TABLE 27-3. Additional Anti-infective Classes[a]

Agent (pronunciation)	Brand Name	Dosage Form	Route
Fluoroquinolones			
Ciprofloxacin (sip roe FLOX a sin)	Ceftraxal	Solution	Otic
	Otiprio	Suspension	Otic
	Ciloxan	Solution, ointment	Ophthalmic
	Cipro	Solution	IV
	Cipro	Tablet	Oral
	ProQuin XR	Extended-release tablet	Oral
Levofloxacin (lee voe FLOX a sin)	Levaquin	Premixed solution, injection solution, oral solution, oral tablet	IV, oral
	Iquix, Quixin	Solution	Ophthalmic
Moxifloxacin (mox i FLOX a sin)	Avelox IV	Premixed solution	IV
	Avelox IV	Tablet	Oral
	Avelox ABC Pack	Tablet	Oral
Ofloxacin (oh FLOX a sin)		Tablet, solution	Oral, otic
	Ocuflox	Solution	Ophthalmic
Delafloxacin (del a FLOX a sin)	Baxdela	Powder for reconstitution	IV
	Baxdela	Tablet	Oral
Aminoglycosides			
Amikacin (am i KAY sin)	—	Solution	IM, IV
Gentamicin (jen ta MYE sin)	—	Solution (concentrated and premixed in NS)	IM, IV, ophthalmic
Neomycin (nee oh MYE sin)	Neo-Fradin	Solution, tablet	Oral
Streptomycin (strep toe MYE sin)	—	Powder for reconstitution	IM, IV
Tobramycin (toe bra MYE sin)	—	Premixed solution, powder for reconstitution, injection solution	IM, IV, ophthalmic
	Tobi	Solution for nebulization	Inhalation
Plazomicin (pla zoe MYE sin)	Zemdri	Solution	IV
Macrolides			
Azithromycin (as ith roe MYE sin)	Zithromax	Powder for reconstitution, powder for oral suspension, tablet	IV, oral
	Zmax	Extended-release microspheres for suspension	Oral
	Zithromax TRI-PAK, Zithromax Z-PAK	Tablet (dose pack)	Oral
Clarithromycin (kla RITH roe mye sin)	Biaxin, Biaxin XL	Tablet, extended-release tablet, suspension	Oral

Continued next page

MEDICATION TABLE 27-3. Additional Anti-infective Classes[a] *(Continued)*

Agent (pronunciation)	Brand Name	Dosage Form	Route
Erythromycin (er ith roe MYE sin)	E.E.S., EryPed, Ery-Tab, PCE	Delayed-release capsule, granules for suspension, powder for suspension, tablet, delayed-release tablet	Oral
	Erythrocin Lactobionate-IV	Powder for reconstitution	IV
	Ilotycin	Ointment	Ophthalmic
	Erythro-RX (USP 100%)	Powder for prescription compounding	RX formulations
	Akne-mycin, Ery	Gel, pads, solution	Topical
Fidaxomicin (fye DAX oh mye sin)	Dificid	Tablet	Oral
Tetracyclines			
Doxycycline (doks i SYE kleen)	Oracea	Capsule, delayed release	Oral
	Ocudox, Oraxyl, Vibramycin	Capsule (hyclate), powder for suspension, syrup	Oral
	Adoxa, Monodox	Capsule, tablet (monohydrate)	Oral
	Doxy 100	Powder for reconstitution	IV
	Alodox, Periostat	Tablet	Oral
	Doryx	Delayed-release tablet	Oral
	Atridox	Extended-release liquid	Subgingival
Minocycline (mi noe SYE kleen)	Minocin	Capsule, powder for reconstitution	Oral, IV
	Dynacin	Tablet	Oral
	Solodyn	Extended-release tablet	Oral
	Arestin	Sustained-release microspheres (powder)	Subgingival
Tetracycline (tet ra SYE kleen)		Capsule	Oral
Tigecycline (tye ge SYE kleen)	Tygacil	Powder for reconstitution	IV
Omadacycline (oh MAD a SYE kleen)	Nuzyra	Tablet, powder for reconstitution	Oral, IV
Eravacycline (ER a va SYE kleen)	Xerava	Powder for reconstitution	IV
Glycopeptides			
Telavancin (tel a VAN sin)	Vibativ	Powder for reconstitution	IV
Vancomycin (van koe MYE sin)	Vancocin	Capsule, premixed solution, powder for reconstitution	Oral, IV
Dalbavancin (dal ba VAN sin)	Dalvance	Powder for reconstitution	IV
Oritavancin (or it a VAN sin)	Orbactiv	Powder for reconstitution	IV

Continued next page

MEDICATION TABLE 27-3. Additional Anti-infective Classes[a] *(Continued)*

Agent (pronunciation)	Brand Name	Dosage Form	Route
Sulfonamides			
Co-trimoxazole (sulfamethoxazole with trimethoprim) (coe try MOX a zole)	—	Injection solution, oral suspension	IV, oral
	Bactrim, Septra	Tablet	Oral
	Bactrim DS, Septra DS	Tablet, double strength	Oral
Sulfacetamide (sul fa SEE ta mide)	Bleph-10, Sulfamide	Solution	Ophthalmic
	Carmol Scalp Treatment, Klaron, Ovace, Rosula, Seb-Prev	Foam, cream, gel, lotion, pad, soap, suspension, shampoo, emulsion, ointment	Topical
Sulfadiazine (sul fa DYE a zeen)	—	Tablet, cream	Oral, Topical
Erythromycin and Sulfisoxazole (er ith roe MYE sin) (sul fi SOX a zole)	E.S.P.	Powder for suspension	Oral
Antimycobacterials			
Clofazamine (kloe FAZ i meen)	Lamprene	Capsule	Oral
Dapsone (DAP sone)	—	Tablet	Oral
Antituberculosis			
Aminosalicylic acid (a mee noe sal i SIL ik) (AS id)	Paser	Delayed-release granules	Oral
Capreomycin (kap ree oh MYE sin)	Capastat	Powder for reconstitution	IV, IM
Cycloserine (sye kloe SER een)	Seromycin	Capsule	Oral
Ethambutol (e THAM byoo tole)	Myambutol	Tablet	Oral
Ethionamide (e thye on A mide)	Trecator	Tablet	Oral
Isoniazid (eye soe NYE a zid)	—	Injection solution, oral solution, tablet, syrup	IM, oral
Pyrazinamide (peer a ZIN a mide)	—	Tablets	Oral
Rifabutin (RIF a byoo tin)	Mycobutin	Capsule	Oral
Rifampin (RIF am pin)	Rifadin	Capsule, powder for reconstitution	Oral, IV
Rifapentine (RIF a pen teen)	Priftin	Tablet	Oral

Continued next page

MEDICATION TABLE 27-3. Additional Anti-infective Classes[a] *(Continued)*

Agent (pronunciation)	Brand Name	Dosage Form	Route
Miscellaneous			
Chloramphenicol (klor am FEN i kol)	—	Powder for reconstitution	IV
Clindamycin (klin da MYE sin)	Cleocin HCl	Capsule	Oral
	Cleocin Pediatric	Granules for solution	Oral
	Cleocin Phosphate	Premixed solution, injection solution, vaginal cream	IV, Topical
Daptomycin (dap toe MYE sin)	Cubicin	Powder for reconstitution	IV
Linezolid (li NE zoh lid)	Zyvox	Premixed solution, powder for oral suspension, tablet	Oral, IV
Tedizolid (ted eye ZOE lid)	Sivextro	Powder for reconstitution, tablet	Oral, IV
Metronidazole (me troe NI da zole)	Flagyl	Capsule, premixed solution, tablet, cream, gel, lotion	Oral, IV, Topical
	Flagyl ER	Extended-release tablet	Oral
Rifaximin (ri FAX i men)	Xifaxan	Tablet	Oral
Quinupristin-dalfopristin (kwi NYOO pris tin) (dal FOE pris tin)	Synercid	Powder for reconstitution	IV
Colistimethate (koe lis ti METH ate)	Coly-Mycin M	Powder for reconstitution	IM, IV
Nitrofurantoin (nye troe fyoor AN toyn)	Furadantin	Capsule	Oral
	Macrobid	Capsule	Oral
	Macrodantin	Suspension	Oral
Fosfomycin (fos foe MYE sin)	Monurol	Packet, powder for reconstitution	Oral, IV
Lefamulin (le FAM ue lin)	Xenleta	Solution, tablet	Oral, IV

IM = intramuscular; IV = intravenous; NS = normal saline.

[a] Pronunciations have been adapted with permission from USP Dictionary of USAN and International Drug Names (USP Dictionary) © 2022.

Chapter 28

Viral Infections

Richard Chan, PharmD, BCPS |
John Flanigan, PharmD |
James Adams, PharmD, BCCCP |
Catherine W. Hebert, PharmD, BCPS

KEY TERMS AND DEFINITIONS

AIDS (acquired immunodeficiency syndrome)—a disease of the human immune system that is caused by the human immunodeficiency virus (HIV) and characterized by a reduction in the numbers of certain immune system cells, thereby rendering the person highly vulnerable to life-threatening opportunistic infections secondary to reduced immune function.

DNA (deoxyribonucleic acid)—the genetic blueprint for all living organisms typically found on chromosomes within the nucleus of human cells but also incorporated into some types of virus particles.

RNA (ribonucleic acid)—a nucleic acid concerned with the synthesis of protein and occurring in the nucleus and cytoplasm of cells but also incorporated into some types of virus particles.

Virus—a microscopic infectious agent, classified as parasitic because it is incapable of reproduction outside an infected living host cell.

DOI 10.37573/9781585286638.028

LEARNING OBJECTIVES

After completing this chapter, you should be able to

1. Define the following:
   - AIDS.
   - DNA.
   - RNA.
   - Virus.

2. Describe common types of viral infections.

3. Differentiate between viral infections treated with antiviral therapy and those whose treatment is restricted to supportive care.

4. Describe the different types of antiviral medications and the targets of action of each.

5. List the major adverse effects, cautions, and drug interactions for antiviral medications.

Viruses are the smallest parasites, ranging from 0.01–0.8 microns (about one tenth the average size of bacteria) and 100–1,000 times smaller than the cells they infect.[1] Unlike bacteria, viruses are not living organisms. They are capsules of genetic material depending completely on living cells (bacterial, plant, or animal) to reproduce, so they are called *obligate* parasites. Viruses have an outer cover of protein and sometimes lipid (fat), referred to as a capsid, and an RNA (ribonucleic acid) or DNA (deoxyribonucleic acid) core. For infection to occur, the virus first attaches to the host cell, then fuses with its cell membrane and enters the cell. The viral DNA or RNA then separates from the outer cover (uncoating) and uses the enzymes and cellular machinery of the host cell to make copies (replicate) of the virus. Most RNA viruses replicate their nucleic acid in the cytoplasm (the material within the cell that is outside the nucleus), whereas most DNA viruses do so in the host cell nucleus. The host cell typically dies, releasing new viruses that infect other host cells. Some infections are asymptomatic or latent. In latent infection, viral RNA or DNA remains in host cells but does not cause disease unless some trigger causes symptoms. This is the case in disease states such as hepatitis. Latency may facilitate person-to-person spreading, as infected individuals do not show signs of illness. Some viruses alter normal cellular machinery, leading to abnormal cellular growth and cancer. These viruses are known as oncogenic viruses.

CASE STUDY

Charles Black is a 74-year-old man who had chills 3 days ago but has since developed a fever, which has lasted more than 48 hours. He complains that he has a terrible headache and is coughing and congested.

The most common types of human viral infections are those affecting the nose, throat, and upper airways, commonly known as upper airway (respiratory) infections (URIs). These include but are not limited to sore throat, the common cold, and sinusitis. Additionally, influenza is a viral infection. Small children often experience croup and inflammation of the windpipe or deeper airways in the lungs. As with other infectious diseases viral respiratory infections are more severe in older patients, infants, and those with lung or heart disorders. Viruses that affect the gastrointestinal (GI) system are known as enteroviruses. Some viruses (such as rabies, West Nile virus, and several different encephalitis viruses) infect the nervous system. Viral infections also develop in the skin, sometimes resulting in warts or other blemishes. Some viral infections are transmitted sexually and through the transfer of blood, whereas others may be inhaled or ingested through the GI tract.

Another group of common viral infections are caused by herpesviruses. Three of them—herpes simplex virus type 1 (HSV-1), herpes simplex virus type 2 (HSV-2), and varicella zoster virus (VZV)—cause infections that produce blisters on the skin or mucus membranes. Another herpesvirus, Epstein-Barr virus (EBV), causes infectious mononucleosis. Cytomegalovirus (CMV) is a cause of serious infections in newborns and in people with weakened immune systems. It can also produce symptoms similar to infectious mononucleosis in people with a healthy immune system. Human herpesviruses 6 and 7 cause a childhood infection called roseola infantum. Human herpesvirus 8 has been implicated as a cause of cancer (Kaposi's sarcoma) in people with AIDS (acquired immunodeficiency syndrome). All of the herpesviruses cause lifelong infection because the virus remains within its host cell in a dormant (latent) state even after the acute (symptomatic) phase of the infection. Sometimes the virus reactivates and produces further episodes of disease. Reactivation may occur rapidly or many years after the initial infection. See Table 28-1.

TABLE 28-1. Common Viruses and Associated Syndromes

Virus	Syndrome
Adenoviruses	Epidemic keratoconjunctivits, diarrhea, hemorrhagic cystitis
Coronaviruses	Severe acute respiratory syndrome (SARS), Middle East respiratory syndrome (MERS), coronavirus disease 2019 (COVID-19)
Coxsackieviruses	Aseptic meningitis, meningoencephalitis
Cytomegalovirus	Retinitis, pneumonia, hepatitis
Echoviruses	Aseptic meningitis, meningoencephalitis
Epstein-Barr virus	Infectious mononucleosis
Flaviviruses	Japanese encephalitis, St. Louis encephalitis, West Nile virus encephalitis, yellow fever, dengue fever
Hantavirus	Hantavirus pulmonary syndrome
Hepatitis A, B, C, D, E	Acute and chronic hepatitis
Herpes simplex virus	Herpes labialis, encephalitis, vulvovaginitis
Human herpesvirus type 6	Roseola infantum
Human papillomavirus	Genital warts, cervical cancer
Influenza viruses, A, B, and C	Influenza, bronchitis, pneumonia, croup
Mumps virus	Parotitis, orchitis, meningoencephalitis
Parainfluenza viruses	Acute bronchitis, pneumonia, croup
Polioviruses	Poliomyelitis (paralytic), aseptic meningitis
Rabies virus	Rabies
Respiratory syncytial virus (RSV)	Lower respiratory illness (infants), mild upper respiratory illness (adults)
Rhinoviruses	Common cold, acute coryza with or without fever
Rubella virus	German measles
Rubeola virus	Measles, encephalomyelitis
Varicella zoster virus	Chickenpox, zoster, shingles
Variola	Smallpox

Viral infections cause a broad constellation of symptoms. The immune responses they elicit are similar to those discussed in Chapter 27 for bacterial infection, including fever and leukocytosis. As with bacterial infections, many viral diseases have a characteristic set of symptoms (eg, chickenpox, measles, influenza). Viral infection presents very similarly to bacterial infection and in many cases it is difficult if not impossible to differentiate based on symptoms alone. For infections that occur in epidemics (such as influenza), the presence of other similar cases may help doctors identify a particular infection. For other viral illnesses, blood tests and cultures (sampling blood, body fluid, or other material taken from an infected area and incubating it to see if anything grows from it) may be done. Blood may be tested for antibodies to viruses or for antigens (proteins on or in viruses that trigger the body's defenses). Techniques known as polymerase chain reaction (PCR) may be used to make many copies of the viral genetic material, enabling doctors to rapidly and accurately identify the virus. Tests must sometimes be done quickly; for instance, when the infection is a serious threat to public health or when symptoms are severe. A sample of blood or other tissues is sometimes examined with an electron microscope, which provides high magnification with clear resolution (as viruses, unlike bacteria, are difficult or impossible to identify through a regular *light* microscope).

TYPES OF VIRUSES

Respiratory Viruses

Many human respiratory infections are caused by adenoviruses, which are DNA viruses commonly acquired by contact with secretions (including finger transmission) from an infected person or by contact with a contaminated object (eg, towel, instrument). Infection may be airborne (particles released by coughing and sneezing) or waterborne. Respiratory or GI viral *shedding* (transmission of infectious viral particles by the infected host) may continue for months, even if infection is asymptomatic, as most are. When infection is symptomatic, many clinical manifestations are possible. The most common syndrome, especially in children, involves fever that tends to be greater than 39°C (102°F) and last more than 5 days. Sore throat, cough, runny nose, or other respiratory symptoms may occur. A separate syndrome involves conjunctivitis (an inflammation in the eye), pharyngitis (sore throat), and fever (pharyngoconjunctival fever). Eye inflammation involving both the conjunctiva and the cornea, termed epidemic keratoconjunctivitis, is sometimes severe and occurs both sporadically and in epidemics. Conjunctivitis is frequently bilateral (affecting both eyes). Periauricular adenopathy—swollen glands in the ear area—may develop. Systemic symptoms and signs are mild or absent. Epidemic keratoconjunctivitis usually resolves within 3 or 4 weeks, although corneal lesions may persist much longer.

Common Cold (Upper Respiratory Infection)

The common cold is an acute, self-limiting viral infection involving upper respiratory symptoms, such as rhinorrhea (runny nose), cough, and sore throat. Most colds are caused by a group of small RNA viruses termed rhinoviruses, which are spread in ways similar to those described for adenoviruses. Others may be due to infection by coronaviruses. URIs and their treatment are considered in detail in Chapter 36.

The most potent deterrent to viral URIs is the presence of specific antibodies in the serum and body fluids, induced by previous exposure to the same or a closely related virus. Susceptibility to colds is not affected by exposure to cold

temperature, host health and nutrition, or upper respiratory tract abnormalities (eg, enlarged tonsils or adenoids). Treatment of the cold is supportive, including antihistamines, decongestants, and antipyretics.

Lower Respiratory Tract Infection

Most children suffer from an acute viral infection of the lower respiratory tract resulting in inflammation of the bronchioles (see Figure 18-1) at least once during their early years, frequently in the winter or early spring.[2] Symptoms are nonspecific and may include irritability and fever, vomiting, and diarrhea, along with cough and breathing difficulties that may resemble asthma. While these infections may be caused by adenoviruses or influenza viruses, among others, the most common agent is respiratory syncytial virus, known as RSV. The infection is usually self-limiting and treatment is symptomatic, using antipyretics to reduce the fever and making sure there is adequate fluid intake to prevent dehydration. Children with more severe symptoms may be hospitalized and treated with oxygen therapy and intravenous (IV) fluids. A few, especially those with underlying heart or lung conditions, may require an aerosol (inhaled) antiviral medication.

CASE?

What common viral illness does Mr. Black most likely have?

Influenza

Influenza is an infection caused by a respiratory virus, influenza A or B. It is characterized by fever, head congestion, cough, headache, and malaise. Symptoms start 1–4 days after infection and can begin suddenly. Chills or a chilly sensation is often the first indication. Fever is common during the first few days, sometimes reaching 39°C (102–103°F). People frequently feel debilitated to the extent they remain in bed for days. Aches and pains are experienced throughout the body, particularly in the back and legs. Headache is often severe, with aching around and behind the eyes. Bright light may make the headache worse. At first, respiratory symptoms may be relatively mild, including a scratchy sore throat, a burning sensation in the chest, a dry cough, and a runny nose. These symptoms may progress and develop into pneumonia, either viral or bacterial. When bacterial pneumonia develops following influenza, it is known as a superinfection. Most symptoms subside after 2 or 3 days; however, they may last for weeks. Pneumonia is most commonly seen among the elderly and those with a heart or lung disorder.

Mortality is possible during epidemics, particularly among high-risk patients (eg, infants; the elderly; or those who are institutionalized, have cardiopulmonary insufficiency, or are in late pregnancy). Diagnosis is usually clinical and depends on local epidemiologic patterns. High-risk patients, their caregivers and household contacts, healthcare practitioners, and all children aged 6–24 months should receive annual influenza vaccination. Antiviral treatments include zanamivir and oseltamivir, as well as amantadine and rimantadine, which will be discussed in the drug therapy section of this chapter.

Hemagglutinin (HA) is a protein on the influenza virus surface that allows it to fuse with the host cell membrane. Neuraminidase (NA), another surface protein, promotes viral dispersion from the infected cell. Relatively minor mutations in HA and NA of influenza A and B result in the frequent emergence of new viral strains (antigenic drift). The result is decreased protection by the antibody generated to the previous strain. In contrast to antigenic drift, a major change in NA or HA occurs in influenza A (antigenic shift) at infrequent intervals (10–40 years during the last century); as a result, the population has no immunity to the new virus, and pandemic (widespread epidemic) influenza may occur.

Influenza is typically diagnosed or at least suspected based on clinical symptoms. Laboratory tests are available to test blood and respiratory secretions for confirmation of influenza infection. These are available in physician offices and hospitals.

Coronaviruses/COVID-19

Coronaviruses have been identified as the cause of multiple respiratory infections, including severe acute respiratory syndrome (SARS), Middle East respiratory syndrome (MERS), and, most notably, coronavirus disease 2019 (COVID-19), resulting in a pandemic. Coronaviruses may affect nonhuman hosts and can be seen in avian hosts. SARS-COV-2 is the virus associated with the COVID-19 pandemic and it is postulated that this virus may be from bats or pangolins. COVID-19 symptoms range broadly, and the severity of the disease can vary heavily from one person to another, from a complete absence of symptoms to severe syndromes requiring hospitalization. Some symptoms associated with COVID-19 include fever, chills, cough, shortness of breath, fatigue, body aches, loss of taste or smell, diarrhea, and rashes. Symptoms may appear anywhere from 2–14 days after exposure to the virus. The COVID-19 pandemic at the time of writing has infected more than 150 million people with more than 3 million deaths worldwide, and more than 500,000 in the United States.

Due to the high transmissibility and mortality of the SARS-COV-2 virus, many different types of medications were tested to help in the treatment of COVID-19. Some of the agents that have been studied include antiviral medications (remdesivir, lopinavir/ritonavir), antimalarial

---

CASE?

After 5 days of getting little relief from taking acetaminophen, Mr. Black has felt increasingly short of breath for the past couple of days. He has a past medical history significant only for chickenpox as a child. In the emergency room, his temperature is 103°F, heart rate = 110 (increased), respiratory rate = 20 (increased), oxygen saturation = 87% (low), chest x-ray demonstrates left lower lobe infiltrate, white blood cell (WBC) count = 21 (increased), and rapid nasal swab for influenza is positive for influenza A. Additionally, he has a rash that developed yesterday. It is located in a band across his lower back and is associated with sharp shooting pains. What common secondary infection does Mr. Black likely have as a result of his influenza infection?

medications (hydroxychloroquine), monoclonal antibodies (tocilizumab, bamlanivimab/etesevimab, casirivimab/imdevimab), and immunomodulators (corticosteroids). The only current medication that is approved by the U.S. Food and Drug Administration (FDA) for the treatment of COVID-19 is remdesivir, an adenosine nucleotide, which is indicated for patients who require hospitalization or have mild to moderate COVID-19 and are at high risk for progression to severe COVID-19. Other therapies to note are dexamethasone, a corticosteroid, which has been studied to reduce mortality in those requiring supplemental oxygen, and tocilizumab, a monoclonal interleukin-6 receptor antagonist, which has shown benefit in patients who exhibit rapid deterioration in their respiratory status.

PRACTICE POINT

Remdesivir may only be administered in healthcare settings in which healthcare providers have immediate access to medications to treat a severe infusion or hypersensitivity reaction, such as anaphylaxis, and the ability to activate the emergency medical system, as necessary.

Accelerated vaccine development for COVID-19 was determined to be instrumental in the fight against the pandemic, and in December 2020, nearly a year after the virus was first noted, a two-shot vaccine was approved by the FDA for the prevention of COVID-19. Clinical trials demonstrated that the vaccine was 95% effective at prevention of COVID-19 after both doses had been given. There are currently strong global efforts to vaccinate all individuals who are willing and able to receive vaccinations. The treatment recommendations for the pandemic are constantly in flux, because of new evidence emerging frequently. Organizations such as the Centers for Disease Control and Prevention (CDC) and the World Health Organization (WHO) are excellent resources for the most up-to-date information on treatment recommendations.

Herpesviruses

Eight different types of herpesviruses infect humans. After initial infection, all herpesviruses remain latent (inactive) within specific host cells and may subsequently reactivate or be shed. Herpesviruses do not survive long outside a host; thus, transmission usually requires contact with blood or sexual fluid, although varicella zoster virus (VZV) may spread by contact with respiratory secretions. Because the virus remains latent, transmission sometimes occurs from asymptomatic infected people.

Herpes simplex virus types 1 and 2 (HSV-1 and HSV-2) are widespread throughout most human populations and cause painful sores and blisters. Cold sores or fever blisters in the mouth or on the lips are most often caused by HSV-1, transmitted by close contact with an infected individual or an object that is contaminated by fluids from that individual. Genital herpes is among the most common sexually transmitted diseases in the United States and, while most often caused by HSV-2 infection, may also be associated with HSV-1. After the initial symptoms (painful blisters that break and become ulcers), the infection becomes latent and can recur throughout the patient's lifetime.

ALERT!

While transmission is more likely to occur while the disease is symptomatic, infected individuals may be continuously contagious even while the disease is latent and no sores or blisters are evident.

One of the most commonly encountered herpesviruses is human herpesvirus type 3 or VZV, the causative organism of chickenpox and shingles. Chickenpox is predominantly a childhood disease caused by initial exposure to the virus. Shingles, also known as herpes zoster, typically presents in older patients. It is caused by reactivation of the VZV contracted at an earlier date. Chickenpox is extremely contagious and spread by droplet contact with an infected individual. Patients typically experience headache, fever, and fatigue as the initial symptoms up to 2 weeks prior to the development of a rash. The rash begins as teardrop-shaped, fluid-filled pouches, known as vesicles, on the face and trunk, and it is extremely itchy. The vesicles erupt (break) and crust over after a couple of days, with new vesicle formation ceasing after 5 days and crusting of vesicles complete by the sixth day. The disease is contagious from 48 hours prior to the development of the rash until final crusting of the rash. Chickenpox is typically a mild disease; however, in adults, newborns, and immunocompromised patients, it can progress to pneumonia and septic shock.

CASE?

What childhood infection may likely be the original cause of Mr. Black's rash?

Shingles, as mentioned earlier, is a reactivation of VZV. When latent, the virus resides in the roots of nerves. Upon reactivation the patient experiences sharp shooting pain in the affected region, followed in 2–3 days by the development of red vesicular lesions (vesicles). Lesions develop for up to 5 days. Typically patients experience only one outbreak of zoster; however, the pain may persist for months to years.

Infection with human herpesvirus type 8 (HHV-8) and EBV are linked to the development of malignancy (cancer). HHV-8 is also known as Kaposi's sarcoma–associated herpesvirus (KSHV) and infections with this agent are most often seen in immunosuppressed patients, especially those with AIDS.

In addition to symptomatic treatment, some antiviral medications (detailed later in this chapter) are active against herpesviruses. Drugs that have activity against herpesviruses include acyclovir, cidofovir, famciclovir, fomivirsen, foscarnet, ganciclovir, idoxuridine, penciclovir, trifluridine, valacyclovir, valganciclovir, and vidarabine. While antiviral therapy can reduce the severity of symptoms, frequency of recurrence, and, possibly, disease transmission, it does not cure the infection.[2] Additionally, vaccines have been developed to protect patients from herpesvirus infections; these are discussed in Chapter 30.

Hepatitis Viruses

Hepatitis is an inflammation of the liver characterized by the widespread death of cells. Noninfectious hepatitis is covered in Chapter 23. Major infectious causes are specific hepatitis viruses A, B, and C. Less common causes include other viral infections (eg, infectious mononucleosis, yellow fever, CMV infection) and leptospirosis (a nonviral parasitic infection). Hepatitis A is spread through the GI tract. It is a self-limiting disease, usually resolving within 2–6 months, and is seldom chronic or fatal.[2] There is no recommended drug treatment for hepatitis A.

ALERT!

Sharing of personal supplies, including toothbrushes, razors, towels, and needles, as well as the use of nonsterile instruments for tattooing and ear piercing, have been implicated in the spread of hepatitis B.[1]

Hepatitis B and C are transmitted via blood or other body fluids. Hepatitis B can even be transmitted from an infected mother to her child during childbirth, as well as sexual activity with an infected partner, which accounts for up to 50% of new cases in the United States.[2]

Hepatitis B infections can be asymptomatic and undetectable except with tests for serum antibodies and may resolve completely in 6 months. Some patients (especially those infected in infancy), however, can progress to a chronic infection, which can be controlled with antivirals but not cured. Patients with chronic infections can be contagious even when they are showing no symptoms. Chronic hepatitis B can result in fatal liver disease and malignancy. Hepatitis C may be the most common blood-borne disease in the United States.[2] Many patients are asymptomatic (but contagious) for long periods, but over 20–30 years develop fatal liver damage. This disease can be controlled and even cured by a combination of antiviral medications.

PRACTICE POINT

Vaccines (discussed in Chapter 30) are available to prevent hepatitis A and B. There is currently no vaccination against hepatitis C.

Enterovirus

Enteroviruses are picornaviruses (pico = small, so these are small RNA viruses). This group includes the poliovirus, coxsackievirus, echovirus, and enterovirus D. Coxsackieviruses and echoviruses are shed in oral secretions, stool, blood, and cerebrospinal fluid and have wide geographic distribution. Enteroviruses cause various diseases, including poliomyelitis and meningitis. Epidemic pleurodynia, hand-foot-and-mouth disease, and herpangina are other diseases caused almost exclusively by enteroviruses.

PRACTICE POINT

Enteroviral diseases/epidemics in the United States occur in the summer and early fall. Antivirals are not used in their therapy, but vaccines are available to prevent some enterovirus infections, such as poliomyelitis.

Rubella Virus

Rubella (German measles) is caused by an RNA virus, which is spread by respiratory droplets through close contact or through the air. It is a contagious viral infection that may produce adenopathy (swollen glands), rash, and sometimes constitutional symptoms, which are usually mild and brief. Infection during early pregnancy can cause spontaneous abortion, stillbirth, or congenital defects, including but not limited to hearing loss, ophthalmologic defects, most commonly cataracts, cardiac abnormalities, and neurologic defects. Diagnosis is clinical and treatment is rarely necessary. Vaccination is effective; hence, only sporadic cases are seen in the United States.

A patient can transmit rubella from asymptomatic infection or from 10 days before until 15 days after the onset of the rash. Congenitally infected infants may transmit rubella for many months after birth. Rubella is less contagious than measles. Immunity appears to be lifelong after natural infection.

Measles Virus

Measles is a viral infection rendered very uncommon in the United States and other developed countries by effective vaccination. It is a highly contagious viral infection most common in children. It is characterized by fever, cough, nasal congestion, conjunctivitis, and a rash consisting of red elevated bumps that usually spreads from the head downward over the body. Koplik's spots, which appear as a dot of white sand on a slightly elevated reddened surface inside the mouth, are also seen. Diagnosis is based on clinical symptoms and treatment is supportive, consisting of acetaminophen or ibuprofen for fever and antihistamines for rash.

Human Immunodeficiency Virus

Human immunodeficiency virus (HIV) infection results from one of two similar agents (HIV-1 and HIV-2) called retroviruses because of the way their RNA works as a template for new DNA in infected host cells. These viruses destroy CD4 lymphocytes (important immune system cells) and impair cell-mediated immunity, increasing the risk of certain infections and cancers.

HIV is spread primarily through sexual contact, although other modes of transmission include parenteral (shared needles or accidental needle sticks, blood transfusion) and childbirth (from mother to child). Initial infection may cause nonspecific febrile illness. The risk of developing subsequent infections is proportional to the level of remaining CD4 lymphocytes. Clinical manifestations range from asymptomatic carriage to AIDS, which is defined by serious opportunistic infections or cancers or a CD4 count of <200/µL. HIV infection can be diagnosed by antibody or antigen testing. Screening should be routinely offered to all adults and adolescents. Treatment aims to suppress HIV replication by using combinations of drugs that inhibit viral enzymes and replication.

ANTIVIRAL MEDICATIONS

Medications targeting viral infection are aimed at numerous different pathways in the viral replication cycle: viral attachment and entry, penetration, uncoating, early protein synthesis, nucleic acid synthesis, late protein synthesis, packaging and assembly of virus, release of virus, viral replication, assimilation of viral particles, and viral shedding. See Figure 28-1 for a description of the actions of various antivirals.

Many different factors come into play in determining the appropriate antiviral medication. As with bacterial infection, knowledge of the most likely pathogens guides empiric choice of antiviral medications. Unlike bacterial infections, treatment for many viral infections (including the common cold, viral gastroenteritis, measles, mild cases of the flu) is supportive. Physicians choose an appropriate antiviral regimen based on patient allergies, age, kidney and liver function, infection site, pregnancy/lactation status, and other disease states and/or drug therapy.

Antiviral medications are divided into the following categories: adamantines, interferons, monoclonal antibodies, NA inhibitors, nucleosides, and nucleotides. These are listed in Medication Table 28-1 (Medication Tables are located at the end of the chapter). An additional category, antiretrovirals, includes medications used mainly against HIV, listed in Medication Table 28-2.

Adamantines

Amantadine (Symmetrel) and its derivative, rimantadine (Flumadine), are cyclic compounds of the adamantine family that inhibit uncoating of the viral RNA within infected host cells, thus preventing replication. These medications have been used for influenza treatment and prophylaxis. The most common side effects are GI and central nervous system (CNS) disturbances (difficulty concentrating, dizziness, insomnia), and in the case of rimantadine, hepatic dysfunction. These are more pronounced in the elderly and in patients with renal insufficiency. Though these medications have activity against influenza A, they are not recommended for treatment or prophylaxis due to high resistance rates. They are only warranted for resistant influenza virus, in conjunction with an NA inhibitor.

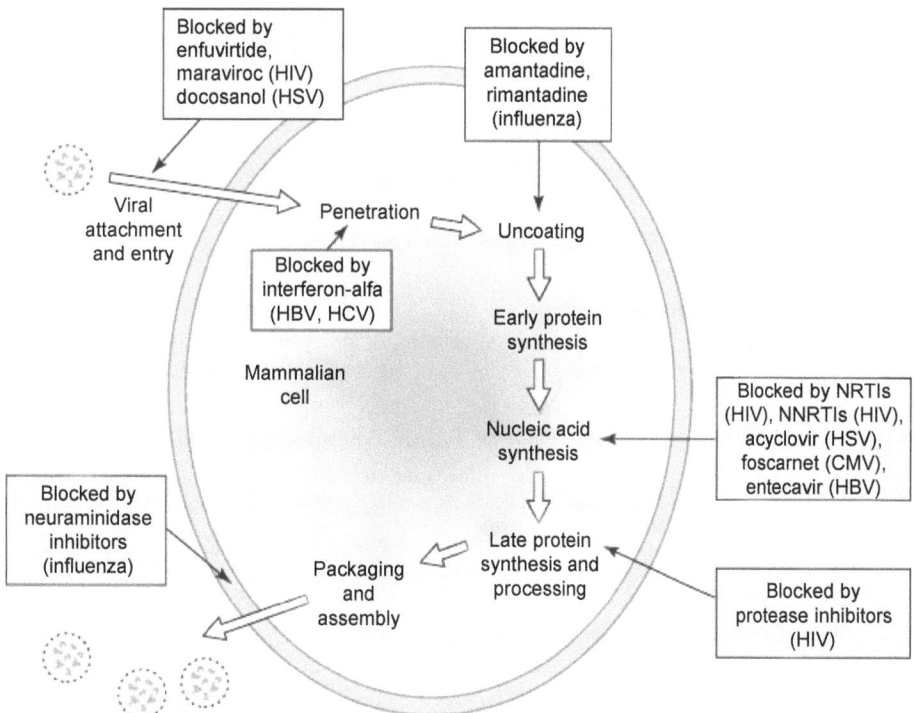

(Source: Modified and reproduced, with permission, from Trevor AT, Katzung BG, Masters SM, eds. *Pharmacology: Examination Board Review*. 6th ed. New York, NY: McGraw Hill, 2002.)

FIGURE 28-1. The viral infection and replication cycle, with sites of antiviral activity. CMV = cytomegalovirus; HBV = hepatitis B virus; HCV = hepatitis C virus; HIV = human immunodeficiency virus; HSV = herpes simplex virus; NNRTI = non-nucleoside reverse transcriptase inhibitor; NRTI = nucleoside reverse transcriptase inhibitor.

CASE?

Does Mr. Black need treatment with either amantadine or rimantadine?

Neuraminidase Inhibitors (Zanamivir, Oseltamivir, Peramivir)

Zanamivir and oseltamivir are inhibitors of NA, which is responsible for the release of influenza virus from infected cells. The release of virus from infected cells is stopped, halting the spread of virus within the respiratory tract. These agents have activity against both influenza A and influenza B. Oseltamivir and zanamivir are easy to administer: zanamivir is a nasal spray and oseltamivir is given orally. They are well tolerated and duration of therapy is 5 days. Peramivir is only available as a solution and is given as an IV infusion. Peramivir may be given as a single dose for patients without complications, or

for up to 10 days in higher-risk patients. Unfortunately, these agents require use within 48 hours of symptom onset to be effective and duration of illness is decreased by only 1–2 days even when they are started appropriately.

Endonuclease Inhibitor (Baloxavir)

Baloxavir Marboxil is an oral pro-drug (must be converted to an active form) of baloxavir, which is an inhibitor of endonuclease. This agent has activity against both influenza A and influenza B by inhibiting viral replication. Baloxavir is a well-tolerated medication and only one dose needs to be given in the treatment of influenza. Like the neuraminidase inhibitors, this medication should be given within 48 hours of influenza symptoms.

CASE?

Should Mr. Black be treated with oseltamivir now?

Interferons

Interferons are cellular messengers responsible for antiviral, immunomodulatory, and antiproliferative activities in the body. Interferon (IFN)-alfa appears to function by inhibiting viral penetration, translation, transcription, protein processing, maturation, and release, as well as enhancing the ability of the body's immune system to eliminate viral particles (virions). Interferons are used to treat chronic hepatitis B, D, and acute hepatitis C. They have also been used experimentally against human papilloma virus (responsible for warts) and West Nile virus.

Comparison of Interferon Forms

Interferon is available in various formulations. Interferon alfa-2b can be administered either subcutaneously or intramuscularly. Interferon alfacon-1 is administered subcutaneously only. The pegylated interferons alfa-2a and alfa-2b are newer agents with longer half-lives suitable for once-weekly dosing. Alfa interferons are eliminated by the kidney, so dosage adjustment is required in patients with renal insufficiency. Liver metabolism is minimal, so dose adjustments are seldom necessary for hepatic insufficiency. Side effects are common, most routinely flu-like syndrome, and/or neuropsychiatric symptoms and immunosuppressive effects (occasionally aplastic anemia).

Nucleosides and Nucleotides

Nucleosides and nucleotides are antiviral medications that interfere with nucleic acid (DNA and/or RNA) synthesis. By inhibiting viral nucleic acid synthesis, they interfere with or prevent viral replication and spread. Acyclovir, ganciclovir, and valganciclovir are all analogs of the nucleoside guanosine. They require a viral enzyme for activation, so they are selectively activated and accumulate in infected cells. Their antiviral activity is accomplished by two mechanisms: competitive inhibition of viral DNA polymerase (where they take the place of the guanosine that is normally used by the virus) and chain termination following assimilation into the viral genome. These medications have activity against herpesvirus, VZV, EBV, and CMV. Intravenous acyclovir is associated with reversible renal toxicity. The main toxicity associated with ganciclovir and valganciclovir is myelosuppression.

Acyclovir was the first agent in this group to be developed. It is active against the herpesviruses, including genital herpes, varicella (chickenpox), and zoster (shingles). It has also been investigated for use in CMV and HSV. Administered by IV or oral routes, it must be given frequently (five times daily or every 4 hours) when used for acute infection. Acyclovir is also available alone or in combination with hydrocortisone as an ointment or cream for the treatment of genital herpes and cold sores.

> ### PRACTICE POINT
>
> *IV acyclovir is dosed based on ideal body weight not actual body weight.*

Other nucleoside analogs that are active against HSV include famciclovir and valacyclovir (oral treatment for genital herpes, cold sores, and shingles) and penciclovir (administered as a cream for cold sores on the lips and face). Ganciclovir is indicated for the treatment of CMV retinitis. It is available in dosage forms administered directly into the eye. Adefovir dipivoxil was initially investigated for the treatment of HIV, but it eventually gained FDA approval for the treatment of hepatitis B infection. Adefovir dipivoxil is a prodrug requiring enzymes in the cell to become active. It inhibits hepatitis B DNA polymerase, resulting in chain termination (halts nucleic acid synthesis). Sixty percent of the drug is absorbed upon oral administration and is unaffected by the presence of food in the stomach (so it may be taken without regard to meals). In contrast to acyclovir, dosage is only once daily. It is renally eliminated, making it safe for patients with severe liver disease. Commonly encountered side effects are headache, diarrhea, abdominal pain, and dose-dependent renal toxicity. Less common, more severe side effects are lactic acidosis and hepatic steatosis. Entecavir is an orally administered guanosine analog that competitively inhibits hepatitis B virus (HBV) replication enzymes. Oral bioavailability approaches 100% but is decreased by food; therefore, entecavir should be taken on an empty stomach. It is excreted by the kidney, so doses are adjusted for patients with renal insufficiency and those on dialysis.

> ### PRACTICE POINT
>
> *Medication guides for antivirals used in the treatment of hepatitis advise patients to avoid alcoholic beverages. Even when there is no drug interaction, alcohol can increase the liver damage caused by the hepatitis infection.*

Cidofovir is a cytosine nucleotide analog with in vitro activity against a variety of viral agents. Unlike acyclovir and similar drugs, cidofovir is transformed to an active form without the need for viral enzymes. Common adverse effects associated with cidofovir are nephrotoxicity, neutropenia, and metabolic acidosis. At the time of this writing, its only approved indication is for the treatment of CMV retinitis in patients with AIDS.

> ## ALERT!
>
> Cidofovir is a hazardous drug and must be prepared and handled as such by pharmacy personnel. This includes reconstitution in a biological safety cabinet and the use of appropriate personal protective garb.

PRACTICE POINT

Even though it is indicated for an eye condition, cidofovir is administered only by IV infusion over 1 hour and never by intraocular injection.

Ribavirin is another guanosine analog that is phosphorylated intracellularly by host cell enzymes. Although its mechanism of action has not been fully explained, it shows antiviral activity against a wide range of viruses, including influenza A and B, parainfluenza, RSV, paramyxoviruses, hepatitis C virus (HCV), and HIV-1. The oral form, currently indicated only for treatment of HCV in combination with an interferon, should be taken with food (meals high in fat increase absorption). Elimination is primarily via the kidneys and dose reduction is needed in cases of renal insufficiency. Hemolytic anemia occurs in up to 20% of patients treated with oral ribavirin. It is associated with depression, fatigue, nausea, and rash.

For RSV infections in infants and children, only inhaled (aerosol) ribavirin (and not the oral form) is indicated. It is generally reserved for hospitalized patients, especially if they also suffer from chronic lung, heart, or immune system deficiencies or diseases. Administration is generally continuous over 12–18 hours daily for 3–7 days.

PRACTICE POINT

Aerosolized ribavirin may only be administered with a special aerosol generator supplied by the medication's manufacturer.

> ## ALERT!
>
> Solutions of ribavirin for aerosol must be prepared in the original vial, and only with sterile water for injection or inhalation containing no preservatives, antimicrobials, or other additives.

> ## ALERT!
>
> Hepatitis exacerbations have been associated with abrupt discontinuation of entecavir and other anti-HBV therapy. Patients should be reminded to consult their physicians before stopping these medications.

Foscarnet (phosphonoformic acid) is an inorganic compound that inhibits viral enzymes directly without requiring activation. It has shown activity against HSV, VZV, CMV, EBV, HHV-6, KSHV, and HIV-1. Its major toxicity is renal function impairment, but it has also been associated with changes in plasma minerals and electrolytes resulting in seizures. Patients receiving this drug are subject to careful monitoring of kidney function and serum electrolytes. Foscarnet is currently indicated only in the treatment of immunocompromised patients with CMV retinitis or certain resistant HSV infections of the skin and mucous membranes. It is administered by IV infusion (not topically).

Letermovir is a viral terminase inhibitor approved for the prophylaxis of CMV.

Tecovirimat is an antiviral medication that has activity against the smallpox virus.

PRACTICE POINT

Foscarnet solutions are chemically incompatible with many IV admixtures, calcium-containing solutions such as Ringer's lactate or total parenteral nutrition. It is physically incompatible with a long list of additional medications, including many anti-infectives, CNS drugs, and others. Pharmacy personnel should be alert to possible incompatibilities and review the package literature before foscarnet is mixed or dispensed.

CASE STUDY

Linda Thorson is a 33-year-old woman and has tested positive for HIV infection. She is 5'9" tall and weighs 112 kg. Her past medical history is notable only for obesity and hyperlipidemia.

CASE?

Ms. Thorson's physician has prescribed lamivudine and zidovudine. What actions do these drugs have on HIV? How long will she have to take them before she is cured?

CASE?

Ms. Thorson has heard she must keep her HIV medications refrigerated. This will be very inconvenient for her, as she must plan to take her zidovudine capsules and lamivudine tablets while she is at work. What will the pharmacy technician tell her?

Antiretroviral Medications

Antiretroviral medications are medications that have activity against HIV. They are categorized by their mechanisms of action. The expected outcome of antiretroviral therapy is not to *cure* HIV infection, but to improve the patients' quality of life by reducing symptoms, maximize immune system functioning, and prevent transmission. This is currently best accomplished by suppression of viral replication, and treatment is generally aimed at that goal.

HIV is a relatively new infection first identified in the last half of the 20th century, and its treatment continues to evolve. The earliest antiretrovirals were the nucleoside reverse transcriptase inhibitors (NRTIs), and the first of these was zidovudine (sometimes still abbreviated AZT for its original name, azidothymidine, which describes its structure). NRTIs, which also include abacavir, emtricitabine, lamivudine, and tenofovir disoproxil fumarate act by inhibition of HIV-1 reverse transcriptase, an enzyme vital to HIV replication. They can also be incorporated into the viral DNA chain to cause early termination (before it is complete). They require an intracellular chemical reaction to become active and have activity against both HIV-1 and HIV-2. The main adverse effects are lactic acidosis, hepatic steatosis (fatty liver), peripheral neuropathy, and pancreatitis. Telbivudine, mentioned among the general antivirals, is classified as an NRTI but is indicated only for chronic HBV (and not currently used for HIV).

PRACTICE POINT

NRTIs must be stored under controlled temperature conditions, with solid oral dosage forms and unreconstituted liquids at 77°F (no lower than 59°F or higher than 86°F). Liquid dosage forms must be refrigerated and unused portions discarded after 30 days.

Tenofovir has a mechanism of action similar to the NRTIs, but because of its chemical structure, it is termed a nucleotide analog reverse transcriptase inhibitor (NtARTI or NtRTI). It also differs because it can have weak effects on some human cell replication enzymes and because it is indicated not only in the treatment of HIV, but also for chronic HBV. Nausea, vomiting, diarrhea, and flatulence are the most frequently experienced adverse events. Lactic acidosis and hepatic steatosis are possible. It may also have effects on bone density and has been associated with kidney damage.

Non-nucleoside reverse transcriptase inhibitors (NNRTIs) bind directly to the HIV-1 enzyme reverse transcriptase, resulting in the blockade of viral protein synthesis. The binding site of NNRTIs is near to but distinct from that affected by NRTIs. Medications in this group include doravirine, efavirenz, etraverine, nevirapine, and rilpivirine. Unlike the NRTI agents, NNRTIs do not require intracellular activation and have little effectiveness against HIV-2. NNRTI resistance occurs rapidly when these drugs are used as monotherapy, so they are usually combined with other agents. Common adverse events are GI distress, elevated liver enzyme levels, skin rash, and occasionally Stevens-Johnson syndrome. They are metabolized by the liver and have many interactions with other medications metabolized in the same way, including anticonvulsants, antifungals, H_2-receptor antagonists, and some antibiotics.

Protease Inhibitors

Protease inhibitors (PIs) are a class of agents that interfere with an important step in the HIV maturation process, causing production of immature, noninfectious viral particles. This group includes atazanavir, darunavir, fosamprenavir, indinavir, nelfinavir, ritonavir, saquinavir, and tipranavir. Unfortunately, resistance is fairly common with these agents, so they are seldom (if ever) used as monotherapy.

The most common adverse reaction to the PIs is GI distress. This class of medications is also associated with a syndrome of central abdominal obesity, buffalo hump (accumulation of fat on back), and breast enlargement. Additionally many patients treated with PIs develop hypertriglyceridemia, hyperlipidemia, and insulin insensitivity. Metabolized via a major liver enzyme responsible for drug metabolism, the PIs have many drug interactions, similar to those listed with the NNRTIs.

Entry Inhibitors

Recall that, for infection to occur, a virus must first attach to the host cell, then fuse with its cell membrane and enter the cell. The antiretrovirals categorized as entry inhibitors act to prevent this step in the process, interfering with the spread of HIV throughout the immune system.

Enfuvirtide is the first representative of this class of antiretroviral agents. It binds to the viral protein envelope, preventing the changes required for fusion with human cellular membranes. It is well tolerated, has no drug interactions, and lacks cross-resistance to other classes of antiretroviral drugs but is only used as part of a multidrug antiretroviral regimen. It requires twice daily subcutaneous (SUBQ) administration and must be reconstituted before use.

PRACTICE POINT

Enfuvirtide is supplied to patients as a kit, which includes vials of lyophilized medication (90 mg), vials of sterile water (1.1 mL), and syringes for use in reconstitution and administration. Patients who have not received prior instruction in preparation and administration will require pharmacist counseling.

ALERT!

Each vial of enfuvirtide is for single use only and unused material (from doses less than 90 mg) must be discarded. If reconstituted in advance (some patients prepare both doses for the day at the same time), the solution must be refrigerated and used within 24 hours.

Maraviroc is unique among currently available antiretrovirals because it does not act on the virus itself, interfering with viral entry by binding with the human cell membrane. It is effective only against certain types of HIV-1 but does not require dose adjustment for renal and hepatic dysfunction. The major side effects of this medication are cough, muscle and joint pain, diarrhea, and increases in liver function tests. Some patients, however, have developed life-threatening liver toxicity, preceded by an allergic reaction. Maraviroc is metabolized by the liver and subsequently has many drug interactions similar to those mentioned with the NNRTIs and PIs.

Integrase Inhibitor

Integrase inhibitors work by blocking integrase, an enzyme required for the HIV particle to combine its genetic material with that of the host cell to continue the replication process.

This group includes raltegravir, dolutegravir, bictegravir, and elvitegravir. The most common side effects are diarrhea, nausea, dizziness, and headache. Because it is metabolized by different liver enzymes from those used by NNRTIs, PIs, and maraviroc, the potential for drug interactions is reduced (though not eliminated).

ALERT!

Patients receiving maraviroc should receive information (pamphlet and/or pharmacist counseling) advising them to seek immediate medical attention if they develop signs or symptoms of hepatitis (abdominal pain, dark urine, yellow-looking eyes or skin, vomiting) or allergic reaction (itching, rash).

PRACTICE POINT

Patients taking rifampin may be prescribed an unusually high dose of raltegravir because rifampin decreases blood levels of the drug.

ANTIRETROVIRAL TREATMENT REGIMENS

The decision to initiate antiretroviral therapy (in some cases soon after diagnosis of HIV infection, in others, only after the patient becomes symptomatic) is one undertaken after serious discussion between the physician and the patient. In all cases, the possible benefits of added length and quality of life must be balanced against the near certainty of adverse effects. The patient must be able to commit to strict adherence to the treatment plan, as lapses can result in accelerated development of viral resistance and a decrease in the variety of treatment options later in the course of the disease. This is difficult to accomplish given the complexity of the regimens, frequency of side effects, cost of therapy, and in some cases changes in the availability of medications.

CASE?

Ms. Thorson's physician explained that her antiretroviral therapy will not cure the HIV infection. Ms. Thorson has read on the Internet that herbal remedies may help and she has asked the pharmacy technician to ring up a bottle of St. John's Wort preparation along with her prescription refills. What should the technician do or say?

All recommended treatment regimens involve combinations of three or more drugs from at least two different categories (eg, two NNRTIs with an NRTI, or two PIs with two NRTIs), all administered on strict schedules over long periods of time (possibly for the rest of the patient's life).[3] Oversight of treatment efficacy by a specialist in HIV is extensive. HIV viral load, CD4 count, complete blood count, and signs and symptoms of opportunistic infection are routinely monitored. In many cases, testing to determine the type of viral mutations conferring resistance to treatment is indicated. To simplify scheduling and increase the patient's ease in adherence, combination products (with two or more antiretrovirals) are sometimes prescribed. These are listed in Medication Table 28-3.

> ### PRACTICE POINT
>
> *Recommended regimens for the treatment of patients infected with HIV are frequently referred to by the acronym HAART (highly active antiretroviral therapy).*

Pre-exposure Prophylaxis

For patients who do not have HIV but may be at high risk for contracting the virus, the use of pre-exposure prophylaxis (PrEP) can be used to reduce the probability of infection. The Centers for Disease Control and Prevention recommends that PrEP be considered in those without HIV who have vaginal or anal sex with a partner who has or may have HIV, those who may share needles or equipment with someone with HIV, and those who have had nonoccupational postexposure prophylaxis (PEP) and continue to engage in high-risk activities. PrEP works by having antiviral medication in the body if and when a person may be exposed to HIV, and helps to halt replication of HIV and stop the virus from spreading. For PrEP it is essential that a person take it every day, otherwise there may not be enough of the medication in their body to prevent the HIV from spreading.[3]

PrEP involves treatment with a combination of two or more antiviral medications with different mechanisms of action. As of this writing, the preparations approved for this type of therapy are oral fixed-dose combinations of emtricitabine and tenofovir. Emtricitabine with tenofovir alafenamide (Descovy) is approved for PrEP to reduce the risk of sexually acquired HIV infection. Emtricitabine with tenofovir disoproxil fumarate (Truvada) is indicated as PrEP for uninfected patients at high risk for acquiring HIV via sexual exposure.

Postexposure Prophylaxis

Because infection with HIV is potentially fatal and there is currently no vaccine available to prevent it, those who have (or may have) been exposed to the virus should receive therapy to prevent infection. This is known as postexposure prophylaxis (PEP). The type of PEP prescribed usually depends on the nature of the exposure.

Occupational (workplace) exposure to HIV occurs when healthcare workers come in contact with materials (blood or body fluids) via needle stick, in the eyes or mouth, or on damaged skin (cuts, chapping, and dermatitis). Although the risk of actual transmission of the HIV virus by such events is very low, the potential harm is so great that PEP is often offered anyway, unless it can be verified that the potentially infective materials are HIV-free. If the source is unknown and the exposed person chooses, a two-drug regimen (usually a PI and an agent from a different class of antiretrovirals) is continued for 4 weeks. If the source of the exposure is known to be HIV-positive, a three-drug regimen (those from the two-drug plan plus an additional agent) is followed.[3]

Nonoccupational exposure to HIV can occur from sexual contact (including assault) with infected (or potentially infected) partners, injection drug use, or other contact with body fluids. PEP for individuals with this type of exposure is chosen on a case-by-case basis, but it generally involves a 4-week HAART regimen.[3]

SUMMARY

A virus is a microscopic infectious agent, classified as parasitic because it is incapable of reproduction outside an infected living *host* cell. It reproduces by using the processes and materials in the cells it infects and spreads when the newly replicated viral particles repeat their infectious processes in new cells. Some viral infections are self-limiting and are treated only with supportive care. Others may be life threatening and require treatment with antiviral medications.

Antiviral medications act by interfering with the processes that allow viruses to enter and infect cells, replicate themselves, or distribute replicated particles to infect new cells. They are generally categorized by their mode of action and/or by the type of viral infections they are used to treat. Many of them have serious side effects, and the risks of these must be balanced against the benefits of therapy with them.

REFERENCES

1. Nester EN, Anderson D, Roberts CE, Jr. *Microbiology: A Human Perspective*. 7th ed. New York, NY: McGraw-Hill; 2012.

2. Anderson PL, Yager, J, Fletcher CV. Human immunodeficiency virus infection. In: DiPiro JT, Talbert RL, Yee GC, et al., eds. *Pharmacotherapy: A Pathophysiologic Approach*. 11th ed. New York, NY: McGraw-Hill; 2020.

3. U.S. National Institutes of Health. Office of AIDS Research. Understanding HIV, Fact Sheets. https://hivinfo.nih.gov/. Accessed May 7, 2021.

CHAPTER RESOURCES

Centers for Disease Control and Prevention. Healthcare Professionals, Antiviral Drugs. https://www.cdc.gov/flu/professionals/antivirals/summary-clinicians.htm. Accessed May 7, 2021.

U.S. National Institutes of Health. COVID-19 Treatment Guidelines. https://www.covid19treatmentguidelines.nih.gov/. Accessed May 7, 2021.

REVIEW QUESTIONS

1. Define and describe a virus.

2. What are the steps in the typical viral infection and replication cycle?

3. Name the members of the herpesvirus group and describe the infections they cause.

4. How do antiviral interferons work and what diseases are they currently used for?

5. Name some of the drug classes that commonly interact with antiretroviral medications. Why are there so many?

MEDICATION TABLES

MEDICATION TABLE 28-1. General Antivirals[a]

Generic Name (pronunciation)*	Brand Name	Dosage Form	Route	Usual Adult Dose	Indications (Viral Infections)[b]	Common Side Effects
Adamantines						
Amantadine (a MAN ta deen)		Capsule, softgel capsule, solution, syrup, tablet	Oral	200 mg daily	Influenza A (treatment and prophylaxis)	CNS depression, impulse control disorders, melanoma, neuroleptic malignant syndrome, suicidal ideation
Rimantadine (ri MAN ta deen)	Flumadine	Tablet	Oral	100 mg twice daily	Influenza A (treatment and prophylaxis)	Insomnia, nervousness, nausea
Neuraminidase Inhibitors						
Oseltamivir (oh sel TAM i vir)	Tamiflu	Capsule, powder for suspension	Oral	Treatment: 75 mg BID, Prophylaxis: 75 mg daily	Influenza A and B	Nausea and vomiting
Zanamivir (za NA mi veer)	Relenza	Powder	Inhalation	10 mg daily	Influenza A and B (treatment and prophylaxis)	Headache, throat discomfort, nasal signs and symptoms, cough, viral infection
Peramivir (pe RA mi veer)	Rapivab	Solution	IV	600 mg daily	Influenza A and B (treatment)	Diarrhea
Endonuclease Inhibitor						
Baloxavir Marboxil (ba LOX A veer mar BOX el)	Xofluza	Tablet	Oral	40–80 mg daily (weight based)	Influenza A and B (treatment)	Diarrhea
Interferons						
Interferon Alfa-2b (in ter FEER on) (AL fa)	Intron A	Powder for reconstitution, solution	IM, SUBQ	Up to 30 million units/m² depending on frequency varies with indication	Chronic HBV, HCV	Autoimmune disease, infectious disorders, ischemic disorders, neuropsychiatric disorders, bone marrow suppression, cerebrovascular events, flu-like symptoms, hepatic effects, hypersensitivity, hypertriglyceridemia, ocular effects, pulmonary effects
Peginterferon Alfa-2a (peg in ter FEER on) (AL fa)	Pegasys	Solution	SUBQ	180 mcg once weekly for 48 weeks	Chronic HBV, HCV	

Continued next page

MEDICATION TABLE 28-1. General Antivirals[a] *(Continued)*

Nucleosides and Nucleotides

Generic Name (pronunciation)*	Brand Name	Dosage Form	Route	Usual Adult Dose	Indications (Viral Infections)[b]	Common Side Effects
Acyclovir (systemic) (ay SYE kloe veer)	Zovirax	Capsule, tablet, oral suspension, powder for reconstitution (injection), injection solution, cream, ointment	Oral, IV, topical	Oral: 1,000–2,400 mg/day in divided doses; IV: 5 mg/kg/dose	Genital herpes, herpes zoster, HSV encephalitis	Malaise, headache, nausea/vomiting, diarrhea
Acyclovir and hydrocortisone (ay SYE kloe veer) (hye droe KOR ti sone)	Xerese	Cream	Topical	Apply 5 times/day for 5 days	Cold sores (HSV)	Dermatologic effects
Adefovir dipivoxil (a DEF o veer)	Hepsera	Tablet	Oral	10 mg daily	Chronic HBV	Headache, abdominal pain, diarrhea, hepatitis exacerbation, weakness, hematuria, rash, flatulence, dyspepsia, back pain, cough rhinitis
Cidofovir (si DOF o veer)		Solution	IV	5 mg/kg once weekly for 2 weeks	CMV retinitis	Chills, fever, headache, pain, alopecia, rash, nausea/vomiting, anemia, weakness, decreased intraocular pressure, renal toxicity, cough, infection
Entecavir (en TE ka veer)	Baraclude	Solution, tablet	Oral	0.5–1 mg daily	Chronic HBV	Peripheral edema, pyrexia, ascites, hematuria, upper respiratory tract infection
Famciclovir (fam SYE kloe veer)	Famvir	Tablet	Oral	500 mg q 8 hr for 7 days (dose and frequency vary with protocol and indication)	Genital herpes, herpes zoster	Headache, nausea, dysmenorrhea, diarrhea, abdominal pain
Ganciclovir (systemic) (gan SYE kloe veer)		Powder for reconstitution	IV	5 mg/kg/dose	CMV retinitis	Thrombocytopenia, leukopenia, anemia, fever, diarrhea, anorexia, vomiting, retinal detachment, sepsis, diaphoresis, blurred vision, ocular irritation
Ganciclovir (topical) (gan SYE kloe veer)	Zirgan	Gel	Ophthalmic	1 drop in affected eye 5 times/day		
	Vitrasert	Intraocular implant	Intravitreal	One implant for 5- to 8-month period		

Continued next page

MEDICATION TABLE 28-1. General Antivirals[a] *(Continued)*

Generic Name (pronunciation)*	Brand Name	Dosage Form	Route	Usual Adult Dose	Indications (Viral Infections)[b]	Common Side Effects
Penciclovir (pen SYE kloe veer)	Denavir	Cream	Topical	Apply q 2 hr for 4 days at first sign or symptom of cold sore	Cold sores (HSV)	Mild erythema
Remdesivir (rem DE si vir)	Veklury	Solution	IV	200 mg IV for 1 dose, then 100 mg once daily for 5–10 days	COVID-19	Infusion reactions, nausea, increased liver function tests (ALT, AST)
Ribavirin (rye ba VYE rin)		Capsule, Tablet	Oral	400–1,200 mg/day in divided doses	Chronic HCV (with interferon)	Anemia, fatigue, headache, insomnia, nausea, anorexia
	Virazole	Powder for reconstitution	Inhalation	20 mg/mL in aerosolizer over 12 hr for 3–7 days	RSV (children only)	
Valacyclovir (val ay SYE kloe veer)	Valtrex	Caplet, tablet	Oral	500–2,000 mg/dose	Genital herpes, herpes zoster, HSV encephalitis	Headache, nausea, abdominal pain, neutropenia, nasopharyngitis, fatigue, depression, rash
Valganciclovir (val gan SYE kloh veer)	Valcyte	Powder for solution, tablet	Oral	900 mg daily	CMV retinitis	Hypertension, fever, headache, insomnia, diarrhea, nausea, vomiting, anemia, tremor, retinal detachment, cough, neuropathy, paresthesia
Miscellaneous Antivirals						
Foscarnet (fos KAR net)	Foscavir	Solution	IV	60–120 mg/kg/day	CMV retinitis, resistant HSV (skin and mucous membranes)	Fever, headache, hypokalemia, hypocalcemia, hypomagnesemia, hypophosphatemia, nausea, vomiting, diarrhea, anemia, granulocytopenia
Letermovir (le term oh vir)	Prevymis	Solution, tablet	IV, oral	480 mg daily	CMV prophylaxis	Nausea, diarrhea, vomiting, peripheral edema, cough, headache, fatigue, abdominal pain
Tecovirimat (TEK oh VIR i mat)	Tpoxx	Capsule Solution	Oral IV	600 mg 2 times/day 200–300 mg q 12 h hours × 14 days	Smallpox	Headache, nausea, abdominal pain, vomiting

CMV = cytomegalovirus; CNS = central nervous system; CPK = creatine phosphokinase; HBC =; HBV = hepatitis B virus; HCV = hepatitis C virus; HSV = herpes simplex virus; IM = intramuscular; IV = intravenous; RSV = respiratory syncytial virus; SUBQ = subcutaneous.

[a] Data from AHFS DI® (Adult and Pediatric). Bethesda, MD: American Society of Health-System Pharmacists.

[b] Some of these agents are also indicated for conditions other than viral infection.

* Lexi-Drugs. Lexicomp. Hudson, OH.

MEDICATION TABLE 28-2. Antiretroviral Agents (Used for HIV)[a]

Generic Name (pronunciation)*	Brand Name	Dosage Form	Route	Usual Dose	Side Effects
Entry and Fusion Inhibitors					
Enfuvirtide (en FYOO vir tide)	Fuzeon	Powder for reconstitution	SUBQ	90 mg twice daily	Fatigue, insomnia, diarrhea, nausea, injection site infection/reactions
Maraviroc (mah RAV er rock)	Selzentry	Tablet	Oral	300 mg twice daily	Fever, rash, upper respiratory infection, cough, dizziness, insomnia, appetite disorders, joint disorders, bronchitis, sinusitis, herpes infection
Protease Inhibitors (PIs)					
Atazanavir (at a za NA veer)	Reyataz	Capsule	Oral	300 mg once daily plus ritonavir 100 mg once daily	Rash, increased cholesterol, nausea, increased bilirubin, increased CPK, cough, jaundice
Darunavir (da ROON a veer)	Prezista	Tablet	Oral	800 mg once daily with ritonavir 100 mg once daily	Hypercholesterolemia, vomiting, diarrhea, headache, rash, hyperglycemia, abdominal pain
Fosamprenavir (FOS am pren a veer)	Lexiva	Suspension, tablet	Oral	1,400 mg; 1,400 mg plus ritonavir 100–200 mg once daily	Rash, diarrhea, pruritus
Indinavir sulfate (in DIN a veer)	Crixivan	Capsule	Oral	800 mg q 8 hr; 800 mg with ritonavir 100–200 mg daily	Abdominal pain, nausea, hyperbilirubinemia, nephrolithiasis
Lopinavir (loe PIN a veer)	Not available as a single entity: see PI combinations	Oral	Only with ritonavir		
Nelfinavir (nel FIN a veer)	Viracept	Tablet	Oral	750 mg 3 times/day	Diarrhea
Ritonavir (ri TOE na veer)	Norvir	Capsule, solution, tablet	Oral	600 mg twice daily	Hypercholesterolemia, triglycerides increased, nausea, diarrhea, vomiting, taste perversion, neuromuscular and skeletal weakness, CPK increase, headache, abdominal pain, anorexia
Tipranavir (tip RA na veer)	Aptivus	Capsule, solution	Oral	500 mg twice daily with ritonavir 200 mg	Rash, hypertriglyceridemia, hypercholesterolemia, diarrhea, fever, fatigue, bleeding, cough

Continued next page

MEDICATION TABLE 28-2. Antiretroviral Agents (Used for HIV)[a] *(Continued)*

Generic Name (pronunciation)*	Brand Name	Dosage Form	Route	Usual Dose	Side Effects
Integrase Inhibitors					
Bictegravir (bik TEG ra vir)	Not available as a single entity; see Reverse Transcriptase Inhibitors combinations	Tablet	Oral with emtricitabine and tenofovir alafenamide		
Dolutegravir (doe loo TEG ra vir)	Tivicay	Tablet	Oral	50 mg twice daily; must be given with another antiretroviral agent; see Reverse Transcriptase Inhibitors combinations	
Elvitegravir (el vi TEG ra vir)	Not available as a single entity; see Reverse Transcriptase Inhibitors combinations	Tablet	Oral with cobicistat, emtricitabine, and tenofovir		
Raltegravir (ral TEG ra veer)	Isentress	Tablet	Oral	400 mg twice daily	Insomnia, headache
Non-Nucleoside Reverse Transcriptase Inhibitors (NNRTIs)					
Doravirine (DOR a VIR een)	Pifeltro	Tablet	Oral	100 mg daily	Nausea, dizziness, fatigue, diarrhea, abdominal pain, insomnia, rash, increased bilirubin
Efavirenz (e fa VEER ens)	Sustiva	Capsule, tablet	Oral	400–600 mg daily	Dizziness, fever, depression, insomnia, anxiety, pain, headache, rash, total cholesterol increase, triglyceride increase, diarrhea, nausea, vomiting, cough
Etravirine (e tra VIR een)	Intelence	Tablet	Oral	200 mg twice daily after meals	Rash, increased total cholesterol, hyperglycemia, nausea
Nevirapine (ne VYE ra peen)	Viramune	Suspension, tablet, extended-release tablet	Oral	200–400 mg daily	Rash
Rilpivirine (ril pi VIR een)	Edurant	Tablet	Oral	25 mg once daily	Depressive disorders

Continued next page

MEDICATION TABLE 28-2. Antiretroviral Agents (Used for HIV)[a] *(Continued)*

Generic Name (pronunciation)*	Brand Name	Dosage Form	Route	Usual Dose	Side Effects
Nucleoside and Nucleotide Reverse Transcriptase Inhibitors (NRTIs)					
Abacavir (a ba KA vir)	Ziagen	Solution, tablet	Oral	300 mg twice daily or 600 mg once daily in combination with other antiretrovirals	Headache, nausea, depression, fever/chills, anxiety, rash, diarrhea, vomiting, musculoskeletal pain
Emtricitabine (em trye SYE ta been)	Emtriva	Capsule, solution	Oral	200 mg daily	Dizziness, headache, fever, insomnia, abnormal dreams, hyperpigmentation, rash, diarrhea, vomiting, nausea, abdominal pain, gastroenteritis, weakness, otitis media, cough, rhinitis, pneumonia, infection
Lamivudine (la MI vyoo deen)	Epivir-HBV, Epivir	Solution, tablet	Oral	300 mg daily	Headache, fatigue, insomnia, nausea, diarrhea, pancreatitis, abdominal pain, vomiting, neutropenia, myalgia, neuropathy, musculoskeletal pain, nasal signs and symptoms, cough, sore throat, infections, dizziness, depression, fever, chills, rash, anorexia, arthralgia
Tenofovir alafenamide (ten OF oh vir) (al a FEN a mide)	Vemlidy	Tablet	Oral	25 mg daily	Insomnia, pain, dizziness, depression, fever, rash, increased triglycerides, abdominal pain, nausea, diarrhea, vomiting, weakness
Tenofovir disoproxil fumarate (ten OF oh vir) (dye soe PROX il) (FUE ma rate)	Viread	Tablet	Oral	300 mg daily	
Zidovudine (zye DOE vyoo deen)	Retrovir	Capsule, injection solution, syrup, tablet	Oral, IV	300 mg twice daily	Headache, malaise, nausea, anorexia, vomiting

CPK = creatine phosphokinase; IV = intravenous; SUBQ = subcutaneous.

[a] Data from AHFS DI® (Adult and Pediatric). Bethesda, MD: American Society of Health-System Pharmacists.

* Lexi-Drugs. Lexicomp. Hudson, OH.

MEDICATION TABLE 28-3. Combination Antiretroviral Products[a]

Generic Name	Doses	Brand Name	Dosage Form	Route
Reverse Transcriptase Inhibitor Combinations				
Efavirenz/emtricitabine/tenofovir (e fa VEER ens) (em trye SYE ta been) (te NOE fo veer)	600 mg/200 mg/300 mg	Atripla	Tablet	Oral
Bictegravir/emtricitabine/tenofovir alafenamide (em trye SYE ta been) (te NOE fo veer) (dye soe PROX il) (FUE ma rate)	50 mg/200 mg/25 mg	Biktarvy	Tablet	Oral
Lamivudine/tenofovir disoproxil fumarate (la MI vyoo deen) (te NOE fo veer) (dye soe PROX il) (FUE ma rate)	300 mg/300 mg	Cimduo	Tablet	Oral
Lamivudine/zidovudine (la MI vyoo deen) (zye DOE vyoo deen)	150 mg/300 mg	Combivir	Tablet	Oral
Emtricitabine/rilpivirine/tenofovir (em trye SYE ta been) (ril pi VIR een) (te NOE fo veer)	200 mg/25 mg/300 mg	Complera	Tablet	Oral
Doravirine/lamivudine/tenofovir disoproxil fumarate (la MI vyoo deen) (te NOE fo veer) (dye soe PROX il) (FUE ma rate)	100 mg/300 mg/300 mg	Delstrigo	Tablet	Oral
Emtricitabine/tenofovir alafenamide	200 mg/25 mg	Descovy	Tablet	Oral
Dolutegravir/lamivudine	50 mg/300 mg	Dovato	Tablet	Oral
Abacavir/lamivudine (a ba KA vir) (la MI vyoo deen)	600 mg/300 mg	Epzicom	Tablet	Oral
Atazanavir/cobicistat	300 mg/150 mg	Evotaz	Tablet	Oral
Elvitegravir/cobicistat/emtricitabine/tenofovir alafenamide	150 mg/150 mg/200 mg/10 mg	Genvoya	Tablet	Oral
Dolutegravir/rilpivirine	50 mg/25 mg	Juluca	Tablet	Oral
Emtricitabine/rilpivirine/tenofovir alafenamide	200 mg/25 mg/25 mg	Odefsey	Tablet	Oral
Darunavir/cobicistat	800 mg/150 mg	Prezcobix	Tablet	Oral
Elvitegravir/cobicistat/emtricitabine/tenofovir disoproxil fumarate	150 mg/150 mg/200 mg/300 mg	Stribild	Tablet	Oral
Efavirenz/lamivudine/tenofovir disoproxil fumarate	600 mg/300 mg/300 mg	Symfi	Tablet	Oral
Efavirenz/lamivudine/tenofovir disoproxil fumarate	400 mg/300 mg/300 mg	Symfi Lo	Tablet	Oral
Darunavir/cobicistat/emtricitabine/tenofovir alafenamide	800 mg/150 mg/200 mg/10 mg	Symtuza	Tablet	Oral
Abacavir/dolutegravir/lamivudine	600 mg/50 mg/300 mg	Triumeq	Tablet	Oral
Abacavir/lamivudine/zidovudine (a ba KA vir) (la MI vyoo deen) (zye DOE vyoo deen)	300 mg/150 mg/300 mg	Trizivir	Tablet	Oral
Emtricitabine/tenofovir (em trye SYE ta been) (te NOE fo veer)	200 mg/300 mg	Truvada	Tablet	Oral
Protease Inhibitor–Based Combinations				
Lopinavir/ritonavir (loe PIN a veer) (ri TOE na veer)	Tablet: 100 mg/25 mg, 200 mg/50 mg Solution: 80 mg/20 mg/mL	Kaletra	Tablet, solution	Oral

[a]Data from AHFS DI® (Adult and Pediatric). Bethesda, MD: American Society of Health-System Pharmacists.

Chapter 29

The Antifungal Agents

Benjamin A. Pontefract, PharmD, BCPS |
Stephanie A. Klepser, PharmD |
Christopher M. Archangeli, MD |
Michael E. Klepser, PharmD, FCCP, FIDP

KEY TERMS AND DEFINITIONS

Aspergillus—a fungus that is widespread in nature and has the potential to cause infection in immunocompromised patients.

Candida—a yeast that can cause a variety of infections in both healthy and immunocompromised patients.

Dermatophytes—fungal pathogens that typically cause skin infections.

Eukaryotic—a cell type that is distinguished by the presence of an internal membrane-bound nucleus and structures (organelles), such as mitochondria and vacuoles.

Fungal—referring to a fungus.

Fungicidal—able to kill fungal cells.

Fungus—a class of spore-forming cellular organisms that obtain nourishment from other living organisms or the byproducts of their decay.

Immunocompromise—a state in which part of the immune system is absent or does not function properly; as a result, the body is unable to properly defend itself from infection.

Mold—a filamentous (threadlike) fungus with colonies that typically appear fuzzy and grow by branching.

Opportunistic pathogen—an organism that is not typically infectious but that is able to cause infection in an immunocompromised host.

DOI 10.37573/9781585286638.029

Postantifungal effect (PAFE)—continued antifungal activity seen even after the antifungal agent has been removed.

Yeast—although technically a yeast is a member of the family Saccharomycetaceae, the term yeast or yeast-like is used to describe fungi that are round or oval, form smooth colonies, and reproduce by budding.

LEARNING OBJECTIVES

After completing this chapter, you should be able to

1. Compare and contrast the mechanisms of action of various classes of antifungal agents.

2. Describe side effects commonly associated with each of the antifungal classes.

3. Describe the drug interaction potential for each class of antifungals.

4. List the formulations available for each antifungal agent.

A fungus is a cellular organism that requires organic compounds, obtained from other living organisms or their decay products, for energy. Fungi (the plural of fungus) can grow in long, branching filaments (threads) that contain multiple cells or as single, round cells. A variety of organisms are classified as fungi, from the familiar mushroom to microscopic yeasts and molds. The latter are the cause of fungal infections and will be the topic of this chapter. Fungi can reproduce sexually, asexually through a process called budding, and through the release of spores. In general, if a fungus is filamentous, it is described as a mold, and if it is a single, rounded cell that reproduces by budding, it is called a yeast. However, some fungi can switch between these two forms, making classification difficult.

CASE STUDY

Ms. Andrews is a 26-year-old female who was recently diagnosed with systemic lupus erythematosus, an autoimmune disorder, and prescribed a high dose (80 mg per day) of oral prednisone (a corticosteroid) to suppress her immune system. Over the past several days, Ms. Andrews has developed a sore throat and difficulty swallowing.

Fungal cells are defined as eukaryotic because, like human cells, they contain a membrane-bound nucleus and membrane-bound organelles (internal structures). This is different from other infectious agents such as bacteria. The fungal cell has a cell membrane, which contains distinctive compounds called sterols. Unlike human cells, but similar to bacterial cells, however, a fungal cell also has a cell wall. The cell wall serves to protect the shape and integrity of the cell and both the wall and the membrane serve as barriers to the entrance of fluids and other materials. Differences between fungal cells and bacterial cells account for some of the differences in treatment between fungal and bacterial infections.

BACKGROUND AND EPIDEMIOLOGY

Significant medical advances have been made over the past several decades in the management of a variety of disease states and conditions. Specifically, advances in the treatment of human immunodeficiency virus infection/acquired immunodeficiency syndrome (HIV/AIDS), oncology (cancer therapy), autoimmune diseases (such as rheumatoid arthritis and systemic lupus erythematosus, discussed in Chapter 13) and transplantation of bone marrow and solid organs mean that now patients suffering these conditions can experience a much longer life expectancy. Therapies utilized to treat these patients (chemotherapy for oncology patients and drugs that suppress the activity of the immune system for transplant patients and those with autoimmune disease) or the disease state itself (HIV/AIDS) often result, however, in a state of significant immunocompromise. In other words, because the immune systems of such patients cannot mount an appropriate protective response against infectious organisms, they are more susceptible not only to typical microbial pathogens, but also to a unique group of opportunistic pathogens (organisms that are not typically infectious but which are able to cause infection in an immunocompromised host). Although opportunistic pathogens seldom infect normal, healthy individuals, they can cause serious illness in patients who are in some state of immune compromise. Fungal infections are a commonly encountered type of opportunistic pathogen among immunocompromised patients.

CASE?

What type of infection is Ms. Andrews likely to have developed?

Healthy individuals can acquire a variety of fungal infections, such as ringworm, endemic fungal infections, and onychomycosis (each of which will be discussed further later in this chapter and at length in Chapter 33). Fungi such as *Candida* and *Aspergillus* species are more likely to infect patients who are immunocompromised. Many effective antifungal agents have been introduced to combat these pathogens. The aim of this chapter is to discuss some of the most commonly utilized antifungal agents and to review some of the fungal infections that are most likely to be clinically encountered.

FUNGAL CELL BIOLOGY

The treatment of fungal infections presents a unique challenge in the development of safe and effective agents. To be effective, an antifungal drug must be able to target and disrupt a critical area of fungal cell biology, which will result in cell damage or death. Additionally, because these agents also come in contact with human cells, the target for antifungal drugs must be a cell component that is unique to fungal cells and absent in human cells. The same principle is used to develop antibacterial agents; however, there are many more biological differences between human and bacterial cells. Because fungal cells, like human cells, are also eukaryotic, there are fewer unique targets for the antifungal agents. This means drugs that harm fungal cells are more likely to have human toxicity, making the development of antifungal agents particularly difficult. Despite this challenge, several successful antifungal agents are available. To understand how antifungal agents work, it is first important to understand a few of the key differences between fungal cell biology and human cell biology.

CASE?

Ms. Andrews's doctor has diagnosed her with oral/esophageal candidiasis, a yeast (fungal) infection. Why would antibiotics like penicillin not be effective for this infection?

A major element differentiating fungal cells is the cell wall, which is absent in human cells and composed of a different material than that of bacterial cells. The cell wall serves to protect the shape and integrity of the cell and serves as a barrier to the influx (entrance) of fluids and other materials. Interfering with components of the cell wall can result in a loss of cell structure, leading to cell damage or cell death. The cell wall is one example of a unique biological target for antifungal agents.

A second difference between human and fungal cells is the composition of the cell membrane. In both cell types, the function of the cell membrane is, among other things, to help regulate the flow of fluids and solutes into and out of the cell. However, although there are many similarities, the composition of the fungal cell membrane differs in some aspects (especially the inclusion of the steroid ergosterol) from human cells, providing another potential target area for antifungal agents. Finally, human and fungal cells contain different enzymes and proteins used to perform critical cell functions. For example, the enzymes used to synthesize the components of the cell membrane in fungal cells differ from those found in human cells, providing yet another potential antifungal target.

CASE?

Ms. Andrews was not sick enough to be admitted to the hospital, but her infection does warrant antifungal therapy. The doctor wants to treat Ms. Andrews at home with an oral antifungal preparation. What antifungals might be prescribed for Ms. Andrews?

THE ANTIFUNGAL AGENTS

Polyenes

The polyenes are a class of antifungal agents that are fungicidal—they have the ability to kill fungal cells. Polyenes bind to ergosterol, a substance that is not part of human cell membranes but is a critical component of fungal cell membranes, which helps to maintain their structure and integrity. The binding of the polyenes to ergosterol disrupts the ability of the fungal cell membrane to prevent the cell's contents from "leaking" out and ultimately results in cell death. Polyene effectiveness is concentration dependent (effectiveness increases with concentration); hence, these agents are more active at higher doses. The polyenes also exhibit a postantifungal effect (PAFE), a continued antifungal activity seen even after they are no longer present, meaning that sustained inhibition of cell growth occurs for a period of time after the drug has been eliminated from the body. Owing to these properties (concentration dependence and PAFE), the most effective dosing strategy would be to use large doses (to maximize the concentration-dependent activity) that are given less frequently (since the PAFE will result in prolonged antifungal activity). However, the toxicity of these agents is often a significant dose-limiting factor. The two polyene agents that are in use clinically are amphotericin B and nystatin.

Amphotericin B

Historically, amphotericin B was considered the "gold standard" for treating serious fungal infections, particularly because of its activity against some difficult-to-treat fungal species. For many clinicians, it is the drug of choice for difficult-to-treat invasive fungal infections. However, dosing problems and significant systemic toxicities have provided clinical challenges for the use of amphotericin B. The development of newer antifungal agents with spectra and activity similar to those of amphotericin B, but without the same issues with administration and toxicity, has caused the use of this agent to fall out of favor.

Although some patients experience no side effects, many patients receiving amphotericin B suffer from severe infusion reactions, such as itching, flushing, fever, shaking chills, and low blood pressure. Other serious systemic effects, such as nephrotoxicity (kidney damage) and electrolyte abnormalities (especially changes in levels of sodium, potassium, and magnesium) can also occur with amphotericin B and warrant frequent laboratory monitoring. Despite its long history of treatment success, many healthcare providers avoid amphotericin B due to its extensive side effect profile (about 80% of patients will develop infusion-related reactions or nephrotoxicity). Today, amphotericin B is only considered in emergencies or when treating pathogens without other effective antifungal options.

Amphotericin B deoxycholate was the first polyene developed and was administered as an intravenous (IV) solution. The potential for infusion-related reactions required that amphotericin B deoxycholate be administered as a slow infusion over at least 2 to 6 hours, often accompanied by premedications such as corticosteroids, acetaminophen, meperidine, and antihistamines to aid in preventing some of its side effects. In an effort to eliminate some of the toxicities associated with amphotericin B deoxycholate (especially nephrotoxicity), several new formulations of amphotericin B were developed: amphotericin B lipid complex (Abelcet®) and amphotericin B liposomal (AmBisome®). Because of their comparable efficacy and lower incidence of serious side effects and adverse reactions, the lipid-based formulations have replaced amphotericin B deoxycholate in most clinical situations. Lipid-based amphotericin B formulations are among the few suspensions currently indicated for IV administration. This is because they are suspensions of liquid globules and contain no solid particulate matter.

> ## ALERT!
>
> The lipid-based amphotericin B formulations are not interchangeable with one another. Confusion between these products could lead to significant dosing errors and potential patient toxicity. (See Medication Table 29-1 for additional information; Medication Tables are located at the end of the chapter).

> ## PRACTICE POINT
>
> *In addition to differences in dosing, differences in product reconstitution, preparation, and stability exist among the amphotericin B products. It is important to read the package insert for each product carefully to ensure that the proper preparation technique and diluent are being utilized.*

Nystatin

Nystatin is the other polyene antifungal agent in current use. It is available in several different formulations and is generally utilized for the treatment of mild or topical *Candida* infections (candidiasis). The oral suspension (500,000 units/5 mL) is commonly used for the treatment of oral or gastrointestinal candidiasis (also referred to as thrush). Patients are instructed to "swish" the suspension in their mouth for as long as possible, and then swallow the dose (usually three to four times daily). Nystatin is not well absorbed into the body following oral administration so most of the dose included in the oral suspension remains in the mouth, throat, and gastrointestinal tract. Thus, the most common side effects from this preparation are stomach upset or diarrhea.

Nystatin is also available as a topical cream, topical ointment, and a topical powder (each 100,000 units/g) for the treatment of *Candida* skin infections. The powder is generally utilized for areas of the body that are known to be moist. Additionally, the nystatin topical cream is also available in combination with the topical corticosteroid triamcinolone. The addition of the corticosteroid is useful for patients with fungal skin infections who are also suffering from bothersome itching. Finally, nystatin is also available as a vaginal tablet for the treatment of vaginal *Candida* infections.

The Azole Antifungals

The azole antifungals work by blocking the fungal enzyme used to produce ergosterol, a critical component of the fungal cell membrane. Without ergosterol, the fungal cell membrane loses its ability to function as a semipermeable barrier between the fungal cell and its external environment—one that allows some fluids and solutes to pass through while stopping others from moving in or out. Without ergosterol, some materials can freely enter and exit the fungal cell, disrupting its functions and equilibrium. Additionally, the enzyme inhibition leads to an accumulation of unused ergosterol precursors, which can become toxic to the fungal cell and impair its functions. In general, the azole antifungals exhibit fungistatic activity against most of the common fungal pathogens (although some agents are fungicidal against some molds). Unlike the polyenes, they do not cause immediate fungal cell death; rather these agents impair the ability of the fungal cell to grow and function normally. Unlike the polyenes, the azole antifungals do not become more effective once doses are increased above a certain threshold so increasing overall time of exposure to these agents is more important than achieving high peak concentrations.

Because the azole antifungals work by inhibiting a critical fungal enzyme, they also have the potential to inhibit human enzymes. In particular, many of the azole antifungals have the ability to inhibit the human liver enzymes that are responsible for the metabolism of many different drugs. As such, there is high potential for drug interactions with the azole antifungals when they are given systemically.

Additionally, because of their effects on the liver, one of the most common side effects of the azole antifungals is an elevation in various liver enzymes.

Although all of the azole antifungals share the same mechanism of action, there is a variety of products in this class that differ both in their indications and how they are administered. There are two broad categories of azole antifungals: the imidazoles and triazoles (named for the number of nitrogen atoms found in the azole ring). The triazole agents have proven to be the superior choice for systemic treatment, but the imidazoles are still in common use for topical treatment and are available in a variety of different preparations (creams, ointments, vaginal applications, etc.). Some of the topical azole products (covered in more detail in Chapter 33) are available over the counter (OTC), while others require a prescription for dispensing. Additionally, some of the topical products are available in combination with topical corticosteroids for patients who have significant itching associated with their infection.

While the topical azole agents are used widely, the five most clinically important azole antifungals that are administered systemically are itraconazole (Sporanox®), fluconazole (Diflucan®), voriconazole (VFEND®) posaconazole (Noxafil®), and isavuconazonium sulfate (Cresemba®).

Itraconazole

Itraconazole is currently available for oral use as a tablet and an oral solution. It has antifungal activity against a variety of *Candida* and *Aspergillus* species. Additionally, it is active against several of the endemic (regional) fungal species and is the first-line treatment in a number of these infections. One of its major drawbacks is inconsistent bioavailability, meaning that when it is administered orally, it is difficult to predict the amount of medication that will be absorbed from the gastrointestinal tract and reach the systemic circulation. For this reason, patients receiving itraconazole may need blood testing to monitor drug concentrations. Itraconazole also has many drug interactions, making its use difficult in patients on interacting agents.

Fluconazole

Fluconazole is available as an oral tablet, oral liquid (suspension), and a solution for intravenous (IV) administration. Compared with itraconazole, the oral bioavailability of fluconazole is much more reliable. For these reasons it is commonly utilized as oral therapy for a variety of uncomplicated *Candida* infections. It has become a mainstay in the treatment of vaginal candidiasis, and because of its long half-life it can be administered for this indication as a one-time oral dose of 150 mg. The IV formulation is also commonly utilized for the treatment of more severe *Candida* infections, such as bloodstream infections or infections of the central nervous system. In addition to its activity against a variety of *Candida* species, fluconazole is also active against a number of the endemic fungi and is sometimes used as an alternative agent in the treatment of these infections. However, fluconazole possesses no antifungal activity against *Aspergillus* species, and some species of *Candida* have developed resistance to fluconazole. Additionally, there are some isolates of *Candida* that have reduced susceptibility to fluconazole.

Voriconazole

Voriconazole is supplied for oral administration (as a tablet and as an oral suspension) as well as for IV administration. While its bioavailability is relatively reliable compared to that of itraconazole, it has a considerable number of clinically significant drug interactions, which present a challenge to its use in some settings. Voriconazole has demonstrated good efficacy against a wide variety of fungal pathogens, including *Candida* species, the endemic fungi, and *Aspergillus* species, as well as several other mold species. While the azoles are generally fungistatic, voriconazole actually possesses fungicidal activity against *Aspergillus* species, making it particularly useful and efficacious for infections by this organism.

Side effects associated with voriconazole are more significant than other azole agents and include temporary vision changes and hallucinations. Because of the side-effect profile and variable absorption, patients treated with voriconazole need to have blood drawn to assess drug concentrations as well as periodic liver function tests.

Posaconazole

Posaconazole is available as an oral delayed-release tablet, oral suspension, or IV solution. The oral tablet has better absorption than the oral suspension, and it is recommended that the oral dosage forms be taken with a meal to enhance bioavailability. Like the other azoles, posaconazole possesses antifungal activity against *Candida* species (including some species that are resistant to fluconazole), as well as activity against a variety of mold species, including *Aspergillus*. Of particular interest is posaconazole's activity against the Mucormycetes, a group of fungal organisms that cause devastating infection in immunocompromised patients and are especially difficult to treat. Patients receiving extended courses (>7 days) of posaconazole need to have blood drawn to assess drug concentrations.

Isavuconazole (Isavuconazonium Sulfate)

Isavuconazole is the newest medication in the azole antifungal family and is available as an oral capsule or IV solution. It is administered as isavuconazonium sulfate, which is metabolized in the body into the active molecule, isavuconazole. Isavuconazole exhibits activity against *Candida* species and *Aspergillus*, and, most notably, *Mucormycetes*. The most common side effect seen is gastrointestinal upset, which is markedly more severe than with other azole antifungals.

The Echinocandins

The echinocandins are the newest class of antifungal agents. They work by inhibiting the fungal enzyme responsible for synthesis of glucan, an essential element of the fungal cell wall. Without glucan, the cell wall loses its ability to regulate water flowing in and out of the cell; this results in cell death. Echinocandins are only available for IV administration and have similar antifungal spectrums of activity. They all have broad activity against *Candida* species, as well as some mold species such as *Aspergillus*. Although they do not have as many significant drug interactions as the azole agents, the echinocandins can cause elevations in human liver enzymes and patients must be monitored regularly for this side effect.

The three echinocandin agents currently available are caspofungin, anidulafungin, and micafungin. All three agents are currently approved for the treatment of *Candida* infections;

however, caspofungin is currently the only agent with an FDA-approved indication for invasive *Aspergillus* infections. Because they have few toxicities, the echinocandins have become the preferred agents for treatment of suspected fungal infections in immunocompromised patients.

> ## ALERT!
>
> Caspofungin and anidulafungin are usually ordered with a double (loading) dose for the first administration, followed by a smaller dose on subsequent days of therapy.

Miscellaneous Antifungals

Terbinafine

Terbinafine is an allylamine antifungal, which works by blocking an enzyme involved in ergosterol synthesis, different from the one affected by the azoles. It is available in a variety of formulations (creams, powders, sprays, etc.) that are applied topically for the treatment of fungal infections of the skin. It is also available as an oral tablet under the trade name Lamisil. Owing to its chemical structure, when terbinafine is administered systemically it accumulates in the fatty tissues, skin, and nails. As a result, it has become a mainstay in the treatment of fungal infections of the nail (onychomycosis), which is difficult to treat with topical antifungals due to their poor penetration into the nail bed.

> ## ALERT!
>
> LOOK-ALIKE/SOUND-ALIKE—The name brand for terbinafine, Lamisil, may look similar to the trade name Lamictal, which is a medication used to treat seizures. Confusing these medications could have serious adverse effects.

> ### PRACTICE POINT
>
> *While most (though not all) topical terbinafine products are available OTC, the oral tablet is prescription only.*

Flucytosine

Flucytosine is an antimetabolite, meaning that its antifungal activity is the result of interference with fungal deoxyribonucleic acid (DNA), ribonucleic acid (RNA), and protein synthesis. Flucytosine was one of the earliest antifungal agents developed; however, owing to some rare but serious side effects, such as bone marrow suppression, central nervous system effects, and liver and kidney toxicity, as well as the emergence of fungal resistance to flucytosine monotherapy (used alone, without other antifungals), its use has now become relatively rare in clinical practice. Although it was once available as an IV formulation, it is now only available for oral administration. Flucytosine possesses antifungal activity against *Candida, Aspergillus*, and *Cryptococcus* species as well as the dermatophytes, fungal pathogens, which cause skin infections. The nonpolyene agents for systemic fungal infections are listed in Medication Table 29-2.

Griseofulvin

Griseofulvin is an oral antifungal agent used primarily for the treatment of fungal infections of the skin, hair, and nails caused by dermatophytes. In particular, it is used commonly for fungal infections of the scalp since it distributes well to the skin and hair follicles. The antifungal activity of griseofulvin is a result of its ability to inhibit fungal mitosis (cell division). There are few side effects associated with griseofulvin, although it can affect the metabolism of other medications, resulting in drug interactions. Because it is available as both a tablet and a pediatric oral suspension, it is commonly prescribed for children with fungal infections of the scalp. Its use and preparations are covered in more detail in Chapter 33 and Medication Table 33-7.

Topical Antifungals

A large variety of antifungal agents are available as topical formulations, including both OTC and prescription products. Many of the azole agents are available as topical formulations, such as creams and powders, as well as products for the treatment of vaginal yeast infections, such as creams, vaginal suppositories, and vaginal tablets. In addition, terbinafine and several other allylamines are available in a variety of topical formulations, such as creams, gels, powders, and spray forms. Nystatin is also available as a cream and an ointment for topical application. As mentioned previously, several topical antifungal agents are also supplied in combination with a corticosteroid to help with itching and inflammation. It is important for clinicians to be aware of the various agents and formulations of topical antifungals when recommending and dispensing a product. Topical antifungals will be discussed in detail in Chapter 33.

FUNGAL INFECTIONS

Candida Infections

Candidiasis describes any variety of opportunistic fungal infections caused by species of the genus *Candida*. The most common *Candida* pathogen in humans is *Candida albicans*. Candidiasis can vary greatly in its severity, presentation, and location. *Candida* infections commonly occur on mucous membranes, including the oral cavity (called thrush), the gastrointestinal tract, and the vagina. *Candida* can also cause skin infections (such as diaper rash). In severe cases, generally in patients with profound immunosuppression or other risk factors, infections of the deep organ systems, such as the liver, heart, bone, lung, and central nervous system, can occur. *Candida* infections can also occur in the bloodstream.

The treatment of *Candida* infections varies based on the clinical presentation, severity of infection, and patient-specific considerations. For infections of the skin and mucous membranes, nystatin or the azoles are generally utilized as first-line therapy. For more severe infections, systemic azole therapy may be used, although resistance to fluconazole among *Candida* species is becoming more common. The echinocandins as well as amphotericin B may also be considered in the treatment of severe *Candida* infections.

Aspergillus Infections

Aspergillosis is the term used to describe infections that may result from inhalation of the spores of *Aspergillus* species (most commonly one of three species: *A. fumigatus*, *A. niger*, or *A. flavus*). Frequently, inhalation exposure to *Aspergillus* can result in an allergic-type reaction, but *Aspergillus* can also result in severe disease if it spreads from the lungs to other parts of the body. Such infections occur in immunocompromised patients and generally either present as a

CASE?

Several months later, Ms. Andrews is admitted to the hospital with persistent cough, shortness of breath, and a widespread rash. She states that she has recently returned from a trip to Phoenix to visit her nephew. What type of infection might be suspected?

pulmonary (lung) infection or as a disseminated (widely spread) infection. Invasive aspergillosis is associated with an overall mortality rate of nearly 60%, and treatment is difficult. Early diagnosis and treatment are imperative in the management of such infections. While amphotericin B was the historical treatment of choice for invasive aspergillosis, newer agents such as voriconazole, posaconazole, and isavuconazole are now recommended over amphotericin B owing to their equal efficacy and fewer side effects.

Endemic Fungal Infections

The term endemic infections refers to infections that are usually diagnosed only among certain populations or in certain regions. The three most important endemic fungal infections in the United States are *Histoplasma capsulatum* (generally found in the eastern United States, especially in the Ohio River Valley), *Coccidioides immitis* (occurring in the southwestern United States and northern Mexico), and *Blastomyces dermatitidis* (found in the eastern United States and Canada). These infections are transmitted through the inhalation of fungal spores. They typically cause pulmonary infections, including pneumonia and pulmonary cavitations (abnormal spaces in the lungs), but the infection can spread to other parts of the body, especially in immunocompromised patients. Treatment of these infections generally involves treatment with antifungal agents but may also include surgical intervention.

CASE?

What treatment might the doctor prescribe for Ms. Andrews's lung condition?

Histoplasmosis

Infection with *Histoplasma capsulatum* (histoplasmosis) occurs following inhalation of the fungal spores and is generally self-limiting and may resolve without treatment. However, in rare cases it may go on to cause acute infections of the lungs and/or disseminated infections (usually in immunocompromised individuals). Mild to moderate pulmonary infections may be treated with itraconazole monotherapy, but in severe cases of acute histoplasmosis, an initial course of IV amphotericin B followed by a prolonged course of itraconazole is warranted. The duration of therapy can range from 6 weeks to 24 months depending on the severity of infection and patient-specific risk factors.

Blastomycosis

Like histoplasmosis, blastomycosis is primarily a pulmonary disease caused by inhalation of *Blastomyces dermatitidis* spores present in the soil but may go on to cause severe disseminated infection in some patients. Although it may resolve without treatment, the clinical manifestations of this infection are more difficult to predict, so it is generally treated, even in otherwise healthy patients. Mild or moderate blastomycosis can be effectively treated with itraconazole (6 months), but for severe infections, IV amphotericin B is the drug of choice, generally in high doses, followed by itraconazole for an additional 6 to 12 months once the patient has stabilized. Fluconazole, voriconazole, or itraconazole may be utilized in the setting of central nervous system involvement or in patients who cannot tolerate amphotericin B therapy.

Coccidioidomycosis

Like the other endemic fungi, coccidioidomycosis results from inhalation of *Coccidioides immitis* spores. Most of these infections will resolve without therapy; therefore, treatment is only recommended for patients who are immunocompromised and at risk for the more severe, disseminated forms of the disease. For patients with severe disease, treatment with fluconazole or itraconazole is recommended. For patients with severe disease and respiratory failure, amphotericin B is utilized as initial therapy followed by itraconazole or fluconazole once the patient is stable. Fluconazole is preferred when the central nervous system is involved. It is recommended that therapy with the azole agent be continued for at least 1 year to try to minimize the risk of relapse.

Cryptococcal Infection

Like the endemic fungi, *Cryptococcus* infection results from the inhalation of the spores of the yeast *Cryptococcus neoformans* or other *Cryptococcus* species. It is of particular concern among immunocompromised patients, such as those with HIV/AIDS or cancer, or those on immunosuppressants following a transplant because of its potential to disseminate and cause central nervous system infection in these populations. The historic treatment of choice for central nervous system involvement is amphotericin B in combination with flucytosine. This combination may be continued for the entire treatment course or may be changed to fluconazole alone after 2 weeks of treatment.

SUMMARY

Owing to an increasing population of immunocompromised patients, the treatment of opportunistic infections caused by fungal pathogens has become an area of much interest over the past several decades. Many antifungal agents are available, diversifying the treatment options for serious systemic fungal infections. Additionally, a number of topical antifungal preparations are available both over the counter (OTC) and with prescription for the management of fungal skin infections. It is essential that the differences among these agents be recognized as they relate to dosing, side effects, drug interactions, compounding, storage, and administration.

CHAPTER RESOURCES

Bennett JE, Dolin R, and Blaser M. *Principles and Practice of Infectious Diseases.* 9th ed. Philadelphia, PA: Elsevier Health Sciences; 2019.

Antifungal Antibiotics [online]. Available at https://www.ncbi.nlm.nih.gov/books/NBK538168/. Accessed June 9, 2022.

Coccidioidomycosis [online]. Available at https://www.ncbi.nlm.nih.gov/books/NBK448161/. Accessed June 9, 2022.

REVIEW QUESTIONS

1. Describe the similarities and differences between fungal and human cells. How do antifungal agents harm the fungus and not the patient?

2. Describe the difference between fungal and bacterial infections. Why are different drugs used to treat them?

3. Patients at risk for fungal infections typically share what characteristic? Why is this important for the acquisition of fungal infections?

4. What are the major toxicities associated with polyene antifungals such as amphotericin B?

5. Which class of antifungal agents has the greatest potential for causing drug-drug interactions? Why?

MEDICATION TABLES

MEDICATION TABLE 29-1. Polyene Antifungal Agents*

Generic Name (pronunciation)	Brand Name	Dosage Form	Route	Usual Dose	Notes
Amphotericin B deoxycholate (am foe TER i sin bee de ok se KO late)	Various generic products	Powder for reconstitution	IV	0.3–1.5 mg/kg daily	1 mg test dose should be given prior to full dose
Amphotericin B lipid complex (am foe TER i sin bee LIP id KOM pleks)	Abelcet	Suspension	IV	3–5 mg/kg daily for most diagnoses	Inline filters are contraindicated; premedication with acetaminophen, diphenhydramine, and/or hydrocortisone is recommended
Amphotericin B liposomal (am foe TER i sin bee lye po SO mal)	AmBisome	Suspension	IV	3–6 mg/kg daily (usual dosage range)	An inline membrane filter (not less than 1 micron) may be used
Nystatin (nye STAT in)	Bio-Statin	Capsule, 1,000,000 units	Oral	1,000,000 units 3–4 times daily	Suspension dosage form is swished in mouth and retained as long as possible before swallowing
	Generics	Tablet, 500,000 units	Oral	500,000 units 3–4 times daily	
	Generics	Suspension, 100,000 units/mL	Oral	400,000 to 600,000 units 4 times daily	
	Nyamic, Nystop,	Cream, ointment, powder, 100,000 units/g	Topical	Apply to affected area as directed	

IV = intravenous.
* Information and pronunciations from Lexicomp. Lexi-Drugs [database]. Hudson, OH: Wolters Kluwer.

MEDICATION TABLE 29-2. Nonpolyene Agents for Systemic Fungal Infections*

Generic Name (pronunciation)	Brand Name	Dosage Form	Route	Usual Dose
Echinocandins				
Anidulafungin (ay nid yoo la FUN jin)	Eraxis	Powder for reconstitution	IV	200 mg on day 1, then 100 mg daily thereafter
Caspofungin (kas poe FUN jin)	Cancidas	Powder for reconstitution	IV	70 mg on day 1, then 50 mg daily thereafter
Micafungin (mi ka FUN gin)	Mycamine	Powder for reconstitution	IV	50–150 mg daily
Imidazoles				
Ketoconazole (kee toe KOE na zole)	Generics	Tablet	Oral	200–400 mg daily
Miconazole (mi KON a zole)	Various	Cream, 2%–4%, suppository, 100 mg, 200 mg	Vaginal	Applicatorful or suppository inserted at bedtime × 3 or 7 days
	Oravig	Dissolving tablet	Buccal	50 mg (1 tablet) to the upper gum region (canine fossa) once daily × 14 days
Triazoles				
Fluconazole (floo KON na zole)	Diflucan	Premixed IV solution, powder for oral suspension, tablet	IV, oral	50–400 mg daily
Isavuconazonium sulfate (eye sa vue koe na ZOE nee um sul FATE)	Cresemba	Powder for reconstitution, capsule	IV, oral	372 mg (200 mg of isavuconazole) every 8 hours for 6 doses followed by 372 mg (200 mg of isavuconazole) daily
Itraconazole (i tra KOE na zole)	Sporanox	Capsule, 100 mg, solution, 10 mg/mL	Oral	200 mg daily, twice daily, or three times a day
	Tolsura	Capsule, 65 mg		130 mg once or twice daily
Posaconazole (poe sa KON a zole)	Noxafil	Premixed IV solution (requires dilution), oral tablet, oral suspension	IV, oral	600–800 mg daily in 3 or 4 divided doses
Voriconazole (vor i KOE na zole)	VFEND	Powder for reconstitution, powder for suspension, tablet	IV, oral	IV: 6 mg/kg every 12 hours × 2 doses, then 4 mg/kg every 12 hours; Oral: 200-300 mg every 12 hours
Antimetabolite				
Flucytosine (floo SYE toe seen)	Ancobon	Capsule	Oral	50–150 mg/kg daily divided every 6 hours
Allylamine Antifungal				
Terbinafine (TER bin a feen)	Generics	Granules, tablet	Oral	250 mg daily or 500 mg twice daily

IV = intravenous.
* Information and pronunciations from Lexicomp. Lexi-Drugs [database]. Hudson, OH: Wolters Kluwer.

Chapter 30

Immunobiologics

Joseph S. Marchiano, PharmD, BCPS, BCGP

KEY TERMS AND DEFINITIONS

Antibody—a molecule developed by the immune system in response to a specific recognized threat, or antigen, that works to trigger immune responses after subsequent exposure to this threat.

Antigen—a substance recognized by the immune system as a threat.

Antitoxin—an antibody that neutralizes a toxic substance, usually obtained from the serum of an animal that has been exposed to the substance.

Biosimilar—an analogue to a biological medication approved by the U.S. Food and Drug Administration that meets regulatory standards regarding its composition, safety, and efficacy relative to its reference product.

Centers for Disease Control and Prevention (CDC)—a U.S. government agency and division of the Department of Health and Human Services whose mission is to "protect America from health, safety and security threats, both foreign and in the U.S. Whether diseases start at home or abroad, are chronic or acute, curable or preventable, human error or deliberate attack, CDC fights disease and supports communities and citizens to do the same."

Immune globulin—an antibody, or a preparation containing antibodies, derived from a human or animal source that has been exposed to one or more antigens that is utilized as a medication. This differs from "immunoglobulin" as "immune globulin" refers specifically to those antibodies or antibody-containing preparations used as medication therapy.

DOI 10.37573/9781585286638.030

Immunoglobulin—An endogenous glycoprotein, also known as an antibody, produced by lymphocyte B-cells as a component of acquired immunity. This differs from "immune globulin" as "immunoglobulin" refers only to antibodies that are endogenous within the body, as opposed to those preparations used as medications.

Immunity—resistance to disease or infection that is usually generated by the response of the body's defense systems. Immunity is often categorized as either *passive* or *active* or, separately, as either *innate* or *acquired*.

- *Passive immunity* comes from the transfer of antibodies into an individual.

- *Active immunity* is a result of the body's own production of antibodies after encountering recognized threats (e.g., antigens).

- *Innate immunity* refers to nonspecific protection against pathogens that is natural to humans from birth, such as the body's external barriers to disease (eg, skin).

- *Acquired immunity* develops only after exposure to a specific recognized threat (eg, antigen).

Immunization—Utilizing targeted medical interventions to provide an individual with immunity to a specific biological threat.

Immunocompromise—a condition in which the function of the immune system is impaired or weakened as a result of illness (eg, acquired immunodeficiency syndrome [AIDS]) or medications (eg, immunosuppressives).

Immunosuppressive—an agent that, intentionally or as an adverse effect, weakens the natural responses of the immune system.

Postexposure prophylaxis—measures taken to prevent illness or infection after a nonimmune individual is exposed to a pathogen that can cause serious or fatal disease (eg, tetanus, diphtheria, hepatitis B). This may include administration of immune sera/immune globulins.

Rejection—an attack by the body's immune system against living cells or tissues that were transplanted or grafted for therapeutic reasons.

Serum (plural is sera)—the liquid portion of blood, or plasma, minus blood cells and clotting factors. An immune serum is a preparation from humans or animals that contains immune globulins/antitoxins and can be administered to confer passive immunity.

Vaccine—a preparation of a killed, weakened, or modified pathogenic agent administered to produce immunity against such agents by stimulating the production of specific antibodies and other immune responses against them.

Vaccine confidence—the trust that patients, their families, and providers have in recommended vaccines and in providers who administer vaccines, as well as in the processes and policies that lead to vaccine development, licensure or authorization, manufacturing, and recommendations for use.

LEARNING OBJECTIVES

After completing this chapter, you should be able to:

1. Recall discussed components of the immune system and classify types of immunity.

2. Recognize different types of immunizations.

3. Explain the value of disease prevention to public health and provide examples of how pharmacy personnel can support public health initiatives.

4. Interpret the CDC vaccination schedule for children and adults.

5. Recall the indications for immunosuppression and identify agents used for such purposes.

6. Define biosimilars and outline the purposes of such products.

THE IMMUNE SYSTEM

Humans are born with a full immune system composed of cells, glands, organs, and fluids located throughout the body to fight invading pathogens (disease-causing organisms). An important step in this fight includes the initial recognition of toxins or invading organisms that enter the body, and our immune system is able to identify specific structures on these invaders known as antigens to perceive them as foreign entities. The immune system is further equipped with several specific and nonspecific means to fight such threats upon recognition. One specific defense is the production of substances called antibodies—molecules targeted against specific recognized antigens. A healthy immune system can produce immense quantities of antibodies to defend against specific attacks every day. Many antibodies disappear once they have helped to destroy the invading antigens, but some cells involved in antibody production remain and become *memory cells*. Memory cells retain the ability to produce a forceful and rapid antibody response if they encounter the antigen again, even after many years. Antibody-based protection from disease by the body's defense system is a form of immunity.

The lymphatic system, which contains the main organs of immunity (called lymphoid organs)—including bone marrow, lymph nodes, the spleen, the thymus gland, and tonsils—is the part of the circulatory system that cleanses body fluids of foreign material as well as old or damaged cells. The fluid contained in this system is known as lymph. White blood cells (WBCs, described in detail in Chapter 25) important to the functioning of the immune system partially reside within lymph and are broken up into several categories of cells. They include the monocytes, eosinophils, basophils, leukocytes, and lymphocytes. Each type has a unique role in helping to protect the body. Lymphocytes develop in either the bone marrow (B-cells) or the thymus (T-cells) before circulating throughout the body. They are named based on where they develop, and each major type of lymphocyte (T-cell and B-cell) helps to provide the body with its ability to respond to immediate insults as well as develop specific immunity in response to recognized threats.

Types of Immunity

Innate immunity is a general, nonspecific protection against pathogens that is natural to humans from birth. Innate immunity includes external barriers, such as the skin and mucous membranes that line the nose, throat, and gastrointestinal tract. These represent the first line of defense in preventing diseases from entering the body. If an outer defensive wall is broken, as when the skin is damaged by a cut or scrape, the body attempts to heal the break quickly while special immune cells on the skin's surface attack any invading bacteria. If a pathogen enters the body despite these external defenses, the innate immune system continues to function by producing a nonspecific inflammatory-based response. Large numbers of WBCs will mobilize, allowing for neutrophils and macrophages to attack the invading threat. As this occurs, chemicals work to call other WBCs to join the defense.

Acquired immunity describes the immune response of the body that is specific to particular organisms or antigens. Therefore, it must develop as a result of exposure and is not present at birth. Once components of the innate immune system mount an initial response, various cells work to generate molecules that specifically target the antigen that has been recognized. Specific antibodies are then released, which trigger powerful reactions against the identified threat. After the antigen has been contained or removed, some of the activated lymphocyte B-cells become *memory cells* that remain in the body and will produce specific antibodies very quickly if the antigen is ever encountered again. Vaccines work by stimulating this response, and immunization occurs by exposing the immune system to a weakened, altered, or destroyed pathogen in order to stimulate the production of *memory cells*. The pathogens present in vaccines are unable to reproduce or cause infection in individuals with a functional immune system. If an individual who has been immunized is exposed to the actual pathogen, the body will be poised to recognize the foreign antigen and quickly attack it with both the innate and adaptive immune system components. This works to prevent the individual from becoming ill. The production of antibodies against a specific entity is known as active immunity.

> ### PRACTICE POINT
>
> *It is important to remember that acquired immunity is pathogen-specific and works only against antigens recognized by the immune system. Someone who has received the measles, mumps, and rubella vaccine will be protected by this acquired immunity against infection due to future exposures to these pathogens, but this protection will not extend to influenza or tetanus. Similarly, vaccination for polio will not protect against varicella or any antigen other than that introduced to the body by the poliovirus vaccine.*

Active immunity can be acquired in two ways: by contracting an infectious disease (eg, chickenpox), or by receiving a vaccination (eg, varicella vaccine). This immunity can be long lasting and sometimes lifelong. Under certain circumstances, antibodies against an antigen can be transferred directly from one person to another. Such a transfer confers passive immunity because an individual's immune system still has not produced its own antibodies. A newborn baby acquires passive immunity from its mother as certain antibodies are passed through the placenta. An individual can also gain passive immunity by receiving antibody-containing blood products such as immune globulins, which may be administered when immediate protection from a specific disease is needed. In addition, antibodies produced in a laboratory that bind to one specific antigenic site, known as *monoclonal* antibodies, may be utilized to confer passive immunity against certain diseases. While the same type of monoclonal antibodies will bind to one specific target, different monoclonal antibodies can be made to target a variety of antigens. This makes monoclonal antibodies a diverse class of medications that have uses related to infections as well as a variety of other medical conditions, depending on the specific agent. Monoclonal antibodies can additionally be designed to target receptors on cancerous cells as antineoplastic agents, and their use in this capacity is more thoroughly reviewed in Chapter 31. The major advantage of passive immunity, regardless of the means through which it is conferred, is that the protection is immediate (in comparison to active immunity, which takes time to develop). Unlike its active counterpart, passive immunity is temporary.

VACCINES AND IMMUNIZATION

Acquired immunity was recognized by people long before the immune system was understood or the agents that caused infection were known. It was noticed that some diseases, like measles or mumps, were often contracted after exposure to someone else who had these illnesses. It was also noted that some individuals who had contracted and recovered from certain communicable diseases did not get them again, even when they had close contact with patients who had the active disease. In the late 18th century, British physician Edward Jenner attempted to take advantage of these observations by exposing several children, including his own, to pus taken from a person with cowpox (a mild disease then common in milkmaids). This process made them immune to smallpox, one of the most widespread and deadly communicable diseases of the time. Jenner, through this therapy, was causing his patients' bodies to produce antibodies against smallpox, which afforded them invaluable protection against such a formidable infection. *Vacca* is the Latin word for cow, so Jenner called his process *vaccination*.[1] At the time, it was a revolutionary concept, and it ultimately proved to be a successful way to confer more consistent immunity in a way that is safer than direct pathogen exposure. The medical community has since refined the process to confer immunity without making the individual ill. Now commonly called

immunization, this therapeutic strategy has worked to eliminate countless fatalities from communicable diseases such as smallpox, poliomyelitis, measles, mumps, rubella, tetanus, diphtheria, pertussis, influenza, pneumonia, hepatitis, and dozens of other threats to humanity.

Despite the availability of vaccines, pneumococcal pneumonia and influenza still result in tens of thousands of deaths each year in the United States among unvaccinated patients. Hepatitis A and B, also preventable by vaccine, cause many additional preventable illnesses and fatalities.[2] It is the responsibility of all healthcare professionals to communicate accurate information related to immunizations to deter the spread of such preventable disease.

Because immunization programs have been very effective in countries like the United States, many people are not familiar with the deadly diseases that have been curtailed by childhood immunizations. Current generations are fortunate to not intimately know the damage that comes from smallpox, polio, or measles infections; this is almost entirely due to successful vaccination programs. In the face of the COVID-19 pandemic, being champions of correct information pertaining to the vaccination process, as well as those immunizations available to offer protection against COVID-19, is an important responsibility of all pharmacy personnel and healthcare professionals.

Vaccines can be separated into several categories based on how they are developed. Certain vaccines contain intact, but weakened, pathogens and are designated as *live-attenuated*. This type is the most likely to result in lifelong immunity after a single dose. While such vaccines are incapable of producing an infection in individuals with an intact immune system, immunosuppressed persons should not receive a *live-attenuated* vaccine without first speaking with their healthcare provider as their immune systems may not be healthy enough to tolerate them. Another category of vaccines contains killed pathogens: these are called *inactivated*. Additional categories of immunizations utilize components of the pathogen to trigger an immune response and may be referred to as *recombinant, conjugate, subunit, or polysaccharide*, depending on the specific part or parts of pathogen(s) used to create the vaccine. Nonlive vaccines are often administered as multiple doses to be sure that they confer long-term immunity. Some of these vaccinations also require doses provided at prescribed intervals long after an initial immunization, called *boosters*, to "remind" the immune system by stimulating the production of additional *memory cells* when the immune response may wane. Examples of *inactivated* immunizations include the vaccine against hepatitis B virus (HBV), which is composed of only the surface proteins of the virus, as well as the vaccine against human papillomavirus (HPV) which is made from the viral protein coat.

Other types of vaccines include those that utilize messenger RNA (mRNA) or an adenovirus vector. mRNA is constantly made by cells throughout the body, and it functions as a blueprint for the creation of many kinds of proteins that allow our bodies to function normally. Therefore, vaccines that utilize mRNA deliver specific instructions to the body's cells so that our cells can manufacture a harmless antigen, which is then recognized by the immune system to produce *memory cells* in the process described above. The mRNA utilized by these vaccines cannot enter the nucleus of cells, which is where DNA is kept, and the mRNA used by the vaccine is destroyed by the cell after it is used to produce the harmless antigen. For these reasons, it is impossible for mRNA vaccines to affect or interact with our DNA. Adenovirus vector vaccines utilize a harmless nonpathogenic virus, which enters our cells and uses the body's natural cellular machinery to produce an antigenic substance. This substance is then recognized by the body's immune system to generate a *memory cell*-based immune response. The components of adenovirus vector vaccines are also incapable of integrating with the DNA found within our cells. Regardless of vaccine type, each product works to confer active immunity without risking the significant harm that may come from exposure to the pathogen in question. Several vaccines against infectious diseases are listed in Medication Table 30-1 (Medication Tables are located at the end of the chapter).

PRACTICE POINT

Several vaccines are available in preparations for infants and children that are different from the preparation available for adults and may not be safely interchanged! One example is the hepatitis B vaccine.

Vaccines have been developed for the prevention of many common and deadly infectious diseases, but there are currently no vaccines for some infections due to the ability of certain viruses to quickly change their antigens. Such change would make the *memory cells* developed by a vaccine unable to produce antibodies against the changed antigens. Currently, human immunodeficiency virus (HIV), hepatitis C, and the common cold do not have vaccines. Research is

progressing, though, related to novel vaccine development for both infectious and certain noninfectious disease states.

Certain bacteria damage the body by producing dangerous products known as toxins. Antibodies against these toxins, however, may eliminate their harmful actions and prevent disease. To stimulate the production of these antibodies, immunization against toxin-producing organisms utilizes a vaccine that contains a harmless version of the toxin, known as a toxoid, thus stimulating the adaptive immune system. Examples of toxoid-containing vaccines are those against diphtheria and tetanus. Such products are listed in Medication Table 30-1, and combined immunizations (ie, single products that contain multiple antigens to stimulate active immunity against multiple pathogens) are presented in Medication Table 30-2.

Immunizations are administered via a variety of routes depending on the preparation used and/or the type of vaccine. The most common routes of administration have historically been by injection: subcutaneous (SUBQ), intradermal, or intramuscular (IM). Most vaccines are given by injection because they may not be well absorbed from the gastrointestinal tract. Rotavirus, cholera, and some typhoid vaccines, however, are given orally in order to produce localized immunity in the bowel; this is the point of entry for these agents in actual infection. Additionally, live-attenuated influenza vaccine has been produced as a nasal spray that is absorbed through the nasal mucosa.

Some immunizations can be administered at the same time as others (some are even mixed together as combination products, such as those described in Medication Table 30-2), while others must be separated by intervals of several weeks. The Centers for Disease Control and Prevention (CDC) publishes annual schedules of recommended vaccinations to prevent diseases for children and adults in the United States (Schedule 30-1 and Schedule 30-2, respectively). The CDC receives recommendations pertaining to vaccinations from a group of experts in the fields of medicine and public health known as the Advisory Committee on Immunization Practices (ACIP). To obtain a full understanding of these schedules, it is vital to visit the CDC's website to read the annotations attached to each set of recommended immunizations and to do so as frequently as these recommendations are updated.[2] Travel abroad may also pose the risk of exposure to infectious agents not normally encountered in the United States, and additional immunizations may therefore be required. Recommendations related to travel vaccinations are provided separately in the CDC's Yellow Book.

SCHEDULE 30-1. Recommended Child and Adolescent Immunization Schedule for ages 18 years or younger, United States, 2022

Vaccine	Birth	1 mo	2 mos	4 mos	6 mos	9 mos	12 mos	15 mos	18 mos	19–23 mos	2–3 yrs	4–6 yrs	7–10 yrs	11–12 yrs	13–15 yrs	16 yrs	17–18 yrs
Hepatitis B (HepB)	1st dose	←— 2nd dose —→			←———————— 3rd dose ————————→												
Rotavirus (RV): RV1 (2-dose series), RV5 (3-dose series)			1st dose	2nd dose	See Notes												
Diphtheria, tetanus, acellular pertussis (DTaP <7 yrs)			1st dose	2nd dose	3rd dose		←——— 4th dose ———→					5th dose					
Haemophilus influenzae type b (Hib)			1st dose	2nd dose	See Notes		3rd or 4th dose, See Notes										
Pneumococcal conjugate (PCV13)			1st dose	2nd dose	3rd dose		←——— 4th dose ———→										
Inactivated poliovirus (IPV <18 yrs)			1st dose	2nd dose	←———————— 3rd dose ————————→							4th dose					
Influenza (IIV4)					Annual vaccination 1 or 2 doses									Annual vaccination 1 dose only			
Influenza (LAIV4)											Annual vaccination 1 or 2 doses			Annual vaccination 1 dose only			
Measles, mumps, rubella (MMR)						See Notes	←——— 1st dose ———→					2nd dose					
Varicella (VAR)							←——— 1st dose ———→					2nd dose					
Hepatitis A (HepA)						See Notes	2-dose series, See Notes										
Tetanus, diphtheria, acellular pertussis (Tdap ≥7 yrs)														1 dose			
Human papillomavirus (HPV)													See Notes	See Notes			
Meningococcal (MenACWY-D ≥9 mos, MenACWY-CRM ≥2 mos, MenACWY-TT ≥2years)								See Notes						1st dose		2nd dose	
Meningococcal B (MenB-4C, MenB-FHbp)															See Notes		
Pneumococcal polysaccharide (PPSV23)														See Notes			
Dengue (DEN4CYD; 9-16 yrs)													Seropositive in endemic areas only (See Notes)				

Legend:

- Range of recommended ages for all children
- Range of recommended ages for catch-up vaccination
- Range of recommended ages for certain high-risk groups
- Recommended vaccination can begin in this age group
- Recommended vaccination based on shared clinical decision-making
- No recommendation/ not applicable

As of this writing, the CDC recommends use of COVID-19 vaccines within the scope of the Emergency Use Authorization or Biologics License Application for the vaccine.[2]

SCHEDULE 30-2. Recommended Adult Immunization Schedule for ages 19 years or older, United States, 2022[2]

Vaccine	19–26 years	27–49 years	50–64 years	≥65 years
Influenza inactivated (IIV4) or Influenza recombinant (RIV4)	1 dose annually			
Influenza live, attenuated (LAIV4)	1 dose annually			
Tetanus, diphtheria, pertussis (Tdap or Td)	1 dose Tdap each pregnancy; 1 dose Td/Tdap for wound management (see notes)			
	1 dose Tdap, then Td or Tdap booster every 10 years			
Measles, mumps, rubella (MMR)	1 or 2 doses depending on indication (if born in 1957 or later)			
Varicella (VAR)	2 doses (if born in 1980 or later)	2 doses		
Zoster recombinant (RZV)	2 doses for immunocompromising conditions (see notes)		2 doses	
Human papillomavirus (HPV)	2 or 3 doses depending on age at initial vaccination or condition	27 through 45 years		
Pneumococcal (PCV15, PCV20, PPSV23)	1 dose PCV15 followed by PPSV23 OR 1 dose PCV20 (see notes)			1 dose PCV15 followed by PPSV23 OR 1 dose PCV20
Hepatitis A (HepA)	2 or 3 doses depending on vaccine			
Hepatitis B (HepB)	2, 3, or 4 doses depending on vaccine or condition			
Meningococcal A, C, W, Y (MenACWY)	1 or 2 doses depending on indication, see notes for booster recommendations			
Meningococcal B (MenB)	19 through 23 years	2 or 3 doses depending on vaccine and indication, see notes for booster recommendations		
Haemophilus influenzae type b (Hib)	1 or 3 doses depending on indication			

Recommended vaccination for adults who meet age requirement, lack documentation of vaccination, or lack evidence of past infection

Recommended vaccination for adults with an additional risk factor or another indication

Recommended vaccination based on shared clinical decision-making

No recommendation/ Not applicable

The CDC reminds us that immunizing individuals contributes to community health, especially by protecting people who cannot be immunized because they are either too young to be vaccinated, cannot be vaccinated for medical reasons, or cannot make an adequate response to vaccination because of poor health or a compromised immune system.[2] Widespread immunization programs can eliminate or reduce the impact of epidemics and disease outbreaks by elevating the overall health of a community.

PHARMACY ROLE

As members of the healthcare community, pharmacy staff members are often involved in initiatives to make immunizations, and accurate information about them, available as widely as possible. Emphasizing reliability and safety are key components of the communication provided related to vaccines. Pharmacy staff can participate in a multitude of activities related to immunization stewardship; these include managing supplies, promoting immunization, and facilitating the administration of vaccines.

Managing the supply of immunizations in the community and in healthcare institutions is a complex process in which pharmacy technicians frequently play a vital role. Because they are biologic products, vaccines and toxoids are frequently issued a short shelf-life; consequently, inventory control, stock rotation, and careful ordering practices are necessary to avoid running out of these important products at an urgent time while simultaneously preventing the waste of funds and product. Records of products received, dispensed, and administered (including lot number and expiration dates) are often maintained in the pharmacy as well.

The application of knowledge to ensure proper vaccine transport and storage is an additional responsibility of everyone in a pharmacy where these products are received, handled, and stocked. Most vaccines must be refrigerated or frozen continuously prior to use, and allowing an immunization to reach a temperature that is outside the range in its labeling (eg, thawing a frozen product, freezing one that should be kept at refrigerated temperatures, letting a product that must be kept cold reach room temperature, or maintaining a vaccine outside of its temperature range) can damage it irretrievably. Inappropriate storage may render a product unable to effectively provide protection to an individual, and such potentially deadly failures of immunization are often difficult to immediately detect. Observing and maintaining the storage conditions on the labeling of each package is always required. Most vaccines must be shipped in an insulated container, and many have an enclosed temperature monitor to verify that they have not been exposed to temperatures outside their recommended storage ranges; reviewing such conditions upon receipt will ensure that vaccinations have not been inappropriately handled in transit. Pharmacy personnel must note the beyond-use date of received products, and immediately place the products in appropriate storage conditions with those expiring first in the most accessible position. The CDC has published a "Vaccine

Storage and Handling Toolkit" which provides updated specific information pertaining to the proper storage of immunizations.[2] The importance of proper vaccine storage and handling is difficult to overstate, especially related to immunizations that need to be stored in unique environments with dynamic supplies available, such as some of those used as vaccines against COVID-19.

Many vaccines require reconstitution before use. It is common for them to be packaged with their own diluents, and, if so, these are the only acceptable agents for the reconstitution process. All reconstitution should be done exactly according to package directions.

PRACTICE POINT

Once reconstituted, vaccines may have only a very short window of time (eg, 30 minutes) within which they can be administered. Make sure to never reconstitute vaccines too far in advance.

ALERT

It is critical to be sure one does not dispense the diluent without reconstituting the vaccine!

Promoting recommended immunizations is an activity in which pharmacy personnel should engage. While knowledge of immunization schedules and vaccine-related informational resources are helpful in ensuring that patients are up to date with vaccination, recent history poses another challenge regarding immunizations related to the public faith in this process that has provided our society with so many remarkable health benefits. Maintaining vaccine confidence requires that pharmacy personnel work toward reaffirming personal and public trust in vaccines, the administrators of immunizations, and regulations surrounding immunizations. Doing so is of paramount importance when considering the monumental impact of immunizations on maintaining public health and, given the time at which this was written, in the use of immunizations in combating the COVID-19 pandemic. While authentic feelings of concern are often at the root of an individual losing vaccine confidence, vaccine confidence can often be maintained or restored by sharing information rooted in the correct interpretation of evidence and connecting this information to

how immunizations may assist in maintaining wellness by safely preventing disease when used as recommended. For a pharmacy professional, it is vital to be aware of the answers to questions about vaccines to increase vaccine confidence, and to be skilled enough to communicate such information in a tactful way to patients who genuinely care about their health and that of their families.

PRACTICE POINT

Patients with low vaccine confidence often care about their health and the health of their families, but they have been incorrectly led to believe that vaccines pose high risks with low benefits. It is key to understand this while having discussions about the safety and efficacy of vaccines, as respectful communication of accurate information must always occur to help boost vaccine confidence.

Several key basics are necessary when presenting information to an individual who is skeptical regarding immunizations. It is often necessary to first recontextualize the benefits of vaccinations for these people. Current generations are extremely fortunate to be reaping the benefit of vaccines without having witnessed many of the reasons why they were created. Diseases such as smallpox, polio, influenza, measles, mumps, rubella, pertussis, tetanus, and many others plagued and killed our ancestors but are relatively rare in the modern era. It is very easy for individuals to not conceptualize vaccines as a cause for why these diseases are more absent and, because these diseases are now uncommon, downplay the danger of these infections. As COVID-19 has manifested as one of the most threatening infectious events in recent history, the impact of an unchecked pandemic has unfortunately become more apparent in modern times, especially to those individuals and families most closely affected by this disease. While changes to day-to-day routines such as mask wearing, social distancing, and limiting social contact are vital means to slow the spread of a potentially life-threatening infection, history and modern data indicate that vaccination is an extremely important tool to assist with ending a pandemic and curtailing avoidable serious health complications brought by COVID-19. It is vital to understand that immunizations have saved countless lives by conferring active immunity against many deadly pathogens, and our society will only be able to remain protected against these diseases and emerging threats if immunization is continued.

Another basic piece of communication corresponds to understanding one of the main roots of losing vaccine confidence: misinformation. Access to virtually unlimited information has emerged, but much of this information is of dubious quality. Numerous web pages, social media groups, and social media posts allow individuals to "confirm" incorrect information or misinterpretation by repeating it; this can make it very challenging to help an individual come to correct conclusions as they are often victims of receiving information from unreliable sources. Encouraging individuals to critically evaluate the sources of their information and specifically stating the value of peer-reviewed literature and conversations with healthcare professionals may inspire realizations regarding the credibility (or lack thereof) of their sources.

In addition to the knowledge and communication of the societal necessity of immunizations, as well as the importance of reliable information sources, understanding the truth regarding common ideas that threaten vaccine confidence is key. Misgivings regarding ingredients, the administration of several vaccines simultaneously, adverse events related to immunizations, and the efficacy of vaccines often permeate conversations about the appropriateness of immunizations.

Knowledge of the purpose and safety of various immunization ingredients is vital to accurately understanding and communicating information related to vaccines. Ingredients that have garnered attention, their uses, and information related to their safety are presented in the following:

- *Formaldehyde* is an essential ingredient utilized to chemically inactivate viruses such as the poliovirus and detoxify bacteria such as *Corynebacterium diphtheriae*, which causes diphtheria, to eliminate the possibility of harm from such pathogens. While toxic in large concentrations (as any medication may be), the amount of formaldehyde in vaccinations is negligible compared to that which the body produces on its own.

- *Aluminum* is present in various immunizations such as the diphtheria toxoid/tetanus toxoid/acellular pertussis (DTaP) vaccine, pneumonia vaccines, and the HBV vaccine. Aluminum functions as an adjuvant in immunizations, which means that it helps boost the immune system's response to the antigen introduced by the vaccine. It has demonstrated safety over six decades of use, and aluminum is commonly encountered in food and water. While hesitant individuals may counter that "ingestion does not equal injection," the absorption of aluminum from immunizations is nonthreatening based on its historically safe use, as well as pharmacokinetic models of metabolism in several age groups (including infants).

- *Fetal calf/bovine* **serum** functions as a nutrient-rich environment that helps to grow virus particles utilized for various immunizations. This serum is also a common laboratory growth medium that works to foster the replication of organisms exposed to it. While this serum is derived from fetal calves, it works as nothing more than a growth environment during the manufacturing of certain immunizations.

- *MF59* is an adjuvant that works to boost the immune system's response to a specific influenza vaccine. It utilizes squalene, which is a natural component of the cholesterol pathway in our bodies, and its safety is well established.

- *AS01B* is another adjuvant utilized in a specific vaccine against shingles. Its two components, *MPL* and *QS-21*, work together to boost the body's ability to fight against the shingles virus antigen introduced by the vaccine. MPL is a fat-like substance, and QS-21 is a compound purified from tree bark.

- *Antibiotics* are utilized to prevent bacterial contamination of immunizations during the manufacturing process and are almost entirely filtered out during the end-stage production of vaccinations. Notably, antibiotics that may trigger allergic reactions in individuals (eg, penicillin agents and sulfa drugs) are not utilized.

- *Thiomersal/Thimerosal* is an ethylated mercury-containing compound utilized as a preservative in some immunizations. It was infamously and incorrectly linked to autism spectrum disorder in a since-discredited study; more recently, multiple nationally sponsored studies have rejected any association between this compound and autism spectrum disorder.[3] It was removed from most immunizations to curb overall mercury exposure despite historical safe use, and individuals still concerned regarding this compound can complete the CDC vaccination recommendations with products entirely free of thiomersal.

Individuals may also express noningredient-related concerns regarding immunizations. Apprehension related to administering multiple vaccines at once is dispelled by the safe use of vaccine combinations dating back to the 1940s, and immunizations that are recommended to be utilized alongside one another are tested in such settings to ensure safety. Some individuals may cite the National Vaccine Injury Compensation Program as evidence that immunizations are malicious or meant to cause harm. It is critical, however, to understand that immunizations are capable of causing rare adverse effects, like all other medications. Such adverse effects may occur following the inappropriate administration of a vaccine, represent an allergic reaction, or be due to the utilization of a vaccine in an individual without a functional immune system. In addition, adverse effects may occur near the timing of an immunization but have no relation to the vaccine itself. A compensation program, contrary to this argument, is evidence of the importance of vaccinations; it exists, in part, to prevent the threat of lawsuits, regardless of merit or immunization causality, from discouraging the production of immunizations.

Some individuals avoid receiving elective immunizations as they do not want to "get sick" from the vaccine. It is important that pharmacy professionals understand the difference between the brief period of fatigue that may follow an immunization and the actual illness in question so that they can explain it to patients. First, it is impossible to contract an illness from a nonlive immunization, as there is nothing in such a product that may confer disease. Live vaccines are weakened, or attenuated, which prevents individuals with a functional immune system from harm; these immunizations, however, are contraindicated in immuno-suppressed individuals because the weakened pathogen may be able to cause harm in such cases. Feeling sick after an immunization may represent an increased period of immune system activity (ie, the reaction associated with antigenic exposure), but this must not be confused with actual infection in individuals with a functional immune system.

The influenza vaccine also receives criticism regarding its utility. Individuals may question its purpose and usefulness related to the CDC's recommendation of one dose each year. This recommendation is rooted in the nature of influenza as a pathogen, for this virus possesses the ability to change its unique antigenic structure over time. Because of this characteristic, the influenza vaccine administered one year may not adequately protect an individual from variations of the virus that may circulate in the future. Scientists work to combat this by developing vaccinations against the most current influenza virus each year; this is why annual vaccination is necessary to confer protection against this deadly pathogen. Various formulations of the influenza vaccine exist, which vary based on the strength of the dose; how many strains of the virus the immunization affords protection against (eg, three strains, or trivalent, vs. four strains, or quadrivalent); whether the virus is live, recombinant, or inactivated; and whether it contains an adjuvant. It is generally recommended that older adults receive a high-dose formulation, but other individuals will likely receive adequate protection with any age-approved vaccine appropriate for their health status. Additionally, individuals with an egg allergy should

still receive the influenza vaccine after consulting their healthcare provider regarding this matter. Annual vaccinations will work to protect both individuals and their close contacts from transmission of this virus each year.

The COVID-19 pandemic has provided yet another reason to emphasize the importance of vaccine confidence, but the recent advances in COVID-19 immunizations have arrived with new challenges in maintaining public trust. Avoiding the potential for serious health consequences related to COVID-19 has driven the consistent production of information during the pandemic, and misinformation has also circulated in this dynamic environment. Because vaccine confidence related to COVID-19 represents an important public health priority, understanding how to communicate reliable facts to dispel misinformation related to vaccination for COVID-19 is critical.

The CDC publishes a frequently updated collection of web pages dedicated to building vaccine confidence related to COVID-19 vaccines and understanding correct information related to common misconceptions related to these immunizations.[4] They recommend several resources and action steps to help affirm COVID-19 vaccine confidence by building trust, empowering healthcare personnel, and engaging communities as well as individuals.

Having successful conversations with friends and family first requires understanding key facts related to COVID-19 vaccines. A fundamentally important truth is the knowledge that COVID-19 vaccines are both safe and effective for use. While concerns may be raised related to the initial use of an Emergency Use Authorization (EUA) for these products as opposed to a more traditional U.S. Food and Drug Administration (FDA) approval, reviewing what an EUA entails provides understanding and confidence related to this part of the vaccination regulatory process. An EUA is a means through which the FDA will allow use of unapproved medical products in an emergency to diagnose, prevent, or treat serious or life-threatening diseases when there are no adequate, approved, or available alternative options. It is paramount to know that, for an EUA to be issued by the FDA for a vaccine, the FDA must decide that any definite or possible benefits of the vaccine outweigh any definite or possible risks. COVID-19 vaccine clinical trials are being held to the high safety and effectiveness standards set by the FDA, and each vaccine provided an EUA by the FDA undergoes three phases of preapproval clinical trial research similar to all other medications. This rigorous process, in addition to intimate knowledge related to how these vaccines work and the evaluation of the manufacturing of these products, factor into the FDA's decision with respect to the appropriateness of issuing an EUA. Postauthorization monitoring is also robust and conducted for each authorized product. Understanding the gravity of an EUA helps to engender vaccine confidence in products assigned such an authorization.

Reviewing the mechanisms related to mRNA vaccination and adenovirus vector vaccination will also help to satisfy concerns related to the safety of these vaccines. As reviewed above, these vaccines provide a blueprint for the body to produce a harmless antigenic protein that confers active immunity to COVID-19. These blueprints are destroyed by cellular machinery after use, and they cannot affect host cell DNA. Therefore, there is no potential for COVID-19 vaccines to alter human DNA. This string of molecular events helps to clarify that it is unlikely that these vaccines may affect fertility; this, in combination with early real-world data, helps to establish the likelihood of safety of these vaccines for those who would like to become pregnant in the future. At the time of writing, the CDC strongly recommends COVID-19 vaccination, if otherwise appropriate, for patients planning a pregnancy, those trying to become pregnant, and in those who might become pregnant in the future. This is related to the risks of COVID-19 in pregnancy which include severe illness, death, and pregnancy complications. The CDC also strongly recommends that pregnant patients receive the COVID-19 vaccine, if otherwise appropriate, related to avoiding the above risks and when considering available data pertaining to the safety and effectiveness of mRNA vaccines. However, as this is a developing area, it is important to refer to current guidelines regarding administration of the COVID-19 vaccine in pregnant patients and to advise patients to discuss such items with their healthcare provider(s). Additionally, further research is being conducted regarding COVID-19 vaccines and pregnancy. Existing data on how these vaccines work also supports that the risk for long-term side effects is very unlikely. Individuals concerned regarding their eligibility for a COVID-19 vaccine are encouraged to discuss this decision with their healthcare professional team. It is worth emphasizing that COVID-19 vaccines cannot give individuals COVID-19 as they only introduce a harmless outer protein of the virus that causes COVID-19 as the antigenic substance.

Expectations regarding how someone might feel after COVID-19 vaccination, and why they may feel this way, are additionally important to understand. As vaccination produces an immune response, symptoms related to such a response (eg, local pain, redness, swelling, tiredness, headache, muscle pain, chills, fever, and nausea) may occur after vaccination. These side effects are likely signs that the body is mounting an immune response and, while they may impact day-to-day activities, they should go away in a few days if experienced at all. Any individual with persistent or troubling side effects should talk to their healthcare professional team, though, for guidance regarding the next best steps or actions to take to safely minimize discomfort.

Additionally, understanding that the production of full immunity related to the formation of *memory cells* occurs approximately two weeks after completing a vaccination series serves as a key feature of COVID-19 vaccines. These vaccines have demonstrated effectiveness in preventing infection related to COVID-19 and, after full vaccination is achieved, individuals may safely reengage in certain activities pursuant to the guidance of national healthcare-related organizations such as the CDC. While COVID-19 vaccines are safe and effective in preventing COVID-19, more information is required with respect to the effectiveness of these vaccines in preventing the spread of COVID-19 from person to person and within a community, the duration of protection afforded by these vaccines (and recommended scheduling for subsequent boosters), how effective these vaccines are against new strains of COVID-19, and how many people must be vaccinated before most people are considered protected from infection (ie, *population immunity*). Staying vigilant with respect to how ongoing, evidence-based studies contribute to the body of knowledge related to COVID-19 vaccination is a key feature of the scientific method and is expected of all pharmacy professionals. Organizations such as the CDC offer regular updates on their web pages to facilitate this process.

Effectively communicating correct information related to COVID-19 vaccines to build vaccine confidence also requires attention related to the conversation itself. Listening to others with an open mind and without judgment helps to establish genuine trust between parties, which will likely make it easier to find common ground and validate one another. Mutual trust and understanding may additionally be created by asking open-ended questions and asking permission to share further information and techniques for finding trustworthy information from reliable sources. It can be impactful to share reasons for getting vaccinated while helping to discover potential motivations that others may have for receiving the vaccination themselves. Finally, helping an individual make a commitment to receive their immunization, and working to make each step of signing up to receive a vaccine as easy as possible, may assist in inspiring vaccine confidence. Ultimately, sharing correct information and reliable sources related to COVID-19 vaccines must be done while respecting and appreciating the concerns of each person.

Pharmacists often administer immunizations. While state laws (pharmacy practice acts) differ in specifics pertaining to such administration, every state in the United States includes pharmacy personnel on the immunization "team."

Pharmacy technicians have usually assisted the pharmacist with administration by ensuring that stocks of immunization supplies are available, in-date, recorded appropriately, communicated successfully, and handled in a manner consistent with approved guidance. Many states require that information pertaining to immunizations be communicated by administering pharmacies to patients' primary care physicians. Ensuring that this infrastructure is present (when required) is an additional element with which pharmacy technicians may assist. Some states permit and encourage appropriately trained pharmacy technicians to administer immunizations, and this practice is likely to become more common in the future.

Sometimes, conferring passive immunity to diseases or toxins is important, and this may be accomplished by directly administering immune globulins or antitoxins to a patient suffering from the impact of a direct immune-related insult. Passive immunity is not long lasting, but it can be accomplished much more immediately than active immunity as it does not require the patient to produce their own agents of adaptive immunity. The use of immune serum can protect individuals who have been recently exposed to a toxin, such as the venom of a poisonous reptile, from some of the dangerous or deadly effects of that toxin; these effects may occur before the immune system can develop its own defenses.

Immune globulins may also be utilized to prevent the effects of incompatible blood types in certain mothers and their fetuses during pregnancy. Some individuals possess blood with an antigen known as Rho(D) and, if a child's blood possesses this while a mother's does not, the mother's immune system may develop antibodies against this component of the baby's blood during pregnancy. This can be fatal for the child. One immune globulin has been designed to prevent the mother from developing antibodies in such cases, and it is utilized in this as well as other Rho(D)-related disease states.

Postexposure prophylaxis includes measures taken to prevent illness or infection after acute exposure of a non-immune individual to a pathogen that can cause serious or fatal disease. This may include administration of specific immune sera/immune globulins. Examples include the hepatitis B immune globulin administered to infants born of HBV-infected mothers, the same immune globulin administered to healthcare workers with needle stick exposures, and the rabies immune globulin administered to a patient who has been bitten by a potentially rabid animal. Normal vaccines to produce active immunity against these antigens are available, but in cases where immediate protection is needed to prevent a suspected insult from causing serious damage, passive immunity may provide a timely advantage.

CASE STUDY

J. R. is a 70-year-old male who presents to the emergency room in late October with cellulitis (skin/tissue inflammation) of his right hand after injuring it while gardening two days ago. He is now experiencing increased pain, redness, and swelling in the injured area. He says he has not seen a physician in the last 20 years and has never received tetanus toxoid-containing vaccines, but he was current with all other immunizations up to that time.

- What pathogens is J. R. protected from as a result of the immunizations he has received leading up to his last physician's visit?

- What vaccination(s) might be indicated for J. R. based on the CDC recommendations for his age group?

- The emergency medicine team suspects that J. R. has been exposed to tetanus and orders both the Td vaccine and tetanus immune globulin due to his lack of a vaccination history for tetanus. Which of these confers passive immunity, thus providing immediate protection? Which will help J. R. build active, long-term immunity to the offending pathogens?

- J. R. initially refuses any immunizations because they will "make him sick" and contain "poison." How would you help to communicate accurate information to ensure that J. R. receives the care he needs?

Some patients are unable to mount an immune response to a pathogen even after vaccine administration. These include those born with deficiencies of their immune systems, patients suffering from serious illness, individuals with certain infections such as HIV, and patients being treated with medications that suppress their immune systems (ie, immunosuppressives). The state where one's immune system is unable to produce a functional defense is known as immunocompromise. Immunocompromised patients are occasionally treated with pooled human immune globulins, which include antibodies to many commonly encountered antigens and vaccine-preventable diseases. Preparations that confer passive immunity against viral infections, toxins, or envenomation, as well as immune-related medication antidotes, are listed in Medication Table 30-3.

ALERT

Look-Alike/Sound-Alike: Do not confuse HBIG (hepatitis B immune globulin) with BabyBIG (botulism immune globulin). They are used in different doses to treat and prevent different disease states in different populations. It is key to also understand the differences and lack of interchangeability between immunizations and immune globulins such as those for varicella, tetanus, and rabies, as well!

PRACTICE POINT

Globulins are protein preparations that often require especially sensitive handling during preparation and delivery. Package inserts should always be consulted for special instructions and precautions to take prior to working with these agents.

IMMUNOSUPPRESSIVES

While the immune system is important in enabling the body to prevent damage by infectious agents and toxins, there are times when its actions are harmful or unwanted.

Sometimes the immune system mistakes the body's own cells and tissues as foreign and attacks them; conditions defined by such actions are known as autoimmune diseases. Autoimmune conditions such as rheumatoid arthritis and systemic lupus erythematosus have been discussed earlier (Chapter 13) and are often treated with medications that intentionally suppress the immune system (ie, immunosuppressives).

It is sometimes necessary for patients whose tissues or organs have been damaged beyond repair by disease or injury to receive similar tissues or organs from others to replace their own. These procedures are called transplants or grafts, and they may involve whole organs (eg, lung, heart, liver, kidney) or tissues (eg, skin, bone marrow). In these cases, the immune system may, albeit correctly, recognize the transplant as foreign and attack it. This phenomenon is known as rejection and can cause failure of the transplant and possibly fatal harm to the transplant recipient. Immunosuppressives are often utilized in this setting to help prevent the incidence of rejection.

PRACTICE POINT

The effectiveness of vaccines may be reduced in immunosuppressed patients. Immunosuppressed patients require earlier vaccinations with certain immunizations while being unable to receive other immunizations (eg, live vaccines) for up to 90 days after immunosuppression. Adequately verifying a patient's medication list prior to vaccination is key!

ALERT

Many immunosuppressives are classified as hazardous drugs, and handling of these medications must follow published standards (eg, USP Chapter 800).

Corticosteroids, discussed in detail in Chapter 9, are effective in suppressing the immune system and may be used to avoid the rejection of transplants, sometimes even while the transplant surgery is still in process. While these medications (eg, IV methylprednisolone and oral prednisolone) have immunosuppressive properties, they are more often utilized in other medical conditions (eg, to decrease inflammation), which makes the risk of immunosuppression an unwanted adverse effect in such instances. Doses of glucocorticoids to prevent rejection are often much higher than doses used for most other medical conditions.

Medications known as antimetabolites (covered in Chapter 31) encompass a broad class that uniformly trick the body into incorporating dysfunctional molecules into chemical reactions required to sustain cell life; this interrupts these critical processes and works to destroy the functionality of the affected cell. Consequently, most antimetabolite medications have uses as anticancer agents. Use of these agents may, however, risk suppressing the immune system as an adverse effect. One antimetabolite, azathioprine, targets specific cells of the immune system, which allows it to be utilized for indications that are not related to cancer. Specifically, it is available as an oral or injectable agent to prevent the rejection of kidney transplants, and it is also used for other immune-related conditions. Because it reduces WBCs, patients taking azathioprine are more susceptible to infection. Azathioprine also bears a black box warning because it increases the risk of malignancy. It is administered with food to decrease the incidence of gastrointestinal side effects.

Much more specific immunosuppressants have been developed during the past several decades. Mycophenolate is one such agent that directly suppresses the immune system by preventing the development of T and B lymphocytes. The hydrochloride (injection) and mofetil, mycophenolic acid, and sodium (oral) preparations may be utilized as a component of an antirejection regimen for cardiac, liver, lung, or kidney transplantation. Although it is a more specific agent, mycophenolate possesses a host of adverse effects due to its interference with widespread cellular processes. These include predisposing a patient to infections, certain blood disorders (eg, anemia), pain, and blood pressure changes. It also possesses a black box warning related to malignancies, serious infections, and fetal toxicity.

PRACTICE POINT

Mycophenolate, especially the mycophenolic acid form, should be administered on an empty stomach (one hour before or two hours after food). Tablets and capsules should be ingested whole without breaking, crushing, opening, or chewing.

PRACTICE POINT

The FDA requires that patients receive a medication guide with each prescription and refill of mycophenolate.

ALERT

Mycophenolate sodium and mycophenolate mofetil are not interchangeable without first consulting the prescriber.

Calcineurin inhibitors are another class of immunosuppressives that decrease immune response by blocking T-cell activity, but they do so by a different mechanism than the antimetabolites. Several of their major side effects are nephrotoxicity (kidney damage) and neurotoxicity (tremors, headache, and even seizures). Infections are always a risk when the immune system is suppressed, and many of these agents consequently have black box warnings related to serious infection.

Cyclosporine (also known as cyclosporin A) is a calcineurin inhibitor available as an intravenous (IV) solution as well as capsules and a solution for oral administration. Oral formulations must be taken on a regular schedule, at the same times every day, and associated with the same meals. Interestingly, cyclosporine is produced under several brand names and is available as either a nonmodified product named SandIMMUNE or a modified product meant to have improved absorption; the modified products are marketed as Gengraf or Neoral. There is also an experimental inhaled product to prevent rejection of lung and bone marrow transplants. Cyclosporine uniquely has a black box warning related to serious elevations in blood pressure and kidney toxicity.

Cyclosporine is metabolized by the liver and has many drug interactions that can either increase blood levels (and risk of toxicity) or decrease them (chancing organ rejection). Some drugs can also have increased effects when taken with cyclosporine. A full medication profile (including herbal supplements) is critical to obtain for every patient taking this medication (and all patients).

Tacrolimus is another calcineurin inhibitor dosed as an IV solution or as several oral forms. It may be dosed once daily or every 12 hours depending on whether the immediate-release or extended-release oral formulation is utilized.

PRACTICE POINTS

- *The different brands and formulations of cyclosporine are not all bioequivalent and may not be used interchangeably. Great care must be taken to ensure that the patient receives the prescribed form of cyclosporine. If a patient is to be converted from one product to another, blood levels and patient response must be monitored professionally.*

- *Dosing syringes used to measure cyclosporine oral solution must be completely dry when used, as even small amounts of water can affect the dose the patient receives.*

- *Cyclosporine oral solutions should be used within 2 months after the original container is opened and should be stored at room temperature (not in the refrigerator).*

- *Cyclosporine oral solutions may be diluted with other liquids (at room temperature) to make them easier to take. SandIMMUNE may be mixed with orange juice or milk (white or chocolate) immediately before administration. Gengraf and Neoral may be diluted with orange or apple juice, but milk is not advised. Patients should choose one kind of diluent and try not to change. Grapefruit juice should be avoided (because of metabolic effects).*

PRACTICE POINT

Sometimes an oral suspension of tacrolimus is extemporaneously compounded using the contents of the capsules in a mixture with simple syrup and Ora-Plus or, alternatively, sterile water, Ora-Plus, and Ora-Sweet. Be sure to follow applicable regulations when handling or compounding such a mixture (eg, USP Chapter 800).

These products cannot be interchanged. Like cyclosporine, it is metabolized in the liver and has many drug interactions, so a complete patient profile is required. In addition to immunosuppression, tacrolimus has an additional black box warning related to increasing the risk of certain malignancies.

ALERT

Look-Alike/Sound-Alike: The brand of cyclosporine known as SandIMMUNE has been confused with Sandostatin (octreotide) used for hypersecretory conditions.

Certain agents, sirolimus and everolimus, change the way T-cells respond to antigenic stimulation by inhibiting a cellular compound known as the mechanistic target of rapamycin (mTOR). Both are administered orally and are used in conjunction with other agents to prevent the rejection of various transplants, depending on the agent. These drugs, like the calcineurin inhibitors above, are metabolized by liver enzymes and have many drug interactions.

PRACTICE POINTS

Sirolimus oral solution is diluted with at least 2 ounces of water or orange juice (no substitutes are acceptable, especially not grapefruit juice) before administration. Everolimus is available as several noninterchangeable brand name products. Zortress is used for transplant patients, Afinitor is predominantly for certain cancers, and Afinitor Disperz is used for specific tuberous sclerosis complex-associated conditions.

A novel type of immunosuppressant is termed a *selective T-cell costimulation blocker* because it prevents certain cells of the immune system from interacting with T-cells. Two medications of this class are belatacept and abatacept. The former is utilized to prevent rejection in kidney and lung transplants, while the latter suppresses the immune system from causing joint inflammation in conditions such as psoriatic and rheumatoid arthritis.

The most common adverse reactions to the T-cell costimulation blockers are infection, anemia, gastrointestinal

ALERT

Many of the immunosuppressants, including azathioprine, everolimus, mycophenolate, sirolimus, and tacrolimus, are mutagenic (may cause cancer) and teratogenic (may cause birth defects). Precautions and safe handling procedures for hazardous substances should be used for the protection of those who prepare, dispense, or administer these medications. Each medication also has specific recommendations regarding contraception use while undergoing immunosuppressive therapy.

PRACTICE POINT

Reconstitution and dilution of belatacept and abatacept must be performed precisely as directed, using only the silicone-free syringe provided with each vial. The vial should not be shaken, and the infusion must be completed within 24 hours of reconstituting the lyophilized powder.

PRACTICE POINT

Premedication with a combination of antihistamines, acetaminophen, and corticosteroids is often used to reduce the side effects of administration of these antibody products.

Several monoclonal antibodies may be used to prevent rejection. One product is available that works against certain receptors on activated T-cells to prevent them from attacking transplanted tissue. This agent, basiliximab, binds to the interleukin-2 (IL-2) complex to elicit its immunosuppressive effect. It is indicated for use in conjunction with other immunosuppressives for preventing various types of organ rejection and, like other antibodies, it is administered intravenously. Side effects include hypertension, headache, tremor, gastrointestinal effects, and infection. It has not been associated with significant drug interactions other than compounded immunosuppression with similar medications.

PRACTICE POINT

Reconstituted basiliximab solutions must be used within 24 hours.

effects, cough, and headache. More concerning reactions are the serious and life-threatening malignancies that involve the lymphatic and central nervous system. There are few drug interactions, except with other agents that affect the immune system.

Several IV antibody preparations have been developed as immunosuppressants. The antithymocyte globulins are *polyclonal* antibodies as they bind to several lymphocyte proteins; *monoclonal* antibodies, however, bind to one target. These antithymocyte globulins are derived from either horse or rabbit tissue and work by binding to the receptors on lymphocytes to prevent them from attacking transplanted tissue. Their main adverse effects are suppression of blood cell formation, anaphylaxis, rash, breathing difficulties, and cardiovascular issues (heart and blood pressure).

A third antibody, muromonab-CD3, is a monoclonal agent specific to the CD3 receptor of the mature human T-cell. It is no longer available due to a voluntary withdrawal from the market.

Rituximab, a monoclonal antibody targeted against a specific complex found on B-lymphocytes known as CD-20, is utilized primarily as an anticancer agent as well as an agent against immune-related joint disorders. It may also assist with rejection in heart transplantation by suppressing the antibody-mediated response produced by B-lymphocytes. Black box warnings for this medication correspond to infusion reactions, mucous membrane reactions, and rare infections. Premedication often occurs with at least acetaminophen and an antihistamine to minimize the risk and severity of infusion reactions. Blood cell suppression, fatigue, lung disease, and cardiac dysfunction represent more common adverse effects. Interactions are similar to other antibodies discussed.

Alemtuzumab is another monoclonal antibody that may be used to combat rejection in heart, lung, or renal transplantation by facilitating the destruction of several immune cells by binding to a specific molecule found on several such cells. Accordingly, it possesses black box warnings related to bone marrow suppression and infection in addition to the possibility of infusion reactions; the latter effect requires premedication to be given prior to infusions similarly to rituximab. This medication risks enhanced immunosuppression when combined with other immunosuppressives, and its use will likely result in headaches and a skin rash.

As discussed in the chapters on the musculoskeletal system (Chapter 13), lower GI (Chapter 22), and dermatologic disorders (Chapter 33), certain immune-related medications target other points to decrease autoimmune activity for nontransplant purposes. Medications such as tofacitinib inhibit an intracellular chain reaction mediated by the Janus kinase (JAK) proteins. Stopping this pathway works to shut down certain immune cells with the goal of treating psoriatic arthritis, rheumatoid arthritis, and ulcerative colitis. Additionally, anakinra is a medication that inhibits the IL-1 receptor to decrease immune-related inflammation in conditions such as rheumatoid arthritis. A last group of monoclonal antibodies, including adalimumab, work to downregulate a mediator of inflammation known as tumor necrosis factor-alpha (TNF-alpha). Such action has proven beneficial in a multitude of musculoskeletal, gastrointestinal, and dermatological conditions. While not utilized for rejection, these medications still predispose patients to infections by generating an immunosuppressive state.

PRACTICE POINT

Patients being treated for autoimmune-related conditions such as rheumatoid arthritis, psoriatic arthritis, ulcerative colitis, and Crohn's disease may be undergoing therapy with immunosuppressive medications. Obtaining an accurate medication list while treating such patients is critical!

The noncorticosteroid immunosuppressive agents that are used as components of regimens to prevent and treat organ rejection are summarized in Medication Table 30-4. Of note, individual agents are often utilized in combination with several other immunosuppressive medications to compose a complete antirejection regimen.

BIOSIMILARS

In recent years, biotechnology and regulation have been used to facilitate the safe production of cost-effective alternatives to certain biologic medications (ie, isolated from natural sources as opposed to chemically synthesized). These alternatives are known as biosimilars. Unlike generically equivalent medications, biosimilar products are biologic agents that possess slight differences from the compound that they mimic; the compound that a biosimilar copies is more formally referred to as a reference product. While these variations initially sound alarming, a biosimilar must be designated by the FDA as "highly similar" to the reference product without possessing "clinically meaningful differences." A "highly similar" product is one that has undergone extensive testing to evaluate the structure, function, and purity of the proposed biosimilar against the reference product. Approved biosimilars must then possess "no clinically meaningful differences" that may stem from any imperfect elements of the comparison, and various clinical tests are often utilized to verify the absence of such differences. In addition, approved biosimilars may be given status as an *interchangeable product*; approved biosimilars may be substituted with the reference product only with physician approval, but those designated as *interchangeable products* by the FDA meet additional standards of similarity that allow them to be substituted for the reference product without prescriber approval (pending state regulations).

Currently approved biosimilars represent several classes of medications, including the aforementioned TNF-alpha inhibitors and anti-CD-20 agents, as well as medications that help the body produce blood cells (eg, colony stimulating factors). Anticancer agents that work against the vascular endothelial growth factor (VEGF) and human epidermal growth receptor 2 (HER2) are also classes of medications with biosimilars.

Biosimilars represent an exciting new wave of medications that may allow costs to be driven down for normally expensive biological products, and the FDA's Purple Book lists approved biosimilars and interchangeable products. Approved biosimilar products as of March 2022 are provided in Medication Table 30-5.

PRACTICE POINT

Biosimilar products share the generic name of their reference product followed by an exclusive four-letter suffix. A biosimilar for the fake generic drug "exampilimab" may therefore be named "exampilimab-rxrx." Biosimilars, in addition to this name, also possess a brand name like most new medications. Be sure to recognize differences between biosimilars and their reference products to avoid dispensing errors!

SUMMARY

The immune system is the body's main defense against disease caused by invading pathogens and the toxins they may produce. While innate immunity is important, acquired immunity enables the body to fight off specific infectious diseases. Active immunity, associated with exposure to pathogenic agents, can be induced by vaccination, which confers protection against specific diseases without causing infection and related consequences. Vaccinations against many diseases have reduced their incidence, eliminated their presence, and improved the quality of life for society in general. Understanding their necessity and safety while communicating such information tactfully is becoming more important each day, especially in the context of the COVID-19 pandemic.

Passive immunity can be conferred by directly transferring antibodies from another source. It is relatively immediate, short-lived, and useful in protecting patients who have been infected or exposed to an acutely dangerous pathogen or toxin to which they have no prior immunity.

In some cases, it is advantageous to suppress the immune system. This is especially true in organ transplantation, when the body's natural response is to attack (reject) the foreign tissue. Using immunosuppressant agents prevents this reaction and allows a transplant to have maximal levels of success. Immunosuppression, while useful in this way, confers a risk of serious adverse effects and alters patients' candidacy for certain immunizations.

Over the next several years, unique and more cost-effective alternatives to many medications, including biologics, will likely emerge. Staying informed on the progression of biosimilar products will ensure that all patients receive the most appropriate medications at all times.

ACKNOWLEDGMENT

The author gratefully acknowledges the contributions of James A. Rapacchietta, PharmD, BCNSP; Mandy J. Hemmert, PharmD; and Jessica P. Tilley, PharmD, in writing the earlier version of this chapter that appears in the first edition.

REFERENCES

1. BBC History. Edward Jenner (1749-1823). http://www.bbc.co.uk/history/historic_figures/jenner_edward.shtml. Accessed March 10, 2022.

2. Centers for Disease Control and Prevention. Vaccines & Immunizations. http://www.cdc.gov/vaccines/. Accessed March 10, 2022.

3. Centers for Disease Control and Prevention. Science Summary: CDC Studies on Thimerosal in Vaccines. https://www.cdc.gov/vaccinesafety/pdf/cdcstudiesonvaccinesandautism.pdf. Accessed March 10, 2022.

4. Building Confidence in COVID-19 Vaccines. Available at https://www.cdc.gov/vaccines/covid-19/vaccinate-with-confidence.html/. Accessed March 10, 2022.

5. Lexicomp. Lexi-Drugs [database]. Hudson, OH: Wolters Kluwer.

6. U.S. Food and Drug Administration. Purple Book: Lists of Licensed Biological Products with Reference Product Exclusivity and Biosimilarity or Interchangeability Evaluations. https://www.fda.gov/drugs/therapeutic-biologics-applications-bla/purple-book-lists-licensed-biological-products-reference-product-exclusivity-and-biosimilarity-or/. Accessed March 10, 2022.

ACTIVITIES FOR REVIEW

1. Describe the differences between innate and acquired immunity versus active and passive immunity.

2. Define the different types of vaccines, and list pertinent differences between these types.

3. Explain how pharmacy personnel can contribute to public health by supporting immunization. List ways for pharmacy personnel to enhance vaccine confidence.

4. Utilize the CDC vaccination schedule to understand vaccinations required for children, adolescents, and adults.

5. Explain why immunosuppression is necessary for patients who have undergone organ transplantation, and name three categories of immunosuppressive medications.

6. Describe how biosimilars differ from generic medications in terms of composition and regulation, and explain the differences between products designated as "biosimilar" or "interchangeable."

MEDICATION TABLES

MEDICATION TABLE 30-1. Immunizations[5]

Vaccine	Category	Brand Name	Dosage Form	Route	Dosing/Schedule	Indications	Notes/Recommendations
Adenovirus (types 4 and 7) vaccine	Live (viral)	N/A	Tablet	Oral	One tablet of each type (type 4 and type 7) by mouth simultaneously as one dose	Immunization against adenovirus types 4 and 7 among military personnel between the ages of 17 and 50	Not commercially available in the United States; routine vaccination not recommended
Anthrax vaccine adsorbed	Inactivated (bacterial)	BioThrax	Injection suspension	IM (preferred), SUBQ	Variable vaccination schedule for preexposure prophylaxis and postexposure prophylaxis	Immunization against *Bacillus anthracis* in persons at high risk for exposure or those already exposed	Routine vaccination not recommended
BCG vaccine	Live (bacterial)	N/A	Injection	Percutaneous	Percutaneous: 0.2–0.3 mL (full-strength dilution); for tuberculosis immunization, conduct post-vaccination tuberculin test in 2–3 mos; if test is negative, repeat vaccination	Immunization against tuberculosis; prevention of leprosy	Recommended for children with negative tuberculin skin test who are continually exposed to *Mycobacterium tuberculosis* and cannot be treated long term or if the exposure is to resistant strains; healthcare workers interacting with a high percentage of patients with resistant *M. tuberculosis* strains
Cholera vaccine	Live (bacterial)	Vaxchora	Reconstituted oral suspension	Oral	100 mL as a single dose at least 10 days prior to possible cholera exposure	Immunization against *Vibrio cholerae* serogroup O1	Recommended for travelers between the ages of 18 and 64 from the United States to an area where cholera is actively transmitted
COVID-19 vaccine (adenovirus vector)	Adenovirus vector vaccine	Janssen COVID-19 Vaccine	Injection suspension	IM	0.5 mL as a single dose initially, followed by a booster dose ≥2 months later	Available based on an FDA Emergency Use Authorization to prevent COVID-19 in persons at least 18 yrs of age as of March 2022	Rare cases of thrombosis-thrombocytopenia syndrome have been reported; this risk has been designated as very low, and the FDA has determined that the benefits of this vaccine outweigh risks

Continued next page

MEDICATION TABLE 30-1. Immunizations[5] (Continued)

Vaccine	Category	Brand Name	Dosage Form	Route	Dosing/Schedule	Indications	Notes/Recommendations
							in individuals aged 18 yrs and older; as of May 2021, ACIP recommends all individuals to receive any age-appropriate COVID-19 vaccine if no contraindications are present; review of storage conditions and steps for administration is key
COVID-19 vaccine (mRNA)	mRNA vaccine	Moderna COVID-19 Vaccine; Comirnaty Pfizer-BioNTech vaccine, Spikevax Moderna vaccine	Injection suspension	IM	Moderna vaccine: 2 doses of 0.5 mL separated by 4–8 weeks; booster 50 mcg dose (volume pending product used) as a single dose ≥5 months after last primary series dose. A second 0.3 mL booster dose may be considered at least 4 months following the first booster dose in all individuals at least 50 years of age and in moderately to severely immunocompromised individuals between 18 and 50 years of age as of March 2022 Pfizer-BioNTech vaccine: 2 doses of 0.3 mL separated by 3–8 weeks; booster 0.3 mL as a single dose ≥5 months after last primary series dose; A second 50 mcg (volume pending product used) booster dose may be considered at least 4 months following the first booster dose in all individuals at least 50 years	COVID-19 prevention: active immunization to prevent COVID-19 in the following persons: ≥5 years of age (Comirnaty [Pfizer-BioNTech vaccine]) or ≥18 years of age (Spikevax [Moderna vaccine]) as of March 2022	As of May 2021, ACIP recommends all individuals to receive any age-appropriate COVID-19 vaccine if no contraindications are present; review of storage conditions and steps for administration is key for each product

Continued next page

MEDICATION TABLE 30-1. Immunizations[5] *(Continued)*

Vaccine	Category	Brand Name	Dosage Form	Route	Dosing/Schedule	Indications	Notes/Recommendations
					of age and in moderately to severely immunocompromised individuals between 18 and 50 years of age as of March 2022		
Dengue tetravalent vaccine	Live (viral)	Dengvaxia	Injection suspension	SUBQ	0.5 mL per dose at 0, 6, and 12 mos	Immunization against dengue fever in individuals with previous laboratory-confirmed dengue disease	Use in individuals between the ages of 9 and 16 living in endemic areas of dengue fever; administration to individuals without previous dengue infection increases the risk of severe dengue complications
Ebola zaire vaccine	Live (viral)	Ervebo	Injection suspension	IM	1 mL as a single dose	Immunization against disease due to *Zaire ebolavirus*	Preexposure vaccination is recommended for individuals at least 18 years of age who are responding to an Ebola virus outbreak, are healthcare professionals working at a federally designated Ebola treatment center, or those working at a biosafety level 4 facility. Protection is not provided against other species of *Ebolavirus* or *Marburgvirus*; duration of protection is unknown; antiviral medication, immune globulin, and/or blood/plasma transfusions may limit effectiveness
Haemophilus b conjugate vaccine	Inactivated (bacterial)	ActHIB, Hiberix, PedvaxHIB	Injection powder for reconstitution; injection suspension	IM	Variable immunization schedule depending on age, product used, immunization history, and health status	Immunization against invasive disease caused by *Haemophilus influenzae* type b	Routine vaccination of all children 2–59 months recommended by the ACIP; unvaccinated individuals with high-risk conditions such

Continued next page

MEDICATION TABLE 30-1. Immunizations[5] (Continued)

Vaccine	Category	Brand Name	Dosage Form	Route	Dosing/Schedule	Indications	Notes/Recommendations
							as anatomical or functional asplenia; all individuals with hematopoietic stem cell transplantation
Hepatitis A virus vaccine	Inactivated (viral)	Havrix, VAQTA	Injection suspension	IM	Varies depending on age and vaccine administered; doses range from 0.5–1 mL based on age	Immunization to HAV in individuals 12 mos of age and older	ACIP recommends routine vaccination with hepatitis A vaccine for all children at 1 year, as well as adults desiring protection or at risk for infection
Hepatitis B vaccine, recombinant	Inactivated (viral)	Engerix-B, Recombivax HB	Injection suspension	IM	Varies depending on age and clinical situation; infants ≥2 kg born to mothers who are negative for the HBV surface antigen should receive three 0.5-mL doses, with the first being within 24 hours of birth, the second at 1–2 mos of age, and the third at 6–18 mos of age (6–12 mos if the environment is one with elevated rates of childhood HBV infection); unvaccinated adolescents between ages 11 and 15 may receive a catch-up 2-dose series with adult Recombivax HB only, with 4 months between doses	Immunization against infection caused by HBV	ACIP recommends routine vaccination for all neonates; all infants and children; all unvaccinated adults at risk or requesting protection from infection; while HBV products may differ by concentration, dosing by volume yields the same equivalent dose between products; different formulations exist for adults and pediatric/adolescent patients
Hepatitis B vaccine, recombinant, adjuvanted	Inactivated (Viral)	Heplisav-B	Injection solution	IM	0.5 mL/dose for 2 total doses administered at least 1 month apart	Immunization against infection caused by HBV in adults	ACIP recommends as an option used to complete a 2-dose series in adults at risk or requesting protection from HBV infection

Continued next page

MEDICATION TABLE 30-1. Immunizations[5] *(Continued)*

Vaccine	Category	Brand Name	Dosage Form	Route	Dosing/Schedule	Indications	Notes/Recommendations
Human papillomavirus vaccine	Inactivated (viral)	Gardasil 9	Injection suspension	IM	0.5 mL at 0, 2, and 6 mos; only 2 doses needed if both administered before 15 yrs of age and 5 mos apart (second dose at 6–12 mos) in individuals without immunocompromising conditions	Utilized for the prevention of several reproductive tract, anal, and head and neck cancers, as well as genital warts caused by several types of human papilloma virus in men and women aged 9–45 yrs	ACIP recommends for all adolescents at age 11–12 yrs (can start at 9 yrs) through 18 yrs. ACIP also recommends for all persons through age 26 yrs and adults between 27 and 45 yrs based on shared decision making between the patient and their healthcare provider team
Influenza virus vaccine inactivated	Inactivated (viral)	Afluria quadrivalent, Fluarix quadrivalent, FluLaval quadrivalent, Fluzone quadrivalent, Fluzone high-dose quadrivalent, Flucelvax quadrivalent, Fluad, Fluad quadrivalent	Injection suspension	IM	0.5 mL/dose (2 doses separated by 4 weeks in children 6 mos-8 yrs who did not receive at least 2 doses previously; one dose per season thereafter)	Active immunity to influenza virus strains contained in the vaccine	ACIP recommends 1 dose IIV, RIV, or LAIV per age and health status annually, ideally in September and October (after initial 2 doses for patients aged 6 mos-8 yrs)
Influenza virus vaccine recombinant	Recombinant (viral) (RIV4)	Flublok quadrivalent	Injection solution	IM	0.5 mL/dose (2 doses separated by 4 weeks in children 6 mos-8 yrs who did not receive at least 2 doses previously; one dose per season thereafter)	Active immunity to influenza virus strains contained in the vaccine	ACIP states that persons at least 18 yrs of age are eligible for RIV in addition to other age-appropriate and health-status-appropriate formulations
Influenza virus vaccine live/attenuated	Live attenuated (viral) (LAIV4)	N/A	Nasal solution	Intranasal	0.2 mL/dose (0.1 mL/nostril)	Active immunity to influenza virus strains contained in the vaccine	ACIP states that healthy, nonpregnant persons without listed contraindications aged 2–49 yrs are eligible for this immunization in

Continued next page

MEDICATION TABLE 30-1. Immunizations[5] (Continued)

Vaccine	Category	Brand Name	Dosage Form	Route	Dosing/Schedule	Indications	Notes/Recommendations
							addition to other age-appropriate and health-status-appropriate formulations; patient may breathe normally during administration
Japanese encephalitis virus vaccine	Inactivated (viral)	Ixiaro	Injection suspension	IM	0.5 mL/dose; a total of two doses given on days 0 and 7 to 28; series should be completed at least 1 wk prior to potential exposure; administer 0.5-mL booster dose at least 1 yr after completion if ongoing exposure	Active immunization against Japanese encephalitis in those at least 2 mos of age	ACIP recommends vaccination for persons spending more than 1 mo in endemic areas, those frequently traveling to endemic areas, or research laboratory workers who may be exposed to the virus
Meningococcal (groups A/C/Y and W-135) diphtheria conjugate vaccine	Inactivated (bacterial)	Menactra (MenACWY-D), MenQuadfi (MenACWY-TT), Menveo (MenACWY-CRM)	Injection solution	IM	0.5 mL/dose given as a 2-dose series at 11–12 yrs then at 16 yrs; special situations require different regimens depending on the selected product and situation	Active immunization of children and adults against invasive meningococcal disease caused by bacterial serogroups A, C, Y, and W-135	ACIP recommends college students should get booster if not previously vaccinated at age 16 or older; certain individuals aged at least 2 mos may require immunization if uniquely susceptible to infection
Meningococcal group B vaccine	Inactivated (bacterial)	Bexsero (MenB-4C), Trumenba (MenB-FHbp)	Injection suspension	IM	Differs based on brand use and patient population	Prevention of meningococcal group B disease	ACIP recommends use for individuals ≥10 yrs at risk for MenB, and for healthy adolescents and young adults between the ages of 16 and 23 based on shared decision making: between the patient and their healthcare provider team (preferred age for vaccination is 16–18 yrs); either product may be used, but they may not be interchanged mid-series

Continued next page

MEDICATION TABLE 30-1. Immunizations[5] *(Continued)*

Vaccine	Category	Brand Name	Dosage Form	Route	Dosing/Schedule	Indications	Notes/Recommendations
Pneumococcal conjugate vaccine (13-Valent) (PCV13)	Inactivated (bacterial)	Prevnar 13	Injection suspension	IM	0.5 mL as a single dose; infants and children 6 wks to 59 mos are given a total of four doses; first at 2 mos of age, the remaining three doses given at 4, 6, and 12–15 mos; variable separate recommendations based on qualifying chronic disease	Immunization of infants, children, adolescents, and adults against invasive disease, otitis media, and pneumonia caused by *Streptococcus pneumoniae* (pending age group)	ACIP recommends routine vaccination for all children aged 2–59 mos; children with certain chronic diseases
Pneumococcal conjugate vaccine (15-valent) (PCV15)	Inactivated (bacterial)	Vaxneuvance	Injection suspension	IM	0.5 mL as a single dose to adults aged at least 65 yrs if no history of pneumococcal conjugate vaccines; variable separate recommendations based on qualifying chronic disease	Active immunization for preventing invasive disease caused by certain *Streptococcus pneumoniae* serotypes in adults at least 18 yrs of age	ACIP recommends for adults aged 65 years or older with no history of receiving a pneumococcal conjugate vaccine or with an unknown vaccination history; and for adults with certain chronic disease states with no history of receiving a pneumococcal conjugate vaccine. Use of PCV15 should be followed with PPSV23, if PPSV23 has not been previously given, at an interval pending the presence of certain chronic disease states.
Pneumococcal conjugate vaccine (20-valent) (PCV20)	Inactivated (bacterial)	Prevnar 20	Injection suspension	IM	0.5 mL as a single dose to adults aged at least 65 yrs if no history of pneumococcal conjugate vaccines; variable separate recommendations based on qualifying chronic disease	Active immunization for preventing pneumonia and invasive disease caused by certain *Streptococcus pneumoniae* serotypes in adults at least 18 years of age	ACIP recommends for adults aged 65 years or older with no history of receiving a pneumococcal conjugate vaccine or with an unknown vaccination history; and for adults with certain chronic disease states with no history of receiving a pneumococcal conjugate vaccine.

Continued next page

MEDICATION TABLE 30-1. Immunizations[5] *(Continued)*

Vaccine	Category	Brand Name	Dosage Form	Route	Dosing/Schedule	Indications	Notes/Recommendations
Pneumococcal polysaccharide vaccine (23-Valent) (PPSV23)	Inactivated (bacterial)	Pneumovax 23	Injection solution	IM; SUBQ	0.5 mL as a single dose at 65 yrs or older pending previous receipt of PCV13 or PCV15 per current ACIP recommendations; variable separate recommendations based on qualifying chronic disease states pending receipt of PCV13 or PCV15 per current ACIP recommendations	Prevention of pneumococcal disease (ie, caused by *S. pneumoniae*) in recommended age/ health status groups	ACIP recommends routine vaccination for adults aged at least 65 if no PPSV23 received after age 65 and no PPSV23 within the past 5 years pending receipt of PCV13 or PCV15 per current ACIP recommendations
Poliovirus vaccine	Inactivated (viral)	IPOL	Injection suspension	IM, SUBQ	4 doses, 0.5 mL each, at ages 2, 4, 6–18 mos, 4–6 yrs; the final dose should be administered on or after the 4th birthday and separated from the previous dose by 6 mos	Active immunization against poliomyelitis caused by poliovirus types 1, 2, and 3	ACIP recommends routine vaccination for all infants and children; certain adults may qualify for immunization at a modified schedule based on previous immunization status and exposure risk
Rabies vaccine	Inactivated (viral)	Imovax Rabies, RabAvert	Injectable; injection suspension	IM	Postexposure for immunocompetent persons not previously immunized: 4 doses (1 mL each) on days 0, 3, 7, 14; in addition to rabies immune globulin with the first dose Preexposure vaccination: three 1-mL doses on days 0, 7, and 21 or 28; regimen changes in those immunocompromised or with previous immunization to rabies	Preexposure and postexposure immunization against rabies	ACIP recommends a primary course of prophylactic immunization for certain persons at risk of infection and postexposure vaccination for an individual assessed by the severity and likelihood vs. the actual risk of acquiring rabies

Continued next page

MEDICATION TABLE 30-1. Immunizations[5] (Continued)

Vaccine	Category	Brand Name	Dosage Form	Route	Dosing/Schedule	Indications	Notes/Recommendations
Rotavirus vaccine	Live (viral)	Rotarix, RotaTeq	Powder for oral suspension; oral solution	Oral	Rotarix: 1 mL/dose at 2 and 4 mos of age RotaTeq: 2 mL/dose at 2, 4, and 6 mos of age	Prevention of rotavirus gastroenteritis in infants and children	ACIP recommends routine vaccination of all infants
Smallpox vaccine	Live (viral)	ACAM2000	Injection powder for reconstitution	Percutaneous (vaccination by scarification multiple-puncture technique only)	A single drop of vaccine suspension and 15 needle punctures (using the same bifurcated needle) into the superficial skin; a trace of blood should appear at vaccination site after 15–20 sec	Active immunization against smallpox disease in persons at high risk for smallpox infection	ACIP recommends routine vaccination for laboratory workers at high risk of exposure, healthcare workers having contact with clinical specimens, persons designated by authorities to investigate smallpox cases with the likelihood of direct patient contact, persons responsible for administering the vaccine, persons exposed to release of the virus, persons likely to have increased contact with infectious materials, or those in close contact for ≥3 hrs with others having suspected or confirmed cases
Typhoid vaccine (inactivated)	Inactivated (bacterial)	Typhim Vi	Injection solution	IM	0.5 mL at least 2 weeks prior to expected exposure; revaccination every 2 yrs with continued exposure	Active immunization against typhoid fever caused by *Salmonella typhi*	Not for routine vaccination; in the United States, use is limited to persons at least 2 years of age traveling to risk areas for *S. typhi* or persons with exposure to the pathogen
Typhoid vaccine (live)	Live (bacterial)	Vivotif	Capsule, enteric coated	Oral	One capsule on alternate days (day 1, 3, 5, and 7) for 4 doses at least 1 wk prior to exposure; repeat every 5 yrs with continued exposure	Active immunization against typhoid fever caused by *Salmonella typhi*	Not for routine vaccination; in the United States, use is limited to persons older than 6 years traveling to risk areas for *S. typhi* or persons with exposure to the pathogen

Continued next page

MEDICATION TABLE 30-1. Immunizations[5] *(Continued)*

Vaccine	Category	Brand Name	Dosage Form	Route	Dosing/Schedule	Indications	Notes/Recommendations
Varicella virus vaccine	Live (viral)	Varivax	Injection	SUBQ	Two doses of 0.5 mL at age 12–15 mos, then 4–6 years; dose 2 may be administered as early as 3 months after dose 1; administer 4–8 wks apart in qualifying adults	Immunization against varicella in children over 12 mos of age and adults without evidence of immunity	ACIP recommends vaccination for all children, adolescents, and adults who do not have evidence of immunity
Yellow fever vaccine	Live (viral)	YF-VAX	Injection powder for reconstitution	SUBQ	One dose (0.5 mL) at least 10 days before travel; booster every 10 yrs for those at an increased risk for disease but is generally not needed	Induction of active immunity against yellow fever virus	ACIP recommends vaccinations primarily for those traveling to or living in areas at risk for yellow fever transmission, traveling to countries that require vaccination for international travel, and laboratory personnel who may be exposed to the yellow fever virus or concentrated preparations of the vaccine; use may be considered in children at least 6 mos of age in unique circumstances
Zoster vaccine (RZV)	Recombinant	Shingrix	Reconstituted suspension	IM	0.5 mL administered as a 2-dose series at 0 and 2–6 mos	Prevention of herpes zoster (shingles) in patients at least 50 yrs of age	ACIP recommends for all adults 50 years or older including those who have received the previous live zoster vaccine (abbreviated as ZVL and previously branded as Zostavax); RZV use is under review in severely immunocompromised individuals; consider delaying until after pregnancy

ACIP = Advisory Committee on Immunization Practices; FDA = U.S. Food and Drug Administration; HAV = hepatitis A virus; HBV = hepatitis B virus; HPV = human papillomavirus; IM = intramuscular; MenB = meningococcal group B; mos = months; N/A = none available; SUBQ = subcutaneous; wks = weeks; yrs = years.

MEDICATION TABLE 30-2. Combined Immunizations[5]

Vaccine	Category	Brand Name	Dosage Form	Route	Dosing/Schedule	Indication	Notes/Recommendations
Diphtheria and tetanus toxoids (Td)	Inactivated (bacterial)	TDVax, Tenivac	Injectable; injection suspension	IM	0.5 mL/dose; administer as a booster every 10 yrs after scheduled Tdap; additionally, a component of catch-up regimen in adults without previous diphtheria, tetanus, and pertussis immunization	Active immunization against diphtheria and tetanus	Abbreviated "Td" as it contains a relatively high amount of Tetanus toxoids and a relatively low amount of diphtheria toxoids; also available with a relatively high amount of both components as a generic formulation for use in selected patients aged 6 wks to <7 yrs; Td may also be used in selected individuals with wounds to confer additional tetanus protection or those with contraindications to pertussis-containing vaccines using a modified schedule
Diphtheria toxoid/ tetanus toxoid/ acellular pertussis vaccine, adsorbed (DTaP/Tdap)	Inactivated (bacterial)	Adacel, Boostrix, Daptacel, Infanrix	Injection suspension	IM	0.5 mL/dose; DTaP: 5 total doses administered at 2, 4, 6, 15–18 mos, and 4-6 yrs Tdap: 1 dose for adolescents/adults (indicated at age 11 or 12 yrs) who have not received a booster dose; one additional dose during each pregnancy during gestational weeks 27–36	Daptacel, Infanrix: active immunization against diphtheria, tetanus, and pertussis from age 6 wks to 6 yrs; Adacel, Boostrix: active booster immunization against such infections	Abbreviated DTaP (Daptacel, Infanrix) as it contains relatively high amounts of Diphtheria toxoids, Tetanus toxoids, and acellular Pertussis; abbreviated Tdap (Adacel, Boostrix) as it contains relatively high amounts of Tetanus toxoids, relatively low amounts of diphtheria toxoids, and acellular pertussis. DTaP is utilized in children to confer initial active immunity, while Tdap is utilized as a booster
Diphtheria, tetanus toxoids, acellular pertussis, hepatitis B (recombinant) and inactivated poliovirus vaccine combined (DTaP/HBV/IPV)	Inactivated (bacterial/viral)	Pediarix	Injection suspension	IM	0.5 mL/dose; administer as a 3-dose series at 2, 4, and 6–18 mos of age in 6- to 8-wk intervals	Active immunization against diphtheria, tetanus, pertussis, hepatitis B virus, and poliomyelitis in children between the ages of 6 wks and 6 yrs	Can be used to satisfy 3 of the 5 DTaP doses, the HBV series, and approved for the first 3 doses of the polio vaccine series; may be used as a component of catch-up immunizations if needed

Continued next page

MEDICATION TABLE 30-2. Combined Immunizations[5] *(Continued)*

Vaccine	Category	Brand Name	Dosage Form	Route	Dosing/Schedule	Indication	Notes/Recommendations
Diphtheria and tetanus toxoids, acellular pertussis, poliovirus, and *Haemophilus* b conjugate vaccine (DTaP/IPV/HiB)	Inactivated (bacterial/viral)	Pentacel	Injection suspension	IM	0.5 mL per dose administered at 2, 4, 6, and 15–18 mos of age (total of 4 doses)	Active immunization against diphtheria, tetanus, pertussis, poliomyelitis, and invasive disease caused by *H. influenzae* type b in children from age 6 wks-4 yrs	Satisfies 4 of the 5 required DTaP doses, the *Haemophilus* B series, and approved for the first 3 doses of polio vaccine; may be used as a component of catch-up immunizations if needed
Diphtheria and tetanus toxoid, acellular pertussis, and poliovirus vaccine (DTaP/IPV)	Inactivated (bacterial/viral)	Kinrix, Quadracel	Injection suspension	IM	0.5 mL as a single dose	Active immunization against diphtheria, tetanus, pertussis, and poliomyelitis in children from age 4–6 yrs	May be used as the fifth dose in the childhood DTaP series and the fourth dose in the childhood IPV series; different products are recommended based on the specific brands utilized for previous doses in each vaccine series
Diphtheria and tetanus toxoids, acellular pertussis, hepatitis B (recombinant), poliovirus (inactivated), and *Haemophilus influenzae* b conjugate (adsorbed) vaccine (DTaP/HBV/IPV/HiB)	Inactivated (bacterial/viral)	Vaxelis	Injection suspension	IM	0.5 mL per dose administered at 2, 4, and 6 mos of age (total of 3 doses)	Active immunization against diphtheria, tetanus, pertussis, hepatitis B, poliomyelitis, and *H. influenzae* type b in infants and children between 6 wks and 4 yrs of age	Use is not recommended for subsequent doses of vaccine series that require additional doses following the 3 doses of this combination vaccine; may be used as a component of catch-up immunizations if needed
Hepatitis A and hepatitis B recombinant vaccine	Inactivated (Viral)	Twinrix	Injection suspension	IM	1 mL per dose given at 0, 1, and 6 mos as a catch-up strategy	Active immunization against disease caused by hepatitis A virus and hepatitis B virus in individuals aged 18 yrs and older	Only approved for persons at least 18 yrs of age; an accelerated regimen is available (3 doses at 0, 7, and 21–30 days, followed by a booster dose at 12 months)

Continued next page

MEDICATION TABLE 30-2. Combined Immunizations[5] *(Continued)*

Vaccine	Category	Brand Name	Dosage Form	Route	Dosing/Schedule	Indication	Notes/Recommendations
Measles, mumps, and rubella virus vaccine	Live (viral)	M-M-R II	Injection powder for reconstitution	SUBQ	Primary immunization: 0.5 mL at 12–15 mos and repeated at 4–6 yrs; the second dose must be at least 4 wks after the first	Active immunization for measles, mumps, and rubella in those at least 12 mos of age	ACIP recommends routine vaccination for all children, adults born 1957 or later without evidence of vaccination or immunity, adults born before 1957 without contraindications, and adults at higher risk for exposure; various catch-up and special-situation administration regimens exist
Measles, mumps, rubella, and varicella virus vaccine (MMRV)	Live (viral)	ProQuad	Injection powder for reconstitution	SUBQ	Primary immunization: 0.5 mL at 12–15 mos and repeated at 4–6 yrs; the second dose must be at least 3 mos after the first	Active immunization for measles, mumps, rubella, and varicella in those 12 mos through 12 yrs of age	Children receiving their first MMR and varicella vaccines between 12 and 47 mos of age are recommended to receive separate vaccines; those receiving their first doses at 48 mos of age or older, or their second dose, are recommended to receive MMRV
Smallpox and monkeypox vaccine	Live (viral)	Jynneos	Injection suspension	SUBQ	2 doses, 0.5 mL each, 4 wks apart	Active immunization against smallpox and monkeypox in adults at least 18 yrs of age at high risk for either infection	FDA approved in 2019, with uncertain availability

ACIP = Advisory Committee on Immunization Practices; DTaP = Diphtheria, Tetanus, and acellular Pertussis; HBV = hepatitis B virus; HiB = *Haemophilus influenzae* type B; IPV = inactivated polio vaccine; Tdap = Tetanus, diphtheria, and acellular pertussis; Td = Tetanus and diphtheria; IM = intramuscular; SUBQ = subcutaneous; mos = months; wks = weeks; yrs = years.

MEDICATION TABLE 30-3. Agents Used for Passive Immunity[5]

Agent	Brand Name	Indication	Route
Ansuvimab	Ebanga	Treatment of infection due to *Zaire ebolavirus* in adult and pediatric patients, including neonates born to a mother who is positive for *Z. ebolavirus* infection	IV
Anthrax immune globulin (human)	Anthrasil	Treatment of inhalational anthrax exposure in adult and pediatric patients in combination with an appropriate antibacterial drug regimen	IV
Antivenin (*Latrodectus mactans*)	N/A	Treatment of patients with moderate to severe symptoms due to *Latrodectus mactans* (black widow spider) envenomation	IM, IV
Antivenin (*Micrurus fulvius*)	N/A	Treatment of envenomation by Eastern coral snake or Texas coral snake	IV
Atoltivimab, Maftivimab, and Odesivimab	Inmazeb	Treatment of infection due to *Z. ebolavirus* in adult and pediatric patients, including neonates born to a mother who is positive for *Z. ebolavirus* infection	IV
Bamlanivimab and Etesevimab	N/A	Authorized for Emergency Use by the FDA in February 2021 for preventing hospitalizations or emergency department visits related to COVID-19 in patients with mild to moderate COVID-19 who are not hospitalized; use per the EUA should be limited to those aged at least 12 years weighing at least 40 kg with a positive COVID-19 viral test and with a designation of being at high risk for progression to severe COVID-19/hospitalization	IV
Bezlotoxumab	Zinplava	To decrease the recurrence of *Clostridioides difficile* infection (CDI) in individuals at least 18 years of age who are being treated with antibiotics for CDI and at a high risk for recurrence of CDI	IV
Botulism antitoxin, heptavalent	N/A	Treatment of symptomatic botulism due to exposure to serotype A, B, C, D, E, F, or G neurotoxin in children or adults	IV
Botulism immune globulin IV	BabyBIG	Treatment of infant botulism due to type A or B toxin	IV
Casirivimab and Imdevimab	N/A	Authorized for Emergency Use by the FDA in November 2020 for preventing hospitalizations or emergency department visits related to COVID-19 in patients with mild to moderate COVID-19 who are not hospitalized; use per the EUA should be limited to those aged at least 12 years weighing at least 40 kg with a positive COVID-19 viral test and with a designation of being at high risk for progression to severe COVID-19/hospitalization	IV
Centruroides immune F(ab')₂ (Equine)	Anascorp	Treatment of envenomation by a scorpion	IV
Crotalidae immune F(ab')₂ (Equine)	Anavip	Treatment of envenomation by a North American rattlesnake	IV
Crotalidae polyvalent immune FAB (Ovine)	CroFab	Management of patients with North American crotalid envenomation (eg, rattlesnakes, copperheads, and cottonmouth/water moccasins)	IV

Continued next page

MEDICATION TABLE 30-3. Agents Used for Passive Immunity[5] (Continued)

Agent	Brand Name	Indication	Route
Cytomegalovirus immune globulin IV–Human	CytoGam	Prophylaxis of cytomegalovirus (CMV) disease related to several solid organ transplants	IV
Digoxin immune Fab	DigiFab	Treatment of serious or life-threatening digoxin intoxication	IV
Diphtheria antitoxin	N/A	Treatment of *Corynebacterium diphtheriae* infection	IM, IV
Hepatitis B immune globulin	HepaGAM B, HyperHEP B, Nabi-HB	Passive prophylactic immunity to hepatitis B following acute exposure to blood, plasma, or serum containing hepatitis B surface antigen (HBsAg); perinatal exposure of infants born to HBsAg-positive mothers; sexual exposure to HBsAg-positive persons; household contact with persons with acute HBV infection	IM, IV
Ibalizumab	Trogarzo	Treatment of human immunodeficiency virus-1 (HIV-1) infection as a component of an antiretroviral regimen in heavily treatment-experienced patients who are infected with a multidrug-resistant HIV-1 infection and whose current therapy is failing	IV
Idarucizumab	Praxbind	Monoclonal antibody reversal agent for dabigatran when emergent reversal is necessary (eg, life-threatening bleeding)	IV
Immune globulin	GamaSTAN (many others for nonpassive immunity indications)	Provision of passive immunity to individuals susceptible to hepatitis A, measles, rubella, and varicella	IM
Obiltoxaximab	N/A	Component of treatment for and prophylaxis against inhalational anthrax	IV
Palivizumab	Synagis	Prevention of serious disease caused by respiratory syncytial virus in selected high-risk pediatric patients	IM
Rabies immune globulin	HyperRAB, HyperRAB S/D, Imogam Rabies-HT, Kedrab	Part of postexposure prophylaxis of persons with rabies exposure	IM, SUBQ (Kedrab)
Raxibacumab	N/A	Component of treatment for and prophylaxis against anthrax exposure	IV
Rh₀(D) immune globulin	HyperRHO S/D, MICRhoGAM Ultra-Filtered Plus, RhoGAM Ultra-Filtered Plus, Rhophylac, WinRho SDF	Suppression of RhD isoimmunization in individuals receiving blood that is RhD-positive who are otherwise RhD-negative; suppression of RhD isoimmunization in RhD-incompatible pregnancies; immune thrombocytopenia in RhD-positive individuals	IM, IV
Tetanus immune globulin (Human)	HyperTET S/D	Prophylaxis against tetanus following injury in individuals with incomplete or uncertain immunization status, or treatment in active infection	IM
Vaccinia immune globulin (IV)	CNJ-016	Treatment of infectious complications of the vaccinia virus	IV
Varicella-zoster immune globulin (human)	Varizig	Prophylaxis against varicella in high-risk individuals ineligible for the varicella vaccine who have been exposed to the virus	IM

EUA = Emergency Use Authorization; IM = intramuscular; IV = intravascular; N/A = none available; SUBQ = subcutaneous.

MEDICATION TABLE 30-4. Immunosuppressive Agents[5]

Agent	Class	Brand Name	Formulation	Route	Selected Indication
Alemtuzumab	Anti-CD52 agent	Campath, Lemtrada	Injection solution	IV (Campath, Lemtrada), SUBQ (Campath)	Induction of immunosuppression in heart (off-label), lung (off-label), and kidney (off-label) transplant; treatment of steroid-resistant renal transplant rejection (off-label)
Antithymocyte globulin (Equine)	Polyclonal antibody	Atgam	Injection solution	IV	Prevention of lung transplant rejection (off-label)
Antithymocyte globulin (Rabbit)	Polyclonal antibody	Thymoglobulin	Injection solution	IV	Prevention of intestinal transplant rejection (off-label) as well as prevention and treatment of lung (off-label), heart (off-label), and kidney transplant rejection
Azathioprine	Antimetabolite	Azasan, Imuran	Injection solution (generic), tablet (Azasan, Imuran, generic)	IV, oral	Prevention of kidney and nonkidney (off-label) transplant rejection
Basiliximab	Monoclonal antibody; interleukin-2 inhibitor	Simulect	Injection solution	IV	Prevention of kidney, heart (off-label), liver (off-label), and lung (off-label) transplant rejection
Belatacept	Selective T-cell costimulation blocker	Nulojix	Injection solution	IV	Prophylaxis of kidney transplant rejection in Epstein-Barr virus–positive recipients, prevention of rejection in lung transplant (off-label)
Cyclosporine	Calcineurin inhibitor	Gengraf, Neoral, SandIMMUNE	Capsule (Gengraf, Neoral, SandIMMUNE, generic), injection solution (SandIMMUNE, generic), oral solution (Gengraf, Neoral, SandIMMUNE, generic)	Oral, IV	Prophylaxis of rejection in heart, liver, kidney, and lung (off-label) transplants
Everolimus	mTOR inhibitor	Zortress (other brand names for nontransplant indications)	Tablet (Zortress, generic)	Oral	Prophylaxis of liver, kidney, heart (off-label), and lung (off-label) transplant rejection

Continued next page

MEDICATION TABLE 30-4. Immunosuppressive Agents[5] (Continued)

Agent	Class	Brand Name	Formulation	Route	Selected Indication
Mycophenolate	Immunosuppressant	CellCept, CellCept IV, Myfortic	Capsule (CellCept, generic), tablet (CellCept, generic), delayed-release tablet (Myfortic, generic), injection solution (CellCept IV, generic), oral suspension (CellCept, generic)	Oral, IV	Prophylaxis of heart (off-label with Myfortic), liver (off-label with Myfortic), kidney, and lung (off-label) transplant rejection
Sirolimus	mTOR inhibitor	Rapamune	Tablet, oral solution	Oral	Prophylaxis of heart (off-label), lung (off-label), and kidney transplant rejection
Rituximab	Anti-CD20 agent	Rituxan	Injection solution	IV	Treatment of rejection in antibody-mediated cardiac transplant (off-label)
Tacrolimus	Calcineurin inhibitor	Astagraf XL, Envarsus XR, Prograf	Capsule (Prograf, generic), capsule extended release (Astagraf XL), oral packet (Prograf), injection solution (Prograf), tablet extended release (Envarsus XR)	Oral, IV, nasogastric tube (contents of IR capsules), sublingual (contents of IR capsules)	Prophylaxis of heart (Prograf), kidney (Astagraf XL, Envarsus XR, Prograf), liver (Prograf), and intestine (off-label) transplant rejection

IR = immediate release; IV = intravenous; SUBQ = subcutaneous.

MEDICATION TABLE 30-5. Biosimilar Agents[6]

Agent	Brand Name	Reference Agent (Brand)	Biosimilar or Interchangeable	Route	Medication Class
Adalimumab-adaz	Hyrimoz	Adalimumab (Humira)	Biosimilar	SUBQ	TNF blocking agent
Adalimumab-adbm	Cyltezo	Adalimumab (Humira)	Interchangeable	SUBQ	TNF blocking agent
Adalimumab-afzb	Abrilada	Adalimumab (Humira)	Biosimilar	SUBQ	TNF blocking agent
Adalimumab-aqvh	Yusimry	Adalimumab (Humira)	Biosimilar	SUBQ	TNF blocking agent
Adalimumab-atto	Amjevita	Adalimumab (Humira)	Biosimilar	SUBQ	TNF blocking agent
Adalimumab-bwwd	Hadlima	Adalimumab (Humira)	Biosimilar	SUBQ	TNF blocking agent
Adalimumab-fkjb	Hulio	Adalimumab (Humira)	Biosimilar	SUBQ	TNF blocking agent
Bevacizumab-awwb	Mvasi	Bevacizumab (Avastin)	Biosimilar	IV	VEGF inhibitor
Bevacizumab-bvzr	Zirabev	Bevacizumab (Avastin)	Biosimilar	IV	VEGF inhibitor
Epoetin alfa-epbx	Retacrit	Epoetin alfa (Epogen/Procrit)	Biosimilar	IV, SUBQ	Colony stimulating factor
Etanercept-szzs	Erelzi	Etanercept (Enbrel)	Biosimilar	SUBQ	TNF blocking agent
Etanercept-ykro	Eticovo	Etanercept (Enbrel)	Biosimilar	SUBQ	TNF blocking agent
Filgrastim-aafi	Nivestym	Filgrastim (Neupogen)	Biosimilar	IV, SUBQ	Colony stimulating factor
Filgrastim-ayow	Releuko	Filgrastim (Neupogen)	Biosimilar	IV, SUBQ	Colony stimulating factor
Filgrastim-sndz	Zarxio	Filgrastim (Neupogen)	Biosimilar	IV, SUBQ	Colony stimulating factor
Infliximab-abda	Renflexis	Infliximab (Remicade)	Biosimilar	IV	TNF blocking agent
Infliximab-axxq	Avsola	Infliximab (Remicade)	Biosimilar	IV	TNF blocking agent
Infliximab-dyyb	Inflectra	Infliximab (Remicade)	Biosimilar	IV	TNF blocking agent
Infliximab-qbtx	Ixifi	Infliximab (Remicade)	Biosimilar	IV	TNF blocking agent
Insulin glargine-aglr	Rezvoglar	Insulin glargine (Lantus)	Biosimilar	SUBQ	Insulin, long-acting
Insulin glargine-yfgn	Semglee	Insulin glargine (Lantus)	Interchangeable	SUBQ	Insulin, long-acting
Pegfilgrastim-apgf	Nyvepria	Pegfilgrastim (Neulasta)	Biosimilar	SUBQ	Colony stimulating factor
Pegfilgrastim-bmez	Ziextenzo	Pegfilgrastim (Neulasta)	Biosimilar	SUBQ	Colony stimulating factor
Pegfilgrastim-cbqv	Udenyca	Pegfilgrastim (Neulasta)	Biosimilar	SUBQ	Colony stimulating factor
Pegfilgrastim-jmdb	Fulphila	Pegfilgrastim (Neulasta)	Biosimilar	SUBQ	Colony stimulating factor
Ranibizumab-nuna	Byooviz	Ranibizumab (Lucentis)	Biosimilar	Intravitreal	Angiogenesis inhibitor
Rituximab-abbs	Truxima	Rituximab (Rituxan)	Biosimilar	IV	Anti-CD20 agent

Continued next page

MEDICATION TABLE 30-5. Biosimilar Agents[6] (Continued)

Agent	Brand Name	Reference Agent (Brand)	Biosimilar or Interchangeable	Route	Medication Class
Rituximab-arrx	Riabni	Rituximab (Rituxan)	Biosimilar	IV	Anti-CD20 agent
Rituximab-pvvr	Ruxience	Rituximab (Rituxan)	Biosimilar	IV	Anti-CD20 agent
Trastuzumab-anns	Kanjinti	Trastuzumab (Herceptin)	Biosimilar	IV	Anti-HER2 agent
Trastuzumab-dkst	Ogivri	Trastuzumab (Herceptin)	Biosimilar	IV	Anti-HER2 agent
Trastuzumab-dttb	Ontruzant	Trastuzumab (Herceptin)	Biosimilar	IV	Anti-HER2 agent
Trastuzumab-pkrb	Herzuma	Trastuzumab (Herceptin)	Biosimilar	IV	Anti-HER2 agent
Trastuzumab-qyyp	Trazimera	Trastuzumab (Herceptin)	Biosimilar	IV	Anti-HER2 agent

HER2 = human epidermal growth factor receptor 2; IV = intravenous; SUBQ = subcutaneous; TNF = tumor necrosis factor; VEGF = vascular endothelial growth factor.

Part 10

ANTINEOPLASTIC AGENTS

Chapter 31

Cancer

Nikola Paulic, PharmD

KEY TERMS AND DEFINITIONS

Adjuvant—describes chemotherapy administered after radiation or surgery.

Antineoplastic—acting to prevent, inhibit, or halt the development of a neoplasm (a tumor).

Apoptosis—programmed cell death.

Benign—noncancerous; a term applied to a growth that does not spread or return if removed.

Body surface area (BSA)—a measurement of the external area of the body, generally expressed in square meters (m^2) and most often calculated from a patient's height and weight rather than actually measured; thought to be a more accurate indicator of the patient's actual size than weight alone.

Cancer—a disease state in which abnormal cells divide without control and are able to invade other tissues.

Carcinoma—cancer that begins in the skin or tissues that cover or line internal organs.

Cytotoxic—describes an agent (cytotoxin) that kills cells.

Cytoprotective—describes an agent that protects cells against damage from cytotoxins.

Emetogenic—causing nausea and vomiting.

Leukemia—cancer that starts in the bone marrow and causes abnormal cells to enter the blood.

Lymphoma—cancer that originates in the lymphatic cells of the immune system.

Malignant—cancerous.

DOI 10.37573/9781585286638.031

Myelosuppression—interference with the bone marrow's functions, especially production of blood cells and platelets.

Necrosis—death of living tissue.

Neoadjuvant—describes chemotherapy administered before radiation therapy or surgery.

Sarcoma—cancer that begins in the connective tissue.

Tumor—a growth or mass of unneeded cells in the body.

LEARNING OBJECTIVES

After completing this chapter, you should be able to

1. List the classes of agents used to treat cancer, including their place in therapy, and give examples of each.

2. Recognize the side effects of different types of chemotherapeutic agents.

3. Define medical terms used in chemotherapy management.

4. List the risk factors for chemotherapy-related nausea and vomiting and discuss medications used in its treatment.

5. Recognize look-alike/sound-alike medications used in treating the oncology patient.

The body consists of cells, which grow, divide, and reproduce according to the influences exerted by natural controls (hormones, enzymes) and external stimuli (chemicals, medications). Body cells are specialized, with functions ranging from the production of hormones (like those in the endocrine system) to attacking outside invaders (like many in the immune system). Normally, old cells that "wear out" or die are replaced and additional cells (like those in the blood and immune system) are produced when the body needs them. Sometimes, however, this natural cycle of cell production, death, and replacement is disrupted. It may be the result of an outside influence (hazardous chemical or drug) or an error in an internal process; often, it occurs when a cell's genetic material has suffered change or damage, called mutation. The outcome can be the formation of additional unneeded cells, which grow and reproduce (proliferate) in an uncontrolled manner not responsive to the body's normal regulation

(eg, by hormones) and sometimes not even resembling the original tissues that produced them. The extra or abnormal cells can form a mass or clump of cells, called a tumor. Another name for a tumor is neoplasm, from the Greek roots for *new (neo)* and *growth (plasia)*.

Some tumors are self-contained. They grow in one place, and while they may cause discomfort or illness because they crowd or interfere with other tissues or even produce natural chemicals in excess of what the body needs, they do not spread to other places or invade body organs and can often be removed and do not return. Such tumors are termed benign and are not cancerous. Other tumors, however, are not as well-behaved. They grow uncontrollably, invade and damage body organs and systems, and may even spread (metastasize), traveling through the blood and lymphatic systems and starting new growths called metastases in other parts of the body. These tumors are termed malignant or metastatic and their spread is called metastasis. While malignant tumors can also be removed, they sometimes grow back, either in the same place or in some other area of the body.

CASE STUDY

Mrs. Sullivan is a 45-year-old female patient who had surgery to remove a tumor from her large intestine.

Cancer is the term used for diseases in which abnormal cells divide without control and are able to invade other tissues. Unlike many other conditions covered in this text (eg, diabetes), cancer is not really a single disease state, but a term that refers to a group of diseases, usually designated by the type of cell or body tissue from or in which it originates. There are more than 100 different types of cancer.[1]

CASE?

Mrs. Sullivan's tumor started in the lining of her colon. What type of neoplasm is this cancer likely to be?

Some cancers are labeled with the name of the organ in which they began, such as prostate cancer, breast cancer, lung cancer, and colorectal cancer. Basal cell cancer is a malignancy of the basal cells of the skin; melanoma originates in the melanocytes of the skin. Lymphoma starts with the cells of the immune system. A more specific designation specifies the type of tissue a cancer represents. Carcinoma is a cancer that begins in the lining around an internal organ. Sarcoma originates in the connective tissue and may have a more descriptive prefix, with osteosarcoma being a bone cancer, myosarcoma a muscle cancer, and liposarcoma a fatty tissue cancer.

Cancers are also sometimes classified based on the type of cell that makes up the malignancy. Neuroendocrine tumors have been diagnosed in several celebrities in recent years. Regardless of where in the body they form, they have this designation because they release hormones in response to nervous system stimulation. A subgroup of these, carcinoid tumors, usually originate in the gastrointestinal (GI) system or lungs but may spread to other body organs.[1]

While all cancers are made of malignant cells and are often referred to as malignancies, they are not necessarily all tumors. Like leukemia, which starts in the blood-cell-forming tissues, some cancers proliferate in a malignant way without forming a solid tumor mass; in the case of leukemia, the extra cells crowd out normal cells in the bone marrow and may circulate in the bloodstream.[2]

More than 1.8 million new cases of cancer are diagnosed each year in the United States.[1] Not all cancer is fatal, but more than 600,000 Americans die from cancer annually.[1] Although people are warned that many things can cause cancer, the National Cancer Institute's (NCI's) list of the most common risk factors includes tobacco, sunlight, ionizing radiation, certain chemicals, some infectious agents, certain hormones, alcohol, poor diet, lack of physical activity, and being overweight.[1] Family history and growing older are also predisposing factors. As the NCI points out, however, most people with risk factors will never develop cancer, but avoiding the risks wherever possible reduces the chance of getting it.

Once diagnosed, most cancers can be treated in some way to reduce their impact, prolong life, or even eliminate them. The branch of medicine devoted to the study and treatment of cancer is oncology, and a doctor who practices in this area is known as an oncologist. The most common cancer treatments involve one or more of the following: surgery (operation to remove the tumor), radiation (x-rays and other high energy used to kill cancer cells and shrink tumors), and medication. Because the medications are chemicals aimed at the cancerous cells (neoplasms), this form of treatment is called antineoplastic chemotherapy. At times, chemotherapy and or radiation therapy may be given before the main treatment (usually surgery) to reduce the tumor size. This is

known as neoadjuvant therapy, which helps to increase the overall chances of success of the main treatment. Likewise, chemotherapy and or radiation therapy can be administered after the main treatment (surgery or radiation), and this is known as adjuvant therapy. It is given to destroy any residual cancerous cells that may have been left behind from the main treatment and reduce the risk of recurrence.

In addition to chemotherapy, another approach in the treatment of cancer is the use of immunotherapy (or biotherapy). Immunotherapies are medications that target specific parts of the immune system to aid in its ability to detect cancer cells, amplify immune responses, slow cancerous growth, and eradicate cancerous cells. Immunotherapy can be given in conjunction with chemotherapy or alone depending on the disease being treated. Since this is a pharmacology text, we will focus on chemotherapy as well as some immunotherapies for the treatment of cancer.

ANTINEOPLASTIC MEDICATIONS

Much of the cancer chemotherapy in current use is cytotoxic, meaning that it kills cells. As noted in Chapter 27, Bacterial Infections, the medications used to kill cells must be more harmful to the unwanted cells (whether bacterial or cancerous) they are intended to destroy than to the normal cells of the body. In general, cancer cells divide more rapidly than most normal cells, and many antineoplastic medications (as well as the radiation therapy mentioned above) target this difference. As a result, tumor cells are more sensitive than most normal cells to the actions of the medications used to treat cancer. Normal cells most likely to be affected by antineoplastic agents are the ones that reproduce the most frequently (scalp hair, white blood cells [WBCs], mouth, and GI lining); this accounts for some of the most common side effects (hair loss, neutropenia, oral ulcers, diarrhea).

Antineoplastic chemotherapy treatments work to disrupt the cell cycle in an attempt to cause enough changes in the cellular makeup that the cell cannot divide, or to damage the cellular makeup enough to cause the cell to die. (These changes can also affect normal cells, the reason for special handling precautions.) Some chemotherapeutic agents are cell-phase specific (meaning they act on cells at a specific stage of growth and division) while others can be given at any time in a cell's life and cause these changes.

Antineoplastic chemotherapy must be precisely dosed to maximize its therapeutic activity and minimize its side effects. Body surface area (BSA) is a measurement of the external area of the body, generally expressed in square meters (m^2) and most often calculated from a patient's height and weight rather than actually measured. Because it is thought to be a more accurate indicator of the patient's actual size than weight alone, it is used in dose calculations for dangerous drugs requiring extra precision, including many cancer chemotherapy agents.

Chemotherapy most often requires a combination of a number of drugs in addition to other treatments such as surgery and radiation therapy. Depending on the type of drug used, it may be administered by mouth, intravenously, or directly into the affected organ. Doses are generally calculated using BSA, resulting in more specific dosing. Antineoplastics are classified by the way they work and how they affect the cancer cell. Usually, chemotherapy will be prescribed as a regimen consisting of a combination of antineoplastic drugs of different types, with different mechanisms of action. We will begin with a discussion of the various classes of agents and move on to how they can be used together for the treatment of various cancers.

Alkylating Agents

An alkylating agent works by binding to DNA, the genetic material of the cell. It interferes with the DNA replication necessary for the cell to grow and divide, slowing or stopping the growth of a tumor. Agents in this group are not cycle specific (see above); they can do their damage at any point in the cell's life cycle. Their action is most evident in fast-growing and replicating cells, but this means they also suppress the cells of normal bone marrow. With increasing doses of alkylating agents, there is usually a corresponding increase in side effects, especially myelosuppression, an interference with the bone marrow's production of blood cells and platelets. Other side effects common to alkylating agents include decreased appetite, hair loss (alopecia), mouth sores (mucositis), and diarrhea. With prolonged use, serious side effects of sterility and secondary cancers have been reported.

Among the first alkylating agents (and antineoplastic therapies overall) were the nitrogen mustards—derivatives of the poisonous gas used in World War I that were noted to suppress production of blood cells in the bone marrow of soldiers who had been exposed. These include chlorambucil, mechlorethamine, and melphalan, as well as two more commonly used agents, cyclophosphamide and ifosfamide. In addition to sharing the side effects common to the other alkylating agents, cyclophosphamide and ifosfamide have a relative emetogenic risk, meaning they may cause nausea and vomiting (N&V) proportional to their prescribed doses. Their most serious and characteristic side effect, however, is

hemorrhagic cystitis, a damaging inflammation of the bladder that can be complicated by serious bleeding. For this reason, patients receiving these drugs are hydrated ahead of time with large volumes of intravenous (IV) and/or oral fluids to dilute the dangerous chemicals they produce, which are toxic to the bladder.

The cytoprotective agent (see Table 31-3) mesna, administered to reduce the damage to normal cells, reacts with the inflammatory byproduct of the alkylating agents to form a stable compound, which can be excreted without causing cystitis. It is always included in regimens containing ifosfamide, and sometimes used with cyclophosphamide therapy as well. Mesna has no antineoplastic activity and few significant side effects. There are no indications for its use either alone or to prevent side effects from other antineoplastics.

PRACTICE POINT

The dose of mesna is based on the dose of ifosfamide. Usually, an IV dose equal to 20% of the ifosfamide dose is administered prior to beginning the ifosfamide infusion and is followed either by additional 20% IV doses at 4 and 8 hours (total 60%) or 40% oral doses at 2 and 6 hours (total 100%). There are other dosing regimens, some even involving mesna mixed and administered with the ifosfamide in the same large-volume bag.

ALERT!

Ifosfamide is never administered without a concurrent order for mesna in the regimen. Mesna must precede or at least accompany the ifosfamide; giving it later reduces its effectiveness.

PRACTICE POINT

Mesna is not cytotoxic and handling it alone (without ifosfamide or cyclophosphamide) does not require any of the precautions necessary for hazardous drugs.

Another type of alkylating agent is a complex incorporating the heavy metal platinum to bind with DNA in the targeted cells. While all the medications in this class have the same mechanism of action, the part of the drug to which the platinum is attached influences the kinds of cancer each is used to treat, and the expected side effects. The original agent in this group, cisplatin, is indicated in treating cancers of the ovary, bladder, and testis, but has been used in regimens to treat many other types of cancers as well. It is considered highly emetogenic and doses are usually preceded by medications to prevent N&V with follow-up treatment over the next 3 to 5 days. Cisplatin can cause severe kidney damage, along with depletion of body potassium and magnesium. To accomplish dilution of the drug in the kidneys, patients generally receive large volumes of fluid both before and after doses. Dosing is adjusted downward for patients with poor kidney function.

ALERT!

Usual doses of cisplatin do not exceed 100 mg/m^2; anything above that must be confirmed with the prescriber and/or against the protocol in use.

PRACTICE POINT

Patient may have orders for 1,000–2,000 mL of normal saline to be administered both before and after cisplatin doses; sometimes potassium chloride and magnesium sulfate are added to these to replace expected losses.

Compared to most other alkylating agents, cisplatin is less myelosuppressive, so decreases in WBCs and platelets are not usually as severe, though anemia may result from long-term dosing regimens. Cisplatin has, however, been linked to nervous system toxicities, including hearing loss and weakness, numbness, or pain in the hands and feet, termed peripheral neuropathy.

Carboplatin also incorporates platinum, and its mechanism of action is similar to that of cisplatin; it is indicated for ovarian cancer, but sometimes is used in treatment regimens for other neoplasms as well. It is less emetogenic, less neurotoxic, and less nephrotoxic than cisplatin but has a higher incidence of myelosuppression (with decreases in WBCs, red blood cells [RBCs], and platelets) and causes more hypersensitivity reactions.

Oxaliplatin is the newest agent of this group and is indicated for colon and colorectal cancers. Like cisplatin, it has been associated with peripheral neuropathy. Neither carboplatin nor oxaliplatin administration requires prehydration with large volumes of fluid. The trade names, dosage forms, routes of administration, usual doses, and indications for these and other alkylating agents (including bendamustine, carmustine, lomustine, busulfan, procarbazine, streptozocin, temozolomide, and thiotepa) are detailed in Medication Table 31-1 (Medication Tables are located at the end of the chapter).

ALERT!

Serious and even fatal hypersensitivity reactions (anaphylaxis) have been associated with administration of platinum compounds.

PRACTICE POINT

Needles and IV sets containing aluminum must not be used in preparation or administration of platinum antineoplastics, as they can react with the medication, causing inactivation and precipitation.

PRACTICE POINT

Oxaliplatin is incompatible with normal saline and must only be diluted in dextrose as any other diluent may cause it to precipitate.

ALERT!

LOOK-ALIKE/SOUND-ALIKE—Cisplatin and carboplatin are look-alike/sound-alike drugs.

Antimetabolites

An antimetabolite is a drug similar to natural cellular chemicals included in DNA and RNA. It works by inhibiting the synthesis of DNA, thus interfering with the division and functioning of cells, because its chemical resemblance enables it to be used by the cell in place of the molecule normally used in a given reaction but with a harmful result. This prevention of normal cell division and reproduction leads to programmed cell death, called apoptosis. Because antimetabolites are not specific to the functions of cancer cells, they are also cytotoxic to rapidly dividing healthy cells, and that is the basis of most of their side effects.[2]

The first group of antimetabolites is termed folate antagonists. When it was discovered that a diet with reduced levels of the B vitamin folic acid led to a decrease in leukemia cell counts, researchers worked to develop a drug treatment that would interfere with the functions of folates in the body. This led to the synthesis of methotrexate, which is chemically similar to folic acid and can replace it in the body processes that produce a form of folate that can be used during DNA synthesis. Methotrexate still plays a significant role as a treatment for sarcoma, leukemias and sometimes breast cancer. Methotrexate is very toxic at high doses. As noted earlier, normal cells are not immune from its effects, although tumor cells seem to retain it in higher concentrations than healthy ones. Methotrexate is less emetogenic than many other chemotherapeutic agents, although dose-related N&V can occur. Serious side effects include myelosuppression, as well as nephrotoxicity (kidney damage), central nervous system (CNS) toxicity, and liver toxicity.

Leucovorin (folinic acid) is the active form of folate in the body and may be administered along with the methotrexate to reduce the myelosuppression and some (though not all) other side effects associated with treatment. It does not appear to prevent some of the toxicities, including those to the liver and kidneys. The use of leucovorin in this way is sometimes termed *leucovorin rescue.*

Pemetrexed is another folic acid antagonist indicated for the treatment of malignant mesothelioma and some lung cancers and used in combination with cisplatin. It works by disrupting folate-dependent metabolic processes essential for the rapid growth of tumors. It is usually scheduled on the first day of a 21-day cycle, as one dose every 3 weeks.

Common side effects include nausea, fatigue, and myelosuppression. Administration has also been associated with skin rash, and many patients are pretreated with an oral corticosteroid (often dexamethasone) the day before and the day of treatment, as well as the day after.

CASE?

Another drug Mrs. Sullivan receives at the oncology center is IV leucovorin. What precautions are necessary when the pharmacy technician prepares and labels this medication?

PRACTICE POINT

Folic acid supplementation (alone or as part of a multiple vitamin) reduces pemetrexed toxicity, and patients are usually instructed to begin this a full week before the first pemetrexed dose. These patients also receive intramuscular (IM) vitamin B_{12} during the week before the first dose and every 9 weeks (with the scheduled pemetrexed dose) thereafter.

CASE?

The third drug (in addition to the leucovorin and oxaliplatin) Mrs. Sullivan receives during her treatment sessions is 5-FU. Is the leucovorin considered a "rescue medication"?

Another group of antimetabolite agents are known as pyrimidine antagonists or analogs because they chemically resemble natural substances known as pyrimidines and replace them in the enzyme reactions that lead to DNA replication. These include fluorouracil (5-FU), capecitabine, and cytarabine. 5-FU is one of the older chemotherapy agents still in use and, since it is distributed generically, is fairly inexpensive (although it has recently been subject to intermittent shortages due to manufacturing delays). 5-FU is used for the treatment of cancers of the breast, pancreas, stomach, colon, skin, and rectum. 5-FU may be applied to the skin via a cream to treat actinic keratoses and is sometimes used for basal cell carcinomas (a type of skin cancer) associated with chronic, prolonged sun exposure and sun damage. Ironically, leucovorin, the agent that is used to "rescue" patients from the effects of methotrexate, is often combined with 5-FU to increase its potency (and, as a result, some of its side effects, too). The most prominent side effects of 5-FU are related to the GI tract, especially lesions of the mouth, known as mucositis, and diarrhea. While it is less likely to cause the most common chemotherapy-associated reactions (nausea, vomiting, and alopecia) compared to many agents, it has been associated with myelosuppression, eye problems, and skin conditions. High doses can also cause cardiac symptoms.

ALERT!

Both 5-FU and capecitabine interact with warfarin to increase its anticoagulant effects and the danger of bleeding if INR (international normalized ratio) is not monitored and doses adjusted. Patients taking phenytoin may also require a decrease in dosage to avoid toxic phenytoin blood levels.

PRACTICE POINT

5-FU is sometimes administered by IV infusion (diluted in a large-volume IV bag of normal saline or 5% dextrose) and sometimes ordered as an IV injection (given undiluted and often prepared in the pharmacy for dispensing in a syringe).

Capecitabine is indicated for breast and colorectal cancer. It is a modified form of 5-FU for oral administration and is converted by the body's enzymes to 5-FU, so it has similar actions and side effects, although it is associated with less myelosuppression. Cytarabine (also known as Ara-C and cytosine arabinoside) is another older antimetabolite still in use. It is a cycle-specific agent, meaning that its action is restricted to proliferating cells. It is indicated for the treatment of leukemias and lymphomas. Side effects include myelosuppression, alopecia, diarrhea, mucositis, rash, and conjunctivitis. Some patients experience flu-like symptoms (muscle pains, fever). It is moderately emetogenic, and neurologic toxicities have been noted.

Gemcitabine is a pyrimidine antimetabolite related to cytarabine and indicated for pancreatic, breast, and some lung cancers. It has fewer side effects than cytarabine and is considered less emetogenic, but it still may cause skin conditions and flu-like symptoms. Another pyrimidine is floxuridine, used to treat cancers of the GI tract.

ALERT!

When cytarabine is being prepared for intrathecal (spinal) administration, only the preservative-free solution (labeled PF) or the liposomal suspension can be used. Technicians must be sure to choose the correct preparation as errors could be fatal.

The final group of antimetabolites is known as purine analogs, after the nucleic acids (purines) they resemble and with which they interfere in cellular processes. These include mercaptopurine, thioguanine, fludarabine, cladribine, and pentostatin. They are used primarily in the treatment of leukemias and are detailed in Medication Table 31-1.

Antitumor Antibiotics

Antitumor (or antineoplastic) antibiotics are derived from microorganisms. They are capable of disrupting cellular functions, primarily blocking cell growth by inhibiting DNA synthesis, and delaying or inhibiting cell division. The anthracycline antibiotics are derived from a fungus. Doxorubicin and daunorubicin are the natural fungal products, while idarubicin and epirubicin are chemically similar compounds.[3] Inside dividing cells, they block important enzymes (topoisomerases) to produce DNA breaks in cells exposed to them, resulting in apoptosis. Anthracyclines are used in the treatment of a variety of cancers, including leukemias (doxorubicin, daunorubicin, idarubicin), breast cancer (doxorubicin and epirubicin), and Hodgkin's disease/lymphomas,

sarcomas, neuroblastoma, thyroid, lung, ovarian, breast, gastric, and bladder cancer (doxorubicin).

The anthracyclines may be highly or moderately emetogenic depending on the dose, and common side effects include myelosuppression, mucositis, and alopecia. The anthracyclines are vesicants, which means they can cause necrosis (death) to living tissue exposed to these agents. For this reason, they must be administered by skilled personnel, and any escape of the medication outside of the vein and into the surrounding tissue, known as extravasation, must be treated immediately to avoid permanent damage.

PRACTICE POINT

Anthracyclines may cause red-orange discoloration of the urine, provided they are chromophores, or chemicals that produce an intense color because of their underlying molecular composition.

While these antineoplastics have long been used to treat a variety of cancers, they have an additional toxic effect that does not appear to be antineoplastic but is, instead, somewhat selective for cardiac muscle tissue. The cardiotoxicity they produce can be *early* (acute) or *late* (delayed). The acute type takes the form of dangerous arrhythmias or pericarditis (inflammation of the tissue surrounding the heart), which can develop during treatment or shortly afterward; it is not necessarily related to the dose. The cardiotoxicity and vesicant properties of the anthracyclines are thought to be related to the creation of free radicals, which are molecular fragments that are highly reactive and have the potential to be damaging to the body's normal cells, particularly the heart muscle.[4] The chronic form can be delayed for months, and its incidence is related to the total (accumulated) dose

---

PRACTICE POINT

The brand name of doxorubicin is Adriamycin, and it represents the A in many of the cancer chemotherapy regimens known by their acronyms, such as the breast cancer regimen AC (Adriamycin and cyclophosphamide).

PRACTICE POINT

Cardiac function is monitored in patients receiving these agents, and immediate discontinuation of treatment may diminish the risk of serious heart damage.

the patient received during the course of therapy and can ultimately result in congestive heart failure.

Dexrazoxane is a cytoprotective agent (see Table 31-3) that reduces the damage by free radicals created in anthracycline exposure. When used as a cardiac protectant, it is administered prior to chemotherapy as a dose 10 times the dose of doxorubicin. If given to reduce tissue damage from extravasation, the dose is based on BSA and administered on 3 consecutive days. While dexrazoxane is a specific antidote for doxorubicin, it has been used with other anthracyclines.[4]

Doxorubicin and daunorubicin are also available as liposomal formulations, with the active drug *encapsulated* in a layer of phospholipids, which lengthen duration of activity and presumably facilitate entrance selectively into tumor cells. This enables lower dosing, with a reduced risk of both vesicant effects and cardiotoxicity.

Bleomycin is an antibiotic agent used in combination chemotherapy regimens to treat Hodgkin's lymphoma and testicular and ovarian cancers. It is only mildly emetogenic and not associated with myelosuppression. Common side effects of this agent include hypersensitivity reactions, flu-like symptoms, and mucositis. Its most serious toxicity is lung damage. Mitoxantrone is an antibiotic agent used to treat prostate cancer and leukemia. (Recall from Chapter 6 that it is also indicated for multiple sclerosis.) Compared with the anthracyclines, mitoxantrone is associated with less heart damage, nausea, and vomiting; it is not a vesicant (although it may cause vein irritation). Side effects are myelosuppression, alopecia, and mucositis. The antitumor antibiotics mentioned above and others are detailed in Medication Table 31-1.

Natural Cytotoxins

In addition to the antibiotics discussed above, some other cytotoxins used to treat cancer are natural products. These agents are derived mostly from plants and include the vinca alkaloids and taxanes, which are active against a wide variety of tumors. They are considered *antimitotics* because they interfere with mitosis (cell division). They are also known as *microtubule-targeting agents* because the cell component with which they interfere is the microtubule. The vinca alkaloids are obtained from the *Vinca rosea* (periwinkle) plant, which was first thought to be useful in the treatment of diabetes. They act by interfering with the dividing cell's separation of chromosomes in preparation for replication; this action and their disruption of other processes results in apoptosis in cells exposed to them. Vincristine can be used for certain leukemias, lymphomas, and sarcomas. Vinblastine can be used used in testicular cancer and lymphomas, as well as Kaposi's sarcoma associated with HIV infection. Vinorelbine is another agent in this class, although it is a synthetic (not natural) analog of the periwinkle derivatives. It is indicated in the treatment of some lung cancers and is also used to treat malignancies of the breast, cervix, and uterus. Vinca alkaloids, while having a relatively low emetogenic effect, are vesicants and are associated with mucositis and myelosuppression. Vinca alkaloids, particularly vincristine, can cause nervous system toxicities, including peripheral neuropathy and damage to motor, sensory, cranial (head), and autonomic nerves. These toxicities result in additional problems including unpleasant sensations, problems with GI motility, facial muscle spasms, and urinary retention. Other toxicities include impaired liver function, hearing, and vision.

The taxanes are another class of naturally derived anticancer agents that bind to internal cell structures, rendering them nonfunctional, inhibiting cell division, and causing apoptosis. Paclitaxel was first extracted from the bark of the Pacific yew (*Taxus brevifolia*, thus the *taxane* designation) during an NCI initiative for screening potentially valuable plant substances.[5] Docetaxel was synthesized from an extract of European yew needles and has activity similar to paclitaxel. Taxanes are used extensively for breast, ovarian, lung, head, and neck tumors.

> ## ALERT!
> Vinca alkaloids have been associated with fatalities when accidentally administered intrathecally (spinal administration). Because the doses are often small volumes given as IV injections, they have been traditionally prepared and dispensed in syringes, which can make them seem like intrathecal rather than IV doses. Vinca alkaloids must carry the warning FOR INTRAVENOUS USE ONLY. FATAL IF GIVEN BY OTHER ROUTES.

Paclitaxel and docetaxel are generally well tolerated and only mildly emetogenic. They are myelosuppressive and associated with hair loss (sometimes over the whole body) and peripheral neuropathy. Paclitaxel can cause muscle and joint aches, mucositis, and cardiac irregularities. Premedication with diphenhydramine, steroids (such as dexamethasone), and a histamine-2 blocker (such as ranitidine) is required before doses of conventional paclitaxel to prevent hypersensitivity reactions, but another dosage form binding the drug to a protein eliminates the need for this. Docetaxel sometimes causes a rash (especially on the hands and arms) and nail disorders. Steroids (usually oral) are generally begun the day prior to a docetaxel dose to reduce fluid retention and prevent edema. Taxanes should only be diluted in PVC-free IV bags and administered via PVC-free tubing due to the risk of leaching plasticizers found within PVC-containing equipment (eg, diethylhexyl phthalate, DEHP).

> ## ALERT!
> The protein-bound form of paclitaxel (Abraxane) has different functional properties than the conventional drug. It must not be substituted for other paclitaxel formulations.

A plant substance known as podophyllotoxin has been chemically modified to produce antineoplastic medications with a mechanism of action similar to the anthracycline antibiotics discussed earlier. Etoposide (VP-16) is used as an IV or orally administered treatment for testicular and lung cancers, and teniposide is administered IV for childhood leukemias. These drugs do not have the cardiac toxicities associated with the anthracyclines but are moderately emetogenic and cause alopecia, mucositis, and hypersensitivity reactions.

Another group of agents derived from plants are the camptothecins. These drugs also block a topoisomerase (although not the same one as the anthracyclines and podophyllotoxins) and are used in the treatment of colon cancer (irinotecan) and ovarian cancer (topotecan). Drugs from this group, along with their brand names, pronunciations, routes of administration, indications, and usual doses, can be found in Medication Table 31-1.

> ## ALERT!
> LOOK-ALIKE/SOUND-ALIKE—Paclitaxel and docetaxel are look-alike/sound-alike drugs.

Hormonal Agents

Hormonal agents have been used to treat several types of cancers. Hormonal therapy interferes at the cellular level with growth stimulatory receptor proteins. The mechanisms of action, however, may differ from one agent to the next. Hormone therapy usually consists of drugs or surgery to decrease the production of male hormones (androgens) or female hormones (estrogens) thereby stopping or limiting the growth of prostate or breast cancer. These cancers are hormone-sensitive or hormone-dependent, meaning that their growth is related to the presence or stimulation of androgens or estrogens. Hormone therapy has the advantage of being specific for tissues that are responsive to hormonal effects and can stop or slow the growth of cancers without having cytotoxicity.

Androgens, estrogens, and agents that mimic or block them have been used in the therapy of malignancies of the prostate, breast, and endometrium (uterine lining). Tests are available to show whether cancer cells have estrogen, progesterone, or testosterone receptors to enable a choice of therapy likely to block the way these hormones stimulate the cancer growth.

There are several groups of hormonal agents used in cancer treatment. The aromatase inhibitors work by blocking the enzyme aromatase. Aromatase enables the body to turn natural androgen into small amounts of estrogen. Three commonly used aromatase inhibitors are anastrozole, exemestane, and letrozole. They are used to treat breast cancers shown to have estrogen receptors *(ER-positive)* and only in postmenopausal women (whose primary source of estrogen is the aromatase-mediated reaction, unlike premenopausal women whose ovaries produce estrogen without the intervention of aromatase). The major side effects of these agents are hot flashes, muscle and joint pain, headache, fatigue, hyperlipidemia, and changes in liver enzyme levels.

PRACTICE POINT

The aromatase inhibitors are also used to treat ovulation disorders; that role was discussed in Chapter 11.

Another type of hormonal therapy is termed antiestrogen and involves interfering with the actions of natural estrogens, often by blocking the receptors to which they attach. This group (used to treat ER-positive breast cancer) includes tamoxifen (also used to prevent breast cancer), fulvestrant, and toremifene (also used for endometrial cancers). Megestrol is a progestin (see Chapter 11) that interferes with normal hormonal activity and is indicated for the treatment of breast and endometrial cancers. Antiestrogens cause hot flashes, fluid retention, weight changes, and depression. Antiandrogens (flutamide, nilutamide, bicalutamide, abiraterone, and abarelix) block the testosterone receptors of prostate cancer cells. Their actions were discussed in detail in Chapter 11. Hormonal cancer treatments are listed in Medication Table 31-1.

Additional hormonal therapies include luteinizing hormone-releasing hormone (LHRH) analogs (goserelin, leuprolide) and antagonists (degarelix). LHRH agents (also known as gonadotropin-releasing hormone [GnRH] agents) work by binding to receptors within the pituitary gland,

ultimately halting the production of testosterone or estrogen through either negative feedback (analogs) or direct blockade (antagonist). These agents are used in advanced breast and prostate cancers. LHRH analogs and antagonists can cause fluid retention, gastrointestinal issues, decreased libido, impotence, and hot flashes.

PRACTICE POINT

Megestrol is also used to stimulate the appetite of oncology patients and thus promote weight gain. When used for this indication, doses are generally much higher than those prescribed for the treatment of breast or endometrial cancer.

Small Molecule Targeted Agents

Intracellular signaling pathways allow cancerous cells to signal growth and trigger division. These pathways rely on enzymes known as kinases that work to transfer a phosphate group from adenosine triphosphate (ATP, known as the energy currency of the cell) to various proteins within the cell, a process known as phosphorylation. This acts as a switch to turn on signaling cascades to start such cellular events as growth and division. At times, these kinases can become mutated and left in the "on" position, causing rapid, uncontrolled growth. Kinase inhibitors work by blocking the site where ATP would normally bind, therefore preventing the switch from turning on. There are various types of kinase inhibitors and most inhibit more than one specific kinase, which leads to stray side effects depending on where they are found. Gene rearrangement tests are conducted to check for the presence of kinase mutations to determine whether a patient may benefit from a specific kinase inhibitor. Almost all kinase inhibitors are taken orally.

In some circumstances, cancerous cells may become resistant to the effects of a kinase inhibitor by reconfiguring the site at which they bind, ultimately preventing the drug from working. This has led to the development of different generations of kinase inhibitors that are able to overcome the resistance developed by certain cancerous cells. For example, crizotinib is a first-generation kinase inhibitor of anaplastic lymphoma kinase (ALK), which is found in certain lymphomas and lung cancers. Over the course of crizotinib therapy, some patients may develop resistance to its effects, at which time they are placed on second or third generations of ALK inhibitors (alectinib, brigatinib, ceritinib, and lorlatinib) that bypass the developed resistance and continue to work accordingly. More information on specific kinase inhibitors and their associated side effects are found in Medication Table 31-2.

Biologic Therapies

Biologic therapies are treatments using substances made from living organisms.[1] Recombinant DNA technology has enabled the manufacture of these substances (or agents with similar action and structure) in laboratories and manufacturing facilities. The type of biologic therapy most frequently used in cancer treatment is immunotherapy, which can actually boost, direct, or restore the body's ability to fight neoplasms.

Monoclonal antibodies are specific antibodies (introduced in Chapter 30) directed against antigens located on the surfaces of tumor cells. Several agents of this type are available to treat various cancers. Because each has a different and very specific target, side effects vary, but fever, chills, and headache occur with many of them, and several are commonly administered after premedication with some combination of acetaminophen, an antihistamine (usually diphenhydramine), and/or a corticosteroid (often dexamethasone). These therapies are identified by the –mab suffix in their names (ie, rituximab, cetuximab, atezolizumab, etc.). Their names also describe the composition of the monoclonal antibody, as follows: (1) chimeric, or constructed utilizing cellular machinery from another mammal—a mouse in most cases (as noted with the –ximab suffix); (2) partially human (ie, humanized), or constructed with nonhuman cellular machinery though more similar in structure to natural human monoclonal antibodies (as noted with the –zumab suffix); and (3) fully human, or constructed with viral machinery that encodes exact copies of human antibodies (as noted with the –umab suffix).[6] The derivations of each monoclonal antibody can help to determine the risk of infusion reactions as those derived from outside sources (ie, chimeric) have a greater chance of causing infusion-related reactions.[6] Some monoclonal antibodies have been associated with serious, even fatal, infusion or other reactions. Monoclonal antibodies used to treat cancer, with their pronunciations, brand names, usual doses, and indications, are listed in Medication Table 31-2.

PRACTICE POINT

Rituximab is a chimeric monoclonal antibody that is known to cause frequent infusion-related reactions (including fatal incidences) particularly with the first infusion. It's strongly recommended that individuals be pretreated with acetaminophen and an antihistamine prior to infusion.

ALERT!

LOOK-ALIKE/SOUND-ALIKE—Rituximab and cetuximab are look-alike/sound-alike drugs.

Cytokines are naturally occurring substances in the immune system. Some suppress immune response, while others stimulate it. Interferons (IFNs) are cytokines that suppress cell proliferation and increase immune system activity against target cells. Their use as antivirals is discussed in Chapter 28, but they are also used in the treatment of some cancers, including hairy cell leukemia, melanoma, chronic myeloid leukemia, and AIDS-related Kaposi's sarcoma.

Interleukins are cytokines that stimulate interferon production as well as increasing the activity of "killer" cells in the immune system. These actions can be directed against tumor cells. While many interleukins have been identified, interleukin-2 (IL-2) is the most widely studied in cancer treatment. Recombinant IL-2 is indicated for the treatment of renal cell carcinoma and metastatic melanoma. A related product, denileukin diftitox combines human IL-2 with portions of the diphtheria toxin molecule and causes apoptosis of certain cells. It is indicated for the treatment of some lymphomas.

As previously mentioned, a subclass of biologic therapy known as immunotherapies has been pivotal in the current approach to treating cancer. Immunotherapies work to invigorate the inherent immune system to seek and destroy

---

PRACTICE POINT

Monoclonal antibodies are biological products that maintain their activity only when handled, stored, and prepared exactly as directed. Most bear warnings that vials and solutions must be handled gently or even the prohibition "DO NOT SHAKE" as shaking can render them inactive.

cancerous cells by upregulating the body's own immune cell activities (particularly T cells). One such target is known as programed cell death protein 1 (PD-1), which is found on normal healthy cells, which ultimately downregulates immune system responses by acting as an inhibitory signal (similar to a key turning off a car).[7] Naturally, PD-1 functions to reduce overreaction in the immune system when it encounters various stimuli. However, PD-1 can be used by cancer cells to hide and evade immune responses that would normally eliminate such abnormal cells. Blocking PD-1 proteins on cancer cells from interacting with immune cells (T and B cells) allows for the detection of cancer cells and triggering of cancer cell death. Immunotherapies may be used as an individual treatment or as part of a regimen in multiple cancers. Examples of such agents and their uses are detailed in Medication Table 31-2.

PRACTICE POINT

Many biotherapies now have available biosimilars that are mistakenly referred to as "generics." Biosimilars are biological products that are highly similar to products already approved by the Food and Drug Administration (FDA), and do not have clinically meaningful differences related to their safety and efficacy.[6] They are not referred to as generics because they are large protein structures and, given their complexity is challenging to make exact copies. The Purple book is a compendium of all known FDA approved and available biosimilars.[8]

Antineoplastic Therapy Regimens

The antineoplastic agents discussed in this chapter are seldom used alone. Cancer chemotherapy generally consists of a regimen, or combination, of medications in specific dose ranges and intervals designed to increase the likelihood of successful therapy, while decreasing the severity of the side effects. Medications from different groups, with different mechanisms of action, are chosen to attack the cancer cells in multiple ways, either simultaneously or sequentially.

There are numerous regimens (with more being developed in clinical trials) available, each of which has been studied for use in specific situations. Some cancer therapy

---

CASE?

Mrs. Sullivan receives three different antineoplastics and has to visit the oncology center 2 days every other week. Why does she need so many drugs and doses?

---

is aimed at a cure, with complete eradication of the cancer. Other therapies are considered palliative and are used to diminish symptoms or even prolong life in patients whose cancers are unlikely to respond to the extent of complete cure. Some antineoplastic regimens are termed adjuvant therapy and are administered to prevent recurrence of disease that has been treated with surgery or radiation. These are often administered cyclically: weekly, every 21 days, monthly, or at some other customized interval (sometimes during only one day of the cycle and sometimes on two or more consecutive days). The interval scheduling is planned in part to allow the bone marrow to recover from a chemotherapy-induced nadir (the point at which blood cell counts are at their lowest). Most cancer treatment regimens and their specific indications can be found in the National Comprehensive Cancer Network® (NCCN) guidelines.[9] The NCCN guidelines are the most up-to-date treatment algorithms and are used extensively in oncologic practices in North America.[9]

CASE?

Mrs. Sullivan had her cancer removed before beginning antineoplastic medications. What is the term for the IV treatment she is receiving at the oncology center?

Chemotherapy regimens are sometimes given distinctive names, such as the Roswell Park Regimen (5-FU with folinic acid) for colorectal cancer, or they simply list the included drugs, such as the carboplatin/pemetrexed regimen for malignant mesothelioma. Many are acronyms that incorporate the first letters in the names (sometimes brand, sometimes generic) of the drugs included, such as FOLFOX6 (folinic acid/fluorouracil/oxaliplatin) for colorectal cancer; TAC (Taxotere–docetaxel/Adriamycin-doxorubicin/cyclophosphamide) for breast cancer; or CHOP (cyclophosphamide/hydroxydaunorubicin–doxorubicin/Oncovin–vincristine/prednisone) for lymphoma.

SIDE EFFECT MANAGEMENT

As emphasized throughout this chapter, antineoplastic medications have many significant side effects. Because therapy must often continue for long periods of time to achieve the goals of treatment, management of these side effects is crucial to both the patient's quality of life and the ability to continue the treatment. Side effects frequently associated with chemotherapy and treated with pharmacologic intervention are N&V, mucositis, and myelosuppression.

Prevention and control of N&V are important parts of many chemotherapy regimens. N&V are unpleasant in themselves but can result in serious consequences, including nutritional depletion, anorexia, deterioration of patients' physical and mental status, decreased ability to function, and withdrawal from potentially useful and curative treatment. Emetogenic potential varies with the agents, and antiemetic therapy is chosen and dosed based on the antineoplastics used. Patients most at risk for hard-to-control N&V from chemotherapy are those who are under 50 years old, female (particularly those with persistent N&V symptoms during pregnancy), those who experienced uncontrolled symptoms during an earlier treatment, those who have a history of motion sickness, or those who have always abstained from alcoholic beverages. Antiemetics and their use in chemotherapy are discussed extensively in Chapter 21, as well as in the NCCN antiemesis guidelines for supportive care.[9]

CASE?

Mrs. Sullivan's physician has ordered a dose of ondansetron 8 mg by mouth twice daily in the weeks she receives chemotherapy. What is the purpose of this additional medication?

The mucosal lining of the GI tract, including the oral mucosa, has a rapid cell turnover rate and is thus highly susceptible to the toxic effects of cytotoxic agents. Oral mucositis describes inflammation of the oral mucosa; when this occurs, the oral cavity becomes red and swollen. Mucositis is managed with topical anesthetics (eg, viscous lidocaine, benzocaine gels, and mouthwash solutions containing diphenhydramine). Kaolin/pectin agents can be used to form a protective barrier and give relief, as well. If oral lesions become irritated or infected, additional management may be indicated. Some options are discussed in Chapter 36.

CASE?

Mrs. Sullivan received chemotherapy on Monday and Tuesday. On Friday, she comes to the pharmacy with a prescription for her sore mouth. Why might her mouth be so swollen? What might the oncologist have prescribed?

Myelosuppression, an interference with the bone marrow's functions, especially the production of blood cells and platelets, is one of the most common toxicities limiting the dose or continuation of therapy for antineoplastic agents. Neutrophils (detailed in Chapter 25) have a relatively short lifespan and are among the first type of cell to be depleted during therapy with myelosuppressive agents; when their count falls too low, patients suffer from neutropenia and are more susceptible to infection. This condition and its treatment are discussed in Chapter 26.

There are many additional adverse effects associated with antineoplastic chemotherapy. It is not unusual for patients receiving antineoplastics to receive preventive medications or to require treatment for the side effects; the prevention or treatment will vary with the regimen being used.

HANDLING CYTOTOXIC MEDICATIONS

Cytotoxic medications and some other antineoplastic agents are hazardous substances, and exposure to them during handling, storage, preparation, delivery, administration, and disposal can pose health risks to pharmacy and medical personnel. These risks include cancer (carcinogenicity), damage to a developing fetus (teratogenicity), fertility impairment (reproductive toxicity), organ toxicity, and damage to DNA (genotoxicity).

Personal protective equipment (PPE), including appropriate gloves, long-sleeved gowns with closed fronts and fitted cuffs, eye and face protection, and shoe coverings, should be worn during the preparation of hazardous agents.[10] The preparation and manipulation of these products in the pharmacy should be accomplished in a closed environment such as a biological safety cabinet or a barrier isolator. Procedures must be in place to treat accidental exposures, and equipment and supplies to clean up after spills must be readily available.

PRACTICE POINT

USP General Chapter provides standards for the safe handling of hazardous drugs to minimize the risk of exposure to healthcare personnel, patients, and the environment. Its standards apply to all healthcare personnel who receive, prepare, administer, transport, or otherwise come in contact with hazardous drugs and all the environments in which they are handled.[10]

CASE?

Mrs. Sullivan's medications include oxaliplatin, leucovorin, 5-FU, ondansetron, and viscous lidocaine. Which of these medications requires special handling, labeling, or disposal precautions? Why?

Cytotoxic preparations dispensed from the pharmacy should always bear a label warning those who will handle or administer them to wear gloves and dispose of them properly. Waste material from preparation and administration must be placed in puncture-proof containers with sealed lids labeled with an appropriate warning.[10]

PRACTICE POINT

Not all antineoplastic chemotherapy is considered hazardous, but technicians must determine ahead of time what precautions are indicated for the medications they are handling.

SUMMARY

Cancer is a disease state in which abnormal cells divide without control and are able to invade other tissues. It can result in serious illness and death, and there are a variety of treatments, including surgery, radiation, and medication. Pharmacotherapy for cancer consists of agents that are intended to kill cancer cells and/or prevent them from multiplying or to enhance the body's ability to fight the disease.

Agents used in chemotherapy frequently have serious side effects, which may limit the administration of an effective dose, and must be managed appropriately. Many of the therapies are hazardous substances and require special handling, labeling, and disposal.

ACKNOWLEDGMENT

The author wishes to acknowledge and thank Allen L. Horne, RPh, author of this chapter in the first edition of this book.

REFERENCES

1. National Cancer Institute at the National Institutes of Health. Available at http://www.cancer.gov/. Accessed June 10, 2022.

2. DiPiro JT, Yee GC, Posey LM, et al., eds. *Pharmacotherapy: A Pathophysiologic Approach.* 11th ed. New York, NY: McGraw-Hill; 2020.

3. Wellstein A. General Principles in the Pharmacotherapy of Cancer. In: Brunton LL, Knollman BC, eds. *Goodman & Gilman's: The Pharmacological Basis of Therapeutics*, 14e. McGraw Hill; 2022. Accessed July 28, 2022 https://accesspharmacy-mhmedical-com.neomed.idm.oclc.org/content.aspx?bookid=3191&sectionid=266700746.

4. Wang RY. Chemotherapeutics. In: Nelson LS, Howland M, Lewin NA, Smith SW, Goldfrank LR, Hoffman RS, eds. *Goldfrank's Toxicologic Emergencies*, 11e. McGraw Hill; 2019. Accessed July 28, 2022. https://accesspharmacy-mhmedical-com.neomed.idm.oclc.org/content.aspx?bookid=2569&sectionid=210272633.

5. Frye DK, Taxane chemotherapy: Advances in treatment for breast cancer. *US Oncological Disease.* 2006;1(1):40-41.

6. Lu R-M, Hwang Y-C, Liu I-J, et al. Development of therapeutic antibodies for the treatment of diseases. *J Biomed Sci.* 2020;27(1). doi:10.1186/s12929-019-0592-z.

7. Messerschmidt JL, Prendergast GC, Messerschmidt GL. How cancers escape immune destruction and mechanisms of action for the new significantly active immune therapies: Helping nonimmunologists decipher recent advances. Oncologist. 2016;21(2):233-243. https://www.ncbi.nlm.nih.gov/pmc/articles/PMC4746082. Accessed June 10, 2022.

8. FDA Purple Book [database]. Silver Spring, MD: U.S. Food and Drug Administration. https://purplebooksearch.fda.gov/. Accessed July 10, 2021.

9. National Comprehensive Cancer Network. Guidelines: Antiemesis. https://www.nccn.org. Accessed June 10, 2022.

10. U. S. Pharmacopeia. USP General Chapter Hazardous Drugs – Handling in Healthcare Settings. https://www.usp.org/compounding/general-chapter-hazardous-drugs-handling-healthcare. Accessed June 23, 2020.

11. Lexi-Drugs [database]. Hudson, OH: Lexicomp; 2021. http://online.lexi.com/. Accessed June 10, 2022.

REVIEW QUESTIONS

1. What is cancer? How does it develop?

2. What are cytotoxic drugs, and why is this type of medication useful in the treatment of cancer?

3. How are hormonal therapies used in the treatment of cancer? Which types of cancer are they usually used to treat?

4. Discuss three common side effects of antineoplastic therapy.

5. Discuss special precautions pharmacy technicians must take in the preparation and handling of some antineoplastic medications and the reasons for these precautions.

MEDICATION TABLES

MEDICATION TABLE 31-1. Cytotoxic and Hormonal Antineoplastic Agents[11]

Generic Name (pronunciation)	Brand Name	Class	Dosage Forms	Route	Common Dose	Indication
Abiraterone (a bir A ter one)	Zytiga, Yonsa	Hormone (antiandrogen)	Tablet	Oral	1,000 mg once daily	Prostate cancer
Anastrozole (an AS troe zole)	Arimidex	Aromatase inhibitor	Tablet	Oral	1 mg daily	Breast cancer
Arsenic trioxide (AR se nik tri OKS id)	Trisenox	Miscellaneous antineoplastic	Solution	IV	0.15 mg/kg/day	Acute promyelocytic leukemia
Asparaginase Erwinia (a SPEAR a ji nase er WIN i ah)	Erwinase	Enzyme	Powder for reconstitution	IV, IM	6,000 units/m^2/dose 3 times/week	Acute lymphoblastic leukemia (ALL)
Azacitidine (ay za SYE ti deen)	Vidaza	Antimetabolite (pyrimidine analog)	Powder for suspension	IV, SUBQ	75 mg/m^2/day for 7 days every 4 weeks	Myelodysplastic syndrome (MDS) Acute myeloid leukemia (AML)
	Onureg		Tablet	Oral	300 mg daily, days 1–14 of 28-day cycle	AML, maintenance
Bendamustine (ben da MUS teen)	Treanda	Alkylating agent	Powder for reconstitution	IV	100 mg/m^2 days 1–2 of 28-day cycle	Chronic lymphocytic leukemia (CLL), progressed indolent B cell non-Hodgkin's lymphoma (NHL)
	Belrapzo, Bendeka		Solution			
Bicalutamide (bye ka LOO ta mide)	Casodex	Hormone (antiandrogen)	Tablet	Oral	50 mg once daily	Prostate cancer
Bleomycin (blee oh MYE sin)		Antibiotic	Powder for reconstitution	IM, IV	10 units/m^2	Squamous cell carcinomas, Hodgkin's lymphoma, testicular cancer
Busulfan (bue SUL fan)	Busulfex, Myleran	Alkylating agent	Injection solution, tablet	IV, oral	4–8 mg/day	Chronic myelogenous leukemia (CML)
Cabazitaxel (ca baz i TAKS el)	Jevtana	Antimitotic (taxane)	Solution	IV	25 mg/m^2/dose once every 3 weeks	Prostate cancer
Capecitabine (ka pe SITE a been)	Xeloda	Antimetabolite (pyrimidine analog)	Tablet	Oral	1,250 mg/m^2 twice daily	Breast and colorectal cancer

Continued next page

MEDICATION TABLE 31-1. Cytotoxic and Hormonal Antineoplastic Agents[11] (Continued)

Generic Name (pronunciation)	Brand Name	Class	Dosage Forms	Route	Common Dose	Indication
Carboplatin (KAR boe pla tin)	Paraplatin	Alkylating agent (platinum complex)	Solution	IV	Calculated using the Calvert formula	Ovarian cancer, breast cancer, NSCLC, small cell lung cancer, head and neck cancer
Carmustine (kar MUS teen)	BiCNU	Alkylating agent	Powder for reconstitution	IV	150–200 mg/m² every 6 weeks	Brain tumors, Hodgkin's lymphoma, multiple myeloma, NHL
	Gliadel		Wafer for implantation	Brain implant	8 wafers surgically placed in the resection cavity	Glioblastoma, newly diagnosed high-grade malignant glioma
Chlorambucil (klor AM byoo sil)	Leukeran	Alkylating agent	Tablet	Oral	0.1 mg/kg/day for 3–6 weeks	CLL, Hodgkin's lymphoma, NHL
Cisplatin (SIS pla tin)	Generics only, formerly Platinol	Alkylating agent (platinum complex)	Injection solution	IV	10–100 mg/m² (variable depending on indication)	Bladder, testicular, ovarian cancer, lung cancer, head and neck cancer
Cladribine (KIA dri been)		Antimetabolite (purine analog)	Injection solution	IV, SUBQ	0.1 mg/kg/day	Hairy cell leukemia
Clofarabine (klo FARE a been)	Clolar	Antimetabolite (purine analog)	Injection solution	IV	Adults ≤21 yrs of age: 52 mg/m²/day on days 1–5 repeated every 2–6 weeks based on tolerability	ALL in children
Cyclophosphamide (sye kloe FOS fa mide)	Formerly Cytoxan	Alkylating agent (nitrogen mustard)	Injection powder for reconstitution, tablet	IV, oral	Varies widely depending on indication	Lymphomas, leukemias, mycosis fungoides, multiple myeloma, neuroblastoma, breast cancer, ovarian cancer
Cytarabine ("Ara-C") (sye TARE a been)	Formerly Cytosar	Antimetabolite (pyrimidine analog)	Injection powder for reconstitution, solution	IV, intrathecal, SUBQ	100 mg/m²/day for 7 days	Leukemias
Dacarbazine ("DTIC") (da KAR ba zeen)		Alkylating agent	Injection powder for reconstitution	IV	250–375 mg/m²/dose	Malignant melanoma, Hodgkin's lymphoma
Dactinomycin (dak ti noe MYE sin)	Cosmegen	Antibiotic	Injection powder for reconstitution	IV	Varies widely depending on indication	Wilms' tumor, sarcomas, ovarian cancer, gestational trophoblastic neoplasm
Daunorubicin (daw noe ROO bi sin)		Antibiotic (anthracycline)	Injection powder for reconstitution	IV	30–60 mg/m²/day	ALL, AML

Continued next page

MEDICATION TABLE 31-1. Cytotoxic and Hormonal Antineoplastic Agents[11] *(Continued)*

Generic Name (pronunciation)	Brand Name	Class	Dosage Forms	Route	Common Dose	Indication
Decitabine (dee SYE ta been)	Dacogen	Antimetabolite (pyrimidine analog)	Injection powder for reconstitution	IV	20 mg/m² over 1 hour once daily for 5 days every 4 weeks	AML, MDS
Degarelix (deg a REL ix)	Firmagon	Hormonal agent (GnRH antagonist)	Injection powder for reconstitution	SUBQ	80 mg every 28 days	Prostate cancer
Docetaxel (doe se TAKS el)		Antimitotic (taxane)	Injection powder for reconstitution, solution	IV	60–100 mg/m² every 3 weeks	Breast cancer, prostate cancer, non-small cell lung cancer (NSCLC), gastric adenocarcinoma, squamous cell head and neck cancer
Doxorubicin (doks oh ROO bi sin)	Adriamycin	Antibiotic (anthracycline)	Injection powder for reconstitution, solution	IV	60 mg/m²/dose every 2 weeks	ALL, AML, lymphomas, soft tissue and bone sarcomas, thyroid cancer, small cell lung cancer, breast cancer, gastric cancer, ovarian cancer, bladder cancer, neuroblastoma, and Wilms' tumor
Doxorubicin liposomal (doks oh ROO bi sin lye po SO mal)	Doxil	Antibiotic (anthracycline)	Suspension	IV	20 mg/m² every 3 weeks	Kaposi's sarcoma, multiple myeloma, ovarian cancer, breast cancer
Epirubicin (ep i ROO bi sin)	Ellence	Antibiotic (anthracycline)	Injection powder for reconstitution, injection solution	IV	Dose varies, 3 or 4 weeks treatment cycles	Breast cancer
Eribulin (er i BUE lin)	Halaven	Antimitotic	Injection solution	IV	1.4 mg/m²/dose on days 1 and 8 of a 21-day treatment cycle	Breast cancer
Estramustine (es tra MUS teen)	Emcyt	Antimitotic	Capsule	Oral	14 mg/kg/day in 3 or 4 divided doses	Prostate cancer
Etoposide (e toe POE side)	Toposar	Antimitotic (podophyllotoxin)	Injection solution	IV	35 mg/m²/day for 5 days every 3-4 weeks	Testicular tumors, small cell lung cancer
	(generics)		Capsule	Oral	70–100 mg/m²/day for 5 days every 3–4 weeks (rounded to the nearest 50 mg)	Small cell lung cancer

Continued next page

MEDICATION TABLE 31-1. Cytotoxic and Hormonal Antineoplastic Agents[11] *(Continued)*

Generic Name (pronunciation)	Brand Name	Class	Dosage Forms	Route	Common Dose	Indication
Etoposide phosphate (e toe POE side FOS fate)	Etopophos	Antimitotic (podophyllotoxin)	Injection solution; formulated without polysorbate 80	IV	50–100 mg/m² days 1–3	Small cell lung cancer, testicular cancer
Exemestane (ex e MES tane)	Aromasin	Aromatase inhibitor	Tablet	Oral	25 mg once daily	Breast cancer (postmenopausal women)
Floxuridine (flox YOOR i deen)		Antimetabolite (pyrimidine analog)	Injection powder for reconstitution	Intra-arterial	0.1–0.6 mg/kg/day continuous intra-arterial administration for 14 days by an implantable pump	Hepatic metastases of colorectal and gastric cancers
Fludarabine (floo DARE a been)		Antimetabolite (purine analog)	Injection powder for reconstitution, injection solution	IV	25–40 mg/m² once daily for 5 days every 28 days	B cell CLL
Fluorouracil (5-FU) (flure oh YOOR a sil)		Antimetabolite (pyrimidine analog)	Injection solution	IV	500 mg/m² once weekly	Carcinomas of the breast, colon, rectum, pancreas, or stomach
Flutamide (FLOO ta mide)	Eulexin	Hormone (antiandrogen)	Capsule	Oral	250 mg 3 times/day	Prostate cancer
Fulvestrant (ful VES trant)	Faslodex	Hormonal agent (estrogen receptor antagonist)	Injection solution	IM	500 mg once monthly	Breast cancer (postmenopausal women)
Gemcitabine (jem SIT a been)	Infugem	Antimetabolite (pyrimidine analog)	Injection solution	IV	1,000 mg/m², weekly in 3 out of 4 weeks	Breast cancer, NSCLC, pancreatic cancer, ovarian cancer
Goserelin (GOE se rel in)	Zoladex	Hormonal agent (GnRH agonist)	Implant	SUBQ	28-day (3.6 mg) or 12-week (10.8 mg) implant	Prostate cancer, breast cancer
Histrelin (his TREL in)	Supprelin LA Vantas	Hormonal agent (GnRH agonist)	Implant	SUBQ	50 mg implant inserted every 12 months	Prostate cancer
Hydroxyurea (hye drox ee yoor EE a)	Droxia, Hydrea, Siklos	Antimetabolite	Capsule, tablet	Oral	20–30 mg/kg once daily	Melanoma, CML, ovarian cancer, squamous cell head and neck cancer, adjunct in the management of sickle cell anemia
Idarubicin (eye da ROO bi sin)	Idamycin PFS	Antibiotic (anthracycline)	Injection solution	IV	12 mg/m²/day for 3 days	AML

Continued next page

MEDICATION TABLE 31-1. Cytotoxic and Hormonal Antineoplastic Agents[11] *(Continued)*

Generic Name (pronunciation)	Brand Name	Class	Dosage Forms	Route	Common Dose	Indication
Ifosfamide (eye FOS fa mide)	Ifex	Alkylating agent (nitrogen mustard)	Injection powder for reconstitution, solution	IV	1,200 mg/m²/day for 5 days every 3 weeks	Testicular cancer
Irinotecan (eye rye no TEE kan)	Camptosar	Antimitotic (camptothecin)	Injection solution	IV	125 mg/m² over 90 minutes on days 1, 8, 15, and 22 of a 6-week treatment cycle	Carcinoma of the colon or rectum
Irinotecan liposomal (eye rye no TEE kan lye po SO mal)	Onyvide	Antimitotic (camptothecin)	Injection	IV	70 mg/m² over 90 minutes once every 2 weeks. NOTE: Not interchangeable with conventional irinotecan	Pancreatic cancer
Ixabepilone (ix ab EP i lone)	Ixempra	Antimitotic	Injection powder for reconstitution	IV	40 mg/m²/dose over 3 hours every 3 weeks	Breast cancer
Letrozole (LET roe zole)	Femara	Aromatase inhibitor	Tablet	Oral	2.5 mg once daily	Breast cancer
Leucovorin (loo koe VOR in) ("Calcium folinate")		Cytoprotective (with methotrexate therapy)	Solution, tablet	IV, oral	15-25 mg every 6 hours × 10 doses beginning 24 hours after methotrexate administration	Reduces methotrexate toxicity
		Enzyme inhibitor (with 5-FU therapy)	Solution	IV	20–200 mg/m² prior to 5-FU	Colorectal cancer
Leuprolide (loo PROE lide)	Eligard, Lupron Depot-Ped, Lupron Depot, Camcevi	Hormonal agent (GnRH agonist)	Injection powder for reconstitution, injection solution, kit	IM, SUBQ	7.5 mg monthly, administered at 1-, 3-, 4-, or 6-month intervals	Prostate cancer
Lomustine (loe MUS teen)	Gleostine	Alkylating agent	Capsule	Oral	130 mg/m² every 6 weeks	Metastatic brain tumors, Hodgkin's disease
Megestrol (me JES trol)		Hormone (progestin)	Suspension, tablet	Oral	Varies widely according to protocols	Breast and endometrial carcinoma; also used as appetite stimulant

Continued next page

MEDICATION TABLE 31-1. Cytotoxic and Hormonal Antineoplastic Agents[11] *(Continued)*

Generic Name (pronunciation)	Brand Name	Class	Dosage Forms	Route	Common Dose	Indication
Melphalan (MEL fa lan)	Evomela, Alkeran	Alkylating agent	Injection powder for reconstitution, tablet	IV, oral	Varies widely depending on indication	Multiple myeloma, ovarian cancer
Mercaptopurine (mer kap toe PURE een)	Purixan	Antimetabolite (purine analog)	Suspension, tablet	Oral	1.5–2.5 mg/kg/day	ALL
Methotrexate (meth oh TREX ate)	Trexall, others	Antimetabolite (antifolate)	Injection powder for reconstitution, injection solution, tablet	IV, IM, oral intrathecal	Varies widely depending on indication	Trophoblastic neoplasms, ALL, meningeal leukemia, breast cancer, head and neck cancer, cutaneous T-cell lymphoma, lung cancer, NHL, osteosarcoma
Mitomycin (mye toe MYE sin)		Antibiotic	Injection powder for reconstitution	IV	20 mg/m² every 6–8 weeks	Adenocarcinoma of the stomach or pancreas
Mitomycin ureteral gel (mye toe MYE sin)	Jelmyto	Antibiotic	Solution, reconstituted	Ureteral instillation	Up to 15 mL (60 mg) weekly × 6 weeks	Urothelial cancer
Mitotane (MYE toe tane)	Lysodren	Adrenal cytotoxic agent	Tablet	Oral	Varies widely depending on indication	Adrenocortical carcinoma
Mitoxantrone (mye toe ZAN trone)		Antibiotic	Injection solution	IV	12 mg/m² once daily for 3 days in 3- to 4-week cycles	Acute nonlymphocytic leukemias (ANLL), prostate cancer, multiple sclerosis
Nelarabine (nel AY re been)	Arranon	Antimetabolite (purine analog)	Injection solution	IV	1,500 mg/m²/dose on days 1, 3, and 5; repeat every 21 days	ALL, lymphoblastic lymphoma
Nilutamide (nye LOO ta mide)	Nilandron	Hormone (antiandrogen)	Tablet	Oral	300 mg once daily	Prostate cancer
Oxaliplatin (ox AL i pla tin)		Alkylating agent (platinum complex)	Injection solution	IV	85 mg/m² every 2 weeks until disease progression or unacceptable toxicity	Colon cancer, colorectal cancer
Paclitaxel (pak li TAX el)	Formerly Taxol	Antimitotic (taxane)	Injection solution	IV	135–175 mg/m² over 3 hours every 3 weeks	Breast, NSCLC and ovarian cancers; AIDS-related Kaposi's sarcoma

Continued next page

MEDICATION TABLE 31-1. Cytotoxic and Hormonal Antineoplastic Agents[11] *(Continued)*

Generic Name (pronunciation)	Brand Name	Class	Dosage Forms	Route	Common Dose	Indication
Paclitaxel protein-bound particles (pak li TAX el)	Abraxane	Antimitotic (taxane)	Suspension for reconstitution	IV	260 mg/m² IV over 30 minutes every 3 weeks	Breast cancer
Pegaspargase (peg AS par jase)	Oncaspar	Enzyme	Injection solution	IM, IV	2,500 units/m² (as part of a chemotherapy regimen), not to be administered more frequently than every 14 days	ALL
Pemetrexed (pem e TREX ed)	Alimta, Pemfexy	Antimetabolite (antifolate)	Injection powder for reconstitution	IV	500 mg/m² on day 1 of each 21-day cycle (in combination with cisplatin)	Malignant pleural mesothelioma, nonsquamous NSCLC
Pentostatin (pen toe STAT in)	Nipent	Antimetabolite (purine analog)	Injection powder for reconstitution	IV	4 mg/m² every 2 weeks	Hairy cell leukemia
Pralatrexate (pral a TREX ate)	Folotyn	Antimetabolite (antifolate)	Injection solution	IV	30 mg/m² once weekly for 6 weeks of a 7-week treatment cycle	Peripheral T-cell lymphoma (PTCL)
Procarbazine (proe KAR ba zeen)	Matulane	Alkylating agent	Capsule	Oral	2–4 mg/kg/day for 7 days then increase to 4–6 mg/kg/day until response is obtained	Hodgkin's disease
Streptozocin (step toe ZOE sin)	Zanosar	Alkylating agent	Injection powder for reconstitution	IV	1–1.4 g/m² weekly for 6 weeks followed by a 4-week rest period	Pancreatic cancer
Tamoxifen (ta MOKS i fen)	Soltamox (formerly Nolvadex)	Hormone (antiestrogen)	Tablet, solution	Oral	20–40 mg/day	Breast cancer
Temozolomide (te moe ZOE loe mide)	Temodar	Alkylating agent	Capsule, injection powder for reconstitution	Oral, IV	100–200 mg/m²/day for 5 days per treatment cycle	Central nervous system (CNS) cancers
Teniposide (ten i POE side)		Antimitotic (podophyllotoxin)	Injection solution	IV	165 mg/m²/dose days 1, 4, 8, and 11 of alternating consolidation cycles	Childhood ALL

Continued next page

MEDICATION TABLE 31-1. Cytotoxic and Hormonal Antineoplastic Agents[11] *(Continued)*

Generic Name (pronunciation)	Brand Name	Class	Dosage Forms	Route	Common Dose	Indication
Thioguanine (thye oh GWAH neen)	Tabloid	Antimetabolite (purine analog)	Tablet	Oral	60 mg/m²/day for 14 days	AML
Thiotepa (thye oh TEP a)	Tepadina	Alkylating agent	Injection powder for reconstitution	Intravesical, IV, intracavitary, intrathecal	Dose and route of administration various depending on indication	Bladder, breast, ovarian cancers
Topotecan (toe poe TEE kan)	Hycamtin	Antimitotic (camptothecin)	Capsule, injection powder for reconstitution, injection solution	IV, oral	1.5 mg/m²/day repeated every 21 days	Ovarian or cervical cancer, small cell lung cancer
Toremifene (tore EM i feen)	Fareston	Hormonal agent (estrogen receptor antagonist)	Tablet	Oral	60 mg once daily	Metastatic breast cancer in postmenopausal women
Triptorelin (trip toe REL in)	Trelstar, Triptodur	Hormonal agent (GnRH agonist)	Injection powder for reconstitution	IM	3.75 mg once every 4 weeks	Prostate cancer
Valrubicin (val ROO bi sin)	Valstar	Antibiotic (anthracycline)	Injection solution	Intravesical	800 mg once weekly (retain for 2 hours) for 6 weeks	Bladder cancer
Vinblastine (vin BLAS teen)	Formerly Velban	Antimitotic (vinca alkaloid)	Injection powder for reconstitution, injection solution	IV	5.5–7.4 mg/m² every 7 days	Hodgkin's and non-Hodgkin's lymphoma, testicular cancer, breast cancer, mycosis fungoides, Kaposi's sarcoma, histiocytosis, choriocarcinoma
Vincristine (vin KRIS teen)	Vincasar PFS (formerly Oncovin)	Antimitotic (vinca alkaloid)	Injection solution	IV	1.4 mg/m²/dose, doses capped at 2 mg/dose according to individual protocol	ALL, lymphomas, Wilms' tumor, neuroblastoma, rhabdomyosarcoma
Vinorelbine (vi NOR el been)		Antimitotic (vinca alkaloid)	Injection solution	IV	30 mg/m²/dose every 7 days	NSCLC

GnRH = gonadotropin-releasing hormone; IM = intramuscular; IV = intravenous; SUBQ = subcutaneous.

MEDICATION TABLE 31-2. Biologic Therapies Used to Treat Cancer[11]

Generic Name (pronunciation)	Brand Name	Class	Dosage Forms	Route	Common Dose	Indication
Abemaciclib (a bem a SYE klib)	Verzenio	Enzyme inhibitor	Tablet	Oral	150 mg or 200 mg twice daily	Breast cancer
Acalabrutinib (a KAL a broo ti nib)	Calquence	Enzyme inhibitor	Capsule	Oral	100 mg every 12 hours	CLL, mantle cell lymphoma
Ado-trastuzumab emtansine (a do tras TU zoo mab em TAN seen)	Kadcyla	Monoclonal antibody-antineoplastic complex	Solution reconstituted	IV	3.6 mg/kg every 3 weeks	Breast cancer
Afatanib (a FA ti nib)	Gilotrif	Enzyme inhibitor	Tablet	Oral	40 mg once daily	NSCLC
Aldesleukin (IL-2) (al des LOO kin)	Proleukin	Biological response modifier	Powder for reconstitution	IV	600,000 International Units/kg every 8 hours	Renal cell carcinoma (RCC), melanoma
Alectinib (al EK ti nib)	Alecensa	Enzyme inhibitor (2nd generation)	Tablet	Oral	600 mg twice daily	NSCLC
Alemtuzumab (al em TOOZ oo mab)	Campath, Lemtrada	Monoclonal antibody	Solution (preservative free)	IV, SUBQ	3 mg/day increased to 30 mg/dose	Lymphomas, prolymphocytic leukemia
Alpelisib (AL pe LIS ib)	Piqray	Enzyme inhibitor	Tablet	Oral	300 mg once daily	Breast cancer
Atezolizumab (ah TEZ oh liz U mab)	Tecentriq	Monclonal antibody	Solution	IV	Flat dose of 840 mg every 2 weeks OR 1,200 mg every 3 weeks OR 1,680 mg every 4 weeks	Breast, lung, or urothelial cancer
Axitinib (ax I ti nib)	Inlyta	Enzyme inhibitor	Tablet	Oral	5–10 mg twice daily	RCC, thyroid cancer
Belinostat (be LIN oh stat)	Beleodaq	Enzyme inhibitor	Solution (preservative free)	IV	1,000 mg/m² once daily on days 1–5 every 21 days	Peripheral T-cell lymphoma
Bevacizumab (be va SIZ yoo mab)	Avastin, Mvasi, Zirabev, Alymsys	Monoclonal antibody	Solution (preservative free)	IV	5 or 10 mg/kg every 2 weeks	Colorectal cancer, NSCLC, glioblastoma, RCC
Bexarotene (bex AIR oh teen)	Targretin	Retinoid	Capsule	Oral	300–400 mg/m²/day	Cutaneous T-cell lymphoma

Continued next page

MEDICATION TABLE 31-2. Biologic Therapies Used to Treat Cancer[11] (*Continued*)

Generic Name (pronunciation)	Brand Name	Class	Dosage Forms	Route	Common Dose	Indication
Binimetinib (bin I ME ti nib)	Mektovi	Enzyme inhibitor	Tablet	Oral	45 mg twice daily	Colorectal cancer, melanoma
Blinatumomab (blin a TOOM oh mab)	Blincyto	Monoclonal antibody	Reconstituted solution	IV	Dose based on weight if ≥45 kg (fixed dose) = Minimal residual disease positive (MRD+): 28 mcg on days 1–28 of 6 week treatment cycle; Relapsed/refractory (RR): 9 mcg daily on days 1–7 followed by 28 mcg days 8–28 of 6 week treatment cycle. Dose based on BSA if <45 kg = Minimal residual disease positive (MRD+): 15 mcg/m²/day (max 28 mcg/day) as a continuous infusion on days 1–28 of 6 week treatment cycle; Relapsed/refractory (RR): 5 mcg/m²/day (max 9 mcg/day) days 1–7 followed by 15 mcg/m²/day (max 28 mcg/day) days 8–28 of 6 week treatment cycle	ALL
Bortezomib (bor TEZ oh mib)	Velcade	Enzyme inhibitor	Powder for reconstitution	IV, SUBQ	1.3 mg/m²	Multiple myeloma, lymphoma
Bosutinib (boe SUE ti nib)	Bosulif	Enzyme inhibitor	Tablet	Oral	400 mg or 500 mg once daily	CML
Brentuximab vedotin (bren TUX i mab ve DOE tin)	Adcetris	Antibody drug conjugate, monoclonal antibody	Powder for reconstitution	IV	1.2–1.8 mg/kg every 2 or 3 weeks	Hodgkins lymphoma, peripheral T-cell lymphoma
Brigatinib (bre GA ti nib)	Alunbrig	Enzyme inhibitor (2nd generation)	Tablet	Oral	180 mg once daily	NSCLC
Cabozantinib (ka boe ZAN ti nib)	Cabometyx, Cometriq	Enzyme inhibitor	Tablet	Oral	60–140 mg once daily	Hepatocellular carcinoma, RCC, thyroid cancer
Carfilzomib (car FILLS oh mib)	Kyprolis	Enzyme inhibitor	Solution	IV	20 mg/m² days 1 and 2, if tolerated increased to 27 mg/m² OR 36 mg/m² OR 56 mg/m² OR 70 mg/m²	Multiple myeloma, Waldenstrom macroglobulinemia

Continued next page

MEDICATION TABLE 31-2. Biologic Therapies Used to Treat Cancer[11] (Continued)

Generic Name (pronunciation)	Brand Name	Class	Dosage Forms	Route	Common Dose	Indication
Ceritinib (Se RI ti nib)	Zykadia	Enzyme inhibitor (2nd generation)	Capsule, tablet	Oral	450 mg once daily	NSCLC
Cetuximab (se TUX i mab)	Erbitux	Monoclonal antibody	Injection solution	IV	Initial dose of 400 mg/m² followed by weekly maintenance dose of 250 mg/m²	Colorectal cancer, squamous cell carcinoma
Copanlisib (koe pan LIS ib)	Aliqopa	Enzyme inhibitor	Tablet	Oral	60 mg on days 1, 8, and 15 of a 28-day treatment cycle	Follicular lymphoma
Crizotinib (kri ZO ti nib)	Xalkori	Enzyme inhibitor (1st generation)	Tablet	Oral	250 mg twice daily	NSCLC
Dabrafenib (da BRAF e nib)	Tafinlar	Enzyme inhibitor	Capsule	Oral	150 mg twice daily	Melanoma, NSCLC, thyroid cancer
Dacomitinib (DAK oh MI ti nib)	Vizimpro	Enzyme inhibitor	Tablet	Oral	45 mg once daily	NSCLC
Daratumumab (dar a TOOM ue mab)	Darzalex	Monoclonal antibody	Injection solution	IV	16 mg/kg once weekly initially	Multiple myeloma
Dasatinib (da SA ti nib)	Sprycel	Enzyme inhibitor	Tablet	Oral	100 mg once daily	Chronic myelogenous leukemia (CML)
Dinutuximab (din ue TUX i mab)	Unituxin	Monoclonal antibody	Injection solution	IV	17.5 mg/m² for 4 consecutive days for maximum 5 cycles	Neuroblastoma
Durvalumab (dur VAL ue mab)	Imfinzi	Monoclonal antibody	Injection solution	IV	10 mg/kg once every 2 weeks	NSCLC, urothelial cancer
Duvelisib (DOO ve LIS ib)	Coptiktra	Enzyme inhibitor	Capsules	Oral	25 mg twice daily	CLL, follicular lymphoma
Elotuzumab (el oh TOOZ ue mab)	Empliciti	Monoclonal antibody	Reconstituted solution	IV	10 mg/kg once weekly initially	Multiple myeloma
Enasidenib (en a SID a nib)	IDHIFA	Enzyme inhibitor	Tablet	Oral	100 mg once daily	Acute myeloid leukemia
Encorafenib (en koe RAF e nib)	Braftovi	Enzyme inhibitor	Capsule	Oral	300 mg or 450 mg once daily	Colorectal cancer, melanoma
Erdafitinib (er da FI ti nib)	Balversa	Enzyme inhibitor	Tablet	Oral	8 mg once daily and increase to dose to 9 mg based on tolerability	Urothelial carcinoma
Erlotinib (er LOE ti nib)	Tarceva	Enzyme inhibitor	Tablet	Oral	150 mg once daily	NSCLC, pancreatic cancer

Continued next page

MEDICATION TABLE 31-2. Biologic Therapies Used to Treat Cancer[11] *(Continued)*

Generic Name (pronunciation)	Brand Name	Class	Dosage Forms	Route	Common Dose	Indication
Everolimus (e ver OH li mus)	Afinitor, Zortress	Enzyme inhibitor	Tablet	Oral	10 mg once daily	Advanced RCC, breast cancer, subependymal giant cell astrocytoma (SEGA), pancreatic neuroendocrine tumors, prophylaxis of organ rejection
Gefitinib (ge FI ti nib)	Iressa	Enzyme inhibitor	Tablet	Oral	250 mg once daily	NSCLC
Gilteritinib (GIL te RI ti nib)	Xospata	Enzyme inhibitor	Tablet	Oral	120 mg once daily	AML
Glasdegib (glas DEG ib)	Daurismo	Hedgehog Pathway inhibitor	Tablet	Oral	100 mg once daily	AML
Ibritumomab (eye bri TOOM oh mab)	Zevalin	Monoclonal antibody	Injection solution	IV	Two-step regimen with rituximab	NHL
Ibrutinib (eye BROO ti nib)	Imbruvica	Enzyme inhibitor	Capsule, tablet	Oral	420 mg or 560 mg once daily	CLL, chronic graft-versus-host disease, mantle cell lymphoma, marginal zone lymphoma, Waldenstrom macroglobulinemia
Idelasib (eye DEL as ib)		Enzyme inhibitor	Tablet	Oral	150 mg twice daily	CLL, follicular B-cell non-Hodgkin's lymphoma, small lymphocytic lymphoma
Ixazomib (ix AZ oh mib)	Ninlaro	Enzyme inhibitor	Capsule	Oral	4 mg once weekly on days 1, 8, and 15 of 28-day treatment	Multiple myeloma
Imatinib (i MAT in ib)	Gleevec	Enzyme inhibitor	Tablet	Oral	400 mg once daily	Gastrointestinal stromal tumors (GIST), chronic myeloid leukemia, acute lymphoblastic leukemia (ALL), aggressive systemic mastocytosis (ASM), dermatofibrosarcoma protuberans (DFSP), hypereosinophilic syndrome (HES), chronic eosinophilic leukemia (CEL), myelodysplastic/myeloproliferative disease (MDS/MPD)

Continued next page

MEDICATION TABLE 31-2. Biologic Therapies Used to Treat Cancer[11] (Continued)

Generic Name (pronunciation)	Brand Name	Class	Dosage Forms	Route	Common Dose	Indication
Interferon alfa-2b (in ter FEER on AL fa)	Intron A	Interferon	Injection powder for reconstitution, injection solution	IM, SUBQ	Dose varies, 6–18 month's duration	Leukemia, malignant melanoma, AIDS-related Kaposi's sarcoma, non-Hodgkin's lymphoma
Ipilimumab (ip i LIM ue mab)	Yervoy	Monoclonal antibody	Injection solution	IV	3 mg/kg every 3 weeks for 4 doses	Metastatic melanoma
Ivosidenib (EYE voe SID e nib)	Tibsovo	Enzyme inhibitor	Tablet	Oral	500 mg once daily	AML
Lapatinib (la PA ti nib)	Tykerb	Enzyme inhibitor	Tablet	Oral	1,250 mg once daily (used as part of a combination therapy)	Metastatic breast cancer
Lenalidomide (len a LID oh mide)	Revlimid	Immunomodulator	Capsule	Oral	10–25 mg once daily for 21 days of a 28-day treatment cycle	Myelodysplastic syndrome (MDS), multiple myeloma
Lenvatinib (len VA ti nib)	Lenvima	Enzyme inhibitor	Capsule	Oral	8–24 mg once daily	Endometrial carcinoma. hepatocellular carcinoma, renal cell carcinoma, thyroid cancer
Lorlatinib (lor LA ti nib)	Lorbrena	Enzyme inhibitor (3rd generation)	Tablet	Oral	100 mg once daily	NSCLC
Midostaurin (mye doe STAW rin)	Rydapt	Enzyme inhibitor	Capsule	Oral	50 mg or 100 mg twice daily	AML, mast cell leukemia, systemic mastocytosis
Mogamulizumab (moe GAM ue LIZ ue mab)	Poteligeo	Monoclonal antibody	Injection solution	IV	1 mg/kg days 1 and 15 of 28-day cycle	Mycosis fungoides, Sezary syndrome
Necitumumab (ne si TOOM oo mab)	Portrazza	Monoclonal antibody		IV	800 mg on days 1 and 8 of a 3-week cycle	Squamous NSCLC
Neratinib (ne RA ti nib)	Nerlynx	Enzyme inhibitor	Tablet	Oral	240 mg once daily	Breast cancer
Nilotinib (nil OT i nib)	Tasigna	Enzyme inhibitor	Capsule	Oral	300 mg twice daily	CML
Niraparib (nye RAP a rib)	Zejula	PARP inhibitor	Capsule	Oral	300 mg once daily	Ovarian, fallopian tube, or primary peritoneal cancer
Nivolumab (nye VOL ue mab)	Opdivo	Monoclonal antibody	Injection solution	IV	240 mg once every 2 weeks or 480 mg once every 4 weeks	Colorectal cancer, head and neck cancer, hepatocellular carcinoma, Hodgkin's lymphoma, melanoma, RCC, small cell lung cancer

Continued next page

MEDICATION TABLE 31-2. Biologic Therapies Used to Treat Cancer[11] *(Continued)*

Generic Name (pronunciation)	Brand Name	Class	Dosage Forms	Route	Common Dose	Indication
Obinutuzumab (oh bi nue TOOZ ue mab)	Gazyva	Monoclonal antibody	Injection solution	IV	1,000 mg once daily	CLL, follicular lymphoma
Ofatumumab (o fa TOOM ue mab)	Arzerra	Monoclonal antibody	Injection solution	IV	Up to 2,000 mg once every 4 weeks for 4 doses	CLL
Osimertinib (oh si mer ti nib)	Tagrisso	Enzyme inhibitor	Tablet	Oral	80 mg once daily	NSCLC
Palbociclib (pal boe SYE klib)	Ibrance	Enzyme inhibitor	Capsule	Oral	125 mg once daily	Breast cancer
Panitumumab (pan i TOOM yoo mab)	Vectibix	Monoclonal antibody	Injection solution	IV	6 mg/kg every 2 weeks	Colorectal cancer
Panobinostat (pan oh BIN oh stat)	Farydak	Enzyme inhibitor	Capsule	Oral	20 mg once every other day for 3 doses every week on weeks 1 and 2 of 21-day cycle	Multiple myeloma
Pazopanib (paz OH pa nib)	Votrient	Enzyme inhibitor	Tablet	Oral	800 mg once daily until disease progression or unacceptable toxicity	RCC
Pembrolizumab (pem broe LIZ ue mab)	Keytruda	Monoclonal antibody	Injection solution	IV	200 mg once every 3 weeks	Cervical cancer, endometrial cancer, esophageal cancer, head and neck cancer, hepatocellualr carcinoma, Hodgkin's lymphoma, melanoma, Merkel cell carcinoma, NSCLC, small cell lung cancer, renal cell carcinoma, urothelial carcinoma
Ponatinib (poe NA ti nib)	Iclusig	Enzyme inhibitor	Tablet	Oral	45 mg once daily	ALL, CML
Ramucirumab (ra mue SIR ue mab)	Cyramza	Monoclonal antibody			8 mg/kg once every 2 weeks or 10 mg/kg on day 1 every 21 days (dose dependent on indication)	Colorectal cancer, gastric cancer, hepatocellualr carcinoma, NSCLC
Regorafenib (re goe RAF e nib)	Stivarga	Enzyme inhibitor	Tablet	Oral	160 mg once daily for first 21 days of 28-day cycle	Colorectal cancer, gastrointestinal stromal tumor, hepatocellular carcinoma
Ribociclib (rye boe SYE klib)	Kisqali	Enzyme inhibitor	Tablet	Oral	600 mg once daily	Breast cancer
Rituximab (ri TUX i mab)	Rituxan, Truxima, Riabni	Monoclonal antibody	Injection solution	IV	375 mg/m^2 in cycle 1, then 500 mg/m^2 on day 1 (every 28 days) of cycles 2-6	NHL, CLL

Continued next page

MEDICATION TABLE 31-2. Biologic Therapies Used to Treat Cancer[11] *(Continued)*

Generic Name (pronunciation)	Brand Name	Class	Dosage Forms	Route	Common Dose	Indication
Rituximab and hyaluronidase (ri TUX i mab & hye al yoor ON i dase)	Rituxan Hycela	Monoclonal antibody	Subcutaneous depot injection	SUBQ	1,400 mg/23,400 units or 1,600 mg/26,800 units	CLL, diffuse large B-cell lymphoma, follicular lymphoma
Romidepsin (roe mi DEP sin)	Istodax	Enzyme inhibitor	Injection powder for reconstitution	IV	14 mg/m^2 days 1, 8, and 15 of a 28-day treatment cycle	Cutaneous T-cell lymphoma (CTCL) and peripheral T-cell lymphoma (PTCL)
Ruxolitinib (rux oh LI ti nib)	Jakafi	Enzyme inhibitor	Tablet	Oral	5–15 mg twice daily	Graft-versus-host disease, myelofibrosis, polycythemia vera
Sonidegib (soe ni DEG ib)	Odomzo	Hedgehog Pathway inhibitor	Capsule	Oral	200 mg once daily	Basal cell carcinoma
Sorafenib (soe RAF e nib)	NexAVAR	Enzyme inhibitor	Tablet	Oral	400 mg twice daily	RCC, hepatocellular cancer
Sunitinib (soo NI ti nib)	Sutent	Enzyme inhibitor	Capsule	Oral	50 mg once daily for 4 weeks of a 6-week treatment cycle	GIST, RCC, pancreatic neuroendocrine tumors
Talazoparib (tal a ZOE pa rib)	Talzenna	PARP inhibitor	Capsule	Oral	1 mg once daily	Breast cancer
Temsirolimus (tem sir OH li mus)	Torisel	Enzyme inhibitor	Injection solution	IV	25 mg once weekly	RCC
Trastuzumab (tras TOO zoo mab)	Herceptin, Kanjinti, Ogivri, Ontruzant, Herzuma	Monoclonal antibody	Injection powder for reconstitution	IV	4 mg/kg infused over 90 minutes	Breast cancer, gastric or gastroesophageal junction adenocarcinoma
Tretinoin (TRET i noe in)	Vesanoid	Retinoid	Capsule	Oral	45 mg/m^2/day in 2 equally divided doses (discontinue 30 days after complete remission or after 90 days of treatment)	APL
Vandetanib (van DET a nib)	Caprelsa	Enzyme inhibitor	Tablet	Oral	300 mg once daily	Thyroid cancer
Vemurafenib (vem ue RAF e nib)	Zelboraf	Enzyme inhibitor	Tablet	Oral	960 mg twice daily	Melanoma, NSCLC
Venetoclax (ven ET oh klax)	Venclexta	BLC-2 inhibitor	Tablet	Oral	400 mg once daily	AML, CLL
Vismodegib (vis moe DEG ib)	Erivedge	Hedgehog Pathway inhibitor	Capsule	Oral	150 mg once daily	Basal cell carcinoma
Vorinostat (vor IN oh stat)	Zolinza	Enzyme inhibitor	Capsule	Oral	400 mg once daily	Cutaneous T-cell lymphoma

IV = intravenous; SUBQ = subcutaneous.

MEDICATION TABLE 31-3. Chemoprotective Agents[11]

Generic Name (pronunciation)	Brand Name	Class	Dosage Forms	Route	Common Dose	Indication
Dexrazoxane (deks ray ZOKS ane)		Chemoprotective	Solution (reconstituted)	IV	10 × dose of doxorubicin	Prevention of doxorubicin cardiotoxicity
	Totect	Antidote	Solution (reconstituted)	IV	1,000 mg/m^2 daily × 2, then 500 mg/m^2 on day 3	Treatment for extravasation of anthracyclines during administration
Mesna (MES na)	Mesnex	Chemoprotective agent	Solution, tablet	IV, oral	IV: 60% of ifosfamide dose in 3 divided doses IV + PO: IV bolus 20% of ifosfamide dose followed by oral administration of 80% of ifosfamide dose in divided doses	Prevention of ifosfamide-induced hemorrhagic cystitis

IV = intravenous; PO = oral.

THE DERMATOLOGIC SYSTEM

Chapter 32

Overview of the Skin and Topical Dosage Forms

Laura A. Perry, PharmD, BCPS |
Lori J. Ernsthausen, PharmD, BCPS

KEY TERMS AND DEFINITIONS

Dermis—the layer of skin beneath the epidermis, which provides structural support to the skin and is composed of blood vessels, nerves, and appendages.

Epidermis—the outermost layer of the skin composed of five layers.

Hypodermis—third layer of skin composed of adipose (fat) tissue.

Integumentary system—the skin and its appendages (hair, glands, nails).

Local—drug effect at site of application.

Melanocytes—cells located in the epidermis responsible for skin color.

Stratum corneum—outermost layer of the epidermis composed of nonliving keratinocytes.

Topical—applied to a surface of the body, such as the skin.

Transdermal—drug transport across or through the skin into the bloodstream.

DOI 10.37573/9781585286638.032

LEARNING OBJECTIVES

After completing this chapter, you should be able to

1. Describe the skin as an organ system:
   a. List the three functionally distinct regions of the skin and describe their function.
   b. Describe the roles of keratinocytes, melanocytes, and Langerhans cells as components of the epidermis.
   c. Define mast cell.
   d. Identify the skin appendages located in the dermis.
   e. Define adipose tissue.

2. Explain how changes in skin thickness, integrity, hydration, and age can alter topical drug absorption.

3. Describe how the vehicle in a topical formulation can influence the absorption of the active drug.

4. Name and describe two types of transdermal preparations.

The skin is the largest organ in the body. Together the skin and its appendages (glands, hair, and nails) are known as the integumentary system. The main function of the skin is to work as a barrier to separate internal body components from the outside environment. This barrier is very important to protect the internal body organs from injury and water loss (dehydration) and to prevent infectious organisms or toxic substances from entering the bloodstream. The following chapter will discuss the structure and function of the skin and how different types of drug therapies work when applied topically.

SKIN STRUCTURE AND FUNCTION

The skin is divided into three main layers known as the epidermis, dermis, and hypodermis (Figure 32-1). The epidermis is the outermost layer of the skin and is composed of several layers (*strata*) of cells. The majority of the cells in the epidermis are known as keratinocytes. Keratinocytes are responsible for the production of keratin, the structural protein of the skin, hair, and nails. Structural changes occur to the keratinocytes as they move from the bottommost layer of the epidermis, the stratum germinativum, to the outermost layer of the epidermis, the stratum corneum. As they move toward the stratum corneum, keratinocytes dry out, die, and are eventually sloughed off. Another major cell type in the epidermis is the melanocyte, found in the stratum germinativum. Melanocytes are responsible for skin color. The third major cell type of the epidermis are the Langerhans cells. These cells are found in the stratum spinosum, the layer above the stratum germinativum. Langerhans cells function to produce an immune response and are involved in the development of allergic reactions on the skin.

The dermis is the second main layer of the skin and is located directly below the epidermis. The dermis is the largest component of the skin structure and is composed of two major cell types: mast cells and fibroblasts. Mast cells

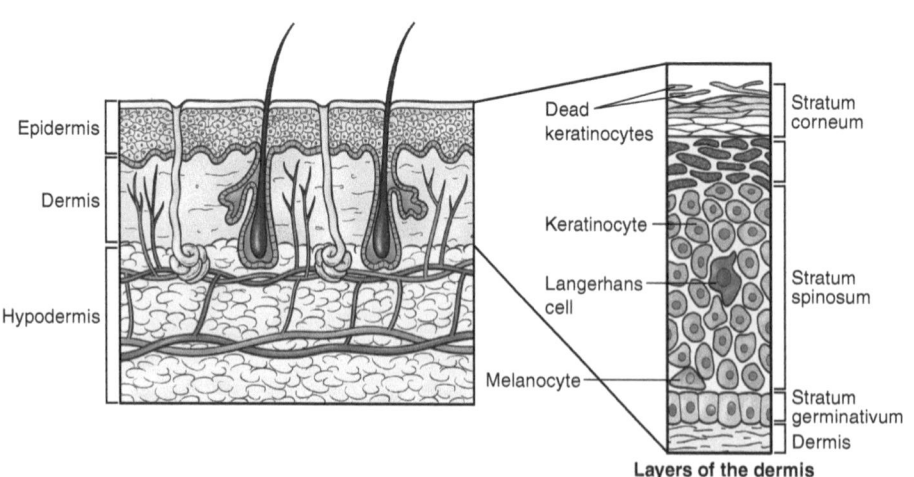

FIGURE 32-1. Skin structure.

are involved in the pathogenesis of allergic skin disorders. Fibroblasts are responsible for the synthesis of elastic fibers and collagen, the structural support components of the skin. Unlike the epidermis, the dermis contains blood vessels, nerves, and appendages. The nerves in the dermis provide the sensation of touch, pain, temperature, and pressure. Appendages located in the dermis are sweat glands, sebaceous glands, and hair follicles. Sebaceous glands secrete sebum, a waxy substance that helps keep the skin moist, and sweat glands secrete toxins and fluids to help maintain body temperature.

The hypodermis is the third main layer of the skin and is located below the dermis. The hypodermis is composed mainly of adipose tissue (fat cells), collagen, and larger blood vessels. The main functions of the hypodermis are to provide cushioning to protect the body from injury and regulation of body temperature.

TOPICAL ADMINISTRATION

CASE STUDY

Mrs. Williams is a 65-year-old woman with seasonal allergies, asthma, psoriasis, and high blood pressure. Her physician is adding a clonidine patch (Catapres-TTS) to her drug regimen to lower her blood pressure. Other topical therapies she is currently using include an ointment and a cream for the management of her psoriasis.

The primary goal of most topical drug preparations is to provide local action on one or more layers of the skin. For example, sunscreen, calamine lotion, keratolytic agents, and topical anti-itch agents are designed to exert their effects on the skin surface to prevent and treat skin disorders. The effects at the site where the preparation is administered are considered local actions. Although some of the active drug in these topical products intended for local uses may reach systemic circulation, typically the amount is subtherapeutic and not of great concern. Systemic agents, on the other hand, such as tablets, capsules, and intravenous (IV) medications, are absorbed or administered directly into the bloodstream and can affect the entire body. Some transdermal products are formulated for systemic absorption, such as fentanyl patches, which provide pain relief throughout the body and not at the site of application. Regardless of the desired site

of action, monitoring the absorption of topical drugs is very important, especially in certain patient populations who may be at risk for serious adverse effects.

CASE?

Is the action of Mrs. William's clonidine patch considered to be local or systemic? How does this action differ from the cream and ointment prescribed for her psoriasis?

SKIN CONDITIONS THAT AFFECT DRUG ABSORPTION

Drugs are absorbed into the skin by a process known as passive diffusion. There are many factors that affect the rate of drug absorption through the skin and into the bloodstream. The first factor is the thickness of the skin. Thick skin will decrease the rate of absorption of drugs, while thin skin will increase the rate of absorption of drugs. This is because the depth of the stratum corneum layer of the epidermis is the rate-limiting barrier to drug absorption. Thick skin, like that on the bottom of the feet, has a very deep stratum corneum layer and thin skin, like that of the scalp, has a very shallow stratum corneum layer. Once the drug moves past the stratum corneum barrier, its molecules easily pass through the dermis and systemic absorption can occur. Therefore, drug absorption will occur more quickly in areas where the skin is thin.

Other factors that affect drug absorption are skin integrity, temperature, and hydration. As mentioned above, the skin is a protective barrier. When a cut or abrasion occurs on the skin, the protective barrier is broken, allowing foreign material to enter the bloodstream. If a drug is placed on an area of broken or inflamed skin, it can bypass the stratum corneum, allowing for quick absorption. In addition to skin integrity, skin temperature and skin hydration also affect drug absorption. Warm, moist skin provides the highest potential for drug absorption. Hydration (addition of moisture) of the stratum corneum increases the space between the skin cells, allowing an open pathway for drugs to move through this skin barrier. Also, moist skin will help to dissolve the drug, allowing for easier passage. Placing bandages or wraps over the skin also prevents water loss, increasing hydration and temperature and allowing for faster drug absorption. Since the goal of topical drug administration is to provide a local action, it is important to recognize what skin conditions increase systemic absorption of these preparations in order to maximize topical effectiveness and avoid adverse effects.

CASE?

Why should Mrs. Williams avoid placing a heating pad over the application site of her patch (or any topical agent)?

DRUG ABSORPTION IN SPECIAL PATIENT POPULATIONS

Systemic absorption of topical preparations should be monitored closely in pediatric and geriatric patients. These populations are at higher risk for systemic toxicity of topically applied drugs for various reasons.

ALERT!

Some over-the-counter (OTC) topical preparations, including rubbing alcohol, antiseptics, and pain relief products have been shown to cause toxicity in newborns. Package instructions limiting use in children below a certain age should be closely observed.

Infants and children have a higher ratio of total body surface area to body mass, which places them at risk for increased exposure to topical agents and high systemic concentrations of drugs. Additionally, infants may not be able to metabolize absorbed drugs effectively due to the immaturity of their organ systems. Along with monitoring infants and children closely, it is also important to monitor pregnant or nursing mothers because topically absorbed drugs may affect the unborn fetus or the nursing infant.

Geriatric patients may also have altered absorption of topical drug preparations. Many changes to the skin occur with increasing age. For example, skin becomes wrinkled, dry, and thinner with age. Thin skin, which has a smaller amount of subcutaneous fat, may increase drug absorption. Also, these normal skin changes place older adults at increased risk of skin injuries. It is important to avoid applying topical drug products to broken or damaged skin.

ALERT!

Just because a topical product is not being ingested or injected into the body does not mean it is safe to use it in ways other than directed by the prescriber or package. Overdoses can still occur and are more likely if products are used in quantities greater than the usual dose or for patients in an age group for which it is not recommended. Consumers purchasing OTC topical products should be reminded to read and follow all package instructions. Patients with prescriptions for medications to be placed on the skin should be reminded that the pharmacist can discuss proper application with them.

Many skin conditions predispose patients to increased topical drug absorption. Examples of these include sunburn (especially after skin peeling), eczema, psoriasis, thermal burns, and chemical peels.

VEHICLES FOR TOPICAL DRUG ADMINISTRATION

There are many formulations available for topical drug administration, such as liquids, creams, gels, ointments, pastes, and powders, as well as some solid dosage forms. Drugs may be applied topically to the skin, mucous membranes, eyes, nose, rectum, and vagina. Often, a drug may be available in several topical dosage forms. Understanding the differences between available vehicles can aid in proper product selection and improve patient adherence.

Ointments are considered semisolid preparations and may be formulated with a variety of bases. Ointments are known for their occlusive (protecting and sealing against water loss) properties and may stay in place better than creams or gels. The emollient property (softening or soothing the skin) of ointments aids in skin hydration and absorption, and the oleaginous (fatty) base improves drug penetration. Ointments are preferred for patients with dry, chapped skin or in disease states such as psoriasis, where the emollient property can help soften the plaques and improve drug delivery. Due to their thicker, oily bases, ointments may discolor clothing and may be more difficult to apply to hairy areas of the skin.

Creams, like ointments, are semisolid dosage forms with emollient effects. However, creams may be more cosmetically pleasing to patients due to their water washable property. Creams are less occlusive than ointments and may be easier to apply. Creams may be used to administer drugs via the vaginal route.

Topical solutions are liquid preparations that contain a drug dissolved in a solvent. Drug particles in a solution disperse very evenly, which allows for uniform dosage when applied. Solutions are less stable than other semisolid dosage forms and should be kept away from light and extreme heat. Solutions or suspensions that are applied topically are often referred to as lotions.

Gels may be preferred by patients for their quick-drying, transparent properties. Gels do not leave a residue on the skin and can be washed off with water. Compared with ointments and creams, gels generally provide faster drug release. Due to their water-soluble bases, gels may be the preferred vehicle for hydrophilic (water-soluble) drugs to optimize their delivery.

The term "paste" refers to an ointment that has a large amount of solid integrated. Pastes are generally stiff and dry and can be applied to areas of skin where oozing or weeping is occurring, as they will absorb secretions. Although pastes are not very occlusive, they remain in place and can protect lesions by serving as a physical barrier.

Powders are finely divided, dry solid dosage forms. Powders intended for topical use should be applied to intact skin for a local effect. Powders are also available for systemic use by mixing in suspensions or solutions for drinking, sprinkling on food, or for compounding into tablets or capsules. Proper dosing and application may be more difficult with powders.

ALERT!

Patients and caregivers applying topical powders should be careful to avoid inhalation of powders, as they can irritate the lungs.

CASE?

Why might patients with thick plaque psoriasis, like Mrs. Williams, prefer topical agents formulated as ointments rather than creams or gel and patients with itching due to an insect bite prefer a cream or gel rather than ointment?

TRANSDERMAL PREPARATIONS

CASE STUDY

Mrs. Smith 53 years old and has begun to experience severe hot flashes and night sweats, along with longer and varying intervals between her menstrual periods. Due to her difficulty in managing these perimenopausal symptoms, her physician has prescribed an estradiol/norethindrone (CombiPatch) transdermal patch.

ALERT!

Many topical preparations are formulated for application to a specific part of the body and are inappropriate for use elsewhere. For example, ointments for application to the skin may have active ingredients identical to those for the eye, but must not be used ophthalmically because ophthalmic preparations must be sterile and may require adjustments in pH or other characteristics of the ointment base to make them suitable for the more delicate tissues of the eye.

The primary goal of transdermal drug administration, unlike topical drug administration, is to achieve and maintain adequate systemic drug concentrations. Transdermal preparations do not target diseases of the skin; rather, they are designed to use the skin as a means for drug absorption. Transdermal patches provide several advantages over oral dosage forms, particularly in those patients who have difficulty swallowing or taking tablets or capsules. Additionally, transdermal semisolids such as nitroglycerin ointment and testosterone gel are available by prescription. Transdermal products are often dosed less frequently than oral forms, which can aid in compliance and may improve disease state control. Transdermal products deliver drugs at a consistent, steady rate, which can avoid side effects that may be due to peaks (high concentrations). First pass metabolism, the breakdown of drugs by the liver, can be avoided with transdermal products because the absorbed drug will not travel to the liver prior to distribution through the body (as oral preparations do). Although the goal of transdermal products is systemic absorption, some products like diclofenac gel are applied to the affected joints of patients with osteoarthritis for pain relief at the site of application. The drug is absorbed through the skin and concentrates in the joint space, rather than the bloodstream.

Although there are several good reasons for choosing a transdermal drug product, there are also several disadvantages. Refer to Table 32-1 for a list of advantages and disadvantages of transdermal drug delivery. The most common adverse effect with transdermal administration is irritation at the site of application. Patients may experience redness, itching, and swelling, which may be caused by the drug, adhesive, or other components of a patch or vehicle. Drug delivery via the transdermal route of administration is limited by certain drug properties, particularly lipophilicity (fat solubility), molecule size, and potency. Lipophilic drugs can more easily move through the skin compared to hydrophilic drugs. Even though lipophilic drugs can move more easily through the stratum corneum, achieving high systemic concentrations can be difficult

using transdermal delivery methods. There are several formulations of drug patches designed to maximize drug delivery and minimize local irritation.

CASE?

What may be the advantage of a twice-weekly patch (CombiPatch) compared to daily oral hormone replacement therapy for Mrs. Smith?

TRANSDERMAL PATCH FORMULATIONS

There are two types of drug patches: matrix or reservoir. See Figures 32-2 and 32-3 for a comparison of the matrix delivery system and the reservoir delivery system. The matrix

TABLE 32-1. Advantages and Disadvantages of Transdermal Delivery

Advantages	Disadvantages
• Steady absorption of drug across skin for consistent serum drug levels • Lack of peak drug concentrations may decrease side effects • Less invasive than intravenous route • Patch is easily removed if toxicity develops • Less frequent administration increases compliance • Alternate route if oral formulation is not tolerated (nausea, stomach upset, unconscious) • Alternate route for drugs that undergo degradation by stomach contents or extensive first pass metabolism	• Local irritation at site of application from drug, adhesive, or other excipients (redness, itching, swelling) • Low permeability of skin limits the number of drugs suitable for this route • Substantial amount of drug left in patch after use leads to potential for exposure to children and pets • Damaged or cut patches may lead to dose dumping

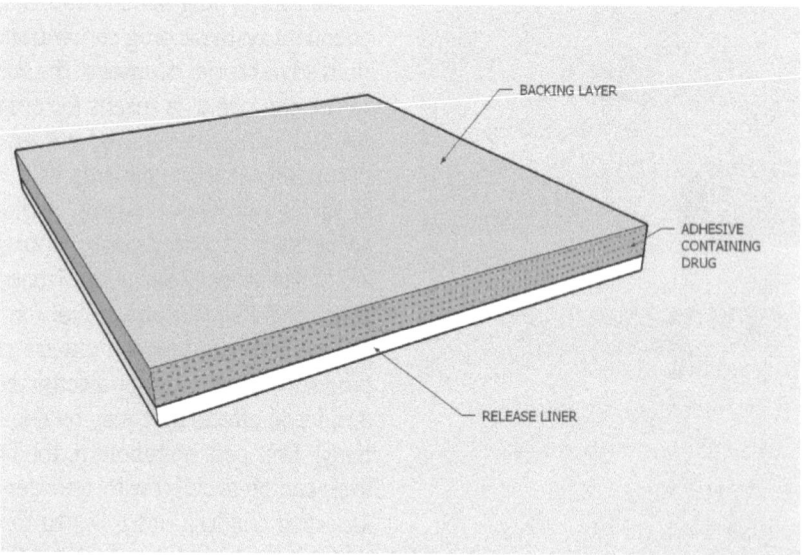

FIGURE 32-2. Matrix delivery system.

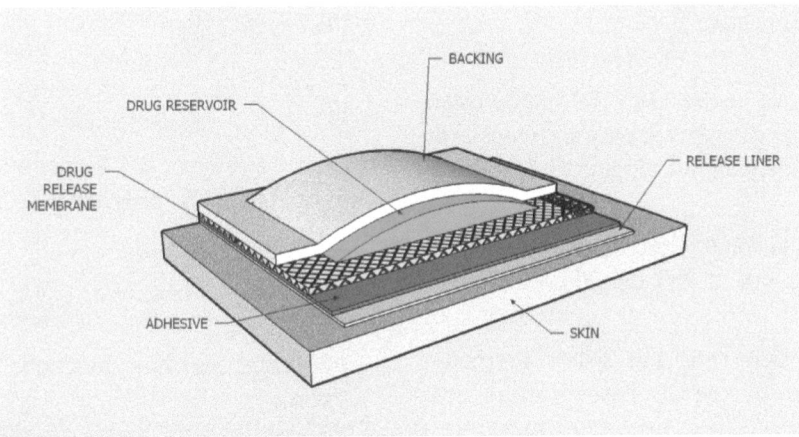

FIGURE 32-3. Reservoir delivery system.

delivery system contains a polymer matrix in which the drug is embedded. The matrix is designed to release drug at a steady rate. These patches tend to be smaller and thinner than reservoir patches. In the reservoir system a membrane is placed between the reservoir, which contains the drug, and the adhesive. The purpose of the membrane is to control the release of drug so constant blood levels can be achieved. As noted in Figures 32-2 and 32-3, both of these delivery systems contain a release liner that protects the patch before use and is removed prior to application.

Transdermal patches may utilize one of several adhesives. Newer pressure-sensitive adhesives, the most commonly used, provide strong adhesion once in contact with the skin, can be removed easily, and tend to produce less skin irritation. Other substances may be incorporated into transdermal patches, such as chemicals that may enhance drug penetration. Compounds that improve hydration, prevent water loss, or remove lipids from the skin may aid in drug delivery (see Medication Table 32-1, located at the end of the chapter).

Patients should be reminded to follow closely the printed instructions for product placement and removal. Some patches may be applied for several hours, while others are intended for week-long use. All patches, regardless of type, should be placed at the recommended application site on clean, dry skin. Periodically changing application sites can minimize skin irritation. Patients should always store patches in the original packaging until use. Cutting or tearing a patch may destroy the polymer matrix or reservoir and may lead to increased drug absorption and adverse effects. The patient should always remove the used patch before placing a new patch on the skin. Active drug will still be present in the used patch and overdosing could occur. Some patches may be discarded in the trash, while others should be flushed down the toilet to prevent accidental exposure or abuse.

PRACTICE POINT

Many transdermal products are intended for uninterrupted use; however, patients using nitroglycerin patches should have a 10- to 12-hour patch-free interval each day. Prescribing directions frequently instruct patients to apply one patch in the morning and remove it before bedtime.

ALERT!

Patients should be reminded not to cut or tear patches as this may lead to increased absorption and possible toxicity.

SUMMARY

Application to the skin provides a convenient method for topical and systemic drug administration. Understanding the skin's structure, drug properties, and available product formulations can aid in the selection of the most appropriate product to maximize drug absorption and minimize potential adverse effects. Transdermal patches offer a unique dosage form for the administration of systemic agents by providing consistent drug levels in the blood, less frequent dosing intervals, and avoiding the need for oral administration. Currently available transdermal patches utilize the matrix or reservoir systems of drug delivery and the patient should always be advised to follow the manufacturer's recommendations for use and disposal.

CHAPTER RESOURCES

Block LH. Medicated topicals. In: Beringer P, DerMarderosian A, Felton L, et al., eds. *Remington: The Science and Practice of Pharmacy*. 22nd ed. Philadelphia, PA: Lippincott & Wilkins; 2013:931-945.

Elder DL, eds. *A Practical Guide to Contemporary Pharmacy Practice and Compounding*. 4th ed. Philadelphia, PA: Wolters Kluwer; 2018.

Law RM, Maibach HI. Skin care and minor dermatologic conditions. In: DiPiro JT, Yee GC, Posey L, et al., eds. *Pharmacotherapy: A Pathophysiologic Approach*. 11th ed. New York, NY: McGraw-Hill Medical; 2019. http://accesspharmacy .mhmedical.com.ezproxy.findlay.edu:2048/content.aspx? bookid=2577&sectionid=219306022. Accessed January 11, 2020.

Saleem MD, Maibach HI, Feldman SR. Principles of topical therapy. In: Kang S, Amagai M, Bruckner AL, et al., eds. *Fitzpatrick's Dermatology in General Medicine*. 9th ed. New York, NY: McGraw-Hill; 2019. http://accessmedicine.mh medical.com.ezproxy.findlay.edu:2048/content.aspx? bookid=2570&sectionid=210413306. Accessed January 11, 2020.

Sewell MJ, Burkhart CN, Morrell DS. Dermatological pharmacology. In: Brunton LL, Hilal-Dandan R, Knollmann BC, eds. *Goodman & Gilman's The Pharmacological Basis of Therapeutics*. 13th ed. New York, NY: McGraw-Hill; 2018. http://accesspharmacy.mhmedical.com.ezproxy.findlay .edu:2048/content.aspx?bookid=2189&sectionid= 165936845. Accessed January 11, 2020.

Wilkosz MF, Bogner RH. Transdermal drug delivery. Part 1: Current status. *US Pharmacist*. 2003;28(4).

REVIEW QUESTIONS

1. Describe the three functionally distinct layers of the skin.

2. Name four factors that affect drug absorption, and describe *how* they affect drug absorption.

3. The manufacturers of IcyHot (7.6% menthol) cream for arthritis recommend not to apply the medication immediately before or after exercise and not to bandage or wrap the area after application. Based on what you have learned about factors of drug absorption, why does the manufacturer make these recommendations?

4. Name two advantages and two disadvantages of transdermal drug administration.

5. Describe the differences between matrix and reservoir delivery systems.

6. How should a patient dispose of a fentanyl patch?

MEDICATION TABLE

MEDICATION TABLE 32-1. Representative Transdermal Patches*

Generic Name (pronunciation)**	Brand Name	Type of Patch	Application	Notes
Pain				
Fentanyl (FEN ta nil)		Reservoir (brand and some generic formulations), matrix (generic formulations)	Replace patch and rotate sites every 72 hours; apply to chest, back, flank, or upper arm	Some patients report differences in efficacy when switching between reservoir and matrix formulations; avoid direct exposure to heat as this may increase fentanyl absorption and potential toxicity; dispose of removed patches by folding sticky sides of the patch together and flush down toilet; remove patch prior to undergoing an MRI
Buprenorphine (byoo pre NOR feen)	Butrans	Matrix	Replace patch and rotate sites every 7 days; apply to upper arm, upper back, upper chest, or side of the chest; do not put a new patch on the same skin area as an old patch for at least 21 days	Dispose used or unused patches using the Patch-Disposal Unit provided in packaging; alternatively, can fold sticky sides of used patches together and flush down the toilet
Lidocaine (LYE doe kane)	Lidoderm, ZTlido	Matrix	Apply 1 to 3 patches to painful area for up to 12 hours in a 24-hour period (12 hours with patch on, 12 hours with patch off)	Available over the counter; may cut patch to fit the exact area of pain; remove patch prior to undergoing an MRI; patch should not get wet
Diclofenac (dye KLOE fen ak)	Flector	Matrix	Apply 1 patch to the most painful area twice a day	Remove patch prior to undergoing an MRI; do not wear when bathing or showering
Attention Deficit Hyperactivity Disorder				
Methylphenidate (meth il FEN i date)	Daytrana	Matrix	Apply to area 2 hours before effect is needed; may wear patch up to 9 hours; apply patch to hip area, alternating sides daily	Dispose of removed patches by folding sticky sides of the patch together and flush down toilet or dispose of in a lidded container.
Smoking Cessation				
Nicotine (NIK oh teen)	Nicoderm CQ, Nicoderm CQ Clear, Habitrol	Reservoir (Nicoderm CQ), matrix (Habitrol)	Replace patch and rotate sites every 16–24 hours; apply to nonhairy skin of upper body	Remove Nicoderm CQ patch prior to undergoing an MRI
Blood Pressure/Angina				
Clonidine (KLOE ni deen)	Catapres-TTS	Reservoir	Replace patch and rotate sites once a week; apply to upper arm or outer chest	Remove patch prior to undergoing an MRI

Continued next page

MEDICATION TABLE 32-1. Representative Transdermal Patches* (Continued)

Generic Name (pronunciation)**	Brand Name	Type of Patch	Application	Notes
Nitroglycerin (nye troe GLI ser in)	Nitro-Dur	Matrix	Apply patch once a day for 12–14 hours (remove patch for the remaining 10–12 hours of each day); apply patch to a nonhairy area and rotate site daily	Remove patch for 10–12 hours in the evening to avoid nitrate tolerance; remove patch prior to undergoing an MRI
Hormones				
Estradiol (es tra DYE ole)	Alora, Climara, Menostar, Minivelle, Vivelle-Dot	Matrix	Climara and Menostar: replace patch and rotate sites once a week; apply to abdomen or buttocks; do not apply to breasts. Alora, Minivelle, Vivelle-Dot: replace patch and rotate sites twice a week; apply to abdomen or buttocks; do not apply to breasts	
Estradiol/norethindrone (es tra DYE ole) (nor ETH in drone)	CombiPatch	Matrix	Replace patch and rotate sites twice a week; apply to lower abdomen; do not apply to breasts	Store refrigerated prior to dispensing; after dispensing, patient may keep at room temperature for up to 6 months
Estradiol/levonorgestrel (es tra DYE ole) (lee voe nor JES trel)	Climara Pro	Matrix	Replace patch and rotate sites once a week; apply to lower abdomen; do not apply to breasts	
Ethinyl estradiol/norelgestromin (ETH in il) (es tra DYE ole) (nor el JES troe min)	Xulane	Matrix	Replace patch and rotate sites once a week for 3 weeks; do not wear a patch on week 4; buttock, abdomen, upper arm, or back; do not apply to breasts	
Testosterone (tes TOS ter one)	Androderm	Reservoir	Replace patch and rotate sites once a day; apply patch at night to back, abdomen, upper arms, and thighs; do not apply to scrotum; do not apply a new patch to the same site for 7 days	Avoid bathing or swimming for at least 3 hours after applying patch
Overactive Bladder				
Oxybutynin (ox i BYOO ti nin)	Oxytrol	Matrix	Replace patch and rotate sites twice a week; apply to abdomen, hips, or buttocks; do not apply a new patch to the same site for 7 days	Available over the counter

Continued next page

MEDICATION TABLE 32-1. Representative Transdermal Patches* *(Continued)*

Generic Name (pronunciation)**	Brand Name	Type of Patch	Application	Notes
Alzheimer's Disease				
Rivastigmine (ri va STIG meen)	Exelon	Matrix	Replace patch and rotate sites daily; apply to upper or lower back, upper arm, or chest; do not apply a new patch to the same site for 14 days	
Parkinson's Disease				
Rotigotine (roe TIG oh teen)	Neupro		Replace patch and rotate sites daily; apply to abdomen, thigh, hip, flank, shoulder, or upper arm; do not apply a new patch to the same site for 14 days	
Major Depressive Disorder				
Selegiline (se LE ji leen)	Emsam	Matrix	Replace patch and rotate sites daily; apply to upper chest, back, abdomen, upper thigh, or outer upper arm	
Motion Sickness				
Scopolamine (skoe POL a meen)	Transderm Scop	Reservoir	Apply 4 hours before needed and replace patch and rotate sites after 3 days; apply to hairless area behind one ear	Remove patch prior to undergoing an MRI; limit contact with water

MRI = magnetic resonance imaging.

* National Library of Medicine, DailyMed. Bethesda, MD: U.S. National Library of Medicine, National Institutes of Health, Health & Human Services; 2021. https://dailymed.nlm.nih.gov/dailymed/. Accessed July 12, 2021

** Pronunciations have been adapted with permission from USP Dictionary of USAN and International Drug Names (USP Dictionary) © 2022.

Chapter 33

Treatment of Dermatologic Disorders

Lori J. Ernsthausen, PharmD, BCPS |
Laura A. Perry, PharmD, BCPS

KEY TERMS AND DEFINITIONS

Acne—a common, chronic, inflammatory skin disorder of the pilosebaceous unit (hair follicle and surrounding sebaceous glands).

Astringent—substance that constricts skin tissue to decrease inflammation, relieve itching, and dry up secretions.

Cellulitis—a common bacterial infection of the skin that occurs after skin trauma or abrasion and is characterized by a nonelevated, red, hot, and painful area of the skin with possible swelling.

Comedo or comedones (plural)—primary acne lesion, thought to be formed by the plugging of the pilosebaceous unit.

Dermatitis—an acute or chronic inflammatory, erythematous (red in color) rash, which may be caused by skin contact with an allergen or irritant.

Emollient—substance that softens or soothes the skin by slowing the evaporation of water.

Folliculitis—inflammation of hair follicles.

Impetigo—a contagious bacterial infection that occurs most commonly on the face of children and is characterized by pus-filled blisters that burst to form a thick yellow crust.

DOI 10.37573/9781585286638.033

Psoriasis—chronic inflammatory skin disorder most commonly characterized by red lesions, or plaques, with silvery-white scales.

Tinea infections—common fungal infections of the skin that occur mostly on areas of the skin that are moist and poorly ventilated, such as the feet or groin.

LEARNING OBJECTIVES

After completing this chapter, you should be able to

1. Define the most common dermatologic disorders.

2. Explain the disease process (pathophysiology) of each dermatologic disorder.

3. Describe nonpharmacologic treatment options for dermatologic disorders.

4. State the brand and generic names of the most widely used medications indicated for dermatologic disorders, along with their routes of administration, dosage forms, and available doses.

5. Explain the mechanism of action and common adverse effects of prescription and nonprescription agents for the treatment of dermatologic disorders.

6. Recognize commonly used treatment regimens for each dermatologic disorder.

The skin, as the largest organ, is subject to many of the same types of disorders as other parts of the body. These include infection, inflammation, and autoimmune disease, although these often cause different symptoms when they affect the dermatologic system. Some diseases that are distinctively considered *skin conditions* are actually caused by a combination of factors. Patients are usually able to see and localize dermatologic problems more easily and specifically than issues involving internal organs, and they frequently seek advice from pharmacists about self-treatment.

ACNE

Acne is characterized by the formation of comedones, or lesions, in the pilosebaceous units of the skin. The pilosebaceous units include the hair follicle and surrounding sebaceous glands. Acne lesions are most commonly found

CASE STUDY

Mr. Josh Jones is an 18-year-old Caucasian male with mild to moderate acne lesions on his face, back, and chest, which have been present for 6 months. Mr. Jones has tried frequent face and body washings with no improvement. He has both open and closed comedones and is known to pick at them, leading to increased redness and irritation. His freshman year of college is quickly approaching and Mr. Jones is anxious to improve his complexion and avoid the embarrassment of his breakouts.

on the face, chest, and back. While these lesions are self-limiting, they may lead to scarring and psychological distress.

Four factors contribute to the formation of comedones: increased sebum production, sloughing of keratinocytes, bacterial growth, and inflammation. An increase in androgen, as seen during puberty, or an increased response to androgen leads to increased sebum production from the sebaceous glands. Increased sebum may result in plugged sebaceous glands and the formation of a comedo. The sloughing or turnover of keratinocytes in the hair follicle is a normal process; however, in acne there is excessive sloughing of the skin cells, which may adhere together and cause blockage of the hair follicle and sebaceous glands, leading to an open comedo or *blackhead*. Blackheads appear dark due to the accumulation of the pigment melanin. *Propionibacterium acnes (P. acnes)*, a bacterium that is normally found in the hair follicle, grows rapidly in the mixture of sebum and keratinocytes. The increased sebum, keratinocyte sloughing, and bacterial proliferation leads to inflammation and the appearance of a closed comedo or *whitehead*. Whiteheads may appear as small, 1–2 mm, white, elevated lesions.

Treatment

Mild acne can be managed with the use of a variety of medications and treatment regimens. Antimicrobials and retinoids are among the most commonly used medication classes for the treatment of acne. The range of treatment regimens include the use of just one medication, a combination of medications, or a combination of medication and nonpharmacologic therapy.

Nonpharmacologic Treatment

Acne management usually begins with nonpharmacologic treatments. Patients should use a mild, nondrying facial soap or nonsoap cleanser twice daily. Excessive washing or scrubbing does not typically reach deep enough into the follicles to remove plugging and should be avoided. Harsh, abrasive products may worsen acne and patients should avoid oil-based cosmetics or shampoos. Clothing, headbands, and helmets may induce irritation, resulting in acne lesions. Avoiding pinching, squeezing, and other manipulation of the lesions is important to reduce the chances of further inflammation or scarring. Changes in diet, through restriction of specific foods, have not been demonstrated to be of benefit in the treatment of acne.

CASE?

What nonpharmacologic treatment options might be appropriate for Mr. Jones?

Pharmacologic Treatment

Topical Agents

Pharmacologic treatment of acne is available in a wide variety of preparations and dosage forms. Some are sold over the counter (OTC) and others are available only by prescription. Medication Table 33-1 summarizes representative products. (Medication Tables are found at the end of the chapter.) One of the most common agents used in the management of mild acne is topical benzoyl peroxide. Although the precise mechanism is unknown, benzoyl peroxide has been shown to have antibacterial activity against *P. acnes*. It also increases keratinocyte turnover and the loosening of follicular plugs, which helps to unclog pores. Benzoyl peroxide is applied topically and is available in a variety of both nonprescription and prescription preparations in concentrations ranging from 1% to 10%. These preparations may cause dryness and irritation, which can sometimes be limited by using products of lower concentration and decreasing the frequency of use. The effectiveness of benzoyl peroxide may be enhanced when used in combination with topical retinoids or topical antibiotics.

Topical retinoids (tretinoin, adapalene, tazarotene, and trifarotene) are used as first-line agents for the treatment of mild acne and are often combined with benzoyl peroxide or topical antimicrobials in moderate acne. Most are prescription products, although adapalene is available OTC in some formulations and strengths. They work by increasing cell turnover in the follicle, thereby promoting unclogging. Adverse effects that may be experienced with topical retinoid use include redness, irritation, dryness, peeling, and photosensitivity (sensitivity to ultraviolet light or sunlight). Patients may experience an initial worsening of their acne with topical retinoid use and may not see significant lesion improvement for several months. Adverse effects may be minimized by initiating treatment with a low potency formulation and titrating to higher potency formulations as needed.

For inhibition of *P. acnes*, topical antimicrobials (clindamycin, erythromycin, and dapsone) may be prescribed in combination with topical retinoids and benzoyl peroxide for the treatment of mild to moderate acne. Each of these antibiotics is formulated in a variety of dosage forms. Adverse effects include dryness, redness, and itching. Although rare and most often associated with oral clindamycin use, diarrhea and pseudomembranous colitis (discussed in Chapter 27) may also occur with topical use.

> ## PRACTICE POINT
>
> *Products containing benzoyl peroxide may stain clothing, bed linens, and hair.*

> ## PRACTICE POINT
>
> *Dapsone may cause temporary yellow or orange skin discoloration when used with benzoyl peroxide.*

Azelaic acid is another (prescription only) topical agent useful in the treatment of mild to moderate acne. It is reserved for patients who are unable to tolerate benzoyl peroxide or topical retinoids. Its mechanism of action includes anti-inflammatory and antibacterial properties, as well as skin-lightening properties that may be useful in treating hyperpigmentation (skin darkening) due to acne. Overall azelaic acid is well tolerated; however, patients may experience burning, itching, stinging, or peeling.

Systemic Agents

Some cases of moderate or severe acne cannot be treated effectively with topical agents. Physicians sometimes prescribe oral antimicrobials (erythromycin, tetracycline, doxycycline, minocycline, and sarecycline) for these patients. Because they

ALERT!

Bacterial resistance is reduced by combining topical erythromycin or clindamycin with benzoyl peroxide, so patients must be reminded that it is important to use both products as directed by their physicians, even if they are using an OTC preparation of benzoyl peroxide.

can limit the colonization and anti-inflammatory properties of *P. acnes*, the oral antimicrobial agents treat and prevent the formation of new acne lesions. Tetracycline, doxycycline, minocycline, and sarecycline can cause gastrointestinal upset and phototoxicity, and all antibiotics mentioned here have drug interactions with antacids and iron. Erythromycin may also cause gastrointestinal disturbances and has many drug interactions. Despite its effectiveness against *P. acnes*, oral clindamycin is rarely used due to the risk of pseudomembranous colitis. Long-term use of oral antibiotics may lead to the development of antibiotic resistance and treatment failure. For this reason, oral antibiotic use is seldom prescribed as monotherapy and is usually limited to short treatment courses.

ALERT!

Prescribers, pharmacies, drug wholesalers, manufacturers, and all patients, male or female, taking isotretinoin must be enrolled in and comply with the iPLEDGE program, a pregnancy prevention and management program. Certain procedures must be followed, including the use of multiple forms of birth control and monthly pregnancy tests. (Prescriptions must be picked up by the patient within 7 days of the test.) For more information, visit the iPLEDGE website (https://www.ipledgeprogram.com).

Isotretinoin is an oral retinoid and is typically reserved for the treatment of acne not responsive to topical and systemic agents. By causing atrophy of the sebaceous gland, decreasing sebum production, inhibiting *P. acnes*, and decreasing inflammation, isotretinoin is considered the most effective agent for the treatment of acne. Furthermore, a 15- to 20-week treatment course may lead to the complete remission of acne lesions. Side effects that are frequently reported with isotretinoin include dryness of the skin, nose, mouth, and eyes (in approximately 90% of patients), peeling skin, itching, photosensitivity, increased triglycerides, increased blood glucose, muscle pain, and depression. The initial cost of treatment with isotretinoin in severe acne may be more expensive than other agents; however, in the long term it may be more cost effective. Isotretinoin is a known teratogen, and its use by pregnant women carries a high risk of severe birth defects such as craniofacial, cardiovascular, thymus, parathyroid gland, and CNS (central nervous system) structure malformations. Spontaneous abortion and premature birth may also occur with fetal exposure.

For female patients with moderate to severe acne, estrogen-containing oral contraceptives are sometimes considered as second-line agents because they decrease sebum production by decreasing androgen levels. The US Food and Drug Administration (FDA) has approved products containing ethinyl estradiol and norgestimate or ethinyl estradiol and norethindrone for the treatment of acne; however, other estrogen-containing contraceptives are considered to be equally effective. Spironolactone, along with its derivative, drospirenone, may also be used for the treatment of acne. Spironolactone and drospirenone are considered to have antiandrogen effects due their ability to block androgen receptors. Drospirenone is found in combination with ethinyl estradiol in the oral contraceptive, Yaz®. Spironolactone, when prescribed for the treatment of acne, is used at high doses (50–200 mg) and may cause hyperkalemia (high potassium in the blood), menstrual irregularities, or breast tenderness.

CASE?

Mr. Jones has not tried any nonprescription or prescription pharmacologic agents for the treatment of his acne. Which pharmacologic agent(s) might be appropriate for his use?

PSORIASIS

Psoriasis is a chronic skin disease characterized by lesions, also called plaques, which are generally well defined, raised, and red to violet in color, and with silvery-white scales

Mrs. Roberts, a 52-year-old woman, presents to the pharmacy complaining of intense itching on her elbows, knees, and hands. She has very defined dark red lesions in these areas covered with white, loose scales. Areas where she has scratched the lesion and removed some of the scales have small scabs where bleeding occurred.

remission, where no lesions are present, lasting from weeks to years. Despite remission, however, psoriasis remains a chronic condition for which there is no cure.

Psoriasis is an autoimmune disorder involving the T cells. Patients with psoriasis have an abnormal number of certain T cells present in the skin. Activation of the T cells by an environmental factor leads to the release of cytokines such as interleukin-2 (IL-2), interferon-γ (IFN-γ), tumor necrosis factor (TNF-α), and others. These cytokines promote inflammation and rapid cell growth, particularly keratinocytes, leading to the development of skin lesions.

(Figure 33-1). Lesions are found most commonly on the scalp, elbows, knees, hands, feet, trunk, and nails and can vary in size from pinpoint to covering large areas of the body. Removal of the scales or trauma to the lesion can lead to bleeding. Patients often complain of intense itching at the site of the plaques.

Approximately 2% of the US population is affected with psoriasis, which is known to have a strong genetic component. Ethnicity may also play a role, with lower prevalence rates among African Americans compared to the general population. Environmental factors such as trauma to the skin, infection, seasonal changes, and medications may trigger the eruption (formation) of new plaques or the worsening of existing plaques. Patients may experience periods of

What information in the case suggests Mrs. Roberts may be suffering from psoriasis?

Treatment

The management of psoriasis centers on modification of the immune response that leads to plaque development. Both nonpharmacologic and pharmacologic therapies may be used and therapies are often combined or alternated. Treatment choice usually depends on the severity of the disease. Mild to moderate psoriasis is typically managed with topical agents,

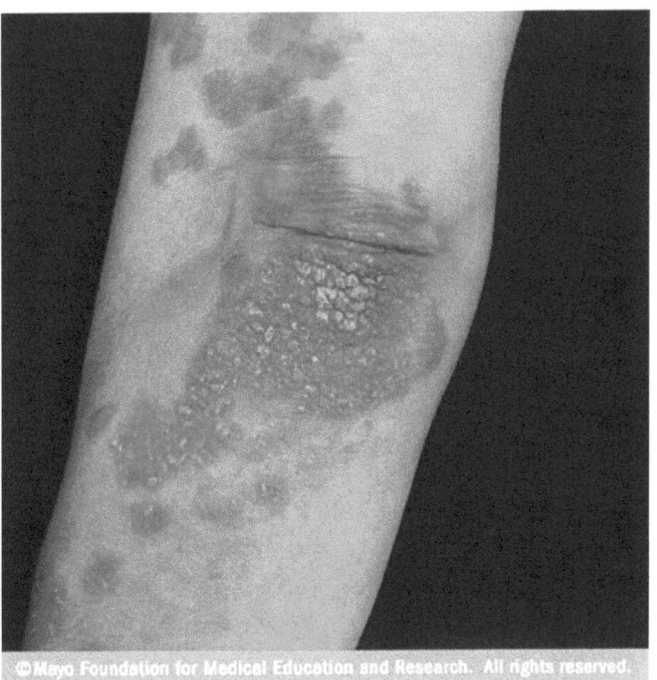

FIGURE 33-1. Psoriasis.

phototherapy, or oral agents, while more severe disease is managed with combination therapy or injectable biologic agents. Disease severity is determined by the percentage of body surface area affected and the effect of psoriasis on the patient's quality of life. The use of biologic agents earlier in disease progression is becoming more common, as these therapies may result in remission (complete clearing of the lesions) and improved quality of life. Combinations of topical agents or topical and oral agents are often used in moderate to severe cases.

Nonpharmacologic Treatment

Nonpharmacologic therapies may provide additional relief for patients with psoriasis, especially when combined with pharmacologic therapies. Emollients are often added to other pharmacologic therapies or used alone during drug-free periods. Their usefulness comes from their ability to hydrate (moisturize) the stratum corneum, minimize water loss, increase skin pliability, and decrease itching. They are most effective when used multiple times per day. Some emollients may cause folliculitis or contact dermatitis.

PRACTICE POINT

Emollients should be applied after showering or bathing. When used with other topical therapies, they should always be applied after (rather than before) the pharmacologic agent.

CASE?

What nonpharmacologic treatment(s) might the pharmacist recommend for Mrs. Roberts?

Phototherapy involves skin exposure to either ultraviolet A (UVA) or ultraviolet B (UVB) rays to help clear skin lesions. A topical pharmacologic agent, usually methoxsalen, may be applied prior to exposure to make the skin more sensitive to UVA rays. Phototherapy is usually prescribed two to three times per week. Adverse effects include nausea, dizziness, headache, increased risk of melanoma, and possibly non-melanoma cancers. Other topical agents are not typically used with PUVA (psoralen and ultraviolet A phototherapy) unless they are applied after treatment. UVB therapies are often used alone, but they may also be used with the topical pharmacologic therapies described later.

Pharmacologic Treatment

Topical corticosteroids are the most commonly used agents for the management of psoriasis. Corticosteroids are classified by their potency from *low* to *very high* (Medication Table 33-2), based on their ability to cause blood vessel constriction. The agents that are the most potent constrictors provide the most anti-inflammatory relief; however, they also have the highest risk for adverse effects and cannot be used for long periods of time. Very-high- and high-potency corticosteroids should be used for the shortest time possible, on the smallest body surface area needed, and may be effective when used as infrequently as 1 or 2 days per week, especially when combined with vitamin D analogues. Lower-potency steroids are safer for use on the face, groin, armpits, and skinfolds and should be used for children or patients who must cover large areas of the body. These products may be applied 2 to 4 times daily. All topical steroids can cause streaks or lines in the skin, known as striae, skin atrophy or thinning, acne, skin infections, and a flushed swelling of the face called rosacea. Long-term use may lead to systemic corticosteroid adverse effects or adrenal suppression. Patients may experience a worsening of psoriasis when discontinuing corticosteroids, an effect known as tachyphylaxis.

In addition to corticosteroids, other treatments for psoriasis include vitamin D analogues, keratolytic agents, oral agents, and biologic agents. Some are for topical use and others are administered for their systemic effects. Medication Table 33-3 details the drugs in each class.

Vitamin D analogues (calcipotriol, calcipotriene) and the topical retinoid tazarotene (discussed with the acne treatments), affect keratinocyte function and alter the immune response. Vitamin D analogues may cause burning and stinging in approximately 10% of patients, which may be lessened by combination therapy with topical corticosteroids. The combination of vitamin D analogues and topical corticosteroids improves psoriasis more than either agent alone. Tazarotene may also cause skin irritation and can be combined with topical corticosteroids. Women using tazarotene should be advised that it is teratogenic.

ALERT!

Acitretin is teratogenic and contraindicated in pregnant women and women who intend to become pregnant within 3 years following discontinuation of treatment.

Acitretin is an oral retinoid that is considered to be a first-line oral agent for the treatment of severe psoriasis. The combination of acitretin with other therapies such as UV light therapy and topical calcipotriol is very effective and may limit adverse effects from either agent. Acitretin is teratogenic and should not be used in anyone who is pregnant or intending to become pregnant at any time during therapy or for up to 3 years after therapy. Concurrent use of alcohol increases the elimination half-life of acitretin; therefore, alcohol should be avoided during therapy and for up to 2 months after treatment. Other adverse effects of acitretin include lipid abnormalities, dry mucous membranes (lips, mouth, eyes, nose, skin), and hepatotoxicity.

ALERT!

Long-term use (>2 years) of cyclosporine may increase the risk of cancer.

Other options for oral treatment of psoriasis include cyclosporine, methotrexate, and other immunosuppressive agents. Methotrexate and cyclosporine therapy are often alternated or rotated to minimize the systemic toxicities of each agent. Cyclosporine is an immunosuppressive agent that inhibits T cell activation and may be used alone or in combination with calcipotriol or methotrexate for the treatment of psoriasis. To limit the risk of toxicity, the dose of cyclosporine should not exceed 5 mg/kg/day and the dose should be decreased if the patient's kidney function is impaired.

ALERT!

Methotrexate is teratogenic and contraindicated in pregnant women.

Methotrexate inhibits T and B cell function and is associated with gastrointestinal side effects such as nausea and vomiting, which can be minimized by dividing the daily dose. Patients taking methotrexate are at risk for bone marrow toxicity, which may present as leukopenia (low white blood cells), anemia (low red blood cells), or thrombocytopenia (low platelets); patients should be monitored through monthly complete blood counts.

Biologic psoriasis therapy is typically used only for severe disease. All of the five FDA-approved agents—

PRACTICE POINT

Oral psoriasis therapies are generally reserved for patients who have failed topical therapy or who have moderate to severe disease.

ALERT!

Because their immune systems may be impaired, patients being treated with biological therapy should not receive live or live attenuated vaccines.

adalimumab, alefacept, etanercept, infliximab, ustekinumab, and secukinumab—are very costly. Though each agent differs in mechanism of action, all modify the T cell activation or response. Biologic agents impair the immune system and place the patient at a higher risk for infection and possibly cancer. For this reason, patients should be evaluated for latent tuberculosis through a tuberculin skin test (PPD) prior to therapy. The adverse effect profiles of the biologic agents vary, as well as their effectiveness in plaque improvement and length or duration of plaque remission.

DERMATITIS

Dermatitis is a general term that refers to an inflammatory condition of the skin. There are many different types of dermatitis; however, this chapter describes the two types of contact dermatitis: irritant and allergic. The difference between these subgroups depends on whether the cause is an antigen (allergic) or irritant. Presentation of an allergen in allergic contact dermatitis triggers an allergic response; however, irritant contact dermatitis is not an allergic response but rather an inflammatory reaction as a result of direct irritation, most commonly due to chemical exposure.

CASE?

If Mrs. Roberts gets a prescription for etanercept to treat her psoriasis, what types of vaccines might not be appropriate for her?

Irritant Contact Dermatitis

CASE STUDY

Jennifer Johnson, a 12-week-old infant, is brought into the pharmacy by her mother. Ms. Johnson is extremely upset because the rash on her daughter's upper thighs and buttocks, which began light pink, has become darker red and appears to be very irritating to the child. The rash appeared 2 days ago and she suspects that her daughter's diaper is not being changed frequently at daycare.

Exposure to chemicals, such as strong acids or bases, detergents, solvents, and oxidizers, may cause irritant dermatitis, which occurs most commonly due to the exposure of unprotected skin in the workplace. Irritant dermatitis may also occur as a result of prolonged skin exposure to urine or feces, which is the cause of diaper dermatitis, a subtype of irritant dermatitis. Exposure to these substances is thought to cause direct damage to the dermal layer of the skin, destroying the skin structure and impairing its function. Damage to the dermal layer increases the risk for further irritation and infection, so prompt, effective treatment is important.

Irritant contact dermatitis most commonly presents as a red, raised, or swollen rash. Papules or blisters are not typically seen in diaper dermatitis or mild cases of irritant dermatitis but may be seen in moderate to severe cases. Patients may complain of irritation, itching, stinging, or burning. The rash may range from light pink with poorly defined edges to dark red with a clear edge.

Nonpharmacologic Treatment

After exposure and throughout treatment, the area should be cleaned with copious amounts of lukewarm water and a mild soap. For cases of diaper dermatitis, the area should be allowed to air dry fully before another diaper is applied and diaper changes should be done as frequently as possible to avoid urine and fecal contact with the skin. Occlusive diapers and clothing over areas of exposure should be avoided, if possible. Patients can be reminded of methods to avoid repeat exposure, such as wearing gloves or other protective clothing.

Pharmacologic Treatment

Skin barriers or protectants, such as zinc oxide, petrolatum, lanolin, and vitamin A and D, form an occlusive barrier between the skin and offending agent to avoid skin irritation. These agents can be applied after every diaper change and discontinued when the rash resolves. Skin protectants are available in a variety of formulations, including creams, ointments, and pastes, and are often combined with moisturizers.

Astringents, such as aluminum acetate and calamine lotion, and topical steroids, such as hydrocortisone cream, may be used to relieve itching in adults. The use of topical steroids should be limited to the lowest potency and to a maximum of a 2-week treatment duration in infants. Antibacterials and antifungals should only be used in cases of infection and only when prescribed by a physician. Adults may experience relief from itching with an oral antihistamine. The FDA has determined that OTC oral antihistamines are neither safe nor effective in children younger than 2 years of age and product labels now recommend against their use in children under the age of 4. Diphenhydramine, hydroxyzine, or doxylamine have sedative effects, which may be useful for intense itching at night, although some patients may experience excitability or restlessness upon administration. The use of topical antihistamines should be avoided due to the risk of an allergic reaction. Medication Table 33-4 lists some representative agents useful in the treatment of dermatitis.

Allergic Contact Dermatitis

CASE STUDY

Aaron Murphy, a 25-year-old male, presents to your pharmacy with complaints of itching and shows you a red, raised rash on his arms. He tells you that he had spent the weekend clearing brush with his father on his family's property while wearing gloves and work boots. He admits his other clothing was just a T-shirt and shorts. He says his rash looks similar to the one he had before when he came into contact with poison ivy while camping.

CASE?

What might the pharmacist recommend for the treatment of baby Johnson's diaper dermatitis?

Allergic contact dermatitis is caused by direct contact with an object, such as a plant, or a fomite (an object that contacted the plant) or by inhalation. Metals, medications, and chemicals can all cause an allergic reaction; however, allergic contact dermatitis is most commonly caused by exposure to urushiol oil, which is found in poison ivy, poison oak, or poison sumac plants. Skin contact and presentation of the antigen leads to an allergic reaction and an inflammatory response in the dermal layers of the skin.

Patients typically present with red, elevated lesions or blisters and intense itching. After the first few days, the lesions may break open and begin to weep and crust. Contact dermatitis is not spread by touching the weeping pustules of an individual with an eruption of contact dermatitis and the disease state is self-limiting, meaning that if untreated, the lesions will clear in approximately 1 to 3 weeks with or without treatment.

CASE?

What information in Mr. Murphy's case supports a diagnosis of allergic contact dermatitis rather than something else?

Nonpharmacologic Treatment

After initial exposure to an antigen, patients should wash skin and clothing immediately using regular soap and laundry detergent. Any objects or tools that may be contaminated should also be cleaned, as urushiol oil, for example, may remain and cause dermatitis on subsequent exposures. Once any remaining antigens have been washed away, cool, soapless showers or the application of a cool, moist compress may relieve the itching associated with allergic dermatitis. The application of harsh or abrasive cleansers is not recommended; only gentle soaps, if needed, should be used. Emollients should be liberally applied after bathing.

Pharmacologic Treatment

Astringents, such as aluminum acetate, witch hazel, calamine, zinc oxide, and sodium bicarbonate, cause a drying effect that helps to soothe weeping or oozing lesions, relieve itching, and decrease inflammation. Patients may apply these agents as soaks, compresses, or other topical products. Examples of these are listed in Medication Table 33-4.

Topical corticosteroids (Medication Table 33-2) decrease inflammation and redness and relieve itching. Hydrocortisone cream or ointment may be applied up to four times daily. To minimize the risk of infection, do not place hydrocortisone ointment over weeping lesions, as it can be occlusive and encourage bacterial growth. Soaking the affected area in a colloidal oatmeal bath (Aveeno®) for 15 to 20 minutes may relieve itching. Keep the bath water running or stirred to avoid clumping and use caution when exiting the bathtub as the bath may be slippery. Following the bath, pat the skin dry, leaving the colloid film on the skin. Oral antihistamines (diphenhydramine, hydroxyzine, doxylamine) may relieve itching, either through the blockade of the histamine (H1) receptor or by sedation. Oral antihistamines may cause dizziness, blurred vision, confusion, and low blood pressure.

CASE?

What treatments, nonpharmacologic and pharmacologic, might the pharmacist recommend for Mr. Murphy?

For patients with moderate to severe allergic contact dermatitis or those who fail to respond to nonprescription therapies, a course of systemic, prescription corticosteroids (prednisone or methylprednisolone, discussed in Chapter 9) may be needed. In severe cases where the rash is widespread or present on the face or genitals, intravenous (IV) or intramuscular (IM) administration of a corticosteroid may provide symptomatic relief.

ALERT!

Topical antihistamines should be avoided in contact dermatitis due to possible worsening of the condition.

SKIN INFECTIONS

CASE STUDY

Mr. Sanchez, a 38-year-old man, went to the doctor because he thought he had an infected spider bite. His leg is red, swollen, and painful to the touch. Upon further examination, however, his doctor diagnosed him with a skin infection.

As described in Chapter 32, one of the main functions of the skin is to act as a barrier. Because the lipid layer of the skin helps to prevent water loss from the epidermis, as well as the slightly acidic and constantly shedding properties exhibited, the skin is typically very resistant to infection. However, in the event that one or more of these protective functions of the skin are disrupted, a skin infection is likely to occur. Most skin infections are a result of a skin puncture or abrasion. However, some people have conditions that predispose them to skin infections. Examples of patients with additional risk factors are persons with very moist skin or an inadequate blood supply to the surface of the skin, or those with diabetes or human-immunodeficiency virus.

Skin infections can be classified as either primary or secondary infections. Primary infections are those that involve previously healthy skin and are usually caused by a single microorganism. If the infection is in an area of previously damaged skin, it is classified as a secondary infection. An example of a secondary infection is an infection developing on a skinned knee or accidental abrasion. Some secondary skin infections may be prevented or treated using OTC preparations such as bacitracin or *double-* or *triple*-antibiotic ointments (see Medication Table 33-5).

PRACTICE POINT

Patients purchasing OTC anti-infective agents for the skin should be made aware of the labeling, which advises them to stop use and contact a healthcare provider if the condition persists longer than 7 days or worsens, or if a rash or other allergic reaction develops.

Skin infections are also classified as complicated or uncomplicated. Complicated skin infections may require surgery to remove part of the damaged skin or may involve patients with a compromised immune system. A variety of microorganisms may cause skin infections, including bacteria, viruses, and fungi. Certain conditions place a person at risk for different microorganisms. For example, someone who plays a contact sport or who frequently uses a locker room may be at a higher risk for both bacterial and fungal infections. Additionally, poor hygiene and improper wound care may also increase the likelihood of developing a bacterial skin infection. Treatment of serious skin infections is typically done on an outpatient basis with topical and oral antimicrobials. Patients who have a fever, appear to be ill, or have a complicated skin infection may be hospitalized and placed on IV antimicrobial therapy.

Bacterial Skin Infections

Cellulitis is a common bacterial skin infection that occurs after a wound from a minor trauma, abrasion, ulcer, or surgery. Insect bites can also cause skin barrier disruption and may lead to subsequent skin infections. Cellulitis is characterized by a nonelevated, erythematous (redness of the skin), hot, and painful area of the skin surface. If left undetected and untreated for an extended period of time, cellulitis is potentially a life-threatening infection requiring hospitalization and IV antibiotics.

Impetigo is another common community-acquired superficial bacterial skin infection. Unlike cellulitis, which is more common in the adult population, impetigo occurs mostly in children 2 to 5 years of age. Other distinguishing factors are that it is highly contagious and is diagnosed by the presence of fluid-filled vesicles (small *pouches*) that develop rapidly into pus-filled blisters. Once these blisters rupture, a golden-yellow crust forms on the skin, which is characteristic of impetigo. Favorable conditions for developing impetigo are hot, humid weather, areas with poor hygiene or crowded living conditions, daycare centers, and schools. Impetigo occurs most commonly on the face and is easily transmitted to other children who are in close contact with one another. Impetigo may resolve spontaneously; however, if left untreated, a secondary cellulitis infection may develop.

Microbiology

Most community-acquired bacterial skin infections, such as cellulitis and impetigo, are caused by *Staphylococcus aureus (S. aureus)* or *Streptococcus pyogenes*. Although both these

Gram-positive bacteria are part of the normal skin flora, they may become pathogenic (infectious) if they are present on the skin in high concentrations and given the opportunity to penetrate the skin barrier. Other types of bacteria, such as other Gram-positive bacteria, Gram-negative bacteria, or anaerobic bacteria, may also cause skin infections but are less common.

Over the past few decades, there has been increasing concern for resistant *S. aureus* infections. Methicillin-resistant *S. aureus* (MRSA) is a particular strain of bacteria that is resistant to the antibiotic class that is used as first-line treatment for bacterial skin infections (antistaphylococcal penicillins). Once found only in hospitals, these resistant infections are now being detected in the community setting.

The treatment of bacterial skin infections involves both pharmacological and nonpharmacological strategies. The goal of antibiotic therapy is to achieve rapid eradication of the bacteria to prevent any additional complications that may arise from a prolonged infection.

ALERT!

Community-acquired MRSA outbreaks are common in correctional facilities, school systems, and among military personnel. Close contact during contact sports and in locker room areas place athletes at the highest risk.

Nonpharmacological Treatment

There are a few different nondrug therapies that can be used to decrease symptoms associated with cellulitis and impetigo. Cool sterile dressings for cellulitis may decrease pain associated with cellulitis. Also, crust removal by soaking the affected skin in soap and water will often help to relieve itching associated with impetigo. Additionally, keeping the wound clean and reinforcing good skin hygiene is essential to prevent the infection from spreading to other areas.

Pharmacological Treatment

Pharmacological treatment includes the use of topical or oral antibiotic medications (listed in Medication Table 33-5). The choice of antibiotic therapy is determined by the severity, location, and causative bacteria, as well as effectiveness and potential side effects of the medications. The most effective antibiotic regimen is one that targets only the most

likely microorganisms. This strategy is essential to prevent the development of antibiotic resistance. Additionally, the use of topical antibiotics may be preferred in some cases to avoid potential side effects from systemic antibiotic therapy. All of the agents used must be effective against *S. aureus* and *S. pyogenes*, the two most common bacterial causes of cellulitis and impetigo.

Systemic Antibiotic Therapy

Oral antibiotics are used most often to treat cellulitis, except for severe cases, which may require IV antibiotic therapy. The most effective systemic (oral or IV) antibiotic classes for cellulitis and impetigo are antistaphylococcal penicillins and first-generation cephalosporins. Both of these antibiotic classes are bacteriocidal (kill the bacteria). The antistaphylococcal penicillins used for cellulitis are nafcillin, oxacillin, and dicloxacillin. The first-generation cephalosporins used for cellulitis are cefazolin and cephalexin. The duration of antibiotic therapy for cellulitis is usually 5 to 10 days. Penicillins and cephalosporins are very well tolerated, with the most common side effects being rash, diarrhea, and stomach upset. A rare but serious adverse effect is diarrhea that can lead to pseudomembranous colitis. Patients should not take penicillins or cephalosporins if they have had a severe allergic reaction to any of the medications contained in these antibiotic classes.

PRACTICE POINT

Nafcillin and cefazolin are IV antibiotics given to patients who are admitted to the hospital with a severe cellulitis infection.

ALERT!

Patients taking oral antibiotics should receive reminders and alerts about the importance of taking their antibiotics as directed and until finished to ensure complete eradication of the infection.

Patients may have an allergy to penicillins and/or cephalosporins. First-generation cephalosporins may be used in patients who have a mild penicillin allergy (rash). If a patient has a severe penicillin allergy (anaphylaxis—a life-threatening condition that involves swelling of the throat and a severe drop in blood pressure) or a cephalosporin allergy, the infection should be treated with vancomycin, linezolid, or clindamycin. Like the penicillins and cephalosporins, vancomycin is bactericidal. Clindamycin, however, is bacteriostatic (inhibits cell growth but does not kill the bacteria).

PRACTICE POINT

Because clindamycin is given orally, it may cause stomach upset. It is important to remind the patient to take clindamycin with food to decrease the occurrence or severity of stomach upset.

In the event a patient fails to respond to one of the above treatment regimens or if a resistant infection (MRSA) is suspected, alternative antibiotics such as vancomycin, linezolid, ceftaroline, sulfamethoxazole/trimethoprim, or clindamycin may be used. Vancomycin, ceftaroline, and linezolid are most effective for MRSA infections. Vancomycin and ceftaroline must be administered intravenously, while linezolid can be given either orally or intravenously. Sulfamethoxazole/trimethoprim and clindamycin may be used to treat susceptible community acquired CA-MRSA isolates. Side effects of sulfamethoxazole/trimethoprim are stomach upset and rash. Patients with a sulfa-allergy should not take sulfamethoxazole/trimethoprim. These antibiotics are discussed more extensively in Chapter 27.

ALERT!

While many topical antibiotic preparations have the same active ingredients as similar preparations for the eye, agents labeled for use on the skin should never be used to treat conditions of the eye.

Topical Antibiotic Therapy

Topical antibiotic therapy may be used to treat impetigo. Although bacitracin, neomycin, and polymyxin administered alone or in combination have been used to treat impetigo, these agents may not be as effective as mupirocin or retapamulin. Mupirocin and retapamulin are as effective as and have fewer side effects than oral therapy for impetigo. In cases when impetigo covers a large area, oral therapy may be preferred due to ease of use. Topical antibiotics are very well tolerated; however, skin irritation may occur.

ALERT!

Topical antibiotic therapy is not used to treat cellulitis.

CASE?

Mr. Sanchez comes to the pharmacy with a prescription for cephalexin 500 mg twice a day for 7 days. He says he has finished the six-pill sample pack his doctor gave him and his infection is much better. He wonders whether it is worth it to get the prescription filled. What should the technician do or say?

Fungal Skin Infections

CASE STUDY

A mother brings her 16-year-old son, Derek, to the pharmacy and tells the pharmacist he has been complaining of a burning, itching sensation, and redness between his toes on both feet. His symptoms have become progressively worse each day since starting football practice about 2 weeks ago. When asked, he says his toenails appear to be normal with no apparent discoloration.

Pathophysiology

Athlete's foot, ringworm, jock itch, and onychomycosis are all types of fungal infections. Named for the area of the body affected, these fungal infections are referred to as dermatophytosis or tinea infections. Most commonly, fungal skin infections are caused by the *Trichophyton, Microsporum,* or *Epidermophyton* genii of the fungi family. These fungi are known as dermatophytes and are able to penetrate

TABLE 33-1. Fungal Skin Infections

Classification	Common Name	Presentation/Symptoms
Tinea pedis	Athlete's foot	Occurs between the toes and on the bottom surface of the foot; usually affects one foot but may affect both feet; characterized as an itching or stinging sensation of the feet with possible fissuring, scaling, and redness
Tinea corporis	Ringworm of the skin	Ring-shaped rash; may be red, crusty, and/or scaly; occurs on any part of the body
Tinea capitis	Ringworm of the scalp	Ring-shaped, red, crusty, and/or scaly rash located on the scalp; most commonly found in children
Tinea cruris	Jock itch	Occurs on the inner part of the thigh and pubic area, often on both sides of the body; characterized as a red, elevated area with possible small, red vesicles, itching, and/or pain; more common in men than women
Tinea unguium	Onychomycoses (fungal infection of toenails or fingernails)	Affects toenails more than fingernails; nails gradually become opaque, thick, rough, yellow, and brittle; the nail may separate from the nail bed and eventually fall off completely

the keratinous areas of the skin, causing various symptoms related to the location of penetration (Table 33-1).

CASE?

What do you think Derek's problem is? Why?

Tinea infections can be spread from person to person, animal to person, or soil to person. Tinea generally presents on areas of the skin that are moist and poorly ventilated, such as the feet and groin area. Prolonged exposure to sweaty clothes, failure to bathe regularly, presence of skin folds, sedentary lifestyle, and bed confinement are all risk factors for the development of fungal infections. Furthermore, certain risk factors, such as older age, family history, immunodeficiency, diabetes, psoriasis, peripheral vascular disease, smoking, nail trauma, and tinea pedis place patients at an increased risk for fungal infections of the nail.

Treatment of fungal skin infections involves both non-pharmacological and pharmacological strategies. The goals of treating fungal skin infections are to provide symptomatic relief, clear the existing infection, and prevent future fungal infections.

Nonpharmacological Treatment

The goal of nondrug therapy is mostly to prevent the spread of the fungal infection to other areas of the body.

One important counseling point for patients is to launder contaminated towels and clothing in hot water to disinfect them. When using a towel, it is important to dry the affected area last or to use a separate towel to dry the infected area. Proper hygiene and daily showers are essential. Other ways to avoid contracting a fungal infection are to wear cotton socks and properly fitting shoes because wool or synthetic fibers trap air and prevent the skin from breathing. Finally, it is important to avoid exposure to infected areas and surfaces. One way to do this is to wear sandals, slippers, or other types of footwear in shower areas of locker rooms and public restrooms.

Pharmacological Treatment

Tinea pedis, tinea corporis, and tinea cruris infections can often be treated with nonprescription topical antifungal agents. Numerous topical antifungal agents are available OTC (listed in Medication Table 33-6). The choice of topical antifungal agent should be patient specific and based on failure of previous topical antifungal therapy, cost, and compliance. Topical antifungals with the fewest daily applications and with the shortest treatment length are recommended for those who may have difficulty complying with other regimens. Directions and duration of use for most topical antifungal agents are to apply sparingly to the affected area twice daily for 2 to 4 weeks. Patients who present with tinea capitis (also known as ringworm of the scalp) or tinea unguium should receive both topical and oral antifungals.

Antifungals—Imidazole Derivatives (azole antifungals)

Clotrimazole, miconazole, ketoconazole, econazole, oxiconazole, sertaconazole, and sulconazole are topical imidazole derivatives that act by inhibiting the synthesis of various components involved in the production of the fungal cell wall, thereby making the cell more permeable. (Refer to Chapter 29 for additional details.) All topical azole antifungals are indicated for tinea pedis, tinea cruris, and tinea corporis. Clotrimazole and miconazole are the most commonly used agents in this class because they are available OTC and in low-cost generic formulations. Ketoconazole, itraconazole, and fluconazole can be used as oral agents for the treatment of tinea capitis.

ALERT!

LOOK-ALIKE/SOUND-ALIKE—Diflucan should not be confused with Diprivan (propofol).

Antifungals—Nonazole Derivatives

Butenafine, terbinafine, and naftifine are topical allylamines that act by inhibiting squalene epoxidase, an enzyme used for production of sterol components of the fungal cell wall, leading to cell death. All topical allylamine derivatives are indicated for tinea pedis, tinea cruris, and tinea corporis. Butenafine and terbinafine are used more often than naftifine because they are available OTC and have low-cost generic formulations. Terbinafine, the only allylamine derivative available in an oral formulation, is the most commonly prescribed medication for onychomycoses.

PRACTICE POINT

Butenafine is the only topical antifungal that has once daily application for tinea infections and may be the best treatment option if compliance with twice daily application is of concern.

Tolnaftate, a nonazole derivative, has a mechanism of action different from the allylamines. Although its mechanism of action is unknown, it is believed to stunt the growth of the fungal cell. Tolnaftate is indicated for the treatment of tinea pedis, tinea cruris, and tinea corporis and is available as an OTC antifungal with a low-cost generic formulation.

Ciclopirox, a nonazole derivative, inhibits the transport of essential elements in the fungal cell, disrupting the synthesis of DNA, RNA, and proteins inside the cell. Ciclopirox is indicated for the topical treatment of tinea pedis, tinea cruris, and tinea corporis. Also, ciclopirox is available in a lacquer solution that can be used for mild onychomycoses infections. Both topical formulations of ciclopirox are by prescription only. Griseofulvin, a nonazole derivative, has a unique mechanism of action different from any other antifungal agent. It is a derivative of penicillin that deposits itself in the keratin of human skin cells to prevent fungal invasion. Although it is an option for oral treatment of tinea infections, its use has fallen out of favor; the newer agents are preferred because of their higher cure rates and lower rates of relapse. As with the other oral antifungal agents, griseofulvin is available only as a prescription.

Overall, topical antifungals are well tolerated. Side effects are rare and may include mild cases of skin irritation, burning, or stinging. There are no known drug-drug interactions with these topical agents because only minimal amounts are absorbed systemically. As mentioned above, the topical antifungal of choice will vary based on each patient's needs. Typically, creams and solutions are the most effective and easiest to use formulations to treat tinea infections. Sprays and powders are often less effective. This may be due to the fact that sprays and powders are not rubbed into the skin adequately after administration. Powders and sprays are most effective for prevention of superficial fungal infections.

Adverse effects with oral antifungals are more common. Nausea, vomiting, and headache are the most common side effects associated with oral antifungal agents. Because they are metabolized in the liver, these agents also have the potential for many drug-drug interactions with other agents metabolized by the liver. Although many drug interactions exist, two of the most significant drug-drug interactions include administration of macrolide antibiotics (erythromycin and clarithromycin) or warfarin with azole antifungals. Patients should be counseled to inform both their pharmacist and their physician of all medications they are taking so they can check for potential serious drug interactions. If antifungals must be administered with a drug known to be metabolized by the liver, the patient should be counseled to watch for side effects of both medications and to inform their physician or pharmacist if these occur. Also, patients should be counseled not to take antacids within 2 hours of taking azole antifungal agents as this may decrease their absorption. Terbinafine may be taken without regard to meals and griseofulvin should be taken with food.

WARTS

Pathophysiology and Presentation

Warts are caused by a virus called human papillomavirus (also known as HPV). They may occur on any skin surface and are common in children. The common wart is also known as verruca vulgaris and is seen most often on the hands. Plantar warts, verruca plantaris, occur on the soles of the feet. Warts can spread from person to person or by indirect exposure to the virus in public showers or swimming pools. The warm water of swimming pools and showers softens the skin layer of the soles of the feet, allowing entry of the virus into the skin. It may take up to 3–4 months for a wart to appear after exposure to the virus.

Warts can appear on any skin surface. Typically, warts are rough and cauliflower like in appearance. They can occur alone or in groups. Over time, warts tend to increase in size. They begin as a lesion with a smooth, skin colored surface.

Common warts are usually asymptomatic. Plantar warts may become painful if they cover a large area of the heel or ball of the foot. While standing, walking, or running, pressure is applied to the plantar wart. If it is a raised lesion, the lesion is forced inward where it can stimulate local nerve endings causing pain and discomfort. Plantar warts are more common in adolescents and adults.

Treatment

Unfortunately, no single therapy has been proven to be effective at clearing warts in every patient. Topical agents and procedures to remove warts can decrease pain and possibly remove warts. It is important to note that warts usually clear spontaneously in 2 to 3 years without treatment. Due to the lack of highly effective treatment options, doing nothing is often the treatment of choice. A painful, disfiguring, or disabling lesion often leads to the decision to treat. The goals of wart treatment are to remove the wart, to avoid scarring, and to prevent the spread of the virus to other areas of the body or to other individuals. Most topical treatments for wart removal are available as nonprescription products, with patient self-treatment being a common approach.

Topical

Topical salicylic acid, a keratolytic agent that breaks down the wart lesion, has been proven as a safe and effective agent for wart removal. Salicylic acid is available in liquids, gels, disks, and patches. Product choice should be individualized based on the size and location of the wart as there is no clear advantage to any product formulation. Plantar warts require a higher concentration of salicylic acid than warts on the hands. Once the salicylic acid is applied, it is important to counsel the patient to practice good hygiene to prevent the spread of the virus. If the wart does not clear in 12 weeks, consultation with a physician is recommended. Additionally, it is recommended that painful plantar warts be treated by a physician.

In the physician's office cryotherapy with liquid nitrogen has been a standard treatment for wart removal. Dimethyl ether and propane (also known as DEMP) is an OTC agent that has also been used to effectively remove warts. The proposed mechanism behind cryotherapy is to irritate the infected tissue to provoke a host immune reaction against the virus. It is recommended to apply the DMEP solution for 20 seconds to freeze the wart, repeating the process in 10 days if the wart does not fall off. Patients should use caution to only apply the cryotherapy solution to the wart and to avoid affecting healthy tissue surrounding the wart.

Imiquimod is a prescription-only topical immune response modifier used for genital warts. Topical imiquimod has demonstrated potential efficacy for nongenital warts; however, high cost limits its use. Systemic and topical retinoids, discussed in the section on acne, are also used for wart removal. Due to the risk of birth defects, retinoid therapy is used as a second-line treatment option. Laser treatments and immunotherapy are options for wart removal that are performed at the physician's office. Laser therapy is as effective as other treatments. Immunotherapy is recommended as a second- or third-line option for treatment-resistant warts. Therapy for warts is summarized in Medication Table 33-7.

Nonpharmacologic

To avoid the spread of warts, patients should wash hands before and after touching the wart surface, avoid contaminating clothing and towels, and avoid walking in bare feet unless the wart is covered. Also, patients should be counseled not to pick at or disrupt the wart surface. This may increase the risk of spreading the virus to other areas.

COLD SORES

Cold sores, like warts, are caused by a virus. Herpes simplex 1 (also known as HSV-1) is the virus known to cause cold sores. Exposure to HSV-1 is usually by direct contact. Once a person is infected, the virus goes through periods of dormancy and reactivation, leaving the individual infected for life. Cold sores commonly occur on the lip but may also occur inside the mouth. Lesions are usually preceded by burning, itching, tingling, and numbness of the area. Next, a papule will form that will evolve into a fluid-filled vesicle that may burst to form crusts. Typically, cold sores last for 10 to 14 days. If the cold sore is not properly cared for, a bacterial infection may occur. Possible triggers for reactivation of HSV-1 are exposure to the sun, stress, fatigue, and menstruation.

CASE?

Rae's dad has chosen to buy Compound W Freeze Off® and Dr. Scholl's® Clear Away® Ultra Thin Discs to treat her warts. How should the pharmacist counsel Rae and her dad about use of these products? Will they likely be effective?

Treatment

Goals for cold sore treatment include relief of discomfort, prevention of secondary bacterial infection, and prevention of viral spread. The mainstay of cold sore treatment is topical skin protectants. Any type of lip balm may be used to keep the cold sore moist to prevent cracking. The only topical medication approved to treat cold sores is docosanol. Topical docosanol inhibits the HSV-1 virus from infecting human cells to prevent viral replication. Docosanol should be applied at the first sign of a cold sore to decrease the size of outbreak. Once the cold sore has erupted, docosanol is of little benefit. Oral antiviral agents, such as acyclovir and valacyclovir, may be used for recurrent cold sores. Other treatment measures are to avoid triggers for activation of the virus and exercise proper hygiene to prevent viral spread. Therapy for cold sores is summarized in Medication Table 33-7.

INFESTATIONS

Head lice and scabies are forms of ectoparasites. Ectoparasites are organisms that live on the outside of the human body, using the human body as a means to survive. The most common symptoms of lice and scabies are itching and skin irritation. Female lice deposit eggs called nits on the hair. After 10 days, the nits hatch and mature to lice in approximately 2 weeks. Lice feed on human blood by piercing the skin with their mouths. Lice can live on clothes and other items. Scabies is caused by an itch mite. Unlike lice, the scabies mite infects areas in between the fingers, back of the knee, armpit, umbilicus, and scrotal areas. Risk factors for lice and scabies are poor personal hygiene and social contact with other persons infected by the parasite.

Nonpharmacological Treatment

Clothing and bedding infected with lice or scabies should be washed in hot water and dried in a dryer to kill remaining lice, nits, or mites. An alternative to washing and drying items is to place them in a sealed plastic bag for at least 2 weeks. It is also recommended to vacuum rugs and furniture. Because lice generally survive for less than 2 days away from the human host, the use of permethrin spray is discouraged. It is highly suggested to avoid the use of permethrin spray to prevent resistant infections. See Medication Table 33-8.

Pharmacological Treatment—Lice

Permethrin (Nix) is the treatment of choice for lice. Available as a nonprescription lotion, permethrin is a readily available option that effectively kills both lice and eggs. Permethrin acts on the nerve cells of the louse to cause paralysis and death. Once applied as directed, permethrin has residual effects for up to 10 days so retreatment is not necessary unless lice reappear. Side effects of permethrin are itching, burning, stinging, and tingling of the skin. Persons who are allergic to chrysanthemums should not use permethrin.

Pyrethrins (Rid) are another nonprescription product to treat lice. Like permethrin, pyrethrins block the nerve impulse of the louse, causing paralysis and death. Unlike permethrin, pyrethrins require a second application 7 to 10 days after the first application to kill any remaining nits that have hatched. When applied in two applications, pyrethrins are as effective as permethrin. Persons who are allergic to chrysanthemums should not use pyrethrins.

Four prescription-only products are available for lice treatment, malathion (Ovide), benzyl alcohol 5% (Ulesfia), spinosad (Natruba), and lindane (Kwell). These agents are reserved for resistant lice infestations. Due to a recent FDA black box warning issued concerning neurotoxicity with lindane (can cause seizures), it is now recommended only as a second-line treatment option. Lindane should not be used in infants or children. Therapy for lice is summarized in Medication Table 33-8.

Pharmacological Treatment—Scabies

Permethrin 5% cream (Elimite) is the treatment of choice for scabies. Lindane may be used as a second-line agent; however, the FDA warning for neurotoxicity limits its use. It is recommended to limit the amount of lindane used to 1 or 2 ounces and to avoid use in infants and children. Therapy for scabies is summarized in Medication Table 33-8.

SUMMARY

The skin is subject to a variety of conditions, both chronic and acute. Many require treatment by physicians and prescription therapies, while others can be effectively managed with over-the-counter (OTC) preparations. The pharmacist can assist patients in deciding whether to seek medical attention or try self-treatment with an OTC product. Technicians should be aware of the importance of pharmacist counseling and recommendations for skin conditions because so many patients assume they can manage without help and it is so easy to make poor choices.

REFERENCES

1. National Library of Medicine, DailyMed. Bethesda, MD: U.S. National Library of Medicine, National Institutes of Health, Health & Human Services; 2021. https://dailymed.nlm.nih.gov/dailymed/. Accessed July 12, 2021.

2. Lexicomp Online, Lexi-Drugs [database]. Waltham, MA: UpToDate, Inc.; 2021. https://online.lexi.com. Accessed July 12, 2021.

3. Fonacier L, Bernstein DI, Pacheco K, et al. Contact dermatitis: A practice parameter—update 2015. *J Allergy Clin Immunol Pract.* 2015;3:S1-S39.

4. Lexicomp Online, AHFS Essentials. Waltham, MA: UpToDate, Inc.; 2021. https://online.lexi.com. Accessed July 12, 2021.

CHAPTER RESOURCES

Mulhem E, Pinelis S. Treatment of nongenital cutaneous warts. *Am Fam Physician.* 2011;84(3):288-293.

Krinsky DL, Ferreri SP, Hemstreet B, et al., eds. *Handbook of Nonprescription Drugs: An Interactive Approach to Self-Care.* 19th ed. Washington DC: American Pharmacists Association; 2019. https://doi-org.ezproxy.findlay.edu/10.21019/9781582122656. Accessed January 11, 2020.

Boehncke W, Schon M. Psoriasis. *Lancet.* 2015;386:983-994.

Weigle N, McBane S. Psoriasis. *Am Fam Physician.* 2013; 87(9):626-633.

DiPiro JT, Yee GC, Posey L, et al., eds. *Pharmacotherapy: A Pathophysiologic Approach.* 11th ed. New York, NY: McGraw-Hill Medical; 2019. http://accesspharmacy.mhmedical.com.ezproxy.findlay.edu:2048/content.aspx?bookid=2577&sectionid=219306022. Accessed January 11, 2020.

Chisholm-Burns MA, Schwinghammer TL, Malone PM, et al., eds. *Pharmacotherapy: Principles & Practice.* New York, NY: McGraw-Hill; 2019. http://ppp.mhmedical.com.ezproxy.findlay.edu:2048/content.aspx?bookid=2440&sectionid=189491584. Accessed January 11, 2020.

iPLEDGE Program. Available at https://www.ipledgeprogram .com/AboutiPLEDGE.aspx. Accessed January 11, 2020.

Stevens DL, Bisno AL, Chambers HF, et al. Practice guidelines for the diagnosis and management of skin and soft tissue infections: 2014 update by the Infectious Diseases Society of America. CID 2014;59(2):e10-52.

REVIEW QUESTIONS

1. What are the four factors that contribute to the formation of comedones?

2. What are at least two important counseling points the pharmacist should discuss with a patient when dispensing benzoyl peroxide for acne treatment? Or topical retinoids?

3. Describe the difference between irritant and allergic dermatitis.

4. Diaper rash, as a type of irritant dermatitis, is most often treated with barrier/protectant products. Why are these agents considered first-line therapy for diaper rash?

5. What corticosteroid potency (low, medium, or high) may be used for psoriasis of the armpit? Justify answer.

6. Treatment of psoriasis with biological agents, such as adalimumab, places the patient at a higher risk of what condition?

7. What two fungal skin infections must be treated with oral antifungal agents?

8. When is docosanol most effective for treating cold sores, those in the early or late stages of development? Explain.

9. Compare and contrast the role of permethrin and pyrethrins for the treatment of lice.

10. Which skin conditions typically require a physician's care rather than self-treatment?

MEDICATION TABLES

MEDICATION TABLE 33-1. Acne Medications[1,2]

CLASS Generic Name (pronunciation)*	Brand Name	Route	Forms	Dose	Regulatory Status	Notes
Topical Agents (Miscellaneous)						
Benzoyl peroxide (BEN zoe il) (per OX ide)	Benzac AC, BenzEFoam, BenzePrO, Benziq, BPO, Clearskin, Desquam-X, Enzoclear, Inova, PanOxyl, Riax, Zaclir	Topical	Cleanser, cream, foam, gel, liquid, lotion, pad, soap, wash	Apply sparingly once daily; dose may be increased gradually to 2–3 times/day until desired effect; if excessive dryness or peeling occurs, reduce dose, frequency, or concentration; if excessive stinging or burning occurs, wash area with mild soap and water	Rx/OTC	May discolor hair and clothing; may increase sensitivity to sunlight
Azelaic acid (ay ze LAY ik) (AS id)	Azelex, Finacea, Finacea Plus	Topical	Cream, gel	Wash and dry skin thoroughly before application; gently massage a thin film into the affected area twice daily (morning and evening); wash hands immediately following application	Rx	
Retinoids						
Tretinoin (TRET i noe in)	Altreno, Atralin, Avita, Refissa, Renova, Retin-A, Retin-A Micro	Topical	Cream, gel	Treatment usually begins with a low concentration and is increased as tolerated; wash area and let dry completely before application; apply once daily in evening to acne lesions; decrease frequency of application if stinging or irritation develops	Rx	May increase sensitivity to sunlight
Adapalene (a DAP a leen)	Differin, Differin XP	Topical	Cream, gel	Cleanse the face gently and dry face completely; apply once daily before bedtime	Rx/OTC	May increase sensitivity to sunlight
Tazarotene (taz AR oh teen)	Arazlo, Fabior, Tazorac	Topical	Cream, gel	Cleanse the face gently and dry face completely; apply a thin film once daily (evening)	Rx	May increase sensitivity to sunlight

Continued next page

MEDICATION TABLE 33-1. Acne Medications[1,2] *(Continued)*

CLASS Generic Name (pronunciation)*	Brand Name	Route	Forms	Dose	Regulatory Status	Notes
Trifarotene (trye FAR oh teen)	Aklief	Topical	Cream	Cleanse the face gently and dry completely; apply a thin film once daily (evening)	Rx	May increase sensitivity to sunlight
Isotretinoin (eye soe TRET i noyn)	Amnesteen, Claravis, Zenatane	Oral	Capsule	0.5–1 mg/kg/day in 2 divided doses	Rx	Used for severe acne; iPLEDGE registration required to decrease risk of birth defects
Antibacterials						
Clindamycin (klin da MYE sin)	Cleocin, Cleocin-T, Clindacin-P Clindagel, Clindesse, Evoclin	Topical, oral	Capsule, gel, lotion, solution, foam	Topical: Apply a thin film once or twice daily (depends on product) Oral: 75–150 mg twice daily	Rx	Oral formulations may cause stomach upset; topical clindamycin is most effective when combined with benzoyl peroxide
Erythromycin (er ith roe MYE sin)	E.E.S., Ery, Erygel, Ery-Tab, Erythrocin	Topical, oral	Tablet, suspension, capsule, gel, ointment, solution	Topical: Apply once or twice daily Oral: 250–500 mg twice daily, followed by 250–500 mg once daily	Rx	Oral formulations may cause stomach upset and increased sensitivity to sunlight; topical erythromycin is most effective when combined with benzoyl peroxide
Dapsone (DAP sone)	Aczone	Topical	Gel	Apply a thin layer to affected areas twice daily	Rx	
Doxycycline (dox i SYE kleen)	Acticlate, Doryx, Morgidox, Vibramycin	Oral	Capsule	50–100 mg twice daily or 100 mg once daily	Rx	May cause stomach upset and increased sensitivity to sunlight
Minocycline (mi noe SYE kleen)	Amzeeq, Zilxi Minocin Solodyn, Minolira, Ximino	Topical Oral	Foam Immediate-release tablet, capsule Extended-release tablet, capsule	Topical: Rub a small amount (eg, cherry size) onto acne-affected area once daily before bedtime Oral immediate-release: 50–100 mg twice daily Oral extended-release: 45–135 mg once daily	Rx	May cause stomach upset, increased sensitivity to sunlight, headache, dizziness, and skin discoloration (blue-gray or brown)

Continued next page

MEDICATION TABLE 33-1. Acne Medications[1,2] *(Continued)*

CLASS Generic Name (pronunciation)*	Brand Name	Route	Forms	Dose	Regulatory Status	Notes
Tetracycline (tet ra SYE kleen)		Oral	Capsule	500 mg twice daily, reduce to 125–500 mg once daily once improvement is noted	Rx	May cause stomach upset and increased sensitivity to sunlight
Sarecycline (sar e SYE kleen)	Seysara	Oral	Tablet	60–150 mg once daily	Rx	May cause stomach upset and increased sensitivity to sunlight
Combination Products						
Adapalene and benzoyl peroxide (a DAP a leen) (BEN zoe il) (per OX ide)	Epiduo	Topical	Gel	Topical; apply once daily to affected areas after skin has been cleaned and dried	Rx	May discolor hair or fabric; may also cause sensitivity to sunlight; daily sunscreen use recommended
Erythromycin and benzoyl peroxide (er ith roe MYE sin) (BEN zoe il) (per OX ide)	Benzamycin	Topical	Gel	Topical; apply twice a day, morning and evening.	Rx	May discolor hair or fabric; may also cause sensitivity to sunlight; daily sunscreen use recommended
Clindamycin and benzoyl peroxide (klin da MYE sin) (BEN zoe il) (per OX ide)	Acanya, BenzaClin, Neuac, Onexton	Topical	Gel	Topical; apply once or twice a day (morning and evening); dosing frequency varies by product	Rx	May discolor hair or fabric; may cause sensitivity to sunlight; daily sunscreen use recommended

* Pronunciations have been adapted with permission from USP Dictionary of USAN and International Drug Names (USP Dictionary) © 2022.

MEDICATION TABLE 33-2. Topical Corticosteroids[1,3]

Potency	Generic Name (pronunciation)*	Brand Name	Dosage Forms	Regulatory Status	Notes
Very High Potency	Augmented betamethasone dipropionate (bay ta METH a sone) (dye PROE pee oh nate)	Diprolene	0.05% ointment, gel, lotion	Rx	Do not discontinue high-potency agents abruptly; treatment duration for high-potency agents should not exceed 2 weeks; avoid use on face, groin, armpits, or skinfolds; do not use occlusive dressings with these agents
	Clobetasol propionate (kloe BAY ta sol) (PROE pee oh nate)	Cormax, Embeline, Embeline E, Temovate, Temovate E, Olux, Olux-E, Clobex, Clobevate	0.05% cream, ointment, gel, foam, lotion, shampoo, scalp application, spray	Rx	
	Diflorasone diacetate (dye FLOR a sone) (DYE a se tate)	ApexiCon, ApexiCon E	0.05% ointment	Rx	
	Fluocinonide (floo oh SIN oh nide)	Vanos	0.1% cream	Rx	
	Halobetasol propionate (hal oh BAY ta sol) (PROE pee oh nate)	Ultravate	0.05% cream, ointment	Rx	
High Potency	Amcinonide (am SIN oh nide)		0.1% cream, ointment, lotion	Rx	Do not use with occlusive dressings
	Augmented betamethasone dipropionate (bay ta METH a sone) (dye PROE pee oh nate)	Diprolene AF	0.05% cream	Rx	
	Betamethasone dipropionate (bay ta METH a sone) (dye PROE pee oh nate)	Diprosone	0.05% ointment, cream	Rx	
	Betamethasone valerate (bay ta METH a sone) (VAL er ate)	Beta-val, Luxiq	0.1% ointment, cream, lotion, foam	Rx	
	Desoximetasone (des ox i MET a sone)	Topicort	0.25% cream, ointment; 0.05% gel	Rx	
	Diflorasone diacetate (dye FLOR a sone) (DYE a se tate)	ApexiCon E, Florone, Psorcon E	0.05% cream	Rx	
	Fluocinonide (floo oh SIN oh nide)	Lidex, Lidex-E	0.05% cream, ointment, gel, solution	Rx	
	Halcinonide (hal SIN oh nide)	Halog	0.1% cream, ointment, solution	Rx	

Continued next page

MEDICATION TABLE 33-2. Topical Corticosteroids[1,3] *(Continued)*

Potency	Generic Name (pronunciation)*	Brand Name	Dosage Forms	Regulatory Status	Notes
Medium Potency	Betamethasone dipropionate (bay ta METH a sone) (dye PROE pee oh nate)		0.05% lotion	Rx	
	Betamethasone valerate (bay ta METH a sone) (VAL er ate)	Beta-Val	0.1% cream, lotion	Rx	
	Clocortolone pivalate (kloe KOR toe lone) (PIV al ate)	Cloderm	0.1% cream	Rx	
	Desoximetasone (des ox i MET a sone)	Topicort LP	0.05% cream	Rx	
	Fluocinolone acetonide (floo oh SIN oh lone) (AS ci tone ide)	Synalar	0.025% cream, ointment	Rx	
	Flurandrenolide (flure an DREN oh lide)	Cordran, Cordran SP	0.05% cream, lotion; 4 mcg/cm2 tape	Rx	
	Fluticasone propionate (floo TIK a sone) (PROE pee oh nate)	Cutivate	0.05% cream, 0.005% ointment	Rx	
	Hydrocortisone butyrate (hye droe KOR ti sone) (BYOO tr ayt)	Locoid, Locoid Lipocream	0.1% cream, ointment, solution	Rx	
	Hydrocortisone valerate (hye doe KOR ti sone) (VAL er ate)	Westcort	0.2% cream, ointment	Rx	
	Mometasone furoate (moe MET a sone) (FUIR o ate)	Elocon	0.1% cream, ointment, lotion	Rx	
	Triamcinolone acetonide (trye am SIN oh lone) (AS ci tone ide)	Kenalog	0.025% cream, ointment, lotion; 0.1% cream, ointment, lotion	Rx	
Low Potency	Alclometasone diproprionate (al kloe MET a sone) (dye PROE pee oh nate)	Aclovate	0.05% cream, ointment	Rx	Low-potency agents are recommended in children or if large areas of the body are to be covered; best agents for use on face
	Desonide (DES oh nide)	DesOwen, Tridesilon, Verdeso	0.05% cream, ointment, lotion, foam	Rx	
	Fluocinolone acetonide (floo oh SIN oh lone) (AS ci tone ide)	Synalar, Capex	0.01% shampoo, solution, cream	Rx	
	Hydrocortisone (hye doe KOR ti sone)		0.5% cream, ointment (OTC); 1% cream, ointment, lotion (some available OTC); 2.5% cream, ointment, lotion, topical solution (prescription only)	Rx/OTC	
	Hydrocortisone acetate (hye doe KOR ti sone)	Corticaine, Lanacort 10	0.5% cream 1% ointment	Rx/OTC	

* Pronunciations have been adapted with permission from USP Dictionary of USAN and International Drug Names (USP Dictionary) © 2022.

MEDICATION TABLE 33-3. Psoriasis Treatments[1,4]

CLASS Generic Name (pronunciation)*	Brand Name	Route	Forms	Dose	Regulatory Status	Notes
Vitamin D Analogues						
Calcipotriene (kal si POE trye een)	Calcitrene, Dovonex, Sorilux	Topical	Ointment, cream, solution	Apply 1–2 times daily to affected areas	Rx	
Calcitriol (kal si TRYE ole)	Vectical	Topical	Ointment	Apply twice daily to affected areas	Rx	
Oral Agents						
Acitretin (a si TRE tin)	Soriatane	PO	Capsule	10–50 mg daily	Rx	Take with food
Methotrexate (meth oh TREX ate)	Rheumatrex, Trexall	PO	Tablet, solution	10–25 mg once weekly	Rx	Monitor complete blood count, liver function tests
Cyclosporine (modified) (SYE kloe spor een)	Gengraf, Neoral	PO	Capsule	Initial dose: 1–3 mg/kg/day, divided twice daily, increase by 0.5 mg/kg/day after 4 weeks if insufficient response up to maximum dose of 4 mg/kg/day	Rx	Monitor blood pressure
Biologic Agents						
Alefacept (a la FA cept)	Amevive	IV, IM	Powder for reconstitution	7.5 mg by rapid IV or 15 mg once weekly IM × 12 weeks	Rx	Must be handled as a hazardous drug; requires monitoring of patient's CD4 counts
Etanercept (et a NER set)	Enbrel	SUBQ	Solution	50 mg twice weekly × 12 weeks, then 50 mg once weekly	Rx	
Adalimumab (a da LIM ue mab)	Humira	SUBQ	Solution	80 mg × 1, then 40 mg every other week starting 1 week after initial dose	Rx	
Infliximab (in FLIX i mab)	Remicade	IV	Solution	5 mg/kg at 0, 2, and 6 weeks, then every 8 weeks	Rx	May premedicate with antihistamines, acetaminophen, and/ or corticosteroids for infusion reactions

Continued next page

MEDICATION TABLE 33-3. Psoriasis Treatments[1,4] *(Continued)*

CLASS Generic Name (pronunciation)*	Brand Name	Route	Forms	Dose	Regulatory Status	Notes
Ustekinumab (us te KIN ue mab)	Stelara	SUBQ	Solution	≤100 kg: 45 mg at 0 and 4 weeks, then every 12 weeks >100 kg: 45 mg or 90 mg at 0 and 4 weeks, then every 12 weeks	Rx	
Secukinumab (sek ue KIN ue mab)	Cosentyx	SUBQ	Solution	300 mg once weekly on weeks 0, 1, 2, 3 and 4, then 300 mg every 4 weeks	Rx	Available in a prefilled syringe that may be self-injected by the patient
Combination Products						
Calcipotriene and betamethasone (kal si POE trye een) (bay ta METH a sone)	Taclonex, Enstilar, Wynzora	Topical	Cream, foam, ointment, suspension	Once daily for up to 4 weeks (foam, ointment) or 8 weeks (cream, suspension)	Rx	Do not apply to >30% of body surface area
Coal tar and salicylic acid (KOLE ta) (sal i SIL ik) (AS id)	Tarsum	Topical	Shampoo	As shampoo: apply to wet hair, leave in for several minutes, then rinse Prior to shampooing: apply to affected areas twice weekly, leave on for 5 minutes, gradually increasing time up to 1 hour, then rinse	OTC	

IV = intravenous; IM = intramuscular; PO = by mouth; SUBQ = subcutaneous.
* Pronunciations have been adapted with permission from USP Dictionary of USAN and International Drug Names (USP Dictionary) © 2022.

MEDICATION TABLE 33-4. Treatment of Dermatitis[1,2]

CLASS Generic Name (pronunciation)*	Brand Name	Route	Forms	Dose	Regulatory Status	Notes
Protectants						
Zinc oxide (zink) (OX ide)	AmeriDerm PeriShield, Ammens Original Medicated, Ammens Shower Fresh, Balmex, Boudreaux's Butt Paste, Desitin Maximum Strength, Desitin Rapid Relief, Dr. Smith's Diaper Rash, PeriGuard, Pharmabase Barrier, Triple Paste	Topical	Aerosol, cream, cream stick, ointment, paste, powder	Apply to affected areas as needed	OTC	Protective ointment to promote healing of chapped skin or diaper rash
Lanolin (LAN oh lin)	Lan-O-Soothe, Lansinoh (also contained in many other compounds such as Lubriderm)	Topical	Cream	Apply to affected areas as needed	OTC	Available with fragrance added or fragrance free
Vitamins A & D	A and D Original, Curad A & D	Topical	Ointment	Apply to affected areas as needed	OTC	
Petrolatum (pet ro LA tum)	Vaseline, many generics	Topical	Jelly	Apply to affected areas as needed	OTC	Not to be used on deep wounds, serious burns, or animal bites
Astringents						
Aluminum acetate (a LOO mi num) (AS e tate)	Burow's solution, Boro-Packs, Pedi-Boro Soak	Topical	Powder, for topical solution	Soak the affected area or dressing in solution (1:40, 1:20, or 1:13 dilution), apply 2-4 times/day for 15-30 min	OTC	
Calamine (KAL a meen)	Caladryl, Calagesic	Topical	Suspension	Apply to affected area as often as needed	OTC	Avoid contact with eyes and mucous membranes
Witch hazel	A.E.R. Traveler, A.E.R. Witch Hazel, Good Sense Medicated, Medi Pads, Preparation H Medicated Wipes, Tucks Anti-Itch	Topical	Liquid, pad, towelette	Apply to anorectal area as needed up to 6 times daily or after each bowel movement	OTC	

Continued next page

MEDICATION TABLE 33-4. Treatment of Dermatitis[1,2] *(Continued)*

CLASS Generic Name (pronunciation)*	Brand Name	Route	Forms	Dose	Regulatory Status	Notes
Representative Emollients						
Ammonium lactate (a MOE nee um) (LAK tate)	AL 12, AmLactin, Geri-Hydrolac, Lac-Hydrin	Topical	Cream, lotion	Apply twice daily to affected area; rub in well	OTC	May cause burning or stinging upon application to abraded skin
Colloidal oatmeal	Aveeno	Topical	Powder	Disperse powder in bathwater	OTC	
Combination Products						
Mixtures of glycerin, mineral oil, petrolatum, lanolin, urea, miscellaneous ingredients	Nivea, Eucerin, Curel, Neutrogena, Lubriderm	Topical	Ointments, creams, lotions	Apply to skin as needed	OTC	

* Pronunciations have been adapted with permission from USP Dictionary of USAN and International Drug Names (USP Dictionary) © 2022.

MEDICATION TABLE 33-5. Preparations to Treat Bacterial Skin Infections[1,2]

CLASS Generic Name (pronunciation)*	Brand Name	Route	Forms	Dose	Rx/OTC	Notes
Topical Antibiotic						
Mupirocin (myoo PEER oh sin)	Bactroban	Topical	Ointment, cream	Apply to lesions 3 times daily	Rx	Impetigo: use for 5–10 days; Secondary skin infection: use for 10 days
Bacitracin (bass i TRAY sin)	Many generics	Topical	Ointment, 500 units/g	Apply to lesions 1–3 times daily	OTC	Stop use and contact a healthcare provider if condition persists >7 days or worsens, or if a rash or other allergic reaction develops
Double antibiotic ointment, polymyxin/bacitracin (pol i MIX in) (bass i TRAY sin)	Polysporin, many generics	Topical	Ointment	Apply to lesions 1–3 times daily	OTC	Stop use and contact a healthcare provider if condition persists >7 days or worsens, or if a rash or other allergic reaction develops
Triple antibiotic ointment, neomycin/polymyxin/bacitracin (nee oh MYE sin) (pol i MIX in) (bass i TRAY sin)	Neosporin	Topical	Ointment	Apply to lesions 1–3 times daily	OTC	Stop use and contact a healthcare provider if condition persists >7 days or worsens, or if a rash or other allergic reaction develops
Pleuromutilin						
Retapamulin (re te PAM ue lin)	Altabax	Topical	Ointment	Apply a thin layer to lesions twice a day	Rx	Only use in children >9 months old; impetigo: use for 5 days
Penicillin						
Dicloxacillin (dye klox a SILL in)		Oral	Capsules	Adults: 250–500 mg 4 times daily for 10 days; Children: 12.5–25 mg/kg/day, divided, 4 times daily for 10 days	Rx	
Nafcillin (naf SILL in) Oxacillin (oks a SILL in)		IV	Vial	Adults: 500–2,000 mg every 4–6 hours; Children: 100–200 mg/kg/day in divided doses every 4–6 hours	Rx	Use IV for severe infections and those unable to take oral medications
Amoxicillin/clavulanate (a mox i SIL in) (KLAV yoo lan ate)	Augmentin	Oral	Tablet, suspension	Adults: 500 mg twice daily for 10 days; Children: 25–45 mg/kg/day, divided, twice daily for 10 days	Rx	

Continued next page

MEDICATION TABLE 33-5. Preparations to Treat Bacterial Skin Infections[1,2] *(Continued)*

CLASS Generic Name (pronunciation)*	Brand Name	Route	Forms	Dose	Rx/OTC	Notes
Cephalosporin						
Cephalexin (sef a LEX in)	Keflex	Oral	Capsule, suspension	Adults: 250–500 mg 4 times daily for 10 days Children: 25–50 mg/kg/day, divided, 2–4 times daily for 10 days	Rx	
Cefazolin (sef A zoe lin)	Ancef	IV	Vial	Adults: 1–2 g every 8 hours Children >1 month: 50–100 mg/kg/day divided every 8 hours	Rx	Use IV for severe infections and those unable to take oral medications
Cefuroxime (se fyoor OX eem)	Ceftin	Oral	Tablet, suspension	Adults: 250–500 mg twice daily for 10 days Children: 20–30 mg/kg/day, divided, twice daily for 10 days	Rx	May use in patients with a mild penicillin allergy (rash)
Ceftaroline (sef TAR oh leen)	Teflaro	IV	Vial	Adults: 600 mg twice daily Children: 12 mg/kg every 8 hours	Rx	Used only in patients with MRSA infections
Macrolide						
Clindamycin (klin da MYE sin)	Cleocin	Oral, IV	Capsule, suspension	Adults: 300–450 mg 3–4 times daily for 10 days Children: 20–40 mg/kg/day, divided, 3–4 times daily for 10 days	Rx	Used for patients with a severe penicillin allergy (anaphylaxis) and in those with community acquired CA-MRSA (high incidence of resistance)
Sulfonamide Derivative						
Sulfamethoxazole/ trimethoprim (sul fa meth OX a zole) (trye METH oh prim)	Septra DS, Bactrim DS	Oral	Tablet	Adult: 1–2 double-strength tablets every 12 hours Children: 8 to 12 mg trimethoprim TMP/kg/day in divided doses every 12 hours	Rx	Unlabeled use for CA-MRSA
Glycopeptide						
Vancomycin (van koe MYE sin)	Vancocin	IV	Vial	15–20 mg/kg/dose every 8–12 hours	Rx	Used only in patients with a severe penicillin allergy (anaphylaxis) or for MRSA infections
Oxazolidinone						
Linezolid (li NE zoh lid)	Zyvox	Oral, IV	Tablet, premixed bag for infusion	Adults: 600 mg every 12 hours Children <11 years: 10 mg/kg every 12 hours	Rx	Used only in patients with MRSA infections

IV = intravenous; MRSA = methicillin-resistant *Staphylococcus aureus*.
*Pronunciations have been adapted with permission from USP Dictionary of USAN and International Drug Names (USP Dictionary) © 2022.

MEDICATION TABLE 33-6. Treatment of Fungal Skin Infections[1,2]

Azoles

CLASS Generic Name (pronunciation)*	Brand Name	Route	Forms	Dose	Regulatory Status	Notes
Clotrimazole (kloe TRIM a zole)	Lotrimin AF, Desenex	Topical	Cream, lotion, solution	Apply topically twice a day for 2–4 weeks	OTC	Effective for athlete's foot, ringworm of the skin, and jock itch
Econazole (e KON na zole)	Spectazole	Topical	Cream	Apply topically once a day for 2–4 weeks	Rx	Effective for athlete's foot, ringworm of the skin, and jock itch
Fluconazole (floo KOE na zole)	Diflucan	Oral	Tablet	Adults: Take 150–200 mg daily for 2–4 weeks Children: not established	Rx	Effective for athlete's foot and infections of the skin and scalp
Miconazole (mi KON a zole)	Lotrimin AF, Micatin, Zeasorb-AF	Topical	Cream, shake powder, liquid spray, spray powder	Apply topically twice a day for 4 weeks	OTC	Effective for athlete's foot, ringworm of the skin, and jock itch
Oxiconazole (ox i KON a zole)	Oxistat	Topical	Cream, lotion	Apply once or twice a day for 2–4 weeks	Rx	Effective for athlete's foot, ringworm of the skin, and jock itch
Sertaconazole (ser ta KON na zole)	Ertaczo	Topical	Cream	Apply twice a day for 4 weeks	Rx	Effective for athlete's foot (FDA-approved indication); also effective for ringworm of the skin, and jock itch (off-label uses)
Sulconazole (sul KON na zole)	Exelderm	Topical	Cream, solution	Apply once or twice a day for 3–4 weeks	Rx	Effective for athlete's foot, ringworm of the skin, and jock itch
Ketoconazole (kee toe KON na zole)	Extina, Nizoral, Nizoral A-D, Xolegel	Topical, oral	Cream, tablet	Topical: apply once daily for 2–6 weeks Oral, adults: 200–400 mg once a day Oral, children ≥2 years: 3.3–6.6 mg/kg/ day as a single dose	Rx/OTC	Topical treatment is effective for athlete's foot, ringworm of the skin, and jock itch; oral treatment is effective for ringworm of the scalp
Itraconazole (it ra KON a zole)	Sporanox	Oral	Capsule, solution	Adult: 200 mg once or twice daily for 5–7 days Children (tinea captitis): 5 mg/kg/dose once daily	Rx	Indicated for toenail fungal infections

Continued next page

MEDICATION TABLE 33-6. Treatment of Fungal Skin Infections[1,2] *(Continued)*

CLASS Generic Name (pronunciation)*	Brand Name	Route	Forms	Dose	Regulatory Status	Notes
Allylamines/Non-Azole						
Butenafine (byoo TEN a feen)	Mentax, Lotrimin Ultra	Topical	Cream	Apply topically once a day for 2–4 weeks	Rx/OTC	Effective for athlete's foot, ringworm of the skin, and jock itch
Naftifine (NAF ti feen)	Naftin	Topical	Cream, gel	Cream: apply once a day for 4 weeks Gel: apply twice a day for 4 weeks	Rx	Effective for athlete's foot, ringworm of the skin, and jock itch
Ciclopirox (sye kloe PEER ox)	Ciclodan, Loprox, Penlac	Topical	Cream, gel, solution	Cream and gel: apply twice a day for 4 weeks Solution: apply one coat daily and allow to dry; apply a new coat over previous coat each day for 7 days, then remove with alcohol and continue cycle; use for a maximum of 48 weeks	Rx	Effective for athlete's foot, ringworm of the skin, jock itch, and onycomycoses
Tolnaftate (tole NAF tate)	Tinactin	Topical	Cream, liquid spray, powder spray, shake powder	Apply twice a day for 2–4 weeks	OTC	Effective for athlete's foot, ringworm of the skin, jock itch, and onycomycoses
Terbinafine (TER bin a feen)	Lamisil AT, Desenex Max, Lamisil	Topical, oral	Cream, liquid spray, tablet	Topical: apply twice a day for 1–2 weeks Oral, adults: 250 mg once daily for 6–12 weeks Oral, children: 62.25–250 mg (based on weight) once daily for 6–12 weeks	Rx/OTC	Topical treatment is effective for athlete's foot, ringworm of the skin, and jock itch; oral treatment is effective for ringworm of the scalp and onycomycoses
Griseofulvin (gri see oh FUL vin)	Grifulvin V, Gris-PEG	Oral	Tablet, suspension	Adult: Grifulvin 500–1,000 mg/day in single or divided doses, Gris-PEG 375 mg/day in single or divided doses; treatment duration 4-6 weeks Children: Grifulvin V 20–25 mg/kg/day in single or divided doses, Gris-PEG 10–15 mg/kg/day in single dose or 2 divided doses; treatment duration 4–6 weeks	Rx	Effective for ringworm of the scalp

FDA = US Food and Drug Administration.
* Pronunciations have been adapted with permission from USP Dictionary of USAN and International Drug Names (USP Dictionary) © 2022.

MEDICATION TABLE 33-7. Treatment of Warts and Viral Skin Infections[1,2]

CLASS Generic Name (pronunciation)*	Brand Name	Route	Forms	Dose	Regulatory Status	Notes
Keratolytic						
Salicylic acid (sal i SIL ik) (AS id)	Compound W, Duofilm, Wart-Off	Topical	Flexible collodion vehicle	Apply to wart once or twice a day for up to 12 weeks	OTC	Common warts
	Clear Away, Dr. Scholl's Clear Away, Compound W One Step Pads	Topical	Embedded pads or discs	Apply and remove pads every 48 hours as needed for up to 12 weeks	OTC	Plantar warts
	Trans-Ver-Sal Adult and Pedi Patch	Topical	Plaster	Apply to wart at bedtime and leave on for at least 8 hours, then remove and discard plaster; repeat daily for up to 12 weeks	OTC	Common warts
Cryotherapy						
Dimethyl ether and propane (DYE meth ill) (EE ther) (PROE pane)	Wartner Wart Removal	Topical		Apply for up to 20 seconds; may repeat in 10 days for up to 3 treatments	OTC	Common and plantar warts
Dimethyl ether, propane, and isobutane (DYE meth ill) (EE ther) (PROE pane) (EYE soe byoo tane)	Compound W Freeze Off, Dr. Scholl's Freeze Away	Topical		Apply for up to 20 seconds; may repeat in 10 days for up to 3 treatments	OTC	Common and plantar warts
Immunologic						
Imiquimod (i mi KWI mod)	Aldara, Zyclara	Topical	Cream	Apply once daily prior to bedtime	Rx	Common warts
Cold Sore Agent						
Docosanol (doe KOE san ole)	Abreva	Topical	Cream	Apply 5 times a day to the affected area until healed	OTC	Indicated only for those ≥12 years of age
Acyclovir (ay SYE kloe veer)	Zovirax	Oral	Tablet	Adults and adolescents: 400 mg three times a day for 5–10 days	Rx	Indicated for the treatment of recurrent herpes labialis (cold sores) for those ≥12 years of age
Valacyclovir (val ay SYE kloe veer)	Valtrex	Oral	Tablet	Adults and adolescents: 1 g twice a day for 5–10 days (initial infection); 2 g twice a day for 1 day (recurrent infection)	Rx	Indicated for the treatment of recurrent herpes labialis (cold sores) for those ≥12 years of age

*Pronunciations have been adapted with permission from USP Dictionary of USAN and International Drug Names (USP Dictionary) © 2022.

MEDICATION TABLE 33-8. Lice and Scabies Preparations[1,2]

CLASS Generic Name (pronunciation)	Brand Name	Route	Forms	Dose	Notes
Antiparasitic					
Synergized pyrethrins (pi RETH rin)	A-200, LiceMD, Pronto Plus, RID®	Topical	Shampoo, spray	Shampoo and lotion: apply shampoo to dry hair and leave in for 10 min; wash and rinse with water; use a fine-tooth comb to remove nits; repeat treatment in 7–10 days Spray: use to remove nits from bedding, not for human use	Lice only
Lindane (LIN dane)	Kwell	Topical	Shampoo, lotion	Lice: apply shampoo to dry hair and massage into hair for 4 minutes, adding small quantities of water to hair until lather forms; rinse hair thoroughly and comb with a fine-tooth comb to remove nits Scabies: apply a thin layer of lotion and massage it on skin; after 8–12 hours, shampoo/bathe to remove the drug	Lice and scabies
Permethrin (per METH rin)	Nix (OTC), Elimite (Rx)	Topical	Lotion, cream, spray	Lice: wash hair with shampoo, rinse, and towel dry; apply a sufficient volume of creme rinse to saturate the hair and scalp; leave on hair for 10 minutes before rinsing off with water; remove remaining nits with a fine-tooth comb; may repeat in 1 week if lice or nits still present Scabies: apply cream from head to toe; leave on for 8–14 hours before washing off with water; may reapply in 1 week if live mites appear Spray: use to remove nits from bedding, not for human use	Lice (lotion) and scabies (cream)
Malathion (mal a THYE on)	Ovide	Topical	Lotion	Sprinkle lotion on dry hair and rub gently until the scalp is thoroughly moistened; allow to dry naturally, leaving it uncovered; after 8–12 hours, wash hair with a nonmedicated shampoo; rinse and use a fine-tooth comb to remove dead lice and eggs; if required, repeat with second application in 7–9 days	Lice only
Spinosad (SPIN oh sad)	Natroba	Topical	Suspension	Shake bottle well; apply to dry scalp and rub gently until the scalp is thoroughly moistened, then apply to dry hair, completely covering scalp and hair; leave on for 10 minutes (start timing treatment after the scalp and hair have been completely covered); the hair should then be rinsed thoroughly with warm water; shampoo may be used immediately after the product is completely rinsed off; if live lice are seen 7 days after the first treatment, repeat with second application; avoid contact with the eyes; nit combing is not required, although a fine-tooth comb may be used to remove treated lice and nits	Lice only
Benzyl alcohol (BEN zil AL ka hol)	Ulesfia	Topical	Lotion	Apply appropriate volume for hair length to dry hair and completely saturate the scalp; leave on for 10 minutes; rinse thoroughly with water; repeat in 7 days	Lice only

* Pronunciations have been adapted with permission from USP Dictionary of USAN and International Drug Names (USP Dictionary) © 2022.

PREPARATIONS FOR THE EYE, EAR, NOSE, AND THROAT

Chapter 34

Ophthalmic Medications

Richard G. Fiscella, PharmD, MPH |
Mary Ann Stuhan, PharmD, RPh

KEY TERMS AND DEFINITIONS

Aqueous humor—the watery fluid produced in the ciliary body and leaving through mainly the trabecular meshwork drain, which provides nutrition to the front of the eye.

Cataract—a clouding of the lens occurring commonly in patients as they age.

Conjunctiva—the clear tissue around the white part (sclera) of the eye.

Conjunctivitis—an inflammation or infection of the conjunctiva.

Cornea—the clear covering over the front of the eye.

Cycloplegia—paralysis of the muscle that holds the lens in place and facilitates dilation of the pupil. Causes a loss of accommodation or ability to focus the lens and sensitivity to light.

Diplopia—double vision.

Glaucoma—an eye condition that can result from increased pressure in the eye, which can cause optic nerve damage and loss of vision.

Intraocular pressure (IOP)—a measurement of pressure in the eye, usually <21 mm Hg. Increases in IOP can lead to glaucoma or blindness.

Iris—the colored part of the eye.

Macula—the focal point on the retina that allows for clear, sharp vision especially when focusing on tasks straight ahead.

Miosis—constriction of the pupil, allowing less light into the eye.

DOI 10.37573/9781585286638.034

Mydriasis—enlargement of the pupil, allowing more light into the eye. May be induced for some eye examination procedures.

Ocular hypertension—an increase in intraocular pressure, which may lead to glaucoma in some patients.

Pupil—the dark space in the middle of the iris that appears black. The pupil dilates and constricts to allow varying amounts of light into the eye.

Retina—the lining in the back of the eyeball that allows light messages to be transmitted to the optic nerve and then the brain.

Sclera—the white, outer part of the eyeball.

LEARNING OBJECTIVES

After completing this chapter, you should be able to

1. Review the anatomy and physiology of the eye.

2. Describe glaucoma and the most commonly used treatment approaches.

3. Describe the causes and symptoms of conjunctivitis, and treatment options.

4. Identify common causes of blindness.

5. Identify medications used in the eye, including their dosage forms, therapeutic effects, most common side effects, and mechanisms of action.

The eye is the organ for sight. Many things can affect the eye, including diabetes, trauma, vision problems, and allergies. Some of these can be improved with treatments, including surgery and medications used in the eye. This chapter discusses these and how ophthalmic medications are used.

ANATOMY OF THE EYE

The eye functions as our organ for sight. Light enters the eye, passing through the transparent cornea, enters the pupil, an open space in the center of the iris, and is refracted through the lens and onto the retina. The retina is attached to the inside back of the eyeball and transmits messages to the optic nerve. The optic nerve carries these light messages to the brain, where they are translated into pictures of what is being seen. These structures are illustrated in Figure 34-1.

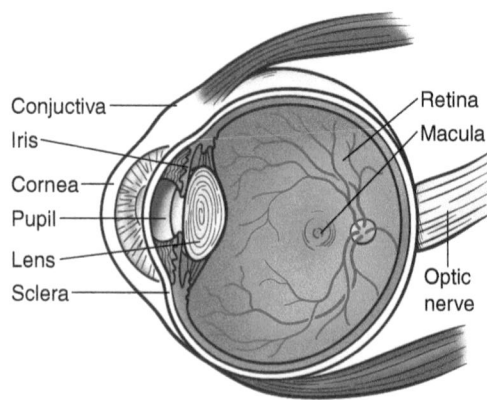

FIGURE 34-1. Anatomy of the eye.

Many problems can occur in this complicated organ and its communication process. Blurry vision is a common occurrence that can have many causes, including vision changes or some medications. One of these vision changes is myopia, or nearsightedness, where the light is focused through the lens to a place in front of the retina instead of on it. This means the person can see objects close up but those at a distance are blurry. The opposite of myopia is farsightedness, where patients can see things far away but items up close are blurry. This occurs when the lens focuses items beyond the back of the retina. Both of these conditions can be improved by corrective lenses and sometimes corrective surgery. Diplopia is double vision, which can occur for various reasons (some minor and some serious). Treatment will depend on the cause. Another common eye condition is presbyopia, where the eye gradually loses the ability to focus on close-up objects. Presbyopia usually occurs as people age, starting in the 40s, and gets worse until around age 60. A cataract is another relatively common eye condition, in which a clouding of the lens occurs as a person ages. As the lens clouds, there is usually a loss in vision. This development is commonly slow, occurring over many years, with a gradual decline in vision. Often, this can be corrected with surgery.

GLAUCOMA

CASE STUDY

Mrs. Griffen has recently been diagnosed with ocular hypertension in both eyes. She hasn't noticed any vision changes yet, but both of her parents had glaucoma and her mother went blind in her 80s.

Aqueous humor, a watery fluid, is produced in the ciliary body and flows from the posterior chamber to the front of the eye or the anterior chamber through the pupil and out mainly through the drain (trabecular meshwork). Aqueous humor provides nutrition to the front of the eye. Intraocular pressure (IOP) reflects the amount of aqueous humor present in the front part of the eye. When the aqueous humor cannot flow out of the eye quickly enough, pressure can start to build and IOP can increase. Normal IOP is less than 21 mm Hg. Anything above that may be considered ocular hypertension.

CASE?

Does Mrs. Griffen have glaucoma?

Glaucoma is the second leading cause of blindness worldwide.[1] It is caused by optic nerve damage, commonly due to elevated IOP, but can occur even when IOP is in the normal range. Patients can have elevated IOP without having glaucoma. There are two main types of glaucoma: open angle and closed angle. Closed-angle glaucoma refers to a physical limitation in the iris where outflow of aqueous humor is mechanically blocked in some way. This occurs in about 10% of glaucoma cases. More commonly, patients have open-angle glaucoma.[2] Open angle means that there is an increase in IOP even though the angle of the iris and cornea appear to be unblocked. There are variations within each of these types.

CASE?

If Mrs. Griffen's initial IOP was 28 mm Hg, what would her IOP goal be?

Most patients with glaucoma start to have certain types of visual field defects that are indications for diagnostic testing (IOP measurements and optic disc examination), although glaucoma can be present with or without increased IOP. The goal of glaucoma treatments is to lower IOP by 20% or more if the disease is more progressed. Often ocular hypertension occurs but may not lead to glaucoma or vision changes; however, the goal in these patients is still to decrease IOP. Treatments include medications, laser surgery, and incisional surgery.

Glaucoma Treatment

Drug treatment is similar for most types of open-angle glaucoma. Several classes of medications are used to treat glaucoma. These include beta-blockers, alpha agonists, carbonic anhydrase inhibitors, prostaglandin analogues, and sympathomimetics, as well as a newer type, rho kinase inhibitors. The classes work in different ways, and can be used in a variety of combinations.

Beta-blockers, already discussed in Chapter 4 ("The Autonomic Nervous System") and Chapter 15 ("Hypertension") work by reducing the production of aqueous humor, therefore reducing IOP because there is less fluid being produced. Beta-blockers can be used chronically (long term). Drugs in this class for ophthalmic use include betaxolol, levobunolol, timolol, carteolol, and metipranolol (see Medication Table 34-1; Medication Tables are located at the end of the chapter). Prostaglandin analogues include bimatoprost, latanoprost, travoprost, and tafluprost. These help to decrease IOP by increasing outflow. Bimatoprost is also approved as the first 10 mcg intracameral (anterior chamber) biodegradable sustained-release implant indicated to reduce IOP in patients with open-angle glaucoma or ocular hypertension.

CASE?

Mrs. Griffen has prescriptions for timolol and pilocarpine eye drops. Is it likely that these will solve her problem and be discontinued next month?

PRACTICE POINT

Latanoprost is stored in the refrigerator until the bottle is opened. Once opened, it can be stored at room temperature for up to 6 weeks.

ALERT!

Prostaglandin analogues used for glaucoma should not be used more than once a day as more frequent use may reduce their IOP-lowering effect.

Cholinergic eye drops include pilocarpine and carbachol. These stimulate cholinergic receptors in the eye and are now considered third or fourth line therapy as described in Chapter 4, cause miosis (decrease in pupil size) and/or open the trabecular meshwork. While this helps to increase outflow of the aqueous humor, cholinergics are now considered third or fourth line therapy. Carbonic anhydrase inhibitors work in the eye by decreasing the production of aqueous humor. Topical preparations for ophthalmic application in this class include brinzolamide and dorzolamide. Oral carbonic anhydrase inhibitors, acetazolamide and methazolamide, can also be used for the treatment of glaucoma but usually have a much higher risk of side effects, including gastrointestinal (GI) effects and blood pressure changes. Sympathomimetics include brimonidine and apraclonidine. They both work at alpha-adrenergic receptors (described in Chapter 4) and decrease the production of aqueous humor, therefore decreasing IOP. Brimonidine also works to increase aqueous humor outflow.

Rho kinase inhibitors are the newest medications indicated for the treatment of glaucoma, and appear to reduce IOP by increasing the outflow of aqueous humor. Netarsudil is currently the only ophthalmic preparation of this type available in the United States.

ALERT!

Administration of prostaglandin analogues should be separated from other eye drop application by at least 5 minutes.

The most common side effects of eye drops used for glaucoma are burning or stinging. Some, like timolol, can be absorbed into the body and affect blood pressure, but this can be minimized by giving only one drop at a time and gently closing the eyes for 3–5 minutes (eyelid closure technique) to minimize systemic absorption.

Beta-blockers, carbonic anhydrase inhibitors, prostaglandin analogues, sympathomimetics, cholinergic drops, and rho kinase inhibitors are typically used in various combinations for the treatment of glaucoma. In closed-angle glaucoma, beta-blockers are used with cholinergic agents like pilocarpine. Patients may receive a laser procedure to lower the IOP. Some eye drops are available in combinations, such as Cosopt, which is dorzolamide and timolol together. Others, such as pilocarpine, are not available in the United States in combination with anything else but can be used with other products as long as there is separation between drop administrations.

CASE?

Mrs. Griffen returns to the pharmacy with a prescription for latanoprost. Does this mean that she should stop using the timolol?

Glaucoma treatment typically begins as a single medication in one eye to assess efficacy and tolerance. Beta-blockers, such as timolol or prostaglandins are usually started first, but brimonidine or topical carbonic anhydrase inhibitors can be used initially in patients who have contraindications to one of the first-line medications. After a few weeks, reassessment is needed to determine the response and tolerance to the initial drug. If there is not enough response, a second drug may be added and assessed after a few more weeks. If a drug cannot be tolerated, changes can be made in the regimen. This is continued until the desired response is seen, or drug therapy is maximized and surgery is the only option left.

MACULAR DEGENERATION

The macula is located in the central part of the retina and helps to give sharp, clear vision when looking straight ahead and performing tasks such as reading or driving. Macular degeneration is a condition in which the macula is slowly destroyed and is often seen in older adults (age-related macular degeneration, AMD). It is classified as either wet or dry. Wet AMD is usually more serious than dry AMD. Wet AMD occurs when new blood vessels behind the retina start to grow under the macula. These new vessels tend to leak fluid and blood, raising the macula from its normal place and quickly damaging it. Dry AMD occurs as some of the cells in the macula start to break down, causing blurred vision in the central vision. Dry AMD can develop slowly over time, whereas wet AMD can occur quickly and damage vision significantly in a short period of time. The first symptom of wet AMD is typically that straight lines appear wavy. The first symptom of dry AMD is typically blurred vision. Treatment for wet AMD most often includes medications injected into the eye to stop blood vessel growth, and laser treatment.

Macular Degeneration Agents

Two types of drugs can be used in macular degeneration. The first type is a vascular endothelial growth factor (VEGF) inhibitor. Anti-VEGF agents have often stabilized and improved vision in patients with wet AMD. Ranibizumab, (Lucentis), aflibercept (Eylea), brolucizumab (BeoVu), and faricimab (Vabysmo) are the anti-VEGF inhibitors currently approved for treatment of wet AMD, and bevicizumab (Avastin) is often used off label. These agents are injected into the eye every 4–6 weeks and slow new blood vessel growth and vision loss. Another type of medication for AMD (not often used) is a choroidal vessel occluder, specifically verteporfin (Visudyne). This medication is given via intravenous (IV) infusion in the doctor's office and a laser may activate the drug in the eye and slow new blood vessel growth. See Medication Table 34-2 for details about these medications.

CASE STUDY

Ms. Arth is a preschool teacher and several of her students have recently had pink eye. She woke up this morning with a matted, crusty left eye. Her conjunctiva looks very bloodshot and her eye feels itchy and dry.

ALERT!

LOOK-ALIKE/SOUND-ALIKE—Over-the-counter eye drops are available in a variety of formulations for different uses, many with similar names. For example, there are currently a dozen different products marketed under the name Visine, including Visine Original for "redness relief" (tetrahydrozoline, a decongestant), Visine for Contacts (wetting/lubrication solution), and Visine Allergy (includes an antihistamine). The label always lists the intended uses and active ingredients of a formulation.

CONJUNCTIVITIS

Conjunctivitis is an inflammation of the conjunctiva or tissue around the eye. This can be caused by irritants like dirt or debris, allergens, bacteria, or viruses. The eye will try to rid itself of anything bothersome by washing it away with tears. Patients with a history of allergic conjunctivitis should avoid allergens when possible; however, ophthalmic antihistamines, mast cell stabilizers, and decongestants can help eye allergy symptoms like itchy or watery eyes. Bacterial conjunctivitis is often treated with antibiotic preparations.

Allergic Conjunctivitis

Antihistamines/Decongestants

Histamine is released from cells when an allergen attaches to the cell and causes vasodilation leading to erythema (redness), stimulation of sensory nerves leading to itching, and increased secretions. Ophthalmic antihistamines work by blocking histamine in the eye and help with symptoms such as itchy or watering eyes. They typically do not cause drowsiness like oral or nasal antihistamines. Many are available over the counter (OTC), but some antihistamine eye drops like azelastine require a prescription. The antihistamine eye drops, along with other treatments for conjunctivitis, are listed in Medication Table 34-3.

ALERT!

Ophthalmic decongestants should not be used for more than 3 days, to reduce the risk of irritation to the eye.

Mast cell stabilizers help to prevent the release of histamine and other inflammatory mediators from the cells. Administered as eye drops, they often have antihistamine action as well. Bepotastine (Bepreve) requires a prescription, but ketotifen, olopatadine, and alcaftadine are available OTC.

ALERT!

Bacterial and viral conjunctivitis can be very contagious. Handwashing and avoiding contact of the hands with the face are important in stopping its spread.

Ophthalmic decongestants work like nasal and oral decongestants in that they cause vasoconstriction. Several decongestants are available OTC and ophthalmic decongestants are the classic ingredients in the well-known Visine Allergy (naphazoline/pheniramine) eye drops.

Infective Conjunctivitis

Bacterial conjunctivitis is an infection, commonly referred to as pink eye, due to the bloodshot appearance of the infected eye. Viral infections can also cause conjunctivitis.

Anti-infective Agents

Antibacterial, antifungal, and antiviral agents are all available in an ophthalmic form to treat eye infections. Antibacterial agents are available from several drug classes, similar to oral and injectable agents: macrolides, quinolones, amino-glycosides, sulfonamides, and others. Some of these, such as ciprofloxacin and bacitracin, are available in both an ointment form and ophthalmic drops. Many of the antivi-ral and antifungal ophthalmic agents work in similar ways to systemic agents but are only available for use in the eye. The most common side effects with anti-infective drops are burning or stinging in the eye after administration. More information on available anti-infective eye drops is available in Medication Table 34-3.

CASE?

Ms. Arth has asked where she can find Visine eye drops on the shelf. What do you think might be the cause of Ms. Arth's eye problem? Should the technician just ring up her Visine or might the pharmacist be consulted for other ideas?

PRACTICE POINT

Eye infections must be diagnosed and treated by a physician. Ophthalmic anti-infectives are available only by prescription.

PRACTICE POINT

An ointment is often prescribed when the medication should be in contact with the eye longer than can be achieved with a drop. Ointments can make vision blurry and should be used after any eye drops.

ALERT!

Contact lenses should not be worn while an eye infection is present and should not be used again until the infection has cleared up, usually 7–10 days after treatment started.

Anti-inflammatory Agents

Nonsteroidal anti-inflammatory agents (NSAIDs) and cor-ticosteroids, discussed in previous chapters, are available as eye drops. NSAIDs can be used to decrease inflammation in the eye and sometimes to aid in the treatment of allergic symptoms. They are also used after eye surgery, like cata-ract surgery, to help decrease the inflammation in the eye. Corticosteroids can be used for similar reasons: conjunc-tivitis, inflammation after surgery, and sometimes allergy symptoms. Other anti-inflammatory agents used in the eye are cyclosporine and lifitegrast, which are prescribed for chronic dry eye. They work by helping to increase tear pro-duction. Agents for ophthalmic inflammation are detailed in Medication Table 34-4.

PRACTICE POINT

Dexamethasone and prednisolone are corticosteroids found in combination with an antibiotic like tobramycin or sulfacetamide, in products such as Tobradex or Blephamide.

CASE?

If Ms. Arth sees a physician, what do you think might be prescribed? Why?

BLEPHAROSPASM AND BLINDNESS

Blepharospasm is a twitch of the eyelid. In some cases, this can be ongoing. Onabotulinum toxin A (Botox) is an intra-muscular injection that helps paralyze the muscle so that it doesn't keep twitching.

Blindness is a condition that can be gradual or immediate and may have many causes. Blindness may also be temporary or permanent. Whether onset is gradual or immediate and temporary or permanent depends on the cause. The leading disease causes of blindness in the United States are glaucoma, diabetic retinopathy, macular degeneration, and cataracts.[3] Accidents may also cause blindness, from incidents such as sports injuries or chemical burns. Other causes of blindness (rare in the United States) may be onchocerciasis (river blind-ness), trachoma, leprosy, and vitamin A deficiency. Many of these, especially cataracts, glaucoma, and macular degeneration, can be treated with surgery and/or medications.

MISCELLANEOUS OPHTHALMIC CONDITIONS AND TREATMENTS

For mild or occasional dry eyes there are eye drops that act like natural tears, usually called artificial tears. They contain compounds such as carboxymethylcellulose or hydroxypropyl cellulose that work as lubricating agents. These can usually be used as often as needed. These and other ophthalmic agents are detailed in Medication Table 34-5.

For diagnostic procedures where the back of the eye is to be examined, mydriasis and/or cycloplegia may be needed. Mydriatics work by dilating the pupil. Cycloplegics cause pupillary dilation and temporarily paralyze the ciliary muscle, which helps the lens to change shape as we focus on objects. Atropine, cyclopentolate, and homatropine are all cycloplegic agents that are used for these purposes. These may cause burning or stinging, as well as temporary vision changes like sensitivity to light and blurry vision or difficulty focusing.

ALERT!

Eye drops are sometimes used in the ear to help treat certain infections, but ear drops should never be used in the eye. For example, Ciloxan (ciprofloxacin 0.3%) ophthalmic solution can be used in the eye or ear, but Cetraxal (ciprofloxacin 0.2%) otic solution should only be used in the ear and never in the eye. Eye drops are specifically buffered and formulated for ophthalmic use because eye tissue is much more sensitive than ear tissue. Using ear drops in the eye causes immediate burning and stinging, redness, and sometimes swelling.

Dosage Forms and Administration of Ophthalmic Agents

Ophthalmic preparations are most commonly available in a solution or suspension formula. Some ophthalmic medications are available as sterile ointments, which allow the medication to have longer contact with the eye because of thicker viscosity of the preparation. Gel-forming solutions, such as Timoptic-XE, have a component that allows a gel to

form on contact with the precorneal tear film. This formulation allows the medication to be in contact with the eye longer before it is washed away by normal tear production.

PRACTICE POINT

Contact lenses should be removed before installing drops into the eye. They should be left out for at least 15 minutes after the dose is applied, and perhaps longer depending on the medication.

ALERT!

All dosage forms applied to the eye must be sterile. If they are compounded in the pharmacy, aseptic technique, sterile ingredients, and sterile dispensing containers are required.

Although ophthalmic products usually have brief instructions for use included, it cannot be assumed that all patients know how to administer them properly. Some physicians and their staff demonstrate application techniques to patients and caregivers, but this is not always the case. Patients purchasing eye drops in the pharmacy, whether OTC or prescription, should always be asked whether they know how to use them, and consultation with the pharmacist may be required to ensure proper administration. When a suspension or gel-forming eye drop and a solution eye drop are used at the same time, the solution eye drop should be instilled first. After 5 minutes, the suspension or gel-forming eye drop can be administered. The suspension or gel-forming eye drop should be used last because it is formulated to stay in the eye for a longer period of time.

ALERT!

Dropper bottles containing ophthalmic suspension preparations must be rolled between the hands prior to administration in order to resuspend active ingredients that may settle with time. Rolling rather than vigorous shaking will prevent the formation of bubbles, which could interfere with proper administration.

SUMMARY

As the eye can have a variety of problems, it can also have a variety of treatments, including medications. Many treatment options exist for glaucoma, including beta-blockers and prostaglandin analogues. Eye allergy symptoms can be improved with antihistamines and mast cell stabilizers. Anti-infective ophthalmic options are many and include drugs that are also used in oral forms. Anti-inflammatory eye drops and corticosteroids help to decrease inflammation in the eye, especially after surgery. Other agents help to lubricate the dry eye or cause mydriasis to aid examinations. Care should be taken to protect the eyes from trauma and permanent vision loss.

ACKNOWLEDGMENT

The authors wish to acknowledge and thank Celtina K. Reinert, PharmD, author of this chapter in the first edition of this book.

REFERENCES

1. Glaucoma Research Foundation. https://www.glaucoma.org/. Accessed July 6, 2021.
2. Fiscella RG, Lesar TS, Owaidhah OA, Edward DP. Glaucoma. In: DiPiro JT, Yee GC, Posey L, et al., eds. *Pharmacotherapy: A Pathophysiologic Approach*. 11th edition. New York, NY: McGraw-Hill; 2020.
3. National Institutes of Health, National Library of Medicine. Medline Plus: Blindness and Vision Loss. http://www.nlm.nih.gov/medlineplus/ency/article/003040.htm. Accessed July 6, 2021.
4. Lexi-Drugs. Lexicomp® [database]. Hudson, OH: Wolters Kluwer. http://online.lexi.com. Accessed July 6, 2021.
5. National Institutes of Health, National Eye Institute. http://www.nei.nih.gov. Accessed April 7, 2022.

REVIEW QUESTIONS

1. What are the leading causes of blindness in the United States? Which are preventable and how?

2. List two classes of medication used as eye drops for the treatment of glaucoma.

3. Name two types of conjunctivitis. List a medication used in the treatment of each type and its mechanism of action.

4. How should patients who are using eye drops deal with contact lenses?

5. Discuss the dosage forms in which ophthalmic medications are available and the considerations for administration of each.

MEDICATION TABLES

MEDICATION TABLE 34-1. Glaucoma Agents[4],a,b

CLASS Generic Name (pronunciation)	Brand Name	Dose
Beta-Blockers		
Betaxolol (be TAX oh lol)	Betoptic-S	0.25% suspension: 1 drop in affected eye twice daily 0.5% solution: 1–2 drops in affected eye twice daily
Carteolol (KAR tee oh lole)	(Generics)	1% solution: 1 drop in affected eye twice daily
Levobunolol (lee voe BYOO noe lole)	(Generics)	0.25%: 1–2 drops in affected eye twice daily 0.5%: 1–2 drops in affected eye daily
Timolol (TYE moe lole)	Timoptic, Betimol	0.25%: 1 drop in affected eye twice daily, increase to 0.5% if needed to increase response, decrease to 1 drop daily if controlled Gel-forming solution 0.25%, 0.5%: 1 drop in affected eye daily
Glaucoma/Prostaglandin Analogues		
Bimatoprost (bi MA toe prost)	Lumigan	0.03% and 0.01%: 1 drop in affected eye every evening
Latanoprost (la TA noe prost)	Xalatan Xelpros	0.005% solution: 1 drop in affected eye every evening 0.005% emulsion: 1 drop in affected eye every evening
Latanoprostene Bunod (la tan oh PROS teen BU nod)[4]	Vyzulta	0.024% solution: 1 drop in affected eye(s) once daily in the evening
Tafluprost (TA floo prost)[4]	Zioptan	0.0015% solution (preservative free): 1 drop in affected eye(s) once daily in the evening
Travoprost (TRA voe prost)	Travatan Z	0.004% solution: 1 dose in affected eye every evening
Sympathomimetics		
Apraclonidine (a pra KLON i deen)	(Generics)	0.5% solution: 1–2 drops in affected eye 3 times daily, separated from other drops by at least 5 min; not commonly used for chronic therapy
Brimonidine (bri MOE ni deen)	Alphagan P	0.1%, 0.15%, 0.2% solution: 1 drop in affected eye 3 times daily, approximately 8 hr apart; may often be administered off label twice daily
Carbonic Anhydrase Inhibitors		
Brinzolamide (brin ZOE la mide)	Azopt	1% suspension: 1 drop in affected eye 3 times daily, separated from other drops by at least 10 min; often prescribed twice daily off label
Dorzolamide (dor ZOLE a mide)	Trusopt	2% solution: 1 drop in affected eye 3 times daily; often prescribed twice daily off label
Cholinergic		
Pilocarpine (pye loe KAR peen)	Isopto Carpine, generics Vuity	1%, 2%, 4%, solution: 1–2 drops in affected eye up to 4 times daily Dose 1 time daily 1.25%, solution: 1 drop daily for presbyopia

a All the agents listed in the table are prescription products.
b Except where otherwise referenced, Pronunciations have been adapted with permission from USP Dictionary of USAN and International Drug Names (USP Dictionary) © 2022.

MEDICATION TABLE 34-2. Treatment of Macular Degeneration[4,a,b]

CLASS Generic Name (pronunciation)	Brand Name	Dose
Intravitreal VEGF Inhibitors		
Aflibercept (a FLIB er sept)[4]	Eylea	2 mg (0.05 mL) once every 4 weeks (monthly) for the first 12 weeks (3 months), followed by 2 mg (0.05 mL) once every 8 weeks (every 2 months)
Brolucizumab (BROE lue SIZ ue mab)[4]	Beovu	6 mg (0.05 mL) once per month (approximately every 25–31 days) for 3 months, followed by 6 mg once every 8 to 12 weeks
Faricimab (far IK I mab)	Vabysmo	6 mg (0.05 mL every 4 weeks) for 4 doses, followed by 6 mg once every 8 to 16 weeks
Ranibizumab (ra ni BIZ oo mab)[4]	Lucentis	0.5 mg once a month (approximately every 28 days); frequency may be reduced (eg, 4–5 injections over 9 months) after the first 3 injections or may be reduced after the first 4 injections to once every 3 months if monthly injections are not feasible
Choroidal Vessel Occluder		
Verteporfin (ver te PORE fin)	Visudyne	Two-step process; first the infusion of verteporfin, then the activation of verteporfin with a nonthermal diode laser; not used commonly for wet AMD

[a] All the agents listed in the table are prescription products. AMD = age-related macular degeneration; VEGF = vascular endothelial growth factor.
[b] Except where otherwise referenced, Pronunciations have been adapted with permission from USP Dictionary of USAN and International Drug Names (USP Dictionary) © 2022.

MEDICATION TABLE 34-3. Conjunctivitis[4,a]

Class Generic Name (pronunciation)	Brand Name	Dose	Regulatory Status
Ophthalmic Antihistamines and/or Mast Cell Stabilizers			
Azelastine (a ZEL as teen)	(Generics)_	0.05%: 1 drop in affected eye twice daily	Rx
Epinastine (ep i NAS tine)	Various generics	0.05%: 1 drop in affected eye twice daily	Rx
Ketotifen (kee toe TYE fen)	Zaditor, Alaway, various others	0.025%: 1 drop in affected eye twice daily, separated by 8–12 hr	OTC
Olopatadine (oh la pat TA deen)	Pataday	0.1%: 1 drop in affected eye twice daily, separated by 6–8 hr 0.2% and 0.7%: 1 drop in affected eye daily	OTC
Ophthalmic Antihistamines/Decongestant Combo			
Pheniramine/naphazoline (fen NIR a meen) (Naf AZ oh leen)	Naphcon-A, Visine products Opcon-A	0.025%/0.3%: 1–2 drops in affected eye up to 4 times daily 0.027%/0.315%: 1 to 2 drops in affected eye(s) up to 4 times daily	OTC
Ophthalmic Mast Cell Stabilizers			
Bepotastine (bep oh TAS teen)	Bepreve	1.5%: 1 drop in affected eye twice daily	Rx
Cromolyn (KROE moe lin)	Various generics	4%: 1–2 drops in affected eye 4–6 times daily	Rx/OTC
Lodoxamide (loe DOX a mide)	Alomide	0.1%: 1–2 drops in affected eye 4 times daily	Rx
Nedocromil (ne doe KROE mil)	Alocril	2%: 1–2 drops in affected eye twice daily	Rx
Ophthalmic Decongestant			
Tetrahydrozoline (tet ra hye DROZ a leen)	Optigene 3, Visine Original	0.05%: 1–2 drops in affected eye 2–4 times daily	OTC
Anti-Infective Agents/Macrolides			
Azithromycin (az ith roe MYE sin)	AzaSite	1%: 1 drop in affected eye twice daily (separated by 8–12 hr) for 2 days, then 1 drop daily for 5 days	Rx
Erythromycin (er ith roe MYE sin)	(Generics)	5 mg/g ointment: apply 0.5-inch ribbon to affected eye 2–6 times/day	Rx

Continued next page

MEDICATION TABLE 34-3. Conjunctivitis[4,a] (Continued)

Class Generic Name (pronunciation)	Brand Name	Dose	Regulatory Status
Representative Anti-Infective Agents: Quinolones			
Besifloxacin (be si FLOX a sin)	Besivance	0.6%: 1 drop in affected eye 3 times daily for 7 days	Rx
Ciprofloxacin (sip roe FLOX a sin)	Ciloxan	0.3% solution: 1–2 drops in affected eye q 2 hr while awake for 2 days then 1–2 drops q 4 hr while awake for 5 days; please note different directions for treating bacterial conjunctivitis and bacterial keratitis 0.3% ointment: apply 0.5-inch ribbon to affected eye 3 times daily for 2 days then twice daily for 5 days	Rx
Gatifloxacin (gat i FLOX a sin)	Zymaxid	0.5%: 1 drop in affected eye q 2 hr while awake for 1 day (max 8 doses/day) then 1 drop in affected eye 2–4 times daily while awake on days 2–7	Rx
Levofloxacin (lee voe FLOX a sin)	(Generics)	0.5%: 1–2 drops in affected eye q 2 hr while awake (max 8 doses per day) for 2 days, then 1-2 drops q 4 hr while awake (max 4 doses/day) for 7 days total	Rx
Moxifloxacin (moxs i FLOX a sin)	Vigamox	Moxeza (0.5%): Instill 1 drop into affected eye(s) 2 times daily for 7 days Vigamox (0.5%): Instill 1 drop into affected eye(s) 3 times daily for 7 days	Rx
Ofloxacin (oh FLOX a sin)	Ocuflox	0.3%: 1–2 drops in affected eye q 2–4 hr while awake for 2 days, then 4 times daily for 5 days; please note different directions for treating bacterial conjunctivitis and corneal ulcer	Rx
Aminoglycosides			
Gentamicin (jen ta MYE sin)	Gentak	0.3% solution: 1–2 drops in affected eye q 4 hr, max 2 drops every hr 0.3% ointment: apply 0.5-inch ribbon to affected eye 2–3 times daily, using q 3–4 hr	Rx
Tobramycin (toe bra MYE sin)	Tobrex	0.3% solution: 1–2 drops in affected eye q 2–4 hr, max 2 drops every hr 0.3% ointment: apply 0.5-inch ribbon to affected eye 2–3 times daily, using q 3–4 hr	Rx
Sulfonamide			
Sulfacetamide sodium (sul fa SEE ta mide) (SOE dee um)	Bleph-10	10%: 1–2 drops in affected eye several times daily, up to q 2–3 hr for 7–10 days 10% ointment: Apply 0.5-inch ribbon into the conjunctival sac of affected eye(s) q 3–4 hr and at bedtime	Rx
Miscellaneous			
Bacitracin, polymixin B (bass i TRAY sin) (pol i MIX in)	Ak-Poly Bac, Polycin	500/10,000 units/g ointment: apply a thin strip to affected eye q 3–4 hr for 7–10 days	Rx
Bacitracin, neomycin, polymixin B (bass i TRAY sin) (nee oh MYE sin) (pol i MIX in)	Neo-Polycin	400/3.5/10,000 units/g ointment: apply 0.5-inch ribbon to affected eye q 3–4 hr for 7–10 days	Rx

Continued next page

MEDICATION TABLE 34-3. Conjunctivitis[4,a] *(Continued)*

Class Generic Name (pronunciation)	Brand Name	Dose	Regulatory Status
Bacitracin, neomycin, polymyxin B, hydrocortisone (bass i TRAY sin) (nee oh MYE sin) (pol i MIX in) (hye droe KOR' ti sone)	Neo-Polycin HC	400/3.5/10,000/10 units/g ointment: apply to inside of lower lid of affected eye(s) q 3 or 4 hr (depending on severity of condition)	Rx
Trimethoprim, polymyxin B (trye METH oh prim) (pol i MIX in)	Polytrim	1 mg/10,000 units/mL: 1 drop in affected eye q 3 hr (max 6 doses/day) for 7–10 days	Rx
Antifungal			
Natamycin (na ta MYE sin)	Natacyn	blepharitis/conjunctivitis: 1 drop in conjunctival sac 4 to 6 times daily keratitis: 1 drop in conjunctival sac every 1 to 2 hours x3–4 days, then 1 drop 6 to 8 times daily for total of 14–21 days	Rx
Antiviral			
Ganciclovir (gan SYE kloe veer)	Zirgan	Gel, ophthalmic, 0.15%: Apply in affected eye 5 times daily (approximately every 3 hours while awake) until corneal ulcer heals, then apply 1 drop 3 times daily for 7 days	Rx
Trifluridine (trye FLURE i deen)	Viroptic	1%: 1 drop in affected eye q 2 hr while awake (max 9 drops/day), until re-epithelialization of corneal ulcer occurs, then use 1 drop q 4 hr while awake for another 7 days; max 21 days of treatment	Rx

[a] Pronunciations have been adapted with permission from USP Dictionary of USAN and International Drug Names (USP Dictionary) © 2022.

MEDICATION TABLE 34-4. Agents for Ophthalmic Inflammation [a]

CLASS Generic Name (pronunciation)	Brand Name	Dose	Regulatory Status
Nonsteroidal Anti-Inflammatory Preparations			
Ketorolac (kee toe ROLE ak)	Acular, Acular LS, Acuvail	0.4%, 0.45%, 0.5%: 1 drop in affected eye 4 times daily	Rx
Nepafenac (ne paf FEN ak)	Nevanac	0.1%: 1 drop in affected eye 3 times daily starting 24 hr before surgery and continuing for 2 wk after surgery 0.3% solution: 1 drop to the affected eye once daily, starting 24 hours prior to surgery; the day of surgery, and continuing for 2 wk after surgery	Rx
Ophthalmic Corticosteroid			
Dexamethasone (dex a METH a sone)	Maxidex, various, many in combination with other agents (AK-Neo Dex, Maxitrol, Ciprodex, Tobradex)	0.1% solution: 1–2 drops in affected eye every hour while awake and q 2 hr during the night, gradually reduce dose to q 3–4 hr then 3–4 times daily	Rx
Difluprednate (dye floo PRED nate)	Durezol	0.05%: 1 drop in affected eye 4 times daily starting 24 hr after surgery, continuing 4 times daily for 2 wk then twice daily for 1 wk then taper off	Rx
Fluorometholone (flure oh METH oh lone)	FML, Flarex	0.1% ointment: apply 0.5-inch ribbon 1–3 times daily, may increase to q 4 hr in initial 24-48 hr 0.25%, 0.1% suspension: 1 drop in affected eye 2–4 times daily, may increase to q 4 hr in initial 24–48 hr	Rx
Loteprednol (loe te PRED nol)	Alrex, Lotemax	(Examples) Alrex 0.2% suspension: 1 drop in affected eye 4 times daily; indicated for allergic conjunctivitis Lotemax 0.5% suspension: 1–2 drops in affected eye 4 times daily, may increase to 1 drop every hour if needed for 1 wk Lotemax 0.5% gel, 0.5% suspension: Instill 1–2 drops into the conjunctival sac of the affected eye(s) 4 times daily beginning 24 hr after surgery and continuing throughout the first 2 wk of the postoperative period	Rx
Prednisolone (pred NISS oh lone)	Pred Forte, Pred Mild	0.12%, 1%: 1–2 drops in affected eye q 1 hr while awake and q 2 hr at night then decrease to 1 drop q 4–6 hr when response obtained	Rx
Anti-Inflammatory, Miscellaneous			
Cyclosporine (SYE kloe spor een)[4]	Restasis	0.05%, 0.1% emulsion: 1 drop in each eye q 12 hr, separate from other drops by 15 min	Rx
	Cequa	0.09% solution: 1 drop in each eye q 12 hr, separate from other drops by 15 min	Rx
Lifitegrast (lif i TEG rast)[4]	Xiidra	5%: 1 drop in each eye q 12 hr, separate from other drops by 15 min	Rx
Blepharospasm			
Onabotulinumtoxin A (o na BOTT you lye num tox in eh)	Botox	100 units: 1.25–2.5 units injected into muscles in upper and lower lid; max dose per site: 5 units, may repeat in 3 mo	Rx

[a] Except where otherwise referenced, Pronunciations have been adapted with permission from USP Dictionary of USAN and International Drug Names (USP Dictionary) © 2022.

MEDICATION TABLE 34-5. Miscellaneous Ophthalmic Preparations[4]

Indication	Generic Name (pronunciation)	Brand Name	Dosage Form	Dose	Regulatory Status
Ophthalmic Lubricants	"Artificial tears"	Various	Ophthalmic solution or ointment	Apply to or place 1–2 drops in affected eye 3–4 times daily as needed for eye dryness/irritation	OTC
	Carboxymethylcellulose (kar box ee meth ill SEL yoo lose)	Refresh, various	Ophthalmic solution	0.25%, 0.5%, 1%: 1–2 drops in affected eye 3–4 times daily	OTC
	Hydroxypropyl cellulose (hye drox ee PROE pil SEL yoo lose)	Lacrisert	Translucent rod ophthalmic insert	5 mg: insert in eye once daily	Rx
	Hydroxypropyl methylcellulose (hye drox ee PROE pil meth ill SEL yoo lose)	GenTeal, various	Ophthalmic solution or gel	0.2%, 0.3%, 0.4%, 0.5%, 2.5%: 1–2 drops in affected eye as needed	Rx/OTC
Cyloplegic Agents	Atropine (A troe peen)	Isopto Atropine	Ophthalmic solution	1%: 1 drop in the conjunctiva 40 min prior to intended maximal dilation time; may repeat up to twice daily as needed	Rx
	Cyclopentolate (sye kloe PEN toe late)	Cyclogyl	Ophthalmic solution	0.5%, 1%, 2%: 1–2 drops now and repeat in 5–10 min; higher concentrations may be needed in heavily pigmented irises	Rx
	Homatropine (hoe MA troe peen)	Homatropaire	Ophthalmic solution	5%: 1–2 drops before procedure, repeat q 5–10 min as needed	Rx

Chapter 35

Ear Medications

Allison R. King, PharmD, FASHP

KEY TERMS AND DEFINITIONS

Auditory—pertaining to hearing and the organs responsible for hearing.

Auricle—the outer portion of the ear; also known as the pinna.

Cerumen—earwax.

Equilibrium—a state of balance referring to the orientation of the body relative to gravity, allowing an individual to maintain coordination and position in space.

Eustachian tube—tube within the middle ear that connects to the pharynx or upper respiratory system.

Ototoxicity—damage to the hearing or balance functions of the ear by drugs or chemicals.

Tinnitus—ringing sound in the ears.

Tympanic membrane—eardrum.

LEARNING OBJECTIVES

After completing this chapter, you should be able to

1. Review the anatomy of the ear.

2. Describe various ear disorders, including signs and symptoms.

3. Identify medications used in the ear to treat cerumen buildup, water-clogged ears, contact dermatitis, and otitis media.

4. List medications that can cause ototoxicity.

5. Describe how to properly administer eardrops.

DOI 10.37573/9781585286638.035

Ear complaints are common and account for more than 1.5% of all doctor visits each year.[1] They can affect people of all ages, but occur more often in pediatric and geriatric patients. The ear is part of the auditory system (which is responsible for hearing and balance), equilibrium, and many communication skills. In order to understand patients' complaints, it is important to understand the anatomy of the ear.

CASE STUDY

A 60-year-old male comes into the pharmacy reporting gradual hearing loss over the past couple of weeks. He reports some pain in the ear that is preventing him from wearing his hearing aid earpiece and from talking on the phone. His ear is also red, swollen, and itchy. Mr. Green states that he has had this problem before and was able to fix it himself using a bobby pin to remove some earwax. He tried the bobby pin trick yesterday but was not successful.

ANATOMY OF THE EAR

The external ear is made up of the auricle, external auditory canal, and tympanic membrane. The auricle has a thin layer of skin, which covers cartilage, whereas the ear lobe has more fatty tissue. The external auditory canal is lubricated with cerumen. The job of the cerumen is to protect the middle ear from infections by trapping dust and other materials, and by providing a waxy, waterproof barrier to defend against pathogens. Cerumen has an acidic pH, which helps to prevent infections from developing. As cerumen collects debris, it is moved outward by jaw movements like talking and chewing. Cerumen darkens as it is exposed to air and may appear light gray, orange, or brown. Its consistency also varies and may be dry and flaky or oily and paste-like.

PRACTICE POINT

Not all earwax has to be removed. Excessive attempts to remove cerumen may damage the external auditory canal. Only cerumen that has moved to the outermost part of the external auditory canal should be removed.

CASE?

Is Mr. Green at risk for having a bacterial or fungal infection, and if so, why?

The external auditory canal is susceptible to collecting moisture, making it a great environment for bacteria and fungus to collect and grow. The defense system for the ear includes the skin, cerumen, acidic pH, and hairs, which line the outer part of the canal. A normal, healthy ear will not allow bacteria and fungus to grow. Breaking or scratching the skin of the auditory canal with objects like fingernails, cotton-tipped applicators (e.g., Q-tips®), or bobby pins creates a door for bacteria and fungus to enter. Ear piercing, sports injuries, and poorly fitted or poorly cleaned hearing aids can also impact the defense system of the ear. Finally, upper respiratory infections and viral infections can break down the defense system of the ear.

The external auditory canal is closed by the tympanic membrane or eardrum, which separates the external ear from the middle ear. This forms a blind cul-de-sac, which can collect moisture. In children, the external auditory canal is shorter, straighter, and flatter. The tympanic membrane is concave and oval, smooth, pearl gray in color, and clear (transparent). It acts as a barrier for the middle ear and is the part of the ear responsible for hearing by transmitting sound waves. When a sound is produced, the tympanic membrane vibrates, causing the three tiny bones (the malleus—*hammer*, stapes—*stirrup*, and incus—*anvil*) within the middle ear to vibrate. The vibration is then transferred to the cochlea, a channel of the inner ear, which is lined with tiny hairs that trigger nerve signals to the brain to register the sound.

PRACTICE POINT

The stapes is considered the smallest bone in the body.

The eustachian tube is also within the middle ear and connects to the pharynx or upper respiratory system. The eustachian tube helps equalize the pressure within the middle ear and allow fluid to drain from the middle ear. When patients experience a cold or viral infection in the nasal cavity, bacteria and viruses can travel through the eustachian tube and contribute to an infection within the ear. Additionally, the eustachian tube tissues can swell, trapping fluid in the middle ear, which can lead to a middle ear

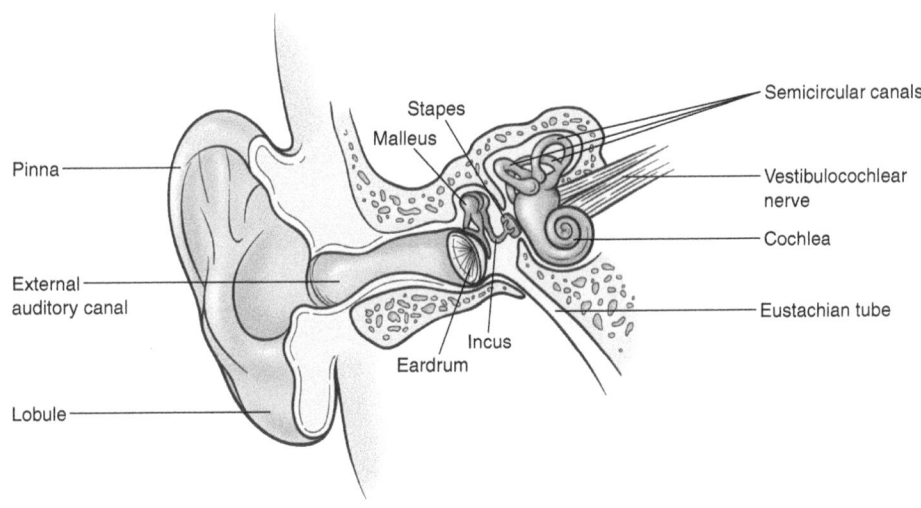

FIGURE 35-1. Anatomy of the ear.

infection. Children are more prone than adults to experience a middle ear infection because their eustachian tubes are shorter. The eustachian tube lengthens downward in adults, which helps to promote drainage.

The inner ear is made up of a series of fluid-filled tubes called the bony labyrinth. The bony labyrinth has three sections: the cochlea, vestibule, and semicircular canals. The cochlea helps with the hearing functions of the ear, is snail shaped, and is lined with tiny hairs (see Figure 35-1). The vestibule connects the cochlea to the semicircular canals and helps with the balance function of the ear. The semicircular canals also help with the balance functions of the ear. Finally, within the inner ear, the vestibulocochlear nerve (cranial nerve VIII) transmits hearing and balance information to the brain. Several conditions, including cerumen buildup, water-clogged ears, contact dermatitis, otitis media, and deafness can impact the hearing or balance functions of the ear or both. Medications can also contribute to hearing loss, both temporarily and permanently. Each condition is described in further detail below.

Cerumen Buildup

Excessive or impacted cerumen affects up to 10% of children, 5% of adults, and more than 30% of older (aged ≥65 years) adults. It is the most common cause of hearing loss at all ages. Narrow or oddly shaped external auditory canals, hearing aids or earplugs, and excessive hair growth in the ear canal make it difficult for people to cycle newly formed cerumen with the older debris-filled cerumen. Additionally, patients may have overactive ceruminous glands, causing excess cerumen production. In older adults, cerumen has less moisture, making it harder to remove. In these situations, the cerumen can become impacted, causing a problem for patients.

When there is excessive or impacted cerumen, patients will complain of fullness or pressure in the ear, possible hearing loss, dull pain or discomfort, dizziness, itching, and/or tinnitus. Efforts to remove the wax with cotton-tipped applicators, bobby pins, fingernails, toothpicks, etc., can actually force the wax further into the ear. Instead, a wet, wrung-out washcloth around a finger may be used to remove the excess cerumen. This method is ineffective once the cerumen is impacted.

The goal of treatment is to soften the cerumen so that it can be removed and prevent any adverse events. Removing the cerumen should correct temporary hearing loss and alleviate any pain the patient may be experiencing. Patients who show signs of infection, have an ear discharge, bleeding, ruptured tympanic membrane, recent ear surgery, tympanostomy tubes (to prevent middle ear fluid accumulation), or are under 12 years of age should be referred to a healthcare practitioner (HCP) first. If the washcloth method does not remove the cerumen buildup, the most effective treatment is often an ear drop like one listed in Medication Table 35-1 (Medication Tables are located at the end of the chapter). Carbamide peroxide 6.5% in anhydrous glycerin is the only nonprescription ear wax softening agent approved by the US Food and Drug Administration (FDA). Carbamide peroxide helps to break down and loosen the cerumen, while glycerin helps to soften the cerumen. This product is available over the counter (OTC) in a variety of brands and packages and is safe for use in adults and children 12 years of age and older. Carbamide drops should stay in the ear canal for several minutes (no longer than 15 minutes) and can be used twice daily for up to 4 days.[1] Common side effects include pain, rash, irritation, tenderness, redness, discharge, and dizziness. Patients developing side effects or whose problem does not resolve within 4 days should be referred to an HCP. Some patients may express a desire to use a rubber otic bulb syringe to remove any remaining cerumen. Specific earwax removal syringes are also widely available, with some claiming to be a safer alternative than a bulb ear syringe. Patients should use these products cautiously so that they insert the syringe tip correctly. Incorrect placement of the syringe tip may lead to otitis media, perforated tympanic membrane, vertigo, otitis media, or tinnitus.

Other treatment options are not recognized by the FDA as approved agents for the removal of earwax and should not be recommended over carbamide peroxide for self-treatment, but some are utilized or prescribed by HCPs when excess cerumen prompts an office visit.

Docusate is an emollient that can soften cerumen; however, it is more commonly used orally as a stool softener. It is more expensive than carbamide and is not available as an OTC product for earwax removal. Patients must cut open the gel cap and insert the liquid contents into the ear according to their HCP's directions. Glycerin, olive oil, and mineral oil are also emollients. They are commonly found in combination with other agents for excessive cerumen. Olive oil has also been used to treat itching and pain in the ear canal, but this is not recommended as self-treatment. Patients experiencing ear pain should be referred to their HCP. Either a 1:1 solution of hydrogen peroxide 3% and warm water or just plain hydrogen peroxide 3% is sometimes recommended or prescribed by HCPs to flush the ear canal to soften or remove excessive cerumen. Overuse of hydrogen peroxide may break down the tissue of the ear canal and lead to infection.

CASE?

Which product might the pharmacist recommend for Mr. Green, and how long should he use the product?

Ear candles are hollow candles made of a fabric tube soaked in beeswax or paraffin or a combination of both. One end is burned while the other is inserted into the ear canal. The FDA has warned patients not to use ear candles because they can cause serious injuries, including burns, broken eardrums, and blockage of the ear canal.[2] Yerba santa and chamomile are two natural products or folk remedies used to treat excessive cerumen. However, there is no published safety and efficacy information on these products. Thus, they are not recommended for use in self-treatment.

Various ear cleaning tools are also available OTC for patients to purchase. Examples include Ototek Loop and Clinere® ear cleaners. Both products are inserted into the outer ear and external auditory canal and bear the risk of injury to the ear canal or tympanic membrane.

Water-Clogged Ears

Water-clogged ears result from excessive moisture in the ear canal, which becomes trapped and cannot escape. Humid climates, sweating, bathing, or incorrect use of solutions to cleanse the ear can result in water-clogged ears. Cerumen can also swell, trapping water in the canal. Some patients are more prone to water-clogged ears because of the shape of their ear canals or excessive cerumen. Often, simple attempts like shaking the head in one direction are not enough to remove the water.

PRACTICE POINT

The use of cotton-tipped applicators on a daily basis after showering can cause abrasions and lead to infections in the ear and is not recommended. Patients should let their ears dry naturally or use a washcloth draped over a finger to dry out the ear.

CASE?

Mr. Green reports that he tried to flush his ear with warm water 1 week ago and was not successful. The next day, he said his ear started itching. Is Mr. Green likely to have water-clogged ears, and if so, what product might the pharmacist recommend?

Patients sometimes complain of a sense of wetness or fullness in the ear and possibly, hearing loss. They may also report pain and itching in the ear canal. The goals of treatment are to remove the water and to prevent recurrences. If patients show signs of infection, ear discharge, bleeding, ruptured tympanic membrane, or have had recent ear surgery, tympanostomy tubes, or are under 12 years of age, they should automatically be referred to their HCP. All patients should also be referred to their HCP prior to any treatment to ensure that their tympanic membrane is not ruptured or a tympanostomy tube is not in place.

Patients wishing to try self-treatment after seeing their HCP should be directed by the pharmacist to tilt the affected ear downward and manipulate the auricle to help remove the excessive water. This can also be done after swimming and bathing to prevent water-clogged ears. A blow dryer may also be used to help dry the ear but should be on the lowest setting and pointed away from the ear. Otherwise, the only FDA-approved treatment is isopropyl alcohol 95% in anhydrous glycerin 5%. Alcohol mixes well with water and acts as a drying agent. Glycerin helps to coat the canal to aid in removal of the water and prevents over-drying from the alcohol. Various OTC products, listed in Medication Table 35-2, containing alcohol, acetic acid, or glycerin are available. A home remedy of 50:50 mixture of household white vinegar and isopropyl alcohol 95% creates an acetic acid solution that has also been used to help dry water-clogged ears, but presents a risk of over-drying the ear.

> ### ALERT!
>
> It is important that patients considering the use of home remedies be warned to use white vinegar and not cider or wine vinegar. Cider and wine vinegars are produced from fruit and contain impurities that could promote bacterial growth.

Patients may also try to prevent water-clogged ears. Options include the use of ear plugs or bathing caps. AquaEars, BioEars, and ClearEars are products that either protect the ears from exposure to water or are intended to absorb water that enters the ear. Lastly, patients may use "waterproofed" cotton balls prior to water exposure to block the ear canal. Cotton balls are "waterproofed" using petroleum jelly.

Water-clogged ears are a separate issue from swimmer's ear. Swimmer's ear is an infection of the outer ear (external otitis), which develops from swimming in polluted water. Although it results from water becoming trapped, as in water-clogged ears, in swimmer's ear, the tissue of the ear begins to break down and eventually leads to an outer ear infection. Prescription medications used to treat external otitis include corticosteroid and antibiotic ear drops. Corticosteroid drops decrease inflammation and help to relieve any pain or itching. Antibiotic drops treat bacterial infection present in the ear. Treatments for otitis are detailed in Medication Table 35-3.

> ### ALERT!
>
> There are no FDA-approved OTC medications for preventing or treating swimmer's ear. In the past, manufacturers may have stated that removing the excess water would prevent breakdown of the ear tissue; however, the FDA no longer allows manufacturers to make statements that their products can prevent swimmer's ear.

Contact Dermatitis

Contact dermatitis or allergic reactions of the external ear can be associated with topical antibacterial ointments, nickel in earrings, poison ivy, and chemicals used to clean hearing aid ear molds. Allergic reactions in the ear are not usually caused by soaps or detergents, which require extended contact to produce an allergic reaction. Most patients will present with itching and redness in the ear. The itching may be so severe that patients will want to stick things in their ears to relieve the pain. Burow's solution (1:40 aluminum acetate) is used to treat contact dermatitis of the ear. It is applied as a wick inserted into the ear canal, kept moist for 24 hours, and then removed.

> ### ALERT!
>
> Eye drops can be used in the ear but ear drops cannot be used in the eye. The tissue in the eye is more sensitive than the ear. Thus, eye drops are gentler than ear drops. The Institute for Safe Medication Practices (ISMP) recommends to "double-check the label on the product—if it says otic, it's for the ear, and if it says ophthalmic, it's for the eye."[3]

Otitis Media

Otitis media is inflammation of the middle ear and is very common in children, especially between the ages of 6 and 18 months. It is the most common reason antibiotic prescriptions are written for children. Otitis media occurs more frequently in the winter months and usually presents after an infection in the nose. An infection of the nasal passageways can result in pressure and buildup into the eustachian tubes, causing them to swell. Swelling of the eustachian tubes can trap bacteria, leading to otitis media. Children have shorter and more horizontal eustachian tubes than adults, making it more difficult for fluid to drain out. Risk factors for otitis media include age less than 2 years, viral respiratory tract infection and the winter season, daycare attendance, young age at first diagnosis, siblings, tobacco smoke exposure, anatomic defects such as cleft palate, pacifier use, lack of breastfeeding, immunodeficiency, and gastroesophageal reflux.

Patients with otitis media will present with fever, ear pain, irritability, ear fullness, and possibly even tugging at the ear and hearing loss. Patients may also report poor sleep, lack of appetite, vomiting, and diarrhea. The goals of treatment are to eliminate the pain and infection in the ear, prevent future infections, and minimize antibiotic use.

Treatment is oral (not locally applied in the ear), usually with high-dose amoxicillin for 10 days. Other drugs given include amoxicillin-clavulanate (Augmentin), cefuroxime, cefpodoxime, and cefdinir. These antibiotics are discussed in detail in Chapter 27. For infections with a fever or for pain control, acetaminophen (Tylenol) and ibuprofen (Advil) can be given to help lower the fever and relieve any pain. Topical anesthetic agents such as benzocaine may also be given, especially in older children. Patients should expect to see an improvement within 72 hours of therapy; however, symptoms may seem worse during the first 24 hours of antibiotics. Some patients may benefit from the application of heat or cold agents, such as a washcloth soaked in very warm water, wrung out, and placed on the external ear for 15 minutes. Finally, in children with recurrent infections, tympanostomy tubes may be placed in the ear. The tubes help to extend the eustachian tubes and promote drainage.

Deafness

Hearing impairment or deafness is a condition in which an individual cannot hear things that other people can hear. Hearing impairment is categorized by the type (conductive, sensorineural, or both), severity, and age of onset. Conductive hearing impairment results from dysfunction in the outer ear, tympanic membrane, or bones of the middle ear, whereas sensorineural hearing impairment results from dysfunction in the inner ear. Most sensorineural impairment result from abnormalities in the hair cells in the cochlea. The severity of hearing impairment is classified by how loud a sound must be before it is detected and can be mild, moderate, severe, or profound.

Major causes of hearing loss include noise, genetic factors, disease, medications, exposure to ototoxic chemicals, and trauma. Noise-induced hearing loss typically affects higher and lower frequencies. Common causes include car stereos, transportation (e.g., airports or freeways), lawn maintenance equipment, gun use, and power tools. The degree of severity depends upon the length of time exposed and the loudness of the sound. Diseases that can result in hearing loss or damage include measles, meningitis, mumps, HIV, AIDS, and otosclerosis, hardening of the stapes (one of the tiniest bones within the inner ear).

Infants born of mothers with chlamydia or syphilis, born prematurely, or born with fetal alcohol syndrome may also experience hearing loss. In addition to medications that cause hearing loss, which are described below, exposure to heavy metals (eg, lead, mercury), solvents (eg, toluene), asphyxiants (eg, carbon monoxide), and pesticides can lead to hearing loss. Often, ototoxic chemical exposure is coupled with noise-induced hearing loss.

Treatment for hearing loss can include the use of sign language, hearing aids, and cochlear implants. Additionally, individuals must also make lifestyle adaptations, such as telecommunications relay services, hearing dogs, and special light devices.

Medications That Cause Ototoxicity

Many drugs can cause ototoxicity or damage to the hearing or balance functions of the ear. The degree of toxicity depends on several factors, including the drug, dose, and location of the damage. Damage can occur in the cochlear and vestibular parts of the inner ear. Cochlear damage will present as hearing loss, whereas with vestibular damage, patients may have hearing loss but also difficulty walking, especially in the dark, and oscillopsia, a sensation that objects are moving or bouncing, seen especially when walking. Patients may experience a full recovery after the drug causing the ototoxicity is stopped but not always. In other cases, the damage may be limited or too small to be noticed. For example, a patient may have high-frequency hearing loss. In extreme situations, the ototoxicity may be permanent.

Medications that cause or contribute to ototoxicity include aminoglycosides (streptomycin, neomycin, kanamycin, amikacin, gentamicin, tobramycin, vancomycin), platinum chemotherapeutic agents (cisplatin, carboplatin), loop diuretics (ethacrynic acid, furosemide), salicylate analgesics

CASE?

Mr. Green's primary care provider would like to start him on furosemide 20 mg daily for his high blood pressure in addition to lisinopril. What, if anything, should be done before he starts the new medication and during the time he receives the new medication?

(aspirin), and quinine. Cancer chemotherapy drugs, especially those containing platinum, can cause tinnitus and hearing loss, which can present immediately or up to several months after finishing treatment. Typically, the hearing loss with platinum chemotherapeutic drugs affects both ears and is permanent. Loop diuretics (such as furosemide) are more likely to cause permanent hearing loss in patients with decreased kidney function and those receiving aminoglycosides. Aspirin in high doses (more than twelve 325-mg tablets daily) can cause tinnitus and temporary hearing loss. Finally, quinine can cause temporary hearing loss. If possible, ototoxic drugs should be avoided in pregnancy, older adults, and individuals with existing hearing loss. If an ototoxic drug must be used, the lowest effective dose should be given and levels should be closely monitored.

Proper Method of Administering Eardrops

To properly administer eardrops, the head should be tilted toward the opposite shoulder. The auricle should be pulled so that the canal is open and visible. Drops should be administered into the canal with the dropper as far into the canal as possible without touching the canal. Patients should lie on their sides for 20 minutes or place a cotton ball blocking the ear canal to maximize drug exposure.[4]

ALERT!

If the dropper for ear drops touches the ear canal, it can become contaminated and allow the patient to get reinfected every time the solution is administered.

SUMMARY

Ear complaints are common, and patients need to understand how easily the external auditory canal can be injured. Patients should be reminded not to use external objects to remove excessive cerumen or water, or alleviate itching. If patient symptoms worsen after 4 days, the patient should be referred to a healthcare provider.

REFERENCES

1. Bandy V. Otic disorders. In: Krinsky DL, Ferreri SP, Hemstreet B, et al., eds. *Handbook of Nonprescription Drugs: An Interactive Approach to Self-Care.* 19th ed. Washington, DC: American Pharmacists Association; 2017:591-606.

2. Don't get burned: Stay away from ear candles. https://www.fda.gov/consumers/consumer-updates/dont-get-burned-stay-away-ear-candles. Accessed January 16, 2020.3. Institute for Safe Medication Practices. "And the 'EYES' have it": Eardrops, that is . . . https://www.ismp.org/resources/and-eyes-have-it-eardrops. Accessed January 16, 2020.

3. "And the 'EYES' Have It": Eardrops, That Is . . . Institute for Safe Medication Practices. Available at https://www.ismp.org/resources/and-eyes-have-it-eardrops. Accessed January 16, 2020.

4. Condren M, Haase MR. Acute otitis media. In: Koda-Kimble MA, Alldredge BK, Corelli RL, et al., eds. *Applied Therapeutics.* 10th ed. Philadelphia, PA: Lippincott Williams & Wilkins; 2013:2304-2306.

5. Lexi-Drugs [database]. Hudson, OH: Wolters Kluwer. Accessed January 27, 2020.

6. AHFS Clinical Drug Information [database]. Bethesda, MD: American Society of Health-System Pharmacists. Accessed March 19, 2020.

CHAPTER RESOURCES

American Society for Deaf Children. http://www.deafchildren.org.

National Association for the Deaf. http://www.nad.org.

REVIEW QUESTIONS

1. What are the functions of the ear and the auditory system?

2. Describe how a sound is transmitted from the ear to the brain.

3. Describe how cerumen is moved out of the ear.

4. What is the most common cause of hearing loss?

5. Which age group is more prone to middle ear infections? Why?

MEDICATION TABLES

TABLE 35-1. Preparations to Clear Excess Cerumen[5,6]

Brand Name	Ingredients	Directions[a,b]	Regulatory Status
Cerumen Buildup			
Auraphene-B, Debrox, various others	Carbamide peroxide 6.5%; anhydrous glycerin	Instill 5–10 drops twice daily for up to 4 days	OTC
NeilMed ClearCanal Earwax Removal System	ClearCanal Carbamide Peroxide Drops: carbamide peroxide 6.5%, glycerin ClearCanal Saline Spray: water, sodium chloride, sodium bicarbonate	Instill 10 drops of Canal Carbamide Peroxide softener as a pretreatment prior to rinsing or as earwax softening drops; maximum use: twice in a week	OTC
Similasan Ear Wax Relief, homeopathic ear drops	Causlicum HPUS 12X, Graphites HPUS 15X, Lachesis HPUS 12X, Lycopodium HPUS 12X, vegetable glycerin	Instill 2–3 drops twice daily for up to 3 days	OTC

[a]All directions based on dosing in affected ear, unless both ears are affected.
[b]All directions for ages 12 and older. For children under 12 years, consult with a healthcare practitioner.

TABLE 35-2. Preparations for Water-Clogged Ears and Earache Relief[5,6]

Brand Name	Ingredients	Directions[a,b]	Regulatory Status
Auro-Dri, Debrox Swimmer's Ear, Swim Ear, many others	Isopropyl alcohol, glycerin	Instill 4 or 5 drops in affected ear	OTC
Similasan Earache Relief Drops	Chamomilla 10X, mercurius solubilis 15X, sulfur 12X	Instill 4–5 drops up to 4 times daily for no more than 2 days	OTC
Highlands Earache Drops	Pulsatilla 30C HPUS, chamomilla 30C HPUS, sulfur 30C HPUS, calcium carbonate 30C HPUS, belladona 30C HPUS, Lycopodium clavatum 30C HPUS	Instill 3–4 drops up to 4 times daily or as needed for ear pain and itching associated with cold and flu and water-clogged ears; recommended for all ages	OTC

[a]All directions based on dosing in affected ear, unless both ears are affected.
[b]All directions for ages 12 and older. For children under 12, consult with a healthcare practitioner.

TABLE 35-3. Preparations for Otitis and Contact Dermatitis[5,6]

Brand Name	Ingredients	Directions[a]	Regulatory Status
External Otitis			
Various generics	Polymyxin B, neomycin, hydrocortisone	Adults 4 drops in affected ear(s) 3 to 4 times daily Pediatric (Limited data in patients < 2 years of age) 3 drops in affected ear(s) 3 to 4 times daily	Rx
Cortisporin-TC	Colistin, neomycin, hydrocortisone, thonzonium	Pediatric (>1 year) • Calibrated dropper: 4 drops 3–4 times daily or • Dropper bottle: 3 drops 3–4 times daily Adult • Calibrated dropper: 5 drops 3–4 times daily or • Dropper bottle: 4 drops 3–4 times daily • Alternatively, a cotton wick saturated with suspension inserted in ear canal every 4 hours; and replaced at least every 24 hours	Rx
Cipro HC Otic (ear)	Ciprofloxacin, hydrocortisone	3 drops twice daily for 7 days For patients ≥ 1 years of age	Rx
Ciprodex (ear)	Ciprofloxacin, dexamethasone	4 drops twice daily for 7 days For patients ≥ 6 months of age	Rx
Otovel (ear)[b]	Ciprofloxacin, fluocinolone	0.25 mL twice daily for 7 days	Rx
Floxin Otic (ear)	Ofloxacin	• Children 6 months to 13 years: 5 drops (or the contents of one single-dose container) once daily for 7 days • >13 years: 10 drops (or the contents of two single-dose containers) once daily for 7 days	Rx
Contact Dermatitis			
Acetasol HC	Acetic acid, propylene glycol, hydrocortisone	Insert saturated wick; keep moist for 24 hours; instill 4–6 drops every 2–3 hours For patients ≥ 3 years of age	OTC

[a] All directions based on dosing in affected ear, unless both ears are affected.
[b] For patients with tympanostomy tubes ≥6 months.

Chapter 36

Mouth, Throat, and Nose Medications

Jamie L. Woodyard, PharmD, BCACP |
Kelly L. Scolaro, PharmD

KEY TERMS AND DEFINITIONS

Anesthetic—medication that reduces pain by numbing the area to which it is applied.

Antihistamine—medication that blocks the histamine receptor to stop allergic reactions and can help dry up nasal secretions.

Antitussive—medication that helps stop coughing.

Decongestant—medication that decreases nasal congestion by causing vasoconstriction.

Expectorant—medication that thins mucus secretions and allows for their removal, usually by coughing.

Larynx—the voice box, connecting the throat to the trachea.

Pharynx—the part of the throat located at the back of the mouth that leads downward toward the esophagus and trachea.

Rhinitis—inflammation or irritation of the nasal tissues, usually causing a runny nose.

Thrush—fungal infection that usually starts as a white, creamy lesion on the inner membranes of the cheeks.

Troche—drug delivery system, which allows for absorption in the mucous membranes of the mouth, usually held between the cheek and gum until dissolved.

DOI 10.37573/9781585286638.036

LEARNING OBJECTIVES

After completing this chapter, you should be able to

1. Describe oral and upper respiratory system anatomy and physiology.

2. Discuss common conditions of the oral cavity and upper respiratory tract.

3. Identify medications used to treat oral conditions, including sore throat.

4. Identify medications used to treat upper respiratory system conditions, including colds, influenza, and allergies.

MOUTH AND THROAT STRUCTURE AND FUNCTION (ANATOMY AND PHYSIOLOGY)

The mouth, or oral cavity, is comprised of the lips, teeth, gingivae (gums), and tongue and is bound by the inner cheek, palate (roof of mouth), and mouth floor.[1] As the entry to the gastrointestinal (GI) tract, the mouth aids in starting the digestive process through salivation and propulsion of food and drink. The pharynx (throat), which is located at the back of the mouth, also propels food into the esophagus. The throat connects the mouth to the upper respiratory system, and both the mouth and throat play a critical role in speech production. The larynx, or voice box, also plays an important role in the production of sound and is located just below the pharynx. Because the mouth and throat are exposed to external influences such as air and food, they are susceptible to many different types of injuries and conditions.

CASE STUDY

Mr. Harrison, a 62-year-old male, calls your pharmacy and complains of sore teeth and bleeding gums. Mr. Harrison has not seen a dentist in several years and states he brushes his teeth every morning. The pain started gradually several months ago, and his gums bleed when he brushes his teeth vigorously. He wants a recommendation to help stop the bleeding and pain.

COMMON CONDITIONS OF THE MOUTH AND THROAT

Cold Sores

Fever blisters, or cold sores, are lesions on the lips or oral mucous membranes caused by the herpes simplex virus type 1 (HSV-1).[2] The sores contain a group of small, fluid-filled blisters that eventually burst, leaving an open sore that oozes and then crusts over. Cold sores are commonly present at the border of the lips and are associated with pain, redness, and discomfort. Additional symptoms include burning, itching, and tingling, which may be felt one day before the visible formation of a lesion. It is estimated that the majority of the population has HSV-1, which is a lifelong infection. The virus typically spreads from person to person through oral secretions containing the virus shared during intimate, though not necessarily sexual, contact. Cold sores are contagious even if the sore cannot be seen and typically heal on their own in two to four weeks. Because the virus never leaves the body, lesions may reappear at varying frequencies.

Canker Sores

Aphthous ulcers, or canker sores, are small lesions inside the mouth.[2] The round or oval sores are covered by a yellow-gray substance, surrounded by a red rim, and most commonly develop on the inner lips and cheek. Patients may have one or multiple canker sores and may develop the lesions frequently or infrequently. The primary symptom associated with canker sores is pain, which may make it difficult to talk and eat. The exact cause of canker sores is unknown and likely multifactorial. Canker sores typically heal on their own within one to two weeks.

Thrush

Thrush is a fungal infection on the mucous membranes in the mouth caused by *Candida albicans*.[2] It appears as creamy white lesions, which can bleed if rubbed and may be painful. Thrush usually starts on the inside of the cheeks or tongue. If untreated, it can spread to the roof of the mouth, throat, and esophagus. Thrush can occur in anyone but is most common in infants, people with dentures, patients using inhaled corticosteroids like inhalers for asthma, or people with weakened immune systems, including those undergoing cancer chemotherapy.

Dry Mouth

Xerostomia, or dry mouth, occurs when a patient's salivary glands do not create enough saliva to keep the mouth moisturized.[2] Hundreds of medications, including some antihistamines discussed later in this chapter and many other over-the-counter (OTC) medications, cause dry mouth as a side effect. Other causes of dry mouth include breathing with an open mouth, snoring, aging, health conditions such as diabetes, radiation treatment or nerve damage to the head or neck, dehydration, and use of tobacco, alcohol, and illegal drugs. In addition to experiencing discomfort, patients with dry mouth may have bad breath and difficulty chewing, swallowing, and speaking. Dry mouth can also lead to tooth decay, gingivitis, and infections such as thrush.

Gingivitis

Gingivitis is the inflammation of the soft, pink gum tissue surrounding each tooth. Gingivitis can cause gum redness, bleeding, swelling, oozing, recession, and discomfort. The most common cause of gingivitis is the buildup of plaque, or bacteria and sugars that adhere to the teeth. If not removed, plaque can harden and turn into tartar, which further promotes an environment in which the bacteria can continue to live. Inadequate oral hygiene leads to this plaque hardening, tartar deposits, and gingivitis. Therefore, proper oral hygiene is recommended to prevent and treat gingivitis. This consists of daily brushing and flossing to remove plaque from the teeth. In addition, professional dental examinations and cleanings are recommended every 6 to 12 months. If untreated, gingivitis can progress to affect other areas supporting the teeth.

CASE?

What do you think is the cause of Mr. Harrison's pain? What has he done (or not done) to contribute to this?

PRACTICE POINT

Good oral hygiene includes regular tooth-brushing, flossing, and routine professional cleanings.

Toothache

A toothache is pain or inflammation in or around a tooth. The primary cause of toothaches is tooth decay, or cavities.[2] A cavity occurs when bacteria in plaque produce an acid that eats through the protective enamel coating on a tooth.[2] Patients may first experience pain from a cavity when eating or drinking something hot or cold. Other causes of toothaches include infection at the root of the tooth or gums, fracture or trauma to a tooth, or teeth breaking through the gums as occurs in teething or the appearance of wisdom teeth.

Sore Throat

Pharyngitis, or sore throat, is inflammation of the pharynx. A sore throat is most commonly caused by a viral infection (see Table 36-1). Other causes include bacterial infection, vocal cord nodules, gastroesophageal reflux disease (GERD), allergies, dry indoor air, environmental irritants like tobacco

TABLE 36-1. Differentiating Respiratory Conditions

Condition	Signs and Symptoms
Allergic rhinitis	Watery eyes; itchy nose, eyes, or throat; repetitive sneezing; nasal congestion; watery rhinorrhea; red, irritated eyes
Asthma	Cough, shortness of breath, wheezing
Bacterial throat infection	Sore throat (moderate to severe pain), fever,* whitish, yellow, or green fluid around tonsils, painful lymph nodes in the neck
Colds	Sore throat (mild to moderate pain), nasal congestion, runny nose, sneezing
Croup	Fever,* rhinitis, and sore throat initially, progressing to cough (may be "barking" cough), high-pitched wheezing, and shortness of breath

Continued next page

TABLE 36-1. Differentiating Respiratory Conditions *(Continued)*

Condition	Signs and Symptoms
COVID-19	Fever,* muscle and joint aches, sore throat, cough, shortness of breath or difficulty breathing, loss of taste or smell, nausea, vomiting, or diarrhea
Influenza	Muscle and joint aches, fever,* sore throat, nonproductive cough, moderate to severe fatigue
Otitis media	Ear popping, fullness, pain, or discharge, hearing loss, dizziness
Pneumonia or bronchitis	Chest tightness, wheezing, shortness of breath, productive cough, changes in sputum color, persistent fever*
Sinusitis	Tenderness over the sinuses, facial pain aggravated by bending down, fever,* tooth pain, halitosis; poor response to decongestants after 7 days
West Nile virus infection	Fever,* headache, fatigue, rash, swollen lymph glands, and eye pain initially, possibly progressing to gastrointestinal distress, central nervous system changes, seizures, or paralysis
Whooping cough	Initial phase (runny nose, mild cough, sneezing) of 1–2 weeks, followed by 1–6 weeks of paroxysmal coughing

* Fever = oral temperature ≥100.4°F (38°C)

smoke, and, rarely, head and neck cancers. Symptoms include pain and/or a scratchy sensation in the throat that often worsens with swallowing or talking. Patients may also experience difficulty swallowing, neck pain or swelling, and hoarseness, which describes a voice that sounds dry, raspy, strained, or has a higher or lower pitch than normal. Hoarseness related to sore throat is due to inflammation of the larynx. The duration of sore throat symptoms depends on the cause. Viral pharyngitis typically resolves within one week and does not require medical treatment. Bacterial pharyngitis, which is most commonly caused by *Streptococcus* bacteria, should be treated with appropriate antibiotic therapy (discussed in Chapter 27).

MEDICATIONS USED FOR COMMON MOUTH AND THROAT CONDITIONS

A variety of medications and formulations are available to treat conditions of the mouth and throat.[3] These are summarized in Medication Table 36-1 (Medication Tables are located at the end of the chapter).

CASE STUDY

Mrs. Swanson, a 35-year-old female, is at the pharmacy asking for advice on what medication to use to help soothe her sore throat. She states the pain just started this morning and is getting worse. She says it hurts when she swallows but she does not have a fever or any other symptoms.

Topical Antivirals

Docosanol and acyclovir are antiviral medications used to treat cold sores by preventing HSV-1 entry and replication within cells. Both medications are available in creams that are applied to the cold sore five times per day. For these to be most effective, they should be started at the first sign of a cold sore (tingling, redness, itching). Patients should wash hands before and after application. Cosmetics should be removed and the area cleaned prior to application. When applying, the cream should be rubbed in gently and completely. Both creams are for external use only and should not be applied directly inside the mouth. Side effects may include drying of the lips or skin, burning, and/or itching.

ALERT!

To prevent the spread of infection, it is important that topical cold sore medications are not shared with others.

Topical Antifungals

Nystatin suspension (liquid) is a prescription antifungal used to treat thrush and other fungal infections of the mouth in infants and adults. All formulations of nystatin, including creams, ointments, powder, tablets, and capsules work to kill fungi by attacking cell membranes, but only nystatin suspension is used for fungal infections of the mouth. Prior to use, it is important to shake the nystatin suspension well.

It is to be swished around the mouth and held in the mouth for several minutes, or as long as possible, and then swallowed. Treatment should be administered four times a day. With infants or children, half the dose is applied to each side of the mouth using a cotton-tipped applicator or dropper. Because nystatin suspension is poorly absorbed into the body, it can be used to treat infections of the intestine and may cause side effects of nausea, stomach pain, vomiting, or diarrhea.

Clotrimazole is another antifungal medication that works like nystatin to prevent or treat thrush. Clotrimazole is available as a lozenge or troche. To treat thrush, the troche is dissolved slowly in the mouth five times a day, typically for 2 weeks. It takes approximately 30 minutes for the troche to dissolve. This slow dissolution is important to make the medication most effective, so patients should not bite or chew the medication troche. One side effect patients may experience is numbness or tingling in the mouth.

Saliva Substitutes

Saliva substitute products are available OTC to temporarily relieve dryness and discomfort associated with dry mouth. These medications are also referred to as artificial saliva and work by moistening the mouth. Many brands and formulations, such as sprays, gels, rinses, and lozenges are available. Saliva substitutes are used as needed and some products may safely be used as frequently as every hour. Patients should avoid food and drink for 15 minutes after using saliva substitutes to make the effects of these medications last longer.

Topical Antibacterials

Chlorhexidine gluconate is a prescription antibacterial mouth rinse used to prevent and treat gingivitis and mouth infections. Chlorhexidine works by slowing the growth of and killing bacteria. Patients using chlorhexidine should first brush and floss normally twice daily. After toothpaste is completely rinsed from the mouth, patients should swish 15 mL (one tablespoon) chlorhexidine for 30 seconds and then spit it out. The cap on the bottle can be used to measure 15 mL. After chlorhexidine use, patients should avoid immediately eating or rinsing with water or other mouthwashes. They should also avoid eating for two to three hours after using. While patients may experience taste alteration or staining of surfaces within the mouth, these side effects are rare.

Hydrogen peroxide–based products provide weak antibacterial effects and can be used to help cleanse areas of minor inflammation, including canker sores. Hydrogen peroxide is available OTC as a gel or solution. Carbamide peroxide, which releases hydrogen peroxide, is also available OTC as a solution. Both hydrogen peroxide and carbamide peroxide are applied to the affected area up to four times daily after meals and at bedtime. After applying the gel or a few drops of the solution, patients should wait two to three minutes and then spit out. Carbamide peroxide and the hydrogen peroxide solution can also be used as mouth rinses, in which case patients should swish the solution for at least one minute prior to spitting out.

ALERT!

While the majority of rinses used to treat mouth conditions should be spit out, there are exceptions to this. It is important patients follow instructions closely for information on how much to apply and whether to spit out or swallow the rinse.

CASE?

What formulation (liquid, lozenge, spray, etc.) might the pharmacist suggest to Mrs. Swanson to use to treat her sore throat? How often should she use it?

Topical Anesthetics

Benzocaine, lidocaine, and phenol are common topical anesthetic medications used to ease pain that accompanies a mouth sore, toothache, or sore throat. These medications numb the area to which they are applied and work by blocking the pain signal as it travels along nerve paths. While these medications do not treat the underlying cause of mouth conditions such as infection or cleanse the area like hydrogen peroxide–containing preparations, they decrease mouth pain and thus discomfort. A variety of formulations, including lozenges, sprays, gels, and solutions, are available (summarized in Medication Table 36-1).

Benzocaine is the most commonly used topical anesthetic, and it is available OTC. Benzocaine gel, liquid, ointment, or spray is applied to the affected area up to four times daily. Phenol is another anesthetic that is available OTC. It is available as lozenges and a solution that can be gargled or sprayed onto the back of the throat. All phenol preparations are used every 2 hours as needed. Lidocaine for oral use is a viscous solution available only with a prescription. Fifteen mL of lidocaine is swished in the mouth and spit out if used to numb pain within the mouth. If used for a sore throat, 15 mL is gargled and swallowed. In either case, lidocaine should not be used more frequently than every 3 hours. Side effects of topical anesthetic use include localized burning, tingling, and itching. While these medications work quickly, generally within seconds, the numbing effect may wear off quickly. Avoiding food or drink for one hour after use can prolong the effect of topical anesthetics.

PRACTICE POINT

Lozenges should be slowly dissolved in the mouth rather than being chewed.

ALERT!

Use of anesthetics should be minimized. Overuse can cause methemoglobinemia, a dangerous condition that impairs oxygen transportation by the blood. Anesthetics should be avoided children under the age of 2 years due to an increased risk of methemoglobinemia in this population.

Oral Analgesics

Analgesic pain relievers such as acetaminophen and anti-inflammatory medications like ibuprofen or naproxen can be taken to reduce pain associated with mouth and throat conditions. These medications are taken by mouth (not applied topically) and were discussed in Chapter 13. In addition to contributing to patient comfort, some of these medications decrease inflammation associated with a sore throat or other mouth conditions.

UPPER RESPIRATORY STRUCTURE AND FUNCTION (ANATOMY AND PHYSIOLOGY)

As discussed in Chapter 18, the upper respiratory system consists of the pharynx, nasopharynx, trachea, nose, and sinuses. The nose acts as a filter for the lungs as it warms, moisturizes, and cleans the air headed to the lungs. The sinuses are hollow areas of the skull that are filled with air. There are four pairs of sinuses: two pairs in the nose, one across the cheeks, and another behind the eyebrows. They help the voice to resonate, reduce the weight of the skull, and insulate the brain. The upper respiratory system is lined with a mucous membrane that secretes mucus. Excess mucus may result in congestion of the nose, sinus pain or pressure, rhinorrhea (a runny nose), or postnasal drip where mucus runs down the back of the throat. Postnasal drip can also cause a sore throat and sometimes a reflexive cough. Because the upper respiratory system is exposed to the open environment it is susceptible to viruses, bacteria, and allergens, which may result in a variety of conditions. See Table 36-1 for common conditions and symptoms.

CASE STUDY

Ms. Floyd, a 45-year-old female, is at the pharmacy asking for help to treat her congestion and cough. She had a sore throat for 2 to 3 days, which went away, and now has had a runny nose for a day or two and a cough at night. This morning she woke up with pressure "around the eyes" (she points to her eyebrows and cheek bones). Her nose was also "clogged." She is on only one medication: lisinopril 20 mg once daily for her high blood pressure.

COMMON CONDITIONS OF THE UPPER RESPIRATORY SYSTEM

Colds

A cold, also known as the common cold, is an acute, self-limiting, viral infection.[4] Most colds are caused by a rhinovirus. Colds may occur at any time of the year, but tend to be more frequent in the winter months. Colds usually start with a sore throat followed by runny nose, congestion, and cough. A typical cold will last 7 to 14 days. Treatments such as decongestants, antitussives, and expectorants can help decrease and manage symptoms but do not cure colds.

Influenza

Influenza, commonly called the flu, is caused by an influenza virus.[4] Influenza can be a serious illness, especially in very young or old people, or those who are pregnant or have other chronic health conditions, such as asthma, diabetes, and heart disease. Symptoms, which develop over several days, are usually fever, chills, runny nose, sore throat, and cough. Influenza also causes muscle and joint achiness, lack of energy, and sometimes headaches. The flu usually lasts 1 to 2 weeks but severe cases may last longer. Yearly influenza vaccines can help prevent infection. Antiviral cures are available (see Chapter 28) but have limitations. Symptomatic treatments commonly used for colds and oral analgesics (refer to Chapter 13 for details on these medications) are frequently used.

Allergies

Allergies can be episodic, intermittent (seasonal), or persistent (perennial). Episodic allergies occur with sudden exposure to an allergen.[5] For example, patients visiting homes with pets may develop allergy symptoms that will resolve when they return to their own homes. Intermittent (seasonal) allergies occur at certain times of the year, usually from a grass pollen or ragweed, and can vary in location based on what plants grow in certain areas of the country. Persistent (perennial) allergies are chronic and may be from indoor allergens (dust mite feces, animal dander, and some mold species) or outdoor allergens like pollution. When an allergen comes in contact with mucous membranes a response mediated by immunoglobulin E, abbreviated IgE, occurs.[5] IgE triggers mast cells to release histamine and other agents that cause inflammation, including rhinitis (inflammation of the nose), and an increase in salivary and bronchial secretions. Symptoms of this response include a runny nose, congestion, sneezing, redness, and itchy eyes or skin. More serious symptoms like wheezing or shortness of breath may indicate a severe allergy, which may require immediate medical attention. Avoidance of allergens is the most effective treatment. This can include staying indoors during peak pollen seasons or away from animals or places where pet dander may be present.[5] If avoidance is not possible, symptomatic treatments may be used to bring relief and improve daily function.[5]

MEDICATIONS USED FOR COMMON UPPER RESPIRATORY CONDITIONS

CASE?

What is the medical description for Ms. Floyd's stuffy nose? What may be causing it?

Decongestants

Decongestants stimulate certain receptors, usually alpha-1 in the sympathetic autonomic nervous system (SANS; discussed in Chapter 4), causing vasoconstriction. This allows the swollen blood vessels to shrink and reduces congestion. Decongestants can be taken orally or applied topically inside the nose with drops or sprays. Medication Table 36-2 provides a summary of these products.[6] Orally administered decongestants act systemically (throughout the body), and the vasoconstriction they cause can increase blood pressure. They may also cause jitteriness or insomnia in some patients and should usually be avoided in the late evening. Pseudoephedrine, a common oral decongestant, is only available for purchase at the pharmacy counter. Pharmacies must track purchases according to state and federal laws.[7] The oral decongestant in the pharmacy aisle is phenylephrine, which is an older decongestant. It is less effective than pseudoephedrine for many patients.

ALERT!

Decongestants are not recommended for children under the age of 4 years.

CASE?

What might the pharmacist recommend for Ms. Floyd's stuffy nose? Why was this particular medication chosen? What information helps to make this decision?

PRACTICE POINT

Because pseudoephedrine can be used in the illegal manufacture of methamphetamine, the federal government restricts how much pseudoephedrine a patient can buy at a time and requires identification for its purchase. Many states have additional laws regulating the sale of pseudoephedrine. Always check your local rules and regulations, as well as your practice site's policies, before selling a patient pseudoephedrine.

Nasal decongestant drops or sprays act locally in the nose with very little or no systemic effects. However, over-use or prolonged use of nasal decongestants for more than 3 to 5 days may cause rebound congestion.[8] The reason why this occurs is not well understood but the result is inflammation of the nasal mucosa and congestion that is resistant to decongestants.[8]

ALERT!

Oral decongestants, even OTC products, can increase blood pressure and should be used cautiously by patients taking antihypertensive medications or those with elevated blood pressure. Nasal decongestants may be a more appropriate treatment option for these patients since nasal decongestants only act locally and are less likely to increase blood pressure like systemic decongestants.

CASE?

If Ms. Floyd also wants something for her cough, what might the pharmacist recommend? Why?

Antitussives

A cough is one of the body's natural ways to help clear the airways. It can be reflexive or done on command. Colds and influenza are frequent causes of short-term coughs. Antitussives work to help stop coughs. Benzonatate is a prescription oral cough medicine, available in capsule form, that numbs the respiratory stretch receptors in the lungs and stops the cough reflex. Other medications work on the cough center in the brain, located in the medulla, which sits at the base of the brain, right at the top of the spinal cord. These include prescription medications like hydrocodone and codeine. These medications are also opiate pain relievers and are controlled substances with abuse potential. To treat a cough, they are typically used in a syrup formulation, but tablet forms are also available. Dextromethorphan (DXM) is a cough medicine that is structurally related to codeine but has less abuse potential. DXM is available OTC. It works in the cough center in the brain and decreases the sensitivity of cough receptors in the lungs. All of these antitussives may cause drowsiness so patients should be counseled to use

caution when driving or doing other activities. Antitussives are listed in Medication Table 36-3.[6]

Expectorants

Guaifenesin is the most commonly used expectorant and is available in OTC and prescription formulations. It works by causing an increase in respiratory tract secretions. This increased volume in secretions decreases the viscosity, or stickiness, of the mucus. Thinner mucus is easier to cough up than thick mucus, making it easier for the patient to expectorate, or cough out, the excess mucus. Consuming an increased amount of water can also aid this action and is recommended with expectorants. While expectorants are commonly used in combination with antitussives, they may not always be needed together. Expectorants are listed in Medication Table 36-3.[6]

Antihistamines

Antihistamines are frequently used by patients with allergies and allergic rhinitis. These medications block the histamine receptor and therefore minimize the allergic response and symptoms like rhinitis, rhinorrhea, and sneezing. Antihistamines are available as oral preparations, topical creams, and nasal inhalations. Oral antihistamines are available with or without a prescription. Azelastine and olopatadine are currently the only antihistamines available for nasal use. See Medication Table 36-4 for a list of these products.[6] Older oral antihistamines, sometimes referred to as first-generation antihistamines, are very drying and commonly cause quite a bit of sedation (drowsiness). Because of this property, they are sometimes used for indications such as motion sickness and as sleep aids. They may also be used in combination with decongestants to treat congestion due to colds or influenza. Newer antihistamines, referred to as second generation, work well for most types of allergy symptoms and do not typically cause as much sedation. They are not effective at treating cold or influenza symptoms. Even when used as a nasal application, antihistamines may cause sedation in many patients.

ALERT!

Older antihistamines are not appropriate for children under 4 years old. Any antihistamine (even nasal preparations) may cause drowsiness but can, paradoxically, make some children hyperactive rather than sleepy.[9]

Corticosteroids

Corticosteroids (discussed in detail in Chapter 8) decrease inflammation and mucosal edema, cause mild vasoconstriction, and help stop mast cell reactions. Because they block the allergic response at multiple points, nasal corticosteroids are considered the best choice to treat rhinitis, sneezing, itchy eyes and nose caused by intermittent and perineal allergies.[5] However, unlike antihistamines and decongestants, which both work fairly quickly after use, corticosteroids may take several days for maximum benefit to be seen. Thus, corticosteroids work best if used as early as possible before the allergic response is triggered or when they are needed for more than 2 to 3 weeks to allow time for maximum efficacy. Nasal corticosteroids are indicated for rhinitis due to allergies and are available by prescription and OTC. Nasal corticosteroid products are listed in Medication Table 36-4.[6]

> **PRACTICE POINT**
>
> *Nasal decongestants are not good options for chronic allergy symptoms because their use is limited to short periods. Nasal corticosteroids can be used for longer periods but may take a few weeks to reach maximum effect.*

Mast Cell Stabilizers

Mast cell stabilizers are useful in treating patients with allergies because they prevent cells from releasing histamine. Cromolyn is a mast cell stabilizer that is available without a prescription for nasal use. Prescription medications like montelukast, a leukotriene inhibitor (discussed in Chapter 19), can also be used for allergy symptoms.

Combination Products

A wide variety of treatment combinations are available OTC. These products provide a convenient way to treat several symptoms with a single preparation, but they must be chosen with care to avoid excessive or needless drug therapy. Many combination products have similar names (e.g., Tylenol Cold, Tylenol Sinus) but different ingredients. Others have the same or similar ingredients but in different dosage forms or strengths. Patients should be reminded to read labels and directions carefully and discuss their questions with the pharmacist. Some representative combinations are listed in Medication Table 36-5.[3,6]

> **PRACTICE POINT**
>
> *By encouraging patients to discuss their symptoms with the pharmacist, technicians can increase the likelihood of the optimal product being chosen—one with the right mix of ingredients to treat the current symptoms—and avoiding dangerous duplications and interactions.*

> **ALERT!**
>
> Many combination products have ingredients that may duplicate those patients are taking in other products or dosage forms. Such duplication (e.g., Tylenol tablets for pain, added to a combination preparation containing acetaminophen, such as Theraflu or Nyquil products) can result in serious toxicity or overdose. Also, some liquid products may contain alcohol which should be avoided in children and adults sensitive to alcohol.

SUMMARY

Anesthetics, antihistamines, decongestants, and corticosteroids can be used to help provide symptomatic relief of symptoms in the nose and throat caused by colds, influenza, and allergies. Gingivitis and mouth pain or irritations can also be treated with topical options such as chlorhexidine gluconate, carbamide peroxide, or topical anesthetics like benzocaine. Antifungal medications can be used to treat thrush topically in the mouth.

ACKNOWLEDGMENT

The authors wish to acknowledge Celtina K. Reinert, PharmD, author of the previous edition of this chapter.

REFERENCES

1. UpToDate. Waltham, MA: Wolters Kluwer; 2020. http://www.uptodate.com. Accessed July 22, 2022.

2. American Dental Association website. http://ada.org. Accessed July 22, 2022.

3. Lexi-Comp. Riverwoods, IL: Wolters Kluwer; 2020. http://online.lexi.com. Accessed June 24, 2022.

4. Centers for Disease Control and Prevention. Common colds: Protect yourself and others. http://www.cdc.gov/features/rhinoviruses/. Accessed June 24, 2022.

5. Dykewicz MS, Wallace DV, Baroody F, et al. Treatment of seasonal allergic rhinitis: An evidence-based focused 2017 guideline update. Ann Allergy Asthma Immunol. 2017;119(6):489-511.e41. doi:10.1016/j.anai.2017.08.012.

6. U.S. Food and Drug Administration. Cold, cough, allergy, bronchodilator, and antiasthmatic drug products for over-the-counter human use. CFR: Code of Federal Regulations. Title 21, Part 341. Updated July 18, 2022. http://www.ecfr.gov/cgi-bin/text-idx?SID=694f58669bc9c396 32fe5305dd2358e6&mc=true&node=pt21.5.341&rgn= div5#se21.5.341_172. Accessed July 22, 2022.

7. U.S. Department of Justice Drug Enforcement Administration. Combat Methamphetamine Epidemic Act 2005. Title VII of USA Patriot Improvement Reauthorization Act of 2005. Pub L No. 109-177. 109th Congress. March 9, 2006. https://www.deadiversion.usdoj.gov/meth/index.html. Accessed June 24, 2022.

8. Mortuaire G, de Gabory L, Francois M, et al. Rebound congestion and rhinitis medicamentosa: Nasal decongestants in clinic practice. Critical review of the literature by a medical panel. Eur Ann Otorhinolaryngol Head Neck Dis. 2013;130(3):137–144. doi:10.1016/j.anorl.2012.09.005.

9. Verbanas, P. For children with colds, doctors are increasingly likely to recommend antihistamines rather than cough and cold medicine. Rutgers Today. July 29, 2019. https://www.rutgers.edu/news/children-colds-doctors -are-increasingly-likely-recommend-antihistamines -rather-cough-and-cold. Accessed June 24, 2022.

REVIEW QUESTIONS

1. Describe what is included in *good oral hygiene*. Why is it important?

2. Most medication rinses used to treat conditions of the mouth and throat are to be spit out. Which medications are exceptions to this and should be swallowed?

3. How long can nasal decongestants be used? What happens if nasal decongestants are used for longer than the recommended time?

4. When is the best time to start using a nasal corticosteroid for allergies? How long should nasal corticosteroids be used?

5. Why is it so important for patients to read the labels of OTC cough, cold, and flu products and follow directions carefully?

MEDICATION TABLES

MEDICATION TABLE 36-1. Topical Medications Used for Mouth and Throat Conditions[3]

Condition	Classification	Active Ingredient	Pronunciation	Brand Name(s)	Dose	Regulatory Status
Cold sore	Antiviral	Docosanol	(doe KOE san ole)	Abreva	10% cream: apply to affected area 5 times daily, start at the first sign of cold sore and continue until healed; if not healed in 10 days, stop use and contact healthcare provider	OTC
	Antiviral	Acyclovir	(ay SYE kloe veer)	Zovirax	5% cream: apply to affected area 5 times daily for 4 days, start at the first sign of cold sore	Rx
Thrush	Antifungal	Nystatin	(nye STAT in)	Generics	100,000 IU/mL suspension: swish and swallow 4 times daily for 7–14 days; doses vary from 200,000-600,000 IU (2–6 mL) depending on factors such as age and infection severity	Rx
	Antifungal	Clotrimazole	(kloe TRIM a zole)	Generics	10 mg troche: dissolve one troche slowly 5 times daily for 14 consecutive days	Rx
Dry mouth	Saliva substitute	Xylitol, Glycerin, plus mix of other ingredients	(ZAHY li tawl) (GLIS er in)	Biotene, ACT Dry Mouth, TheraBreath, others	Spray: spray directly into mouth; do not rinse Gel: apply on tongue and spread evenly Rinse: rinse in mouth for 30 seconds; some products should be spit out whereas others are safe to swallow Lozenge: dissolve one lozenge in the mouth slowly; allow lozenge to move around	OTC
Gingivitis	Antibacterial	Chlorhexidine	(klor HEX i deen)	Periogard, Peridex	0.12% solution: swish 15 mL (½ oz) for 30 seconds, then spit out twice daily after brushing and flossing; wait at least 2 hours to eat after using	Rx

Continued next page

MEDICATION TABLE 36-1. Topical Medications Used for Mouth and Throat Conditions[3] *(Continued)*

Condition	Classification	Active Ingredient	Pronunciation	Brand Name(s)	Dose	Regulatory Status
Mouth irritation	Antibacterial	Hydrogen peroxide	(HYE droe jen) (per OX ide)	Peroxyl	1.5% solution: use 10 mL up to 4 times daily; swish in mouth over affected area(s) for at least 1 minute before spitting; do not swallow 1.5% gel: apply small amount of gel to affected area(s) up to 4 times daily; allow to sit for at least 1 minute and spit out	OTC
	Anti-inflammatory	Carbamide peroxide	(KAR ba mide) (per OX ide)	Generics	10% liquid: apply several drops to affected area 4 times daily after meals and at bedtime; spit out after a few minutes; to use as a rinse, place 10-20 drops onto the tongue, swish for at least 1 minute, and spit out	OTC
Mouth irritation or pain	Anesthetic	Benzocaine	(BEN zoe kane)	Anbesol, Orajel	10%-20% topical gel, liquid, ointment, spray: apply thin layer to area up to 4 times daily 15 mg lozenge: allow 1 lozenge to dissolve slowly in mouth; may repeat every 2 hours as needed; do not chew	OTC
	Anesthetic	Lidocaine	(LYE doe kane)	Generics	2% viscous solution: swish and spit with 15 mL (½ oz) every 3-8 hours (max 8 doses/24 hours)	Rx
	Anesthetic	Phenol	(FEE nol)	Chloraseptic	14.5–29 mg lozenges: use 1–2 lozenges every 2 hours as needed 1.4% spray: use 1 spray to affected area; let sit in place for at least 15 seconds, then spit out; use every 2 hours as needed 1.4% gargle: spray onto throat, gargle 15 seconds and spit out; may repeat every 2 hours	OTC

MEDICATION TABLE 36-2. Medications Used for Congestion[6]

Classification	Active Ingredient	Pronunciation[3]	Brand Name	Dose	Regulatory Status
Oral decongestant	Pseudoephedrine	(soo doe e FED rin)	Sudafed	30 mg tablets: 1–2 tablets every 4–6 hours; max 240 mg/day 120 mg 12-hour extended-release tablets: 1 tablet every 12 hours; max 2 tablets/day 240 mg 24-hour extended-release tablets: 1 tablet every 24 hours	OTC
	Phenylephrine	(fen il EF rin)	Sudafed PE	10 mg tablets: 1 every 4–6 hours; max 60 mg/day	OTC
Nasal decongestant	Naphazoline	(naf AZ oh leen)	Privine	0.05% drops or spray: use 1–2 drops/sprays in each nostril every 6 hours	OTC
	Oxymetazoline	(ok see met AZ oh leen)	Afrin	0.05% solution: use 2–3 sprays in each nostril twice daily	OTC
	Phenylephrine	(fen il EF rin)	Neo-Synephrine	0.25% or 0.5% drops or spray: use 1–2 drops/sprays in each nostril every 4 hours as needed	OTC
	Propylhexedrine	(proe pil HEX e dreen)	Benzedrex	0.4–0.5 mg: use 2 sprays in each nostril not more than every 2 hours	OTC

MEDICATION TABLE 36-3. Medications Used for Cough[6]

Classification	Active Ingredient	Pronunciation[3]	Brand Name	Dose	Regulatory Status
Antitussive	Benzonatate	(ben ZOE na tate)	Generics	100–200 mg 3 times daily as needed for cough	Rx
	Dextromethorphan	(dex troe meth OR fan)	Delsym, various	10–20 mg every 4 hours; 30 mg every 6–8 hours; or 60 mg extended release every 12 hours; max 120 mg/day	OTC
	Codeine	(KOE deen)	Various, ingredient in combination with guaifenesin; products frequently labeled "AC"	10–20 mg every 4–6 hours as needed; max 120 mg/day in guaifenesin antitussive/expectorant combinations	combined with guaifenesin, schedule V)
Expectorant	Guaifenesin	(gwye FEN e sin)	Mucinex, Tussin, various others	200–400 mg every 4 hours; max 2,400 mg/day 600–1200 mg extended release every 12 hours; max 2,400 mg/day	Rx, OTC

MEDICATION TABLE 36-4. Medications Used for Allergy Symptoms[6]

Classification	Active Ingredient	Pronunciation[3]	Brand Name	Dose	Regulatory Status
Oral antihistamine/ first generation	Diphenhydramine	(dye fen HYE dra meen)	Benadryl	25 mg: 1–2 every 6–8 hours	OTC
	Carbinoxamine	(kar bi NOX a meen)	Karbinal ER; RyVent	4 mg: 1–2 tablets 3–4 times daily	Rx
	Chlorpheniramine	(klor fen IR a meen)	Chlor-Trimeton	4 mg every 4– hours; max 24 mg/day	OTC
	Clemastine	(KLEM as teen)	Generics	2.68 mg: 0.5–1 tablet 2–3 times daily; max 3 tablets/day	OTC
Oral antihistamine/ second generation	Cetirizine	(se TI ra zeen)	Zyrtec	10 mg: 1 tablet daily	OTC
	Loratadine	(lor AT a deen)	Claritin	10 mg: 1 tablet daily	OTC
	Fexofenadine	(fex oh FEN a deen)	Allegra	60 mg: 1 tablet twice daily 180 mg: 1 tablet daily	OTC
	Levocetirizine	(lee voe se TIR i zeen)	Xyzal	5 mg: 1 tablet daily	OTC
	Desloratadine	(des lor AT a deen)	Clarinex	5 mg: 1 tablet daily	Rx
Nasal antihistamines	Azelastine	(a ZEL as teen)	Astepro Allergy	0.15%: use 1–2 sprays in each nostril every 12 hours or 2 sprays in each nostril daily (maximum 4 sprays/nostril in 24 hours)	OTC
	Olopatadine	(oh loe PAT a deen)	Patanase	(0.6%) 2 sprays in each nostril twice daily	Rx
Nasal mast cell stabilizer	Cromolyn	(KROE moe lin)	Nasalcrom	40 mg/mL: 1 spray in each nostril 3–4 times daily (max 6 uses/day)	OTC

Continued next page

MEDICATION TABLE 36-4. Medications Used for Allergy Symptoms[6] *(Continued)*

Classification	Active Ingredient	Pronunciation[3]	Brand Name	Dose	Regulatory Status
Nasal corticosteroid	Beclomethasone	(be kloe METH a sone)	Beconase AQ, QNASL	42 mcg: 1–2 sprays in each nostril twice daily	Rx
	Budesonide	(byoo DES oh nide)	Generics	32 mcg: 1 spray in each nostril daily	OTC
	Ciclesonide	(sye KLES oh nide)	Omnaris, Zetonna	50 mcg: 2 sprays in each nostril once daily 37 mcg: 1 spray in each nostril once daily	Rx
	Flunisolide	(floo NISS oh lide)	Generics	50 mcg: 2 sprays in each nostril 2–3 times daily	Rx
	Fluticasone	(floo TIK a sone)	Flonase, Flonase Sensimist, others	50 mcg (Flonase): 1–2 sprays in each nostril once daily 27.5 mcg (Sensimist): 1–2 sprays in each nostril once daily	Rx, OTC (depending on dosage form)
	Mometasone	(moe MET a sone)	Generics	50 mcg: 2 sprays in each nostril daily	Rx
	Triamcinolone	(trye am SIN oh lone)	Nasacort	55 mcg: 2 sprays in each nostril daily	OTC
Nasal moisturizer	Sodium chloride (sometimes with additional ingredients such as aloe, glycerin, or benzalkonium chloride)	(SOE dee um) (KLOR ide)	Rhinaris, SalineX, Breathe Free, Ocean	0.2%–0.9% solution or spray: 2–6 drops/sprays in each nostril every 2 hours, as often as needed	OTC
			Rhinaris, Entsol	Intranasal gel: apply a small amount of gel into each nostril every 4 hours as needed	OTC

MEDICATION TABLE 36-5. Select Over-the-Counter Combination Products for Upper Respiratory Conditions[3]

Product(s)	Analgesic	Antihistamine	Antitussive	Decongestant	Expectorant
Maximum Strength Mucinex Fast-Max Cold, Flu & Sore Throat Caplets; Robitussin Maximum Strength Severe Multi-Symptom Cough Cold + Flu Liquid; Tylenol Cold + Flu Severe Caplets; Tylenol Cold + Mucus Severe COOL BURST Liquid	Acetaminophen (a seet a MIN oh fen)		Dextromethorphan (dex troe meth OR fan)	Phenylephrine (fen il EF rin)	Guaifenesin (gwye FEN e sin)
Zyrtec-D		Cetirizine (se TI ra zeen)		Pseudoephedrine (soo doe e FED rin)	
Sudafed PE Head Congestion + Pain	Ibuprofen (eye byoo PROE fen)			Phenylephrine (fen il EF rin)	
Advil Cold & Sinus	Ibuprofen (eye byoo PROE fen)			Pseudoephedrine (soo doe e FED rin)	
Aleve-D Sinus & Cold	Naproxen (na PROX en)			Pseudoephedrine (soo doe e FED rin)	
Alka-Seltzer Plus Severe Cold Sparkling Original Powerfast Fizz	Aspirin (AS pir in)	Chlorpheniramine (klor fen IR a meen)		Phenylephrine (fen il EF rin)	
Contac Cold + Flu Night	Acetaminophen (a seet a MIN oh fen)	Chlorpheniramine (klor fen IR a meen) in caplets; doxylamine (dox IL a meen) in liquid		Phenylephrine (fen il EF rin)	
Theraflu Nighttime Multi-Symptom Severe Cold	Acetaminophen (a seet a MIN oh fen)	Diphenhydramine (dye fen HYE dra meen)		Phenylephrine (fen il EF rin)	
NyQuil Cold & Flu Nighttime Relief	Acetaminophen (a seet a MIN oh fen)	Doxylamine (dox IL a meen)	Dextromethorphan (dex troe meth OR fan)		
DayQuil Cold & Flu	Acetaminophen (a seet a MIN oh fen)		Dextromethorphan (dex troe meth OR fan)	Phenylephrine (fen il EF rin)	

Note: Page numbers for Key Terms and Definitions are in bold. Page numbers followed by *f* refer to figures; those followed by *b* refer to boxes; those followed by *t* refer to tables; and those followed by *mt* refer to Medication Tables.

DOI 10.37573/9781585286638.IDX